| metoclopramide HCl | midazolam HCl | morphine sulfate | nalbuphine HCl | pentazocine lactate | pentobarbital Na | perphenazine | phenobarbital Na | prochlorperazine edisylate | promazine HCl | promethazine HCl | ranitidine HCl | scopolamine HBr | secobarbital Na | sodium bicarbonate | thiethylperazine maleate | thiopental Na | |
|---|---|---|---|---|---|---|---|---|---|---|---|---|---|---|---|---|---|
| P | Y | P | Y | P | P | Y | | P | P | P | Y | P | | | | | atropine sulfate |
| | Y | Y | | Y | N | | N | | | | | Y | N | | | N | benzquinamide HCl |
| | Y | Y | | Y | N | Y | | Y | | Y | | Y | | | Y | | butorphanol tartrate |
| P | Y | P | | P | N | Y | | Y | P | P | Y | Y | | | | N | chlorpromazine HCl |
| | Y | Y | Y | Y | N | Y | | Y | Y | Y | | Y | N | | | | cimetidine HCl |
| | | | | | | | | | | | | | | | | | codeine phosphate |
| P | N | P | | P | N | Y | | N | N | N | Y | P | | | | N | dimenhydrinate |
| Y | Y | P | | P | N | Y | | P | P | P | Y | P | | | | N | diphenhydramine HCl |
| P | Y | P | Y | P | N | Y | | P | P | P | | P | | | | | droperidol |
| P | Y | P | | P | N | Y | | P | P | P | Y | P | | | | | fentanyl citrate |
| | Y | Y | | N | N | | | Y | Y | Y | Y | Y | N | N | | N | glycopyrrolate |
| P(5) | | N* | | N | | | P(5) | | | N | | | | | | | heparin Na |
| | Y | | Y | Y | | | | N* | | Y | Y | Y | | | Y | | hydromorphone HCl |
| P | Y | Y | Y | Y | N | | | P | P | P | N | Y | | | | | hydroxyzine HCl |
| P | Y | N | | P | N | P | | P | P | Y | Y | P | | | | N | meperidine HCl |
| ■ | Y | P | | P | | P | | P | P | P | Y | P | | N | | | metoclopramide HCl |
| Y | ■ | Y | Y | | N | N | | N | Y | Y | N | Y | | | Y | | midazolam HCl |
| P | Y | ■ | | P | N* | Y | | P* | P | P* | Y | P | | | | N | morphine sulfate |
| | Y | | ■ | | N | | | Y | | Y | Y | Y | | | Y | | nalbuphine HCl |
| P | | P | | ■ | N | Y | | P | Y | Y | Y | P | | | | | pentazocine lactate |
| | N | N* | N | N | ■ | | | N | N | N | | Y | | Y | | Y | pentobarbital Na |
| P | N | Y | | Y | N | ■ | | Y | | | | Y | | | | | perphenazine |
| | | | | | | | ■ | | | | N | | | | | | phenobarbital Na |
| P | N | P* | Y | P | N | | | ■ | P | P | Y | P | | | | N | prochlorperazine edisylate |
| P | Y | P | | Y | N | | | P | ■ | P | P | | | | | | promazine HCl |
| P | Y | P* | Y | Y | N | | | P | P | ■ | Y | P | | | | N | promethazine HCl |
| Y | N | Y | Y | Y | | | Y | N | Y | P | ■ | | | | Y | | ranitidine HCl |
| P | Y | P | Y | P | Y | | | P | | P | Y | ■ | | | | Y | scopolamine HBr |
| | | | | | | | | | | | | | ■ | | | | secobarbital Na |
| N | | | | Y | | | | | | | | | | ■ | | N | sodium bicarbonate |
| | Y | | Y | | | | | | | | Y | | | | ■ | | thiethylperazine maleate |
| | | N | | | Y | | | N | | N | | Y | | N | | ■ | thiopental Na |

lowed by a list of selected combination products in which these drugs are found. Specific information on each drug is arranged under the following headings: *How Supplied; Action; Onset, Peak, Duration; Indications & Dosage; Adverse Reactions; Interactions; Contraindications; Nursing Considerations;* and *Patient Teaching.*

In each drug entry, the drug's generic name is immediately followed by an alphabetized list of its brand names. A trade name followed by an open diamond (◊) indicates a drug that is available in preparations that do not require a prescription. Brands available *only* in Canada are designated with a dagger (†); those available *only* in Australia, with a double dagger (‡). A brand name with no symbol is available in the United States, Canada, and possibly Australia. The mention of a brand name in no way implies endorsement of that product or guarantees its legality.

*Alcohol and Tartrazine Content*

Many liquid drug preparations for oral use contain alcohol. Although the slight sedative effect that alcohol produces is not harmful in most patients — and can sometimes be beneficial — alcohol ingestion can be undesirable and even dangerous in some circumstances. Alcohol-containing oral drugs should be given very cautiously, if at all, to patients who are:

● concomitantly taking potent CNS depressants, such as barbiturates

● taking drugs that may produce a disulfiram-type reaction (such as chlorpropamide or metronidazole)

● taking disulfiram as part of a treatment program for their alcoholism. Such patients, upon ingestion of alcohol, will exhibit severe symptoms that may include blurred vision, confusion, dyspnea, flushing, sweating, and tachycardia.

To help prevent inadvertent exposure to alcohol, the text signals alcohol content with a single asterisk (*) after each brand of a liquid preparation that may contain it. In many of the preparations so marked, the alcohol content is small. Nevertheless, these drugs should be avoided in patients who are susceptible to adverse effects upon exposure to alcohol.

Tartrazine dye, also known as FD&C Yellow No. 5, is a common coloring agent in some foods and drugs. Usually harmless, it can provoke a severe reaction in susceptible persons. For this reason, most drug manufacturers have begun to eliminate tartrazine from their products, but many drugs still contain it.

The incidence of tartrazine sensitivity is approximately 1 in 10,000 in the general population but somewhat higher in persons with asthma or sensitivity to aspirin. Why this is so is unknown. The most common symptoms of tartrazine sensitivity are urticaria, rhinorrhea, asthma, and angioedema. Acutely sensitive persons may develop allergic vascular purpura, tachycardia, dyspnea, and chest pain. These allergic symptoms typically subside spontaneously upon discontinuation of the tartrazine-containing drug but may require treatment with antihistamines or epinephrine.

Avoiding exposure to tartrazine is not simply a matter of avoiding yellow-colored drugs because this substance may be present in many other color blends, such as turquoise, green, and maroon. This text signals tartrazine content with a double asterisk (**) after each brand that may contain it. If you suspect tartrazine sensitivity in a patient receiving such a drug, inform the doctor and contact the manufacturer to determine which dosage forms contain tartrazine.

*Controlled Substance Schedules*

If a drug is a controlled substance, that is indicated (example: Controlled Substance Schedule II). Drugs regu-

# 1

## How to use *Nursing97 Drug Handbook*

*Nursing97 Drug Handbook* is meant to fill a very special need. It represents a joint effort by pharmacists and nurses to provide the nursing profession with drug information that focuses on what nurses need to know. With this in mind, it emphasizes clinical aspects and does not attempt to replace detailed pharmacology texts. Also, the information is arranged in a format designed to make it readily accessible.

### New features in this edition
The 1997 edition contains several new features to enhance nursing knowledge and skills:
• A "New Drug" logo before a generic drug name indicates that the drug was approved by the FDA within the past year.
• Adverse reactions are now classified four ways to enhance patient safety even more than before (see "Adverse Reactions" later in this chapter for details).
• A new Patient Teaching section gathers all patient-oriented instructions under one heading (see "Patient Teaching" later in this chapter for details).
• A new "Alert" logo identifies situations that could jeopardize patient safety and suggests ways to avoid harm.
• *Nursing97 DrugDisk* (inside back cover) lets the user take two continuing education tests (and earn 9.5 contact hours), learn and perform dosage calculations, and print out concise instructions for the patient on more than 700 commonly prescribed drugs.

### Introductory chapters
Chapter 2 explains, in a general way, how drugs work. It also tells about adverse reactions and gives general guidelines about drug use in pregnancy and the presence of drugs in breast milk. Chapters 3 and 4 discuss the unique problems of administering drugs to children and elderly patients and offer guidelines to minimize problems in these areas. Chapter 5 discusses drug therapy as it relates to the nursing process.

### Therapeutic class chapters
In chapters 6 to 98, all drugs are classified according to their approved therapeutic uses. Drugs with multiple therapeutic uses are classified according to their most common use; they are also listed (with a cross-reference to the major drug entry) in drug groups that share their secondary applications. For example, nadolol, a beta-adrenergic blocker, is described in the chapter that covers antianginals because its major therapeutic application is the management of angina pectoris; because it is less commonly used to treat hypertension, it is also listed among the generic drugs grouped as antihypertensives, with a cross-reference to Chapter 22, Antianginals.

Such classification by therapeutic use offers several advantages. It helps the reader identify an unknown drug by its clinical application alone. At the same time, it automatically identifies all other drugs that share the same use and provides easy comparison of their dosages and effects. In this way, it quickly identifies potential pharmacotherapeutic alternatives for patients who cannot tolerate or fail to respond to a particular drug.

Each chapter, representing a major therapeutic use, begins with an alphabetical list of the generic drugs described in that chapter. This is fol-

**A.H. Robins Company**
Micro-K Extencaps®

**Roxane Laboratories, Inc.**
Roxicet™

**Rugby Laboratories, Inc.**
dicyclomine hydrochloride

**Sandoz Pharmaceuticals
Corporation**
DynaCirc®
Fiorinal® with Codeine
Pamelor®

**Schein Pharmaceutical,
Inc.**
nortriptyline hydrochloride

**Schering-Plough
Corporation**
Claritin®
K-Dur®
Theo-Dur®

**G.D. Searle & Company**
Ambien®
Calan®
Daypro®

**SmithKline Beecham
Pharmaceuticals**
Amoxil®
Augmentin®
Compazine®
Compazine® Spansule®
Dyazide®
Paxil®
Relafen®
Tagamet®

**Solvay Pharmaceuticals,
Inc.**
Orasone®

**The Upjohn Company**
Ansaid®
Deltasone®
Glynase®
Halcion®
Micronase®
Motrin®
Ogen®
Provera®
Xanax®

**U.S. Pharmaceuticals
Group
Pfizer Inc.**
Cardura®
Glucotrol®
Glucotrol XL™
Norvasc®
Procardia XL®
Zithromax®
Zoloft®

**Warner-Lambert
Company**
Accupril®
Dilantin®
Dilantin® Kapseals®
gemfibrozil
Lopid®
Nitrostat®

**Watson Laboratories, Inc.**
hydrocodone bitartrate and
acetaminophen

**Wyeth-Ayerst Laboratories**
Ativan®
Effexor®
Inderal®
Lodine®
Oruvail®
Premarin®

**Zeneca Pharmaceuticals**
Nolvadex®
Tenormin®
Zestril®

# ACKNOWLEDGMENTS

*We would like to thank the following companies for granting us permission to include their drugs in the full-color photoguide.*

**Abbott Laboratories**
Biaxin®
Depakote®
Depakote® Sprinkle
E.E.S.®
Ery-Tab®
Erythrocin Stearate
 Filmtab®
Erythromycin Base
 Filmtab®
Hytrin®
PCE®

**Astra Merck**
Prilosec®

**Astra USA**
Toprol XL™

**Bristol-Myers Squibb Company**
BuSpar®
Capoten®
Cefzil®
cephalexin
Duricef®
Estrace®
Pravachol®
Sumycin®
Trimox®
Veetids®

**Daniels Pharmaceuticals, Inc.**
Levoxyl®

**Dupont/Merck**
Coumadin®
Percocet®
Sinemet®
Sinemet® CR

**Eli Lilly and Company**
Axid®
Ceclor®
Darvocet-N® 100
Lorabid®
Prozac®

**ESI/Lederle Generics**
atenolol

**Ethex Corporation**
potassium chloride

**Forest Pharmaceutical, Inc.**
Lorcet® 10/650

**Glaxo Wellcome Inc.**
Ceftin®
Lanoxin®
Zantac®
Zantac® EFFERdose®
Zovirax®

**Goldline Laboratories, Inc.**
verapamil hydrochloride

**Hoechst Marion Roussel, Inc.**
Altace®
Carafate®
Cardizem®
Cardizem® CD
Cardizem® SR®
DiaBeta®
Lasix®
Seldane®
Seldane-D®
Trental®

**Hoffman-La Roche, Inc.**
Bumex®
Klonopin®
Naprosyn®
Toradol®
Valium®

**Janssen Pharmaceutical, Inc.**
Hismanal®
Propulsid®

**Knoll Pharmaceutical Company**
E-Mycin®
ibuprofen
Synthroid®
Vicodin®
Vicodin ES®

**Lederle Laboratories**
Suprax®
Verelan®

**Lemmon Company**
acetaminophen and codeine
 (300 mg/30 mg)
Cotrim® D.S.

**MD Pharmaceutical, Inc.**
methylphenidate
 hydrochloride

**Merck & Co., Inc.**
Mevacor®
Pepcid®
Prinivil®
Vasotec®
Zocor®

**Miles, Inc.**
Adalat®
Cipro®

**Mylan Pharmaceuticals Inc.**
amitriptyline hydrochloride
cimetidine
cyclobenzaprine
 hydrochloride
doxepin hydrochloride
furosemide
glipizide
naproxen
propoxyphene napsylate
 with acetaminophen

**Novopharm USA Inc., Division of Novopharm Limited**
amoxicillin trihydrate

**Ortho/McNeil Pharmaceutical**
Floxin®
Tylenol® with Codeine
 No. 3
Ultram®

**Pfizer Inc.**
Diflucan®

**Proctor and Gamble Pharmaceuticals**
Macrobid®

**Purepac Pharmaceutical Co.**
acetaminophen and codeine
 (300 mg/60 mg)

**Rhône-Poulenc Rorer Pharmaceuticals Inc.**
Dilacor XR®
Lozol®
Slo-bid® Gyrocaps®

# CONSULTANTS, REVIEWERS, AND ADVISORS

*At the time of publication, the clinical consultants, pharmacy reviewers, and advisors held the following positions.*

## Clinical Consultants

**Marlene Ciranowicz, RN, MSN, CDE**
Independent Consultant
Dresher, Pa.

**Michael R. Cohen, RPh, MS, FASHP**
President
Institute for Safe Medication Practices
Warminster, Pa.

**Robert A. Cohen, RPh**
Pharmacist
Norristown, Pa.

**Nancy S. Gould, RPh**
Assistant Director
Pharmacy Department
Doylestown (Pa.) Hospital

**Barbara McVan, RN**
Independent Consultant
Lansdale, Pa.

**Kenneth Wieland, RPh, PharmD**
Director of Pharmacy
Chestnut Hill (Pa.) Hospital

## Pharmacy Reviewers

**James Camamo, PharmD**
Clinical Pharmacist
University Medical Center
Tucson, Ariz.

**Lawrence P. Carey, PharmD**
Clinical Pharmacist
Thomas Jefferson Home Infusion
Service
Philadelphia

**Sandra L. Chase, PharmD, BS**
Clinical Pharmacist
Drug Use Policy and Medical
Information
Thomas Jefferson University Hospital
Philadelphia

**R. Kevin Coleman, PharmD**
Oncology Pharmacist
St. Jude Children's Research Hospital
Memphis

**Beth Anne Logsdon, PharmD**
Pediatric Pharmacotherapy Resident
LeBonheur Children's Medical Center
Memphis

**Marie Maloney, PharmD**
Clinical Pharmacist
University Medical Center
Tucson, Ariz.

**Jan E. Markind, RPh, PharmD**
Drug Information Specialist
University of Illinois at Chicago

**Frank J. Massaro, PharmD**
Pharmacy Clinical Coordinator
New England Medical Center
Boston

**George Melko, PharmD**
Clinical Pharmacist
Thomas Jefferson Home Infusion Service
Philadelphia

**Nancy Moneymaker, PharmD**
Clinical Pharmacist
St. Jude Children's Research Hospital
Memphis

**Christine V. O'Neill, RPh, PharmD**
Clinical Pharmacy Specialist
Hematology/Oncology
New England Medical Center
Boston

**Leslie N. Schechter, PharmD**
Clinical Pharmacist
Transplant and Surgery
Thomas Jefferson University Hospital
Philadelphia

**Tracy L. Skaer, PharmD, BPharm**
Assistant Professor of Pharmacy Practice
College of Pharmacy
Washington State University
Pullman

**Gregg S. Teitel, PharmD**
Freelance Writer/Editor
Doylestown, Pa.

**Peggy S. Wimmer, PharmD**
Pharmacy Resident
St. Jude Children's Research Hospital
Memphis

## Topical Drugs

## Nutritional Drugs

## Miscellaneous Drug Categories

## Appendices and Index

**Nursing97 DrugDisk** ......................... inside back cover

## Autonomic Nervous System Drugs

## Respiratory Tract Drugs

## Gastrointestinal Tract Drugs

## Photoguide to Tablets and Capsules ............ follows p. 662

## Hormonal Drugs

# CONTENTS

lated under the jurisdiction of the Controlled Substances Act of 1970 are divided into the following groups, or schedules:

● Schedule I (C-I): High abuse potential and no accepted medical use — for example, heroin, marijuana, and LSD.

● Schedule II (C-II): High abuse potential with severe dependence liability — for example, narcotics, amphetamines, dronabinol, and some barbiturates.

● Schedule III (C-III): Less abuse potential than schedule II drugs and moderate dependence liability — for example, nonbarbiturate sedatives, nonamphetamine stimulants, and limited amounts of certain narcotics.

● Schedule IV (C-IV): Less abuse potential than schedule III drugs and limited dependence liability — for example, some sedatives, antianxiety agents, nonnarcotic analgesics.

● Schedule V (C-V): Limited abuse potential. Primarily small amounts of narcotics, such as codeine, used as antitussives or antidiarrheals. Under federal law, limited quantities of certain C-V drugs may be purchased without a prescription directly from a pharmacist if allowed under specific state statutes. The purchaser must be at least age 18 and must furnish suitable identification. All such transactions must be recorded by the dispensing pharmacist.

*Pregnancy Risk Category*
Each systemically absorbed drug has been assigned a pregnancy risk category based upon available clinical and preclinical information. The Pregnancy Risk Category parallels the five Pregnancy Categories (A, B, C, D, and X) assigned by the Food and Drug Administration to reflect a drug's potential to cause birth defects. Although drugs are best avoided during pregnancy, this rating system permits rapid assessment of the risk-benefit

ratio should drug administration to a pregnant woman become necessary. Drugs in category A are generally considered safe to use in pregnancy; drugs in category X are generally contraindicated.

● A: Adequate studies in pregnant women have failed to show a risk to the fetus.

● B: Animal studies have not shown a risk to the fetus, but controlled studies have not been conducted in pregnant women; or animal studies have shown an adverse effect on the fetus, but adequate studies in pregnant women have not shown a risk to the fetus.

● C: Animal studies have shown an adverse effect on the fetus, but adequate studies have not been conducted in humans. The benefits from use in pregnant women may be acceptable despite potential risks.

● D: The drug may cause risk to the human fetus, but the potential benefits of use in pregnant women may be acceptable despite the risks.

● X: Studies in animals or humans show fetal abnormalities, or adverse reaction reports indicate evidence of fetal risk. The risks involved clearly outweigh potential benefits.

● NR: Not rated.

*How Supplied*
This section lists the preparations available for each drug (for example, tablets, capsules, solutions for injection), specifying available dosage forms and strengths. Dosage strengths available *only* in Canada are designated with a dagger (†); those available *only* in Australia, with a double dagger (‡). Preparations that do not require a prescription are marked with an open diamond (◇).

*Action*
This section succinctly describes the mechanism of action — that is, how the drug provides its therapeutic ef-

fect. For example, although all antihypertensives lower blood pressure, they don't all do so by the same pharmacologic process.

### Onset, Peak, Duration
This section describes the onset, peak (described in terms of effect or peak blood level), and duration of drug action for each route of administration, if data are available or applicable. Values listed are for patients with normal renal function, unless specified otherwise.

### Indications & Dosage
This section lists general dosage information for adults (including recommended geriatric dosages, when available) and children, as applicable. Children's dosages are usually indicated in terms of mg/kg daily. Dosage instructions reflect current clinical trends in therapeutics and can't be considered as absolute and universal recommendations. For individual application, dosage instructions must be considered in light of the patient's clinical condition.

### Adverse Reactions
This section lists the adverse reactions to each drug by body system. The most common adverse reactions (those experienced by at least 10% of people taking the drug in clinical trials) are in *italic* type; less common reactions are in roman type; life-threatening reactions are in ***bold italic*** type; and reactions that are both common and life-threatening are in **BOLD CAPITAL LETTERS**.

### Interactions
This section lists each drug's confirmed, *clinically significant* interactions with other drugs (additive effects, potentiated effects, and antagonistic effects) or foods, with specific suggestions for avoiding dangerous drug or food interactions (for exam-

ple, by reducing doses or monitoring food intake). Drug interactions are listed under the drug that is adversely affected. For example, magnesium trisilicate, an ingredient in antacids, interacts with tetracycline to cause decreased absorption of tetracycline. Therefore, this interaction is listed under tetracycline. To check on the possible effects of using two or more drugs simultaneously, refer to the interaction entry for *each* of the drugs in question.

### Contraindications
This section lists any conditions, especially diseases, in which the use of the drug is undesirable.

### Nursing Considerations
This section lists recommendations for cautious use, followed by other useful information, such as monitoring techniques and suggestions for prevention and treatment of adverse reactions. Also included are suggestions for patient comfort and for preparing, administering, and storing each drug. Recommendations for I.V. use are highlighted by **boldface** type.

### Patient Teaching
This section focuses on explaining the drug's purpose, promoting compliance, and ensuring proper use and storage of the drug. It also includes instructions for preventing or minimizing adverse reactions.

### Photoguide to tablets and capsules
To make drug identification easier for nurses and to enhance patient safety, *Nursing97 Drug Handbook* offers a full-color photoguide to the most commonly prescribed tablets and capsules. Shown in actual size, the drugs are arranged alphabetically for quick reference, along with their most common dosage strengths. Page references to the drugs appear in boldface type in the Index.

## A guide to abbreviations

| | |
|---|---|
| **ACE** | angiotensin-converting enzyme |
| **ADH** | antidiuretic hormone |
| **AIDS** | acquired immunodeficiency syndrome |
| **ALT** | alanine aminotransferase |
| **AST** | aspartate aminotransferase |
| **AV** | atrioventricular |
| **b.i.d.** | twice daily |
| **BUN** | blood urea nitrogen |
| **cAMP** | cyclic 3′, 5′ adenosine monophosphate |
| **CBC** | complete blood count |
| **CHF** | congestive heart failure |
| **CK** | creatine kinase |
| **CMV** | cytomegalovirus |
| **CNS** | central nervous system |
| **COPD** | chronic obstructive pulmonary disease |
| **CSF** | cerebrospinal fluid |
| **CV** | cardiovascular |
| **CVA** | cerebrovascular accident |
| **$D_5W$** | dextrose 5% in water |
| **DNA** | deoxyribonucleic acid |
| **ECG** | electrocardiogram |
| **EEG** | electroencephalogram |
| **EENT** | eyes, ears, nose, throat |
| **FDA** | Food and Drug Administration |
| **g** | gram |
| **G** | gauge |
| **GFR** | glomerular filtration rate |
| **GI** | gastrointestinal |
| **GU** | genitourinary |
| **G6PD** | glucose-6-phosphate dehydrogenase |
| **$H_1$** | histamine$_1$ |
| **$H_2$** | histamine$_2$ |
| **HIV** | human immunodeficiency virus |
| **h.s.** | at bedtime |
| **I.D.** | intradermal |
| **I.M.** | intramuscular |
| **IND** | investigational new drug |
| **IPPB** | intermittent positive-pressure breathing |
| **IU** | international unit |
| **I.V.** | intravenous |

| | |
|---|---|
| **kg** | kilogram |
| **M** | molar |
| **$m^2$** | square meter |
| **MAO** | monoamine oxidase |
| **mcg** | microgram |
| **mEq** | milliequivalent |
| **mg** | milligram |
| **MI** | myocardial infarction |
| **ml** | milliliter |
| **$mm^3$** | cubic millimeter |
| **Na** | sodium |
| **NaCl** | sodium chloride |
| **NSAID** | nonsteroidal anti-inflammatory drug |
| **OTC** | over the counter |
| **PABA** | para-aminobenzoic acid |
| **P.O.** | by mouth |
| **P.R.** | by rectum |
| **p.r.n.** | as needed |
| **PT** | prothrombin time |
| **PTT** | partial thromboplastin time |
| **PVCs** | premature ventricular contractions |
| **q** | every |
| **q.d.** | every day |
| **q.i.d.** | four times daily |
| **q.o.d.** | every other day |
| **RBC** | red blood cell |
| **RDA** | recommended daily allowance |
| **REM** | rapid eye movement |
| **RNA** | ribonucleic acid |
| **RSV** | respiratory syncytial virus |
| **SA** | sinoatrial |
| **S.C.** | subcutaneous |
| **SIADH** | syndrome of inappropriate antidiuretic hormone |
| **S.L.** | sublingual |
| **$T_3$** | triiodothyronine |
| **$T_4$** | thyroxine |
| **t.i.d.** | three times daily |
| **UCE** | urea cycle enzymopathy |
| **USP** | United States Pharmacopeia |
| **WBC** | white blood cell |

# 2

# Drug actions, reactions, and interactions

Administration of any drug provokes a series of physicochemical events within the body. The first event, when a drug combines with cellular drug receptors, is known as the drug action. What follows as a result of this action of the drug is known as the drug effect. Depending on the number of different cellular drug receptors affected by a given drug, a drug effect can be local, systemic, or both. Obviously, a local effect follows application to the skin; however, transdermal absorption can produce systemic effects. Moreover, local effects can follow systemic absorption. For example, the antipeptic ulcer drug cimetidine acts solely by blocking histamine receptor cells in the parietal cells of the stomach. This is known as a local drug effect because the drug action is sharply limited to one area and does not spread to other parts of the body. On the other hand, diphenhydramine produces a systemic effect in that it blocks histamine receptors in widespread areas of the body. In other words, local drug effects are specific to a limited number of organ systems, whereas systemic drug effects are generalized and affect different and diverse organ systems.

## Four important drug properties
### 1. Absorption
Before a drug can act within the body, it must be absorbed into the bloodstream — usually after oral administration, the most frequently used route. Before a drug contained in a tablet or capsule can be absorbed, the dosage form must disintegrate — that is, break into smaller particles. Then these smaller particles can dissolve in gastric juices. Only after so dissolving can a drug be absorbed. Most absorption of orally administered drugs occurs in the small intestine, where the mucosal villi provide extensive surface area. Once absorbed and circulated in the bloodstream, it is bioavailable, or ready to produce a drug effect. Whether such absorption is complete or partial depends on several factors: the drug's physicochemical effects, its dosage form, its route of administration, its interactions with other substances in the GI tract, and various patient characteristics. These same factors also determine the speed of absorption. Thus, oral solutions and elixirs, which bypass the need for disintegration and dissolution, are usually absorbed more rapidly. Some tablets have enteric coatings that prevent disintegration in the acidic environment of the stomach; others may have coatings of varying thickness that delay release of the drug.

Drugs administered intramuscularly must first be absorbed through the muscle into the bloodstream. Rectal suppositories must dissolve to be absorbed through the rectal mucosa. Drugs administered intravenously, which are injected directly into the bloodstream, are completely and immediately bioavailable.

### 2. Distribution
After absorption, a drug moves from the bloodstream into various fluids and tissues within the body; this is distribution. Individual patient variations can greatly alter the amount of drug that is distributed throughout the body. For example, in an edematous patient, a given dose must be distributed to a larger volume than in a nonedematous patient; the amount of drug must sometimes be increased to account for this. Remember, the dose

should be decreased when the edema is corrected. Conversely, in an extremely dehydrated patient, the drug will be distributed to a much smaller volume, so the dose must then be decreased. The total area to which a drug is distributed is known as volume of distribution. Patients who are particularly obese may present another problem when considering drug distribution. Some drugs—such as digoxin, gentamicin, and tobramycin—are not well distributed to fatty tissue. Therefore, dosing based on actual body weight may lead to overdose and serious toxicity. In some cases, dosing must be based on lean body weight, which may be estimated from actuarial tables that give average weight range for height.

### 3. Metabolism

Most drugs are metabolized in the liver. Hepatic diseases may affect one or more of the metabolic functions of the liver. Therefore, in patients with hepatic disease, the metabolism of a drug may be increased, decreased, or unchanged. Clearly, all patients with hepatic disease must be monitored closely for drug effect and toxicity.

The rate at which a drug is metabolized varies with the individual. In some patients, drugs are metabolized so quickly that their blood and tissue levels prove therapeutically inadequate. In others, the rate of metabolism is so slow that ordinary doses can produce toxic results.

### 4. Excretion

The body eliminates drugs by metabolism (usually hepatic) and excretion (usually renal). Drug excretion refers to the movement of a drug or its metabolites from the tissues back into circulation and from the circulation into the organs of excretion. Although most drugs are excreted by the kidneys, some drugs can be eliminated via the lungs, exocrine glands (sweat, salivary, or mammary), kidneys, liver, skin, and intestinal tract. Drugs may also be removed artificially by direct interventions, such as peritoneal dialysis or hemodialysis.

### Other modifying factors

An important factor that influences a drug's action and effect is its *binding to plasma proteins,* especially albumin, and other tissue components. Because only a free, unbound drug can act in the body, such binding greatly influences effectiveness and duration of effect.

The *patient's age* is another important factor. Elderly patients usually have decreased hepatic function, less muscle mass, and diminished renal function. Consequently, they need lower doses and sometimes longer dosage intervals to avoid toxicity. With similar consequences, neonates have underdeveloped metabolic enzyme systems and inadequate renal function. They need highly individualized dosages and careful monitoring.

*Underlying disease* can also markedly affect drug action and effect. For example, acidosis may cause insulin resistance. Genetic diseases, such as G6PD deficiency and hepatic porphyria, may turn drugs into toxins with serious consequences. Patients with G6PD deficiency may develop hemolytic anemia when given sulfonamides or a number of other drugs. A genetically susceptible patient can develop an acute porphyria attack if given a barbiturate. Also, patients who have highly active hepatic enzyme systems (for example, rapid acetylators), when treated with isoniazid, can develop hepatitis from the rapid intrahepatic buildup of a toxic metabolite.

### Things to consider about administration

- *Dosage forms do matter.* Some tablets and capsules are too large to be easily swallowed by very ill patients.

You may then request an oral solution or elixir of the same drug, but bear in mind that because a liquid is more easily and completely absorbed, it produces higher blood levels than a tablet. When a potentially toxic drug (such as digoxin) is given, the increased amount absorbed could cause toxicity. Sometimes a change in dosage form requires a change in dosage.

• *Routes of administration are not therapeutically interchangeable.* For example, phenytoin is readily absorbed orally but is slowly and erratically absorbed intramuscularly. On the other hand, gentamicin must be given parenterally because oral administration yields inadequate blood levels to treat systemic infections.

• *Improper storage can alter a drug's potency.* Most drugs should be stored in tight containers protected from direct sunlight and extremes in temperature and humidity that can cause them to deteriorate. Some may require special storage conditions, such as refrigeration.

• *The timing of drug administration can be important.* Sometimes, giving an oral drug during or shortly after mealtime decreases the amount of drug absorbed. This is not clinically significant with most drugs and may in fact be desirable with irritating drugs, such as aspirin. But penicillins and tetracyclines should not be scheduled for administration at mealtimes because certain foods can inactivate them. If in doubt about the effect of food on a certain drug, check with the pharmacist.

• *Consider the patient's age, height, and weight.* The doctor will need this information when calculating the dosage for many drugs. It should be accurately recorded on the patient's chart. This chart should also include current laboratory data, especially renal and liver function studies, so the doctor can adjust the dosage as needed.

• *Watch for metabolic changes.* Monitor for any physiologic change (depressed respiratory function, acidosis or alkalosis) that might alter drug effect.

• *Know the patient's history.* Whenever possible, obtain a comprehensive family history from the patient or his family. Ask about past reactions to drugs, possible genetic traits that might alter drug response, and the current use of other drugs. Multiple drug therapy can cause drug interactions that can dramatically change the effects of many drugs.

## Drug interactions

When one drug administered in combination with or shortly after another drug alters the effect of one or both drugs, this is known as a drug interaction. Usually, the effect of one drug is increased or decreased. For instance, one drug may inhibit or stimulate the metabolism or excretion of the other, or it may release another from plasma protein-binding sites, freeing it for further action.

Combination therapy is based on drug interaction. One drug, for example, may be given to potentiate another. Probenecid, which blocks the excretion of penicillin, is sometimes given with penicillin to maintain adequate blood levels of penicillin for a longer period. Often, two drugs with similar actions are given together precisely because of the additive effect that results. For instance, aspirin and codeine, both analgesics, are often given in combination because together they provide greater pain relief than either alone.

Drug interactions are sometimes used to prevent or antagonize certain adverse reactions. Hydrochlorothiazide and spironolactone, both diuretics, are often administered in combination because the former is potassium-depleting, whereas the latter is potassium-sparing.

But not all drug interactions are

beneficial. Multiple drugs can interact to produce effects that are often undesirable and sometimes hazardous. Harmful drug interactions decrease efficacy or increase toxicity. A hypertensive patient well controlled with guanethidine may see his blood pressure rise to its former high level if he takes the antidepressant amitriptyline at the same time. Such a drug effect is known as antagonism. Drug combinations that produce these effects should be avoided if possible. Another kind of inhibiting effect occurs when a tetracycline drug is administered with calcium- or magnesium-containing drugs or foods (such as antacids or milk). These combine with tetracycline in the GI tract and cause inadequate absorption of tetracycline.

**Adverse reactions**

Any drug effect other than what is therapeutically intended can be called an adverse reaction. It may be expected and benign or unexpected and potentially harmful. Mild, but *predictable,* adverse reactions are sometimes called side effects. Drowsiness caused by antihistamines is an example of this. During hay fever season, a patient may have to contend with this drowsiness to get relief from hay fever symptoms. In such a case, the dosage may be adjusted up or down to balance therapeutic effects with side effects.

An adverse reaction may be tolerated for a necessary therapeutic effect, or it may be hazardous and unacceptable and require discontinuation of the drug. Some adverse reactions subside with continued use. As an example, the drowsiness associated with methyldopa and the orthostatic hypotension associated with prazosin usually subside after several days, as the patient develops a tolerance to these effects. But many adverse reactions are dosage-related and lessen or disappear only if the dosage is reduced.

Although most adverse reactions are not therapeutically desirable, an occasional one can be put to clinical use. An outstanding example of this is the drowsiness associated with diphenhydramine, which makes it clinically useful as a mild hypnotic.

Hypersensitivity, a term sometimes used interchangeably with drug allergy, is the result of an antigen-antibody immune reaction that occurs in the body when a drug is given to a susceptible patient. One of the most dangerous of all drug hypersensitivities is penicillin allergy. In its severest form, penicillin anaphylaxis can rapidly become fatal.

Rarely, idiosyncratic reactions occur. These are highly unpredictable, individual, and unusual. Probably the best known idiosyncratic drug reaction is the aplastic anemia caused by the antibiotic chloramphenicol. This reaction appears in only 1 out of 40,000 patients, but when it does, it can be fatal. A more common idiosyncratic reaction is extreme sensitivity to very low doses of a drug, or insensitivity to higher-than-normal doses.

To deal with adverse reactions correctly, you need to be alert to even minor changes in the patient's clinical status. Such minor changes may be an early warning of pending toxicity. Listen to the patient's complaints about his reactions to a drug, and consider each complaint objectively. You may be able to reduce adverse reactions in several ways. Obviously, dosage reduction often helps. But often so does a simple rescheduling of the same dose. For example, pseudoephedrine may produce stimulation that will be no problem if it's given early in the day; similarly, the drowsiness that occurs with antihistamines or tranquilizers can be totally harmless if the dose is given at bedtime. Most important, your patient needs to be told what adverse reactions to expect so he won't become worried or even stop taking the drug on his own. Of course, the patient should report any unusual or unexpected adverse reactions to the doctor.

Recognizing drug allergies or serious idiosyncratic reactions can sometimes be lifesaving. Ask each patient about drugs he is taking or has taken in the past and what, if any, unusual reactions he experienced from taking them. If a patient claims to be allergic to a drug, ask him to tell you exactly what happens when he takes it. He may be calling a harmless side effect such as upset stomach an allergic reaction, or he may have a true tendency toward anaphylaxis. In either case, you and the doctor need to know this. Of course, you must record and report any clinical changes throughout the patient's hospital stay. If you suspect a severe adverse reaction, withhold the drug until you can check with the pharmacist and the doctor.

## Toxic reactions
Chronic drug toxicities are generally caused by the cumulative effect and resulting buildup of the drug in the body. These effects may be extensions of the desired therapeutic effect. For example, guanethidine-induced norepinephrine depletion produces a desired antihypertensive effect, but in larger doses, this action often produces orthostatic hypotension.

Drug toxicities typically occur when drug blood levels rise due to impaired metabolism or excretion. For example, blood levels of theophylline rise when hepatic dysfunction impairs metabolism of the drug. Similarly, digoxin toxicity can follow impaired renal function because digoxin is eliminated from the body almost exclusively by the kidneys (via glomerular filtration). Of course, toxic blood levels also follow excessive dosage. Aspirin tinnitus is usually a sign that the safe dose has been exceeded.

Most drug toxicities are predictable and dosage-related; fortunately, most are also readily reversible upon dosage adjustment. So be sure to monitor patients carefully for physiologic changes that might alter drug effect. Watch especially for impaired hepatic and renal function. Warn the patient about signs of pending toxicity, and tell him what to do if a toxic reaction occurs. Also, be sure to emphasize the importance of taking a drug exactly as prescribed. Warn the patient about serious problems that could arise if he changes the dose or the schedule for taking it.

## Drugs and pregnancy
Ever since the thalidomide tragedy of the late 1950s — when thousands of malformed infants were born after their mothers used this mild sedative-hypnotic during pregnancy — use of drugs during pregnancy has been a source of serious medical concern and controversy. To identify drugs that may cause such teratogenic effects, preclinical drug studies always include tests on pregnant laboratory animals. These tests point out gross teratogenicity but do not clearly establish safety. Because different species react to drugs in different ways, animal studies do not rule out possible teratogenic effects in humans. For example, the preliminary studies on thalidomide gave no warning of teratogenic effects, and it was subsequently released for general use in Europe.

What about the placental barrier? Once thought to protect the fetus from drug effects, the placenta isn't actually much of a barrier at all. Except for drugs with exceptionally large molecular structure, almost every drug administered to a pregnant woman crosses the placenta and enters the fetal circulation. An example of a drug with a large molecular size is heparin, the injectable anticoagulant. Theoretically, then, heparin could be used in a pregnant woman without fear of harming the fetus — but even heparin carries a warning for cautious use in pregnancy. Conversely, just because a drug crosses the placenta doesn't necessarily mean it's harmful to the fetus.

Actually, only one factor — stage of fetal development — seems clearly related to exaggerated risk during pregnancy. During two stages of pregnancy — the first and the third trimesters — the fetus is especially vulnerable to damage from maternal use of drugs. During these times, *all* drugs should be given with extreme caution.

The most sensitive period for drug-induced fetal malformation is the first trimester, when fetal organs are differentiating (organogenesis). During this time, *all* drugs should be withheld unless doing so would jeopardize the mother's health. Theoretically, during this sensitive time, even aspirin could harm the fetus. So, strongly advise your patient to avoid *all* self-prescribed drugs during early pregnancy. The other time of special fetal sensitivity to drugs is the last trimester. The reason? At birth, when separated from his mother, the neonate must rely on his own metabolism to eliminate any remaining drug. Because his detoxifying systems are not fully developed, any residual drug may take a long time to be metabolized — and thus may induce prolonged toxic reactions. Consequently, drugs should be used only when absolutely necessary during the last 3 months of pregnancy.

Of course, in many circumstances, pregnant women must continue to take certain drugs. For example, a woman with a seizure disorder that is well controlled with an anticonvulsant should continue to take the drug even during pregnancy. Similarly, a pregnant woman with a bacterial infection must receive antibiotics. In such cases, the potential risk to the fetus is outweighed by the mother's need. The relative risk to the fetus is expressed by the drug's pregnancy risk category (see Chapter 1).

Following these general guidelines can prevent indiscriminate and potentially harmful use of drugs in pregnancy:

● Before a drug is prescribed for a woman of childbearing age, she should be asked the date of her last menstrual period and whether she may be pregnant. If a drug is a known teratogen (for example, isotretinoin), some manufacturers may recommend special precautions to ensure that the drug not be given to a female of childbearing age until pregnancy is ruled out.

● Especially during the first and the third trimesters, a pregnant patient should avoid *all* drugs except those *essential* to maintain the pregnancy or maternal health.

● Topical drugs are not exempt from the warning against indiscriminate use during pregnancy. Many topically applied drugs can be absorbed in large enough amounts to be harmful to the fetus.

● When a pregnant patient needs *any* drug, the doctor should prescribe the *safest* possible drug in the *lowest* possible dose to minimize any harmful effect to the fetus.

● Every pregnant patient should check with her doctor before taking *any* drug.

**Drugs and lactation**

Most drugs a mother takes appear in breast milk. Drug levels in breast milk tend to be high when blood levels are high — generally, shortly after taking each dose. Therefore, the mother should be advised to breast-feed *before* taking medication, not *after*.

Nevertheless, with very few exceptions, a mother who wishes to breast-feed may continue to do so with her doctor's permission. However, breast-feeding should be temporarily interrupted and replaced with bottle-feeding when the mother must take tetracyclines, chloramphenicol, sulfonamides (during first 2 weeks postpartum), oral anticoagulants, iodine-containing drugs, or antineoplastics.

To protect her infant, a breast-feeding mother should avoid taking drugs indiscriminately. If she needs to take a drug, she should first check with her doctor to be sure of taking the safest drug at the lowest dose.

## What to teach patients about proper use of drugs

The following general guidelines will help to ensure that the patient gets maximal therapeutic benefits and avoids adverse reactions, accidental overdose, or potentially harmful changes in effectiveness:

• Store drugs in their original containers, at room temperature (unless directed otherwise), in places that are not accessible to children or exposed to sunlight. Avoid storage in the bathroom medicine cabinet or the glove compartment or trunk of an automobile, where extremes of temperature and humidity will cause them to deteriorate.

• Learn the trade name and generic name of any drug you are taking. Be sure to tell doctors, dentists, or other health care professionals you see regularly that you are taking it. Before taking any drug, be sure you have informed your doctor, nurse, or pharmacist about any unusual reactions you've had to drugs in the past and about your allergies to foods and other substances, any special medical problems, and any drugs you've taken over the last few weeks, including any OTC drugs.

• Always read the label before taking any drug, and take the drug exactly as prescribed at the recommended dosage and for the duration of treatment. Never share prescription drugs.

• When using a drug prescribed for occasional or prolonged use, check the container for an expiration date.

• To avoid potentially harmful changes in effectiveness, do not change brands of a drug without medical approval. Certain generic preparations are not precisely equivalent in effect to brand-name preparations of the same drug.

• Never mix different drugs in a single container, and don't remove any drug from its original container or remove the label. Relying on your memory to identify a drug and specific directions for its use is hazardous.

• Discard any drugs that are outdated or no longer needed.

• Before you have any surgery (including dental surgery), tell the doctor about all the drugs that you have been taking.

• Be sure to tell the doctor, nurse, or pharmacist about any adverse reactions you've experienced while taking a drug.

• If you or someone else has taken an overdose, call your doctor, poison control center, or pharmacist immediately. Keep syrup of ipecac in your home to induce vomiting, but induce vomiting only if one of these professionals advises you to do so.

• Try to have all your prescriptions filled at the same pharmacy so that the pharmacist can identify and warn against potentially harmful drug interactions. Inform the pharmacist of any OTC drugs you're taking.

# 3

# Drug therapy in children

A child's absorption, distribution, metabolism, and excretion processes undergo profound changes that affect drug dosage. To ensure optimal drug effect and minimal toxicity, consider these factors when administering drugs to a child.

## Absorption

Drug absorption in children depends on the form of the drug; its physical properties; other drugs or substances, such as food, taken simultaneously; physiologic changes; and concurrent disease.

● The pH of neonatal gastric fluid is neutral or slightly acidic and becomes more acidic as the infant matures. This affects drug absorption. For example, nafcillin and penicillin G are better absorbed in an infant than in an adult because of low gastric acidity.

● Various infant formulas or milk products may increase gastric pH and impede absorption of acidic drugs. So, if possible, give a child oral medications on an empty stomach.

● Gastric emptying time and transit time through the small intestine — which is longer in children than in adults — can affect absorption. Also, intestinal hypermotility (as in diarrhea) can diminish the drug's absorption.

● A child's comparatively thin epidermis allows increased absorption of topical drugs.

## Distribution

As with absorption, changes in body weight and physiology during childhood can significantly influence a drug's distribution and effects. In a premature infant, body fluid makes up about 85% of total body weight; in a full-term infant, 55% to 70%; and in an adult, 50% to 55%. Extracellular fluid (mostly blood) constitutes 40% of a neonate's body weight, compared with 20% in an adult. Intracellular fluid remains fairly constant throughout life and has little effect on drug dosage.

Extracellular fluid volume influences a water-soluble drug's concentration and effect because most drugs travel through extracellular fluid to reach their receptors. Children have a larger proportion of fluid to solid body weight, so their distribution area is proportionately greater.

Because the proportion of fat to lean body mass increases with age, the distribution of fat-soluble drugs is more limited in children than adults. As a result, a drug's lipid or water solubility affects the dosage for a child.

### Binding to plasma proteins

As the result of a decrease in albumin concentration or intermolecular attraction between drug and plasma protein, many drugs are less bound to plasma proteins in infants than in adults.

Furthermore, preparations that bind plasma proteins may displace endogenous compounds, such as bilirubin or free fatty acids. Conversely, an endogenous compound may displace a weakly bound drug. For example, displacement of bound bilirubin can cause a rise in unbound bilirubin, which can lead to increased risk of kernicterus at normal bilirubin levels.

Since only an unbound, or free, drug has a pharmacologic effect, any alteration in ratio of a protein-bound to an unbound active drug can greatly influence its effect.

Several diseases and disorders, such as nephrotic syndrome and malnutrition, can also decrease plasma protein and increase the concentration of an unbound drug, intensifying the drug's effect or producing toxicity.

## Metabolism

A neonate's ability to metabolize a drug depends on the integrity of the hepatic enzyme system, the intrauterine exposure to the drug, and the nature of the drug itself.

Certain metabolic mechanisms are underdeveloped in neonates. Glucuronidation is a metabolic process that renders most drugs more water soluble, thereby facilitating renal excretion. This process is insufficiently developed to permit full pediatric doses until the infant is 1 month old. Because of this, the use of chloramphenicol in a neonate may cause gray syndrome, illustrating the infant's inability to metabolize the drug. Use of chloramphenicol in neonates, therefore, requires decreased dosage (25 mg/kg/day) and monitoring of blood levels.

Conversely, intrauterine exposure to drugs may induce precocious development of hepatic enzyme mechanisms, increasing the infant's capacity to metabolize potentially harmful substances.

Older children can metabolize some drugs (theophylline, for example) more rapidly than adults. This ability may come from their increased hepatic metabolic activity. Larger doses than those recommended for adults may be required.

Also, preparations given concurrently to a child may alter hepatic metabolism and induce production of hepatic enzymes. Phenobarbital, for example, can induce hepatic enzyme production and accelerate metabolism of drugs given concurrently.

## Excretion

Renal excretion of a drug is the net effect of glomerular filtration, active tubular secretion, and passive tubular reabsorption. Because so many drugs are excreted in the urine, the degree of renal development or presence of renal disease can profoundly affect a child's dosage requirements.

If a child is unable to excrete a drug renally, drug accumulation and possible toxicity may result unless the dosage is reduced.

Physiologically, an infant's kidneys differ from an adult's in that they have:

• high resistance to blood flow and receive a smaller proportion of cardiac output
• incomplete glomerular and tubular development and short, incomplete loops of Henle (A child's glomerular filtration reaches adult values between ages 2½ to 5 months; his tubular secretion may reach adult values between ages 7 to 12 months.)
• low glomerular filtration rate (Penicillins are eliminated by this route.)
• decreased ability to concentrate urine or reabsorb various filtered compounds
• reduced ability of the proximal tubules to secrete organic acids.

Both children and adults have diurnal variations in urine pH that correlate with sleep-awake patterns.

## Calculating and monitoring pediatric dosages

When calculating pediatric dosages, don't use formulas that modify adult dosages: A child is not a scaled-down version of an adult. Pediatric dosages should be calculated on the basis of either body weight (mg/kg) or body surface area (mg/m²).

• Reevaluate dosages at regular intervals to ensure necessary adjustments as the child develops.
• Although body surface area provides a useful standard for adults and older children, don't use it in premature or full-term infants. Use the body weight method instead.

- Don't exceed the maximum adult dosage when calculating amounts per kilogram of body weight (except with certain drugs, such as theophylline, if indicated).
- Obtain an accurate maternal drug history — prescription and nonprescription drugs, vitamins, and herbs or other health foods taken during pregnancy.
- Drugs passed through breast milk can also have adverse effects on the breast-feeding infant. Before a drug is prescribed for a breast-feeding mother, the potential effects on the infant should be investigated. For example, sulfonamides given to a breast-feeding mother for a urinary tract infection appear in breast milk and may cause kernicterus at lower-than-normal levels of unconjugated bilirubin. Also, high concentrations of isoniazid appear in breast milk. Since this drug is metabolized by the liver, an infant's immature hepatic enzyme mechanisms cannot metabolize the drug, and the infant may suffer CNS toxicity.

## Oral medications
- *When giving oral medication to an infant,* administer it in liquid form if possible. For accuracy, measure and give the preparation by syringe; never use a vial or cup.
- Lift the patient's head to prevent aspiration of the medication, and press down on his chin to prevent choking.
- You may also place the drug in a nipple and allow the infant to suck the contents.
- *If the patient is a toddler,* explain how you're going to give him the medication. If possible, have the parents enlist the child's cooperation.
- Don't mix medication with food or call it "candy," even if it has a pleasant taste.
- Let the child drink liquid medication from a calibrated medication cup rather than from a spoon: It's easier and more accurate. If the preparation is available only in tablet form, crush it and mix it with a compatible syrup. (Check with the pharmacist to verify that the tablet can be crushed without compromising its effectiveness.)
- *If the patient is an older child* who can swallow a tablet or capsule by himself, have him place the medication on the back of his tongue and swallow it with water or fruit juice. Remember, milk or milk products may interfere with drug absorption.

## I.V. infusions
When administering I.V. infusions to children, note the following special considerations.

*Protecting the insertion site*
In infants, use a peripheral vein or a scalp vein in the temporal region for I.V. infusions. The scalp vein is safest in that the needle is not likely to be dislodged; however, the head must be shaved around the site. Temporary disfigurement may also result from the needle and infiltrated fluids. For these reasons, the scalp veins are not used as frequently today as they were in the past.

The extremities are the most accessible insertion sites; however, since patients tend to move about, take these precautions:
- Protect the insertion site to prevent catheter or needle dislodgment.
- Use a padded arm board to minimize dislodgment. Remove the arm board during range-of-motion exercises.
- Place the clamp out of the child's reach; if extension tubing is used to allow the child greater mobility, securely tape the connection.
- Restrain the child only when necessary.
- To allay anxiety, give a simple explanation to the child who must be restrained while asleep.

*Maintaining flow rate and fluid balance*

While administering an I.V. infusion to a child, monitor flow rate and check the patient's condition and insertion site at least hourly — more frequently if indicated.

Adjust the flow rate only while the patient is composed; crying and emotional upset can constrict blood vessels. Flow rate may vary if a pump isn't used. Flow should be adequate because some drugs (calcium, for example) can be very irritating at low flow rates. Infants, small children, and children with compromised cardiopulmonary status are particularly vulnerable to fluid overload with I.V. medication administration. To prevent this problem and help ensure that a limited amount of fluid is infused in a controlled manner, use a volume-control set (a volume-control device in the I.V. tubing) and an infusion pump or a syringe. Do not place more than 2 hours worth of I.V. fluid at a time in the volume-control set.

## I.M. injections

I.M. injections are preferred when the drug cannot be given by other parenteral routes and rapid absorption is necessary.

• In children under age 2, the vastus lateralis muscle is the preferred injection site; in older children, either the ventrogluteal area or the gluteus medius muscle can be used.

• To determine correct needle size, consider the patient's age, muscle mass, and nutritional status and the drug's viscosity; record and rotate injection sites.

• Explain to the patient that the injection will hurt, but that the medication will help him. Restrain him during the injection, if needed, and comfort him afterward.

## Topical medications and inhalants

• Use ear drops warmed to room temperature; cold drops can cause considerable pain and possibly vertigo.

• To administer drops, turn the patient on his side, with the affected ear up. If he is under age 3, pull the pinna down and back; if he is age 3 or over, pull the pinna up and back.

• Avoid using inhalants in very young children: obtaining their cooperation is difficult.

• Before attempting to administer medication through a metered-dose nebulizer to an older child, explain the inhaler to him. Then have him hold the nebulizer upside down and close his lips around the mouthpiece. Have him exhale, pinch his nostrils shut and, when he starts to inhale, release one dose of medication into his mouth. Tell the patient to continue inhaling until his lungs feel full.

• Most inhaled agents are not useful if taken orally; therefore, if you doubt the patient's ability to use the inhalant correctly, don't use it.

• Use topical corticosteroids with caution because chronic steroid use in children has been associated with delayed growth. When topical corticosteroids are used on the diaper area of infants, avoid covering this area with plastic or rubber pants, which will act as an occlusive dressing and enhance systemic absorption.

## Parenteral nutrition

I.V. nutrition is given to patients who can't or won't take adequate food orally and patients with hypermetabolic conditions who need supplementation. The latter group includes premature infants and children who have burns or other major trauma, intractable diarrhea, malabsorption syndromes, GI abnormalities, emotional disorders (such as anorexia nervosa), and congenital abnormalities.

Before fat emulsions are administered to infants and children, however, potential benefits must be weighed against possible risks.

Fats—supplied as 10% or 20% emulsions—are administered both peripherally and centrally. Their use is limited by the child's ability to metabolize them. An infant or a child with a diseased liver cannot efficiently metabolize fats, for example.

Some fats, however, must be supplied both to prevent essential fatty acid deficiency and to permit normal growth and development. A minimum of calories (2% to 4%) must be supplied as linoleic acid—an essential fatty acid found in lipids. In infants, fats are essential for normal neurologic development.

Nevertheless, fat solutions may decrease oxygen perfusion and may adversely affect children with pulmonary disease. This risk can be minimized by supplying only the minimum fat needed for essential fatty acid requirements and not the usual intake of 40% to 50% of the child's total calories.

Fatty acids can also displace bilirubin bound to serum albumin, causing a rise in free, unconjugated bilirubin and an increased risk of kernicterus. However, fat solutions may interfere with some bilirubin assays and cause falsely elevated levels. To avoid this complication, a blood sample should be drawn 4 hours after infusion of the lipid emulsion; or if the emulsion is introduced over 24 hours, the blood sample should be centrifuged before the assay is performed.

# 4

# Drug therapy in elderly patients

If you're providing drug therapy for elderly patients, you'll want to understand physiologic and pharmacokinetic changes that may alter appropriate drug dosage or cause common adverse reactions or compliance problems in elderly patients.

## Physiologic changes affecting drug action

As a person ages, gradual physiologic changes occur. Some of these age-related changes may alter the therapeutic and toxic effects of medications.

### Body composition

Proportions of fat, lean tissue, and water in the body change with age. Total body mass and lean body mass tend to decrease; the proportion of body fat tends to increase.

Varying from person to person, these changes in body composition affect the relationship between a drug's concentration and distribution in the body.

For example, a water-soluble drug, such as gentamicin, is not distributed to fat. Since there's relatively less lean tissue in an elderly person, more drug remains in the blood.

### GI function

In elderly patients, decreases in gastric acid secretion and GI motility slow the emptying of stomach contents and the movement of intestinal contents through the entire tract. Furthermore, research suggests that elderly patients may have more difficulty absorbing medications. This is a particularly significant problem with drugs having a narrow therapeutic range, such as digoxin, in which any change in absorption can be crucial.

### Hepatic function

The liver's ability to metabolize certain drugs decreases with age. This is caused by diminished blood flow to the liver, which results from the age-related decrease in cardiac output and from the diminished activity of certain liver enzymes. When an elderly patient takes certain sleep medications, such as secobarbital, the liver's reduced ability to metabolize the drug may produce a hangover effect the next morning.

Decreased hepatic function may cause:
• more intense drug effects due to higher blood levels
• longer-lasting drug effects due to prolonged blood concentrations
• greater incidence of drug toxicity.

### Renal function

Although an elderly person's renal function is usually sufficient to eliminate excess body fluid and waste, the ability to eliminate some medications may be reduced by 50% or more.

Many medications commonly used by elderly patients, such as digoxin, are excreted primarily through the kidneys. If the kidneys' ability to excrete the drug is decreased, high blood concentrations may result. Digoxin toxicity, therefore, is relatively common in elderly patients who are not receiving a reduced digoxin dosage that accommodates decreased renal function.

Drug dosages can be modified to compensate for age-related decreases in renal function. Aided by laboratory tests, such as blood urea nitrogen and serum creatinine, doctors may adjust medication dosages so the patient receives the expected therapeutic benefits without the risk of toxicity. Observe your patient for signs of toxicity. A patient taking digoxin, for example, may experience anorexia, nausea, vomiting, or confusion.

## Adverse drug reactions

Compared with younger people, elderly patients experience twice as many adverse drug reactions relating to greater drug consumption, poor compliance, and physiologic changes.

Signs and symptoms of adverse drug reactions — confusion, weakness, and lethargy — are often mistakenly attributed to senility or disease. If the adverse reaction isn't identified, the patient may continue to receive the drug. Furthermore, he may receive unnecessary additional medication to treat complications caused by the original medication. This can sometimes result in a pattern of inappropriate and excessive medication use.

Although any medication can cause adverse reactions, most of the serious reactions in the elderly are caused by relatively few medications. Be particularly alert for toxicities resulting from diuretics, antihypertensives, digoxin, corticosteroids, sleeping aids, and nonprescription drugs.

### Diuretic toxicity

Because total body water content decreases with age, normal dosages of potassium-wasting diuretics, such as hydrochlorothiazide and furosemide, may result in fluid loss and even dehydration in an elderly patient.

These diuretics may deplete serum potassium, causing weakness in the patient, and they may raise blood uric acid and glucose levels, complicating preexisting gout and diabetes mellitus.

### Antihypertensive toxicity

Many elderly people experience lightheadedness or fainting when using antihypertensive medications, partly in response to atherosclerosis and decreased elasticity of the blood vessels. Antihypertensive drugs lower blood pressure too rapidly, resulting in insufficient blood flow to the brain. This may cause dizziness, fainting, or even stroke.

Consequently, dosages of antihypertensive drugs must be carefully individualized. In elderly patients, too aggressive treatment of high blood pressure may do more harm than good, so treatment goals should be reasonable. Although bringing blood pressure down to 120/85 mm Hg may be appropriate in a young hypertensive patient, a more reasonable goal for an elderly hypertensive patient might be 150/95 mm Hg.

### Digoxin toxicity

As the body's renal function and rate of excretion decline, digoxin concentrations in the blood may build to toxic levels, causing nausea, vomiting, diarrhea, and — most serious — cardiac arrhythmias. Try to prevent severe toxicity by observing your patient for early signs, such as appetite loss, confusion, or depression.

### Corticosteroid toxicity

Elderly patients on corticosteroids may experience short-term effects, including fluid retention and psychological manifestations ranging from mild euphoria to acute psychotic reactions. Long-term toxic effects, such as osteoporosis, can be especially severe in elderly patients who have been taking prednisone or related steroidal compounds for months or even years. To prevent serious toxicity, carefully monitor patients on long-term regimens. Observe them for subtle changes in appearance, mood, and mobility, as well as for signs of impaired healing and fluid and electrolyte disturbances.

### Sleeping aid toxicity

Sedatives or sleeping aids, such as

flurazepam, may cause excessive sedation or residual drowsiness. Keep in mind that ingestion of alcohol may exaggerate such depressant effects, even if the sleeping aid was taken the previous evening.

*Nonprescription drug toxicity*
When aspirin and aspirin-containing analgesics are used in moderation, toxicity is minimal, but prolonged ingestion may cause GI irritation and gradual blood loss resulting in severe anemia. Although anemia from chronic aspirin consumption can affect all age-groups, elderly patients may be less able to compensate because of their already reduced iron stores.

Laxatives may cause diarrhea in elderly patients who are extremely sensitive to such drugs as bisacodyl. Chronic oral use of mineral oil as a lubricating laxative may result in lipid pneumonia from aspiration of small residual oil droplets in the patient's mouth.

**Patient noncompliance**
Poor compliance can be a problem with patients of any age. However, in elderly patients, specific factors linked to aging—such as diminished visual acuity, hearing loss, forgetfulness, the common need for multiple drug therapy, and various socioeconomic factors—can combine to make compliance a special problem. Approximately one-third of elderly patients fail to comply with their prescribed drug therapy. They may fail to take prescribed doses or to follow the correct schedule or they may take medications prescribed for previous disorders, discontinue medications prematurely, or use p.r.n. medications indiscriminately.

Review your patient's medication regimen with him. Make sure he understands the medication amount and the time and frequency of doses.

Also, explain how he should take each medication—that is, with food or water or by itself.

Give your patient whatever help you can to avoid drug therapy problems, and refer him to the doctor or pharmacist if he needs further information.

# 5

# Drug therapy and the nursing process

The nursing process guides nursing decisions about drug administration to ensure the patient's safety and meet medical and legal standards. This five-step process provides thorough assessment, appropriate nursing diagnosis, effective planning, correct interventions, and constant evaluation.

## First step: Assessment

During assessment, the nurse focuses on direct data collection by:
- obtaining a drug history from the patient, parent, spouse, or companion
- reviewing the patient's medical history
- performing a physical examination
- obtaining and interpreting relevant laboratory or diagnostic test results.

### Drug history

Data collection begins at admission to the hospital or in an outpatient setting with specific questions about the patient's background, including allergies, medical history, habits, socioeconomic status, lifestyle and beliefs, and sensory deficits. These aspects of the patient's background can significantly influence drug therapy.

### Allergies

The patient's allergy profile includes reactions to both drugs and food. Information about allergic reactions must specify the drug; a description of the reaction; its situation, time, and setting; and any contributing factors. Examples of contributing factors include concurrent use of stimulants, tobacco, alcohol, or illegal drugs or a significant change in nutritional patterns. Asking the patient to describe his allergic reaction is especially important to help determine whether the patient reacts adversely or simply dislikes taking the drug.

Allergies to foods can also affect drug therapy. For example, allergies to shellfish can contraindicate use of drugs that contain iodine or are by-products of shellfish. Allergies to eggs are significant in patients who are to receive vaccines, which are commonly derived from chick embryos.

### Prescription drugs

The patient's drug history should explore the following:
- the reason for using the drug
- the patient's knowledge of the appropriate dosage
- the patient's knowledge about determining effectiveness of the drug (if appropriate), potential adverse effects, what to do about adverse effects, and when to contact the doctor
- route of administration
- the pattern of administration at home
- use of OTC drugs
- cognitive status.

Note any special monitoring the patient must perform, such as blood glucose monitoring before insulin administration or checking radial pulse rate before taking digoxin. Make sure the patient is performing such procedures correctly and that the results are within acceptable limits.

Discuss the effects of drug therapy with the patient and determine if new symptoms or unpredicted adverse reactions have developed. Noting the patient's pattern of administration may provide insight into why a particular drug regimen succeeds or fails.

### OTC drugs

A comprehensive drug history should

also list any OTC drugs the patient is taking. Many OTC drugs can inhibit or potentiate the effects of a prescribed drug. For example, aspirin potentiates the anticoagulant effects of warfarin.

OTC drugs include a wide range of products from common aspirin and nutritional supplements to various sprays and cleaning agents. The patient may not think of these as drugs, so the nurse may have to name types of products to get an accurate response.

Dosage and frequency of use are just as important as the type of OTC product. One aspirin tablet taken once a day may have no effect on concomitant drug therapy; however, a higher dosage (such as that used for arthritis) could profoundly influence therapy.

*Medical history*
In gathering the medical history, note any chronic diseases or disorders the patient may have and record the following information for each:
• date of diagnosis
• initial prescribed treatment
• current treatment
• the doctor in charge.

Careful attention to this part of the medical history can uncover one of the most important problems with drug therapy — conflicting and incompatible drug regimens. The patient who does not have a family doctor to oversee and coordinate all care may seek the care of several specialists who may prescribe drug treatment without knowing what other drugs the patient is taking. A carefully detailed medical history can uncover such problems. The nurse who identifies such conflicting or overlapping drug therapy must call them to the appropriate doctor's attention and then teach the patient about the importance of informing caregivers about all drugs he is taking.

*Habits*
Carefully consider dietary habits and the nontherapeutic use of drugs.

Certain foods can directly affect the effectiveness of many drugs. For example, a person who is taking the anticoagulant warfarin should not increase his intake of green leafy vegetables because they contain levels of vitamin K that can antagonize the drug's anticoagulant effect.

Nontherapeutic use of drugs can profoundly affect a patient's health and impair the effectiveness of drug therapy. Consider the possible use of alcohol, tobacco, caffeine, and illegal drugs, such as marijuana, cocaine, and heroin. For example, if the patient uses alcohol, note the frequency of use, the amount, and the type of alcohol consumed. Carefully document the intake of stimulants, such as caffeine, because they significantly affect a patient's cardiovascular status and nervous system. Record the type of stimulant, the frequency of intake, and the amount consumed.

For the patient who uses tobacco, document the following information:
• the number of years the patient has used tobacco
• the kind of tobacco the patient smokes (cigarettes, cigar, or pipe) or chews
• how many cigarettes or cigars the patient smokes per day or how much and how long he chews tobacco daily
• the brand of tobacco the patient smokes or chews.

Defining the patient's use of illegal drugs may be difficult. However, the nurse who suspects such use should encourage the patient to discuss it honestly, emphasizing that these drugs have profound effects that may cause serious drug interactions. If the patient admits using illegal drugs, document the drug, the amount and frequency of use, and the route of administration.

*Socioeconomic status*

Note the patient's age, educational level, occupation, and insurance coverage. These factors may be significant to compliance and to an effective plan of care. The patient's age, for example, can determine whom to include in the care (parents or other family members) and the level of information that is appropriate for teaching the patient.

Knowing the patient's educational background and occupation helps you select interventions at an appropriate level, plan a drug regimen that fits the patient's daily routine, and encourage compliance. Knowing the patient's insurance status may help you anticipate the need for financial assistance and counseling. Remember that noncompliance commonly results from inability to afford medications.

*Lifestyle and beliefs*

Support systems, marital status, childbearing status, attitudes toward health and health care, use of the health care system, and daily patterns of activities all affect the plan of care and patient compliance. For example, an 18-year-old single parent who is a high-school dropout on medical assistance and has no family support will probably require more teaching and support to gain a commitment and compliance than a 40-year-old affluent professional who has family support, can understand why she needs the drug, and can readily pay for it.

*Sensory deficits*

Any sensory deficit can significantly shape an appropriate plan of care. For example, impaired vision, paralysis of one or more extremities, loss of a limb, or loss of sensation in an extremity can impair the patient's ability to administer a subcutaneous injection, break a scored tablet, or open a medication container. Color blindness may cause difficulty in distinguishing between two medications. Hearing impairment can complicate effective patient instruction. Any sensory deficit requires careful consideration in any plan of prescribed drug therapy.

*Clinical status*

Two other factors can profoundly influence drug therapy: the patient's cognitive status and the systemic effects of the prescribed drugs. A patient's intact cognitive abilities ensure that he can understand and implement the actions necessary for compliance. During the interview, note if the patient is alert and oriented, if he is able to interact appropriately with people, and if his conversation is appropriate. Consider whether the patient can think clearly and express his thoughts coherently. Finally, check both short-term and long-term memory because the patient needs both to follow a specified drug regimen. If such evaluation identifies a cognitive deficit, determine the probable cause, which can range from a transient drug-related effect to permanent neurologic impairment, and then determine whether or not the patient can carry out the prescribed drug regimen. If not, the nurse must find another way to ensure that the patient receives the prescribed therapy.

After completing the drug history, perform a physical examination to assess those body systems that may be affected by a particular drug the patient is taking or that may be prescribed. Every drug has a desired effect on a body system, but it may have an undesired effect on another. For example, chemotherapeutic agents destroy cancerous cells, but they also affect normal cells and typically cause the patient to experience hair loss, diarrhea, or nausea. Therefore, examine the patient for expected drug effects; also closely monitor the patient for potentially harmful adverse effects.

## Second step: Formulating a nursing diagnosis

Using information gathered during assessment, define any potential or actual drug-related problems by formulating each in a relevant nursing diagnosis. The most common problem statements related to drug therapy are *Knowledge deficit, Noncompliance,* and *Altered Health Maintenance.*

## Third step: Planning

Nursing diagnoses provide the framework for planning interventions and outcome criteria (patient goals).

*Outcome criteria*
Outcome criteria state the desired patient behaviors or responses that should result from nursing care. Such criteria should be measurable and objective, concise, realistic for the patient, and attainable by nursing management. They should also express patient behavior in terms of expectations and specify a time frame. A typical outcome statement is "Before discharge, the patient verbalizes major adverse effects related to his chemotherapy."

## Fourth step: Intervention

After developing the outcome criteria, the nurse determines the interventions needed to help the patient reach the desired behavior or goals. Drug-related interventions may focus on patient teaching for a drug's action, adverse effects, scheduling, steps to avoid or treat a drug reaction, or drug administration techniques.

Appropriate interventions related to drug therapy will also include administration procedures and techniques, legal and ethical concerns, patient teaching, and any concerns related to special groups of patients (geriatric, pediatric, pregnant, or breast-feeding patients). Such interventions may be independent nursing actions, such as turning a bedridden patient every 2 hours, or may be nursing actions that require a doctor's order.

## Fifth step: Evaluation

The final component of the nursing process, evaluation, is a formal and systematic process for determining the effectiveness of nursing care. This process enables the nurse to determine whether outcome criteria were met and thereby make informed decisions about subsequent interventions. For example, if the patient experienced relief of headache within 1 hour after the nurse administered a p.r.n. analgesic, the outcome criterion was met. If the headache was the same or worse, the outcome criterion was not met and requires a new assessment. This may result in a new plan of care or may yield new data that invalidate the nursing diagnosis or suggest new nursing interventions that are more specific or more acceptable to the patient. This assessment could lead to a higher dosage, a different analgesic, or a reevaluation of the cause.

Evaluation enables the nurse to design and implement a revised plan of care, to continuously reevaluate outcome criteria, and to plan again until each nursing diagnosis is successfully completed.

# 6

# Amebicides and antiprotozoals

**atovaquone**
**chloroquine hydrochloride**
(See Chapter 9, ANTIMALARIALS.)
**chloroquine phosphate**
(See Chapter 9, ANTIMALARIALS.)
**eflornithine hydrochloride**
**iodoquinol**
**metronidazole**
**metronidazole hydrochloride**
**paromomycin sulfate**
**pentamidine isethionate**

## COMBINATION PRODUCTS
None.

---

## atovaquone
Mepron

*Pregnancy Risk Category: C*

### HOW SUPPLIED
*Suspension:* 750 mg/5 ml

### ACTION
Unknown. Appears to interfere with electron transport in protozoal mitochondria, inhibiting enzymes needed for the synthesis of nucleic acids and adenosine triphosphate.

### ONSET, PEAK, DURATION
Onset and duration unknown. Two peak plasma levels occur after an oral dose, suggesting enterohepatic recycling. The first occurs after 1 to 8 hours; the second occurs after 1 to 4 days.

### INDICATIONS & DOSAGE
*Mild to moderate* Pneumocystis carinii *pneumonia in patients who cannot tolerate co-trimoxazole* –
**Adults:** 750 mg P.O. b.i.d. with food for 21 days.

### ADVERSE REACTIONS
**CNS:** *headache, insomnia,* asthenia, anxiety, dizziness.
**EENT:** *cough,* sinusitis, rhinitis, taste perversion.
**GI:** *nausea, diarrhea, vomiting,* constipation, *abdominal pain,* anorexia, dyspepsia.
**Skin:** *rash,* pruritus, *diaphoresis.*
**Other:** *fever, oral monilia, pain,* hypoglycemia, hypotension.

### INTERACTIONS
*Rifampin, rifabutin:* decreases atovaquone's steady state concentration. Do not administer concurrently if possible.

### CONTRAINDICATIONS
Contraindicated in patients with hypersensitivity to the drug.

### NURSING CONSIDERATIONS
• Use cautiously in breast-feeding patients. In animal studies, substantial amounts of drug were excreted in breast milk.
• Because drug is highly bound to plasma protein (greater than 99.9%), also use cautiously with other highly protein-bound drugs.
• Because of the risk of other concurrent pulmonary infections, monitor patients closely during therapy.

### ☑ PATIENT TEACHING
• Instruct patient to take drug with meals because food enhances absorption significantly.

---

## eflornithine hydrochloride (DFMO)
Ornidyl

*Pregnancy Risk Category: C*

---

## HOW SUPPLIED
*Injection (concentrate):* 200 mg/ml

## ACTION
Specifically and irreversibly inhibits the enzyme ornithine decarboxylase and limits the availability of substrate for certain amines necessary for cell differentiation and division.

## ONSET, PEAK, DURATION
Onset immediate with I.V. infusion. Serum levels peak immediately after an I.V. infusion. Duration unknown.

## INDICATIONS & DOSAGE
*Meningoencephalitic stage of* Trypanosoma brucei gambiense *(sleeping sickness)* –
**Adults:** 100 mg/kg by I.V. infusion over at least 45 minutes q 6 hours for 14 days.

## ADVERSE REACTIONS
**CNS:** *seizures,* hearing impairment, dizziness, headache, asthenia.
**GI:** diarrhea, vomiting, abdominal pain, anorexia.
**Hematologic:** *anemia, leukopenia, thrombocytopenia, myelosupression,* eosinophilia.
**Other:** facial edema, alopecia.

## INTERACTIONS
None significant.

## CONTRAINDICATIONS
Contraindicated in patients with hypersensitivity to the drug.

## NURSING CONSIDERATIONS
• Use cautiously in patients with impaired renal function because most (about 80%) of the drug is excreted unchanged in the urine.
• Keep in mind that myelosuppression is a common and serious adverse reaction that is reversible when therapy is discontinued. Close patient monitoring is essential. Perform CBC and platelet counts before initiation of therapy, twice weekly during therapy, and weekly after the drug is discontinued until hematologic parameters return to pretreatment levels.
• Impose seizure precautions because seizures occurred in about 8% of patients receiving the drug during clinical trials.
• Obtain serial audiograms when feasible. Some patients have experienced hearing impairment.
• Monitor the patient for at least 24 months after treatment.
• **I.V. use:** Know that the infusion concentrate is hypertonic and must be diluted before administration. Dilute with sterile water for injection and follow strict aseptic technique. To prepare infusion, dilute one part drug to four parts sterile water for injection by adding 25 ml (5,000 mg or 5 g) of the concentrate to each of four bags containing 100 ml of sterile water. After dilution, the final concentration of each bag will be 5,000 mg/125 ml or 40 mg/ml. Use within 24 hours.
• Administer infusion over 45 minutes. Do not administer other drugs with the infusion.
• To minimize the risk of microbial growth, store diluted drug in refrigerator (39° F [4° C]).
• Be aware that the undiluted concentrate may be stored at room temperature (below 86° F [30° C]), but protect from light and freezing.

☑ **PATIENT TEACHING**
• Instruct patient to report hearing changes and other adverse reactions.

---

# iodoquinol (diiodohydroxyquin)
Diodoquin†, Diquinol, Yodoquinol, Yodoxin

*Pregnancy Risk Category: C*

## HOW SUPPLIED
*Tablets:* 210 mg, 650 mg
*Powder:* 25 g

---

## ACTION
Unknown. It is an iodine derivative with amebicidal activity in the intestinal lumen.

## ONSET, PEAK, DURATION
Unknown.

## INDICATIONS & DOSAGE
*Intestinal amebiasis –*
**Adults:** 630 to 650 mg P.O. t.i.d. after meals for 20 days. Total daily dosage should not exceed 1.95 g.
**Children:** usual dosage is 30 to 40 mg/kg of body weight daily in two to three divided doses for 20 days.
Additional doses should not be repeated before a resting interval of 2 to 3 weeks.

## ADVERSE REACTIONS
**CNS:** vertigo, headache, peripheral neuropathy.
**EENT:** optic neuritis, optic atrophy.
**GI:** anorexia, vomiting, abdominal cramps, diarrhea, anal irritation and itching.
**Skin:** pruritus, hives, papular and pustular eruptions, urticaria, bullae.
**Other:** thyroid enlargement, fever, chills.

## INTERACTIONS
None significant.

## CONTRAINDICATIONS
Contraindicated in patients with hypersensitivity to 8-hydroxyquinoline derivatives or iodine-containing preparations. Iodoquinol causes liver damage in such patients. Also contraindicated in patients with hepatic or renal disease or preexisting optic neuropathy.

## NURSING CONSIDERATIONS
● Use cautiously in patients with thyroid diseases.
● If the patient has difficulty swallowing, crush tablets and mix with applesauce or chocolate syrup.
● Record fluid intake and output and color and amount of stools. Send warm specimens to laboratory for analysis.
● Watch for diarrhea during the first 2 or 3 days; notify the doctor if diarrhea continues.
● Be aware that iodoquinol may interfere with thyroid function tests for up to 6 months after drug discontinuation.

## ☑ PATIENT TEACHING
● Recommend that the patient have periodic ophthalmic examinations during treatment.
● Advise the patient not to discontinue the drug prematurely. Tell him to notify the doctor if rash occurs.
● To help prevent reinfestation, teach the patient about the need for personal hygiene, especially good hand-washing technique. Encourage the patient not to prepare food for others until stools are negative.

# metronidazole
Apo-Metronidazole†, Flagyl, Metric-21, Metrogyl‡, Metrozine‡, Neo-Metric†, Novonidazol†, PMS Metronidazole†, Protostat, Trikacide†

# metronidazole hydrochloride
Flagyl I.V. RTU, Metro I.V., Novonidazol†

*Pregnancy Risk Category: B*

## HOW SUPPLIED
*Tablets:* 200 mg‡, 250 mg, 375 mg, 400 mg‡, 500 mg
*Oral suspension (benzoyl metronidazole):* 200 mg/5 ml‡
*Injection:* 500 mg/100 ml ready to use
*Powder for injection:* 500-mg single-dose vials

## ACTION
A direct-acting trichomonacide and amebicide that works at both intestinal and extraintestinal sites. It is

thought to enter the cells of microorganisms that contain nitroreductase. Unstable compounds are then formed that bind to DNA and inhibit synthesis, causing cell death.

## ONSET, PEAK, DURATION
Onset occurs immediately after I.V. infusion, unknown after oral administration. Peak plasma levels occur immediately after I.V. infusion and within 1 to 2 hours of oral administration. Duration unknown.

## INDICATIONS & DOSAGE
*Amebic hepatic abscess –*
**Adults:** 500 to 750 mg P.O. t.i.d. for 5 to 10 days.
**Children:** 35 to 50 mg/kg daily (in three doses) for 10 days.
*Intestinal amebiasis –*
**Adults:** 750 mg P.O. t.i.d. for 5 to 10 days.
**Children:** 35 to 50 mg/kg daily (in three doses) for 10 days. Therapy followed with oral iodoquinol.
*Trichomoniasis –*
**Adults:** 250 mg P.O. t.i.d. for 7 days or 2 g P.O. in single dose (may give the 2-g dose in two 1-g doses, each on the same day); 4 to 6 weeks should elapse between courses of therapy.
**Children:** 5 mg/kg dose P.O. t.i.d. for 7 days.
*Refractory trichomoniasis –*
**Adults:** 250 mg P.O. b.i.d. for 10 days.
*Bacterial infections caused by anaerobic microorganisms –*
**Adults:** loading dose is 15 mg/kg I.V. infused over 1 hour (approximately 1 g for a 70-kg adult). Maintenance dose is 7.5 mg/kg I.V. or P.O. q 6 hours (approximately 500 mg for a 70-kg adult). The first maintenance dose should be administered 6 hours after the loading dose. Maximum dosage not to exceed 4 g daily.
*Giardiasis –*
**Adults:** 250 mg P.O. t.i.d. for 5 to 7 days or 2 g P.O. once daily for 3 days.

**Children:** 5 mg/kg P.O. t.i.d. for 5 to 7 days.
*Prevention of postoperative infection in contaminated or potentially contaminated colorectal surgery –*
**Adults:** 15 mg/kg I.V. infused over 30 to 60 minutes and completed approximately 1 hour before surgery. Then, 7.5 mg/kg I.V. infused over 30 to 60 minutes at 6 and 12 hours after the initial dose.

## ADVERSE REACTIONS
**CNS:** vertigo, headache, ataxia, dizziness, syncope, incoordination, confusion, irritability, depression, weakness, insomnia, *seizures,* peripheral neuropathy.
**CV:** ECG change (flattened T wave), edema (with I.V. RTU preparation).
**GI:** abdominal cramping, stomatitis, epigastric distress, nausea, vomiting, anorexia, diarrhea, constipation, proctitis, dry mouth.
**GU:** darkened urine, polyuria, dysuria, cystitis, decreased libido, dyspareunia, dryness of vagina and vulva, vaginal candidiasis.
**Hematologic:** transient leukopenia, neutropenia.
**Skin:** flushing, rash.
**Other:** overgrowth of nonsusceptible organisms, especially *Candida* (glossitis, furry tongue); metallic taste; fever; thrombophlebitis after I.V. infusion; fleeting joint pains, sometimes resembling serum sickness.

## INTERACTIONS
*Cimetidine:* increased risk of metronidazole toxicity because of inhibited hepatic metabolism. Monitor closely.
*Disulfiram:* acute psychoses and confusional states. Don't use together.
*Ethanol:* disulfiram-like reaction (nausea, vomiting, headache, cramps, flushing). Don't use together.
*Lithium:* increased lithium levels resulting in possible toxicity. Monitor serum lithium levels closely.

---

Reactions may be *common,* uncommon, *life-threatening,* or COMMON AND LIFE-THREATENING.

*Oral anticoagulants:* increased anticoagulant effects. Monitor closely.
*Phenytoin, phenobarbital:* decreased metronidazole effectiveness because of increased hepatic clearance. Monitor closely.

## CONTRAINDICATIONS
Contraindicated in patients with hypersensitivity to the drug or other nitroimidazole derivatives.

## NURSING CONSIDERATIONS
● Use cautiously in patients with a history of blood dyscrasia or CNS disorder and in patients with retinal or visual field changes. Also use cautiously in patients with hepatic disease or alcoholism and in conjunction with known hepatotoxic drugs.
● If indicated during pregnancy for trichomoniasis, be aware that the 7-day regimen is preferred over the 2-g single-dose regimen.
● Give oral form with meals to minimize GI distress.
● **I.V. use:** Keep in mind that no preparation is necessary for RTU (ready to use). To prepare lyophilized vials of metronidazole, add 4.4 ml of sterile water for injection, bacteriostatic water for injection, sterile 0.9% sodium chloride for injection, or bacteriostatic 0.9% sodium chloride for injection. The reconstituted drug contains 100 mg/ml. Add the contents of the vial to 100 ml of $D_5W$, lactated Ringer's injection, or 0.9% sodium chloride for a final concentration of 5 mg/ml. The resulting highly acidic solution must be neutralized before administering. Carefully add 5 mEq sodium bicarbonate for each 500 mg metronidazole; carbon dioxide gas will form that may need to be vented.
● *Alert:* Infuse drug over at least 1 hour. Don't give I.V. push.
● Don't refrigerate the neutralized diluted solution. Precipitation may occur. If Flagyl I.V. RTU is refrigerated, crystals may form. These will disappear after the solution is gently warmed to room temperature.
● Observe carefully for edema, especially in patients also receiving corticosteroids because Flagyl I.V. RTU may cause sodium retention.
● Record number and character of stools when used in the treatment of amebiasis. Metronidazole should be used only after *Trichomonas vaginalis* has been confirmed by wet smear or culture or *Entamoeba histolytica* has been identified. Asymptomatic sexual partners of patients being treated for *T. vaginalis* infection should be treated simultaneously to avoid reinfection.

☑ **PATIENT TEACHING**
● Instruct the patient to take oral form with food to minimize adverse GI reactions.
● Inform the patient that sexual partners should be treated simultaneously to avoid reinfection.
● Instruct the patient in proper hygiene.
● Tell the patient to avoid alcohol or alcohol-containing medications during therapy and for at least 48 hours after therapy is completed.
● Tell the patient metallic taste and dark or red-brown urine may occur.

# paromomycin sulfate
Humatin
*Pregnancy Risk Category: NR*

## HOW SUPPLIED
*Capsules:* 250 mg

## ACTION
Unknown but it acts as an intestinal amebicide. It appears to inhibit protein synthesis in susceptible bacteria at the 30S segment of the ribosome.

## ONSET, PEAK, DURATION
Unknown.

## INDICATIONS & DOSAGE

*Intestinal amebiasis, acute and chronic —*

**Adults and children:** 25 to 35 mg/kg daily P.O. in three doses with meals for 5 to 10 days.

*Tapeworms (fish, beef, pork, dog) —*

**Adults:** 1 g P.O. q 15 minutes for four doses.

**Children:** 11 mg/kg P.O. q 15 minutes for four doses.

## ADVERSE REACTIONS

**CNS:** headache, vertigo.

**EENT:** ototoxicity (potential).

**GI:** anorexia, nausea, vomiting, epigastric pain and burning, abdominal cramps, diarrhea, increased motility, steatorrhea, pruritus ani, malabsorption syndrome.

**GU:** hematuria, *nephrotoxicity* (potential).

**Hematologic:** eosinophilia.

**Skin:** rash, exanthema.

**Other:** overgrowth of nonsusceptible organisms.

## INTERACTIONS

None significant.

## CONTRAINDICATIONS

Contraindicated in patients with hypersensitivity to the drug and in those with impaired renal function or intestinal obstruction.

## NURSING CONSIDERATIONS

• Use cautiously in patients with ulcerative lesions of the bowel to avoid inadvertent absorption and resulting renal toxicity. Poorly absorbed orally, but will accumulate in patients with renal impairment or ulcerative lesions.

• Ask about history of sensitivity to drug before giving first dose.

• Administer with meals.

• Be aware that criterion of cure is absence of amebae in stools examined weekly for 6 weeks after treatment and thereafter at monthly intervals for 2 years. Examine stools of family members or suspected contacts.

• Be aware that patient should avoid high doses or prolonged therapy.

• Watch for signs of superinfection (continued fever and other signs of new infections, especially monilial infections).

• Notify doctor if ringing in ears, hearing impairment, or dizziness occurs.

## ☑ PATIENT TEACHING

• Instruct patient to take drug with meals.

• To help prevent reinfestation, teach patient about the need for personal hygiene, especially good hand-washing technique.

• Instruct patient to refrain from preparing food for others until stools are negative.

---

# pentamidine isethionate
NebuPent, Pentacarinat, Pentam 300, Pneumopent

*Pregnancy Risk Category: C*

## HOW SUPPLIED

*Injection:* 300-mg vial
*Aerosol:* 300-mg vial

## ACTION

Interferes with biosynthesis of DNA, RNA, phospholipids, and proteins in susceptible organisms.

## ONSET, PEAK, DURATION

Unknown except peak serum levels occur ½ to 1 hour after I.M. injection, immediately after I.V. infusion.

## INDICATIONS & DOSAGE

*Pneumocystis carinii pneumonia —*

**Adults and children:** 4 mg/kg I.V. or I.M. once daily for 14 days.

*Prevention of P. carinii pneumonia in high-risk individuals —*

**Adults:** 300 mg by inhalation (using a

---

Respirgard II nebulizer) once every 4 weeks.

## ADVERSE REACTIONS
**CNS:** confusion, hallucinations, *fatigue, dizziness,* headache.
**CV:** *hypotension, ventricular tachycardia,* chest pain.
**GI:** *nausea, metallic taste, decreased appetite, pharyngitis, vomiting,* diarrhea, abdominal pain, anorexia, bad taste in mouth.
**GU:** *elevated serum creatinine,* **acute renal failure.**
**Hematologic:** leukopenia, ***thrombocytopenia,*** anemia.
**Hepatic:** elevated liver function tests.
**Respiratory:** *cough, bronchospasm, shortness of breath,* pneumothorax.
**Skin:** *rash,* Stevens-Johnson syndrome.
**Other:** *hypoglycemia,* hypocalcemia, *sterile abscess, pain or induration at injection site, congestion, night sweats, chills,* edema, myalgia.

## INTERACTIONS
*Aminoglycosides, amphotericin B, capreomycin, cisplatin, colistin, methoxyflurane, polymyxin B, vancomycin:* increased risk of nephrotoxicity.

## CONTRAINDICATIONS
Contraindicated in patients with a history of an anaphylactic reaction to the drug.

## NURSING CONSIDERATIONS
● Use cautiously in patients with hypertension, hypotension, hypoglycemia, hypocalcemia, leukopenia, thrombocytopenia, anemia, or hepatic or renal dysfunction.
● Administer the aerosol form only by the Respirgard II nebulizer manufactured by Marquest. Dosage recommendations are based on the particle size and delivery rate of this device. To administer aerosol, mix the contents of one vial in 6 ml of sterile water for injection. *Do not* use 0.9%

sodium chloride solution because it will cause precipitation. Do not mix with other drugs.
● Do not use low-pressure (less than 20 psi) compressors. The flow rate should be 5 to 7 liters/minute from a 40- to 50-psi air or oxygen source.
● **I.V. use:** Reconstitute drug with 3 ml of sterile water for injection. Then dilute in 50 to 250 ml of $D_5W$. Inject over at least 60 minutes.
● *Alert:* To minimize risk of hypotension, infuse drug slowly with the patient lying down. Closely monitor blood pressure.
● For I.M. injection, reconstitute drug with 3 ml of sterile water for a solution containing 100 mg/ml; administer deeply. Expect pain and induration to occur.
● Monitor blood glucose, serum calcium, serum creatinine, and BUN levels daily. After parenteral administration, blood glucose level may decrease initially; hypoglycemia may be severe in 5% to 10% of patients. This may be followed by hyperglycemia and insulin-dependent diabetes mellitus, which may be permanent.
● In patients with AIDS, be aware that pentamidine may produce less severe adverse reactions than co-trimoxazole, the alternative treatment, and may be the treatment of choice.

### ☑ PATIENT TEACHING
● Instruct the patient to use the aerosol device until the chamber is empty, which may take up to 45 minutes.
● Warn the patient that I.M. injection is painful.

---

*Liquid form contains alcohol.  **May contain tartrazine.  †Canada only.  ‡Australia only.  ◊OTC.

# 7

# Anthelmintics

mebendazole
niclosamide
oxamniquine
piperazine adipate
praziquantel
pyrantel embonate
pyrantel pamoate
thiabendazole

**COMBINATION PRODUCTS**
None.

## mebendazole
Vermox
*Pregnancy Risk Category: C*

**HOW SUPPLIED**
*Tablets (chewable):* 100 mg
*Oral suspension:* 100 mg/5 ml‡

**ACTION**
Selectively and irreversibly inhibits uptake of glucose and other nutrients in susceptible helminths.

**ONSET, PEAK, DURATION**
Onset unknown. Plasma levels peak in 2 to 5 hours. Duration varies.

**INDICATIONS & DOSAGE**
*Pinworm*—
**Adults and children over 2 years:**
100 mg P.O. as a single dose; repeated if infection persists 3 weeks later.
*Roundworm, whipworm, hookworm*—
**Adults and children over 2 years:**
100 mg P.O. b.i.d. for 3 days; repeated if infection persists 3 weeks later.

**ADVERSE REACTIONS**
**GI:** occasional, transient abdominal pain and diarrhea in massive infection and expulsion of worms.
**Other:** fever.

**INTERACTIONS**
*Cimetidine:* increased plasma concentrations of mebendazole. Monitor closely.

**CONTRAINDICATIONS**
Contraindicated in patients with hypersensitivity to the drug.

**NURSING CONSIDERATIONS**
• Be aware that tablets may be chewed, swallowed whole, or crushed and mixed with food.
• Administer the drug to all family members, as prescribed, to decrease the risk of spreading the infection.
• Know that no dietary restrictions, laxatives, or enemas are necessary.

☑ **PATIENT TEACHING**
• Teach the patient about personal hygiene, especially good hand-washing technique. Advise him to refrain from preparing food for others.
• To avoid reinfection, teach the patient to wash perianal area daily, to change undergarments and bedclothes daily, and to wash hands and clean fingernails before meals and after bowel movements.

## niclosamide
Niclocide, Yomesan‡
*Pregnancy Risk Category: B*

**HOW SUPPLIED**
*Tablets (chewable):* 500 mg

**ACTION**
Inhibits oxidative phosphorylation in tapeworms.

**ONSET, PEAK, DURATION**
Unknown.

---

Reactions may be *common,* uncommon, *life-threatening,* or COMMON AND LIFE-THREATENING.

## INDICATIONS & DOSAGE

*Tapeworms (fish, beef, and pork)* –
**Adults:** 4 tablets (2 g) chewed thoroughly as a single dose.
**Children over 2 years and more than 34 kg:** 3 tablets (1.5 g) chewed thoroughly as a single dose.
**Children over 2 years and 11 to 34 kg:** 2 tablets (1 g) chewed thoroughly as a single dose.
*Dwarf tapeworm* –
**Adults:** 4 tablets chewed thoroughly, daily for 7 days.
**Children over 2 years and more than 34 kg:** 3 tablets (1.5 g) chewed thoroughly on the first day, then 2 tablets (1 g) daily for the next 6 days.
**Children over 2 years and 11 to 34 kg:** 2 tablets (1 g) chewed thoroughly on the first day, then 1 (0.5 g) tablet daily for the next 6 days.

## ADVERSE REACTIONS

**CNS:** drowsiness, dizziness, headache, weakness.
**EENT:** oral irritation, bad taste in mouth.
**GI:** nausea, vomiting, anorexia, diarrhea, abdominal discomfort, constipation, rectal bleeding.
**Skin:** rash, pruritus ani.

## INTERACTIONS

None significant.

## CONTRAINDICATIONS

Contraindicated in patients with hypersensitivity to the drug.

## NURSING CONSIDERATIONS

• Expect to administer an antiemetic before treatment as ordered. Many clinicians also give a laxative 2 hours after a dose to expel the killed worms and prevent migration of ova into the stomach.
• When treating dwarf tapeworms, urge the patient to drink fruit juices. This helps to eliminate the accumulated intestinal mucus under which the tapeworms lodge.

• **Alert:** Be aware that the patient is not cured until stools have been negative for tapeworms for at least 3 months.

## ☑ PATIENT TEACHING

• Instruct the patient to take tablets as a single dose after breakfast.
• Instruct the patient to chew tablets thoroughly and to wash down with water; for children, crush and mix the tablets with water or applesauce.
• Teach the patient about personal hygiene, especially good hand-washing technique. Advise him to refrain from preparing food for others.

# oxamniquine
Vansil

*Pregnancy Risk Category: C*

## HOW SUPPLIED

*Capsules:* 250 mg

## ACTION

Unknown although it reduces the egg load of *Schistosoma mansoni*.

## ONSET, PEAK, DURATION

Onset and duration unknown. Plasma levels peak within 1 to 1½ hours.

## INDICATIONS & DOSAGE

*Schistosomiasis caused by* S. mansoni, *Western Hemisphere strains* –
**Adults and children over 30 kg:** 12 to 15 mg/kg as a single oral dose.
**Children under 30 kg:** 10 mg/kg P.O., followed by 10 mg/kg P.O. 2 to 8 hours later.
*Schistosomiasis caused by* S. mansoni, *East and Central African strains* –
**Adults and children:** 30 mg/kg given as a single oral dose or in two equally divided doses over 1 to 2 days.
*Schistosomiasis caused by* S. mansoni, *in Sudan, Uganda, and Zaire* –
**Adults and children:** 40 mg/kg given as a single oral dose or in two equally divided doses over 1 to 2 days.

*Schistosomiasis caused by* S. mansoni, *in Egypt, South Africa, and Zimbabwe* –
**Adults and children:** 60 mg/kg given as 15 mg/kg b.i.d. for 2 days or 20 mg/kg b.i.d. for 3 days.

## ADVERSE REACTIONS
**CNS:** *epileptiform seizures, dizziness, drowsiness,* headache.
**GI:** nausea, vomiting, abdominal pain, anorexia.
**Skin:** urticaria.

## INTERACTIONS
None significant.

## CONTRAINDICATIONS
Contraindicated in patients with hypersensitivity to the drug.

## NURSING CONSIDERATIONS
• Use cautiously in patients with a history of epilepsy; in rare cases, seizures have been observed within the first few hours after ingestion.
• Administer drug after meals to improve GI tolerance.
• Keep in mind that although *S. mansoni* infection is rare in the United States and Canada, travelers or immigrants from such areas as Puerto Rico, Latin America, and Africa may have contracted the infection from contaminated water.

## ☑ PATIENT TEACHING
• Tell the patient to take drug after meals.
• Warn the patient that oxamniquine may cause urine to turn red.
• Instruct the patient to avoid hazardous activities during treatment.

---

## piperazine adipate
Entacyl†

*Pregnancy Risk Category: NR*

## HOW SUPPLIED
*Oral suspension:* 600 mg/5 ml†
*Granules:* 2 g/packet†

## ACTION
Blocks neuromuscular action, paralyzing the worm and causing its expulsion by normal peristalsis.

## ONSET, PEAK, DURATION
Onset and duration vary. Peak concentration occurs in 2 to 4 hours.

## INDICATIONS & DOSAGE
*Enterobiasis (pinworm)* –
**Adults and children:** 65 mg/kg P.O. daily for 7 to 8 days. Maximum daily dosage is 2.5 g. Alternatively, adults 2 g P.O. daily for 7 days, and children 1 g/m² P.O. daily for 7 days.
  Some clinicians order according to body weight:
**Children under 7 kg:** 250 mg P.O. daily for 7 days.
**Children 7 to 14 kg:** 500 mg P.O. daily for 7 days.
**Children 14 to 27 kg:** 1 g P.O. daily for 7 days.
**Children over 27 kg and adults:** 2 g P.O. daily for 7 days.
*Ascariasis (roundworm)* –
**Adults:** 3.5 g P.O. in single doses for 2 consecutive days.
**Children:** 75 mg/kg or 2 g/m² P.O. daily for 2 consecutive days. Maximum daily dosage is 3.5 g.
  Alternatively, dosage given according to body weight:
**Children under 14 kg:** 1 g P.O. daily for 2 days.
**Children 14 to 23 kg:** 2 g P.O. daily for 2 days.
**Children 23 to 45 kg:** 3 g P.O. daily for 2 days.
**Children over 45 kg and adults:** 3.5 g P.O. daily for 2 days.
  Some clinicians continue treatment for 4 days in patients with massive infestation. Treatment may be repeated in 1 week if necessary.

## ADVERSE REACTIONS
**CNS:** ataxia, tremor, choreiform movements, muscular weakness, myoclonus, hyporeflexia, paresthesia,

*seizures,* sense of detachment, EEG abnormalities, memory defect, headache, vertigo.
**EENT:** nystagmus, blurred vision, paralytic strabismus, cataracts with visual impairment, lacrimation, rhinorrhea.
**GI:** nausea, vomiting, diarrhea, abdominal cramps.
**Skin:** urticaria, photodermatitis, *erythema multiforme,* purpura, eczematous skin reactions.
**Other:** arthralgia, fever, bronchospasm, *hemolytic anemia.*

### INTERACTIONS
*Pyrantel pamoate:* possible antagonism. Don't administer together.

### CONTRAINDICATIONS
Contraindicated in patients with hypersensitivity to the drug and in those with hepatic or renal impairment or seizure disorders.

### NURSING CONSIDERATIONS
• Use cautiously in patients with severe malnutrition or anemia.
• Monitor the patient for CNS or GI reactions; be prepared to discontinue the drug if any occur.
• Be aware that no diet restrictions, laxatives, or enemas are necessary.
• Be aware that drug should be administered to all family members, as prescribed, to decrease risk of spreading infection.
• Be aware that because of potential neurotoxicity, prolonged or repeated treatment (especially in children) should be avoided.

### ☑ PATIENT TEACHING
• Tell the patient to take the drug on empty stomach to promote absorption.
• Teach the patient about personal hygiene, especially good hand-washing technique. To avoid reinfection, teach the patient to wash perianal area, to change undergarments and bedclothes daily, and to wash hands and clean fingernails before meals and after

bowel movements. Instruct the patient to disinfect toilet facilities daily.
• Advise the patient to refrain from preparing food for others.

## praziquantel
Biltricide

*Pregnancy Risk Category: B*

### HOW SUPPLIED
*Tablets:* 600 mg

### ACTION
Causes a contraction of schistosomes by a specific effect on the permeability of the cell membrane.

### ONSET, PEAK, DURATION
Onset and duration unknown. Peak serum concentration occurs in 1 to 3 hours.

### INDICATIONS & DOSAGE
*Schistosomiasis caused by* Schistosoma mekongi, S. japonicum, S. mansoni, *and* S. haematobium —
**Adults and children 4 years and older:** 20 mg/kg P.O. t.i.d. as a 1-day treatment. The interval between doses should be 4 to 6 hours.
*Clonorchiasis caused by* Clonorchis sinensis, *opisthorchiasis caused by* Opisthorchis viverrini —
**Adults and children 4 years and older:** 25 mg/kg t.i.d. as a 1-day treatment.

### ADVERSE REACTIONS
**CNS:** malaise, headache, dizziness.
**GI:** abdominal discomfort, nausea.
**Skin:** urticaria.
**Other:** fever.

### INTERACTIONS
None significant.

### CONTRAINDICATIONS
Contraindicated in patients with hypersensitivity to the drug and in those with ocular cysticercosis because de-

---

*Liquid form contains alcohol.   **May contain tartrazine.   †Canada only.   ‡Australia only.   ◊OTC.

struction of the eye parasite may cause permanent eye damage.

## NURSING CONSIDERATIONS
• Keep in mind that praziquantel is effective for several different species of *Schistosoma* and may also be effective against liver flukes.
• For overdose, a fast-acting laxative is given.

☑ **PATIENT TEACHING**
• Advise the patient to take the tablet during meals and to wash down the unchewed tablet.
• Warn the patient that the tablets taste bitter. Keeping them in the mouth may cause gagging or vomiting.
• Tell the patient to avoid hazardous activities on the day of treatment and the day after because praziquantel may produce drowsiness.

---

## pyrantel embonate
Anthel‡, Combantrin‡, Early Bird‡

## pyrantel pamoate
Antiminth, Combantrin†, Reese's Pinworm Medicine

*Pregnancy Risk Category: NR*

## HOW SUPPLIED
**pyrantel embonate**
*Tablets:* 125 mg‡, 250 mg‡
*Oral suspension:* 50 mg/ml‡
*Squares (chocolate-flavored):* 100 mg‡
**pyrantel pamoate**
*Tablets:* 125 mg†
*Oral suspension:* 50 mg/ml

## ACTION
Blocks neuromuscular action, paralyzing the worm and causing its expulsion by normal peristalsis.

## ONSET, PEAK, DURATION
Onset is highly variable. Plasma levels peak within 1 to 3 hours. Duration varies with GI transit time and extent of infestation.

## INDICATIONS & DOSAGE
*Roundworm and pinworm –*
**Adults and children over 2 years:**
11 mg/kg P.O. as a single dose. Maximum dosage is 1 g. For pinworm, dosage should be repeated in 2 weeks.

## ADVERSE REACTIONS
**CNS:** headache, dizziness, drowsiness, insomnia.
**GI:** anorexia, nausea, vomiting, gastralgia, abdominal cramps, diarrhea, tenesmus.
**Hepatic:** transient elevation of AST.
**Skin:** rash.
**Other:** fever, weakness.

## INTERACTIONS
*Piperazine salts:* possible antagonism; don't give together.

## CONTRAINDICATIONS
Contraindicated in patients with hypersensitivity to the drug.

## NURSING CONSIDERATIONS
• Use cautiously in patients with severe malnutrition or anemia or in patients with hepatic dysfunction.
• Be aware that no diet restrictions, laxatives, or enemas are needed.
• Be aware that drug should be given to all family members.

☑ **PATIENT TEACHING**
• Advise the patient that pyrantel may be taken with food, milk, or fruit juices. Shake suspension well.
• Teach the patient about personal hygiene, especially good hand-washing technique. To avoid reinfection, teach the patient to wash perianal area daily, to change undergarments and bedclothes daily, and to wash hands and clean fingernails before meals and after bowel movements.
• Advise him to refrain from preparing food for others.

---

Reactions may be *common*, uncommon, *life-threatening*, or **COMMON AND LIFE-THREATENING**.

# thiabendazole
Mintezol

*Pregnancy Risk Category: C*

## HOW SUPPLIED
*Tablets (chewable):* 500 mg
*Oral suspension:* 500 mg/5 ml

## ACTION
Unknown, but the drug appears to inhibit the helminth-specific enzyme fumarate reductase.

## ONSET, PEAK, DURATION
Onset and duration unknown. Plasma levels peak in 1 to 2 hours.

## INDICATIONS & DOSAGE
*Cutaneous infestations with larva migrans (creeping eruption) –*
**Adults and children:** 25 mg/kg P.O. b.i.d. for 2 to 5 days. Maximum dosage is 3 g daily. If lesions persist after 2 days, course is repeated.
*Pinworm –*
**Adults and children:** 25 mg/kg P.O. in 2 doses daily for 1 day; repeated in 7 days.
*Roundworm, threadworm, whipworm –*
**Adults and children:** 25 mg/kg P.O. in 2 doses daily for 2 successive days.
*Trichinosis –*
**Adults and children:** 25 mg/kg P.O. in 2 doses daily for 2 to 4 successive days.

## ADVERSE REACTIONS
**CNS:** impaired mental alertness, impaired coordination, numbness, seizures, *drowsiness, fatigue,* giddiness, *headache,* dizziness.
**CV:** *hypotension.*
**EENT:** tinnitus, blurry vision, dry mouth and eyes, xanthopsia.
**GI:** *anorexia, nausea, vomiting,* diarrhea, epigastric distress, cholestasis.
**GU:** hematuria, enuresis, crystalluria, malodorous urine.
**Hematologic:** leukopenia.
**Hepatic:** *jaundice, parenchymal liver damage.*

**Skin:** *rash, pruritus, erythema multiforme, Stevens-Johnson syndrome.*
**Other:** lymphadenopathy, fever, flushing, chills, *angioedema, anaphylaxis.*

## INTERACTIONS
*Theophylline:* may impair hepatic metabolism of theophylline, increasing risk of toxicity. Monitor patient closely.

## CONTRAINDICATIONS
Contraindicated in patients with hypersensitivity to the drug.

## NURSING CONSIDERATIONS
• Use cautiously in patients with hepatic or renal dysfunction, severe malnutrition, and anemia and in patients who are vomiting.
• Be aware that drug should be administered to all family members, as prescribed, to prevent risk of spreading infection.
• Be aware that no dietary restrictions, laxatives, or enemas are necessary. However, know that supportive therapy is indicated for anemic, dehydrated, or malnourished patients.

## ☑ PATIENT TEACHING
• Teach the patient to take drug after meals. For oral suspension, shake before measuring dose. For tablets, advise patient to chew before swallowing.
• Advise the patient to avoid hazardous activities, such as driving, because drug may cause drowsiness.
• Teach the patient about personal hygiene, especially good hand-washing technique. To avoid reinfection, teach the patient to wash perianal area daily, change undergarments and bedclothes daily, and wash hands and clean fingernails before meals and after bowel movements. Tell him not to prepare food for others during infestation.

---

*Liquid form contains alcohol. **May contain tartrazine. †Canada only. ‡Australia only. ◇OTC.

amphotericin B
fluconazole
flucytosine
griseofulvin microsize
griseofulvin ultramicrosize
itraconazole
ketoconazole
miconazole
nystatin

**COMBINATION PRODUCTS**
None.

---

## amphotericin B
Fungilin Oral‡, Fungizone
Intravenous

*Pregnancy Risk Category: B*

### HOW SUPPLIED
*Tablets:* 100 mg‡
*Oral suspension:* 100 mg/ml‡
*Lozenges:* 10 mg‡
*Injection:* 50-mg lyophilized cake

### ACTION
Unknown. Probably acts by binding to sterol in the fungal cell membrane, altering cell permeability and allowing leakage of intracellular components.

### ONSET, PEAK, DURATION
Onset is immediate and serum levels peak immediately after I.V. infusion. Onset, peak, and duration are unknown after oral administration.

### INDICATIONS & DOSAGE
*Systemic fungal infections (histoplasmosis, coccidioidomycosis, blastomycosis, cryptococcosis, disseminated moniliasis, aspergillosis, phycomycosis), meningitis –*
**Adults:** initially, 1 mg in 250 ml of D₅W infused over 2 to 4 hours; or 0.25 mg/kg daily by slow infusion over 6 hours. Daily dosage is gradually increased to maximum 1 mg/kg daily. If drug is discontinued for 1 week or more, drug is resumed with initial dose and increased gradually.
*Infections of the GI tract caused by* Candida albicans –
**Adults:** 100 mg P.O. q.i.d. for 2 weeks.
*Oral and perioral candidal infections –*
**Adults:** 1 lozenge q.i.d. for 7 to 14 days. Lozenge should be allowed to dissolve slowly.

### ADVERSE REACTIONS
**CNS:** *headache,* peripheral neuropathy, **seizures.**
**CV:** hypotension, **cardiac arrhythmias, asystole,** hypertension.
**EENT:** hearing loss, tinnitus, transient vertigo, blurred vision, diplopia.
**GI:** *anorexia, weight loss, nausea, vomiting, dyspepsia, diarrhea, epigastric pain, cramping,* melena, **hemorrhagic gastroenteritis.**
**GU:** *abnormal renal function with hypokalemia, azotemia, hyposthenuria, renal tubular acidosis, nephrocalcinosis;* with large doses –**permanent renal impairment,** anuria, oliguria.
**Hematologic:** *normochromic, normocytic anemia,* **thrombocytopenia,** leukopenia, **agranulocytosis,** eosinophilia, leukocytosis.
**Hepatic:** hepatitis, jaundice, **acute liver failure.**
**Respiratory:** dyspnea, tachypnea, bronchospasm, wheezing.
**Skin:** maculopapular rash, pruritus (without rash).
**Other:** arthralgia, tissue damage with extravasation, *phlebitis, thrombophlebitis, pain at injection site,* myalgia, *fever, chills, malaise, generalized pain,* flushing, **anaphylactoid reactions.**

---

Reactions may be *common,* uncommon, *life-threatening,* or **COMMON AND LIFE-THREATENING.**

## INTERACTIONS

*Corticosteroids:* enhanced potassium depletion. Monitor serum potassium levels.

*Digitalis glycosides:* increased risk of digitalis toxicity in potassium-depleted patients. Monitor closely.

*Flucytosine:* synergistic effect; may cause increased toxicity of flucytosine. Monitor closely.

*Other nephrotoxic drugs, such as antibiotics or antineoplastic agents:* may cause additive renal toxicity. Administer cautiously.

## CONTRAINDICATIONS

Contraindicated in patients with hypersensitivity to the drug.

## NURSING CONSIDERATIONS

• Use cautiously in patients with impaired renal function.

• **Alert:** To reduce severe adverse reactions, be aware that the patient may receive premedication with antipyretics, antihistamines, antiemetics, or small doses of corticosteroids; addition of phosphate buffer and heparin to the solution; and alternate-day schedule. For severe reactions, discontinue drug and notify doctor.

• Give parenterally only in hospitalized patients, under close supervision, when diagnosis of potentially fatal fungal infection has been confirmed.

• Monitor fluid intake and output; report change in urine appearance or volume. Monitor BUN and serum creatinine (or creatinine clearance) at least weekly. Kidney damage is typically reversible if drug is stopped at first sign of dysfunction.

• Obtain liver and renal function studies weekly, if ordered. If BUN exceeds 40 mg/100 ml, or if serum creatinine exceeds 3 mg/100 ml, doctor may reduce or stop drug until renal function improves. Monitor CBC weekly. Drug may be stopped if alkaline phosphatase or bilirubin levels increase.

• Monitor potassium levels closely, and report signs of hypokalemia. Check calcium and magnesium levels twice weekly, as ordered.

• **I.V. use:** Be prepared to give initial test dose as prescribed. 1 mg is added to 50 to 250 ml of $D_5W$ and infused over 20 to 30 minutes; monitor the patient's pulse, respiratory rate, temperature, and blood pressure for at least 4 hours.

• Use an infusion pump and in-line filter with mean pore diameter larger than 1 micron. Infuse over 6 hours; rapid infusion may cause cardiovascular collapse.

• Choose I.V. sites in distal veins. If veins become thrombosed, alternate administration sites.

• Monitor vital signs every 30 minutes; fever, shaking chills, and hypotension may appear 1 to 2 hours after start of I.V. infusion and should subside within 4 hours of stopping drug.

• Be aware that reconstituted solution is stable for 1 week under refrigeration or 24 hours at room temperature. It has 8-hour stability in room light.

• Give antibiotics separately; don't mix or piggyback with amphotericin B.

• Know that amphotericin B seems to be compatible with limited amounts of heparin sodium, hydrocortisone sodium succinate, and methylprednisolone sodium succinate.

• Store the dry form at 2° to 8° C (35.6° to 46.4° F). Protect from light. Reconstitute with 10 ml of sterile water only. To avoid precipitation, do not mix with solutions containing sodium chloride, other electrolytes, or bacteriostatic agents such as benzyl alcohol. Do not use if solution contains precipitate or foreign matter.

## ☑ PATIENT TEACHING

• Warn the patient of possible discomfort at I.V. site and of other potential adverse reactions. Instruct the patient to report signs and symptoms of hypersensitivity immediately.

---

*Liquid form contains alcohol.  **May contain tartrazine.  †Canada only.  ‡Australia only.  ◇OTC.

- Inform patient that therapy may take several months. Stress importance of compliance and recommended follow-up.

---

# fluconazole
Diflucan

*Pregnancy Risk Category: C*

## HOW SUPPLIED
*Tablets:* 50 mg, 100 mg, 150 mg, 200 mg
*Powder for oral suspension:* 10 mg/ml, 40 mg/ml
*Injection:* 200 mg/100 ml, 400 mg/200 ml

## ACTION
Inhibits fungal cytochrome P-450 (responsible for fungal sterol synthesis) and weakens fungal cell walls.

## ONSET, PEAK, DURATION
Onset immediate with I.V. administration; unknown with oral administration. Peak serum levels occur immediately after I.V. infusion, 1 to 2 hours after oral administration. Duration unknown.

## INDICATIONS & DOSAGE
*Oropharyngeal candidiasis –*
**Adults:** 200 mg P.O. or I.V. on first day, followed by 100 mg once daily. Therapy should last at least 2 weeks.
*Esophageal candidiasis –*
**Adults:** 200 mg P.O. or I.V. on the first day, followed by 100 mg once daily. Higher doses (up to 400 mg daily) have been used, depending on the patient's condition and tolerance of treatment. Patients should receive the drug for at least 3 weeks and for 2 weeks after symptoms resolve.
*Systemic candidiasis –*
**Adults:** 400 mg P.O. or I.V. on the first day, followed by 200 mg once daily. Treatment should continue for at least 4 weeks or for 2 weeks after symptoms resolve.

*Cryptococcal meningitis –*
**Adults:** 400 mg P.O. or I.V. on the first day, followed by 200 mg once daily. Higher doses (up to 400 mg daily) may be used. Treatment should continue for 10 to 12 weeks after CSF cultures are negative.
*Prevention of candidiasis in bone marrow transplant –*
**Adults:** 400 mg P.O. or I.V. once daily. Start prophylaxis several days before anticipated granulocytopenia. Continue therapy for 7 days after the neutrophil count rises above 1,000 cells/mm$^3$.
*Suppression of relapse of cryptococcal meningitis in patients with AIDS –*
**Adults:** 200 mg P.O. or I.V. daily.

In patients with renal failure: If creatinine clearance is 21 to 50 ml/minute, dosage is reduced by 50%. If creatinine clearance is 11 to 20 ml/minute, dosage is reduced by 75%. Patients receiving regular hemodialysis treatment should receive the usual dose after each dialysis session.

## ADVERSE REACTIONS
**CNS:** headache.
**GI:** *nausea,* vomiting, abdominal pain, diarrhea.
**Hepatic:** *hepatotoxicity* (rare), elevated liver enzymes.
**Skin:** rash, *Stevens-Johnson syndrome* (rare).
**Other:** *anaphylaxis.*

## INTERACTIONS
*Cyclosporine, phenytoin:* may increase plasma concentrations of these drugs. Monitor serum cyclosporine or phenytoin levels.
*Isoniazid, phenytoin, rifampin, valproic acid, oral sulfonylureas:* increased incidence of elevated hepatic transaminases. Monitor closely.
*Oral antidiabetic agents (tolbutamide, glyburide, glipizide):* may increase plasma concentrations of these drugs. Monitor for enhanced hypoglycemic effect.

---

Reactions may be *common,* uncommon, *life-threatening,* or COMMON AND LIFE-THREATENING.

*Rifampin:* enhanced metabolism of fluconazole. Monitor for lack of response.
*Warfarin:* increased risk of bleeding. Monitor PT.

## CONTRAINDICATIONS
Contraindicated in patients with hypersensitivity to the drug.

## NURSING CONSIDERATIONS
• Use cautiously in patients with hypersensitivity to other antifungal azole compounds; no information exists regarding cross-sensitivity.
• Do not remove protective overwrap from I.V. bags until just before use, to ensure product sterility. The plastic container may show some opacity from moisture absorbed during sterilization. This is normal, doesn't affect the drug, and diminishes over time.
• **I.V. use:** Administer by continuous infusion at a rate not to exceed 200 mg/hour. Use an infusion pump. To prevent air embolism, do not connect in series with other infusions. Do not add any other drugs to the solution.
• Periodically monitor liver function during prolonged therapy, as ordered. Although adverse hepatic effects are rare, they can be serious.
• If the patient develops mild rash, monitor closely. Discontinue drug if lesions progress and notify doctor.
• Be aware that the incidence of adverse reactions appears to be greater in HIV-infected patients.
• Be aware that safety and effectiveness in children have not been established, but a few children ages 3 to 13 years have received 3 to 6 mg/kg/day.

## ☑ PATIENT TEACHING
• Instruct the patient to take medication exactly as directed, even after he feels better.
• Tell the patient to shake oral suspension in its container before measuring each dose.

• Instruct the patient to report adverse reactions promptly.

---

# flucytosine
# (5-fluorocytosine, 5-FC)
Ancobon, Ancotil†

*Pregnancy Risk Category: C*

## HOW SUPPLIED
*Capsules:* 250 mg, 500 mg

## ACTION
Unknown. Appears to penetrate fungal cells and cause defective protein synthesis.

## ONSET, PEAK, DURATION
Onset and duration unknown. Serum levels peak 1 to 2 hours after oral dose.

## INDICATIONS & DOSAGE
*Severe fungal infections caused by susceptible strains of* Candida *(including septicemia, endocarditis, urinary tract and pulmonary infections) and* Cryptococcus *(meningitis, pulmonary infection, and possible urinary tract infections)* –
**Adults and children over 50 kg:** 50 to 150 mg/kg daily P.O. q 6 hours.
**Adults and children under 50 kg:** 1.5 to 4.5 g/m$^2$/day P.O. in four divided doses.
   Severe infections, such as meningitis, may require doses up to 250 mg/kg.

## ADVERSE REACTIONS
**CNS:** headache, vertigo, sedation, fatigue, weakness, confusion, hallucinations, psychosis, ataxia, hearing loss, paresthesia, parkinsonism, peripheral neuropathy.
**CV:** *cardiac arrest.*
**GI:** nausea, vomiting, diarrhea, abdominal pain, emesis, dry mouth, duodenal ulcer, *hemorrhage,* ulcerative colitis.
**GU:** azotemia, elevated creatinine and BUN levels, crystalluria, *renal failure.*

---

*Liquid form contains alcohol.   **May contain tartrazine.   †Canada only.   ‡Australia only.   ◇OTC.

**Hematologic:** anemia, *leukopenia, bone marrow suppression, thrombocytopenia,* eosinophilia, *agranulocytosis, aplastic anemia.*
**Hepatic:** elevated liver enzymes, elevated serum alkaline phosphatase, jaundice.
**Respiratory:** *respiratory arrest,* chest pain, dyspnea.
**Skin:** occasional rash, pruritus, urticaria, photosensitivity.
**Other:** hypoglycemia, hypokalemia.

## INTERACTIONS
*Amphotericin B:* synergistic effects and possibly enhanced toxicity when used together. Monitor closely.

## CONTRAINDICATIONS
Contraindicated in patients with hypersensitivity to the drug.

## NURSING CONSIDERATIONS
• Use with extreme caution in patients with impaired hepatic or renal function or bone marrow suppression.
• Obtain hematologic tests and renal and liver function studies, as ordered. Ensure that susceptibility tests establishing that organism is flucytosine-sensitive are on the chart.
• Administer capsules over 15 minutes to reduce adverse GI reactions.
• Monitor blood, liver, and renal function studies frequently during therapy; obtain susceptibility tests weekly, as ordered, to monitor drug resistance.
• Monitor fluid intake and output; report any marked change.
• If possible, regularly perform blood level assays of drug, as ordered, to maintain flucytosine at therapeutic level (25 to 120 mcg/ml). Higher blood levels may be toxic.

## ☑ PATIENT TEACHING
• Inform the patient that therapeutic response may take weeks or months.
• Instruct the patient to report adverse reactions promptly.

# griseofulvin microsize
Fulcin‡, Fulvicin-U/F, Grifulvin V, Grisactin, Grisovin‡, Grisovin 500‡, Grisovin-FP

# griseofulvin ultramicrosize
Fulvicin P/G, Grisactin Ultra, Griseostatin‡, Gris-PEG

*Pregnancy Risk Category: NR*

## HOW SUPPLIED
**griseofulvin microsize**
*Tablets:* 250 mg, 500 mg
*Capsules:* 125 mg, 250 mg
*Oral suspension:* 125 mg/5ml
**griseofulvin ultramicrosize**
*Tablets:* 125 mg, 165 mg, 250 mg, 330 mg

## ACTION
Arrests fungal cell activity by disrupting its mitotic spindle structure.

## ONSET, PEAK, DURATION
Onset and duration unknown. Serum levels peak 4 to 8 hours after oral dose.

## INDICATIONS & DOSAGE
*Ringworm infections of skin, hair, nails (tinea corporis, tinea capitis) when caused by* Trichophyton, Microsporum, *or* Epidermophyton —
**Adults:** 500 mg (microsize) P.O. daily in single or divided doses. Severe infections may require up to 1 g daily. Alternatively, 330 to 375 mg ultramicrosize daily in single or divided doses.
*Tinea pedis and tinea unguium —*
**Adults:** 0.75 to 1 g of microsize P.O. daily. Alternatively, 660 to 750 mg of ultramicrosize P.O. daily in divided doses.
**Children:** 11 mg/kg/day of microsize P.O. Alternatively, 7.3 mg/kg/day of ultramicrosize.

## ADVERSE REACTIONS
**CNS:** headache (in early stages of treatment), transient decrease in hearing, fatigue with large doses, occa-

Reactions may be *common,* uncommon, *life-threatening,* or COMMON AND LIFE-THREATENING.

sional mental confusion, impaired performance of routine activities, psychotic symptoms, dizziness, insomnia, paresthesias of the hands and feet after extended therapy.
**GI:** nausea, vomiting, flatulence, diarrhea, epigastric distress, ***bleeding.***
**GU:** proteinuria.
**Hematologic:** leukopenia, ***granulocytopenia*** (requires discontinuation of drug), porphyria.
**Hepatic:** ***hepatic toxicity.***
**Skin:** *rash, urticaria,* photosensitivity, angioneurotic edema.
**Other:** oral thrush, hypersensitivity reactions (rash), menstrual irregularities, lupus erythematosus.

## INTERACTIONS
*Coumarin anticoagulants:* decreased effectiveness. Monitor PT when used concurrently.
*Ethanol:* may cause tachycardia, diaphoresis, and flushing. Avoid ethanol.
*Oral contraceptives:* decreased effectiveness. Suggest alternative methods of contraception.
*Phenobarbital:* decreased griseofulvin blood levels due to decreased absorption or increased metabolism. Avoid using together or administer griseofulvin t.i.d.

## CONTRAINDICATIONS
● Contraindicated in those with hypersensitivity to drug and in those with porphyria or hepatocellular failure.
● Also contraindicated in pregnant patients or women who intend to become pregnant during therapy.

## NURSING CONSIDERATIONS
● Use cautiously in penicillin-sensitive patients.
● ***Alert:*** Because of potential toxicity, know that drug is used only when topical treatment fails.
● Obtain laboratory tests as ordered to confirm diagnosis. Continue drug until clinical and laboratory examinations confirm eradication.

● Be aware that because griseofulvin ultramicrosize is dispersed in polyethylene glycol, it is absorbed more rapidly and completely than microsize preparations and is effective at one-half to two-thirds the usual griseofulvin dose.
● Administer after a high-fat meal to enhance absorption and minimize GI distress.
● Assess hematologic, renal, and hepatic function periodically during prolonged therapy, as ordered.
● Keep in mind that effective treatment of tinea pedis may require concomitant use of a topical agent.

☑ **PATIENT TEACHING**
● Tell the patient to take drug after a high-fat meal.
● Advise him that prolonged treatment may be needed to control infection and prevent relapse, even if symptoms abate in first few days of therapy. Tell him to keep skin clean and dry and to maintain good hygiene.
● Tell him to avoid intense sunlight.

# itraconazole
Sporanox

*Pregnancy Risk Category: C*

## HOW SUPPLIED
*Capsules:* 100 mg

## ACTION
Interferes with fungal cell-wall synthesis by inhibiting the formation of ergosterol, a vital component, and increasing cell-wall permeability that makes the fungus susceptible to osmotic instability.

## ONSET, PEAK, DURATION
Unknown.

## INDICATIONS & DOSAGE
*Pulmonary and extrapulmonary blastomycosis; histoplasmosis –*
**Adults:** 200 mg P.O. daily. Dosage

increased as needed and tolerated in 100-mg increments to a maximum of 400 mg daily. Dosages that exceed 200 mg daily should be given in two divided doses. Treatment should continue for a minimum of 3 months. In life-threatening illness, a loading dose of 200 mg t.i.d. is given for 3 days.
*Aspergillosis*—
**Adults:** 200 to 400 mg P.O. daily.
*Onychomycosis (fungal nail disease) from dermatophytes of toenail*—
**Adults:** 200 mg P.O. once daily for 12 consecutive weeks.

## ADVERSE REACTIONS
**CNS:** headache, dizziness, somnolence.
**CV:** hypertension.
**GI:** *nausea,* vomiting, diarrhea, abdominal pain, anorexia.
**GU:** albuminuria.
**Hepatic:** impaired hepatic function.
**Skin:** rash, pruritus.
**Other:** edema, fatigue, fever, malaise, decreased libido, hypokalemia, impotence.

## INTERACTIONS
*Cyclosporine, digoxin:* possible increased plasma levels of these drugs. Monitor plasma levels closely.
*$H_2$-receptor antagonists, antacids, rifampin, phenytoin:* possible lowered itraconazole plasma levels. Avoid concomitant use.
*Isoniazid:* may decrease plasma levels of itraconazole. Monitor closely.
*Oral anticoagulants:* possible enhanced anticoagulant effects. Monitor PT closely.
*Oral antidiabetic agents:* similar antifungals have caused hypoglycemia. Monitor blood glucose levels closely.
*Terfenadine, astemizole:* inhibited metabolism of these antihistamines, resulting in elevated blood levels and risk of serious cardiac toxicity. Never administer together.

## CONTRAINDICATIONS
Contraindicated in patients with hypersensitivity to the drug, in patients receiving terfenadine or astemizole, and in breast-feeding patients because drug is excreted in breast milk.

## NURSING CONSIDERATIONS
• Use cautiously in patients with hypochlorhydria because they may not absorb the drug as readily as patients with normal gastric acidity. Because hypochlorhydria can accompany HIV infection, also use cautiously in HIV-infected patients.
• Use cautiously in patients receiving other highly bound medications because itraconazole and its metabolites are more than 99% bound to plasma proteins.
• Perform baseline liver function tests, as ordered, and monitor periodically.

## ☑ PATIENT TEACHING
• Teach the patient to recognize and report the signs and symptoms of liver disease (anorexia, dark urine, pale stools, unusual fatigue, or jaundice).
• Tell the patient to take drug with food to ensure maximal absorption.

---

# ketoconazole
Nizoral

*Pregnancy Risk Category: C*

## HOW SUPPLIED
*Tablets:* 200 mg
*Oral suspension:* 100 mg/5 ml†

## ACTION
Inhibits purine transport and DNA, RNA, and protein synthesis; increases cell-wall permeability, making the fungus more susceptible to osmotic pressure.

## ONSET, PEAK, DURATION
Onset and duration unknown. Serum levels peak 1 to 2 hours after oral dose.

---

Reactions may be *common,* uncommon, *life-threatening,* or COMMON AND LIFE-THREATENING.

## INDICATIONS & DOSAGE

*Systemic candidiasis, chronic muco-candidiasis, oral thrush, candiduria, coccidioidomycosis, histoplasmosis, chromomycosis, and paracoccidioido-mycosis; severe cutaneous dermatophyte infections resistant to therapy with topical or oral griseofulvin—*
**Adults and children over 40 kg:** initially, 200 mg P.O. daily in a single dose. Dosage may be increased to 400 mg once daily in patients who don't respond to lower dosage.
**Children 2 years and over:** 3.3 to 6.6 mg/kg P.O. daily as a single dose.

## ADVERSE REACTIONS

**CNS:** headache, nervousness, dizziness, somnolence, photophobia, *suicidal tendencies,* severe depression.
**GI:** *nausea, vomiting,* abdominal pain, diarrhea.
**Hematologic:** *thrombocytopenia,* hemolytic anemia, leukopenia.
**Hepatic:** elevated liver enzymes, or *fatal hepatotoxicity.*
**Skin:** pruritus.
**Other:** gynecomastia with tenderness, fever, chills, impotence.

## INTERACTIONS

*Antacids, anticholinergics, H₂ blockers:* decreased absorption of ketoconazole. Wait at least 2 hours after ketoconazole dose before administering these drugs.
*Astemizole, terfenadine:* may increase plasma levels of these drugs, precipitating CV events. Monitor closely.
*Cisapride:* may cause ventricular arrhythmias. Avoid concomitant use.
*Rifampin, isoniazid:* increased ketoconazole metabolism. Monitor for decreased antifungal effect.

## CONTRAINDICATIONS

Contraindicated in patients with hypersensitivity to the drug and in those taking terfenadine or astemizole.

## NURSING CONSIDERATIONS

● Use cautiously in patients with hepatic disease and in those who are taking other hepatotoxic drugs.
● Because of the potential for serious hepatotoxicity, be aware that ketoconazole should not be used for less serious conditions, such as fungus infections of the skin or nails.
● Monitor for elevated liver enzymes and nausea that does not subside, as well as for unusual fatigue, jaundice, dark urine, or pale stools—all signs of possible hepatotoxicity.
● Keep in mind that much larger doses (up to 800 mg/day) can be used to treat fungal meningitis and intracerebral fungal lesions.

## ☑ PATIENT TEACHING

● Instruct the patient with achlorhydria to dissolve each tablet in 4 ml aqueous solution of 0.2 N hydrochloric acid, sip the mixture through a glass or plastic straw (to avoid contact with teeth), and end the procedure with a glass of water because ketoconazole requires gastric acidity for dissolution and absorption.
● Make sure the patient understands that treatment should be continued until all clinical and laboratory tests indicate that active fungal infection has subsided. If drug is discontinued too soon, infection will recur. Minimum treatment for candidiasis is 7 to 14 days; for other systemic fungal infections, 6 months; for resistant dermatophyte infections, at least 4 weeks.
● Reassure the patient that, although nausea is common early in therapy, it will subside. To minimize nausea, divide the daily dosage into two doses or take it with meals.

## miconazole
Monistat I.V.
*Pregnancy Risk Category: C*

## HOW SUPPLIED
*Injection:* 10 mg/ml

---

*Liquid form contains alcohol.  **May contain tartrazine.  †Canada only.  ‡Australia only.  ◇OTC.

## ACTION
Inhibits purine transport and DNA, RNA, and protein synthesis; increases cell-wall permeability, making the fungus more susceptible to osmotic pressure.

## ONSET, PEAK, DURATION
Onset immediate. Plasma levels peak immediately after I.V. infusion. Duration unknown.

## INDICATIONS & DOSAGE
*Systemic fungal infections (coccidioidomycosis, candidiasis, cryptococcosis, paracoccidioidomycosis), chronic mucocutaneous candidiasis –*
**Adults:** 200 to 3,600 mg/day I.V. Dosages may vary with diagnosis and with infective agent. Daily dosage may be divided over 3 infusions, 200 to 1,200 mg per infusion. Dilute in at least 200 ml of 0.9% sodium chloride. Repeated courses may be needed because of relapse or reinfection.
**Children 1 year and over:** 20 to 40 mg/kg/day I.V. Do not exceed 15 mg/kg per infusion.
*Fungal meningitis –*
**Adults:** 20 mg intrathecally as adjunct to I.V. administration, q 3 to 7 days.

## ADVERSE REACTIONS
**CNS:** dizziness, drowsiness.
**GI:** *nausea,* vomiting, diarrhea.
**Hematologic:** transient decrease in hematocrit, ***thrombocytopenia.***
**Skin:** *pruritic rash.*
**Other:** ***anaphylactoid reactions,*** *fever, chills,* transient decrease in serum sodium, *phlebitis at injection site.*

## INTERACTIONS
*Oral anticoagulants:* enhanced anticoagulant effect. Monitor closely.

## CONTRAINDICATIONS
Contraindicated in patients with hypersensitivity to the drug.

## NURSING CONSIDERATIONS
● Use cautiously because the drug is dissolved in a vehicle containing polyoxyl 35 castor oil, a substance known to cause anaphylactoid reactions. Give the first dose under continuous medical supervision with emergency resuscitative equipment immediately available. Subsequent doses may be administered on an outpatient basis in selected patients.
● To lessen adverse GI reactions, do not administer at mealtimes.
● Know that premedication with an antiemetic may lessen nausea and vomiting.
● **I.V. use:** Be aware that I.V. miconazole has been replaced largely by newer drugs that are better tolerated.
● Dilute infusion with at least 200 ml of 0.9% sodium chloride solution and infuse over 30 to 60 minutes.
● ***Alert:*** Rapid I.V. injection of undiluted miconazole may produce arrhythmias.
● For intrathecal use, administer drug undiluted using a subcutaneous intrathecal (Ommaya) reservoir. Alternatively, drug may be given by lumbar or cisternal puncture.
● Monitor levels of hemoglobin, hematocrit, electrolytes, and lipids regularly. Transient elevations in serum cholesterol and triglycerides may be caused by castor oil vehicle.
● In treatment of fungal meningitis and urinary bladder infections, assist with supplemental intrathecal administration and bladder irrigation, respectively.

## ☑ PATIENT TEACHING
● Inform the patient that pruritic rash, which may be controlled with diphenhydramine, may persist for weeks after drug is discontinued.
● Inform the patient that adequate therapeutic response may take weeks or months. Stress importance of compliance with drug therapy and follow-up.

---

Reactions may be *common,* uncommon, *life-threatening,* or COMMON AND LIFE-THREATENING.

- Instruct the patient to report adverse reactions promptly.
- Advise the patient to avoid performing hazardous activities if drowsiness or dizziness occurs.

---

## nystatin
Mycostatin*, Nadostine†, Nilstat, Nystex*

*Pregnancy Risk Category: NR*

### HOW SUPPLIED
*Tablets:* 500,000 units
*Oral suspension:* 100,000 units/ml
*Vaginal suppositories:* 100,000 units

### ACTION
Unknown. Probably acts by binding to sterols in fungal cell membrane, altering cell permeability and allowing leakage of intracellular components.

### ONSET, PEAK, DURATION
Not applicable; drug is not absorbed.

### INDICATIONS & DOSAGE
*GI infections –*
**Adults:** 500,000 to 1 million units as oral tablets t.i.d.
*Oral, vaginal, and intestinal infections caused by* Candida albicans (Monilia) *and other* Candida *species –*
**Adults:** 400,000 to 600,000 units oral suspension q.i.d. for oral candidiasis.
**Children and infants over 3 months:** 250,000 to 500,000 units oral suspension q.i.d.
**Neonates and premature infants:** 100,000 units oral suspension q.i.d.
*Vaginal infections –*
**Adults:** 100,000 units, as vaginal tablets, inserted high into vagina, daily or b.i.d. for 14 days.

### ADVERSE REACTIONS
**GI:** transient nausea, vomiting, diarrhea (usually with large oral dosage).

### INTERACTIONS
None significant.

### CONTRAINDICATIONS
Contraindicated in patients with hypersensitivity to the drug.

### NURSING CONSIDERATIONS
- Keep in mind that nystatin is not effective against systemic infections.
- Know that vaginal tablets can be used by pregnant patients up to 6 weeks before term to treat maternal infection that may cause thrush in neonates.
- For treatment of oral candidiasis (thrush): After the mouth is clean of food debris, have the patient hold suspension in mouth for several minutes before swallowing. When treating infants, swab medication on oral mucosa. Immunosuppressed patients are sometimes instructed by the doctor to suck on vaginal tablets (100,000 units) because this provides prolonged contact with oral mucosa.

### ☑ PATIENT TEACHING
- Advise the patient to continue medication for at least 2 days after symptoms disappear. Consult the doctor for exact length of therapy.
- Instruct the patient to continue therapy during menstruation.
- Explain that predisposing factors of vaginal infection include use of antibiotics, oral contraceptives, and corticosteroids; diabetes; reinfection by sexual partner; and tight-fitting panty hose. Encourage the patient to use cotton (not synthetic) underpants.
- Instruct the patient in careful hygiene for affected areas, including cleaning perineal area from front to back after defecation.
- Advise the patient to report redness, swelling, or irritation.
- Tell the patient that overusing mouthwash or wearing poorly fitting dentures, especially in older patients, may promote infection.

---

*Liquid form contains alcohol.   **May contain tartrazine.   †Canada only.   ‡Australia only.   ◇OTC.

# 9

## Antimalarials

chloroquine hydrochloride
chloroquine phosphate
chloroquine sulfate
doxycycline
(See Chapter 14, TETRACYCLINES.)
hydroxychloroquine sulfate
mefloquine hydrochloride
primaquine phosphate
pyrimethamine
pyrimethamine with sulfadoxine

### COMBINATION PRODUCTS
ARALEN PHOSPHATE WITH PRIMA-QUINE PHOSPHATE: chloroquine phosphate 500 mg (300 mg base) and primaquine phosphate 79 mg (45 mg base).

### chloroquine hydrochloride
Aralen HCl, Chlorquin‡

### chloroquine phosphate
Aralen Phosphate, Chlorquin‡

### chloroquine sulfate
Nivaquine‡

*Pregnancy Risk Category: NR*

### HOW SUPPLIED
**chloroquine hydrochloride**
*Injection:* 50 mg/ml (40-mg/ml base)
**chloroquine phosphate**
*Tablets:* 250 mg (150-mg base), 500 mg (300-mg base)
**chloroquine sulfate**
*Tablets:* 200 mg (150-mg base)
*Syrup:* 68 mg (50-mg base)/5 ml

### ACTION
Unknown. As an antimalarial, chloroquine may bind to and alter the properties of DNA in susceptible parasites.

### ONSET, PEAK, DURATION
Onset and duration unknown. Peak levels occur 30 minutes after parenteral administration and within 1 to 3 hours after oral administration.

### INDICATIONS & DOSAGE
*Acute malarial attacks caused by* Plasmodium vivax, P. malariae, P. ovale, *and susceptible strains of* P. falciparum—
**Adults:** initially, 600 mg (base) P.O., then 300 mg at 6, 24, and 48 hours. Or 160 to 200 mg (base) I.M. initially; repeated in 6 hours p.r.n. Patient should be switched to oral therapy as soon as possible.
**Children:** initially, 10 mg (base)/kg P.O., then 5 mg (base)/kg at 6, 24, and 48 hours (do not exceed adult dose). Or 5 mg (base)/kg I.M. initially; repeated in 6 hours p.r.n. Do not exceed 10 mg (base)/kg/24 hours. Patient should be switched to oral therapy as soon as possible.
*Malaria prophylaxis—*
**Adults and children:** 5 mg (base)/kg P.O. (not to exceed 300 mg) weekly on the same day (begun 2 weeks before probable exposure and continued for 4 to 6 weeks after leaving endemic area). If treatment begins after exposure, the initial dose is doubled (600 mg for adults, 10 mg/kg for children) in 2 divided doses P.O. 6 hours apart.
*Extraintestinal amebiasis—*
**Adults:** 1 g (600-mg base) chloroquine phosphate P.O. daily for 2 days; then 500 mg (300-mg base) daily for at least 2 weeks. Treatment is usually combined with an intestinal amebicide.
**Children:** 16 mg/kg chloroquine phosphate (10 mg/kg base) P.O. once daily for 2 to 3 weeks. Maximum dos-

---

Reactions may be *common,* uncommon, *life-threatening,* or **COMMON AND LIFE-THREATENING.**

age is 500 mg chloroquine phosphate (300-mg base) daily.

## ADVERSE REACTIONS

**CNS:** mild and transient headache, psychic stimulation, *seizures,* dizziness, neuropathy.

**CV:** hypotension, ECG changes.

**EENT:** visual disturbances (blurred vision; difficulty in focusing; reversible corneal changes; typically irreversible, sometimes progressive or delayed retinal changes, such as narrowing of arterioles; macular lesions; pallor of optic disk; optic atrophy; patchy retinal pigmentation, typically leading to blindness); ototoxicity (nerve deafness, vertigo, tinnitus).

**GI:** anorexia, abdominal cramps, diarrhea, nausea, vomiting, stomatitis.

**Hematologic:** *agranulocytosis, aplastic anemia,* hemolytic anemia, *thrombocytopenia.*

**Skin:** pruritus, lichen planus eruptions, skin and mucosal pigmentary changes, pleomorphic skin eruptions.

## INTERACTIONS

*Cimetidine:* decreased hepatic metabolism of chloroquine. Monitor for toxicity.

*Magnesium and aluminum salts, kaolin:* decreased GI absorption. Separate administration times.

## CONTRAINDICATIONS

Contraindicated in patients with hypersensitivity to the drug and in those with retinal or visual field changes or porphyria.

## NURSING CONSIDERATIONS

● Use with extreme caution in patients with severe GI, neurologic, or blood disorders.

● Use cautiously in patients with hepatic disease or alcoholism because drug concentrates in liver, and in those with G6PD deficiency or pso-

riasis because drug may exacerbate these conditions.

● Ensure baseline and periodic ophthalmic examinations are performed. Check periodically for ocular muscle weakness after long-term use.

● Assist patient with obtaining audiometric examinations before, during, and after therapy, especially if long-term.

● Monitor CBCs and liver function studies periodically during long-term therapy as ordered; if a severe blood disorder not attributable to the disease develops, drug may need to be discontinued.

● *Alert:* Monitor the patient for possible overdose, which can quickly lead to toxic symptoms: headache, drowsiness, visual disturbances, cardiovascular collapse, and seizures, followed by cardiopulmonary arrest. Children are extremely susceptible to toxicity; avoid long-term treatment.

## ☑ PATIENT TEACHING

● To enhance compliance for prophylaxis, advise the patient to take drug immediately before or after meals on same day each week.

● Instruct the patient to avoid excessive sun exposure to prevent exacerbation of drug-induced dermatoses.

● Tell the patient to report adverse reactions promptly, especially blurred vision, increased sensitivity to light, or muscle weakness.

---

## hydroxychloroquine sulfate
Plaquenil

*Pregnancy Risk Category: NR*

## HOW SUPPLIED
*Tablets:* 200 mg (155-mg base)

## ACTION
Unknown. May bind to and alter the properties of DNA in susceptible organisms.

---

## ONSET, PEAK, DURATION
Onset and duration unknown. Plasma levels peak within 2 to 4½ hours.

## INDICATIONS & DOSAGE
*Suppressive prophylaxis of malaria attacks caused by* Plasmodium vivax, P. malariae, P. ovale, *and susceptible strains of* P. falciparum —
**Adults and children:** for suppression — 5 mg (base)/kg P.O. (not to exceed 310 mg) weekly on same day of the week (begin 2 weeks before entering and continue for 8 weeks after leaving endemic area). If not started before exposure, initial dose is doubled (620 mg for adults, 10 mg/kg for children) in 2 divided doses P.O. 6 hours apart.
*Acute malarial attacks —*
**Adults:** initially, 800 mg (sulfate) P.O., then 400 mg after 6 to 8 hours, then 400 mg daily for 2 days (total 2 g sulfate salt).
**Children:** 13 mg/kg (sulfate) P.O., then 6.5 mg/kg 6 hours later, then 6.5 mg/kg daily for 2 days.
*Lupus erythematosus (chronic discoid and systemic) —*
**Adults:** 400 mg (sulfate) P.O. daily or b.i.d., continued for several weeks or months, depending on response. Prolonged maintenance dosage — 200 to 400 mg (sulfate) daily.
*Rheumatoid arthritis —*
**Adults:** initially, 400 to 600 mg (sulfate) P.O. daily. When good response occurs (usually in 4 to 12 weeks), dosage is cut in half.

## ADVERSE REACTIONS
**CNS:** irritability, nightmares, ataxia, *seizures,* psychosis, vertigo, nystagmus, dizziness, hypoactive deep tendon reflexes, ataxia, lassitude, skeletal muscle weakness, headache.
**EENT:** visual disturbances (blurred vision; difficulty in focusing; reversible corneal changes; typically irreversible, sometimes progressive or delayed retinal changes, such as narrowing of arterioles; macular lesions; pallor of optic disk; optic atrophy; visual field defects; patchy retinal pigmentation, commonly leading to blindness), ototoxicity (irreversible nerve deafness, tinnitus, labyrinthitis).
**GI:** anorexia, abdominal cramps, diarrhea, nausea, vomiting.
**Hematologic:** *agranulocytosis, leukopenia, thrombocytopenia, hemolysis in patients with G6PD deficiency, aplastic anemia.*
**Skin:** pruritus, lichen planus eruptions, skin and mucosal pigmentary changes, pleomorphic skin eruptions.
**Other:** weight loss, alopecia, bleaching of hair.

## INTERACTIONS
*Cimetidine:* decreased hepatic metabolism of hydroxychloroquine. Monitor for toxicity.
*Magnesium and aluminum salts, kaolin:* decreased GI absorption. Separate administration times.

## CONTRAINDICATIONS
Contraindicated in patients with hypersensitivity to the drug, in long-term therapy for children, and in patients with retinal or visual field changes or porphyria.

## NURSING CONSIDERATIONS
• Use with extreme caution in patients with severe GI, neurologic, or blood disorders.
• Use cautiously in patients with hepatic disease or alcoholism because drug concentrates in liver, and in those with G6PD deficiency or psoriasis because drug may exacerbate these conditions.
• Ensure baseline and periodic ophthalmic examinations are performed. Check periodically for ocular muscle weakness after long-term use.
• Assist patient with obtaining audiometric examinations before, during, and after therapy, especially if long-term.

Reactions may be *common,* uncommon, *life-threatening,* or COMMON AND LIFE-THREATENING.

• Monitor CBCs and liver function studies periodically during long-term therapy, as ordered; if severe blood disorder not attributable to disease develops, drug may need to be discontinued.

• **Alert:** Monitor the patient for possible overdose, which can quickly lead to toxic symptoms: headache, drowsiness, visual disturbances, cardiovascular collapse, and seizures, followed by cardiopulmonary arrest. Children are extremely susceptible to toxicity; long-term treatment should be avoided.

☑ **PATIENT TEACHING**

• To enhance compliance for prophylaxis, advise the patient to take hydroxychloroquine immediately before or after meals on same day each week.

• Instruct the patient to report adverse reactions promptly.

---

## mefloquine hydrochloride
Lariam

*Pregnancy Risk Category: C*

### HOW SUPPLIED
*Tablets:* 250 mg

### ACTION
Unknown. Antimalarial activity may be related to its ability to form complexes with hemin.

### ONSET, PEAK, DURATION
Onset and duration unknown. Time to peak concentrations is 7 to 24 hours.

### INDICATIONS & DOSAGE
*Acute malaria infections caused by mefloquine-sensitive strains of* Plasmodium falciparum *or* P. vivax —
**Adults:** 1,250 mg P.O. as a single dose. Patients with *P. vivax* infections should receive subsequent therapy with primaquine or other 8-amino-

quinolines to avoid relapse after treatment of the initial infection.
*Malaria prophylaxis* —
**Adults:** 250 mg P.O. once weekly. Prophylaxis should be initiated 1 week before entering endemic area and continued for 4 weeks after returning. If the patient returns to an area without malaria after a prolonged stay in an endemic area, prophylaxis should end after three doses.

### ADVERSE REACTIONS
**CNS:** dizziness, syncope, headache, psychotic manifestations, hallucinations, confusion, anxiety, fatigue, vertigo, depression, *seizures.*
**CV:** extrasystoles.
**EENT:** tinnitus, visual disturbances.
**GI:** loss of appetite, vomiting, *nausea,* loose stools, diarrhea, abdominal discomfort or pain.
**Skin:** rash.
**Other:** fever, chills, myalgia.

### INTERACTIONS
*Quinine, chloroquine:* increased risk of seizures.
*Quinine, quinidine, beta-adrenergic blockers:* ECG abnormalities and cardiac arrest may occur. Avoid concomitant use.
*Valproic acid:* decreased valproic acid blood levels and loss of seizure control at start of mefloquine therapy. Monitor anticonvulsant blood levels.

### CONTRAINDICATIONS
Contraindicated in patients with hypersensitivity to mefloquine or related compounds.

### NURSING CONSIDERATIONS
• Use cautiously in patients with cardiac disease or seizure disorders.
• Because the health risks from concomitant administration of quinine and mefloquine are great, be aware that mefloquine therapy should not begin sooner than 12 hours after the last dose of quinine or quinidine.

---

*Liquid form contains alcohol. **May contain tartrazine. †Canada only. ‡Australia only. ◇OTC.

• Keep in mind that patients with *P. vivax* infections are at high risk for relapse because the drug does not eliminate the hepatic phase (exoerythrocytic parasites). Follow-up therapy with primaquine is advisable.

• Monitor liver function tests periodically as ordered.

• In cases of suspected overdose, induce vomiting or perform gastric lavage as appropriate because of potential for cardiotoxicity. Animal studies reveal that mefloquine has cardiac actions similar to quinidine and quinine.

☑ **PATIENT TEACHING**

• Advise the patient to take the drug on the same day of the week when using it for prophylaxis.

• Tell the patient not to take the drug on an empty stomach and always to take it with a full glass (at least 8 oz [240 ml]) of water.

• Advise the patient to use caution when performing activities that require alertness and coordination because dizziness, disturbed sense of balance, and neuropsychiatric reactions may occur.

• Instruct the patient taking mefloquine prophylactically to discontinue the drug if signs or symptoms of impending toxicity, such as unexplained anxiety, depression, confusion, or restlessness, occur and to notify the doctor.

• Advise the patient undergoing long-term therapy to have periodic ophthalmic examinations because ocular lesions have been noted in laboratory animals.

# primaquine phosphate
*Pregnancy Risk Category: NR*

**HOW SUPPLIED**
*Tablets:* 7.5 mg (base)‡, 15 mg (base)

**ACTION**
Unknown. It may be effective because of the drug's ability to bind to and alter the properties of DNA.

**ONSET, PEAK, DURATION**
Onset and duration unknown. Plasma levels peak in 2 to 3 hours.

**INDICATIONS & DOSAGE**
*Radical cure of relapsing* Plasmodium vivax *malaria, eliminating symptoms and infection completely; prevention of relapse* –
**Adults:** 15 mg (base) P.O. daily for 14 days. (A 26.3-mg tablet provides 15 mg of base.)
**Children:** 0.5 mg/kg/day (0.3 mg base/kg/day; maximum 15 mg/base/dose) P.O. for 14 days.

**ADVERSE REACTIONS**
**GI:** nausea, vomiting, epigastric distress, abdominal cramps.
**Hematologic:** leukopenia, *hemolytic anemia in G6PD deficiency,* methemoglobinemia in NADH methemoglobin reductase deficiency.

**INTERACTIONS**
*Magnesium and aluminum salts:* decreased GI absorption. Separate administration times.
*Quinacrine:* enhanced toxicity of primaquine. Don't use together.

**CONTRAINDICATIONS**
Contraindicated in patients with systemic diseases in which granulocytopenia may develop (such as lupus erythematosus or rheumatoid arthritis) and in those taking bone marrow suppressants and potentially hemolytic drugs.

**NURSING CONSIDERATIONS**
• Use cautiously in patients with previous idiosyncratic reaction (manifested by hemolytic anemia, methemoglobinemia, or leukopenia); in those with a family or personal his-

tory of favism; and in those with erythrocytic G6PD deficiency or NADH methemoglobin reductase deficiency.
• Administer drug with meals.
• Keep in mind that when administering the drug, a fast-acting antimalarial (such as chloroquine) is used to reduce possibility of drug-resistant strains.
• Obtain frequent blood studies and urine examinations as ordered in light-skinned patients taking more than 30 mg (base) daily, dark-skinned patients taking more than 15 mg (base) daily, and patients with severe anemia or suspected sensitivity.
• Monitor patient for sudden fall in hemoglobin concentration, erythrocyte or leukocyte count, or marked darkening of the urine, which suggests impending hemolytic reactions. Discontinue drug immediately and notify the doctor.

☑ **PATIENT TEACHING**
• Instruct patient to take drug with meals to minimize stomach upset. If stomach upset (nausea, vomiting, or stomach pain) persists, tell patient to notify doctor.
• Tell patient to stop drug therapy and notify doctor immediately if marked darkening of urine occurs.
• Stress to patient the importance of completing full course of therapy.

---

## pyrimethamine
Daraprim

## pyrimethamine with sulfadoxine
Fansidar

*Pregnancy Risk Category: C*

**HOW SUPPLIED**
**pyrimethamine**
*Tablets:* 25 mg

**pyrimethamine with sulfadoxine**
*Tablets:* pyrimethamine 25 mg, sulfadoxine 500 mg

**ACTION**
Inhibits the enzyme dihydrofolate reductase, thereby impeding reduction of dihydrofolic acid to tetrahydrofolic acid. Sulfadoxine competitively inhibits use of PABA.

**ONSET, PEAK, DURATION**
Onset and duration unknown. When administered alone, pyrimethamine serum levels peak 2 to 6 hours after oral dose. When given as the combination product, serum pyrimethamine levels peak 1½ to 8 hours and sulfadoxine levels peak 2½ to 6 hours after oral dose.

**INDICATIONS & DOSAGE**
*Malaria prophylaxis and transmission control (pyrimethamine)* –
**Adults and children 10 years and older:** 25 mg P.O. weekly.
**Children 4 to 10 years:** 12.5 mg P.O. weekly.
**Children under 4 years:** 6.25 mg P.O. weekly.
   Needs to be continued in all age-groups at least 10 weeks after leaving endemic areas.
*Acute attacks of malaria (Fansidar)* –
**Adults and children 14 years and older:** 2 to 3 tablets as a single dose, either alone or in sequence with quinine or primaquine.
**Children 9 to 14 years:** 2 tablets.
**Children 4 to 8 years:** 1 tablet.
**Children under 4 years:** ½ tablet.
*Malaria prophylaxis (Fansidar)* –
**Adults and children 14 years and older:** 1 tablet weekly, or 2 tablets q 2 weeks.
**Children 9 to 14 years:** ¾ tablet weekly, or 1½ tablets q 2 weeks.
**Children 4 to 8 years:** ½ tablet weekly, or 1 tablet q 2 weeks.
**Children under 4 years:** ¼ tablet weekly, or ½ tablet q 2 weeks.

---

*Acute attacks of malaria (pyrimethamine)* –
**Adults and children 15 years and older:** 25 mg P.O. daily for 2 days.
**Children under 15 years:** 12.5 mg P.O. daily for 2 days.

Not recommended alone in nonimmune patients; should be used with faster-acting antimalarials, such as chloroquine, for 2 days to initiate transmission control and suppressive cure.

*Toxoplasmosis (pyrimethamine)* –
**Adults:** initially, 100 mg P.O., then 25 mg P.O. daily for 4 to 5 weeks; at the same time, 1 g sulfadiazine is given P.O. q 6 hours.
**Children:** initially, 1 mg/kg P.O. (not to exceed 100 mg) in two equally divided doses for 2 to 4 days, then 0.5 mg/kg daily for 4 weeks, along with 100 mg sulfadiazine/kg P.O. daily, divided q 6 hours.

**ADVERSE REACTIONS**
**GI:** anorexia, vomiting, atrophic glossitis.
**Hematologic:** *agranulocytosis, aplastic anemia,* megaloblastic anemia, leukopenia, *thrombocytopenia, pancytopenia.*
*Note:* Adverse drug reactions related to sulfadiazine are similar to sulfonamides.

**INTERACTIONS**
*Folic acid and PABA:* decreased antitoxoplasmic effects. May require dosage adjustment.
*Sulfonamides, co-trimoxazole, methotrexate:* increased risk of bone marrow suppression. Don't use together.

**CONTRAINDICATIONS**
• Pyrimethamine is contraindicated in patients with hypersensitivity to the drug and in patients with megaloblastic anemia caused by folic acid deficiency. Fansidar is contraindicated in patients with porphyria because it contains sulfadoxine, a sulfonamide.

• Repeated use of Fansidar is contraindicated in patients with severe renal insufficiency, marked liver parenchymal damage or blood dyscrasias, known hypersensitivity to pyrimethamine or sulfonamides, documented megaloblastic anemia due to folate deficiency; in infants under 2 months; in pregnancy at term; and during breast-feeding.

**NURSING CONSIDERATIONS**
• Use cautiously in patients with impaired hepatic or renal function, severe allergy or bronchial asthma, G6PD deficiency, or seizure disorders (smaller doses may be needed) and after treatment with chloroquine.
• Obtain twice-weekly blood counts, including platelets, as ordered, for the patient with toxoplasmosis because dosages used approach toxic levels. If signs of folic acid or folinic acid deficiency develop, dosage should be reduced or discontinued while the patient receives parenteral folinic acid (leucovorin) until blood counts become normal.
• Keep in mind that, when used to treat toxoplasmosis in patients with AIDS, therapy may be lifelong.
• Because of the possibility of severe skin reactions, keep in mind that Fansidar should be used only in areas where chloroquine-resistant malaria is prevalent and only if the traveler plans to stay longer than 3 weeks.

☑ **PATIENT TEACHING**
• Instruct the patient to take drug with meals to minimize GI distress.
• Inform the patient with toxoplasmosis of the importance of frequent laboratory studies and compliance with therapy. Tell the patient of potential need for long-term therapy.
• Warn the patient taking Fansidar to stop drug and notify doctor at first sign of rash.
• Tell him to take first prophylactic dose 1 to 2 days before traveling.

Reactions may be *common,* uncommon, *life-threatening,* or **COMMON AND LIFE-THREATENING.**

# 10

## Antituberculars and antileprotics

aminosalicylate sodium
capreomycin sulfate
clofazimine
cycloserine
dapsone
ethambutol hydrochloride
ethionamide
isoniazid
pyrazinamide
rifampin
streptomycin sulfate
(See Chapter 11, AMINOGLYCOSIDES.)

## COMBINATION PRODUCTS

RIFAMATE: isoniazid 150 mg and rifampin 300 mg.
RIFATER: isoniazid 50 mg, rifampin 120 mg, and pyrazinamide 300 mg.
RIMACTANE/INH DUAL PACK: thirty 300-mg isoniazid tablets and sixty 300-mg rifampin capsules.

---

## aminosalicylate sodium (para-amino salicylate, PAS)
Nemasol Sodium†, Sodium P.A.S.

*Pregnancy Risk Category: NR*

### HOW SUPPLIED
*Tablets:* 500 mg

### ACTION
Unknown. Believed to suppress growth and reproduction of *Mycobacterium tuberculosis* by competitively inhibiting the formation of folic acid.

### ONSET, PEAK, DURATION
Onset and duration unknown. Serum levels peak within 1 to 2 hours.

### INDICATIONS & DOSAGE
*Adjunctive treatment of tuberculosis –*
**Adults:** 4 g P.O. q 8 hours, or 5 to 6 g q 12 hours. Maximum daily dosage is 20 g. Must be taken with other antituberculars.
**Children:** 50 to 75 mg/kg P.O. q 6 hours or 66.7 to 100 mg/kg q 8 hours. Maximum daily dosage is 12 g. Must be taken with other antituberculars.

### ADVERSE REACTIONS
**GI:** *abdominal pain, nausea, vomiting, diarrhea,* anorexia.
**Hematologic:** hemolytic anemia, leukopenia, *agranulocytosis, thrombocytopenia.*
**Hepatic:** *hepatitis*, jaundice.
**Skin:** eruptions of various types.
**Other:** *hypersensitivity reactions (fever),* mononucleosis-like syndrome, goiter or myxedema (with long-term therapy), encephalopathy.

### INTERACTIONS
*Aminobenzoate derivatives:* decreased absorption of aminosalicylate sodium from the GI tract. Avoid concomitant use.
*Cyanocobalamin (vitamin B$_{12}$):* decreased absorption of vitamin B$_{12}$ from the GI tract. Provide parenteral supplement as ordered.
*Digoxin:* may cause decreased absorption of digoxin. Monitor closely.
*Probenecid, sulfinpyrazone:* decreased excretion of aminosalicylate sodium, resulting in toxicity. Monitor closely.
*Rifampin:* may impair the absorption of rifampin. Separate administration times by at least 6 hours.
*Warfarin, other anticoagulants:* enhanced anticoagulant effect. Monitor for bleeding.

### CONTRAINDICATIONS
Contraindicated in patients with hypersensitivity to the drug, other salicylates, or sulfonamides.

## NURSING CONSIDERATIONS

• Use cautiously in patients with peptic ulcer or other GI disease and in patients with CHF. Also use cautiously in patients who may become pregnant because the drug may be teratogenic.
• Be aware that urine glucose determinations may be false-positive with copper sulfate tests (Benedict's solution, Clinitest); glucose enzymatic tests (Clinistix, Tes-Tape) are not affected.

☑ **PATIENT TEACHING**
• Advise the patient to take the drug with meals or antacids to minimize GI adverse effects. Children may tolerate this drug better than adults.
• Tell the patient to report back pain; pain during urination; unusual bruising or bleeding; fever or sore throat; yellow eyes, sclera, or skin; or severe joint pain.
• Encourage the patient to comply with therapy, which may last several months.
• Instruct the patient to store drug away from heat, humidity, or direct sunlight. Tell the patient not to take tablets that are discolored.

---

## capreomycin sulfate
Capastat Sulfate

*Pregnancy Risk Category: C*

### HOW SUPPLIED
*Injection:* 1 g/vial

### ACTION
Unknown.

### ONSET, PEAK, DURATION
Onset and duration unknown. Plasma levels peak 1 to 2 hours after I.M. injection.

### INDICATIONS & DOSAGE
*Adjunctive treatment of tuberculosis* –
**Adults:** 15 mg/kg/day up to 1 g I.M. daily injected deeply into large muscle mass for 60 to 120 days; then 1 g two to three times weekly for 18 to 24 months. Maximum dosage should not exceed 20 mg/kg/day. Must be given in conjunction with another antitubercular.

### ADVERSE REACTIONS
**EENT:** *ototoxicity,* innitus, vertigo, hearing loss.
**GU:** *nephrotoxicity (elevated BUN).*
**Hematologic:** eosinophilia, leukocytosis, leukopenia, *thrombocytopenia.*
**Other:** *hypersensitivity reactions* (with concomitant use of other antituberculars), urticaria, maculopapular rashes, hepatotoxicity, pain, induration, excessive bleeding, and sterile abscesses at injection site, hypokalemia.

### INTERACTIONS
*Nephrotoxic or ototoxic drugs such as aminoglycosides, colistin, polymyxin B, or vancomycin:* increased risk of additive toxicity. Avoid concomitant use.
*Nondepolarizing neuromuscular blockers:* Neuromuscular blockade may be enhanced by concurrent capreomycin due to a synergistic effect on myoneural function. Monitor closely.

### CONTRAINDICATIONS
Contraindicated in patients with hypersensitivity to the drug.

### NURSING CONSIDERATIONS
• Use with extreme caution in patients receiving other ototoxic or nephrotoxic drugs.
• Use cautiously in patients with impaired renal function, history of allergies, or hearing impairment.
• Assess patient's hearing before beginning therapy. Evaluate patient's hearing every 1 to 2 weeks afterward. Notify the doctor if the patient complains of tinnitus, vertigo, or hearing impairment.

---

Reactions may be *common,* uncommon, *life-threatening,* or COMMON AND LIFE-THREATENING.

• Assess patient's renal function before beginning therapy. Monitor renal function during therapy; notify the doctor if function diminishes. In renal impairment, dosage must be reduced.

• Be aware that capreomycin is considered a "second-line" drug in the treatment of tuberculosis and should always be administered with other antituberculars to prevent the development of resistant organisms.

• To prepare solution, add 2 ml of 0.9% sodium chloride or sterile water for injection to powder to obtain a 1-g dose; add 2.15 ml for a 350 mg/ml concentration; 2.63 ml for a 300 mg/ml concentration; 3.3 ml for a 250 mg/ml concentration; and 4.3 ml for a 200 mg/ml concentration. Wait 2 to 3 minutes for complete dissolution.

• Be aware that straw- or dark-colored solution after reconstitution does not indicate a loss in potency. Do not administer solutions that contain a precipitate.

• *Alert:* Give deep I.M. to minimize local reactions. Apply ice to injection site p.r.n. for pain. Know that drug is never given I.V. because this route may cause neuromuscular blockade.

• Monitor serum potassium levels regularly as ordered.

## ☑ PATIENT TEACHING

• Instruct a family member or friend how to prepare drug and administer an I.M. injection. Tell them not to use any solution that contains a precipitate. However, reassure them that straw- or dark-colored solution may be used.

• Warn the patient that injection may be painful, and suggest applying ice to injection site p.r.n. for pain.

• Instruct the patient to report adverse reactions promptly.

• Stress the importance of recommended laboratory tests to monitor for adverse reactions.

# clofazimine
Lamprene

*Pregnancy Risk Category: C*

## HOW SUPPLIED
*Capsules:* 50 mg, 100 mg

## ACTION
Unknown. Thought to inhibit mycobacterial growth by binding preferentially to mycobacterial DNA. Also has anti-inflammatory effects that suppress skin reactions of erythema nodosum leprosum.

## ONSET, PEAK, DURATION
Onset and duration unknown. With long-term therapy, time to peak concentration is 1 to 6 hours.

## INDICATIONS & DOSAGE
*Dapsone-resistant leprosy (Hansen's disease)* –
**Adults:** 100 mg P.O. daily in combination with other antileprotics for 3 years. Then, clofazimine *alone,* 100 mg daily.
*Erythema nodosum leprosum* –
**Adults:** 100 to 200 mg P.O. daily for up to 3 months. Dosage is tapered to 100 mg daily as soon as possible. Dosages above 200 mg daily are not recommended.

## ADVERSE REACTIONS
**EENT:** *conjunctival and corneal pigmentation, dryness, burning, itching, irritation.*
**GI:** *epigastric pain, diarrhea, nausea, vomiting, GI intolerance, **bowel obstruction, GI bleeding.***
**Skin:** *pink to brownish black pigmentation, ichthyosis and dryness*, rash, pruritus.
**Other:** ***splenic infarction***, discolored body fluids and excrement.

---

*Liquid form contains alcohol.  **May contain tartrazine.  †Canada only.  ‡Australia only.  ◇OTC.

## INTERACTIONS
*Dapsone:* impaired anti-inflammatory effects of clofazimine; no intervention appears necessary.
*Isoniazid:* may decrease skin levels and increase serum and urine levels of clofazimine. Monitor for decreased effectiveness.
*Rifampin:* decreased rifampin bioavailability. Monitor for decreased effectiveness.

## CONTRAINDICATIONS
None known.

## NURSING CONSIDERATIONS
• Use cautiously in patients with GI dysfunction, such as abdominal pain and diarrhea.
• Be aware that doses that exceed 100 mg daily should be given for as short a period as possible and only under close medical supervision.
• If the patient complains of colic, burning abdominal pain, or any other GI symptom, report this to the doctor, who may reduce the dose or increase the interval between doses.

## ☑ PATIENT TEACHING
• Advise the patient to take the drug with meals or milk.
• Warn the patient that clofazimine may discolor skin, body fluids, and excrement. The color ranges from red to brownish black. Reassure the patient that the unsightly skin discoloration is reversible but may not disappear until several months or years after drug treatment ends.
• Tell the patient to apply skin oil or cream to help reverse skin dryness or ichthyosis.

---

## cycloserine
Seromycin

*Pregnancy Risk Category: C*

## HOW SUPPLIED
*Capsules:* 250 mg

## ACTION
Inhibits cell-wall biosynthesis by interfering with the bacterial use of amino acids. Action may be bacteriostatic or bactericidal, depending on the concentration of the drug attained at the site of infection and the susceptibility of the infecting organism.

## ONSET, PEAK, DURATION
Onset and duration unknown. Serum levels peak 3 to 4 hours after oral dose.

## INDICATIONS & DOSAGE
*Adjunctive treatment in pulmonary or extrapulmonary tuberculosis –*
**Adults:** initially, 250 mg P.O. q 12 hours for 2 weeks; then, if blood levels are below 25 to 30 mcg/ml and no toxicity has developed, dose is increased to 250 mg q 8 hours for 2 weeks. If optimum blood levels are still not achieved and no toxicity has developed, then dose is increased to 250 mg q 6 hours. Maximum dosage is 1 g/day. If CNS toxicity occurs, drug is discontinued for 1 week, then resumed at 250 mg daily for 2 weeks. If no serious toxic effects occur, dosage is increased by 250-mg increments q 10 days until blood level of 25 to 30 mcg/ml is obtained.

## ADVERSE REACTIONS
**CNS:** *seizures*, drowsiness, somnolence, headache, tremor, dysarthria, vertigo, confusion, loss of memory, *possible suicidal tendencies*, psychosis, hyperirritability, paresthesia, paresis, hyperreflexia, *coma*.
**CV:** sudden CHF.
**Other:** hypersensitivity reactions (allergic dermatitis), elevated transaminase level.

## INTERACTIONS
*Ethanol or ethionamide:* increased risk of CNS toxicity (seizures); monitor patient closely.

---

Reactions may be *common,* uncommon, *life-threatening,* or COMMON AND LIFE-THREATENING.

*Isoniazid:* CNS toxicity (dizziness or drowsiness); monitor patient closely.

## CONTRAINDICATIONS
Contraindicated in patients with hypersensitivity to the drug and in those with seizure disorders, depression or severe anxiety, psychosis, severe renal insufficiency, or excessive concurrent use of alcohol.

## NURSING CONSIDERATIONS
• Use cautiously in patients with impaired renal function; reduced dosage is required.
• Obtain specimen for culture and sensitivity tests before therapy begins and periodically thereafter to detect possible resistance.
• Know that cycloserine is considered a "second-line" drug in the treatment of tuberculosis and should always be administered with other antituberculars to prevent the development of resistant organisms.
• Monitor serum cycloserine levels periodically as ordered, especially in patients receiving high doses (more than 500 mg daily) because toxic reactions may occur with blood levels above 30 mcg/ml.
• Monitor results of hematologic tests and renal and liver function studies.
• Observe for psychotic symptoms, hallucinations, and possible suicidal tendencies.
• Administer pyridoxine, anticonvulsants, tranquilizers, or sedatives, as ordered, to relieve adverse reactions.

## ☑ PATIENT TEACHING
• Warn the patient to avoid alcohol, which may cause serious neurologic reactions.
• Advise the patient not to perform hazardous activities if drowsiness occurs.
• Tell the patient to report adverse reactions promptly because dosage adjustment may be necessary or other medications may be prescribed to relieve adverse reactions.

# dapsone
Avlosulfon†, Dapsone 100‡
*Pregnancy Risk Category: C*

## HOW SUPPLIED
*Tablets:* 25 mg, 100 mg

## ACTION
Unknown. May inhibit folic acid biosynthesis in susceptible organisms.

## ONSET, PEAK, DURATION
Onset and duration unknown. Plasma levels peak 4 to 8 hours after oral dose.

## INDICATIONS & DOSAGE
*All forms of leprosy (Hansen's disease) —*
**Adults:** 100 mg P.O. daily, indefinitely; give with rifampin 600 mg daily for 6 months.
**Children:** 1.4 mg/kg P.O. daily for a minimum of 3 years.
*Dermatitis herpetiformis —*
**Adults:** 50 mg P.O. daily; increased to 300 mg daily as needed.

## ADVERSE REACTIONS.
**CNS:** insomnia, psychosis, headache, paresthesia, peripheral neuropathy, vertigo.
**EENT:** tinnitus, blurred vision.
**GI:** anorexia, abdominal pain, nausea, vomiting.
**GU:** albuminuria, nephrotic syndrome, renal papillary necrosis.
**Hematologic:** *hemolytic anemia* (dose-related), *agranulocytosis, apastic anemia.*
**Skin:** lupus erythematosus, phototoxity, *exfoliative dermatitis, toxic erythema, erythema multiforme, toxic epidermal necrolysis, morbiliform and scarlatiniform reactions, urticaria, erythema nodosum.*
**Other:** fever, tachycardia, pancreati-

---

tis, male infertility, pulmonary eosinophilia, infectious mononucleosis-like syndrome, *sulfone syndrome (fever, malaise, jaundice* [with hepatic necrosis], *exfoliative dermatitis, lymphadenopathy, methhemoglobinemia, hemolytic anemia).*

## INTERACTIONS
*Activated charcoal:* may decrease dapsone's GI absorption and enterohepatic recycling. Monitor closely.
*Didanosine:* possible therapeutic failure of dapsone, leading to an increase in infection. Avoid concomitant use.
*Folic acid antagonists, such as methotrexate:* increased risk of adverse hematologic reactions. Avoid concomitant use.
*PABA:* PABA may antagonize the effect of dapsone by interfering with the primary mechanism of action. Monitor for lack of efficacy.
*Probenecid:* probenecid reduces urinary excretion of dapsone metabolites, increasing plasma concentrations. Monitor closely.
*Rifampin:* increased hepatic metabolism of dapsone. Monitor for lack of efficacy.
*Trimethoprim:* increased serum levels of both drugs may occur, possibly increasing the pharmacologic and toxic effects of each drug. Monitor closely.

## CONTRAINDICATIONS
Contraindicated in patients with hypersensitivity to the drug.

## NURSING CONSIDERATIONS
• Use cautiously in patients with chronic renal, hepatic, or CV disease; refractory types of anemia; and G6PD deficiency.
• Obtain CBC before therapy to establish a baseline value, as ordered. Monitor CBC weekly for the first month, monthly for 6 months, and semiannually thereafter.
• Be prepared to reduce or temporarily discontinue dapsone if hemoglobin

falls below 9 g/dl, WBC count falls below 5,000/mm³, or RBC count falls below 2.5 million/mm³ or remains low.
• If generalized, diffuse dermatitis occurs, notify doctor and prepare to interrupt therapy.
• Administer antihistamines as ordered to combat dapsone-induced allergic dermatitis.
• Monitor for signs and symptoms of erythema nodosum reaction, which may occur during therapy as a result of *Mycobacterium leprae* bacilli (malaise, fever, painful inflammatory induration in the skin and mucosa, iritis, and neuritis). In severe cases, therapy should be stopped and glucocorticoids given cautiously.

## ☑ PATIENT TEACHING
• *Alert:* Instruct the breast-feeding patient to report cyanosis in infant, which indicates high sulfone level.
• Tell the patient to avoid prolonged exposure to sunlight or sunlamps as dapsone may cause photosensitivity.
• Inform the patient of need for long-term therapy. Stress importance of compliance with drug therapy.

# ethambutol hydrochloride
Etibi†, Myambutol

*Pregnancy Risk Category: NR*

## HOW SUPPLIED
*Tablets:* 100 mg, 400 mg

## ACTION
Unknown. Appears to interfere with the synthesis of one or more metabolites of susceptible bacteria, altering cellular metabolism during cell division (bacteriostatic).

## ONSET, PEAK, DURATION
Onset and duration unknown. Plasma levels peak within 2 to 4 hours after oral dose.

## INDICATIONS & DOSAGE
*Adjunctive treatment in pulmonary tuberculosis –*
**Adults and children over 13 years:** for patients who have not received previous antitubercular therapy, 15 mg/kg P.O. daily in a single dose.
**Re-treatment:** 25 mg/kg P.O. daily as a single dose for 60 days with at least one other antitubercular; then decreased to 15 mg/kg/day as a single dose.

## ADVERSE REACTIONS
**CNS:** headache, dizziness, mental confusion, possible hallucinations, peripheral neuritis (numbness and tingling of extremities).
**EENT:** optic neuritis (related to dose and duration of treatment).
**GI:** anorexia, nausea, vomiting, abdominal pain, GI upset.
**Skin:** dermatitis, pruritus, toxic epidermal necrolysis.
**Other:** *anaphylactoid reactions*, fever, malaise, bloody sputum, *thrombocytopenia*, joint pain, elevated uric acid level, precipitation of acute gout, abnormal liver function tests.

## INTERACTIONS
*Aluminum salts:* may delay and reduce absorption of ethambutol. Separate administration times by several hours.

## CONTRAINDICATIONS
Contraindicated in patients with hypersensitivity to the drug, in those with optic neuritis, and in children under 13 years.

## NURSING CONSIDERATIONS
● Use cautiously in patients with impaired renal function, cataracts, recurrent eye inflammations, gout, and diabetic retinopathy.
● Perform visual acuity and color discrimination tests before and during therapy.
● Obtain AST and ALT levels before

therapy, and monitor these levels every 3 to 4 weeks, as ordered.
● Anticipate dosage reduction in patients with impaired renal function.
● Know that ethambutol should always be administered with other antituberculars to prevent the development of resistant organisms.
● Monitor serum uric acid level as ordered; observe the patient for signs of gout.

## ☑ PATIENT TEACHING
● Reassure the patient that visual disturbances will generally disappear several weeks to months after drug is stopped.
● Inform the patient that drug is administered concurrently with other antituberculars.
● Stress importance of compliance with drug therapy.

---

# ethionamide
Trecator-SC
*Pregnancy Risk Category: NR*

## HOW SUPPLIED
*Tablets:* 250 mg

## ACTION
Unknown. Probably inhibits peptide synthesis.

## ONSET, PEAK, DURATION
Onset and duration unknown. Plasma levels peak in approximately 1.8 hours.

## INDICATIONS & DOSAGE
*Adjunctive treatment in pulmonary or extrapulmonary tuberculosis (when primary therapy with streptomycin or isoniazid cannot be used or has failed) –*
**Adults:** 500 mg to 1 g P.O. daily in divided doses. Concomitant administration of other antituberculars and pyridoxine recommended.
**Children:** 15 to 20 mg/kg P.O. daily

in three to four doses. Maximum dosage is 1 g daily.

## ADVERSE REACTIONS
**CNS:** *depression, asthenia, drowsiness*, peripheral neuritis and neuropathy, olfactory disturbances, blurred vision, diplopia, optic neuritis, dizziness, headache, restlessness, psychosis.
**CV:** postural hypotension.
**GI:** *anorexia, nausea, vomiting*, metallic taste, diarrhea, stomatitis.
**Hematologic:** *thrombocytopenia*.
**Hepatic:** jaundice, *hepatitis*, elevated AST and ALT levels.
**Skin:** rash, acne, alopecia.
**Other:** gynecomastia, impotence, menorrhagia, increased difficulty managing diabetes mellitus.

## INTERACTIONS
None significant.

## CONTRAINDICATIONS
Contraindicated in patients with hypersensitivity to the drug or severe liver damage.

## NURSING CONSIDERATIONS
• Use cautiously in patients with diabetes mellitus.
• Obtain culture and sensitivity tests, as ordered, before starting therapy.
• Remember that ethionamide should always be administered with other antituberculars to prevent the development of resistant organisms.
• Give with meals or antacids to minimize GI effects. The patient may require an antiemetic.
• Monitor hepatic function every 2 to 4 weeks.
• If rash occurs, withhold drug and notify doctor; condition may progress to exfoliative dermatitis.
• Be aware that pyridoxine may be ordered to prevent neuropathy.

## ☑ PATIENT TEACHING
• Instruct the patient to take this drug exactly as prescribed; warn against discontinuing drug without the doctor's consent.
• Tell the patient to take drug with meals or antacids to minimize stomach upset.
• Warn the patient against excessive alcohol ingestion, which may make him more vulnerable to liver damage.
• Stress importance of compliance with drug therapy.

---

# isoniazid (isonicotinic acid hydride, INH)
Isotamine†, Laniazid, Nydrazid**
PMS Isoniazid†

*Pregnancy Risk Category: NR*

## HOW SUPPLIED
*Tablets:* 50 mg, 100 mg, 300 mg
*Oral solution:* 50 mg/5 ml
*Injection:* 100 mg/ml

## ACTION
Unknown. Appears to inhibit cell-wall biosynthesis by interfering with lipid and DNA synthesis (bactericidal).

## ONSET, PEAK, DURATION
Onset and duration unknown. Plasma levels peak within 1 to 2 hours after oral or I.M. administration.

## INDICATIONS & DOSAGE
*Actively growing tubercle bacilli –*
**Adults:** 5 mg/kg P.O. or I.M. daily in a single dose, up to 300 mg/day, continued for 6 months to 2 years.
**Infants and children:** 10 to 20 mg/kg P.O. or I.M. daily in a single dose, up to 300 to 500 mg/day, continued long enough to prevent relapse. Concomitant administration of at least one other antitubercular is recommended.
*Prevention of tubercle bacilli in those exposed to tuberculosis or those with positive skin test whose chest X-rays and bacteriologic studies are consis-*

---

*tent with nonprogressive tuberculosis—*

**Adults:** 300 mg P.O. daily in a single dose, continued for 6 months to 1 year.

**Infants and children:** 10 mg/kg P.O. daily in a single dose, up to 300 mg/day, continued for 1 year.

## ADVERSE REACTIONS

**CNS:** *peripheral neuropathy* (dose-related and especially in patients who are malnourished, alcoholic, diabetic, or slow acetylators), usually preceded by paresthesia of hands and feet, seizures, toxic encephalopathy, optic neuritis and atropy, memory impairment, toxic psychosis.

**GI:** nausea, vomiting, epigastric distress.

**Hematologic:** *agranulocytosis*, hemolytic anemia, *aplastic anemia*, eosinophilia, *thrombocytopenia*, sideroblastic anemia.

**Hepatic:** *hepatitis* (occasionally severe and sometimes fatal, especially in elderly patients), jaundice, *elevated serum transaminase levels*, bilirubinemia.

**Other:** rheumatic and lupuslike syndromes, hypersensitivity reactions (fever, rash, lymphadenopathy, vasculitis), hyperglycemia, metabolic acidosis, pyridoxine deficiency, hypocalcemia, hypophosphatemia, gynecomastia, irritation at I.M. injection site.

## INTERACTIONS

*Aluminum-containing antacids and laxatives:* may decrease the rate and amount of isoniazid absorbed. Give isoniazid at least 1 hour before antacid or laxative.

*Benzodiazepines:* isoniazid may inhibit the metabolic clearance of benzodiazepines that undergo oxidative metabolism (diazepam, triazolam), possibly increasing the activity of the benzodiazepine. Monitor closely.

*Carbamazepine, halothane:* increased risk of isoniazid hepatotoxicity. Use together cautiously.

*Corticosteroids:* may decrease therapeutic effectiveness of isoniazid. Monitor need for larger isoniazid dose.

*Cycloserine, meperidine:* may increase CNS adverse reactions and hypotension (meperidine only). Institute safety precautions.

*Disulfiram:* may cause neurologic symptoms, including changes in behavior and coordination. Avoid concomitant use.

*Enflurane:* in rapid acetylators of isoniazid, high output renal failure may occur due to nephrotoxic concentrations of inorganic fluoride. Monitor renal function.

*Ethanol:* may be associated with increased incidence of isoniazid-related hepatitis. Avoid concomitant use.

*Ketoconazole:* serum concentrations of ketoconazole may be decreased. Monitor for lack of efficacy.

*Oral anticoagulants:* anticoagulant activity may be enhanced. Monitor PT closely.

*Phenytoin, carbamazepine:* increased plasma levels of these anticonvulsants. Monitor closely.

## CONTRAINDICATIONS

Contraindicated in patients with acute hepatic disease or isoniazid-associated liver damage.

## NURSING CONSIDERATIONS

● Use cautiously in patients with chronic non-isoniazid-associated liver disease, seizure disorders (especially in those taking phenytoin), severe renal impairment, and chronic alcoholism and in elderly patients.

● Be aware that isoniazid should always be administered with other antituberculars to prevent the development of resistant organisms.

● Keep in mind that isoniazid pharmacokinetics may vary among patients because its metabolism occurs

---

*Liquid form contains alcohol.  **May contain tartrazine.  †Canada only.  ‡Australia only.  ◇OTC.

in the liver by genetically controlled acetylation. Fast acetylators metabolize the drug up to five times as fast as slow acetylators. About 50% of blacks and whites are slow acetylators; over 80% of Chinese, Japanese, and Eskimos are fast acetylators.

● Monitor hepatic function closely for changes.

● Administer pyridoxine, as ordered, to prevent peripheral neuropathy, especially in malnourished patients.

### ☑ PATIENT TEACHING

● Instruct the patient to take this drug exactly as prescribed; warn against discontinuing drug without the doctor's consent.

● Advise the patient to take with food if GI irritation occurs.

● Tell the patient to notify the doctor immediately if symptoms of liver impairment occur (loss of appetite, fatigue, malaise, jaundice, dark urine).

● Advise the patient to avoid alcoholic beverages while taking this drug. Also tell the patient to avoid certain foods (fish such as skipjack and tuna and tyramine-containing products such as aged cheese, beer, and chocolate) because drug has some monoamine oxidase inhibitor activity.

● Encourage the patient to fully comply with treatment, which may take months or years.

## pyrazinamide
pms Pyrazinamide†, Tebrazid†, Zinamide‡

*Pregnancy Risk Category: C*

### HOW SUPPLIED
*Tablets:* 500 mg

### ACTION
Unknown.

### ONSET, PEAK, DURATION
Onset and duration unknown. Serum levels peak in 1 to 2 hours.

### INDICATIONS & DOSAGE
*Adjunctive treatment of tuberculosis (when primary and secondary antituberculars cannot be used or have failed) –*
**Adults:** 15 to 30 mg/kg P.O. once daily. Maximum dosage is 2 g daily. Alternatively when compliance is a problem, 50 to 70 mg/kg (based on lean body mass) P.O. twice weekly.

### ADVERSE REACTIONS
**GI:** anorexia, nausea, vomiting.
**GU:** dysuria.
**Hematologic:** sideroblastic anemia, *thrombocytopenia*.
**Skin:** rash, urticaria, pruritis, photosensitivity.
**Other:** malaise, fever, porphyria, hyperuricemia and gout, interstitial nephritis, *arthralgia, myalgia, hepatitis*.

### INTERACTIONS
None significant.

### CONTRAINDICATIONS
Contraindicated in patients with hypersensitivity to the drug, severe hepatic disease, or acute gout.

### NURSING CONSIDERATIONS
● Use cautiously in patients with diabetes mellitus, renal failure, or gout.

● Be aware that pyrazinamide should always be administered with other antituberculars to prevent the development of resistant organisms.

● Know that drug is administered for the initial 2 months of a 6-month or longer treatment regimen for drug susceptible patients. Patients with concomitant HIV infection may require longer courses of therapy.

● Keep in mind that a reduced dosage is needed in patients with renal impairment because nearly 100% of the drug is excreted in urine.

● Question doses that exceed 35 mg/kg because they may cause liver damage.

- Monitor hematopoietic studies and serum uric acid levels, as ordered.
- Monitor liver function studies; assess for jaundice and liver tenderness or enlargement before and frequently during therapy.
- Watch closely for signs of gout and of liver impairment (anorexia, fatigue, malaise, jaundice, dark urine, and liver tenderness). Notify the doctor at once.
- When used with surgical management of tuberculosis, pyrazinamide is started 1 to 2 weeks before surgery and continued for 4 to 6 weeks postoperatively.

☑ **PATIENT TEACHING**
- Inform the patient that other antituberculars will be required concomitantly.
- Instruct the patient to report adverse reactions promptly.
- Stress importance of compliance with drug therapy. If daily therapy poses a problem for the patient, tell him to ask doctor about twice-weekly dosing.

---

## rifampin (rifampicin)
Rifadin, Rifadin IV, Rimactane, Rimycin‡, Rofact†

*Pregnancy Risk Category: C*

### HOW SUPPLIED
*Capsules:* 150 mg, 300 mg
*Injection:* 600 mg

### ACTION
Inhibits DNA-dependent RNA polymerase, thus impairing RNA synthesis (bactericidal).

### ONSET, PEAK, DURATION
Onset and duration unknown. Serum levels peak 2 to 4 hours after oral dose.

### INDICATIONS & DOSAGE
*Pulmonary tuberculosis –*
**Adults:** 600 mg P.O. or I.V. daily in single dose 1 hour before or 2 hours after meals.
**Children over 5 years:** 10 to 20 mg/kg P.O. or I.V. daily in single dose 1 hour before or 2 hours after meals. Maximum dosage is 600 mg daily. Concomitant administration with other antituberculars is recommended.
*Meningococcal carriers –*
**Adults:** 600 mg P.O. or I.V. b.i.d. for 2 days, or 600 mg P.O. or I.V. once daily for 4 days.
**Children 1 month to 12 years:** 10 mg/kg P.O. or I.V. b.i.d. for 2 days, not to exceed 600 mg/day, or 10 to 20 mg/kg once daily for 4 days.
**Neonates:** 5 mg/kg P.O. or I.V. b.i.d. for 2 days.
*Prophylaxis of* Haemophilus influenzae *type b –*
**Adults and children:** 20 mg/kg P.O. daily for 4 days, not to exceed 600 mg/day.

### ADVERSE REACTIONS
**CNS:** headache, fatigue, drowsiness, behavioral changes, dizziness, mental confusion, generalized numbness.
**GI:** epigastric distress, anorexia, nausea, vomiting, abdominal pain, diarrhea, flatulence, sore mouth and tongue, pseudomembranous colitis, pancreatitis.
**GU:** hemoglobinuria, hematuria, and *acute renal failure.*
**Hematologic:** eosinophilia, *thrombocytopenia*, transient leukopenia, hemolytic anemia.
**Hepatic:** *hepatotoxicity, transient abnormalities in liver function tests.*
**Skin:** pruritus, urticaria, rash.
**Other:** flulike syndrome, discoloration of body fluids, hyperuricemia, shortness of breath, wheezing, *shock*, ataxia, osteomalacia, visual disturbances, exudative conjunctivitis, por-

---

phyria exacerbation, menstrual disturbances.

## INTERACTIONS

*Anticoagulants, corticosteroids, cyclosporine, digitalis glycosides, quinidine, oral contraceptives, sulfonylureas, dapsone, narcotics, analgesics, methadone, barbiturates, diazepam, verapamil, beta-adrenergic blockers, clofibrate, progestins, disopyramide, mexiletine, theophylline, chloramphenicol, anticonvulsants:* reduced effectiveness of these drugs. Monitor closely.

*Ethanol:* may increase risk of hepatotoxicity and should be avoided.

*Halothane:* may increase risk of hepatotoxicity of both drugs. Monitor liver function closely.

*Ketoconazole, para-aminosalicylate sodium:* may interfere with absorption of rifampin. Give these drugs 8 to 12 hours apart.

*Probenecid:* may increase rifampin levels. Use cautiously.

## CONTRAINDICATIONS

Contraindicated in patients with hypersensitivity to the drug.

## NURSING CONSIDERATIONS

● Use cautiously in patients with liver disease.

● Be aware that concomitant treatment with at least one other antitubercular is recommended.

● Give 1 hour before or 2 hours after meals for optimal absorption; however, if GI irritation occurs, the patient may take rifampin with meals.

● **I.V. use:** Reconstitute vial with 10 ml of sterile water for injection to make a solution containing 60 mg/ml. Add to 100 ml of D₅W and infuse over 30 minutes, or add to 500 ml of D₅W and infuse over 3 hours. When dextrose is contraindicated, drug may be diluted with 0.9% sodium chloride for injection. Do not use other I.V. solutions.

● Monitor hepatic function, hematopoietic studies, and serum uric acid levels, as ordered.

● Watch closely for signs of hepatic impairment and, if present, report them to the doctor.

● May cause hemorrhage in neonates of rifampin-treated mothers.

## ☑ PATIENT TEACHING

● Instruct the patient who develops drug-induced GI upset to take drug with meals.

● Warn the patient about drowsiness and possible red-orange discoloration of urine, feces, saliva, sweat, sputum, and tears. Soft contact lenses may be permanently stained.

● Advise the patient to avoid alcoholic beverages while taking this drug.

# 11

# Aminoglycosides

**amikacin sulfate**
**gentamicin sulfate**
**kanamycin sulfate**
**neomycin sulfate**
**netilmicin sulfate**
**streptomycin sulfate**
**tobramycin sulfate**

**COMBINATION PRODUCTS**
NEOSPORIN G.U. IRRIGANT: 40 mg
neomycin sulfate and 200,000 units
polymixin B sulfate/ml.

## amikacin sulfate
Amikin

*Pregnancy Risk Category: D*

**HOW SUPPLIED**
*Injection:* 50 mg/ml, 250 mg/ml

**ACTION**
Inhibits protein synthesis by binding
directly to the 30S ribosomal subunit.
Generally bactericidal.

**ONSET, PEAK, DURATION**
Onset immediate after I.V. infusion;
unknown after I.M. injection. Peak
serum levels occur immediately after
I.V. infusion, 1 hour after I.M. injection. Measurable serum levels persist
for 8 to 12 hours.

**INDICATIONS & DOSAGE**
*Serious infections caused by sensitive
strains of* Pseudomonas aeruginosa,
Escherichia coli, Proteus, Klebsiella,
Serratia, Enterobacter, Acinetobacter, Providencia, Citrobacter, Staphylococcus; *meningitis* —
**Adults and children:** 15 mg/kg/day
divided q 8 to 12 hours I.M. or I.V.
infusion (in 100 to 200 ml of $D_5W$ or
0.9% sodium chloride solution run in
over 30 to 60 minutes).

**Neonates:** initially, loading dose of
10 mg/kg I.V., followed by 7.5 mg/kg
q 12 hours.
*Uncomplicated urinary tract infection* —
**Adults:** 250 mg I.M. or I.V. b.i.d.
*In impaired renal function* —
**Adults:** initially, 7.5 mg/kg. Subsequent doses and frequency determined by blood amikacin levels and
renal function studies.

**ADVERSE REACTIONS**
**CNS:** *neuromuscular blockade.*
**EENT:** *ototoxicity.*
**GU:** *nephrotoxicity, azotemia.*
**Other:** arthralgia, acute muscular pa-
ralysis.

**INTERACTIONS**
*Cephalothin:* increased nephrotoxicity. Use together cautiously.
*Dimenhydrinate:* may mask symptoms of ototoxicity. Use with caution.
*General anesthetics, neuromuscular
blockers:* may potentiate neuromuscular blockade.
*Indomethacin:* may increase serum
trough and peak levels of amikacin.
Monitor serum amikacin level closely.
*I.V. loop diuretics (such as furose-
mide):* increased ototoxicity. Use cautiously.
*Other aminoglycosides, acyclovir,
amphotericin B, cisplatin, methoxyflurane, vancomycin:* increased nephrotoxicity. Use together cautiously.
*Parenteral penicillins (such as ticar-
cillin):* amikacin inactivation in vitro.
Don't mix together.

**CONTRAINDICATIONS**
Contraindicated in patients with hypersensitivity to the drug or other
aminoglycosides.

---

*Liquid form contains alcohol.   **May contain tartrazine.   †Canada only.   ‡Australia only.   ◇OTC.

## NURSING CONSIDERATIONS

• Use cautiously in patients with impaired renal function or neuromuscular disorders, in neonates and infants, and in elderly patients.
• Obtain specimen for culture and sensitivity tests before first dose. Therapy may begin pending results.
• Evaluate patient's hearing before and during therapy. Notify the doctor if the patient complains of tinnitus, vertigo, or hearing loss.
• Weigh the patient and review renal function studies before therapy begins.
• **I.V. use:** After I.V. infusion, flush line with 0.9% sodium chloride solution or $D_5W$.
• Obtain blood for peak amikacin level 1 hour after I.M. injection and 30 minutes to 1 hour after infusion ends; for trough levels, draw blood just before next dose. Don't collect blood in a heparinized tube; heparin is incompatible with aminoglycosides.
• Be aware that peak blood levels above 35 mcg/ml and trough levels above 10 mcg/ml may be associated with a higher incidence of toxicity.
• Monitor renal function (output, specific gravity, urinalysis, BUN and creatinine levels, and creatinine clearance). Notify the doctor of signs of decreasing renal function.
• Watch for superinfection (continued fever and other signs of new infection, especially of upper respiratory tract).
• Keep in mind that therapy is usually continued for 7 to 10 days. If no response occurs after 3 to 5 days, therapy may be stopped and new specimens obtained for culture and sensitivity testing.

## ☑ PATIENT TEACHING

• Instruct patient to report adverse reactions promptly.
• Encourage adequate fluid intake.

# gentamicin sulfate

Cidomycin†‡, Garamycin,
Gentamicin Sulfate ADD-Vantage,
Jenamicin

*Pregnancy Risk Category: NR*

## HOW SUPPLIED

*Injection:* 40 mg/ml (adult), 10 mg/ml (pediatric), 2 mg/ml (intrathecal)
*I.V. infusion (premixed):* 40 mg, 60 mg, 70 mg, 80 mg, 90 mg, 100 mg, available in 0.9% sodium chloride solution

## ACTION

Inhibits protein synthesis by binding directly to the 30S ribosomal subunit. Usually bactericidal.

## ONSET, PEAK, DURATION

Onset immediate after I.V. administration, unknown after I.M. administration. Peak serum levels occur in 30 to 90 minutes. Duration unknown.

## INDICATIONS & DOSAGE

*Serious infections caused by sensitive strains of* Pseudomonas aeruginosa, Escherichia coli, Proteus, Klebsiella, Serratia, Enterobacter, Citrobacter, Staphylococcus—
**Adults:** 3 mg/kg daily in divided doses I.M. or I.V. infusion q 8 hours (in 50 to 200 ml of 0.9% sodium chloride solution or $D_5W$ infused over 30 minutes to 2 hours). For life-threatening infections, the patient may receive up to 5 mg/kg daily in three to four divided doses.
**Children:** 2 to 2.5 mg/kg q 8 hours I.M. or by I.V. infusion.
**Neonates over 1 week or infants:** 7.5 mg/kg daily in divided doses q 8 hours.
**Neonates under 1 week and preterm infants:** 2.5 mg/kg I.V. q 12 hours.
*Meningitis—*
**Adults:** systemic therapy as above; or 4 to 8 mg intrathecally daily.

---

Reactions may be *common*, uncommon, **life-threatening**, or **COMMON AND LIFE-THREATENING**.

**Children and infants over
3 months:** systemic therapy as above;
or 1 to 2 mg intrathecally daily.
*Endocarditis prophylaxis for GI or
GU procedure or surgery –*
**Adults:** 1.5 mg/kg I.M. or I.V. 30
minutes before procedure or surgery.
Maximum dosage is 80 mg. Given
with ampicillin (vancomycin in peni-
cillin-allergic patients). Repeated in
8 hours.
**Children:** 2 mg/kg I.M. or I.V. 30
minutes before procedure or surgery.
Maximum dosage is 80 mg. Given
with ampicillin (vancomycin in peni-
cillin-allergic patients). After 8
hours, half the initial dose is given.
*After hemodialysis to maintain thera-
peutic blood levels –*
**Adults:** 1 to 1.7 mg/kg I.M. or by I.V.
infusion after each dialysis.
**Children:** 2 to 2.5 mg/kg I.M. or by
I.V. infusion after each dialysis.

**ADVERSE REACTIONS**
**CNS:** headache, lethargy, encephalopa-
thy, confusion, dizziness, *seizures,*
numbness, peripheral neuropathy.
**CV:** hypotension.
**EENT:** *ototoxicity,* blurred vision.
**GI:** vomiting, nausea.
**GU:** *nephrotoxicity.*
**Hematologic:** anemia, eosinophilia,
leukopenia, *thrombocytopenia,* gran-
ulocytopenia.
**Respiratory:** apnea.
**Skin:** rash, urticaria, pruritus, tin-
gling.
**Other:** fever, muscle twitching,
myasthenia gravislike syndrome, *ana-
phylaxis,* pain at injection site.

**INTERACTIONS**
*Cephalothin:* increased nephrotoxicity. Use together cautiously.
*Dimenhydrinate:* may mask symptoms of ototoxicity. Use with caution.
*General anesthetics, neuromuscular
blockers:* may potentiate neuromuscular blockade.
*Indomethacin:* may increase serum

peak and trough levels of gentamicin.
Monitor serum gentamicin levels
closely.
*I.V. loop diuretics (such as furose-
mide):* increased ototoxicity. Use cautiously.
*Other aminoglycosides, amphotericin
B, acyclovir, cisplatin, methoxyflurane, vancomycin:* increased ototoxicity and nephrotoxicity. Use together
cautiously.
*Parenteral penicillins (such as ampi-
cillin and ticarcillin):* gentamicin inactivation in vitro. Don't mix together.

**CONTRAINDICATIONS**
Contraindicated in patients with hypersensitivity to the drug or other
aminoglycosides.

**NURSING CONSIDERATIONS**
● Use cautiously in neonates, infants,
elderly patients, and patients with impaired renal function or neuromuscular disorders.
● Obtain specimen for culture and
sensitivity tests before first dose.
● Evaluate patient's hearing before
and during therapy. Notify the doctor
if the patient complains of tinnitus,
vertigo, or hearing loss.
● Weigh the patient and review renal
function studies before therapy begins.
● **I.V. use:** When giving by intermittent I.V. infusion, dilute with 50 to
200 ml of $D_5W$ or 0.9% sodium chloride injection and infuse over 30 minutes to 2 hours. After completing I.V.
infusion, flush the line with 0.9% sodium chloride solution or $D_5W$.
● Use preservative-free formulations
of gentamicin when intrathecal route
is ordered.
● Obtain blood for peak gentamicin
level 1 hour after I.M. injection and
30 minutes to 1 hour after I.V. infusion; for trough levels, draw blood
just before next dose. Don't collect
blood in a heparinized tube; heparin
is incompatible with aminoglycosides.

---

*Liquid form contains alcohol.   **May contain tartrazine.   †Canada only.   ‡Australia only.   ◇OTC.

- Be aware that peak blood levels above 12 mcg/ml and trough levels above 2 mcg/ml may be associated with higher incidence of toxicity.
- Monitor renal function (output, specific gravity, urinalysis, BUN and creatinine levels, and creatinine clearance). Notify the doctor of signs of decreasing renal function.
- Know that hemodialysis (8 hours) removes up to 50% of drug from blood.
- Watch for superinfection (continued fever and other signs of new infection, especially of upper respiratory tract).
- Know that therapy usually continues for 7 to 10 days. If no response occurs in 3 to 5 days, therapy may be stopped and new specimens obtained for culture and sensitivity testing.

☑ **PATIENT TEACHING**
- Instruct patient to report adverse reactions promptly.
- Encourage adequate fluid intake.
- Caution patient not to perform hazardous activities if adverse CNS reactions occur.

# kanamycin sulfate
Kanasig‡, Kantrex

*Pregnancy Risk Category: D*

**HOW SUPPLIED**
*Capsules:* 500 mg
*Injection:* 37.5 mg/ml (pediatric), 250 mg/ml, 333 mg/ml

**ACTION**
Inhibits protein synthesis by binding directly to the 30S ribosomal subunit. Generally bactericidal.

**ONSET, PEAK, DURATION**
Onset immediate after I.V. infusion, unknown after I.M. or oral administration. Peak serum levels occur immediately after I.V. infusion, 1 hour after I.M. injection. Measurable serum levels persist for 8 to 12 hours.

**INDICATIONS & DOSAGE**
*Serious infections caused by sensitive strains of* Escherichia coli, Proteus, Enterobacter aerogenes, Klebsiella pneumoniae, Serratia marcescens, Acinetobacter—
**Adults and children with normal renal function:** 15 mg/kg/day divided q 8 to 12 hours I.M. or I.V. Maximum daily dosage is 1.5 g.
**Neonates:** 15 mg/kg/day divided q 12 hours I.M. or I.V.
*Adjunct treatment in hepatic coma—*
**Adults:** 8 to 12 g P.O. daily in divided doses.
*Preoperative bowel sterilization—*
**Adults:** 1 g P.O. q 1 hour for four doses, then q 4 hours for four doses; or 1 g P.O. q 1 hour for four doses, then q 6 hours for 36 to 72 hours.
*Intraperitoneal irrigation—*
500 mg in 20 ml sterile distilled water instilled via catheter into wound after patient has recovered from anesthesia and neuromuscular blocker effects.
*Wound irrigation—*
Up to 2.5 mg/ml in 0.9% sodium chloride solution.
*Inhalation—*
250 mg diluted with 3 ml of 0.9% sodium chloride solution via nebulizer two to four times per day.

**ADVERSE REACTIONS**
**CNS:** *neuromuscular blockade.*
**EENT:** *ototoxicity.*
**GU:** *nephrotoxicity.*
**Respiratory:** apnea.
**Other:** pain at injection site, acute muscular paralysis.

**INTERACTIONS**
*Cephalothin:* increased nephrotoxicity. Use together cautiously.
*Dimenhydrinate:* may mask symptoms of ototoxicity. Use with caution.
*General anesthetics, neuromuscular blockers:* may potentiate neuromuscular blockade.
*I.V. loop diuretics (such as furose-*

---

Reactions may be *common,* uncommon, *life-threatening,* or **COMMON AND LIFE-THREATENING.**

*mide):* increased ototoxicity. Use cautiously.

*Other aminoglycosides, acyclovir, amphotericin B, cisplatin, methoxyflurane, vancomycin:* increased nephrotoxicity. Don't use together.

*Parenteral penicillins (such as ticarcillin):* kanamycin inactivation in vitro. Don't mix together.

## CONTRAINDICATIONS

Contraindicated for oral use in patients with intestinal obstruction and in treatment of systemic infection. Also contraindicated in patients with hypersensitivity to the drug or other aminoglycosides.

## NURSING CONSIDERATIONS

● Use cautiously in patients with impaired renal function or neuromuscular disorders and in elderly patients.
● Obtain specimen for culture and sensitivity tests before first dose. Therapy may begin pending results.
● Evaluate the patient's hearing before and during therapy. Notify the doctor if the patient complains of tinnitus, vertigo, or hearing loss.
● Weigh the patient and review renal function studies before therapy.
● Know that darkening of vials during shelf life does not indicate loss of potency.
● **I.V. use:** Dilute 500 mg of the drug with 200 ml of 0.9% sodium chloride solution or $D_5W$ and infuse over 30 to 60 minutes.
● For I.M. administration, inject deeply into upper outer quadrant of buttocks. Rotate injection sites.
● Obtain peak and trough levels as ordered. Be aware that peak blood levels over 30 mcg/ml and trough levels over 10 mcg/ml may be associated with increased incidence of toxicity.
● Monitor renal function (output, specific gravity, urinalysis, BUN and creatinine levels, and creatinine clearance). Notify the doctor of signs of decreasing renal function.

● Watch for superinfection (continued fever and other signs of new infection, especially of upper respiratory tract).
● Know that if no response occurs in 3 to 5 days, therapy may be stopped and new specimens obtained for culture and sensitivity testing.

## ☑ PATIENT TEACHING

● Instruct patient to report adverse reactions promptly.
● Encourage adequate fluid intake.

---

## neomycin sulfate
Mycifradin, Neo-fradin, Neosulf‡, Neo-Tabs

*Pregnancy Risk Category: NR*

### HOW SUPPLIED
*Tablets:* 500 mg
*Oral solution:* 125 mg/5 ml

### ACTION
Inhibits protein synthesis by binding directly to the 30S ribosomal subunit. Generally bactericidal.

### ONSET, PEAK, DURATION
Onset unknown. Peak plasma levels occur in 1 to 4 hours. The drug is usually detectable in plasma for about 8 hours.

### INDICATIONS & DOSAGE
*Infectious diarrhea caused by enteropathogenic* Escherichia coli —
**Adults:** 50 mg/kg daily P.O. in four divided doses for 2 to 3 days.
**Children:** 50 to 100 mg/kg daily P.O. divided q 4 to 6 hours for 2 to 3 days.
*Suppression of intestinal bacteria preoperatively —*
**Adults:** 1 g P.O. q 1 hour for four doses, then 1 g q 4 hours for the balance of the 24 hours. A saline cathartic should precede therapy.
**Children:** 40 to 100 mg/kg daily P.O. divided q 4 to 6 hours. First dose should follow saline cathartic.

---

*Adjunct treatment in hepatic coma –*
**Adults:** 1 to 3 g P.O. q.i.d. for 5 to 6 days; or 200 ml of 1% solution or 100 ml of 2% solution as enema retained for 20 to 60 minutes q 6 hours.

## ADVERSE REACTIONS
**EENT:** *ototoxicity.*
**GI:** nausea, vomiting, diarrhea, malabsorption syndrome, *Clostridium difficile*-associated colitis.
**GU:** *nephrotoxicity.*

## INTERACTIONS
*Cephalothin:* increased nephrotoxicity. Use together cautiously.
*Digoxin:* decreased digoxin absorption. Monitor closely.
*Dimenhydrinate:* may mask symptoms of ototoxicity. Use with caution.
*I.V. loop diuretics (such as furosemide):* increased ototoxicity. Use cautiously.
*Oral anticoagulants:* inhibited vitamin K-producing bacteria; may potentiate anticoagulant effect.
*Other aminoglycosides, acyclovir, amphotericin B, cisplatin, methoxyflurane, vancomycin:* increased nephrotoxicity. Use together cautiously.

## CONTRAINDICATIONS
Contraindicated in patients with hypersensitivity to other aminoglycosides and in those with intestinal obstruction.

## NURSING CONSIDERATIONS
• Use cautiously in patients with impaired renal function, neuromuscular disorders, or ulcerative bowel lesions and in elderly patients. Never administer parenterally.
• Monitor renal function (output, specific gravity, urinalysis, BUN and creatinine levels, and creatinine clearance). Notify the doctor of signs of decreasing renal function.
• Evaluate patient's hearing before and during prolonged therapy. Notify the doctor if the patient complains of

tinnitus, vertigo, or hearing loss. Onset of deafness may occur several weeks after drug is stopped.
• Watch for superinfection (fever or other signs of new infection).
• In adjunctive treatment of hepatic coma, decrease the patient's dietary protein, and assess neurologic status frequently during therapy.
• For preoperative disinfection, provide a low-residue diet and a cathartic immediately before oral administration of neomycin, as ordered.
• Keep in mind that the ototoxic and nephrotoxic properties of neomycin limit its usefulness.
• Know that neomycin is nonabsorbable at the recommended dosage. However, more than 4 g/day may be systemically absorbed and lead to nephrotoxicity.
• Be aware that drug is available in combination with polymyxin B as a urinary bladder irrigant.

☑ **PATIENT TEACHING**
• Instruct patient to report adverse reactions promptly.
• Encourage adequate fluid intake.

---

# netilmicin sulfate
Netromycin

*Pregnancy Risk Category: D*

## HOW SUPPLIED
*Injection:* 25 mg/ml†, 50 mg/ml†, 100 mg/ml

## ACTION
Inhibits protein synthesis by binding directly to the 30S ribosomal subunit. Generally bactericidal.

## ONSET, PEAK, DURATION
Onset immediate after I.V. infusion, unknown after I.M. injection. Peak serum levels occur immediately after I.V. infusion, ½ to 1 hour after I.M. injection. Measurable serum levels persist for 8 to 12 hours.

## INDICATIONS & DOSAGE

*Serious infections caused by sensitive strains of* Pseudomonas aeruginosa, Escherichia coli, Proteus, Klebsiella, Serratia, Enterobacter, Citrobacter, Staphylococcus—

**Adults and children over 12 years:** 3 to 6.5 mg/kg/day by I.M. injection or I.V. infusion. May be given q 12 hours to treat serious urinary tract infections (UTIs) and q 8 to 12 hours to treat serious systemic infections.

**Infants and children 6 weeks to 12 years:** 5.5 to 8 mg/kg/day by I.M. injection or I.V. infusion given either as 1.8 to 2.7 mg/kg q 8 hours or as 2.7 to 4 mg/kg q 12 hours.

**Neonates under 6 weeks:** 4 to 6.5 mg/kg/day by I.M. injection or I.V. infusion given as 2 to 3.25 mg/kg q 12 hours.

*Complicated UTIs—*

**Adults (normal renal function):** 3 to 4 mg/kg/day by I.M. injection or I.V. infusion divided into two equal doses given q 12 hours.

## ADVERSE REACTIONS

**CNS:** *neuromuscular blockade,* encephalopathy, *seizures,* dizziness, numbness, peripheral neuropathy.
**EENT:** *ototoxicity.*
**GU:** *nephrotoxicity.*
**Respiratory:** apnea.
**Other:** muscle twitching, myasthenia gravislike syndrome, skin tingling.

## INTERACTIONS

*Cephalothin:* increased nephrotoxicity. Use together cautiously.
*Dimenhydrinate:* may mask symptoms of ototoxicity. Use cautiously.
*General anesthetics, neuromuscular blockers:* may potentiate neuromuscular blockade.
*I.V. loop diuretics (such as furosemide):* increased ototoxicity. Use cautiously.
*Other aminoglycosides, acyclovir, amphotericin B, cisplatin, methoxy-*
*flurane, vancomycin:* increased nephrotoxicity. Use together cautiously.
*Parenteral penicillins (such as ticarcillin):* netilmicin inactivation. Don't mix together.

## CONTRAINDICATIONS

Contraindicated in patients with hypersensitivity to the drug or other aminoglycosides.

## NURSING CONSIDERATIONS

• Use cautiously in patients with impaired renal function or neuromuscular disorders and in neonates, infants, and elderly patients. Commercially available form contains sulfites, which may cause an allergic reaction in certain individuals.
• Obtain specimen for culture and sensitivity tests before first dose. Therapy may begin pending results.
• Weigh the patient and review renal function studies before therapy begins.
• Evaluate the patient's hearing before and during therapy. Notify the doctor if the patient complains of tinnitus, vertigo, or hearing loss. However, some studies show that this drug is less ototoxic than other aminoglycosides.
• **I.V. use:** After completing I.V. infusion, flush the line with 0.9% sodium chloride solution or $D_5W$.
• Obtain blood for peak level 1 hour after I.M. injection and ½ to 1 hour after infusion ends; for trough levels, draw blood just before next dose. Don't draw blood in a heparinized tube because heparin is incompatible with aminoglycosides.
• Be aware that blood levels above 16 mcg/ml and trough levels above 4 mcg/ml may be associated with higher incidence of toxicity.
• Monitor renal function (output, specific gravity, urinalysis, BUN and creatinine levels, and creatinine clearance) as ordered. Notify the doctor of signs of decreasing renal function.
• Watch for superinfection (continued

fever and other signs of new infection, especially of upper respiratory tract).
• Know that therapy usually continues for 7 to 10 days. If no response occurs in 3 to 5 days, therapy may be stopped and new specimens obtained for culture and sensitivity testing.

☑ **PATIENT TEACHING**
• Instruct patient to report adverse reactions promptly.
• Caution patient not to perform hazardous activities if dizziness occurs.
• Encourage adequate fluid intake.

---

## streptomycin sulfate
*Pregnancy Risk Category: D*

**HOW SUPPLIED**
*Injection:* 1 g/2.5 ml ampules

**ACTION**
Inhibits protein synthesis by binding directly to the 30S ribosomal subunit. Generally bactericidal.

**ONSET, PEAK, DURATION**
Onset and duration unknown. Serum levels peak 1 to 2 hours after I.M. injection.

**INDICATIONS & DOSAGE**
*Streptococcal endocarditis –*
**Adults:** 1 g q 12 hours I.M. for 1 week, then 500 mg q 12 hours for 1 week, given with penicillin. Patients over 60 years should receive 500 mg I.M. q 12 hours for entire 2 weeks.
*Primary and adjunctive treatment in tuberculosis –*
**Adults:** 1 g or 15 mg/kg I.M. daily for 2 to 3 months, then 1 g two or three times a week.
**Children:** 20 to 40 mg/kg I.M. daily in divided doses injected deeply into large muscle mass. Given concurrently with other antitubercular agents, but *not* with capreomycin. Continued until sputum specimen becomes negative.

*Enterococcal endocarditis –*
**Adults:** 1 g I.M. q 12 hours for 2 weeks, then 500 mg I.M. q 12 hours for 4 weeks, given with penicillin.
*Tularemia –*
**Adults:** 1 to 2 g I.M. daily in divided doses injected deep into upper outer quadrant of buttocks. Continued until patient is afebrile for 5 to 7 days.

**ADVERSE REACTIONS**
**CNS:** *neuromuscular blockade.*
**EENT:** *ototoxicity.*
**GI:** vomiting, nausea.
**GU:** some nephrotoxicity (not as frequently as with other aminoglycosides).
**Hematologic:** eosinophilia, leukopenia, *thrombocytopenia.*
**Respiratory:** apnea.
**Skin:** *exfoliative dermatitis.*
**Other:** hypersensitivity reactions (rash, fever, urticaria, angioedema), *anaphylaxis.*

**INTERACTIONS**
*Cephalothin:* increased nephrotoxicity. Use together cautiously.
*Dimenhydrinate:* may mask symptoms of streptomycin-induced ototoxicity. Use together cautiously.
*General anesthetics, neuromuscular blockers:* may potentiate neuromuscular blockade.
*I.V. loop diuretics (such as furosemide):* increased ototoxicity. Use together cautiously.
*Other aminoglycosides, acyclovir, amphotericin B, cisplatin, methoxyflurane, vancomycin:* increased nephrotoxicity. Use together cautiously.

**CONTRAINDICATIONS**
Contraindicated in patients with hypersensitivity to the drug or other aminoglycosides and in patients with labyrinthine disease. Never administer I.V.

---

Reactions may be *common,* uncommon, *life-threatening,* or COMMON AND LIFE-THREATENING.

## NURSING CONSIDERATIONS

• Use cautiously in patients with impaired renal function or neuromuscular disorders and in elderly patients.
• Obtain specimen for culture and sensitivity tests before first dose except when treating tuberculosis. Therapy may begin pending results.
• Evaluate patient's hearing before therapy and for 6 months afterward. Notify the doctor if the patient complains of hearing loss, roaring noises, or fullness in ears.
• Protect hands when preparing because drug is irritating.
• For I.M. administration, inject deeply into upper outer quadrant of buttocks. Rotate injection sites.
• Obtain blood for peak streptomycin level 1 to 2 hours after I.M. injection; for trough levels, draw blood just before next dose. Don't use a heparinized tube because heparin is incompatible with aminoglycosides.
• Watch for signs of superinfection (continued fever and other signs of new infections).
• Be aware that in primary treatment of tuberculosis, streptomycin is discontinued when sputum becomes negative.

### ☑ PATIENT TEACHING

• Instruct patient to report adverse reactions promptly.
• Encourage adequate fluid intake.
• Emphasize the need for blood tests to monitor streptomycin levels and determine the effectiveness of therapy.

---

## tobramycin sulfate
Nebcin

*Pregnancy Risk Category: D*

### HOW SUPPLIED

*Injection:* 40 mg/ml, 10 mg/ml (pediatric)
*Powder for injection:* 30 mg/ml after reconstitution
*Premixed parenteral injection for I.V.*

*infusion:* 60 mg or 80 mg in 0.9% sodium chloride solution

### ACTION

Inhibits protein synthesis by binding directly to the 30S ribosomal subunit. Generally bactericidal.

### ONSET, PEAK, DURATION

Onset immediate after I.V. infusion, unknown after I.M. injection. Peak serum levels occur immediately after I.V. infusion, 30 to 90 minutes after I.M. injection. Measurable serum levels persist for about 8 hours after I.M. or I.V. administration.

### INDICATIONS & DOSAGE

*Serious infections caused by sensitive strains of* Escherichia coli, Proteus, Klebsiella, Enterobacter, Serratia, Morganella morganii, Staphylococcus aureus, Pseudomonas, Citrobacter, Providencia—
**Adults:** 3 mg/kg I.M. or I.V. daily divided q 8 hours. Up to 5 mg/kg daily divided q 6 to 8 hours for life-threatening infections.
**Children:** 6 to 7.5 mg/kg I.M. or I.V. daily in three or four equally divided doses.
**Neonates under 1 week or premature infants:** up to 4 mg/kg/day I.V. or I.M. in two equal doses q 12 hours.

### ADVERSE REACTIONS

**CNS:** headache, lethargy, confusion, disorientation.
**EENT:** *ototoxicity.*
**GI:** vomiting, nausea, diarrhea.
**GU:** *nephrotoxicity.*
**Hematologic:** anemia, eosinophilia, leukopenia, thrombocytopenia, granulocytopenia.
**Other:** fever, rash, urticaria, pruritus.

### INTERACTIONS

*Cephalothin:* increased nephrotoxicity. Use together cautiously.

---

*Liquid form contains alcohol.  **May contain tartrazine.  †Canada only.  ‡Australia only.  ◇OTC.

*Dimenhydrinate:* may mask symptoms of ototoxicity. Use with caution.
*General anesthetics, neuromuscular blockers:* may potentiate neuromuscular blockade.
*I.V. loop diuretics (such as furosemide):* increased ototoxicity. Use together cautiously.
*Other aminoglycosides, acyclovir, amphotericin B, cisplatin, methoxyflurane, vancomycin:* increased nephrotoxicity. Use together cautiously.
*Parenteral penicillins (such as ticarcillin):* tobramycin inactivation in vitro. Don't mix together.

## CONTRAINDICATIONS
Contraindicated in patients with hypersensitivity to the drug or other aminoglycosides.

## NURSING CONSIDERATIONS
• Use cautiously in patients with impaired renal function or neuromuscular disorders and in elderly patients.
• Obtain specimen for culture and sensitivity tests before first dose. Therapy may begin pending results.
• Weigh the patient and review renal function studies before therapy.
• Evaluate patient's hearing before and during therapy. Notify the doctor if the patient complains of tinnitus, vertigo, or hearing loss.
• **I.V. use:** Dilute in 50 to 100 ml of 0.9% sodium chloride solution or $D_5W$ for adults and in less volume for children. Infuse over 20 to 60 minutes. After I.V. infusion, flush line with 0.9% sodium chloride solution or $D_5W$.
• Obtain blood for peak level 1 hour after I.M. injection and ½ to 1 hour after infusion ends; draw blood for trough level just before next dose. Don't collect blood in a heparinized tube because heparin is incompatible with aminoglycosides.
• *Alert:* Be aware that blood levels over 12 mcg/ml and trough levels

above 2 mcg/ml may be associated with increased incidence of toxicity.
• Monitor renal function (output, specific gravity, urinalysis, BUN and creatinine levels, and creatinine clearance). Notify the doctor of signs of decreasing renal function.
• Watch for signs of superinfection (continued fever and other signs of new infections).
• Be aware that if no response occurs in 3 to 5 days, therapy may be stopped and new specimens obtained for culture and sensitivity testing.

## ☑ PATIENT TEACHING
• Instruct patient to report adverse reactions promptly.
• Caution patient not to perform hazardous activities if adverse CNS reactions occur.
• Encourage adequate fluid intake.

---

# 12

## Penicillins

amoxicillin/clavulanate
  potassium
amoxicillin trihydrate
ampicillin
ampicillin sodium
ampicillin trihydrate
ampicillin sodium/sulbactam
  sodium
bacampicillin hydrochloride
carbenicillin indanyl sodium
cloxacillin sodium
dicloxacillin sodium
methicillin sodium
mezlocillin sodium
nafcillin sodium
oxacillin sodium
penicillin G benzathine
penicillin G potassium
penicillin G procaine
penicillin G sodium
penicillin V
penicillin V potassium
piperacillin sodium
piperacillin sodium and
  tazobactam sodium
ticarcillin disodium
ticarcillin disodium/clavulanate
  potassium

### COMBINATION PRODUCTS
AUGMENTIN, CLAVULIN†: amoxicillin 250 mg and clavulanate potassium
125 mg per tablet; amoxicillin 500 mg
and clavulanate potassium 125 mg per
tablet; amoxicillin 125 mg and clavulanate potassium 31.5 mg per chewable tablet; amoxicillin 250 mg and
clavulanate potassium 62.5 mg per
chewable tablet; amoxicillin 125 mg
and clavulanate potassium 31.5 mg
per 5 ml oral suspension; amoxicillin
250 mg and clavulanate potassium
62.5 mg per 5 ml oral suspension.
POLYCILLIN-PRB: ampicillin trihydrate 3.5 g and probenecid 1 g per
bottle.

PRINCIPEN WITH PROBENECID: ampicillin trihydrate 3.5 g and probenecid 1 g per bottle.

---

## amoxicillin/clavulanate potassium (amoxycillin/clavulanate potassium)
Augmentin, Clavulin†

*Pregnancy Risk Category: B*

### HOW SUPPLIED
*Tablets (chewable):* 125 mg amoxicillin trihydrate, 31.25 mg clavulanic
acid; 250 mg amoxicillin trihydrate,
62.5 mg clavulanic acid
*Tablets (film-coated):* 250 mg amoxicillin trihydrate, 125 mg clavulanic
acid; 500 mg amoxicillin trihydrate,
125 mg clavulanic acid
*Oral suspension:* 125 mg amoxicillin
trihydrate and 31.25 mg clavulanic
acid/5 ml (after reconstitution); 250
mg amoxicillin trihydrate and 62.5
mg clavulanic acid/5 ml (after reconstitution)

### ACTION
An aminopenicillin that prevents bacterial cell-wall synthesis during replication. Clavulanic acid increases
amoxicillin effectiveness by inactivating beta lactamases, which destroy
amoxicillin.

### ONSET, PEAK, DURATION
Onset unknown. Serum levels peak in
1 to 2½ hours. Serum concentrations
are usually low or undetectable 6 to 8
hours after oral administration.

### INDICATIONS & DOSAGE
*Lower respiratory infections, otitis
media, sinusitis, skin and skin-structure infections, and urinary tract infections caused by susceptible strains*

---

*Liquid form contains alcohol. **May contain tartrazine. †Canada only. ‡Australia only. ◇OTC.

of gram-positive and gram-negative organisms –

**Adults:** 250 mg (based on the amoxicillin component) P.O. q 8 hours. For more severe infections, 500 mg q 8 hours.
**Children:** 20 to 40 mg/kg (based on the amoxicillin component) P.O. daily in divided doses q 8 hours.

## ADVERSE REACTIONS
**CNS:** agitation, anxiety, insomnia, confusion, behavioral changes, dizziness.
**GI:** *nausea,* vomiting, *diarrhea,* indigestion, gastritis, stomatitis, glossitis, black "hairy" tongue, enterocolitis, pseudomembranous colitis.
**Hematologic:** anemia, ***thrombocytopenia,*** thrombocytopenic purpura, eosinophilia, leukopenia, ***agranulocytosis.***
**Other:** hypersensitivity reactions (erythematous maculopapular rash, urticaria, ***anaphylaxis***), overgrowth of nonsusceptible organisms, vaginitis.

## INTERACTIONS
*Allopurinol:* increased incidence of rash.
*Oral contraceptives:* efficacy of oral contraceptives may be decreased. Additional form of contraception recommended during penicillin therapy.
*Probenecid:* increased blood levels of amoxicillin and other penicillins. Probenecid may be used for this purpose.

## CONTRAINDICATIONS
Contraindicated in patients with hypersensitivity to the drug or other penicillins and in those with a previous history of amoxicillin-associated cholestatic jaundice or hepatic dysfunction.

## NURSING CONSIDERATIONS
• Use cautiously in patients with other drug allergies, especially to cephalosporins (possible cross-sensitivity), and in those with mononucleosis (high incidence of maculopapular rash).
• Before giving, ask the patient about any allergic reactions to penicillin. However, a negative history of penicillin allergy is no guarantee against an allergic reaction.
• Obtain specimen for culture and sensitivity tests before first dose. Therapy may begin pending results.
• Give drug at least 1 hour before bacteriostatic antibiotics.
• Observe closely. With large doses and prolonged therapy, bacterial or fungal superinfection may occur, especially in elderly, debilitated, or immunosuppressed patients.
• *Alert:* Know that both the "250" and "500" tablets contain the same amount of clavulanic acid (125 mg). Therefore, two "250" tablets are not equivalent to one "500" tablet.
• Be aware that this drug combination is particularly useful in clinical settings with high prevalence of amoxicillin-resistant organisms.
• After reconstitution, refrigerate the oral suspension; discard after 10 days.
• Know that urine glucose determinations may be false-positive with copper sulfate tests (Benedict's solution, Clinitest); glucose enzymatic tests (Clinistix, Tes-Tape) are not affected.

## ☑ PATIENT TEACHING
• Tell the patient to take entire quantity of drug exactly as prescribed, even after he feels better.
• Instruct him to take drug with food to prevent GI upset. If he's taking the oral suspension, tell him to keep drug refrigerated, to shake it well before administration, and to discard any remaining drug after 10 days.
• Tell the patient to call doctor if a rash occurs. A rash is a sign of an allergic reaction.

---

## amoxicillin trihydrate (amoxycillin trihydrate)

Alphamox‡, Amoxil, Apo-Amoxi†, Cilamox‡, Ibiamox‡, Larotid, Moxacin‡, Novamoxin†, Nu-Amoxi†, Polymox, Trimox, Wymox

*Pregnancy Risk Category: NR*

### HOW SUPPLIED
*Tablets (chewable):* 125 mg, 250 mg
*Capsules:* 250 mg, 500 mg
*Oral suspension:* 50 mg/ml (pediatric drops), 125 mg/5 ml, 250 mg/5 ml (after reconstitution)

### ACTION
An aminopenicillin that inhibits cell-wall synthesis during bacterial multiplication; bacteria resist amoxicillin by producing penicillinases — enzymes that hydrolyze amoxicillin.

### ONSET, PEAK, DURATION
Onset unknown. Serum levels peak within 1 to 2 hours. Serum concentrations are usually low or undetectable 6 to 8 hours after oral administration.

### INDICATIONS & DOSAGE
*Systemic infections, acute and chronic urinary tract infections caused by susceptible strains of gram-positive and gram-negative organisms —*
**Adults and children 20 kg or over:** 250 to 500 mg P.O. q 8 hours.
**Children under 20 kg:** 20 mg/kg P.O. daily in divided doses q 8 hours; in severe infection, 40 mg/kg P.O. daily in divided doses q 8 hours or 500 mg to 1 g/m² P.O. in divided doses q 8 hours.
*Uncomplicated gonorrhea —*
**Adults and children over 45 kg:** 3 g P.O. with 1 g probenecid given as a single dose.
*Endocarditis prophylaxis for dental procedures —*
**Adults:** initially, 3 g P.O. 1 hour before procedure; then 1.5 g 6 hours later.

**Children:** initially, 50 mg/kg P.O. 1 hour before procedure; then half the initial dose 6 hours later.

### ADVERSE REACTIONS
**CNS:** lethargy, hallucinations, *seizures,* anxiety, confusion, agitation, depression, dizziness, fatigue.
**GI:** *nausea,* vomiting, *diarrhea,* glossitis, stomatitis, gastritis, abdominal pain, enterocolitis, pseudomembranous colitis, black "hairy" tongue.
**GU:** interstitial nephritis, nephropathy.
**Hematologic:** anemia, *thrombocytopenia,* thrombocytopenic purpura, eosinophilia, leukopenia, hemolytic anemia, *agranulocytosis.*
**Other:** hypersensitivity reactions (erythematous maculopapular rash, urticaria, *anaphylaxis*), overgrowth of nonsusceptible organisms, vaginitis.

### INTERACTIONS
*Allopurinol:* increased incidence of rash.
*Oral contraceptives:* efficacy of oral contraceptives may be decreased. Additional form of contraception recommended during penicillin therapy.
*Probenecid:* increased blood levels of amoxicillin and other penicillins. Probenecid may be used for this purpose.

### CONTRAINDICATIONS
Contraindicated in patients with hypersensitivity to the drug or other penicillins.

### NURSING CONSIDERATIONS
● Use cautiously in patients with other drug allergies, especially to cephalosporins (possible cross-sensitivity) and in those with mononucleosis (high incidence of maculopapular rash).
● Before giving, ask the patient about any allergic reactions to penicillin. However, a negative history of penicillin allergy is no guarantee against an allergic reaction.
● Obtain specimen for culture and

sensitivity tests before first dose. Therapy may begin pending results.
• Give amoxicillin at least 1 hour before bacteriostatic antibiotics.
• Observe closely. With large doses and prolonged therapy, bacterial or fungal superinfection may occur, especially in elderly, debilitated, or immunosuppressed patients.
• Store Trimox oral suspension at room temperature for up to 2 weeks. Be sure to check individual product labels for storage information.
• Be aware that urine glucose determinations may be false-positive with copper sulfate tests (Benedict's solution, Clinitest); glucose enzymatic tests (Clinistix, Tes-Tape) are not affected.
• Keep in mind that amoxicillin generally causes diarrhea less often than ampicillin.

☑ **PATIENT TEACHING**
• Tell the patient to take entire quantity of medication exactly as prescribed, even after he feels better.
• Tell him to take drug with food.
• Warn the patient never to use leftover amoxicillin for a new illness or to share it with family and friends.
• Tell the patient to call the doctor if rash, fever, or chills develop. A rash is the most common allergic reaction, especially when the patient is also taking allopurinol.

# ampicillin
Apo-Ampi†, Novo Ampicillin†, Nu-Ampi†, Omnipen, Principen

# ampicillin sodium
Ampicin†, Ampicyn Injection‡, Omnipen-N, Penbritin†, Polycillin-N, Totacillin-N

# ampicillin trihydrate
Ampicyn Oral‡, D-Amp, Omnipen, Penbritin‡, Polycillin, Principen-250, Principen-500, Totacillin

*Pregnancy Risk Category: B*

## HOW SUPPLIED
*Capsules:* 250 mg, 500 mg
*Oral suspension:* 100 mg/ml (pediatric drops), 125 mg/5 ml, 250 mg/5 ml, 500 mg/5 ml (after reconstitution)
*Injection:* 125 mg, 250 mg, 500 mg, 1 g, 2 g
*Infusion:* 500 mg, 1 g, 2 g
*Pharmacy bulk package:* 10-g vial

## ACTION
An aminopenicillin that inhibits cell-wall synthesis during microorganism multiplication; bacteria resist ampicillin by producing penicillinases — enzymes that hydrolyze ampicillin.

## ONSET, PEAK, DURATION
Onset immediate after I.V. administration, unknown after I.M. injection. Peak plasma levels occur immediately after I.V. administration, within 1 hour of I.M. administration, and within 2 hours of oral administration. Serum levels are usually low or undetectable 6 to 8 hours after oral administration.

## INDICATIONS & DOSAGE
*Systemic infections and acute and chronic urinary tract infections caused by susceptible strains of gram-positive and gram-negative organisms—*
**Adults and children 20 kg or over:** 250 to 500 mg P.O. q 6 hours; or 2 to 12 g I.M. or I.V. daily, in divided doses q 4 to 6 hours.
**Children 20 kg or less:** 50 to 100 mg/kg P.O. daily, in divided doses q 6 hours; or 100 to 200 mg/kg I.M. or I.V. daily, in divided doses q 6 hours.
*Meningitis—*
**Adults:** 8 to 14 g I.V. daily in divided doses q 3 to 4 hours.

---

Reactions may be *common,* uncommon, *life-threatening,* or COMMON AND LIFE-THREATENING.

**Children:** up to 300 mg/kg I.V. daily in divided doses q 3 to 4 hours.
*Uncomplicated gonorrhea –*
**Adults and children over 45 kg:** 3.5 g P.O. with 1 g probenecid given as a single dose.
*Endocarditis prophylaxis for dental procedures –*
**Adults:** 1 to 2 g I.M. or I.V. with gentamicin 30 minutes before procedure; repeated 6 hours after initial dose.
**Children** 50 mg/kg I.M. or I.V. with gentamicin 2 mg/kg 30 minutes before procedure; half the initial dose is given 6 hours later.

## ADVERSE REACTIONS
**CNS:** lethargy, hallucinations, *seizures,* anxiety, confusion, agitation, depression, dizziness, fatigue.
**GI:** *nausea,* vomiting, *diarrhea,* glossitis, stomatitis, gastritis, abdominal pain, enterocolitis, pseudomembranous colitis, black "hairy" tongue.
**GU:** interstitial nephritis, nephropathy.
**Hematologic:** anemia, *thrombocytopenia,* thrombocytopenic purpura, eosinophilia, leukopenia, hemolytic anemia, *agranulocytosis.*
**Other:** hypersensitivity reactions (erythematous maculopapular rash, urticaria, *anaphylaxis*), overgrowth of nonsusceptible organisms, pain at injection site, vein irritation, thrombophlebitis, vaginitis.

## INTERACTIONS
*Allopurinol:* increased incidence of rash.
*Oral contraceptives:* efficacy of oral contraceptives may be decreased. Additional form of contraception recommended during penicillin therapy.
*Probenecid:* increased blood levels of ampicillin and other penicillins. Probenecid may be used for this purpose.

## CONTRAINDICATIONS
Contraindicated in patients with hypersensitivity to the drug or other penicillins.

## NURSING CONSIDERATIONS
● Use cautiously in patients with other drug allergies, especially to cephalosporins (possible cross-sensitivity), or in those with mononucleosis (high incidence of maculopapular rash).
● Before giving, ask the patient about any allergic reactions to penicillin. However, a negative history of penicillin allergy is no guarantee against a future allergic reaction.
● Obtain specimen for culture and sensitivity tests before first dose. Therapy may begin pending results.
● **I.V. use:** For I.V. injection, reconstitute with bacteriostatic water for injection. Use 5 ml for the 125-mg, 250-mg, or 500-mg vials; 7.4 ml for the 1-g vials; or 14.8 ml for the 2-g vials. Give direct I.V. injections over 3 to 5 minutes for doses of 500 mg or less; over 10 to 15 minutes for larger doses. Don't exceed a rate of 100 mg/ minute. Alternatively, dilute in 50 to 100 ml of 0.9% sodium chloride for injection and give by intermittent infusion over 15 to 30 minutes.
● *Alert:* Don't mix with solutions containing dextrose or fructose because these solutions promote rapid breakdown of ampicillin.
● Use initial dilution within 1 hour. Follow manufacturer's directions for stability data when ampicillin is further diluted for I.V. infusion.
● Give I.V. intermittently to prevent vein irritation. Change site every 48 hours.
● Give the drug I.M. or I.V. only if prescribed and the infection is severe or if patient can't take oral dose.
● Give 1 to 2 hours before or 2 to 3 hours after meals. When given orally, drug may cause GI disturbances. Food may interfere with absorption.
● Give ampicillin at least 1 hour before bacteriostatic antibiotics.
● Observe closely. With large doses or prolonged therapy, bacterial or fungal superinfection may occur, espe-

---

*Liquid form contains alcohol. **May contain tartrazine. †Canada only. ‡Australia only. ◊OTC.

cially in elderly, debilitated, or immunosuppressed patients.
• Know that dosage should be altered in patients with impaired renal function.
• Be aware that in pediatric meningitis, ampicillin may be given concurrently with parenteral chloramphenicol for 24 hours pending cultures.
• Keep in mind that urine glucose determinations may be false-positive with copper sulfate tests (Benedict's solution, Clinitest); glucose enzymatic tests (Clinistix, Tes-Tape) are not affected.

☑ **PATIENT TEACHING**
• Tell the patient to take entire quantity of medication exactly as prescribed, even after he feels better.
• Instruct the patient to take oral form on an empty stomach.
• Tell the patient to call the doctor if rash, fever, or chills develop. A rash is the most common allergic reaction, especially if the patient is also taking allopurinol.
• Warn the patient never to use leftover ampicillin for a new illness or to share it with family and friends.
• Instruct the patient to report discomfort at I.V. injection site.

## ampicillin sodium/ sulbactam sodium
Unasyn

*Pregnancy Risk Category: B*

### HOW SUPPLIED
*Injection:* vials and piggyback vials containing 1.5 g (1 g ampicillin sodium with 0.5 g sulbactam sodium) and 3 g (2 g ampicillin sodium with 1 g sulbactam sodium)
*Pharmacy bulk package:* 15 g (10g ampicillin sodium with 5 g sulbactam sodium)

### ACTION
Ampicillin (an aminopenicillin) inhibits cell-wall synthesis during microorganism multiplication; sulbactam inactivates bacterial beta-lactamase, which inactivates ampicillin and causes bacterial resistance to it.

### ONSET, PEAK, DURATION
Onset immediate after I.V. administration, unknown after I.M. injection. Peak serum levels occur immediately after I.V. administration, unknown after I.M. injection. Duration unknown.

### INDICATIONS & DOSAGE
*Intra-abdominal, gynecologic, and skin-structure infections caused by susceptible strains—*
**Adults:** dosage expressed as total drug (each 1.5-g vial contains 1 g ampicillin sodium and 0.5 g sulbactam sodium)—1.5 to 3 g I.M. or I.V. q 6 hours. Maximum daily dosage is 4 g sulbactam (12 g of combined drugs).

### ADVERSE REACTIONS
**GI:** *nausea,* vomiting, *diarrhea,* glossitis, stomatitis, gastritis, black "hairy" tongue, enterocolitis, pseudomembranous colitis.
**Hematologic:** anemia, ***thrombocytopenia,*** thrombocytopenic purpura, eosinophilia, leukopenia, ***agranulocytosis.***
**Other:** hypersensitivity reactions (erythematous maculopapular rash, urticaria, ***anaphylaxis***), ***overgrowth of nonsusceptible organisms,*** pain at injection site, vein irritation, thrombophlebitis.

### INTERACTIONS
*Allopurinol:* increased incidence of rash.
*Oral contraceptives:* efficacy of oral contraceptives may be decreased. Additional form of contraception recommended during penicillin therapy.
*Probenecid:* increased levels of ampi-

---

Reactions may be *common,* uncommon, ***life-threatening,*** or **COMMON AND LIFE-THREATENING.**

cillin. Probenecid may be used for this purpose.

## CONTRAINDICATIONS
Contraindicated in patients with hypersensitivity to the drug or other penicillins.

## NURSING CONSIDERATIONS
• Use cautiously in patients with other drug allergies, especially to cephalosporins (possible cross-sensitivity), or in those with mononucleosis (high incidence of maculopapular rash).
• Before giving, ask the patient about any allergic reactions to penicillin. However, a negative history of penicillin allergy is no guarantee against a future allergic reaction.
• Obtain specimen for culture and sensitivity tests before first dose. Therapy may begin pending results.
• **I.V. use:** When preparing I.V. injection, reconstitute powder with any of the following diluents: 0.9% sodium chloride solution, sterile water for injection, D₅W, lactated Ringer's injection, ⅙ M sodium lactate, dextrose 5% and 0.45% sodium chloride for injection, and 10% invert sugar. Stability varies with diluent, temperature, and concentration of solution.
• After reconstitution, allow vials to stand for a few minutes for foam to dissipate. This will permit visual inspection of contents for particles.
• Give I.V. dose by slow injection (over 10 to 15 minutes), or dilute in 50 to 100 ml of a compatible diluent, and infuse over 15 to 30 minutes. If permitted, give intermittently to prevent vein irritation. Change site every 48 hours.
• When giving I.V., don't add or mix with other drugs because they might prove incompatible.
• For I.M. injection, reconstitute with sterile water for injection or 0.5% or 2% lidocaine hydrochloride injection. Add 3.2 ml to a 1.5-g vial

(or 6.4 ml to a 3-g vial) to yield a concentration of 375 mg/ml. Administer deeply.
• Give drug at least 1 hour before bacteriostatic antibiotics.
• Observe closely. With large doses and prolonged therapy, bacterial or fungal superinfection may occur, especially in elderly, debilitated, or immunosuppressed patients.
• Know that dosage should be altered in patients with impaired renal function.
• Keep in mind that urine glucose determinations may be false-positive with copper sulfate tests (Benedict's solution, Clinitest); glucose enzymatic tests (Clinistix, Tes-Tape) are not affected.

## ☑ PATIENT TEACHING
• Tell the patient to report a rash, fever, or chills. A rash is the most common allergic reaction.
• Also tell the patient to report discomfort at I.V. insertion site.
• Warn the patient that I.M. injection may cause pain at injection site.

---

# bacampicillin hydrochloride
Penglobet, Spectrobid

*Pregnancy Risk Category: B*

## HOW SUPPLIED
*Tablets:* 400 mg

## ACTION
An aminopenicillin that inhibits cell-wall synthesis during microorganism multiplication; bacteria resist bacampicillin by producing penicillinases — enzymes that hydrolyze its active form (ampicillin) when drug is absorbed in GI tract.

## ONSET, PEAK, DURATION
Onset unknown. Plasma levels peak within 30 to 90 minutes. Serum con-

---

centrations are usually low or undetectable 6 to 8 hours later.

## INDICATIONS & DOSAGE

*Upper respiratory tract infections and otitis media caused by streptococci, pneumococci, staphylococci, and* Haemophilus influenzae; *urinary tract infections caused by* Escherichia coli, Proteus mirabilis, *and* Enterococcus faecalis; *skin infections caused by streptococci and susceptible staphylococci* –

**Adults and children over 25 kg: 400 mg P.O. q 12 hours.**

**Children 25 kg or less: 25 mg/kg/day P.O. in divided doses q 12 hours.**

*Lower respiratory tract infections; other severe infections* –

**Adults and children over 25 kg: 800 mg P.O. q 12 hours.**

**Children 25 kg or less: 50 mg/kg/day P.O. in divided doses q 12 hours.**

*Gonorrhea* –

Adults: 1.6 g P.O. plus 1 g probenecid given as a single dose.

## ADVERSE REACTIONS

**GI:** *nausea,* vomiting, *diarrhea,* glossitis, stomatitis, epigastric upset, black "hairy" tongue, enterocolitis, pseudomembranous colitis.

**Hematologic:** anemia, ***thrombocytopenia,*** thrombocytopenic purpura, eosinophilia, leukopenia, ***agranulocytosis.***

**Other:** hypersensitivity reactions (erythematous maculopapular rash, urticaria, ***anaphylaxis***), overgrowth of nonsusceptible organisms.

## INTERACTIONS

*Allopurinol:* increased incidence of rash.

*Disulfiram:* possible disulfiram-alcohol reaction. Do not give together.

*Oral contraceptives:* efficacy of oral contraceptives may be decreased. Additional form of contraception recommended during penicillin therapy.

*Probenecid:* increased blood levels of bacampicillin or other penicillins. Probenecid may be used for this purpose.

## CONTRAINDICATIONS

Contraindicated in patients with hypersensitivity to the drug or other penicillins.

## NURSING CONSIDERATIONS

• Use cautiously in patients with other drug allergies, especially to cephalosporins (possible cross-sensitivity), or in those with mononucleosis (high incidence of maculopapular rash).

• Before giving, ask the patient about any allergic reactions to penicillin. However, a negative history of penicillin allergy is no guarantee against an allergic reaction.

• Obtain specimen for culture and sensitivity tests before first dose. Therapy may begin pending results.

• Unlike ampicillin, administer bacampicillin with meals without fear of diminished drug absorption.

• Give bacampicillin at least 1 hour before bacteriostatic antibiotics.

• Observe closely. With large doses and prolonged therapy, bacterial or fungal superinfection may occur, especially in elderly, debilitated, or immunosuppressed patients.

• Know that diarrhea may occur less frequently with bacampicillin than with ampicillin.

• Be aware that bacampicillin is specially formulated to cause high blood levels of antibiotic when administered twice daily.

• Keep in mind that urine glucose determinations may be false-positive with copper sulfate tests (Benedict's solution, Clinitest); glucose enzymatic tests (Clinistix, Tes-Tape) are not affected.

## ☑ PATIENT TEACHING

• Tell the patient to take entire quantity of medication as prescribed, even after he feels better.

---

Reactions may be *common,* uncommon, ***life-threatening,*** or COMMON AND LIFE-THREATENING.

• Inform the patient that drug may be taken with or without food.
• Warn the patient never to use left-over bacampicillin for a new illness or to share it with family and friends.
• Tell the patient to call the doctor if rash, fever, or chills develop. A rash is the most common allergic reaction.

---

## carbenicillin indanyl sodium
Geocillin, Geopen Oral†

*Pregnancy Risk Category: B*

### HOW SUPPLIED
*Tablets:* 382 mg

### ACTION
An extended-spectrum penicillin that inhibits cell-wall synthesis during microorganism multiplication; bacteria resist carbenicillin by producing penicillinases — enzymes that hydrolyze its active form.

### ONSET, PEAK, DURATION
Onset unknown. Serum levels peak within 30 minutes. Serum carbenicillin concentrations are generally low or undetectable 6 hours after a dose.

### INDICATIONS & DOSAGE
*Urinary tract infection and prostatitis caused by susceptible strains of gram-negative organisms—*
**Adults:** 382 to 764 mg P.O. q.i.d.

### ADVERSE REACTIONS
**GI:** *nausea,* vomiting, *diarrhea, flatulence, abdominal cramps, unpleasant taste,* glossitis, dry mouth, furry tongue.
**Hematologic:** leukopenia, neutropenia, eosinophilia, ***hemolytic anemia, thrombocytopenia.***
**Other:** hypersensitivity reactions (rash, urticaria, pruritus, ***anaphylaxis***), overgrowth of nonsusceptible organisms.

### INTERACTIONS
*Oral contraceptives:* efficacy of oral contraceptives may be decreased. Additional form of contraception recommended during penicillin therapy.

### CONTRAINDICATIONS
Contraindicated in patients with hypersensitivity to the drug or other penicillins.

### NURSING CONSIDERATIONS
• Use cautiously in patients with other drug allergies, especially to cephalosporins (possible cross-sensitivity).
• Before giving, ask the patient about any allergic reactions to penicillin. However, a negative history of penicillin allergy is no guarantee against a future allergic reaction.
• Obtain specimen for culture and sensitivity tests before first dose. Therapy may begin pending results.
• Know that drug is used only in patients whose creatinine clearance values are 10 ml/minute or more.
• Give 1 to 2 hours before or 2 to 3 hours after meals because food may interfere with absorption.
• Observe closely. With large doses or prolonged therapy, bacterial or fungal superinfection may occur, especially in elderly, debilitated, or immunosuppressed patients.
• Keep in mind that urine glucose determinations may be false-positive with copper sulfate tests (Benedict's solution, Clinitest); glucose enzymatic tests (Clinistix, Tes-Tape) are not affected.
• Be aware that carbenicillin may interfere with direct results of Coombs' test and tests for serum uric acid.

### ☑ PATIENT TEACHING
• Tell the patient to take all of the medication exactly as prescribed, even after he feels better.
• Instruct the patient to take drug on an empty stomach.

---

• Tell the patient to call the doctor if rash, fever, or chills develop. A rash is the most common allergic reaction.
• Warn the patient never to use left-over carbenicillin for a new illness or to share it with family and friends.

---

## cloxacillin sodium
Alclox‡, Apo-Cloxi†, Austrastaph‡, Cloxapen, Novo-Cloxin†, Nu-Cloxi†, Orbenin†, Orbenin Injection‡, Tegopen

*Pregnancy Risk Category: B*

### HOW SUPPLIED
*Capsules:* 250 mg, 500 mg
*Oral solution:* 125 mg/5 ml (after reconstitution)

### ACTION
A penicillinase-resistant penicillin that inhibits cell-wall synthesis during microorganism multiplication; bacteria resist penicillins by producing penicillinases—enzymes that convert penicillins to inactive penicilloic acid. Cloxacillin resists these enzymes.

### ONSET, PEAK, DURATION
Onset unknown. Plasma levels peak within 2 hours. Drug concentrations are generally low 6 hours after a dose.

### INDICATIONS & DOSAGE
*Systemic infections caused by penicillinase-producing staphylococci—*
**Adults and children over 20 kg:** 250 to 500 mg P.O. q 6 hours.
**Children 20 kg or less:** 50 to 100 mg/kg P.O. daily, in divided doses q 6 hours.

### ADVERSE REACTIONS
**CNS:** lethargy, hallucinations, *seizures,* anxiety, confusion, agitation, depression, dizziness, fatigue.
**GI:** *nausea,* vomiting, *epigastric distress, diarrhea,* enterocolitis, pseudomembranous colitis, black "hairy" tongue, abdominal pain.
**GU:** interstitial nephritis, nephropathy.
**Hematologic:** eosinophilia, anemia, *thrombocytopenia,* eosinophilia, leukopenia, hemolytic anemia, *agranulocytosis.*
**Other:** hypersensitivity reactions (rash, urticaria, chills, fever, sneezing, wheezing, *anaphylaxis*), intrahepatic cholestasis, overgrowth of non-susceptible organisms.

### INTERACTIONS
*Oral contraceptives:* efficacy of oral contraceptives may be decreased. Additional form of contraception recommended during penicillin therapy.
*Probenecid:* increased blood levels of cloxacillin and other penicillins. Probenecid may be used for this purpose.

### CONTRAINDICATIONS
Contraindicated in patients with hypersensitivity to the drug or other penicillins.

### NURSING CONSIDERATIONS
• Use cautiously in patients with other drug allergies, especially to cephalosporins (possible cross-sensitivity), or in those with mononucleosis (high incidence of maculopapular rash).
• Before giving, ask the patient about any allergic reactions to penicillin. However, a negative history of penicillin allergy is no guarantee against a future allergic reaction.
• Obtain specimen for culture and sensitivity tests before first dose. Therapy may begin pending results.
• Give 1 to 2 hours before or 2 to 3 hours after meals. Drug may cause GI disturbances. Food may interfere with its absorption.
• Give cloxacillin at least 1 hour before bacteriostatic antibiotics.
• As ordered, periodically assess renal, hepatic, and hematopoietic function in patients receiving long-term therapy.
• Observe closely. With large doses

---

Reactions may be *common,* uncommon, *life-threatening,* or COMMON AND LIFE-THREATENING.

and prolonged therapy, bacterial or fungal superinfection may occur, especially in elderly, debilitated, or immunosuppressed patients.
• Keep in mind that cloxacillin may falsely elevate or cause false-positive results with certain tests for urine or serum proteins.

☑ **PATIENT TEACHING**
• Tell the patient to take entire quantity of medication exactly as prescribed, even after he feels better.
• Instruct the patient to take drug on an empty stomach.
• Tell the patient to call the doctor if rash, fever, or chills develop. A rash is the most common allergic reaction.
• *Alert:* Instruct the patient to take each dose with a full glass of water, not with fruit juice or carbonated beverage, because their acid will inactivate the drug.
• Warn the patient never to use leftover cloxacillin for a new illness or to share it with family and friends.

## diclovacillin sodium
Dycill, Dynapen, Pathocil
*Pregnancy Risk Category: NR*

**HOW SUPPLIED**
*Capsules:* 250 mg, 500 mg
*Oral suspension:* 62.5 mg/5 ml (after reconstitution)

**ACTION**
A penicillinase-resistant penicillin that inhibits cell-wall synthesis during microorganism multiplication; bacteria resist penicillins by producing penicillinases — enzymes that convert penicillins to inactive penicilloic acid. Dicloxacillin resists these enzymes.

**ONSET, PEAK, DURATION**
Onset unknown. Plasma levels peak within 2 hours. Drug concentrations are generally low 6 hours after a dose.

**INDICATIONS & DOSAGE**
*Systemic infections caused by penicillinase-producing staphylococci —*
**Adults and children over 40 kg:** 125 to 250 mg P.O. q 6 hours.
**Children 40 kg or less:** 25 to 50 mg/kg P.O. daily, in divided doses q 6 hours.

**ADVERSE REACTIONS**
**CNS:** neuromuscular irritability, *seizures,* lethargy, hallucinations, anxiety, confusion, agitation, depression, dizziness, fatigue.
**GI:** *nausea,* vomiting, *epigastric distress,* flatulence, *diarrhea,* enterocolitis, pseudomembranous colitis, black "hairy" tongue, abdominal pain.
**GU:** interstitial nephritis, nephropathy.
**Hematologic:** eosinophilia, anemia, *thrombocytopenia,* eosinophilia, leukopenia, hemolytic anemia, *agranulocytosis.*
**Other:** hypersensitivity reactions (pruritus, urticaria, rash, *anaphylaxis*), overgrowth of nonsusceptible organisms.

**INTERACTIONS**
*Oral contraceptives:* efficacy of oral contraceptives may be decreased. Additional form of contraception recommended during penicillin therapy.
*Probenecid:* increased blood levels of dicloxacillin and other penicillins. Probenecid may be used for this purpose.

**CONTRAINDICATIONS**
Contraindicated in patients with hypersensitivity to the drug or other penicillins.

**NURSING CONSIDERATIONS**
• Use cautiously in patients with other drug allergies, especially to cephalosporins (possible cross-sensitivity), or in those with mononucleosis (high incidence of maculopapular rash).
• Before giving, ask the patient about

---

*Liquid form contains alcohol. **May contain tartrazine. †Canada only. ‡Australia only. ◊OTC.

any allergic reactions to penicillin. However, a negative history of penicillin allergy is no guarantee against a future allergic reaction.

• Obtain specimen for culture and sensitivity tests before first dose. Therapy may begin pending results.

• Give 1 to 2 hours before or 2 to 3 hours after meals. Drug may cause GI disturbances. Food may interfere with absorption.

• Give dicloxacillin at least 1 hour before bacteriostatic antibiotics.

• As ordered, periodically assess renal, hepatic, and hematopoietic function in patients receiving long-term therapy.

• Observe closely. With large doses and prolonged therapy, bacterial or fungal superinfection may occur, especially in elderly, debilitated, or immunosuppressed patients.

☑ **PATIENT TEACHING**
• Tell the patient to take entire quantity of medication exactly as prescribed, even after he feels better.

• Instruct the patient to take drug on an empty stomach.

• Tell the patient to call the doctor if rash, fever, or chills develop. A rash is the most common allergic reaction.

• Warn the patient never to use leftover dicloxacillin for a new illness or to share it with family and friends.

## methicillin sodium
Metin‡, Staphcillin

*Pregnancy Risk Category: B*

### HOW SUPPLIED
*Injection:* 1 g, 4 g
*I.V. infusion piggyback:* 1 g
*Pharmacy bulk package:* 10 g

### ACTION
A penicillinase-resistant penicillin that inhibits cell-wall synthesis during microorganism multiplication; bacteria resist penicillins by producing penicilli-

nases – enzymes that convert penicillins to inactive penicilloic acid. Methicillin resists these enzymes.

### ONSET, PEAK, DURATION
Onset immediate after I.V. administration, unknown after I.M. administration. Peak serum levels occur immediately after I.V. infusion, within 30 to 60 minutes of I.M. injection. Drug concentrations undetectable 6 hours after an I.M. dose.

### INDICATIONS & DOSAGE
*Systemic infections caused by penicillinase-producing staphylococci –*
**Adults and children over 40 kg:** 4 to 12 g I.M. or I.V. daily, in divided doses q 4 to 6 hours.
**Children 40 kg and less:** 100 to 300 mg/kg I.M. or I.V. daily, in divided doses q 4 to 6 hours.

### ADVERSE REACTIONS
**CNS:** neuropathy, *seizures,* lethargy, hallucinations, anxiety, confusion, agitation, depression, dizziness, fatigue.
**GI:** glossitis, stomatitis, nausea, vomiting, enterocolitis, pseudomembranous colitis.
**Hematologic:** *agranulocytosis, eosinophilia,* hemolytic anemia, transient neutropenia, anemia, leukopenia, *thrombocytopenia.*
**GU:** interstitial nephritis, nephropathy.
**Other:** hypersensitivity reactions (chills, fever, edema, rash, urticaria, *anaphylaxis*), overgrowth of nonsusceptible organisms, vein irritation, thrombophlebitis.

### INTERACTIONS
*Oral contraceptives:* efficacy of oral contraceptives may be decreased. Additional form of contraception recommended during penicillin therapy.
*Probenecid:* increased blood levels of methicillin and other penicillins. Probenecid may be used for this purpose.

---

Reactions may be *common,* uncommon, *life-threatening,* or COMMON AND LIFE-THREATENING.

## CONTRAINDICATIONS

Contraindicated in patients with hypersensitivity to the drug or other penicillins.

## NURSING CONSIDERATIONS

• Use cautiously in patients with other drug allergies, especially to cephalosporins (possible cross-sensitivity), and in infants.
• Before giving, ask the patient about any allergic reactions to penicillin. However, a negative history of penicillin allergy is no guarantee against a future allergic reaction.
• Obtain specimen for culture and sensitivity tests before first dose. Therapy may begin pending results.
• **I.V. use:** Reconstitute vials with sterile water for injection or 0.9% sodium chloride for injection. For 1-g vials, use 1.5 ml of diluent; for 4-g vials, 5.7 ml of diluent; and for 6-g vials, 8.6 ml of diluent. For direct injection, further dilute each 500 mg drug with 35 ml of 0.9% sodium chloride for injection and inject at a rate of 10 ml/minute into the tubing of a free-flowing compatible I.V. solution. For intermittent infusion, dilute to a maximum concentration of 2 to 20 mg/ml and infuse over 20 to 30 minutes.
• Give I.V. intermittently to prevent vein irritation. Change site every 48 hours.
• For I.M. administration, inject reconstituted drug deeply into the gluteus maximus to avoid sciatic nerve injury.
• Give methicillin at least 1 hour before bacteriostatic antibiotics.
• Assess hepatic, renal, and hematopoietic function in patients receiving long-term therapy.
• Closely monitor renal function. Urinalysis should be done frequently to detect interstitial nephritis.
• **Alert:** Institute seizure precautions. Patients with high blood levels of this drug may develop seizures.
• Observe closely. With large doses and prolonged therapy, bacterial or fungal superinfection may occur, especially in elderly, debilitated, or immunosuppressed patients.

## ☑ PATIENT TEACHING

• Instruct patient to report adverse reactions promptly.
• Tell patient to alert nurse if discomfort occurs at I.V. site. Explain that if medication is ordered to be given 4 times a day the nurse will need to give one dose during the night.

# mezlocillin sodium
Mezlin

*Pregnancy Risk Category: B*

## HOW SUPPLIED

*Injection:* 1 g, 2 g, 3 g, 4 g
*Pharmacy bulk package:* 20 g

## ACTION

An extended-spectrum penicillin that inhibits cell-wall synthesis during microorganism multiplication; bacteria resist mezlocillin by producing penicillinases — enzymes that hydrolyze mezlocillin.

## ONSET, PEAK, DURATION

Onset immediate after I.V. administration, unknown after I.M. injection. Peak serum levels occur immediately after I.V. administration, within 45 to 90 minutes of I.M. injection. Duration unknown.

## INDICATIONS & DOSAGE

*Systemic infections caused by susceptible strains of gram-positive and especially gram-negative organisms (including* Proteus *and* Pseudomonas aeruginosa*) —*
**Adults:** 200 to 300 mg/kg daily I.V. or I.M. in four to six divided doses. Usual dose is 3 g q 4 hours or 4 g q 6 hours. For very serious infections, up to 24 g daily may be administered.
**Children up to 12 years:** 50 mg/kg

q 4 hours by I.V. infusion or direct I.V. injection.

## ADVERSE REACTIONS
**CNS:** neuromuscular irritability, *seizures.*
**GI:** nausea, diarrhea, vomiting, abnormal taste sensation, pseudomembranous colitis.
**GU:** interstitial nephritis.
**Hematologic:** *bleeding* (with high doses), neutropenia, *thrombocytopenia,* eosinophilia, leukopenia, *hemolytic anemia.*
**Other:** hypersensitivity reactions (*anaphylaxis,* edema, fever, chills, rash, pruritus, urticaria), overgrowth of nonsusceptible organisms, *hypokalemia,* pain at injection site, vein irritation, phlebitis.

## INTERACTIONS
*Aminoglycoside antibiotics (such as amikacin, gentamicin and tobramycin):* chemically incompatible. Don't mix together in I.V. solution. Give 1 hour apart, especially in patients with renal insufficiency.
*Oral contraceptives:* efficacy of oral contraceptives may be decreased. Additional form of contraception recommended during penicillin therapy.
*Probenecid:* increased blood levels of mezlocillin. Probenecid may be used for this purpose.

## CONTRAINDICATIONS
Contraindicated in patients with hypersensitivity to the drug or other penicillins.

## NURSING CONSIDERATIONS
• Use cautiously in patients with other drug allergies, especially to cephalosporins (possible cross-sensitivity), or in those with bleeding tendencies, uremia, or hypokalemia.
• Before giving, ask the patient about any allergic reactions to penicillin. A negative history of penicillin allergy,

however, is no guarantee against future allergic reaction.
• Obtain specimen for culture and sensitivity tests before first dose. Therapy may begin pending results.
• **I.V. use:** Reconstitute vials with at least 10 ml/g of drug using sterile water for injection, $D_5W$, or 0.9% sodium chloride for injection. Solutions with a concentration not exceeding 10% may be given by direct injection over 3 to 5 minutes. Alternatively, dilute in about 50 to 100 ml of suitable I.V. solution, and give by intermittent infusion over 30 minutes.
• Give I.V. intermittently to prevent vein irritation. Change site every 48 hours.
• When giving I.M., don't give more than 2 g per injection. Inject deeply and slowly (12 to 15 seconds) into the body of a large muscle.
• Give mezlocillin at least 1 hour before bacteriostatic antibiotics.
• Check CBC and platelet counts frequently, as ordered. Drug may cause thrombocytopenia.
• Monitor serum potassium level.
• **Alert:** Institute seizure precautions. Patients with high serum levels of this drug may have seizures.
• Observe closely. With large doses and prolonged therapy, bacterial or fungal superinfection may occur, especially in elderly, debilitated, or immunosuppressed patients.
• Be aware that dosage should be altered in patients with impaired renal function.
• Be aware that drug is almost always used with another antibiotic, such as gentamicin.
• Be aware that mezlocillin may interfere with positive direct antiglobulin (Coomb's) test results. Drug may also interfere with certain tests for serum and urine proteins; tests that use bromphenol blue (Albustix, Albutest) are not affected.

---

Reactions may be *common,* uncommon, *life-threatening,* or **COMMON AND LIFE-THREATENING.**

## ☑ PATIENT TEACHING
● Instruct patient to report adverse reactions promptly.
● Tell patient to alert nurse if discomfort occurs at I.V. site.
● Caution patient to limit salt intake during mezlocillin therapy because of drug's high sodium content.

---

## nafcillin sodium
Nafcil, Nallpen, Unipen

*Pregnancy Risk Category: B*

### HOW SUPPLIED
*Capsules:* 250 mg
*Oral solution:* 250 mg/5 ml (after reconstitution)
*Injection:* 500 mg, 1 g, 2 g
*I.V. infusion piggyback:* 1 g, 2 g
*Pharmacy bulk package:* 10 g

### ACTION
A penicillinase-resistant penicillin that inhibits cell-wall synthesis during microorganism multiplication; bacteria resist penicillins by producing penicillinases — enzymes that hydrolyze penicillins. Nafcillin resists these enzymes.

### ONSET, PEAK, DURATION
Onset immediate after I.V. administration, unknown after I.M. injection. Peak serum levels occur immediately after I.V. administration, within ½ to 1 hour of I.M. injection, ½ to 2 hours after oral administration. Duration unknown.

### INDICATIONS & DOSAGE
*Systemic infections caused by penicillinase-producing staphylococci* —
**Adults:** 250 to 500 mg P.O. q 4 to 6 hours (more severe infections may be treated with 1 g P.O. q 4 to 6 hours); or with 2 to 12 g I.M. or I.V. daily in divided doses q 4 to 6 hours.
**Children older than 1 month:** 50 to 100 mg/kg P.O. daily, in divided doses q 6 hours; or 100 to 200 mg/kg I.M. or I.V. daily in divided doses q 4 to 6 hours.

### ADVERSE REACTIONS
**GI:** *nausea,* vomiting, diarrhea.
**Hematologic:** transient leukopenia, neutropenia, granulocytopenia, *thrombocytopenia* with high doses.
**Other:** hypersensitivity reactions (chills, fever, rash, pruritus, urticaria, *anaphylaxis*), vein irritation, thrombophlebitis.

### INTERACTIONS
*Aminoglycosides:* synergistic effect; monitor closely. Chemical and physical incompatibility; do not mix together in same I.V. solution.
*Oral contraceptives:* efficacy of oral contraceptives may be decreased. Additional form of contraception recommended during penicillin therapy.
*Probenecid:* increased blood levels of nafcillin. Probenecid may be used for this purpose.
*Rifampin:* dose-dependent antagonism. Monitor closely.
*Warfarin:* increased risk of bleeding when used with I.V. nafcillin. Monitor closely.

### CONTRAINDICATIONS
Contraindicated in patients with hypersensitivity to the drug or other penicillins.

### NURSING CONSIDERATIONS
● Use cautiously in patients with other drug allergies, especially to cephalosporins (possible cross-sensitivity), or in those with GI distress.
● Before giving, ask the patient about any allergic reactions to penicillin. However, a negative history of penicillin allergy is no guarantee against a future allergic reaction.
● Obtain specimen for culture and sensitivity tests before first dose. Therapy may begin pending results.
● Give 1 to 2 hours before or 2 to 3 hours after meals. When given orally,

---

drug may cause GI disturbances. Food may interfere with absorption.

• **I.V. use:** Reconstitute piggyback containers according to manufacturer's instructions. Reconstitute 500-mg, 1-g, or 2-g vials with sterile water for injection, $D_5W$, or 0.9% sodium chloride for injection. Add 1.7 ml for each 500 mg of drug. Reconstituted drug may be given I.M. Alternatively, dilute with 15 to 30 ml of sterile water for injection or 0.45% or 0.9% sodium chloride for injection, and give by direct injection into a vein or into the tubing of a free-flowing I.V. solution over 5 to 10 minutes. Or dilute drug to a concentration of 2 to 40 mg/ml, and give by intermittent I.V. infusion over 30 to 60 minutes.

• Avoid continuous I.V. infusions to prevent vein irritation. Change site every 48 hours.

• Give nafcillin at least 1 hour before bacteriostatic antibiotics.

• Observe closely. With large doses and prolonged therapy, bacterial or fungal superinfection may occur, especially in elderly, debilitated, or immunosuppressed patients.

• Keep in mind that nafcillin may cause false-positive results with certain tests for urine or serum proteins.

☑ **PATIENT TEACHING**
• Tell the patient to take entire quantity of medication exactly as prescribed, even after he feels better.
• Instruct the patient to take oral form of drug on an empty stomach.
• Tell the patient to call the doctor if rash, fever, or chills develop. A rash is the most common allergic reaction.

---

## oxacillin sodium
Bactocill, Prostaphlin

*Pregnancy Risk Category: B*

**HOW SUPPLIED**
*Capsules:* 250 mg, 500 mg
*Oral solution:* 250 mg/5 ml (after reconstitution)
*Injection:* 250 mg, 500 mg, 1 g, 2 g, 4 g
*I.V. infusion:* 1 g, 2 g, 4 g
*Pharmacy bulk package:* 4 g, 10 g

**ACTION**
A penicillinase-resistant penicillin that inhibits cell-wall synthesis during microorganism multiplication; bacteria resist penicillins by producing penicillinases — enzymes that convert penicillins to inactive penicilloic acid. Oxacillin resists these enzymes.

**ONSET, PEAK, DURATION**
Onset immediate after I.V. administration, unknown after I.M. injection. Peak serum levels occur immediately after I.V. administration, within ½ to 2 hours of oral dose, within ½ hour of an I.M. dose. Duration unknown.

**INDICATIONS & DOSAGE**
*Systemic infections caused by penicillinase-producing staphylococci —*
**Adults and children over 40 kg:** 500 mg P.O. q 4 to 6 hours; or 2 to 12 g I.M. or I.V. daily, in divided doses q 4 to 6 hours.
**Children 40 kg or less:** 50 to 100 mg/kg P.O. daily, in divided doses q 6 hours; or 100 to 200 mg/kg I.M. or I.V. daily, in divided doses q 4 to 6 hours.

**ADVERSE REACTIONS**
**CNS:** neuropathy, neuromuscular irritability, *seizures,* lethargy, hallucinations, anxiety, confusion, agitation, depression, dizziness, fatigue.
**GI:** oral lesions, nausea, vomiting, diarrhea, enterocolitis, pseudomembranous colitis.
**GU:** interstitial nephritis, nephropathy.
**Hematologic:** granulocytopenia, *thrombocytopenia,* eosinophilia, *hemolytic anemia,* neutropenia, anemia, *agranulocytosis.*

---

Reactions may be *common,* uncommon, *life-threatening,* or COMMON AND LIFE-THREATENING.

**Other:** hypersensitivity reactions (fever, chills, rash, urticaria, ***anaphylaxis***), overgrowth of nonsusceptible organisms, elevated liver enzymes, *thrombophlebitis.*

## INTERACTIONS
*Aminoglycosides:* possible synergistic effect; monitor closely. Chemical and physical incompatibility; do not mix together in the same I.V. solution.
*Oral contraceptives:* efficacy of oral contraceptives may be decreased. Additional form of contraception recommended during penicillin therapy.
*Probenecid:* increased blood levels of oxacillin and other penicillins. Probenecid may be used for this purpose.
*Rifampin:* possible antagonism. Monitor closely.

## CONTRAINDICATIONS
Contraindicated in patients with hypersensitivity to the drug or other penicillins.

## NURSING CONSIDERATIONS
● Use cautiously in patients with other drug allergies, especially to cephalosporins (possible cross-sensitivity); in neonates; and in infants.
● Before giving, ask the patient about any allergic reactions to penicillin. However, a negative history of penicillin allergy is no guarantee against a future allergic reaction.
● Obtain specimen for culture and sensitivity tests before first dose. Therapy may begin pending results.
● **I.V. use:** For direct I.V. injection, reconstitute vials with sterile water for injection or 0.9% sodium chloride for injection. Use 5 ml of diluent for a 250- or 500-mg vial, 10 ml of diluent for a 1-g vial, 20 ml of diluent for a 2-g vial, or 40 ml of diluent for a 4-g vial. When the solution is clear, withdraw the ordered dose and inject over 10 minutes. When giving by piggyback injection, reconstitute the 1-g piggyback vial with 20 to 100 ml of diluent; reconstitute the 2-g vial with 19 to 99 ml of diluent. For intermittent infusion, further dilute the drug to a concentration of 5 to 40 mg/ml.
● To prevent vein irritation, avoid continuous infusions. Change site every 48 hours.
● Give the drug I.M. or I.V. only if ordered and the infection is severe or if the patient can't take oral dose.
● Give 1 to 2 hours before or 2 to 3 hours after meals. When given orally, drug may cause GI disturbances. Food may interfere with absorption.
● Give oxacillin at least 1 hour before bacteriostatic antibiotics.
● Monitor periodic liver function studies; watch for elevated AST and ALT levels.
● Observe closely. With large doses and prolonged therapy, bacterial or fungal superinfection may occur, especially in elderly, debilitated, or immunosuppressed patients.
● Keep in mind that oxacillin may falsely elevate or cause false-positive results with certain tests for urine or serum proteins.

☑ **PATIENT TEACHING**
● Tell the patient to take entire quantity of medication exactly as prescribed, even after he feels better.
● Instruct the patient to take drug on an empty stomach.
● Tell the patient to call the doctor if rash, fever, or chills develop. A rash is the most common allergic reaction.

## penicillin G benzathine (benzylpenicillin benzathine)
Bicillin L-A, Permapen
*Pregnancy Risk Category: B*

## HOW SUPPLIED
*Injection:* 300,000 units/ml, 600,000 units/ml

---

*Liquid form contains alcohol. **May contain tartrazine. †Canada only. ‡Australia only. ◊OTC.

## ACTION
A natural penicillin that inhibits cell-wall synthesis during microorganism multiplication; bacteria resist penicillins by producing penicillinases — enzymes that convert penicillins to inactive penicilloic acid.

## ONSET, PEAK, DURATION
Onset unknown. Serum levels peak 13 to 24 hours after I.M. injection. Detectable in serum 1 to 4 weeks after I.M. injection.

## INDICATIONS & DOSAGE
*Congenital syphilis* –
**Children under 2 years:** 50,000 units/kg I.M. as a single dose.
*Group A streptococcal upper respiratory infections* –
**Adults:** 1.2 million units I.M. as a single injection.
**Children over 27 kg:** 900,000 units I.M. as a single injection.
**Children under 27 kg:** 300,000 to 600,000 units I.M. as a single injection.
*Prophylaxis of poststreptococcal rheumatic fever* –
**Adults and children:** 1.2 million units I.M. once monthly or 600,000 units twice monthly.
*Syphilis of less than 1 year's duration* –
**Adults:** 2.4 million units I.M. as a single dose.
*Syphilis of more than 1 year's duration* –
**Adults:** 2.4 million units I.M. weekly for 3 successive weeks.

## ADVERSE REACTIONS
**CNS:** neuropathy, *seizures* (with high doses), lethargy, hallucinations, anxiety, confusion, agitation, depression, dizziness, fatigue.
**GI:** nausea, vomiting, enterocolitis, pseudomembranous colitis.
**GU:** interstitial nephritis, nephropathy.
**Hematologic:** eosinophilia, hemo-lytic anemia, *thrombocytopenia,* leukopenia, anemia, *agranulocytosis.*
**Other:** hypersensitivity reactions (maculopapular and *exfoliative dermatitis,* chills, fever, edema, *anaphylaxis*), pain and sterile abscess at injection site.

## INTERACTIONS
*Aminoglycosides:* physical and chemical incompatibility. Administer separately.
*Colestipol:* decreased serum concentrations of penicillin G benzathine. Administer penicillin G benzathine 1 hour before or 4 hours after colestipol.
*Oral contraceptives:* efficacy of oral contraceptives may be decreased. Additional form of contraception recommended during penicillin therapy.
*Probenecid:* increased blood levels of penicillin. Probenecid may be used for this purpose.

## CONTRAINDICATIONS
Contraindicated in patients with hypersensitivity to the drug or other penicillins.

## NURSING CONSIDERATIONS
• Use cautiously in patients with other drug allergies, especially to cephalosporins (possible cross-sensitivity).
• Before giving, ask the patient about any allergic reactions to penicillin. However, a negative history of penicillin allergy is no guarantee against a future allergic reaction.
• Obtain specimen for culture and sensitivity tests before first dose. Therapy may begin pending results.
• Shake medication well before injection.
• **Alert:** Never give I.V. — inadvertent I.V. administration has caused cardiac arrest and death.
• Inject deeply into upper outer quadrant of buttocks in adults; in midlateral thigh in infants and small chil-

dren. Avoid injection into or near major nerves or blood vessels to prevent permanent neurovascular damage.
• Give penicillin G benzathine at least 1 hour before bacteriostatic antibiotics.
• Know that drug's extremely slow absorption time makes allergic reactions difficult to treat.
• Observe closely. With large doses and prolonged therapy, bacterial or fungal superinfection may occur, especially in elderly, debilitated, or immunosuppressed patients.

☑ **PATIENT TEACHING**
• Tell the patient to report adverse reactions promptly. Fever and eosinophilia are the most common reactions.
• Warn the patient that I.M. injection may be painful but that ice applied to the site may ease discomfort.

---

## penicillin G potassium (benzylpenicillin potassium)
Megacillin†, Pfizerpen

*Pregnancy Risk Category: B*

### HOW SUPPLIED
*Tablets:* 500,000 units†
*Oral suspension:* 250,000 units†, 500,000 units†
*Injection:* 1 million units, 5 million units, 10 million units, 20 million units

### ACTION
A natural penicillin that inhibits cell-wall synthesis during microorganism multiplication; bacteria resist penicillins by producing penicillinases — enzymes that convert penicillins to inactive penicilloic acid.

### ONSET, PEAK, DURATION
Onset immediate after I.V. infusion, unknown after oral dose and I.M. injection. Peak serum levels occur immediately after I.V. infusion, within

15 to 30 minutes of I.M. injection, within ½ to 1 hour of oral dose. Duration unknown.

### INDICATIONS & DOSAGE
*Moderate to severe systemic infection* –
**Adults:** highly individualized; 1.6 to 3.2 million units P.O. daily in divided doses q 6 hours; 1.2 to 24 million units I.M. or I.V. daily in divided doses q 4 hours.
**Children:** 25,000 to 100,000 units/kg P.O. daily in divided doses q 6 hours; or 25,000 to 300,000 units/kg I.M. or I.V. daily in divided doses q 4 hours.

### ADVERSE REACTIONS
**CNS:** neuropathy, *seizures* (with high doses), lethargy, hallucinations, anxiety, confusion, agitation, depression, dizziness, fatigue.
**GI:** nausea, vomiting, enterocolitis, pseudomembranous colitis.
**GU:** interstitial nephritis, nephropathy.
**Hematologic:** *hemolytic anemia,* leukopenia, *thrombocytopenia,* anemia, eosinophilia, *agranulocytosis.*
**Other:** hypersensitivity reactions (rash, urticaria, maculopapular eruptions, *exfoliative dermatitis,* chills, fever, edema, *anaphylaxis*), overgrowth of nonsusceptible organisms, possible severe potassium poisoning with high doses (hyperreflexia, *seizures, coma*), thrombophlebitis, pain at injection site.

### INTERACTIONS
*Aminoglycosides:* physical and chemical incompatibility. Administer separately.
*Colestipol:* decreased serum concentrations of penicillin G potassium. Administer penicillin G potassium 1 hour before or 4 hours after colestipol.
*Oral contraceptives:* efficacy of oral contraceptives may be decreased. Additional form of contraception recommended during penicillin therapy.
*Potassium-sparing diuretics:* possible

---

*Liquid form contains alcohol.   \*\*May contain tartrazine.   †Canada only.   ‡Australia only.   ◇OTC.

increased risk of hyperkalemia. Do not use together.
*Probenecid:* increased blood levels of penicillin. Probenecid may be used for this purpose.

**CONTRAINDICATIONS**
Contraindicated in patients with hypersensitivity to the drug or other penicillins.

**NURSING CONSIDERATIONS**
• Use cautiously in patients with other drug allergies, especially to cephalosporins (possible cross-sensitivity).
• Before giving, ask the patient about any allergic reactions to penicillin. However, a negative history of penicillin allergy is no guarantee against a future allergic reaction.
• Obtain specimen for culture and sensitivity tests before first dose. Therapy may begin pending results.
• **I.V. use:** Reconstitute vials with sterile water for injection, $D_5W$, or 0.9% sodium chloride for injection. Volume of diluent varies with manufacturer.
• Give a continuous I.V. infusion when large doses are required (10 million units or more). Otherwise, give via intermittent I.V. infusion over 1 to 2 hours.
• For I.M. injection, administer deeply into large muscle; may be extremely painful.
• Give 1 to 2 hours before or 2 to 3 hours after meals. When given orally, drug may cause GI disturbances. Food may interfere with absorption.
• Give penicillin G potassium at least 1 hour before bacteriostatic antibiotics.
• Monitor renal function closely. Patients with poor renal function are predisposed to high blood levels.
• Monitor serum potassium and sodium levels closely in patients receiving more than 10 million units I.V. daily.
• Observe closely. With large doses

and prolonged therapy, bacterial or fungal superinfection may occur, especially in elderly, debilitated, or immunosuppressed patients.
• *Alert:* Institute seizure precautions. Patients with high blood levels of this drug may develop seizures.

☑ **PATIENT TEACHING**
• Tell the patient taking oral form to take entire amount exactly as prescribed, even after he feels better.
• Instruct patient to take oral drug on empty stomach.
• Warn patient never to use leftover penicillin for a new illness or to share penicillin with family and friends.
• Tell the patient to call the doctor if rash, fever, or chills develop. A rash is the most common allergic reaction.
• Warn patient that I.M. injection may be painful but that ice applied to the site may help alleviate discomfort.

---

# penicillin G procaine (benzylpenicillin procaine)
Ayercillin†, Crysticillin 300 A.S., Wycillin

*Pregnancy Risk Category: B*

**HOW SUPPLIED**
*Injection:* 300,000 units/ml, 500,000 units/ml, 600,000 units/ml

**ACTION**
A natural penicillin that inhibits cell-wall synthesis during microorganism multiplication; bacteria resist penicillins by producing penicillinases — enzymes that convert penicillins to inactive penicilloic acid.

**ONSET, PEAK, DURATION**
Onset unknown. Serum levels peak 1 to 4 hours after I.M. dose. Drug persists in serum for 1 to 2 days; after high doses, for 5 days.

---

Reactions may be *common,* uncommon, *life-threatening,* or **COMMON AND LIFE-THREATENING.**

## INDICATIONS & DOSAGE

*Moderate to severe systemic infection—*
**Adults:** 600,000 to 1.2 million units
I.M. daily in a single dose.
**Children over 1 month:** 25,000 to
50,000 units/kg I.M. daily in a single
dose.
*Uncomplicated gonorrhea—*
**Adults and children over 12 years:**
1 g probenecid; after 30 minutes, 4.8
million units of penicillin G procaine
I.M., divided between two injection
sites.
*Pneumococcal pneumonia—*
**Adults and children over 12 years:**
600,000 units to 1.2 million units
I.M. daily for 7 to 10 days.

## ADVERSE REACTIONS

**CNS:** *seizures,* lethargy, hallucinations, anxiety, confusion, agitation,
depression, dizziness, fatigue.
**GI:** nausea, vomiting, enterocolitis,
pseudomembranous colitis.
**GU:** interstitial nephritis, nephropathy.
**Hematologic:** *thrombocytopenia, hemolytic anemia,* leukopenia, anemia,
eosinophilia, *agranulocytosis.*
**Other:** arthralgia, hypersensitivity
reactions (rash, urticaria, chills, fever, edema, prostration, *anaphylaxis*), overgrowth of nonsusceptible
organisms.

## INTERACTIONS

*Aminoglycosides:* physical and chemical incompatibility. Administer separately.
*Colestipol:* decreased serum concentrations of penicillin G procaine. Administer penicillin G procaine 1 hour
before or 4 hours after colestipol.
*Oral contraceptives:* efficacy of oral
contraceptives may be decreased. Additional form of contraception recommended during penicillin therapy.
*Probenecid:* increased blood levels of
penicillin. Probenecid may be used
for this purpose.

## CONTRAINDICATIONS

Contraindicated in patients with hypersensitivity to the drug or other
penicillins.

## NURSING CONSIDERATIONS

● Use cautiously in patients with
other drug allergies, especially to
cephalosporins (possible cross-sensitivity). Some formulations contain
sulfites, which may cause allergic reactions in sensitive persons.
● Before giving, ask the patient about
any allergic reactions to penicillin.
However, a negative history of penicillin allergy is no guarantee against a
future allergic reaction.
● Obtain specimen for culture and
sensitivity tests before first dose.
Therapy may begin pending results.
● Give deep I.M. in upper outer quadrant of buttocks in adults; in midlateral
thigh in small children. Do not give
subcutaneously. Don't massage injection site. Avoid injection near major
nerves or blood vessels to prevent permanent neurovascular damage.
● *Alert:* Never give I.V.—inadvertent
I.V. administration has caused death
from CNS toxicity caused by procaine.
● Give penicillin G procaine at least
1 hour before bacteriostatic antibiotics.
● Know that because of drug's slow
absorption rate, allergic reactions are
hard to treat.
● Monitor renal and hematopoietic
function periodically, as ordered.
● Observe closely. With large doses
and prolonged therapy, bacterial or
fungal superinfection may occur, especially in elderly, debilitated, or immunosuppressed patients.

### ☑ PATIENT TEACHING

● Tell the patient to report adverse reactions promptly. A rash is the most
common allergic reaction.
● Warn the patient that I.M. injection
may be painful but that ice applied to
the site may help alleviate discomfort.

---

*Liquid form contains alcohol.   **May contain tartrazine.   †Canada only.   ‡Australia only.   ◇OTC.

# penicillin G sodium (benzylpenicillin sodium)
Crystapen†

*Pregnancy Risk Category: B*

## HOW SUPPLIED
*Injection:* 5 million-units vial

## ACTION
A natural penicillin that inhibits cell-wall synthesis during active multiplication; bacteria resist penicillins by producing penicillinases — enzymes that convert penicillins to inactive penicilloic acid.

## ONSET, PEAK, DURATION
Onset immediate after I.V. administration, unknown after I.M. injection. Peak serum levels occur 15 to 30 minutes after I.M. injection, immediately after I.V. administration. Duration unknown.

## INDICATIONS & DOSAGE
*Moderate to severe systemic infection —*
**Adults:** 1.2 to 24 million units daily I.M. or I.V. in divided doses q 4 to 6 hours.
**Children:** 25,000 to 300,000 units/kg daily I.M. or I.V. in divided doses q 4 to 6 hours.
*Endocarditis prophylaxis for dental surgery —*
**Adults and children over 27 kg:** 2 million units I.V. or I.M. 30 to 60 minutes before procedure; then 1 million units 6 hours later.

## ADVERSE REACTIONS
**CNS:** neuropathy, *seizures,* lethargy, hallucinations, anxiety, confusion, agitation, depression, dizziness, fatigue.
**CV:** *CHF* (with high doses).
**GI:** nausea, vomiting, enterocolitis, pseudomembranous colitis.
**GU:** interstitial colitis, nephropathy.
**Hematologic:** hemolytic anemia, leukopenia, *thrombocytopenia, agranulocytosis,* anemia, eosinophilia.
**Other:** arthralgia, hypersensitivity reactions (*exfoliative dermatitis,* urticaria, *anaphylaxis*), overgrowth of nonsusceptible organisms, vein irritation, pain at injection site, thrombophlebitis.

## INTERACTIONS
*Aminoglycosides:* physical and chemical incompatibility. Administer separately.
*Colestipol:* decreased serum concentrations of penicillin G sodium. Administer penicillin G sodium 1 hour before or 4 hours after colestipol.
*Oral contraceptives:* efficacy of oral contraceptives may be decreased. Additional form of contraception recommended during penicillin therapy.
*Probenecid:* increased blood levels of penicillin. Probenecid may be used for this purpose.

## CONTRAINDICATIONS
Contraindicated in patients with hypersensitivity to the drug or other penicillins and in patients on sodium-restricted diets.

## NURSING CONSIDERATIONS
• Use cautiously in patients with other drug allergies, especially to cephalosporins (possible cross-allergenicity).
• Before giving, ask the patient about any allergic reactions to penicillin. However, a negative history of penicillin allergy is no guarantee against a future allergic reaction.
• Obtain specimen for culture and sensitivity tests before first dose. Therapy may begin pending results.
• **I.V. use:** Reconstitute vials with sterile water for injection, 0.9% sodium chloride for injection, or $D_5W$. Check manufacturer's instructions for volume of diluent necessary to produce desired drug concentration.
• For patients receiving 10 million

---

Reactions may be *common,* uncommon, *life-threatening,* or COMMON AND LIFE-THREATENING.

units of drug or more daily, dilute in 1 to 2 liters of compatible solution, and administer over 24 hours. Otherwise, give by intermittent I.V. infusion: Dilute drug in 50 to 100 ml, and give over 1 to 2 hours q 4 to 6 hours.
• In neonates and children, give divided doses over 15 to 30 minutes.
• Give penicillin G sodium at least 1 hour before bacteriostatic antibiotics.
• Observe closely. With large doses and prolonged therapy, bacterial or fungal superinfection may occur, especially in elderly, debilitated, or immunosuppressed patients.
• **Alert:** Institute seizure precautions. Patients with high blood levels of this drug may develop seizures.

### ☑ PATIENT TEACHING
• Tell patient to report adverse reactions promptly.
• Instruct patient to alert nurse if discomfort occurs at I.V. site.
• Warn patient receiving I.M. injection that the injection may be painful but that ice applied to site may help alleviate discomfort.

## penicillin V (phenoxymethylpenicillin)

## penicillin V potassium (phenoxymethylpenicillin potassium)
Abbocillin VK‡, Apo-Pen-VK†, Beepen-VK, Betapen-VK, Cilicane VK‡, Ledercillin VK, Nadopen-V-200†, Nadopen-V-400†, Nadopen-VK†, NovoPen-VK†, Nu-Pen VK†, Pen Vee, Pen Vee K, PVF K†, PVK‡, Robicillin VK, V-Cillin K, Veetids**

*Pregnancy Risk Category: B*

### HOW SUPPLIED
**penicillin V**
*Tablets:* 250 mg, 500 mg
*Oral suspension:* 125 mg/5 ml, 250 mg/5 ml (after reconstitution)

**penicillin V potassium**
*Tablets:* 125 mg, 250 mg, 500 mg
*Tablets (film-coated):* 250 mg, 500 mg
*Capsules:* 250 mg‡
*Oral suspension:* 125 mg/5 ml, 250 mg/5 ml (after reconstitution)

### ACTION
A natural penicillin that inhibits cell-wall synthesis during microorganism multiplication; bacteria resist penicillins by producing penicillinases — enzymes that convert penicillins to inactive penicilloic acid.

### ONSET, PEAK, DURATION
Onset and duration unknown. Serum levels peak within 30 to 60 minutes.

### INDICATIONS & DOSAGE
*Mild to moderate systemic infections –*
**Adults:** 250 to 500 mg (400,000 to 800,000 units) P.O. q 6 hours.
**Children:** 15 to 50 mg/kg (25,000 to 90,000 units/kg) P.O. daily, in divided doses q 6 to 8 hours.
*Endocarditis prophylaxis for dental surgery –*
**Adults:** 2 g P.O. 30 to 60 minutes before procedure; then 1 g 6 hours after.
**Children under 30 kg:** half of the adult dose.

### ADVERSE REACTIONS
**CNS:** neuropathy.
**GI:** *epigastric distress,* vomiting, diarrhea, *nausea,* black "hairy" tongue.
**GU:** nephropathy.
**Hematologic:** eosinophilia, hemolytic anemia, leukopenia, ***thrombocytopenia.***
**Other:** hypersensitivity reactions (rash, urticaria, fever, laryngeal edema, ***anaphylaxis***), overgrowth of nonsusceptible organisms.

### INTERACTIONS
*Oral contraceptives:* efficacy of oral contraceptives may be decreased. Ad-

---

*Liquid form contains alcohol.   **May contain tartrazine.   †Canada only.   ‡Australia only.   ◇OTC.

ditional form of contraception recommended during penicillin therapy.
*Probenecid:* increased blood levels of penicillin. Probenecid may be used for this purpose.

## CONTRAINDICATIONS
Contraindicated in patients with hypersensitivity to the drug or other penicillins.

## NURSING CONSIDERATIONS
• Use cautiously in patients with other drug allergies, especially to cephalosporins (possible cross-sensitivity), or in those with GI disturbances.
• Before giving, ask the patient about any allergic reactions to penicillins. However, a negative history of penicillin allergy is no guarantee against a future allergic reaction.
• Obtain specimen for culture and sensitivity tests before first dose. Therapy may begin pending results.
• Give penicillin V at least 1 hour before bacteriostatic antibiotics.
• As ordered, periodically assess renal and hematopoietic function in patients receiving long-term therapy.
• Observe closely. With large doses and prolonged therapy, bacterial or fungal superinfection may occur, especially in elderly, debilitated, or immunosuppressed patients.
• Be aware that The American Heart Association considers amoxicillin the preferred agent for endocarditis prophylaxis because GI absorption is better and serum levels are sustained longer. Penicillin V is considered an alternative agent.

## ☑ PATIENT TEACHING
• Tell the patient to take entire quantity of medication exactly as prescribed, even after he feels better.
• Tell the patient to take drug with food if stomach upset occurs.
• Warn patient never to use leftover penicillin for a new illness or to share penicillin with family and friends.
• Tell the patient to call the doctor if rash, fever, or chills develop. A rash is the most common allergic reaction.

# piperacillin sodium
Pipracil, Pipril‡

*Pregnancy Risk Category: B*

## HOW SUPPLIED
*Injection:* 2 g, 3 g, 4 g
*Pharmacy bulk package:* 40 g

## ACTION
Extended-spectrum penicillin that inhibits cell-wall synthesis during microorganism multiplication; bacteria resist penicillins by producing penicillinases — enzymes that convert penicillins to inactive penicilloic acid.

## ONSET, PEAK, DURATION
Onset immediate after I.V. administration, unknown after I.M. injection. Peak serum levels occur immediately after I.V. administration, within 30 to 50 minutes of I.M. dose. Duration unknown.

## INDICATIONS & DOSAGE
*Systemic infections caused by susceptible strains of gram-positive and especially gram-negative organisms (including* Proteus *and* Pseudomonas aeruginosa) —
**Adults and children over 12 years:** 100 to 300 mg/kg daily in divided doses q 4 to 6 hours I.V. or I.M.
*Prophylaxis of surgical infections —*
**Adults:** 2 g I.V., given 30 to 60 minutes before surgery. Dose may be repeated during surgery and once or twice more after surgery.

## ADVERSE REACTIONS
**CNS:** *seizures,* headache, dizziness, fatigue.
**GI:** nausea, diarrhea, vomiting, pseudomembranous colitis.

---

Reactions may be *common,* uncommon, *life-threatening,* or **COMMON AND LIFE-THREATENING.**

**GU:** interstitial nephritis.
**Hematologic:** *bleeding* (with high doses), neutropenia, eosinophilia, leukopenia, **thrombocytopenia**.
**Other:** *hypokalemia,* hypersensitivity reactions (edema, fever, chills, rash, pruritus, urticaria, **anaphylaxis**), overgrowth of nonsusceptible organisms, pain at injection site, vein irritation, phlebitis, prolonged muscle relaxation.

## INTERACTIONS

*Aminoglycoside antibiotics (such as gentamicin and tobramycin):* chemically incompatible. Don't mix in the same I.V. container.
*Oral contraceptives:* efficacy of oral contraceptives may be decreased. Additional form of contraception recommended during penicillin therapy.
*Probenecid:* increased blood levels of piperacillin. Probenecid may be used for this purpose.

## CONTRAINDICATIONS

Contraindicated in patients with hypersensitivity to the drug or other penicillins.

## NURSING CONSIDERATIONS

• Use cautiously in patients with other drug allergies, especially to cephalosporins (possible cross-sensitivity), or in those with bleeding tendencies, uremia, and hypokalemia.
• Before giving, ask the patient about any allergic reactions to penicillin. However, a negative history of penicillin allergy is no guarantee against a future allergic reaction.
• Obtain specimen for culture and sensitivity tests before first dose. Therapy may begin pending results.
• **I.V. use:** Reconstitute each gram of drug with 5 ml of diluent, such as sterile or bacteriostatic water for injection, 0.9% sodium chloride for injection (with or without preservative), $D_5W$, or dextrose 5% in 0.9% sodium chloride for injection. Shake until dissolved. Inject reconstituted solution directly into a vein or into the tubing of a free-flowing I.V. solution over 3 to 5 minutes. Alternatively, dilute with at least 50 ml of a compatible I.V. solution, and give by intermittent infusion over 30 minutes.
• Avoid continuous infusions to prevent vein irritation. Change site every 48 hours.
• For I.M. injection, reconstitute with sterile or bacteriostatic water for injection, 0.9% sodium chloride for injection (with or without preservative), or 0.5% to 1% lidocaine hydrochloride. Add 2 ml of diluent for each gram of drug. Final solution will contain 1 g/2.5 ml.
• Give piperacillin at least 1 hour before bacteriostatic antibiotics.
• Check CBC and platelet counts frequently, as ordered. Drug may cause thrombocytopenia.
• Monitor serum potassium level.
• **Alert:** Institute seizure precautions. Patients with high serum levels of this drug may have seizures.
• Observe closely. With large doses and prolonged therapy, bacterial or fungal superinfection may occur, especially in elderly, debilitated, or immunosuppressed patients.
• Know that dosage should be altered in patients with impaired renal function.
• Be aware that patients with cystic fibrosis tend to be most susceptible to fever or rash.
• Be aware that drug may be better suited for patients on sodium-free diets than ticarcillin (piperacillin contains 1.85 mEq of sodium/g).
• Keep in mind that piperacillin is typically used with another antibiotic, such as gentamicin.

## ☑ PATIENT TEACHING

• Tell patient to report adverse reactions promptly.
• Instruct patient receiving drug I.V. to report discomfort at I.V. site.

---

• Advise patient to limit salt intake during drug therapy because drug contains 1.98 mEq of sodium/g.

---

## piperacillin sodium and tazobactam sodium
Zosyn

*Pregnancy Risk Category: B*

### HOW SUPPLIED
*Powder for injection:* 2 g piperacillin and 0.25 g tazobactam per vial, 3 g piperacillin and 0.375 g tazobactam per vial, 4 g piperacillin and 0.5 g tazobactam per vial
*Pharmacy bulk package:* 40.5 g

### ACTION
Piperacillin is an extended-spectrum penicillin that inhibits cell-wall synthesis during microorganism multiplication; tazobactam increases piperacillin's effectiveness by inactivating beta lactamases, which destroy penicillins.

### ONSET, PEAK, DURATION
Onset immediate after I.V. infusion. Plasma levels peak immediately after I.V. infusion. Duration unknown.

### INDICATIONS & DOSAGE
*Appendicitis (complicated by rupture or abscess) and peritonitis caused by* Escherichia coli, Bacteroides fragilis, B. ovatus, B. thetaiotaomicron, *or* B. vulgatus; *skin and skin-structure infections caused by* Staphylococcus aureus; *postpartum endometritis or pelvic inflammatory disease caused by* E. coli; *moderately severe community-acquired pneumonia caused by* Haemophilus influenzae –
**Adults:** 3 g piperacillin and 0.375 g tazobactam I.V. q 6 hours.
*In patients with renal impairment –*
**Adults:** if creatinine clearance is 20 to 40 ml/minute, 2 g piperacillin and 0.25 g tazobactam I.V. q 6 hours. If creatinine clearance is below 20 ml/minute, 2 g piperacillin and 0.25 g tazobactam I.V. q 8 hours.

### ADVERSE REACTIONS
**CNS:** *headache, insomnia,* agitation, dizziness, anxiety.
**CV:** hypertension, tachycardia, chest pain, edema.
**EENT:** rhinitis.
**GI:** *diarrhea, nausea, constipation,* vomiting, dyspepsia, stool changes, abdominal pain.
**GU:** interstitial nephritis.
**Hematologic:** leukopenia, anemia, eosinophilia, ***thrombocytopenia.***
**Respiratory:** dyspnea.
**Skin:** rash (including maculopapular, bullous, urticarial, and eczematoid), pruritus.
**Other:** fever; pain; moniliasis; inflammation, phlebitis at I.V. site; ***anaphylaxis.***

### INTERACTIONS
*Aminoglycoside antibiotics (such as amikacin, gentamicin and tobramycin):* chemically incompatible. Don't mix in the same I.V. container.
*Oral contraceptives:* efficacy of oral contraceptives may be decreased. Additional form of contraception recommended during penicillin therapy.
*Probenecid:* increased blood levels of piperacillin. Probenecid may be used for this purpose.
*Vercuronium:* prolongation of neuromuscular blockage. Monitor closely.

### CONTRAINDICATIONS
Contraindicated in patients with hypersensitivity to the drug or other penicillins.

### NURSING CONSIDERATIONS
• Use cautiously in patients with other drug allergies, especially to cephalosporins (possible cross-sensitivity), or in those with bleeding tendencies, uremia, and hypokalemia.
• Obtain specimen for culture and

---

sensitivity tests before first dose. Therapy may begin pending results.

- **I.V. use:** Reconstitute each gram of piperacillin with 5 ml of diluent, such as sterile or bacteriostatic water for injection, 0.9% sodium chloride for injection, bacteriostatic 0.9% sodium chloride for injection, $D_5W$, dextrose 5% in 0.9% sodium chloride for injection, or dextran 6% in 0.9% sodium chloride for injection. Don't use lactated Ringer's injection. Shake until dissolved. Further dilute to a final volume of 50 ml before infusion.
- Infuse over at least 30 minutes. Discontinue any primary infusion during administration if possible. Don't mix with other drugs.
- Use drug immediately after reconstitution. Discard unused drug after 24 hours if stored at room temperature; 48 hours if refrigerated. Once diluted, drug is stable in I.V. bags for 24 hours at room temperature or 1 week if refrigerated.
- Change I.V. site every 48 hours.
- Because hemodialysis removes 6% of the piperacillin dose and 21% of the tazobactam dose, be aware that supplemental doses may be needed after hemodialysis.
- With large doses and prolonged therapy, bacterial and fungal superinfection may occur, especially in elderly, debilitated, or immunosuppressed patients.

☑ **PATIENT TEACHING**
- Tell patient to report adverse reactions promptly.
- Instruct patient to alert nurse if discomfort occurs at I.V. site.

## ticarcillin disodium
Ticar, Ticillin‡

*Pregnancy Risk Category: NR*

**HOW SUPPLIED**
*Injection:* 1 g, 3 g, 6 g
*I.V. infusion:* 3 g

*Pharmacy bulk package:* 20 g, 30 g

**ACTION**
An extended-spectrum penicillin that inhibits cell-wall synthesis during microorganism multiplication; bacteria resist penicillins by producing penicillinases—enzymes that convert penicillins to inactive penicilloic acid.

**ONSET, PEAK, DURATION**
Onset immediate after I.V. administration, unknown after I.M. injection. Peak serum levels occur immediately after I.V. administration, within 30 to 75 minutes of I.M. injection. Duration unknown.

**INDICATIONS & DOSAGE**
*Severe systemic infections caused by susceptible strains of gram-positive and especially gram-negative organisms (including* Pseudomonas *and* Proteus)—
**Adults:** 18 g I.V. or I.M. daily, in divided doses q 4 to 6 hours.
**Children:** 50 to 300 mg/kg I.V. or I.M. daily, in divided doses q 4 to 6 hours.

**ADVERSE REACTIONS**
**CNS:** *seizures,* neuromuscular excitability.
**GI:** nausea, diarrhea, vomiting, pseudomembranous colitis.
**Hematologic:** leukopenia, neutropenia, eosinophilia, *thrombocytopenia,* hemolytic anemia.
**Other:** hypersensitivity reactions (rash, pruritus, urticaria, chills, fever, edema, *anaphylaxis*), overgrowth of nonsusceptible organisms, hypokalemia, pain at injection site, vein irritation, phlebitis.

**INTERACTIONS**
*Aminoglycoside antibiotics (such as amikacin, gentamicin and tobramycin):* chemically incompatible. Don't mix in the same I.V. container.
*Lithium:* altered renal elimination of

---

*Liquid form contains alcohol. **May contain tartrazine. †Canada only. ‡Australia only. ◊OTC.

lithium. Monitor serum lithium levels closely.

*Oral contraceptives:* efficacy of oral contraceptives may be decreased. Additional form of contraception recommended during penicillin therapy.

*Probenecid:* increased blood levels of ticarcillin and other penicillins. Probenecid may be used for this purpose.

## CONTRAINDICATIONS
Contraindicated in patients with hypersensitivity to the drug or other penicillins.

## NURSING CONSIDERATIONS
• Use cautiously in patients with other drug allergies, especially to cephalosporins (possible cross-sensitivity), or in those with impaired renal function, hemorrhagic conditions, hypokalemia, or sodium restrictions (contains 5.2 to 6.5 mEq sodium/g).

• Before giving, ask the patient about any allergic reactions to penicillin. However, a negative history of penicillin allergy is no guarantee against a future allergic reaction.

• Obtain specimen for culture and sensitivity tests before first dose. Therapy may begin pending results.

• **I.V. use:** Reconstitute vials using $D_5W$, 0.9% sodium chloride injection, sterile water for injection, or other compatible solution. Add 4 ml of diluent for each gram of drug. Further dilute to a maximum concentration of 50 mg/ml, and inject slowly directly into a vein or into the tubing of a free-flowing I.V. solution. Alternatively, dilute to a concentration of 10 to 100 mg/ml, and give by intermittent infusion over 30 to 120 minutes in adults or 10 to 20 minutes in neonates.

• Avoid continuous infusion to prevent vein irritation. Change site every 48 hours.

• For I.M. injection, reconstitute vials using sterile water for injection, 0.9% sodium chloride for injection, or lidocaine 1% (without epinephrine). Use 2 ml diluent for each gram of drug. Give deep I.M. into large muscle. Don't exceed 2 g per injection.

• Give ticarcillin at least 1 hour before bacteriostatic antibiotics.

• Monitor serum potassium.

• Check CBC and platelet counts frequently, as ordered. Drug may cause thrombocytopenia.

• **Alert:** Institute seizure precautions. Patients with high blood levels of ticarcillin may develop seizures.

• Be aware that ticarcillin is typically used with another antibiotic, such as gentamicin.

• Observe closely. With large doses and prolonged therapy, bacterial or fungal superinfection may occur, especially in elderly, debilitated, or immunosuppressed patients.

• Know that dosage should be decreased in patients with impaired renal function.

☑ **PATIENT TEACHING**
• Tell patient to report adverse reactions promptly.

• Instruct patient to alert nurse if discomfort occurs at I.V. insertion site.

---

## ticarcillin disodium/ clavulanate potassium
Timentin

*Pregnancy Risk Category: B*

## HOW SUPPLIED
*Injection:* 3 g ticarcillin and 100 mg clavulanic acid
*Pharmacy bulk package:* 31 g

## ACTION
Ticarcillin is an extended-spectrum penicillin that inhibits cell-wall synthesis during microorganism replication; clavulanic acid increases ticarcillin's effectiveness by inactivating beta lactamases, which destroy ticarcillin.

---

Reactions may be *common,* uncommon, *life-threatening,* or COMMON AND LIFE-THREATENING.

## ONSET, PEAK, DURATION
Onset immediate after I.V. infusion. Peak serum levels occur immediately after I.V. infusion. Duration unknown.

## INDICATIONS & DOSAGE
*Lower respiratory tract, urinary tract, bone and joint, and skin and skin-structure infections and septicemia when caused by beta-lactamase-producing strains of bacteria or by ticarcillin-susceptible organisms –*
**Adults:** 3.1 g (3 g ticarcillin and 100 mg clavulanate acid) administered by I.V. infusion q 4 to 6 hours.

## ADVERSE REACTIONS
**CNS:** *seizures,* neuromuscular excitability, headache, giddiness.
**GI:** nausea, diarrhea, stomatitis, vomiting, epigastric pain, flatulence, pseudomembranous colitis, taste and smell disturbances.
**Hematologic:** leukopenia, neutropenia, eosinophilia, *thrombocytopenia,* hemolytic anemia, anemia.
**Other:** hypersensitivity reactions (rash, pruritus, urticaria, chills, fever, edema, *anaphylaxis*), overgrowth of nonsusceptible organisms, hypokalemia, pain at injection site, vein irritation, phlebitis.

## INTERACTIONS
*Aminoglycoside antibiotics (such as amikacin, gentamicin and tobramycin):* chemically incompatible. Don't mix in the same I.V. container.
*Oral contraceptives:* efficacy of oral cntraceptives may be decreased. Additional form of contraception recommended during penicillin therapy.
*Probenecid:* increased blood levels of ticarcillin. Probenecid may be used for this purpose.

## CONTRAINDICATIONS
Contraindicated in patients with hypersensitivity to the drug or other penicillins.

## NURSING CONSIDERATIONS
● Use cautiously in patients with other drug allergies, especially to cephalosporins (possible cross-sensitivity), and in those with impaired renal function, hemorrhagic condition, hypokalemia, or sodium restrictions (contains 4.5 mEq sodium/g).
● Before giving, ask the patient about any allergic reactions to penicillin. However, a negative history of penicillin allergy is no guarantee against a future allergic reaction.
● Obtain specimen for culture and sensitivity tests before first dose. Therapy may begin pending results.
● **I.V. use:** Reconstitute drug with 13 ml of sterile water for injection or 0.9% sodium chloride for injection. Further dilute to a maximum of 10 to 100 mg/ml (based on ticarcillin component), and administer by I.V. infusion over 30 minutes. In fluid-restricted patients, dilute to a maximum of 48 mg/ml if using $D_5W$, 43 mg/ml if using 0.9% sodium chloride for injection, or 86 mg/ml if using sterile water for injection.
● Give drug at least 1 hour before bacteriostatic antibiotics.
● Check CBC and platelet counts frequently, as ordered. Drug may cause thrombocytopenia.
● Observe closely. With large doses and prolonged therapy, bacterial or fungal superinfection may occur, especially in elderly, debilitated, or immunosuppressed patients.
● Know that dosage should be decreased in patients with impaired renal function.

## ☑ PATIENT TEACHING
● Tell patient to report adverse reactions promptly.
● Instruct patient to alert nurse if discomfort occurs at I.V. site.
● Advise patient to limit salt intake during drug therapy because of high sodium content.

---

# 13

# Cephalosporins

cefaclor
cefadroxil monohydrate
cefamandole nafate
cefazolin sodium
cefepime hydrochloride
cefixime
cefmetazole sodium
cefonicid sodium
cefoperazone sodium
cefotaxime sodium
cefotetan disodium
cefoxitin sodium
cefpodoxime proxetil
cefprozil
ceftazidime
ceftizoxime sodium
ceftriaxone sodium
cefuroxime axetil
cefuroxime sodium
cephalexin hydrochloride
cephalexin monohydrate
cephalothin sodium
cephapirin sodium
cephradine
loracarbef

**COMBINATION PRODUCTS**
None.

## cefaclor

Ceclor

*Pregnancy Risk Category: B*

**HOW SUPPLIED**
*Capsules:* 250 mg, 500 mg
*Oral suspension:* 125 mg/5 ml, 250 mg/5 ml, 187 mg/5 ml, 375 mg/5 ml

**ACTION**
A second-generation cephalosporin that inhibits cell-wall synthesis, promoting osmotic instability; usually bactericidal.

**ONSET, PEAK, DURATION**
Onset and duration unknown. Peak levels occur within 30 to 60 minutes.

**INDICATIONS & DOSAGE**
*Respiratory or urinary tract, skin, and soft-tissue infections and otitis media caused by* Haemophilus influenzae, Streptococcus pneumoniae, S. pyogenes, Escherichia coli, Proteus mirabilis, Klebsiella *species, and* staphylococci –
**Adults:** 250 to 500 mg P.O. q 8 hours. For pharyngitis or otitis media, daily dosage may be given in two equally divided doses q 12 hours.
**Children:** 20 mg/kg daily P.O. in divided doses q 8 hours. For pharyngitis or otitis media, daily dosage may be given in two equally divided doses q 12 hours. In more serious infections, 40 mg/kg daily are recommended, not to exceed 1 g daily.

**ADVERSE REACTIONS**
**CNS:** dizziness, headache, somnolence, malaise.
**GI:** *nausea,* vomiting, *diarrhea,* anorexia, dyspepsia, abdominal cramps, pseudomembranous colitis, oral candidiasis.
**GU:** vaginal moniliasis, vaginitis.
**Hematologic:** transient leukopenia, anemia, eosinophilia, ***thrombocytopenia,*** lymphocytosis.
**Skin:** *maculopapular rash,* dermatitis, pruritus.
**Other:** hypersensitivity reactions (serum sickness, ***anaphylaxis***), fever, transient increases in liver enzymes.

**INTERACTIONS**
*Chloramphenicol:* antagonistic effect. Do not use together.
*Probenecid:* may inhibit excretion and increase blood levels of cefaclor.

---

Reactions may be *common,* uncommon, *life-threatening,* or COMMON AND LIFE-THREATENING.

## CONTRAINDICATIONS
Contraindicated in patients with hypersensitivity to other cephalosporins.

## NURSING CONSIDERATIONS
• Use cautiously in patients with impaired renal function or a history of sensitivity to penicillin and in breast-feeding women.
• Obtain specimen for culture and sensitivity tests before first dose. Therapy may begin pending results.
• With large doses or prolonged therapy, monitor for superinfection, especially in high-risk patients.
• Store reconstituted suspension in refrigerator. Stable for 14 days if refrigerated. Shake well before using.
• Keep in mind that 40% to 75% of those receiving cephalosporins show a false-positive direct Coombs' test.
• Be aware that urine glucose determinations may be false-positive with copper sulfate tests (Clinitest); glucose enzymatic tests (Clinistix, Tes-Tape) are not affected.

## ☑ PATIENT TEACHING
• Tell the patient to take entire amount of medication exactly as prescribed, even after he feels better.
• Tell the patient that drug may be taken with meals. If suspension is used, instruct the patient to shake container well before measuring dose and to keep the drug refrigerated.
• Tell the patient to call the doctor if rash develops.

---

## cefadroxil monohydrate
Duricef, Ultracef

*Pregnancy Risk Category: B*

## HOW SUPPLIED
*Tablets:* 1 g
*Capsules:* 500 mg
*Oral suspension:* 125 mg/5 ml, 250 mg/5 ml, 500 mg/5 ml

## ACTION
A first-generation cephalosporin that inhibits cell-wall synthesis, promoting osmotic instability; usually bactericidal.

## ONSET, PEAK, DURATION
Onset and duration unknown. Serum levels peak within 1 to 2 hours after an oral dose.

## INDICATIONS & DOSAGE
*Urinary tract infections caused by* Escherichia coli, Proteus mirabilis, *and* Klebsiella *species; skin and soft-tissue infections caused by Staphylococci and Streptococci; and pharyngitis or tonsillitis caused by group A beta-hemolytic streptococci –*
**Adults:** 500 mg to 2 g P.O. daily, depending on infection being treated. Usually given once daily or b.i.d.
**Children:** 30 mg/kg P.O. daily in two divided doses.

## ADVERSE REACTIONS
**CNS:** *seizures.*
**GI:** pseudomembranous colitis, *nausea,* vomiting, *diarrhea,* glossitis, abdominal cramps, oral candidiasis.
**GU:** genital pruritus, moniliasis, vaginitis, renal dysfunction.
**Hematologic:** transient neutropenia, eosinophilia, leukopenia, anemia, *agranulocytosis, thrombocytopenia.*
**Skin:** *maculopapular and erythematous rashes,* urticaria.
**Other:** hypersensitivity reactions (serum sickness, *anaphylaxis,* angioedema), transient increases in liver enzymes, dyspnea, fever.

## INTERACTIONS
*Probenecid:* may inhibit excretion and increase blood levels of cefadroxil.

## CONTRAINDICATIONS
Contraindicated in patients with hypersensitivity to the drug or other cephalosporins.

---

## NURSING CONSIDERATIONS

• Use cautiously in patients with a history of sensitivity to penicillin or in breast-feeding women. Also use cautiously in patients with impaired renal function; dosage adjustments may be necessary.
• Obtain specimen for culture and sensitivity tests before first dose. Therapy may begin pending results.
• Be aware that if creatinine clearance is below 50 ml/minute, dosage interval should be lengthened so drug doesn't accumulate.
• With large doses or prolonged therapy, monitor for superinfection, especially in high-risk patients.
• Keep in mind that 40% to 75% of those receiving cephalosporins show a false-positive direct Coombs' test.
• Be aware that urine glucose determinations may be false-positive with copper sulfate tests (Clinitest); glucose enzymatic tests (Clinistix, Tes-Tape) are not affected.

## ☑ PATIENT TEACHING

• Tell patient to take drug with food or milk to lessen GI discomfort.
• Tell the patient to take entire amount of medication exactly as prescribed, even after he feels better.
• Advise the patient to call the doctor if rash develops.

## cefamandole nafate
Mandol

*Pregnancy Risk Category: B*

## HOW SUPPLIED
*Injection:* 1 g, 2 g
*Pharmacy bulk package:* 10 g

## ACTION
A second-generation cephalosporin that inhibits cell-wall synthesis, promoting osmotic instability; usually bactericidal.

## ONSET, PEAK, DURATION
Onset immediate after I.V. administration, unknown after I.M. injection. Peak serum levels occur ½ to 2 hours after I.M. injection, immediately after I.V. administration. Duration unknown.

## INDICATIONS & DOSAGE
*Perioperative prophylaxis in contaminated surgery –*
**Adults:** 1 to 2 g I.M. or I.V. 30 to 60 minutes before surgery; then 1 to 2 g I.M. or I.V. q 6 hours for 24 hours.
**Children 3 months and older:** 12.5 to 25 mg/kg I.M. or I.V. 30 to 60 minutes before surgery; then 12.5 to 25 mg/kg I.M. or I.V. q 6 hours for 24 hours.
• *Alert:* In cases where infection could be devastating, prophylaxis may be continued for 3 days.
*Serious infections of respiratory and GU tracts; skin, soft-tissue, bone, and joint infections; septicemia; and peritonitis caused by* Escherichia coli *and other coliform bacteria,* Staphylococcus aureus *(penicillinase- and nonpenicillinase-producing),* S. epidermidis, *group A beta-hemolytic streptococci,* Klebsiella, Haemophilus influenzae, Proteus mirabilis, *and* Enterobacter –
**Adults:** 500 mg to 1 g q 4 to 8 hours. In life-threatening infections, up to 2 g q 4 hours may be needed.
**Infants and children:** 50 to 100 mg/kg daily in equally divided doses q 4 to 8 hours. May be increased to total daily dosage of 150 mg/kg, not to exceed maximum adult dosage.

## ADVERSE REACTIONS
**GI:** pseudomembranous colitis, nausea, vomiting, *diarrhea,* oral candidiasis.
**Hematologic:** eosinophilia.
**Skin:** *maculopapular and erythematous rashes,* urticaria.
**Other:** hypersensitivity reactions (serum sickness, *anaphylaxis*); transient increases in liver enzymes; at in-

---

Reactions may be *common,* uncommon, *life-threatening,* or COMMON AND LIFE-THREATENING.

jection site — *pain, induration, sterile abscesses,* temperature elevation, tissue sloughing; with I.V. injection — *phlebitis, thrombophlebitis.*

## INTERACTIONS
*Aminoglycosides:* incompatible when mixed together. Administer at a different site.
*Aspirin, oral anticoagulants:* increased risk of bleeding. Monitor for bleeding.
*Ethanol:* possible disulfiram-like reaction. Warn patient not to drink alcohol for several days after discontinuing cefamandole.
*Probenecid:* may inhibit excretion and increase serum levels of cefamandole. Sometimes used for this effect.

## CONTRAINDICATIONS
Contraindicated in patients with hypersensitivity to the drug or other cephalosporins.

## NURSING CONSIDERATIONS
• Use cautiously in patients with a history of sensitivity to penicillin and in breast-feeding women. Also use cautiously and with dosage adjustments in patients with renal failure.
• Obtain specimen for culture and sensitivity tests before first dose. Therapy may begin pending results.
• **I.V. use:** Reconstitute 1 g with 10 ml of sterile water for injection, $D_5W$, or 0.9% sodium chloride for injection. To give by direct injection, inject into a large vein or into the tubing of a free-flowing I.V. solution over 3 to 5 minutes. If using sterile water, dilute to 20 ml to avoid giving a hypertonic solution.
• After reconstitution, remember that drug is stable for 24 hours at room temperature; for 96 hours under refrigeration.
• For intermittent injection, dilute to 100 ml with a compatible solution.
• Don't mix with I.V. infusions con-

taining calcium ions (chemically incompatible).
• For I.M. administration, inject deeply into a large muscle mass, such as the gluteus maximus or the lateral aspect of the thigh.
• With large doses or prolonged therapy, monitor for superinfection, especially in high-risk patients.
• Monitor for signs of bleeding. The chemical structure of this drug includes the methylthiotetrazole side chain that has been associated with bleeding disorders. Vitamin K can promptly reverse bleeding if it occurs.
• Know that from 40% to 75% of patients receiving cephalosporins show a false-positive direct Coombs' test.
• Keep in mind that urine glucose determinations may be false-positive with copper sulfate tests (Clinitest); glucose enzymatic tests (Clinistix, Tes-Tape) are not affected.

☑ **PATIENT TEACHING**
• Instruct patient to report adverse reactions promptly.
• Tell patient to alert nurse if discomfort occurs at I.V. injection site.

## cefazolin sodium
Ancef, Kefzol, Zolicef

*Pregnancy Risk Category: B*

## HOW SUPPLIED
*Injection (parenteral):* 500 mg, 1 g
*Infusion:* 500 mg/50 ml vial, 500 mg/ 100 ml vial
*Pharmacy bulk package:* 5 g, 10 g, 20 g

## ACTION
A first-generation cephalosporin that inhibits cell-wall synthesis, promoting osmotic instability; usually bactericidal.

## ONSET, PEAK, DURATION
Onset immediate after I.V. administration, unknown after I.M. injection.

---

Plasma levels peak within 1 to 2 hours after I.M. injection, immediately after I.V. administration. Duration unknown.

## INDICATIONS & DOSAGE
*Perioperative prophylaxis in contaminated surgery* –
**Adults:** 1 g I.M. or I.V. 30 to 60 minutes before surgery; then 0.5 to 1 g I.M. or I.V. q 6 to 8 hours for 24 hours. In long operations (over 2 hours), another 0.5 to 1 g dose may be administered intraoperatively.

*Note:* In cases where infection would be devastating, prophylaxis may be continued for 3 to 5 days.
*Serious infections of respiratory, biliary, and GU tracts; skin, soft-tissue, bone, and joint infections; septicemia; and endocarditis caused by* Escherichia coli, *Enterobacteriaceae, gonococci,* Haemophilus influenzae, Klebsiella, Proteus mirabilis, Staphylococcus aureus, Streptococcus pneumoniae, *and group A beta-hemolytic streptococci* –
**Adults:** 250 mg I.M. or I.V. q 8 hours to 1.5 g q 6 hours. Maximum 12 g/day in life-threatening situations.
**Children over 1 month:** 25 to 50 mg/kg or 1.25 g/m² daily I.M. or I.V. in three or four divided doses. In severe infections, dosage may be increased to 100 mg/kg/day.

## ADVERSE REACTIONS
**GI:** pseudomembranous colitis, nausea, anorexia, vomiting, *diarrhea,* glossitis, dyspepsia, abdominal cramps, anal pruritus, oral candidiasis.
**GU:** genital pruritus and moniliasis, vaginitis.
**Hematologic:** neutropenia, leukopenia, eosinophilia, *thrombocytopenia.*
**Skin:** *maculopapular and erythematous rashes, urticaria, pruritus.*
**Other:** hypersensitivity reactions (serum sickness, *anaphylaxis*); transient increases in liver enzymes; Ste-

vens-Johnson syndrome; at injection site – *pain, induration, sterile abscesses, tissue sloughing;* with I.V. injection – *phlebitis, thrombophlebitis.*

## INTERACTIONS
*Probenecid:* may inhibit excretion and increase blood levels of cefazolin.

## CONTRAINDICATIONS
Contraindicated in patients with hypersensitivity to other cephalosporins.

## NURSING CONSIDERATIONS
• Use cautiously in patients with a history of sensitivity to penicillin and in breast-feeding women. Also use cautiously and with dosage adjustments in patients with renal failure.
• Obtain specimen for culture and sensitivity tests before first dose. Therapy may begin pending results.
• Be aware that dose and dosing interval will be adjusted if creatinine clearance is below 55 ml/minute.
• **I.V. use:** Reconstitute with sterile water, bacteriostatic water, or 0.9% sodium chloride solution as follows: 2 ml to 500-mg vial; 2.5 ml to 1-g vial. Shake well until dissolved. Resultant concentration: 225 mg/ml or 330 mg/ml, respectively.
• Know that reconstituted cefazolin is stable for 24 hours at room temperature or 96 hours under refrigeration.
• For direct injection, further dilute Ancef with 5 ml or Kefzol with 10 ml, of sterile water for injection. Inject into a large vein or into the tubing of a free-flowing I.V. solution over 3 to 5 minutes. For intermittent infusion, add reconstituted drug to 50 to 100 ml of compatible solution or use premixed solution. Commercially available frozen solutions of cefazolin in $D_5W$ should be given only by intermittent or continuous I.V. infusion.
• Alternate injection sites if I.V. therapy lasts longer than 3 days. Use of small I.V. needles in larger available veins may be preferable.

---

Reactions may be *common,* uncommon, *life-threatening,* or **COMMON AND LIFE-THREATENING.**

• After reconstitution, inject I.M. drug without further dilution (this drug is not as painful as other cephalosporins). Injection should be given deeply into a large muscle mass, such as the gluteus maximus or lateral aspect of the thigh.

• With large doses or prolonged therapy, monitor for superinfection, especially in high-risk patients.

• Keep in mind that 40% to 75% of those receiving cephalosporins show a false-positive direct Coombs' test.

• Be aware that urine glucose determinations may be false-positive with copper sulfate tests (Clinitest); glucose enzymatic tests (Clinistix, Tes-Tape) are not affected.

### ☑ PATIENT TEACHING
• Instruct patient to report adverse reactions promptly.
• Tell patient to alert nurse if discomfort occurs at I.V. injection site.

▼ *NEW DRUG*

## cefepime hydrochloride
Maxipime

*Pregnancy Risk Category: B*

### HOW SUPPLIED
*Injection:* 500 mg/15 ml vial, 1 g/100 ml piggyback bottle, 1 g/ADD-Vantage vial, 1 g/15 ml vial, 2 g/100 ml piggyback bottle, 2 g/20 ml vial

### ACTION
A fourth-generation cephalosporin that inhibits bacterial cell-wall synthesis, promotes osmotic instability, and destroys bacteria.

### ONSET, PEAK, DURATION
Onset occurs within 30 minutes. Peak levels occur in 1 to 2 hours. Duration is unknown.

### INDICATIONS & DOSAGE
*Mild to moderate urinary tract infections caused by* Escherichia coli, Klebsiella pneumoniae, *or* Proteus mirabilis, *including cases associated with concurrent bacteremia with these microorganisms —*
**Adults and children 12 years and older:** 0.5 to 1 g I.M. (I.M. route used only for infections caused by *E. coli*) or I.V infused over 30 minutes q 12 hours for 7 to 10 days.
*Severe urinary tract infections, including pyelonephritis, caused by* E. coli *or* K. pneumoniae —
**Adults and children 12 years and older:** 2 g I.V. infused over 30 minutes q 12 hours for 10 days.
*Moderate to severe pneumonia caused by* Streptococcus pneumoniae, Pseudomonas aeruginosa, K. pneumoniae, *or* Enterobacter *species —*
**Adults and children 12 years and older:** 1 to 2 g I.V. infused over 30 minutes q 12 hours for 10 days.
*Moderate to severe skin infections, uncomplicated skin infections, and skin structure infections caused by* Staphylococcus aureus *(methicillin-susceptible strains only) or* Streptococcus pyogenes —
**Adults and children 12 years and older:** 2 g I.V. infused over 30 minutes q 12 hours for 10 days.

### ADVERSE REACTIONS
**CNS:** headache.
**GI:** colitis, diarrhea, nausea, vomiting, oral moniliasis.
**GU:** vaginitis.
**Skin:** rash, pruritus, urticaria.
**Other:** phlebitis, pain, inflammation, fever.

### INTERACTIONS
*Aminoglycosides:* may increase risk of nephrotoxicity and ototoxicity. Monitor renal and hearing functions closely.
*Potent diuretics such as furosemide:* may increase risk of nephrotoxicity. Monitor renal function closely.

*Liquid form contains alcohol.  **May contain tartrazine.  †Canada only.  ‡Australia only.  ◇OTC.

## CONTRAINDICATIONS

Contraindicated in patients with hypersensitivity to the drug, other cephalosporins, penicillins, or other beta-lactam antibiotics.

## NURSING CONSIDERATIONS

● Use cautiously in patients with renal impairment, poor nutrition, or history of gastrointestinal disease (particularly colitis); in those receiving a protracted course of antimicrobial therapy; and in breast-feeding women.
● Safety of drug in children under age 12 has not been established.
● Obtain culture and sensitivity tests before first dose, if appropriate. Therapy may begin pending results.
● Dosage adjustment is necessary in patients with impaired renal function.
● **I.V. use:** Follow manufacturer's guidelines closely when reconstituting drug. Variations occur in constituting drug for administration, depending on concentration of drug ordered and how drug is packaged (piggyback vial, ADD-Vantage vial, or regular vial). Also be aware that the type of diluent used for constitution varies, depending on the product used. Use only solutions recommended by the manufacturer. The resulting solution should be administered over about 30 minutes.
● Intermittent I.V. infusion with a Y-type administration set can be accomplished with compatible solutions. However, during infusion of a solution containing cefepime, discontinuing the other solution is recommended.
● For I.M. administration, constitute the drug using sterile water for injection, 0.9% sodium chloride for injection, 5% dextrose injection, 0.5% or 1% lidocaine hydrochloride or bacteriostatic water for injection with parabens or benzyl alcohol. Follow the manufacturer's guidelines for quantity of diluent to use.
● Inspect solution for particulate matter before administration. The powder and its solutions tend to darken, depending on storage conditions. Product potency is not adversely affected when stored as recommended.
● Monitor the patient for superinfection. Drug may cause overgrowth of nonsusceptible bacteria or fungi.
● Be aware that many cephalosporins can reduce prothrombin activity. Patients at risk include those with renal or hepatic impairment or poor nutrition and those receiving prolonged cefepime therapy. Monitor prothrombin time in these patients as ordered. Administer exogenous vitamin K as indicated and ordered.
● Be aware that positive direct Coombs' test may occur during treatment with cefepime.

☑ **PATIENT TEACHING**
● Warn patient receiving drug I.M. that pain may occur at injection site.
● Instruct patient to report adverse reactions promptly.

---

# cefixime
Suprax

*Pregnancy Risk Category: B*

## HOW SUPPLIED

*Tablets:* 200 mg, 400 mg
*Oral suspension:* 100 mg/5 ml (after reconstitution)

## ACTION

A third-generation cephalosporin that inhibits cell-wall synthesis, promoting osmotic instability; usually bactericidal.

## ONSET, PEAK, DURATION

Onset and duration unknown. Serum levels peak within 3.1 to 4.4 hours after an oral dose. Peak serum concentrations are approximately 15% to 50% higher when administered as oral suspension rather than tablets.

---

## INDICATIONS & DOSAGE
*Uncomplicated urinary tract infections caused by* Escherichia coli *and* Proteus mirabilis; *otitis media caused by* Haemophilus influenzae *(beta-lactamase positive and negative strains)*, Moraxella (Branhamella) catarrhalis, *and* Streptococcus pyogenes; *pharyngitis and tonsillitis caused by* S. pyogenes; *acute bronchitis and acute exacerbations of chronic bronchitis caused by* S. pneumoniae *and* H. influenzae *(beta-lactamase positive and negative strains)* –
**Adults and children over 12 years or weighing over 50 kg:** 400 mg/day P.O. as a single 400-mg tablet or 200 mg q 12 hours.
**Children 12 years and younger or weighing 50 kg or less:** 8 mg/kg/day suspension P.O. as a single daily dose or 4 mg/kg q 12 hours.
*Uncomplicated gonorrhea caused by* Neisseria gonorrhoeae –
**Adults:** 400 mg P.O. as a single dose.

## ADVERSE REACTIONS
**CNS:** headache, dizziness.
**GI:** *diarrhea,* loose stools, abdominal pain, nausea, vomiting, dyspepsia, flatulence, pseudomembranous colitis, diarrhea.
**GU:** genital pruritus, vaginitis, genital candidiasis, transient increases in BUN and serum creatinine levels.
**Hematologic:** *thrombocytopenia,* leukopenia, eosinophilia.
**Skin:** pruritus, rash, urticaria, erythema multiforme, Stevens-Johnson syndrome.
**Other:** drug fever, transient increases in liver enzymes, hypersensitivity reactions (serum sickness, *anaphylaxis*).

## INTERACTIONS
*Probenecid:* may inhibit excretion and increase blood levels of cefixime. Use together cautiously.
*Salicylates:* may displace cefixime from plasma protein-binding sites. Clinical significance is unknown.

## CONTRAINDICATIONS
Contraindicated in patients with hypersensitivity to the drug or other cephalosporins.

## NURSING CONSIDERATIONS
● *Alert:* Use cautiously and with reduced dosage in patients with renal dysfunction; reduced dosage is necessary in patients with creatinine clearance below 60 ml/minute.
● Also use cautiously in patients with a history of sensitivity to penicillin and in breast-feeding women.
● Obtain specimen for culture and sensitivity tests before first dose. Therapy may begin pending results.
● To prepare oral suspension: add required amount of water to powder in two portions. Shake well after each addition. After mixing, suspension is stable for 14 days. No need to refrigerate, but keep tightly closed. Shake well before using.
● With large doses or prolonged therapy, monitor for superinfection, especially in high-risk patients.
● Know that from 40% to 75% of patients receiving cephalosporins show a false-positive direct Coombs' test.
● Keep in mind that urine glucose determinations may be false-positive with copper sulfate tests (Clinitest); glucose enzymatic tests (Clinistix, Tes-Tape) are not affected.

## ☑ PATIENT TEACHING
● Tell the patient to take all of the medication prescribed, even after he feels better.
● Instruct the patient using oral suspension to shake container before measuring dose. Tell him suspension does not need to be refrigerated.
● Tell the patient to call the doctor if rash develops.

---

*Liquid form contains alcohol. **May contain tartrazine. †Canada only. ‡Australia only. ◇OTC.

# cefmetazole sodium (cefmetazone)
Zefazone

*Pregnancy Risk Category: B*

## HOW SUPPLIED
*Injection:* 1 g, 2 g

## ACTION
A semisynthetic cephamycin antibiotic pharmacologically similar to second-generation cephalosporins that inhibits cell-wall synthesis, promoting osmotic instability; usually bactericidal.

## ONSET, PEAK, DURATION
Onset and duration unknown. Plasma levels peak immediately after I.V. administration.

## INDICATIONS & DOSAGE
*Lower respiratory tract infections caused by* Streptococcus pneumoniae, Staphylococcus aureus *(penicillinase- and non-penicillinase-producing strains),* Escherichia coli, *and* Haemophilus influenzae *(non-penicillinase-producing strains); intra-abdominal infections caused by* E. coli *or* Bacteroides fragilis; *skin and skin-structure infections caused by* S. aureus *(penicillinase- and non-penicillinase-producing strains),* S. epidermidis, Streptococcus pyogenes, S. agalactiae, E. coli, Proteus mirabilis, Klebsiella pneumoniae, *and* B. fragilis—
**Adults:** 2 g I.V. q 6 to 12 hours for 5 to 14 days.
*Urinary tract infections caused by* E. coli—
**Adults:** 2 g I.V. q 12 hours.
*Prophylaxis in patients undergoing vaginal hysterectomy—*
**Adults:** 2 g I.V. 30 to 90 minutes before surgery as a single dose; or 1 g I.V. 30 to 90 minutes before surgery, repeated in 8 and 16 hours.
*Prophylaxis in patients undergoing abdominal hysterectomy—*

**Adults:** 1 g I.V. 30 to 90 minutes before surgery, repeated in 8 and 16 hours.
*Prophylaxis in patients undergoing cesarean section—*
**Adults:** 2 g I.V. as a single dose after clamping cord; or 1 g I.V. after clamping cord, repeated in 8 and 16 hours.
*Prophylaxis in patients undergoing colorectal surgery—*
**Adults:** 2 g I.V. as a single dose 30 to 90 minutes before surgery. Some clinicians follow with additional 2-g doses in 8 and 16 hours.
*Prophylaxis in high-risk patients undergoing cholecystectomy—*
**Adults:** 1 g I.V. 30 to 90 minutes before surgery, repeated in 8 and 16 hours.

## ADVERSE REACTIONS
**CNS:** headache, hot flashes.
**CV:** *shock,* hypotension.
**EENT:** epistaxis.
**GI:** nausea, vomiting, *diarrhea,* epigastric pain, pseudomembranous colitis, candidiasis, bleeding.
**GU:** vaginitis.
**Respiratory:** pleural effusion, dyspnea, respiratory distress.
**Skin:** rash, pruritus, generalized erythema.
**Other:** fever, bacterial or fungal superinfection, hypersensitivity reactions (serum sickness, *anaphylaxis*), altered color perception, pain at injection site, phlebitis, thrombophlebitis, joint pain and inflammation.

## INTERACTIONS
*Aminoglycosides:* potential increased risk of nephrotoxicity. Monitor closely.
*Ethanol:* possible disulfiram-like reaction. Should be avoided for 24 hours before and after administration of cefmetazole.
*Probenecid:* may inhibit excretion and increase blood levels of cefmetazole. Sometimes used for this effect.

---

Reactions may be *common,* uncommon, *life-threatening,* or COMMON AND LIFE-THREATENING.

## CONTRAINDICATIONS

Contraindicated in patients with hypersensitivity to the drug or other cephalosporins.

## NURSING CONSIDERATIONS

• Use cautiously in patients with a history of sensitivity to penicillin and in breast-feeding women.
• Obtain specimen for culture and sensitivity tests before first dose. Therapy may begin pending results.
• **I.V. use:** Reconstitute with bacteriostatic water for injection, sterile water for injection, or 0.9% sodium chloride for injection. After reconstitution, drug may be further diluted to concentrations ranging from 1 to 20 mg/ml by adding it to 0.9% sodium chloride injection, D₅W, or lactated Ringer's injection. Reconstituted or dilute solutions are stable for 24 hours at room temperature (77° F [25° C]) or 1 week if refrigerated at 46° F (8° C).
• Monitor patient for bacterial and fungal superinfections. Prolonged use may result in overgrowth of nonsusceptible organisms.
• Monitor PT in patients at risk (from renal or hepatic impairment, malnutrition, or prolonged therapy), as ordered. The chemical structure of this drug includes the methylthiotetrazole side chain that has been associated with bleeding disorders. However, such bleeding has not been reported with this drug.
• Know that from 40% to 75% of patients receiving cephalosporins show a false-positive direct Coombs' test.
• Keep in mind that urine glucose determinations may be false-positive with copper sulfate tests (Clinitest); glucose enzymatic tests (Clinistix, Tes-Tape) are not affected.

## ☑ PATIENT TEACHING

• Tell patient to report adverse reactions promptly.
• Instruct patient to alert nurse if discomfort occurs at I.V. insertion site.

# cefonicid sodium
Monocid

*Pregnancy Risk Category: B*

## HOW SUPPLIED

*Injection:* 500 mg, 1 g
*Infusion:* 1 g/100 ml
*Pharmacy bulk package:* 10 g

## ACTION

A second-generation cephalosporin that inhibits cell-wall synthesis, promoting osmotic instability; usually bactericidal.

## ONSET, PEAK, DURATION

Onset immediate after I.V. administration, unknown after I.M. injection. Plasma levels peak within 1 to 2 hours after I.M. injection, immediately after I.V. administration. Duration unknown.

## INDICATIONS & DOSAGE

*Perioperative prophylaxis in contaminated surgery –*
**Adults:** 1 g I.M. or I.V. 30 to 60 minutes before surgery; then 1 g I.M. or I.V. daily for 2 days after surgery.
*Serious infections of the lower respiratory and urinary tracts, skin and skin-structure infections, septicemia, bone and joint infections, and preoperative prophylaxis. Susceptible microorganisms include* Streptococcus pneumoniae, Klebsiella pneumoniae, Escherichia coli, Haemophilus influenzae, Proteus mirabilis, Staphylococcus aureus, S. epidermidis, *and* Streptococcus pyogenes –
**Adults:** usual dosage is 1 g I.V. or I.M. q 24 hours; in life-threatening infections, 2 g q 24 hours.

## ADVERSE REACTIONS

**CNS:** dizziness, headache, malaise, paresthesia.
**GI:** pseudomembranous colitis, diarrhea.

---

*Liquid form contains alcohol. **May contain tartrazine. †Canada only. ‡Australia only. ◊OTC.

**GU:** *acute renal failure,* interstitial nephritis.

**Hematologic:** neutropenia, leukopenia, eosinophilia, anemia, thrombocytosis, *thrombocytopenia.*

**Skin:** *maculopapular and erythematous rashes,* urticaria.

**Other:** hypersensitivity reactions (serum sickness, *anaphylaxis*); at injection site—*pain, induration, sterile abscesses, tissue sloughing;* with I.V. injection—*phlebitis, thrombophlebitis,* fever, myalgia.

## INTERACTIONS
*Probenecid:* may inhibit excretion and increase blood levels of cefonicid. Use together cautiously.

## CONTRAINDICATIONS
Contraindicated in patients with hypersensitivity to the drug or other cephalosporins.

## NURSING CONSIDERATIONS
• Use cautiously in patients with a history of sensitivity to penicillin and breast-feeding women. Also use cautiously and with dosage adjustments in patients with renal failure.
• Obtain specimen for culture and sensitivity tests before first dose. Therapy may begin pending results.
• Be aware that dosing interval will be adjusted for patients with renal impairment.
• **I.V. use:** Reconstitute 500-mg vial with 2 ml of sterile water for injection (yields a concentration of 220 mg/ml) and 1-g vial with 2.5 ml of sterile water for injection (yields a concentration of 325 mg/ml). Shake well. Reconstitute piggyback vials with 50 to 100 ml of sterile water for injection, bacteriostatic water for injection, or 0.9% sodium chloride solution.
• For I.M. use, when administering 2-g I.M. doses once daily, divide the dose equally and inject deeply into large muscle masses, such as the glu-

teus maximus or the lateral aspect of the thigh.
• With large doses or prolonged therapy, monitor for superinfection, especially in high-risk patients.
• Be aware that the chemical structure of this drug includes the methylthiotetrazole side chain that has been associated with bleeding disorders. However, such bleeding has not been reported with this drug.
• Know that from 40% to 75% of patients receiving cephalosporins show a false-positive direct Coombs' test.
• Keep in mind that urine glucose determinations may be false-positive with copper sulfate tests (Clinitest); glucose enzymatic tests (Clinistix, Tes-Tape) are not affected.

## ☑ PATIENT TEACHING
• Tell patient to report adverse reactions promptly.
• Instruct patient to alert nurse if discomfort is felt at I.V. insertion site.

---

# cefoperazone sodium
Cefobid

*Pregnancy Risk Category: B*

## HOW SUPPLIED
*Infusion:* 1 g, 2 g piggyback
*Parenteral:* 1 g, 2 g
*Pharmacy bulk package:* 10-g vial

## ACTION
A third-generation cephalosporin that inhibits cell-wall synthesis, promoting osmotic instability; usually bactericidal.

## ONSET, PEAK, DURATION
Onset immediate after I.V. administration, unknown after I.M. injection. Serum levels peak in 1 to 2 hours after I.M. injection, immediately after I.V. administration. Duration unknown.

---

## INDICATIONS & DOSAGE

*Serious infections of the respiratory tract; intra-abdominal, gynecologic, and skin infections; bacteremia; and septicemia. Susceptible microorganisms include* Streptococcus pneumoniae *and* S. pyogenes; Staphylococcus aureus *(penicillinase- and non-penicillinase-producing) and* S. epidermidis; *enterococci;* Escherichia coli; Klebsiella; Haemophilus influenzae; Enterobacter; Citrobacter; Proteus; *some* Pseudomonas, *including* P. aeruginosa; *and* Bacteroides fragilis —
**Adults:** usual dosage is 1 to 2 g q 12 hours I.M. or I.V. In severe infections or in infections caused by less sensitive organisms, the total daily dosage or frequency may be increased up to 16 g/day in certain situations.

## ADVERSE REACTIONS

**GI:** pseudomembranous colitis, nausea, vomiting, *diarrhea.*
**Hematologic:** transient neutropenia, *eosinophilia,* anemia, hypoprothrombinemia, bleeding.
**Skin:** *maculopapular and erythematous rashes, urticaria.*
**Other:** mildly elevated liver enzymes; hypersensitivity reactions (serum sickness, *anaphylaxis*); at injection site — *pain, induration, sterile abscesses, temperature elevation, tissue sloughing;* with I.V. injection — *phlebitis, thrombophlebitis,* drug fever.

## INTERACTIONS

*Ethanol:* possible disulfiram-like reaction. Warn patients not to drink alcohol for several days after discontinuing cefoperazone.
*Probenecid:* may inhibit excretion and increase blood levels of cefoperazone. Use together cautiously.

## CONTRAINDICATIONS

Contraindicated in patients with hypersensitivity to the drug or other cephalosporins.

## NURSING CONSIDERATIONS

● Use cautiously in patients with impaired renal function or with a history of sensitivity to penicillin. Also use cautiously in breast-feeding women.
● Doses of 4 g/day should be given cautiously to patients with hepatic disease or biliary obstruction. Higher dosages require monitoring of serum levels.
● Obtain specimen for culture and sensitivity tests before first dose. Therapy may begin pending results.
● **I.V. use:** Reconstitute 1- or 2-g vial with a minimum of 2.8 ml of compatible I.V. solution; the manufacturer recommends using 5 ml/g. Give by direct injection into a large vein or into the tubing of a free-flowing I.V. solution over 3 to 5 minutes. When giving by intermittent infusion, add reconstituted drug to 20 to 40 ml of a compatible I.V. solution and infuse over 15 to 30 minutes.
● To prepare drug for I.M. injection: using the 1-g vial, dissolve drug with 2 ml of sterile water for injection; then add 0.6 ml of 2% lidocaine hydrochloride for a final concentration of 333 mg/ml. Alternatively, dissolve drug with 2.8 ml of sterile water for injection; then add 1 ml of 2% lidocaine hydrochloride for a final concentration of 250 mg/ml. When using the 2-g vial, dissolve drug with 3.8 ml of sterile water for injection; then add 1.2 ml of 2% lidocaine hydrochloride for a final concentration of 333 mg/ml. Alternatively, dissolve drug with 5.4 ml of sterile water for injection; then add 1.8 ml of 2% lidocaine hydrochloride for a final concentration of 250 mg/ml.
● For I.M. administration, inject deeply into a large muscle mass, such as the gluteus maximus or the lateral aspect of the thigh.
● With large doses or prolonged therapy, monitor for superinfection, especially in high-risk patients.
● Monitor PT regularly. The chemi-

cal structure of this drug includes the methylthiotetrazole side chain that has been associated with bleeding disorders. Vitamin K promptly reverses bleeding if it occurs.

• **Alert:** Monitor serum drug concentrations closely in patients with hepatic disease or biliary obstruction. Because of high degree of biliary excretion, serum concentrations increase in these patients.

• Know that from 40% to 75% of patients receiving cephalosporins show a false-positive direct Coombs' test.

• Keep in mind urine glucose determinations may be false-positive with copper sulfate tests (Clinitest); glucose enzymatic tests (Clinistix, Tes-Tape) are not affected.

☑ **PATIENT TEACHING**
• Tell patient to report adverse reactions promptly.
• Instruct patient to alert nurse if discomfort occurs at I.V. insertion site.

## cefotaxime sodium
Claforan

*Pregnancy Risk Category: B*

### HOW SUPPLIED
*Injection:* 500 mg, 1 g, 2 g
*Infusion:* 1 g, 2 g
*Pharmacy bulk package:* 10-g vial

### ACTION
A third-generation cephalosporin that inhibits cell-wall synthesis, promoting osmotic instability; usually bactericidal.

### ONSET, PEAK, DURATION
Onset immediate after I.V. administration, unknown after I.M. injection. Serum levels peak 30 minutes after I.M. injection, immediately after I.V. administration. Duration unknown.

### INDICATIONS & DOSAGE
*Perioperative prophylaxis in contaminated surgery –*
**Adults:** 1 g I.M. or I.V. 30 to 60 minutes before surgery. Patients undergoing bowel surgery should receive preoperative mechanical bowel cleansing and a nonabsorbable anti-infective agent such as neomycin. Patients undergoing cesarean section should receive 1 g I.M. or I.V. as soon as the umbilical cord is clamped, then 1 g I.M. or I.V. 6 and 12 hours later.
*Serious infections of the lower respiratory and urinary tracts, CNS, skin, bone, and joints; gynecologic and intra-abdominal infections; bacteremia; and septicemia. Susceptible microorganisms include streptococci, including* Streptococcus pneumoniae *and* S. pyogenes; Staphylococcus aureus *(penicillinase- and non-penicillinase-producing) and* S. epidermidis; Escherichia coli; Klebsiella; Haemophilus influenzae; Serratia marcescens; Pseudomonas *species, including* P. aeruginosa; Enterobacter; Proteus; *and* Peptostreptococcus –
**Adults:** usual dose is 1 g I.V. or I.M. q 6 to 8 hours. Up to 12 g daily can be given in life-threatening infections.
**Children weighing 50 kg or more:** the usual adult dose, but dosage should not exceed 12 g daily.
**Children 1 month to 12 years weighing less than 50 kg:** 50 to 180 mg/kg/day I.M. or I.V. in four to six divided doses.
**Neonates to 1 week:** 50 mg/kg I.V. q 12 hours.
**Neonates 1 to 4 weeks:** 50 mg/kg I.V. q 6 to 8 hours.

### ADVERSE REACTIONS
**CNS:** headache.
**GI:** pseudomembranous colitis, nausea, vomiting, *diarrhea.*
**GU:** vaginitis, moniliasis, interstitial nephritis.
**Hematologic:** transient neutropenia,

---

eosinophilia, hemolytic anemia, ***thrombocytopenia, agranulocytosis.*** **Skin:** *maculopapular and erythematous rashes, urticaria.*
**Other:** hypersensitivity reactions (serum sickness, ***anaphylaxis***); transient increases in liver enzymes; elevated temperature; at injection site — *pain, induration, sterile abscesses, temperature elevation, tissue sloughing;* with I.V. injection — *phlebitis, thrombophlebitis.*

## INTERACTIONS
*Aminoglycosides:* may increase risk of nephrotoxicity. Monitor closely.
*Probenecid:* may inhibit excretion and increase blood levels of cefotaxime. Use together cautiously.

## CONTRAINDICATIONS
Contraindicated in patients with hypersensitivity to the drug or other cephalosporins.

## NURSING CONSIDERATIONS
• Use cautiously in patients with a history of sensitivity to penicillin and in breast-feeding women. Also use cautiously and with dosage adjustments in patients with renal failure.
• Obtain specimen for culture and sensitivity tests before first dose. Therapy may begin pending results.
• **I.V. use:** For direct injection, reconstitute 500-mg, 1-g, or 2-g vials with 10 ml of sterile water for injection. Solutions containing 1 g/14 ml are isotonic. Inject drug into a large vein or into the tubing of a free-flowing I.V. solution over 3 to 5 minutes.
• For I.V. infusion, reconstitute infusion vials with 50 to 100 ml of D₅W or 0.9% sodium chloride solution. Infuse drug over 20 to 30 minutes. Interrupt flow of primary I.V. solution during infusion.
• For I.M. administration, inject deeply into a large muscle mass, such as the gluteus maximus or the lateral aspect of the thigh.

• With large doses or prolonged therapy, monitor for superinfection, especially in high-risk patients.
• Know that from 40% to 75% of patients receiving cephalosporins show a false-positive direct Coomb's test.
• Keep in mind that urine glucose determinations may be false-positive with copper sulfate tests (Clinitest); glucose enzymatic tests (Clinistix, Tes-Tape) are not affected.

## ☑ PATIENT TEACHING
• Tell patient to report adverse reactions promptly.
• Instruct patient to alert nurse if discomfort occurs at I.V. insertion site.

# cefotetan disodium
Cefotan

*Pregnancy Risk Category: B*

## HOW SUPPLIED
*Injection:* 1 g, 2 g
*Infusion:* 1 g, 2 g piggyback
*Pharmacy bulk package:* 10-g vial

## ACTION
A semisynthetic cephamycin antibiotic that is pharmacologically similar to the second-generation cephalosporins. Inhibits cell-wall synthesis, promoting osmotic instability; usually bactericidal.

## ONSET, PEAK, DURATION
Onset immediate after I.V. administration, unknown after I.M. injection. Peak serum levels occur 1½ to 3 hours after I.M. injection, immediately after I.V. administration. Duration unknown.

## INDICATIONS & DOSAGE
*Serious urinary tract and lower respiratory tract infections and gynecologic, skin and skin-structure, intraabdominal, and bone and joint infections caused by susceptible strepto-*cocci, Staphylococcus aureus *(penicil-*

*linase- and non-penicillinase-producing) and* S. epidermidis, Escherichia coli, Klebsiella, Enterobacter, Proteus, Haemophilus influenzae, Neisseria gonorrhoeae, *and* Bacteroides, *including* B. fragilis; *and perioperative prophylaxis* –
**Adults:** 1 to 2 g I.V. or I.M. q 12 hours for 5 to 10 days. Up to 6 g daily in life-threatening infections.

## ADVERSE REACTIONS
**GI:** pseudomembranous colitis, nausea, *diarrhea.*
**GU:** nephrotoxicity.
**Hematologic:** transient neutropenia, eosinophilia, hemolytic anemia, hypoprothrombinemia, bleeding, thrombocytosis, *agranulocytosis, thrombocytopenia.*
**Skin:** *maculopapular and erythematous rashes, urticaria.*
**Other:** hypersensitivity reactions (serum sickness, *anaphylaxis*); transient increases in liver enzymes; elevated temperature; at injection site – *pain, induration, sterile abscesses, tissue sloughing;* with I.V. injection – *phlebitis, thrombophlebitis.*

## INTERACTIONS
*Aminoglycosides:* possible synergistic effect and possible increased risk of nephrotoxicity. Use with caution.
*Ethanol:* possible disulfiram-like reaction. Warn patients not to drink alcohol for several days after discontinuing cefotetan.
*Probenecid:* may inhibit excretion and increase blood levels of cefotetan. Sometimes used for this effect.

## CONTRAINDICATIONS
Contraindicated in patients with hypersensitivity to the drug or other cephalosporins.

## NURSING CONSIDERATIONS
● Use cautiously in patients with a history of sensitivity to penicillin and in breast-feeding women. Also use

cautiously and with dosage adjustments in patients with renal failure.
● Obtain specimen for culture and sensitivity tests before first dose. Therapy may begin pending results.
● **I.V. use:** Reconstitute with sterile water for injection. Then may be mixed with 50 to 100 ml of $D_5W$ or 0.9% sodium chloride solution. Interrupt flow of primary I.V. solution during cefotetan infusion.
● Reconstitute I.M. injection with sterile water or bacteriostatic water for injection, 0.9% sodium chloride for injection, or 0.5% or 1% lidocaine hydrochloride. Shake to dissolve and let stand until clear.
● Know that reconstituted solution is stable for 24 hours at room temperature or 96 hours if refrigerated.
● With large doses or prolonged therapy, monitor for superinfection, especially in high-risk patients.
● Know that the chemical structure of this drug includes the methylthiotetrazole side chain that has been associated with bleeding disorders. However, such bleeding has not been reported with this drug.
● Be aware that 40% to 75% of those receiving cephalosporins show a false-positive direct Coombs' test.
● Keep in mind that urine glucose determinations may be false-positive with copper sulfate tests (Clinitest); glucose enzymatic tests (Clinistix, Tes-Tape) are not affected.

☑ **PATIENT TEACHING**
● Tell patient to report adverse reactions promptly.
● Instruct patient to alert nurse if discomfort occurs at I.V. site.

## cefoxitin sodium
Mefoxin

*Pregnancy Risk Category: B*

---

Reactions may be *common,* uncommon, *life-threatening,* or COMMON AND LIFE-THREATENING.

## HOW SUPPLIED
*Injection:* 1 g, 2 g
*Infusion:* 1 g, 2 g in 50-ml or 100-ml container
*Pharmacy bulk package:* 10 g

## ACTION
A semisynthetic cephamycin antibiotic that is pharmacologically similar to the second-generation cephalosporins. Inhibits cell-wall synthesis, promoting osmotic instability; usually bactericidal.

## ONSET, PEAK, DURATION
Onset immediate after I.V. administration, unknown after I.M. injection. Serum levels peak occur within 20 to 30 minutes after I.M. injection, immediately after I.V. administration. Duration unknown.

## INDICATIONS & DOSAGE
*Serious infections of respiratory and GU tracts, skin, soft-tissue, bone, and joint infections, and bloodstream and intra-abdominal infections caused by susceptible* Escherichia coli *and other coliform bacteria,* Staphylococcus aureus *(penicillinase- and non-penicillinase-producing) and* S. epidermidis, streptococci, Klebsiella, Haemophilus influenzae, *and* Bacteroides, *including* B. fragilis; *and perioperative prophylaxis* –
**Adults:** 1 to 2 g q 6 to 8 hours for uncomplicated infections. Up to 12 g daily in life-threatening infections.
**Children over 3 months:** 80 to 160 mg/kg daily given in four to six equally divided doses. Maximum daily dose is 12 g.
*Prophylactic use in surgery* –
**Adults:** 2 g I.M. or I.V. 30 to 60 minutes before surgery, then 2 g I.M. or I.V. q 6 hours for 24 hours (72 hours after prosthetic arthroplasty).
**Children 3 months or older:** 30 to 40 mg/kg I.M. or I.V. 30 to 60 minutes before surgery, then 30 to 40 mg/kg

q 6 hours for 24 hours (72 hours after prosthetic arthroplasty).

## ADVERSE REACTIONS
**CV:** hypotension.
**GI:** pseudomembranous colitis, nausea, vomiting, *diarrhea.*
**GU:** *acute renal failure.*
**Hematologic:** transient neutropenia, eosinophilia, *hemolytic anemia,* anemia, *thrombocytopenia.*
**Skin:** *maculopapular and erythematous rashes, urticaria,* exfoliative dermatitis.
**Other:** hypersensitivity reactions (serum sickness, *anaphylaxis*); transient increases in liver enzymes; elevated temperature; at injection site – *pain, induration, sterile abscesses, tissue sloughing;* with I.V. injection – *phlebitis, thrombophlebitis,* dyspnea.

## INTERACTIONS
*Nephrotoxic agents:* possible increased risk of nephrotoxicity. Monitor closely.
*Probenecid:* may inhibit excretion and increase blood levels of cefoxitin. Sometimes used for this effect.

## CONTRAINDICATIONS
Contraindicated in patients with hypersensitivity to the drug or other cephalosporins.

## NURSING CONSIDERATIONS
• Use cautiously in patients with a history of sensitivity to penicillin and in breast-feeding women. Also use cautiously and with dosage adjustments in patients with renal failure.
• Obtain specimen for culture and sensitivity tests before first dose. Therapy may begin pending results.
• **I.V. use:** Reconstitute 1 g with at least 10 ml of sterile water for injection and 2 g with 10 to 20 ml of sterile water for injection. Solutions of dextrose 5% and 0.9% sodium chloride for injection can also be used. For direct injection, inject drug into a large

---

*Liquid form contains alcohol.   **May contain tartrazine.   †Canada only.   ‡Australia only.   ◇OTC.

vein or into the tubing of a free-flowing I.V. solution over 3 to 5 minutes. For intermittent infusion, add reconstituted drug to 50 or 100 ml of dextrose 5% or 10% in water or 0.9% sodium chloride injection. Interrupt flow of primary I.V. solution during infusion.

• Reconstitute I.M. injection with 0.5% or 1% lidocaine hydrochloride (without epinephrine) to minimize pain. Inject deeply into a large muscle mass, such as the gluteus maximus or the lateral aspect of the thigh.

• After reconstitution, store for 24 hours at room temperature or 1 week under refrigeration.

• Assess I.V. site frequently. Such use has been linked to development of thrombophlebitis.

• With large doses or prolonged therapy, monitor for superinfection, especially in high-risk patients.

• Be aware that 40% to 75% of those receiving cephalosporins show a false-positive direct Coombs' test.

• Keep in mind that urine glucose determinations may be false-positive with copper sulfate tests (Clinitest); glucose enzymatic tests (Clinistix, Tes-Tape) are not affected.

☑ **PATIENT TEACHING**
• Tell patient to report adverse reactions promptly.
• Instruct patient to alert nurse if discomfort is felt at I.V. site.

---

## cefpodoxime proxetil
Vantin

*Pregnancy Risk Category: B*

**HOW SUPPLIED**
*Tablets (film-coated):* 100 mg, 200 mg
*Oral suspension:* 50 mg/5 ml, 100 mg/5 ml in 100-ml bottles

**ACTION**
A second-generation cephalosporin that inhibits cell-wall synthesis, pro-

moting osmotic instability; usually bactericidal.

**ONSET, PEAK, DURATION**
Onset and duration unknown. Serum levels peak in 2 to 3 hours after an oral dose.

**INDICATIONS & DOSAGE**
*Acute, community-acquired pneumonia caused by non-beta-lactamase-producing strains of* Haemophilus influenzae *or* Streptococcus pneumoniae —
**Adults and children 13 years and older:** 200 mg P.O. q 12 hours for 14 days.
*Acute bacterial exacerbation of chronic bronchitis caused by S. pneumoniae, H. influenzae (non-beta-lactamase-producing strains only), or* Moraxella (Branhamella) catarrhalis —
**Adults and children 13 years and older:** 200 mg P.O. q 12 hours for 10 days.
*Uncomplicated gonorrhea in men and women; rectal gonococcal infections in women —*
**Adults and children 13 years and older:** 200 mg P.O. as a single dose. Follow with doxycycline 100 mg P.O. b.i.d. for 7 days.
*Uncomplicated skin and skin-structure infections caused by* Staphylococcus aureus *or* Streptococcus pyogenes —
**Adults and children 13 years and older:** 400 mg P.O. q 12 hours for 7 to 14 days.
*Acute otitis media caused by* S. pneumoniae, H. influenzae, *or* M. catarrhalis —
**Children 6 months and over:** 5 mg/kg (not to exceed 200 mg) P.O. q 12 hours for 10 days.
*Pharyngitis or tonsillitis caused by* S. pyogenes —
**Adults:** 100 mg P.O. q 12 hours for 10 days.
**Children 6 months and over:** 5 mg/kg (not to exceed 100 mg) P.O. q 12 hours for 10 days.

---

Reactions may be *common,* uncommon, ***life-threatening,*** or **COMMON AND LIFE-THREATENING.**

*Uncomplicated urinary tract infections caused by* Escherichia coli, Klebsiella pneumoniae, Proteus mirabilis, *or* Staphylococcus saprophyticus—

**Adults:** 100 mg P.O. q 12 hours for 7 days.

In patients with renal failure: Know that when creatinine clearance is below 30 ml/minute, dosage interval should be increased to q 24 hours. Patients receiving dialysis should get the drug three times weekly after dialysis.

## ADVERSE REACTIONS
**CNS:** headache.
**GI:** *diarrhea,* nausea, vomiting, abdominal pain.
**GU:** vaginal fungal infections.
**Skin:** rash.
**Other:** hypersensitivity reactions *(anaphylaxis).*

## INTERACTIONS
*Antacids, H₂ antagonists:* decreased absorption of cefpodoxime. Avoid concomitant use.
*Probenecid:* decreased excretion of cefpodoxime. Monitor for toxicity.

## CONTRAINDICATIONS
Contraindicated in patients with hypersensitivity to the drug or other cephalosporins. Safety and efficacy in children under age 6 months have not been established.

## NURSING CONSIDERATIONS
• Use cautiously in patients with a history of penicillin hypersensitivity because of the risk of cross-sensitivity and in patients receiving nephrotoxic drugs because other cephalosporins have been shown to have nephrotoxic potential. Because drug is excreted in human breast milk, also use cautiously in breast-feeding women.
• Obtain specimen for culture and sensitivity tests before first dose. Therapy may begin pending results.
• Administer drug with food to en-hance absorption. Shake suspension well before using.
• Store suspension in the refrigerator (36° to 46° F [2° to 8° C]). Discard unused portion after 14 days.
• Monitor for superinfection. Drug may cause overgrowth of nonsusceptible bacteria or fungi.
• Know that from 40% to 75% of patients receiving cephalosporins show a false-positive direct Coombs' test.
• Keep in mind that urine glucose determinations may be false-positive with copper sulfate tests (Clinitest); glucose enzymatic tests (Clinistix, Tes-Tape) are not affected.

## ☑ PATIENT TEACHING
• Tell the patient to take all of the medication prescribed, even after he feels better.
• Instruct the patient to take drug with food. If the patient is using suspension, tell him to shake container before measuring dose and to keep it refrigerated.
• Tell the patient to call doctor if rash develops.

# cefprozil
Cefzil

*Pregnancy Risk Category: B*

## HOW SUPPLIED
*Tablets:* 250 mg, 500 mg
*Oral suspension:* 125 mg/5 ml, 250 mg/5 ml

## ACTION
A second-generation cephalosporin that interferes with cell-wall synthesis during microorganism replication, leading to osmotic instability and cell lysis (bactericidal).

## ONSET, PEAK, DURATION
Onset and duration unknown. Serum levels peak within 1½ hours after an oral dose.

---

## INDICATIONS & DOSAGE

*Pharyngitis or tonsillitis caused by* Streptococcus pyogenes —
**Adults and children 13 years and older:** 500 mg P.O. daily for at least 10 days.

*Otitis media caused by* S. pneumoniae, Haemophilus influenzae, *and* Moraxella (Branhamella) catarrhalis —
**Infants and children 6 months to 12 years:** 15 mg/kg P.O. q 12 hours for 10 days.

*Secondary bacterial infections of acute bronchitis and acute bacterial exacerbation of chronic bronchitis caused by* S. pneumoniae, H. influenzae, *and* M. catarrhalis —
**Adults and children 13 years and older:** 500 mg P.O. q 12 hours for 10 days.

*Uncomplicated skin and skin-structure infections caused by* Staphylococcus aureus *and* S. pyogenes —
**Adults and children 13 years and older:** 250 mg P.O. b.i.d., or 500 mg daily to b.i.d.

## ADVERSE REACTIONS

**CNS:** dizziness, hyperactivity, headache, nervousness, insomnia, confusion, somnolence.
**GI:** *diarrhea, nausea,* vomiting, abdominal pain.
**GU:** elevated BUN level, elevated serum creatinine level, genital pruritus, vaginitis.
**Hematologic:** decreased leukocyte count, eosinophilia.
**Hepatic:** elevated liver enzymes, cholestatic jaundice (rare).
**Skin:** rash, urticaria, diaper rash.
**Other:** superinfection, hypersensitivity reactions (serum sickness, *anaphylaxis*).

## INTERACTIONS

*Aminoglycosides:* potential increased risk of nephrotoxicity. Monitor closely.
*Probenecid:* may inhibit excretion and increase blood levels of cefprozil. Use together cautiously.

## CONTRAINDICATIONS

Contraindicated in patients with hypersensitivity to the drug or other cephalosporins.

## NURSING CONSIDERATIONS

• Use cautiously in patients with a history of sensitivity to penicillin and in breast-feeding women. Also use cautiously in patients with impaired hepatic or renal function.
• **Alert:** Know that patients with creatinine clearance less than 30 ml/minute should receive 50% of usual dose.
• Obtain specimen for culture and sensitivity tests before first dose. Therapy may begin pending results.
• Administer after hemodialysis treatment is completed; drug is removed by hemodialysis.
• Know that from 40% to 75% of patients receiving cephalosporins show a false-positive direct Coombs' test.
• Keep in mind that urine glucose determinations may be false-positive with copper sulfate tests (Clinitest); glucose enzymatic tests (Clinistix, Tes-Tape) are not affected.
• Monitor for superinfection. May cause overgrowth of nonsusceptible bacteria or fungi.

## ☑ PATIENT TEACHING

• Tell the patient to take all of the medication as prescribed, even after he feels better.
• Tell the patient to shake suspension well before measuring dose.
• Tell the patient that oral suspensions contain the drug in a bubble-gum flavored form to improve palatability and promote compliance in children. Tell him to refrigerate reconstituted suspension and to discard unused drug after 14 days.
• Tell the patient to notify doctor if rash occurs.

# ceftazidime

Ceptaz, Fortaz, Tazicef, Tazidime

*Pregnancy Risk Category: B*

## HOW SUPPLIED

*Injection (with sodium carbonate):*
500 mg, 1 g, 2 g; 6 g (pharmacy bulk package)
*Injection (with arginine):* 1 g, 2 g; 6 g, 10 g (pharmacy bulk package)
*Infusion:* 1 g, 2 g in 50-ml and 100-ml vials (premixed)

## ACTION

A third-generation cephalosporin that inhibits cell-wall synthesis, promoting osmotic instability; usually bactericidal.

## ONSET, PEAK, DURATION

Onset immediate after I.V. administration, unknown after I.M. injection. Peak serum levels occur within 1 hour after I.M. injection, immediately after I.V. administration. In women, peak serum concentrations may be lower after I.M. injection into the gluteus maximus than into the vastus lateralis. Duration unknown.

## INDICATIONS & DOSAGE

*Serious infections of the lower respiratory and urinary tracts; gynecologic, intra-abdominal, CNS, and skin infections; bacteremia; and septicemia. Among susceptible microorganisms are streptococci, including* Streptococcus pneumoniae *and* S. pyogenes; Staphylococcus aureus *(penicillinase- and non-penicillinase-producing);* Escherichia coli; Klebsiella; Proteus; Enterobacter; Haemophilus influenzae; Pseudomonas; *and some strains of* Bacteroides —
**Adults and children 12 years and older:** 1 g I.V. or I.M. q 8 to 12 hours; up to 6 g daily in life-threatening infections.
**Children 1 month to 12 years:** 30 to 50 mg/kg I.V. q 8 hours.

**Neonates 0 to 4 weeks:** 30 mg/kg I.V. q 12 hours.

## ADVERSE REACTIONS

**CNS:** headache, dizziness, paresthesia, *seizures.*
**GI:** pseudomembranous colitis, nausea, vomiting, diarrhea, candidiasis, abdominal cramps.
**GU:** vaginitis.
**Hematologic:** eosinophilia; thrombocytosis, leukopenia, hemolytic anemia, *agranulocytosis, thrombocytopenia.*
**Skin:** *maculopapular and erythematous rashes, urticaria.*
**Other:** hypersensitivity reactions (serum sickness, *anaphylaxis*); transient elevation in liver enzymes; at injection site — *pain, induration, sterile abscesses, tissue sloughing;* with I.V. injection — *phlebitis, thrombophlebitis.*

## INTERACTIONS

*Aminoglycosides:* additive or synergistic effect against some strains of *P. aeruginosa* and Enterobacteriaceae.
*Chloramphenicol:* antagonistic effect. Avoid concomitant use.

## CONTRAINDICATIONS

Contraindicated in patients with hypersensitivity to the drug or other cephalosporins.

## NURSING CONSIDERATIONS

• Use cautiously in patients with a history of sensitivity to penicillin and in breast-feeding women. Also use cautiously and with dosage adjustments in patients with renal failure.
• Obtain specimen for culture and sensitivity tests before first dose. Therapy may begin pending results.
• **I.V. use:** Reconstitute sodium carbonate-containing solutions with sterile water for injection. Add 5 ml to a 500-mg vial; 10 ml to a 1-g or 2-g vial. Shake well to dissolve drug. Carbon dioxide is released during dissolution, and positive pressure will de-

velop in the vial. Reconstitute arginine-containing solutions with 10 ml of sterile water for injection. This formulation won't release gas bubbles. Each brand of ceftazidime includes specific instructions for reconstitution. Read and follow these instructions carefully.

• For I.M. administration, inject deeply into a large muscle mass, such as the gluteus maximus or the lateral aspect of the thigh.

• With large doses or prolonged therapy, monitor for superinfection, especially in high-risk patients.

• **Alert:** Keep in mind that commercially available preparations contain either sodium carbonate (Fortaz, Magnacef, Tazicef, Tazidime) or arginine (Ceptaz, Pentacef) to facilitate dissolution of drug. Safety and efficacy of arginine-containing solutions in children 12 years and under have not been established.

• Be aware that 40% to 75% of those receiving cephalosporins show a false-positive direct Coombs' test.

• Keep in mind that urine glucose determinations may be false-positive with copper sulfate tests (Clinitest); glucose enzymatic tests (Clinistix, Tes-Tape) are not affected.

• Know that ceftazidime is removed by hemodialysis; a supplemental dose of the drug is indicated after each dialysis period, as ordered.

☑ **PATIENT TEACHING**
• Tell patient to report adverse drug reactions promptly.
• Instruct patient to alert nurse if discomfort is felt at I.V. insertion site.

---

## ceftizoxime sodium
Cefizox

*Pregnancy Risk Category: B*

### HOW SUPPLIED
*Injection:* 500 mg, 1 g, 2 g
*Infusion:* 1 g, 2 g in 100-mg vials or in 50 ml of $D_5W$
*Pharmacy bulk package:* 10 g

### ACTION
A third-generation cephalosporin that inhibits cell-wall synthesis, promoting osmotic instability; usually bactericidal.

### ONSET, PEAK, DURATION
Onset immediate after I.V. administration, unknown after I.M. injection. Serum levels peak ½ to 1½ hours after I.M. injection, immediately after I.V. administration. Duration unknown.

### INDICATIONS & DOSAGE
*Serious infections of the lower respiratory and urinary tracts, gynecologic infections, bacteremia, septicemia, meningitis, intra-abdominal infections, bone and joint infections, and skin infections. Among susceptible microorganisms are streptococci, including* Streptococcus pneumoniae *and* S. pyogenes; Staphylococcus aureus *(penicillinase- and non-penicillinase-producing) and* S. epidermidis; Escherichia coli; Klebsiella; Haemophilus influenzae; Enterobacter; Proteus; *some* Pseudomonas; *and* Peptostreptococcus—
**Adults:** usual dosage is 1 to 2 g I.V. or I.M. q 8 to 12 hours. In life-threatening infections, up to 2 g q 4 hours.
**Children over 6 months:** 33 to 50 mg/kg I.V. q 6 to 8 hours. For serious infections, up to 200 mg/kg/day in divided doses may be used. Don't exceed 12 g/day.

### ADVERSE REACTIONS
**GI:** pseudomembranous colitis, nausea, anorexia, vomiting, *diarrhea*.
**GU:** vaginitis.
**Hematologic:** transient neutropenia, eosinophilia, hemolytic anemia,

---

Reactions may be *common*, uncommon, *life-threatening*, or COMMON AND LIFE-THREATENING.

thrombocytosis, anemia, ***thrombocytopenia.***
**Skin:** *maculopapular and erythematous rashes, urticaria.*
**Other:** hypersensitivity reactions (serum sickness, ***anaphylaxis***); dyspnea; elevated temperature; at injection site—*pain, induration, sterile abscesses, tissue sloughing;* with I.V. injection—*phlebitis, thrombophlebitis,* transient elevation in liver enzymes.

## INTERACTIONS
*Probenecid:* may inhibit excretion and increase blood levels of ceftizoxime. Sometimes used for this effect.

## CONTRAINDICATIONS
Contraindicated in patients with hypersensitivity to ceftizoxime or other cephalosporins.

## NURSING CONSIDERATIONS
● Use cautiously in patients with a history of sensitivity to penicillin and in breast-feeding women. Also use cautiously and with dosage adjustments in patients with renal failure.
● Obtain specimen for culture and sensitivity tests before first dose. Therapy may begin pending results.
● **I.V. use:** To reconstitute powder, add 5 ml of sterile water to a 500-mg vial, 10 ml to a 1-g vial, or 20 ml to a 2-g vial. Reconstitute piggyback vials with 50 to 100 ml of 0.9% sodium chloride solution or D₅W. Shake well.
● For I.M. administration, inject deeply into a large muscle mass, such as the gluteus maximus or the lateral aspect of the thigh. Larger doses (2 g) should be divided and administered at two separate sites.
● With large doses or prolonged therapy, monitor for superinfection, especially in high-risk patients.
● Know that from 40% to 75% of patients receiving cephalosporins show a false-positive direct Coombs' test.
● Keep in mind that urine glucose determinations may be false-positive

with copper sulfate tests (Clinitest); glucose enzymatic tests (Clinistix, Tes-Tape) are not affected.

## ☑ PATIENT TEACHING
● Tell patient to report adverse reactions promptly.
● Instruct patient to alert nurse if discomfort is felt at I.V. site.

# ceftriaxone sodium
Rocephin
*Pregnancy Risk Category: B*

## HOW SUPPLIED
*Injection:* 250 mg, 500 mg, 1 g, 2 g
*Infusion:* 1 g, 2 g
*Pharmacy bulk package:* 10 g

## ACTION
A third-generation cephalosporin that inhibits cell-wall synthesis, promoting osmotic instability; usually bactericidal.

## ONSET, PEAK, DURATION
Onset immediate after I.V. administration, unknown after I.M. injection. Peak serum levels occur 1½ to 4 hours after I.M. injection, immediately after I.V. administration. Duration unknown.

## INDICATIONS & DOSAGE
*Uncomplicated gonococcal vulvovaginitis, urethritis, or proctitis*—
**Adults:** 250 mg I.M. as a single dose, followed with 100 mg of doxycycline P.O. q 12 hours for 7 days.
**Children:** 125 mg I.M. as a single dose.
*Serious infections of the lower respiratory and urinary tracts; gynecologic, bone and joint, intra-abdominal, and skin infections; bacteremia; septicemia; and Lyme disease caused by such susceptible microorganisms as streptococci, including* Streptococcus pneumoniae *and* S. pyogenes; Staphylococcus aureus *(penicillinase- and non-peni-*

*cillinase-producing) and* S. epidermidis; Escherichia coli; Klebsiella; Haemophilus influenzae; Neisseria meningitidis; N. gonorrhoeae; Enterobacter; Proteus; Peptostreptococcus, Pseudomonas; *and* Serratia marcescens —

**Adults and children over 12 years:** 1 to 2 g I.M. or I.V. daily or in equally divided doses b.i.d. Total daily dosage should not exceed 4 g.

**Children 12 years and under:** 50 to 75 mg/kg, not to exceed 2 g/day, given in divided doses q 12 hours.

*Meningitis* —

**Adults and children:** 100 mg/kg given in divided doses q 12 hours. May give loading dose of 75 mg/kg, not to exceed 4 g.

*Preoperative prophylaxis* —

**Adults:** 1 g I.V. as a single dose ½ to 2 hours before surgery.

## ADVERSE REACTIONS

**CNS:** headache, dizziness.
**GI:** pseudomembranous colitis, nausea, vomiting, diarrhea.
**GU:** genital pruritus, moniliasis, elevated BUN levels.
**Hematologic:** eosinophilia, thrombocytosis, leukopenia.
**Skin:** pain, induration, tenderness at injection site; phlebitis; *rash;* pruritus.
**Other:** hypersensitivity reactions (serum sickness, *anaphylaxis*), elevated temperature, chills.

## INTERACTIONS

*Aminoglycosides:* additive or synergistic effect against some strains of *P. aeruginosa* and Enterobacteriaceae.
*Probenecid:* high doses (1 or 2 g/day) may enhance hepatic clearance of ceftriaxone and shorten its half-life. Avoid concomitant use.

## CONTRAINDICATIONS

Contraindicated in patients with hypersensitivity to ceftriaxone or other cephalosporins.

## NURSING CONSIDERATIONS

• Use cautiously in patients with a history of sensitivity to penicillin and in breast-feeding women.
• Obtain specimen for culture and sensitivity tests before first dose. Therapy may begin pending results.
• **I.V. use:** Reconstitute with sterile water for injection, 0.9% sodium chloride injection, dextrose 5% or 10% injection, or a combination of sodium chloride and dextrose injection and other compatible solutions. Reconstitute by adding 2.4 ml of diluent to the 250-mg vial, 4.8 ml to the 500-mg vial, 9.6 ml to the 1-g vial, and 19.2 ml to the 2-g vial. All reconstituted solutions yield a concentration that averages 100 mg/ml. After reconstitution, dilute further for intermittent infusion to desired concentration. I.V. dilutions are stable for 24 hours at room temperature.
• For I.M. administration, inject deeply into a large muscle mass, such as the gluteus maximus or the lateral aspect of the thigh.
• With large doses or prolonged therapy, monitor for superinfection, especially in high-risk patients.
• Know that from 40% to 75% of patients receiving cephalosporins show a false-positive direct Coombs' test.
• Keep in mind that urine glucose determinations may be false-positive with copper sulfate tests (Clinitest); glucose enzymatic tests (Clinistix, Tes-Tape) are not affected.
• Be aware that drug is commonly used in home antibiotic programs for outpatient treatment of serious infections, such as osteomyelitis.

☑ **PATIENT TEACHING**
• Tell patient to report adverse reactions promptly.
• Instruct patient to alert nurse if discomfort occurs at I.V. insertion site.
• Teach home care patient and family how to prepare and administer drug.
• If home care patient is a diabetic

---

who is testing his urine for glucose, tell him drug may affect results of copper sulfate tests; instead he should use an enzymatic test.

---

## cefuroxime axetil
Ceftin

## cefuroxime sodium
Kefurox, Zinacef

*Pregnancy Risk Category: B*

### HOW SUPPLIED
**cefuroxime axetil**
*Tablets:* 125 mg, 250 mg, 500 mg
*Suspension:* 125 mg/5 ml
**cefuroxime sodium**
*Injection:* 750 mg, 1.5 g
*Infusion:* 750 mg, 1.5 g premixed, frozen solution
*Pharmacy bulk package:* 7.5 g

### ACTION
A second-generation cephalosporin that inhibits cell-wall synthesis, promoting osmotic instability; usually bactericidal.

### ONSET, PEAK, DURATION
Onset is immediate after I.V. administration, unknown after oral and I.M. administration. Peak serum levels occur within 2 hours after oral administration, 15 to 60 minutes after I.M. injection, immediately after I.V. administration. Duration unknown.

### INDICATIONS & DOSAGE
*Injectable form is for serious infections of the lower respiratory and urinary tracts; skin and skin-structure infections; bone and joint infections; septicemia; meningitis; and gonorrhea; and for perioperative prophylaxis; oral form is used to treat otitis media, pharyngitis, tonsillitis, infections of the urinary and lower respiratory tracts, and skin and skin-structure infections. Among susceptible organisms are* Streptococcus pneumo-

niae *and* S. pyogenes, Haemophilus influenzae, Klebsiella, Staphylococcus aureus, Escherichia coli, Moraxella catarrhalis *(including beta-lactamase-producing strains),* Enterobacter, *and* Neisseria gonorrhoeae —
**Adults and children 12 years and older:** usual dosage of cefuroxime sodium is 750 mg to 1.5 g I.M. or I.V. q 8 hours for 5 to 10 days. For life-threatening infections and infections caused by less susceptible organisms, 1.5 g I.M. or I.V. q 6 hours; for bacterial meningitis, up to 3 g I.V. q 8 hours.

Alternatively, administer 250 mg of cefuroxime axetil P.O. q 12 hours. For severe infections, dosage may be increased to 500 mg q 12 hours.
**Children and infants over 3 months:** 50 to 100 mg/kg/day of cefuroxime sodium I.M. or I.V. in equally divided doses q 6 to 8 hours. Higher doses are administered when treating meningitis. Alternatively, 125 mg of cefuroxime axetil P.O. q 12 hours; for bacterial meningitis, 200 to 240 mg/kg I.V. in divided doses q 6 to 8 hours.
*Uncomplicated urinary tract infection —*
**Adults:** 125 to 250 mg P.O. q 12 hours.
*Otitis media —*
**Children under 2 years:** 125 mg P.O. q 12 hours.
**Children 2 years and over:** 250 mg P.O. q 12 hours.
*Perioperative prophylaxis —*
**Adults:** 1.5 g I.V. 30 to 60 minutes before surgery; in lengthy operations, 750 mg I.V. or I.M. q 8 hours. For open-heart surgery, 1.5 g I.V. at induction of anesthesia and then q 12 hours for a total dosage of 6 g.

### ADVERSE REACTIONS
**GI:** pseudomembranous colitis, nausea, anorexia, vomiting, *diarrhea.*
**Hematologic:** transient neutropenia, eosinophilia, *hemolytic anemia, thrombocytopenia,* decreased hemoglobin and hematocrit levels.

---

*Liquid form contains alcohol. **May contain tartrazine. †Canada only. ‡Australia only. ◇OTC.

**Skin:** *maculopapular and erythematous rashes, urticaria.*

**Other:** transient increases in liver enzymes; hypersensitivity reactions (serum sickness, **anaphylaxis**); at injection site—*pain, induration, sterile abscesses, temperature elevation, tissue sloughing;* with I.V. injection—*phlebitis, thrombophlebitis.*

## INTERACTIONS
*Diuretics:* increased risk of adverse renal reactions. Monitor closely.
*Probenecid:* may inhibit excretion and increase blood levels of cefuroxime. Sometimes used for this effect.

## CONTRAINDICATIONS
Contraindicated in patients with hypersensitivity to cefuroxime or other cephalosporins.

## NURSING CONSIDERATIONS
• Use cautiously in patients with history of sensitivity to penicillin and in breast-feeding women. Also use cautiously and with reduced dosage in patients with impaired renal function.
• Obtain specimen for culture and sensitivity tests before first dose. Therapy may begin pending results.
• **I.V. use:** For each 750-mg vial of Kefurox, reconstitute with 9 ml of sterile water for injection. Withdraw 8 ml from the vial for the proper dose. For each 1.5-g vial of Kefurox, reconstitute with 16 ml of sterile water for injection; withdraw entire contents of vial for a dose. For each 750-mg vial of Zinacef, reconstitute with 8 ml of sterile water for injection; for each 1.5-g vial, reconstitute with 16 ml. In each case, withdraw entire contents of vial for a dose.
• To give by direct injection, inject into a large vein or into the tubing of a free-flowing I.V. solution over 3 to 5 minutes.
• For intermittent infusion, add reconstituted drug to 100 ml D₅W, 0.9% sodium chloride for injection, or other compatible I.V. solution. Infuse over 15 to 60 minutes.
• For I.M. administration, inject deeply into a large muscle mass, such as the gluteus maximus or the lateral aspect of the thigh.
• Know that absorption of cefuroxime axetil is enhanced by food.
• Keep in mind that cefuroxime axetil is available only in tablet form, which may be crushed for patients who cannot swallow tablets. Tablets may be allowed to dissolve in small amounts of apple, orange, or grape juice or chocolate milk. However, the drug has a bitter taste that is difficult to mask, even with food.
• With large doses or prolonged therapy, monitor for superinfection, especially in high-risk patients.
• Know that from 40% to 75% of patients receiving cephalosporins show a false-positive direct Coombs' test.
• Keep in mind that urine glucose determinations may be false-positive with copper sulfate tests (Clinitest); glucose enzymatic tests (Clinistix, Tes-Tape) are not affected.

## ☑ PATIENT TEACHING
• Tell the patient to take all of the medication as prescribed, even after he feels better.
• Instruct the patient to take oral form with food. If patient has difficulty swallowing tablets, tell him how to dissolve or crush tablets but warn him that the bitter taste that results is hard to mask, even with food. If suspension is being use, tell patient to shake container well before measuring dose.
• Tell the patient to notify doctor if rash occurs.
• Instruct the patient receiving drug I.V. to alert nurse if discomfort occurs at I.V. insertion site.

# cephalexin hydrochloride
Keftab

# cephalexin monohydrate
Apo-Cephalex†, Bio-cef, Cefanex, Ceporex†‡, C-Lexin, Keflex, Novo-Lexin†, Nu-Cephalex†‡

*Pregnancy Risk Category: B*

## HOW SUPPLIED
**cephalexin hydrochloride**
*Tablets:* 250 mg, 500 mg
**cephalexin monohydrate**
*Tablets:* 250 mg, 500 mg, 1 g
*Capsules:* 250 mg, 500 mg
*Oral suspension:* 100 mg/5 ml, 125 mg/5 ml, 250 mg/5 ml

## ACTION
A first-generation cephalosporin that inhibits cell-wall synthesis, promoting osmotic instability; usually bactericidal.

## ONSET, PEAK, DURATION
Onset unknown. Serum levels peak within 1 hour. Duration unknown.

## INDICATIONS & DOSAGE
*Respiratory tract, GI tract, skin, soft-tissue, bone, and joint infections and otitis media caused by* Escherichia coli *and other coliform bacteria,* group A beta-hemolytic streptococci, Haemophilus influenzae, Klebsiella, Moraxella (Branhamella) catarrhalis, Proteus mirabilis, Streptococcus pneumoniae, *and staphylococci*—
**Adults:** 250 mg to 1 g P.O. q 6 hours.
**Children:** 6 to 12 mg/kg P.O. q 6 hours (monohydrate only). Maximum 25 mg/kg q 6 hours.

## ADVERSE REACTIONS
**CNS:** dizziness, headache, fatigue, agitation, confusion, hallucinations.
**GI:** pseudomembranous colitis, *nausea, anorexia,* vomiting, *diarrhea,* gastritis, glossitis, dyspepsia, abdominal pain, anal pruritus, tenesmus, oral candidiasis.
**GU:** genital pruritus and moniliasis, vaginitis, interstitial nephritis.
**Hematologic:** neutropenia, eosinophilia, anemia, *thrombocytopenia.*
**Skin:** *maculopapular and erythematous rashes,* urticaria.
**Other:** transient increases in liver enzymes, hypersensitivity reactions (serum sickness, *anaphylaxis*), arthritis, arthralgia, joint pain.

## INTERACTIONS
*Probenecid:* may increase blood levels of cephalosporins. Sometimes used for this effect.

## CONTRAINDICATIONS
Contraindicated in patients with hypersensitivity to cephalosporins.

## NURSING CONSIDERATIONS
● Use cautiously in breast-feeding women and in patients with impaired renal function or history of sensitivity to penicillin.
● Ask the patient if he's had any reaction to cephalosporin or penicillin therapy before giving first dose.
● Obtain specimen for culture and sensitivity tests before first dose. Therapy may begin pending results.
● To prepare oral suspension: Add required amount of water to powder in two portions. Shake well after each addition. After mixing, store in refrigerator. The mixture will remain stable for 14 days without significant loss of potency. Keep tightly closed and shake well before using.
● With large doses or prolonged therapy, monitor for superinfection, especially in high-risk patients.
● Know that from 40% to 75% of patients receiving cephalosporins show a false-positive direct Coombs' test, but in only a few of them does this indicate hemolytic anemia.
● Keep in mind that urine glucose determinations may be false-positive with copper sulfate tests (Clinitest);

---

*Liquid form contains alcohol.   **May contain tartrazine.   †Canada only.   ‡Australia only.   ◇OTC.

glucose enzymatic tests (Clinistix, Tes-Tape) are not affected.
• Know that group A beta-hemolytic streptococcal infections should be treated for a minimum of 10 days.

☑ **PATIENT TEACHING**
• Tell the patient to take all of the medication exactly as prescribed, even after he feels better.
• Tell the patient to take drug with food or milk to lessen GI discomfort. If patient is taking suspension form, instruct him to shake container well before measuring dose and to store in refrigerator.
• Instruct the patient to call the doctor if rash develops.

---

## cephalothin sodium
Ceporacin†‡, Keflin

*Pregnancy Risk Category: B*

### HOW SUPPLIED
*Injection:* 1 g, 2 g, 4 g
*Infusion:* 1 g/50 ml, 2 g/50 ml, 1 g/dl, 2 g/dl
*Pharmacy bulk package:* 20 g

### ACTION
A first-generation cephalosporin that inhibits cell-wall synthesis, promoting osmotic instability; usually bactericidal.

### ONSET, PEAK, DURATION
Onset immediate after I.V. administration, unknown after I.M. injection. Serum levels peak within 30 minutes of I.M. injection, immediately after I.V. administration. Duration unknown.

### INDICATIONS & DOSAGE
*Serious infections of respiratory, GU, or GI tract; skin and soft-tissue infections (including peritonitis); bone and joint infections; septicemia; and endocarditis caused by such susceptible organisms as* Escherichia coli *and other* coliform bacteria, Enterobacteriaceae, enterococci, gonococci, group A beta-hemolytic streptococci, Haemophilus influenzae, Klebsiella, Proteus mirabilis, Salmonella, Staphylococcus aureus, Shigella, Streptococcus pneumoniae and S. viridans, and staphylococci; and perioperative prophylaxis—
**Adults:** 500 mg to 1 g I.M. or I.V. (or intraperitoneally) q 4 to 6 hours; in life-threatening infections, up to 2 g q 4 hours.
**Children:** 80 to 160 mg/kg/day I.V. in divided doses q 4 or 6 hours. Dose should be proportionately less in accordance with age, weight, and severity of infection.
*Perioperative prophylaxis in contaminated or potentially contaminated surgery—*
**Adults:** 1 to 2 g I.V. 30 to 60 minutes before surgery and 1 to 2 g q 6 hours postoperatively for 24 hours.
**Children:** 20 to 30 mg/kg I.V. 30 to 60 minutes before surgery and q 6 hours postoperatively for 24 hours

### ADVERSE REACTIONS
**CNS:** headache, malaise, paresthesia, dizziness.
**GI:** pseudomembranous colitis, nausea, anorexia, vomiting, *diarrhea,* dyspepsia, abdominal cramps.
**GU:** nephrotoxicity, genital pruritus and moniliasis.
**Hematologic:** transient neutropenia, eosinophilia, *hemolytic anemia, thrombocytopenia.*
**Skin:** *maculopapular and erythematous rashes, urticaria.*
**Other:** transient increases in liver enzymes; hypersensitivity reactions (serum sickness, *anaphylaxis*); at injection site—*pain, induration, sterile abscesses, tissue sloughing;* with I.V. injection—*phlebitis, thrombophlebitis.*

---

Reactions may be *common,* uncommon, *life-threatening,* or COMMON AND LIFE-THREATENING.

## INTERACTIONS
*Probenecid:* may increase blood levels of cephalosporins. Use together cautiously.

## CONTRAINDICATIONS
Contraindicated in patients with hypersensitivity to cephalothin or other cephalosporins.

## NURSING CONSIDERATIONS
● Use cautiously in patients with impaired renal function and in those with a history of sensitivity to penicillin. Also use cautiously in breast-feeding women.
● Obtain specimen for culture and sensitivity tests before first dose. Therapy may begin pending results.
● **I.V. use:** When giving this drug I.V., check frequently for vein irritation and phlebitis. Alternate injection sites if I.V. therapy lasts longer than 3 days. Use of small I.V. needles in larger available veins may be preferable. Addition of a small concentration of heparin (100 units) or hydrocortisone (10 to 25 mg) may reduce incidence of phlebitis.
● Dilute contents of 2-g vial with at least 20 ml of sterile water for injection, dextrose 5% for injection, or 0.9% sodium chloride for injection and add to one of following I.V. solutions: dextrose 5% for injection, dextrose 5% in lactated Ringer's injection, Ionosol B in D₅W, lactated Ringer's injection, Normosol-N in D₅W, Plasma-Lyte injection, Plasma-Lyte-N injection in dextrose 5%, Ringer's injection, or Plasma-Lyte-N in 0.9% sodium chloride for injection. Choose solution and fluid volume according to patient's fluid and electrolyte status.
● Know that I.V. route is preferable in severe or life-threatening infections.
● For I.M. administration, reconstitute each gram of cephalothin sodium with 4 ml of sterile water for injection, providing 500 mg in each 2.2 ml. If vial contents don't dissolve

completely, add an additional 0.2 to 0.4 ml of diluent, and warm contents slightly. Inject deeply into a large muscle mass, such as the gluteus maximus or the lateral aspect of the thigh.
● **Alert:** Avoid I.M. route if possible; drug causes severe pain when administered I.M.
● With large doses or prolonged therapy, monitor for superinfection, especially in high-risk patients.
● Know that from 40% to 75% of patients receiving cephalosporins show a false-positive direct Coombs' test; only a few of these indicate hemolytic anemia.
● Keep in mind that urine glucose determinations may be false-positive with copper sulfate tests (Clinitest); glucose enzymatic tests (Clinistix, Tes-Tape) are not affected.

☑ **PATIENT TEACHING**
● Tell patient to report adverse reactions promptly.
● Instruct patient to alert nurse if discomfort occurs at I.V. insertion site.
● Warn patient receiving drug I.M. that injection is painful but that application of ice to site may help to relieve discomfort.

---

## cephapirin sodium
Cefadyl

*Pregnancy Risk Category: B*

## HOW SUPPLIED
*Injection:* 500-mg, 1-g, 2-g vials; 1-g, 2-g, 4-g piggyback vials
*Pharmacy bulk package:* 20 g

## ACTION
Synthetic first-generation cephalosporin that inhibits cell-wall synthesis, promoting osmotic instability; usually bactericidal.

---

## ONSET, PEAK, DURATION
Onset immediate after I.V. administration, unknown after I.M. injection. Serum levels peak within 30 minutes of I.M. injection, immediately after I.V. administration. Duration unknown.

## INDICATIONS & DOSAGE
*Perioperative prophylaxis in contaminated or potentially contaminated surgery* –
**Adults:** 1 to 2 g I.M. or I.V. 30 to 60 minutes before surgery; then 1 to 2 g I.M. or I.V. q 6 hours for 24 hours. In procedures longer than 2 hours, additional doses may be given during surgery. In cases where infection would be devastating, prophylaxis may be continued for 3 to 5 days.
*Serious infections of respiratory, GU, or GI tract; skin and soft-tissue infections; bone and joint infections (including osteomyelitis); septicemia; and endocarditis caused by* Streptococcus pneumoniae, Escherichia coli, *group A beta-hemolytic streptococci,* Haemophilus influenzae, Klebsiella, Proteus mirabilis, Staphylococcus aureus, *and* Streptococcus viridans –
**Adults:** 500 mg to 1 g I.M. or I.V. q 4 to 6 hours. In life-threatening infections, up to 12 g/day may be used.
**Children over 3 months:** 10 to 20 mg/kg I.V. or I.M. q 6 hours; dose depends on age, weight, and severity of infection.

Patients with reduced renal function may be treated adequately with a lower dose (7.5 to 15 mg/kg q 12 hours), depending on causative organism and severity of function. Patients with severely reduced renal function who are scheduled for dialysis should receive same dose just before dialysis and q 12 hours thereafter.

## ADVERSE REACTIONS
**CNS:** dizziness, headache, malaise, paresthesia.
**GI:** pseudomembranous colitis, nausea, anorexia, vomiting, *diarrhea,* abdominal cramps, oral candidiasis.
**GU:** genital pruritus and moniliasis, vaginitis.
**Hematologic:** transient neutropenia, eosinophilia, anemia, ***thrombocytopenia.***
**Skin:** *maculopapular and erythematous rashes, urticaria.*
**Other:** transient increases in liver enzymes; hypersensitivity reactions (serum sickness, ***anaphylaxis***); at injection site –*pain, induration, sterile abscesses, tissue sloughing;* with I.V. injection –*phlebitis, thrombophlebitis.*

## INTERACTIONS
*Probenecid:* may increase blood levels of cephalosporins. Sometimes used for this effect.

## CONTRAINDICATIONS
Contraindicated in patients with hypersensitivity to cephapirin or other cephalosporins.

## NURSING CONSIDERATIONS
• Use cautiously in patients with a history of sensitivity to penicillin and in breast-feeding women.
• Obtain specimen for culture and sensitivity tests before first dose. Therapy may begin pending results.
• **I.V. use:** Prepare I.V. infusion using dextrose for injection, sodium chloride for injection, or bacteriostatic water for injection as diluent: 20 ml yields 1 g/10 ml; 50 ml yields 1 g/25 ml; 100 ml yields 1 g/50 ml.
• When using I.V. infusion with Y-tubing, dilute 4-g vial with 40 ml of diluent. During infusion of cephapirin solution, stop the flow of the other solution. Check volume of cephapirin solution carefully so that calculated dose is infused.
• When giving this drug I.V., check frequently for vein irritation and phlebitis. Alternate injection sites if I.V. therapy lasts longer than 3 days. Use

of small I.V. needles in the larger available veins may be preferable.

• For I.M. use, reconstitute 1-g vial with 2 ml of sterile water for injection or bacteriostatic water for injection so that 1.2 ml contains 500 mg of cephapirin. Prepare patient for painful I.M. injection. Inject deeply into a large muscle mass, such as the gluteus maximus or the lateral aspect of the thigh.

• Store reconstituted cephapirin for 10 days under refrigeration and for 24 hours at room temperature.

• With large doses or prolonged therapy, monitor for superinfection, especially in high-risk patients.

• Know that from 40% to 75% of patients receiving cephalosporins show a false-positive direct Coombs' test, but in only a few of them does this indicate hemolytic anemia.

• Keep in mind that urine glucose determinations may be false-positive with copper sulfate tests (Clinitest); glucose enzymatic tests (Clinistix, Tes-Tape) are not affected.

☑ **PATIENT TEACHING**
• Tell patient to report adverse reactions promptly.
• Instruct patient to alert nurse if discomfort occurs at I.V. insertion site.
• Warn patient receiving drug I.M. that injection is painful but that application of site to site may help to relieve discomfort.

## cephradine
Velosef**

*Pregnancy Risk Category: B*

### HOW SUPPLIED
*Capsules:* 250 mg, 500 mg
*Oral suspension:* 125 mg/5 ml, 250 mg/5 ml

### ACTION
First-generation cephalosporin that inhibits cell-wall synthesis, promot-

ing osmotic instability; usually bactericidal.

### ONSET, PEAK, DURATION
Onset and duration unknown. Serum levels peak within 1 hour after oral dose.

### INDICATIONS & DOSAGE
*Serious infections of respiratory, GU, or GI tract; skin and soft-tissue infections; bone and joint infections; septicemia; endocarditis; and otitis media caused by such susceptible organisms as* Escherichia coli *and other coliform bacteria, group A beta-hemolytic streptococci,* Haemophilus influenzae, Klebsiella, Proteus mirabilis, Staphylococcus aureus, Streptococcus pneumoniae, S. viridans, *and staphylococci; and perioperative prophylaxis –*
**Adults:** 250 to 500 mg P.O. q 6 hours.
**Children over 9 months:** 25 to 50 mg/kg P.O. daily in divided doses.
*Otitis media –*
75 to 100 mg/kg P.O. daily. Don't exceed 4 g daily.

All patients, regardless of age and weight, may be given larger doses (up to 1 g q.i.d.) for severe or chronic infections.

### ADVERSE REACTIONS
**CNS:** dizziness, headache, malaise, paresthesia.
**GI:** pseudomembranous colitis, *nausea, anorexia,* vomiting, heartburn, abdominal cramps, *diarrhea,* oral candidiasis.
**GU:** genital pruritus and moniliasis, vaginitis.
**Hematologic:** transient neutropenia, eosinophilia, ***thrombocytopenia.***
**Skin:** *maculopapular and erythematous rashes, urticaria.*
**Other:** transient increases in liver enzymes, hypersensitivity reactions (serum sickness, ***anaphylaxis***).

---

*Liquid form contains alcohol.   **May contain tartrazine.   †Canada only.   ‡Australia only.   ◇OTC.

## INTERACTIONS

*Probenecid:* may increase blood levels of cephalosporins. Sometimes used for this effect.

## CONTRAINDICATIONS

Contraindicated in patients with hypersensitivity to cephradine and to other cephalosporins.

## NURSING CONSIDERATIONS

• Use cautiously in patients with impaired renal function or with a history of sensitivity to penicillin. Also use cautiously in breast-feeding women.
• Obtain specimen for culture and sensitivity tests before first dose. Therapy may begin pending results.
• Know that group A beta-hemolytic streptococcal infections should be treated for a minimum of 10 days.
• Be aware that from 40% to 75% of patients receiving cephalosporins show a false-positive direct Coombs' test, but only a few indicate hemolytic anemia.
• Keep in mind that urine glucose determinations may be false-positive with copper sulfate tests (Clinitest); glucose enzymatic tests (Clinistix, Tes-Tape) are not affected.
• With large doses or prolonged therapy, monitor for superinfection, especially in high-risk patients.

## ☑ PATIENT TEACHING

• Tell the patient to take all of the medication as prescribed, even after he feels better.
• Tell the patient to take drug with food or milk to lessen GI discomfort. If patient is taking suspension form tell him to shake it well before measuring dose.
• Tell the patient to notify doctor if rash occurs.

# loracarbef
Lorabid
*Pregnancy Risk Category: B*

## HOW SUPPLIED

*Pulvules:* 200 mg, 400 mg
*Powder for oral suspension:* 100 mg/5 ml, 200 mg/5 ml in 50-ml and 100-ml bottles

## ACTION

A synthetic beta-lactam antibiotic of the carbacephem class with actions similar to the second-generation cephalosporins. Inhibits cell-wall synthesis, promoting osmotic instability; usually bactericidal.

## ONSET, PEAK, DURATION

Onset and duration unknown. Serum levels peak ½ to 1 hour after an oral dose.

## INDICATIONS & DOSAGE

*Secondary bacterial infections of acute bronchitis –*
**Adults:** 200 to 400 mg P.O. q 12 hours for 7 days.
*Acute bacterial exacerbations of chronic bronchitis –*
**Adults:** 400 mg P.O. q 12 hours for 7 days.
*Pneumonia –*
**Adults:** 400 mg P.O. q 12 hours for 14 days.
*Pharyngitis, sinusitis, or tonsillitis –*
**Adults:** 200 to 400 mg P.O. q 12 hours for 10 days.
**Children:** 15 mg/kg P.O. daily in divided doses q 12 hours for 10 days.
*Acute otitis media –*
**Children:** 30 mg/kg (oral suspension) P.O. daily in divided doses q 12 hours for 10 days.
*Uncomplicated skin and skin-structure infections –*
**Adults:** 200 mg P.O. q 12 hours for 7 days.
*Impetigo –*

---

Reactions may be *common,* uncommon, *life-threatening*, or COMMON AND LIFE-THREATENING.

**Children:** 15 mg/kg P.O. daily in divided doses q 12 hours for 7 days.
*Uncomplicated cystitis –*
**Adults:** 200 mg P.O. daily for 7 days.
*Uncomplicated pyelonephritis –*
**Adults:** 400 mg P.O. q 12 hours for 14 days.

Patients with a creatinine clearance greater than or equal to 50 ml/minute don't require dose and interval changes. Patients with a creatinine clearance of 10 to 49 ml/minute should receive half of the usual dose at the same interval; with a creatinine clearance below 10 ml/minute, the usual dose q 3 to 5 days. Hemodialysis patients require another dose after dialysis.

## ADVERSE REACTIONS
**CNS:** headache, somnolence, nervousness, insomnia, dizziness.
**CV:** vasodilation.
**GI:** diarrhea, nausea, vomiting, abdominal pain, anorexia, pseudomembranous colitis.
**GU:** vaginal candidiasis or moniliasis, transient increases in BUN and creatinine levels.
**Hematologic:** *transient thrombocytopenia,* leukopenia, eosinophilia.
**Skin:** rash, urticaria, pruritus, *erythema multiforme.*
**Other:** hypersensitivity reactions, including *anaphylaxis;* transient elevations in AST, ALT, and alkaline phosphatase levels.

## INTERACTIONS
*Probenecid:* decreased excretion of loracarbef, causing increased plasma levels. Monitor for toxicity.

## CONTRAINDICATIONS
Contraindicated in patients with hypersensitivity to the drug or other cephalosporins and in patients with diarrhea caused by pseudomembranous colitis.

## NURSING CONSIDERATIONS
• Use cautiously in pregnant or breast-feeding women. Safety and efficacy have not been established in infants under 6 months.
• Obtain specimen for culture and sensitivity tests before first dose. Therapy may begin pending results.
• To reconstitute powder for oral suspension, add 30 ml of water in two portions to the 50-ml bottle or 60 ml of water in two portions to the 100-ml bottle; shake after each addition.
• After reconstitution, store oral suspension for 14 days at room temperature (59° to 86° F [15° to 30° C]).
• Monitor for superinfection. May cause overgrowth of nonsusceptible bacteria or fungi.
• *Alert:* Monitor the patient for seizures. Beta-lactam antibiotics may trigger seizures in susceptible patients, especially when given without dosage modification to those with renal impairment. If seizures occur, discontinue drug and notify the doctor. Administer anticonvulsants as ordered.
• For otitis media, remember that the more rapidly absorbed oral suspension produces higher peak plasma levels than do the capsules.
• Know that from 40% to 75% of patients receiving cephalosporins show a false-positive direct Coombs' test; in only a few of them does this indicate hemolytic anemia.

## ☑ PATIENT TEACHING
• Tell the patient to take all of the medication prescribed, even after he feels better.
• Tell the patient to take drug on an empty stomach, at least 1 hour before or 2 hours after meals. Tell him to shake container of suspension well before measuring dose.
• Instruct the patient to discard unused portion after 14 days.
• Instruct the patient to notify doctor if rash appears.

---

*Liquid form contains alcohol. **May contain tartrazine. †Canada only. ‡Australia only. ◊OTC.

demeclocycline hydrochloride
doxycycline
doxycycline calcium
doxycycline hyclate
doxycycline hydrochloride
doxycycline monohydrate
minocycline hydrochloride
oxytetracycline hydrochloride
tetracycline hydrochloride

## COMBINATION PRODUCTS
UROBIOTIC-250: oxytetracycline hydrochloride 250 mg, sulfamethizole 250 mg, and phenazopyridine hydrochloride 50 mg.

---

## demeclocycline hydrochloride
Declomycin, Ledermycin‡

*Pregnancy Risk Category: NR*

### HOW SUPPLIED
*Film coated tablets:* 150 mg, 300 mg
*Capsules:* 150 mg

### ACTION
Unknown. Thought to exert bacteriostatic effect by binding to the 30S ribosomal subunit of microorganisms, thus inhibiting protein synthesis.

### ONSET, PEAK, DURATION
Onset and duration unknown. Serum levels peak within 3 to 4 hours after oral dose.

### INDICATIONS & DOSAGE
*Infections caused by susceptible gram-negative and gram-positive organisms, including* Haemophilus ducreyi, Rickettsiae, Mycoplasma pneumoniae, Yersinia pestis, Campylobacter fetus. *Also indicated for the organism causing psittacosis, lymphogranuloma venereum, granuloma inguinale, relapsing fever, and trachoma* –
**Adults:** 150 mg P.O. q 6 hours or 300 mg P.O. q 12 hours.
**Children over 8 years:** 6 to 12 mg/kg P.O. daily, in divided doses q 6 to 12 hours.
*Gonorrhea* –
**Adults:** initially, 600 mg P.O.; then 300 mg P.O. q 12 hours for 4 days (total 3 g).

### ADVERSE REACTIONS
**CNS:** *intracranial hypertension (pseudotumor cerebri),* dizziness.
**CV:** pericarditis.
**EENT:** dysphagia, glossitis, tinnitus, visual disturbances.
**GI:** anorexia, *nausea, vomiting, diarrhea,* enterocolitis, anogenital inflammation, pancreatitis.
**Hematologic:** neutropenia, eosinophilia, **thrombocytopenia, hemolytic anemia.**
**Skin:** *maculopapular and erythematous rashes, photosensitivity, increased pigmentation, urticaria.*
**Other:** hypersensitivity reactions **(anaphylaxis),** elevated liver enzymes, *increased BUN level,* diabetes insipidus syndrome (polyuria, polydipsia, weakness), permanent tooth discoloration or bone growth retardation if used in children under 8 years.

### INTERACTIONS
*Antacids (including sodium bicarbonate) and laxatives containing aluminum, magnesium, or calcium; antidiarrheals; food, milk, or other dairy products:* decreased antibiotic absorption. Give antibiotic 1 hour before or 2 hours after any of the above.
*Ferrous sulfate and other iron products, zinc:* decreased antibiotic ab-

---

Reactions may be *common,* uncommon, *life-threatening,* or COMMON AND LIFE-THREATENING.

sorption. Give antibiotic 3 hours after or 2 hours before iron administration.
*Methoxyflurane:* may cause nephrotoxicity with tetracyclines. Monitor carefully.
*Oral anticoagulants:* increased anticoagulant effect. Monitor PT and adjust dosage as ordered.
*Oral contraceptives:* decreased contraceptive effectiveness and increased risk of breakthrough bleeding. Use a nonhormonal birth control method.
*Penicillins:* may interfere with bactericidal action of penicillins. Avoid using together.

## CONTRAINDICATIONS
Contraindicated in patients with hypersensitivity to the drug or other tetracyclines.

## NURSING CONSIDERATIONS
Use cautiously in patients with impaired renal or hepatic function. Use of these drugs during last half of pregnancy and in children under 8 years may cause permanent discoloration of teeth, enamel defects, and bone growth retardation.
● Obtain specimen for culture and sensitivity tests before first dose. Therapy may begin pending test results.
● *Alert:* Check expiration date. Outdated or deteriorated tetracyclines have been associated with reversible nephrotoxicity (Fanconi's syndrome).
● Don't expose these drugs to light or heat; store in tight container.
● With large doses or prolonged therapy, monitor for superinfection, especially in high-risk patients.
● Check the patient's tongue for signs of monilia infection. Stress good oral hygiene.
● Be aware that demeclocycline may cause false-negative reading of glucose enzymatic tests (Clinistix, Tes-Tape).

## ☑ PATIENT TEACHING
● Instruct the patient to take entire amount of medication, exactly as prescribed, even after he feels better.
● Explain to the patient that drug's effectiveness is reduced when taken with milk or other dairy products, food, antacids, or iron products. Tell him to take each dose with a full glass of water on an empty stomach, at least 1 hour before or 2 hours after meals. Also tell him to take drug at least 1 hour before bedtime to prevent esophagitis.
● Warn the patient to avoid direct sunlight and ultraviolet light. A sunscreen may help prevent photosensitivity reactions. Photosensitivity persists for some time after discontinuation of drug.

# doxycycline
Doxylin‡, Vibramycin

# doxycycline calcium
Vibramycin

# doxycycline hyclate
Apo-Doxy†, Doryx, Doxy-Caps, Doxy 100, Doxy 200, Doxycin†, Monodox, Novodoxylin†, Vibramycin, Vibra-Tabs

# doxycycline hydrochloride
Cyclidox‡, Doryx‡, Vibramycin‡, Vibra-Tabs 50‡

# doxycycline monohydrate
Monodox, Vibramycin

*Pregnancy Risk Category: D*

## HOW SUPPLIED
**doxycycline**
*Tablets:* 50 mg‡, 100 mg‡
*Oral suspension:* 25 mg/5 ml
**doxycycline calcium**
*Oral suspension:* 50 mg/5ml
**doxycycline hyclate**
*Tablets:* 100 mg
*Capsules:* 50 mg, 100 mg

---

*Liquid form contains alcohol. **May contain tartrazine. †Canada only. ‡Australia only. ◊OTC.

*Capsules (coated pellets):* 100 mg
*Injection:* 100 mg, 200 mg
**doxycycline hydrochloride**
*Tablets:* 50 mg‡, 100 mg‡
*Capsules:* 50 mg‡, 100 mg‡, 250 mg‡
*Injection:* 100 mg‡
**doxycycline monohydrate**
*Capsules:* 50 mg, 100 mg
*Oral suspension:* 25 mg/5ml

## ACTION
Unknown. Thought to exert bacteriostatic effect by binding to the 30S ribosomal subunit of microorganisms,
thus inhibiting protein synthesis.

## ONSET, PEAK, DURATION
Onset immediate after I.V. administration, unknown after oral administration. Serum levels peak within 1½
to 4 hours after oral dose; not clearly
defined for I.V. use. Duration unknown.

## INDICATIONS & DOSAGE
*Infections caused by sensitive gram-
negative and gram-positive organisms, including* Rickettsiae, Chlamydia, *and* Mycoplasma, *and the organisms that cause trachoma and Lyme
disease–*
**Adults and children 45 kg and over:**
100 mg P.O. q 12 hours on first day,
then 100 mg P.O. daily; or 200 mg
I.V. on first day in one or two infusions, then 100 to 200 mg I.V. daily.
**Children over 8 years and under 45
kg:** 4.4 mg/kg P.O. or I.V. daily, in
divided doses q 12 hours on first day;
then 2.2 to 4.4 mg/kg daily.
Give I.V. infusion slowly (minimum 1 hour). Infusion must be completed within 12 hours (within 6 hours
in lactated Ringer's solution or dextrose 5% in lactated Ringer's solution).
*Gonorrhea in patients allergic to peni-
cillin–*
**Adults:** 100 mg P.O. b.i.d. for 7 days.
*Primary or secondary syphilis in pa-
tients allergic to penicillin–*

**Adults:** 300 mg P.O. daily in divided
doses for at least 10 days.
*Uncomplicated urethral, endocervi-
cal, or rectal infections caused by*
Chlamydia trachomatis *or* Ureaplasma urealyticum–
**Adults:** 100 mg P.O. b.i.d. for at least
7 days.
*Prophylaxis of malaria–*
**Adults:** 100 mg P.O. daily.
**Children over 8 years:** 2 mg/kg P.O.
once daily. Dosage should not exceed
adult dose.
*Note:* Prophylaxis should begin 1 to
2 days before travel to malarious area
and be continued throughout travel
and for 4 weeks afterward.

## ADVERSE REACTIONS
**CNS:** *intracranial hypertension
(pseudotumor cerebri).*
**CV:** pericarditis.
**EENT:** glossitis, dysphagia.
**GI:** anorexia, *epigastric distress, nausea,* vomiting, *diarrhea,* oral candidiasis, enterocolitis, anogenital inflammation.
**Hematologic:** neutropenia, eosinophilia, ***thrombocytopenia,*** hemolytic
anemia.
**Skin:** *maculopapular and erythematous rashes, photosensitivity, increased pigmentation,* urticaria.
**Other:** hypersensitivity reactions
*(anaphylaxis);* elevated liver enzymes; permanent discoloration of
teeth, enamel defects, bone growth
retardation if used in children under 8
years; superinfection; thrombophlebitis.

## INTERACTIONS
*Antacids (including sodium bicarbon-
ate) and laxatives containing aluminum, magnesium, or calcium; antidiarrheals:* decreased antibiotic absorption. Give antibiotic 1 hour before or
2 hours after any of the above.
*Ferrous sulfate and other iron prod-
ucts, zinc:* decreased antibiotic ab-

sorption. Give drug 3 hours after or 2 hours before iron administration.
*Methoxyflurane:* may cause nephrotoxicity with tetracyclines. Monitor carefully.
*Oral anticoagulants:* increased anticoagulant effect. Monitor PT and adjust dosage as ordered.
*Oral contraceptives:* decreased contraceptive effectiveness and increased risk of breakthrough bleeding. Use a nonhormonal form of birth control.
*Penicillins:* may interfere with bactericidal action of penicillins. Avoid using together.
*Phenobarbital, carbamazepine, alcohol:* decreased antibiotic effect. Avoid if possible.

## CONTRAINDICATIONS
Contraindicated in patients with hypersensitivity to the drug or other tetracyclines.

## NURSING CONSIDERATIONS
● Use cautiously in patients with impaired renal or hepatic function. Use of these drugs during last half of pregnancy and in children under 8 years may cause permanent discoloration of teeth, enamel defects, and bone growth retardation.
● Obtain specimen for culture and sensitivity tests before first dose. Therapy may begin pending test results.
● **Alert:** Check expiration date. Outdated or deteriorated tetracyclines have been associated with reversible nephrotoxicity (Fanconi's syndrome).
● Administer with milk or food if adverse GI reactions develop.
● **I.V. use:** Reconstitute powder for injection with sterile water for injection. Use 10 ml in 100-mg vial and 20 ml in 200-mg vial. Dilute solution to 100 to 1,000 ml for I.V. infusion. Avoid extravasation. Don't infuse solutions that are more concentrated than 1 mg/ml. Infusion time varies with dose, but usually ranges from 1

to 4 hours. Monitor I.V. infusion site for signs of thrombophlebitis, which may occur with I.V. administration.
● Don't expose drug to light or heat. Protect it from sunlight during infusion.
● Know that reconstituted injectable solution is stable for 72 hours if refrigerated.
● Be alert that parenteral form may cause false-positive reading of copper sulfate tests (Clinitest). All forms may cause false-negative reading of glucose enzymatic tests (Clinistix, Tes-Tape).
● With large doses or prolonged therapy, monitor for superinfection, especially in high-risk patients.
● Check the patient's tongue for signs of fungal infection. Stress good oral hygiene.

### ☑ PATIENT TEACHING
● Tell the patient to take entire amount of medication exactly as prescribed, even after he feels better.
● Instruct the patient to report adverse reactions promptly. If drug is being administered I.V., tell patient to alert nurse if discomfort occurs at I.V site.
● Tell the patient to take oral forms of drug with food or milk if stomach upset occurs. Also advise patient not to take oral tablets or capsules within 1 hour of bedtime because of possible dysphagia.
● Tell the patient to use a sunscreen and avoid strong sunlight during therapy to prevent photosensitivity reactions.

## minocycline hydrochloride
Dynacin, Minocin*, Minomycin‡, Minomycin IV‡
*Pregnancy Risk Category: D*

## HOW SUPPLIED
*Tablets (film-coated):* 50 mg, 100 mg
*Capsules:* 50 mg, 100 mg

*Oral suspension:* 50 mg/5 ml
*Injection:* 100 mg

## ACTION
Unknown. Thought to exert bacterio-static effect by binding to the 30S ribosomal subunit of microorganisms, thus inhibiting protein synthesis.

## ONSET, PEAK, DURATION
Onset immediate after I.V. administration, unknown after oral administration. Serum levels peak immediately after I.V. administration, within 1 to 4 hours after oral dose. Duration unknown.

## INDICATIONS & DOSAGE
*Infections caused by sensitive gram-negative and gram-positive organisms, trachoma, amebiasis* —
**Adults:** 200 mg I.V.; then 100 mg I.V. q 12 hours. Not to exceed 400 mg/day. Or 200 mg P.O. initially; then 100 mg P.O. q 12 hours. Some clinicians use 100 or 200 mg P.O. initially, followed by 50 mg q.i.d.
**Children over 8 years:** initially, 4 mg/kg P.O. or I.V., followed by 2 mg/kg q 12 hours.
　Given I.V. in 500- to 1,000-ml solution without calcium and administered over 6 hours.
*Gonorrhea in patients sensitive to penicillin* —
**Adults:** initially, 200 mg P.O.; then 100 mg q 12 hours for at least 4 days.
*Syphilis in patients sensitive to penicillin* —
**Adults:** initially, 200 mg P.O.; then 100 mg q 12 hours for 10 to 15 days.
*Meningococcal carrier state* —
100 mg P.O. q 12 hours for 5 days.
*Uncomplicated urethral, endocervical, or rectal infection caused by* Chlamydia trachomatis *or* Ureaplasma urealyticum —
**Adults:** 100 mg P.O. b.i.d. for at least 7 days.
*Uncomplicated gonococcal urethritis in men* —

**Adults:** 100 mg P.O. b.i.d. for 5 days.

## ADVERSE REACTIONS
**CNS:** headache, *intracranial hypertension (pseudotumor cerebri)*, light-headedness, dizziness, vertigo.
**CV:** pericarditis.
**EENT:** dysphagia, glossitis.
**GI:** *anorexia,* epigastric distress, oral candidiasis, *nausea,* vomiting, *diarrhea,* enterocolitis, inflammatory lesions in anogenital region.
**Hematologic:** neutropenia, eosinophilia, *thrombocytopenia,* hemolytic anemia.
**Skin:** *maculopapular and erythematous rashes, photosensitivity, increased pigmentation, urticaria.*
**Other:** hypersensitivity reactions *(anaphylaxis)*; elevated liver enzymes; increased BUN level; permanent discoloration of teeth, enamel defects, and bone growth retardation if used in children under 8 years; superinfection; *thrombophlebitis.*

## INTERACTIONS
*Antacids (including sodium bicarbonate) and laxatives containing aluminum, magnesium, or calcium; antidiarrheals:* decreased antibiotic absorption. Give antibiotic 1 hour before or 2 hours after any of the above.
*Ferrous sulfate and other iron products, zinc:* decreased antibiotic absorption. Give drug 3 hours after or 2 hours before iron administration.
*Methoxyflurane:* may cause nephrotoxicity with tetracyclines. Monitor carefully.
*Oral anticoagulants:* increased anticoagulant effect. Monitor PT and adjust dosage as ordered.
*Oral contraceptives:* decreased contraceptive effectiveness and increased risk of breakthrough bleeding. Use a nonhormonal form of birth control.
*Penicillins:* may interfere with bactericidal action of penicillins. Avoid using together.

---

Reactions may be *common,* uncommon, *life-threatening,* or COMMON AND LIFE-THREATENING.

## CONTRAINDICATIONS
Contraindicated in patients with hypersensitivity to the drug or other tetracyclines.

## NURSING CONSIDERATIONS
• Use cautiously in patients with impaired renal or hepatic function. Use of these drugs during last half of pregnancy and in children under 8 years may cause permanent discoloration of teeth, enamel defects, and bone growth retardation.
• Obtain specimen for culture and sensitivity tests before first dose. Therapy may begin pending test results.
• *Alert:* Check expiration date. Outdated or deteriorated tetracyclines have been associated with reversible nephrotoxicity (Fanconi's syndrome).
• Don't expose these drugs to light or heat. Keep cap tightly closed.
• **I.V. use:** Reconstitute 100-mg of powder with 5-ml of sterile water for injection, with further dilution of 500 to 1,000 ml for I.V. infusion. Stable for 24 hours at room temperature.
• Be aware that patient may develop thrombophlebitis with I.V. administration of this drug. Avoid extravasation. Switch to oral therapy as soon as possible.
• With large doses or prolonged therapy, monitor for superinfection, especially in high-risk patients.
• Check the patient's tongue for signs of monilia infection. Stress good oral hygiene.
• Be aware that the drug may cause tooth discoloration in young adults. Observe for brown pigmentation, and inform the doctor if it occurs.
• Know that parenteral form may cause false-positive reading of copper sulfate tests (Clinitest). All forms may cause false-negative reading of glucose enzymatic tests (Clinistix, Tes-Tape).

## ☑ PATIENT TEACHING
• Tell the patient to take entire amount of medication exactly as prescribed, even after he feels better.
• Tell the patient to take oral form of drug with a full glass of water. Drug may be taken with food. Tell patient not to take within 1 hour of bedtime to avoid esophagitis.
• Warn the patient to avoid driving or other hazardous tasks until the adverse CNS effects of the drug are known.
• Warn the patient to avoid direct sunlight and ultraviolet light. A sunscreen may help prevent photosensitivity reactions.

# oxytetracycline hydrochloride
Terramycin

*Pregnancy Risk Category: NR*

## HOW SUPPLIED
*Capsules:* 250 mg
*Injection:* 50 mg/ml, 125 mg/ml (with lidocaine 2%)

## ACTION
Unknown. Thought to exert bacteriostatic effect by binding to the 30S ribosomal subunit of microorganisms, thus inhibiting protein synthesis.

## ONSET, PEAK, DURATION
Onset and duration unknown. Serum levels peak within 2 to 4 hours after oral dose, unknown after I.M. injection.

## INDICATIONS & DOSAGE
*Infections caused by sensitive gram-negative and gram-positive organisms, trachoma, rickettsiae –*
**Adults:** 1 to 2 g P.O. in four divided doses, 100 mg I.M. q 8 to 12 hours, or 250 mg I.M. as a single dose.
**Children over 8 years:** 25 to 50 mg/kg P.O. daily, in divided doses q 6

---

*Liquid form contains alcohol.   **May contain tartrazine.   †Canada only.   ‡Australia only.   ◊OTC.

hours; 15 to 25 mg/kg I.M. daily, in divided doses q 8 to 12 hours.
*Brucellosis –*
**Adults:** 500 mg P.O. q.i.d. for 3 weeks combined with 1 g of streptomycin I.M. q 12 hours first week, once daily second week.
*Syphilis in patients sensitive to penicillin –*
**Adults:** 30 to 40 g total dosage P.O., divided equally over 10 to 15 days.
*Gonorrhea in patients sensitive to penicillin –*
**Adults:** initially, 1.5 g P.O., followed by 0.5 g q.i.d., for a total of 9 g.

## ADVERSE REACTIONS
**CNS:** *intracranial hypertension (pseudotumor cerebri).*
**CV:** pericarditis.
**EENT:** dysphagia, glossitis.
**GI:** *anorexia, nausea,* vomiting, *diarrhea,* oral candidiasis, enterocolitis, stomatitis.
**GU:** *proctitis, anogenital inflammation,* vaginitis.
**Hematologic:** neutropenia, eosinophilia.
**Skin:** *maculopapular and erythematous rashes, urticaria, photosensitivity, increased pigmentation.*
**Other:** hypersensitivity reactions *(anaphylaxis);* elevated liver enzymes; permanent discoloration of teeth, enamel defects, and bone growth retardation if used in children under 8 years; superinfection; increased BUN levels; *irritation after I.M. injection; thrombophlebitis.*

## INTERACTIONS
*Antacids (including sodium bicarbonate) and laxatives containing aluminum, magnesium, or calcium; antidiarrheals; food, milk, or other dairy products:* decreased antibiotic absorption. Give antibiotic 1 hour before or 2 hours after any of the above.
*Ferrous sulfate and other iron products, zinc:* decreased antibiotic ab-

sorption. Give antibiotic 3 hours after or 2 hours before iron administration.
*Methoxyflurane:* may cause nephrotoxicity with tetracyclines. Monitor carefully.
*Oral anticoagulants:* increased anticoagulant effect. Monitor PT and adjust dosage as ordered.
*Oral contraceptives:* decreased contraceptive effectiveness and increased risk of breakthrough bleeding. Use a nonhormonal form of birth control.
*Penicillins:* may interfere with bactericidal action of penicillins. Avoid using together.

## CONTRAINDICATIONS
Contraindicated in patients with hypersensitivity to the drug or other tetracyclines.

## NURSING CONSIDERATIONS
• Use cautiously in patients with impaired renal or hepatic function. Use of these drugs during last half of pregnancy and in children under 8 years may cause permanent discoloration of teeth, enamel defects, and bone growth retardation.
• Obtain specimen for culture and sensitivity tests before first dose. Therapy may begin pending test results.
• *Alert:* Check expiration date. Outdated or deteriorated oxytetracyclines have been associated with reversible nephrotoxicity (Fanconi's syndrome).
• Don't expose these drugs to light or heat.
• For I.M. administration, inject deeply into a large muscle mass. Rotate sites. I.M. preparations contain a local anesthetic; ask the patient about hypersensitivity reactions to local anesthetics.
• With large doses or prolonged therapy, monitor for superinfection, especially in high-risk patients.
• Check the patient's tongue for signs of fungal infection. Stress good oral hygiene.

---

Reactions may be *common,* uncommon, *life-threatening,* or **COMMON AND LIFE-THREATENING.**

• Know that parenteral form may cause false-positive reading of copper sulfate tests (Clinitest). All forms may cause false-negative reading of glucose enzymatic tests (Clinistix, Tes-Tape).

☑ **PATIENT TEACHING**
• Tell the patient to take entire amount of medication exactly as prescribed, even after he feels better.
• Explain to the patient that oral drug's effectiveness is reduced when taken with milk or other dairy products, food, antacids, or iron products. Tell him to take each dose with a full glass of water on an empty stomach, at least 1 hour before or 2 hours after meals. Also tell him to take drug at least 1 hour before bedtime to prevent esophagitis.
• Warn the patient that I.M. injection may be painful.
• Warn the patient to avoid direct sunlight and ultraviolet light. A sunscreen may help prevent photosensitivity reactions. Photosensitivity persists for considerable time after discontinuation of drug.

---

**tetracycline hydrochloride**
Achromycin V, Ala-Tet, Apo-Tetra†, Austramycin V‡, Hostacycline P‡, Nor-Tet, Novotetra†, Panmycin**, Panmycin P‡, Robitet, Sumycin, Teline, Tetracap, Tetralan, Tetralean†, Tetram

*Pregnancy Risk Category: NR*

**HOW SUPPLIED**
*Tablets:* 250 mg, 500 mg
*Capsules:* 100 mg, 250 mg, 500 mg
*Oral suspension:* 125 mg/5 ml

**ACTION**
Unknown. Thought to exert bacteriostatic effect by binding to the 30S ribosomal subunit of microorganisms, thus inhibiting protein synthesis.

**ONSET, PEAK, DURATION**
Onset and duration unknown. Serum levels peak within 2 to 4 hours.

**INDICATIONS & DOSAGE**
*Infections caused by sensitive gram-negative and gram-positive organisms, including Rickettsiae, Chlamydia, Mycoplasma, and organisms that cause trachoma –*
**Adults:** 250 to 500 mg P.O. q 6 hours.
**Children over 8 years:** 25 to 50 mg/kg P.O. daily, in divided doses q 6 hours.
*Uncomplicated urethral, endocervical, or rectal infection caused by* Chlamydia trachomatis –
**Adults:** 500 mg P.O. q.i.d. for at least 7 days.
*Brucellosis –*
**Adults:** 500 mg P.O. q 6 hours for 3 weeks combined with 1 g of streptomycin I.M. q 12 hours first week; daily, the second week.
*Gonorrhea in patients sensitive to penicillin –*
**Adults:** initially, 1.5 g P.O.; then 500 mg q 6 hours for a total dose of 9 g.
*Syphilis in patients sensitive to penicillin –*
**Adults:** total of 30 to 40 g P.O. in equally divided doses over 10 to 15 days.
*Acne –*
**Adults and adolescents:** initially, 250 mg P.O. q 6 hours; then 125 to 500 mg daily or q.o.d.

**ADVERSE REACTIONS**
**CNS:** dizziness, headache, *intracranial hypertension (pseudotumor cerebri).*
**CV:** pericarditis.
**EENT:** sore throat, glossitis, dysphagia.
**GI:** anorexia, *epigastric distress, nausea,* vomiting, *diarrhea,* esophagitis, oral candidiasis, stomatitis, enterocolitis, inflammatory lesions in anogenital region.

---

**Hematologic:** neutropenia, eosinophilia.

**Skin:** *candidal superinfection, maculopapular and erythematous rashes, urticaria, photosensitivity, increased pigmentation.*

**Other:** hypersensitivity reactions, elevated liver enzymes, *increased BUN levels, permanent discoloration of teeth, enamel defects, and retardation of bone growth if used in children under 8 years.*

## INTERACTIONS
*Antacids (including sodium bicarbonate) and laxatives containing aluminum, magnesium, or calcium; antidiarrheals containing kaolin, pectin, or bismuth subsalicylate; food, milk, or other dairy products:* decreased antibiotic absorption. Give antibiotic 1 hour before or 2 hours after any of the above.

*Ferrous sulfate and other iron products, zinc:* decreased antibiotic absorption. Give tetracyclines 3 hours after or 2 hours before iron administration.

*Lithium carbonate:* may alter serum lithium levels.

*Methoxyflurane:* may cause severe nephrotoxicity with tetracyclines. Monitor carefully.

*Oral anticoagulants:* potentiated anticoagulant effects. Monitor PT and adjust anticoagulant dosage as ordered.

*Oral contraceptives:* decreased contraceptive effectiveness and increased risk of breakthrough bleeding. Use a nonhormonal form of birth control.

*Penicillins:* may interfere with bactericidal action of penicillins. Avoid using together.

## CONTRAINDICATIONS
Contraindicated in patients with hypersensitivity to tetracyclines.

## NURSING CONSIDERATIONS
● Use with extreme caution in patients with impaired renal or hepatic function. Also use with extreme caution (if at all) during last half of pregnancy and in children under 8 years because drug may cause permanent discoloration of teeth, enamel defects, and bone growth retardation.

● Obtain specimen for culture and sensitivity tests before giving first dose. Therapy may begin pending test results.

● *Alert:* Check expiration date. Outdated or deteriorated tetracyclines have been associated with reversible nephrotoxicity (Fanconi's syndrome).

● Don't expose drug to light or heat.

● With large doses or prolonged therapy, monitor for superinfection, especially in high-risk patients.

● Check the patient's tongue for signs of monilia infection. Stress good oral hygiene.

● Know that drug may cause false-negative reading with glucose enzymatic tests (Clinistix, Tes-Tape).

## ☑ PATIENT TEACHING
● Tell the patient to take drug exactly as prescribed, even after he feels better, and to take entire amount prescribed.

● Explain to the patient that effectiveness is reduced when taken with milk or other dairy products, food, antacids, or iron products. Tell him to take each dose with a full glass of water on an empty stomach, at least 1 hour before or 2 hours after meals. Also tell him to take it at least 1 hour before bedtime to prevent esophagitis.

● Warn the patient to avoid direct sunlight and ultraviolet light. A sunscreen may help prevent photosensitivity reactions. Photosensitivity persists after discontinuation of drug.

---

Reactions may be *common,* uncommon, ***life-threatening,*** or **COMMON AND LIFE-THREATENING.**

# 15

# Sulfonamides

co-trimoxazole
sulfadiazine
sulfamethoxazole
sulfisoxazole
sulfisoxazole acetyl

## COMBINATION PRODUCTS

AZO GANTANOL, AZO SULFAMETH-
OXAZOLE†, URO GANTANOL†:
sulfamethoxazole 500 mg and phenazopyridine hydrochloride 100 mg.
AZO GANTRISIN, AZO SULFISOXA-
ZOLE: sulfisoxazole 500 mg and phenazopyridine hydrochloride 50 mg.
PEDIAZOLE: sulfisoxazole 600 mg
and erythromycin ethylsuccinate 200
mg per 5 ml.
TRIPLE SULFA: sulfadiazine 167 mg,
sulfamerazine 167 mg, and sulfa-
methazine 167 mg.

## co-trimoxazole
(sulfamethoxazole-
trimethoprim)

Apo-Sulfatrim†, Apo-Sulfatrim DS†,
Bactrim*, Bactrim DS, Bactrim I.V.
Infusion, Cotrim, Cotrim D.S.,
Novotrimel†, Novotrimel DS†,
Protrin†, Protrin DF†, Resprim‡,
Roubac†, Roubac DS†, Septra*,
Septra DS, Septra I.V. Infusion,
Septrin‡, SMZ-TMP, Sulfatrim,
Sulmeprim, Trib‡, Uroplus DS,
Uroplus SS

*Pregnancy Risk Category: C
(contraindicated at term)*

## HOW SUPPLIED

*Tablets:* trimethoprim 80 mg and sulfamethoxazole 400 mg; trimethoprim
160 mg and sulfamethoxazole 800 mg
*Oral suspension:* trimethoprim 40 mg
and sulfamethoxazole 200 mg/5 ml
*Injection:* trimethoprim 16 mg and
sulfamethoxazole 80 mg/ml (5 ml/am-
pule)

## ACTION

Sulfamethoxazole inhibits formation
of dihydrofolic acid from PABA; trimethoprim inhibits dihydrofolate reductase. Both decrease bacterial folic
acid synthesis.

## ONSET, PEAK, DURATION

Onset immediate after I.V. administration, unknown after oral administration. Serum levels peak 1 to 4
hours after an oral dose or immediately after an I.V. infusion. Duration
unknown.

## INDICATIONS & DOSAGE

*Urinary tract infections (UTIs) and
shigellosis —*
**Adults:** 160 mg trimethoprim/800 mg
sulfamethoxazole (double strength
tablet) P.O. q 12 hours for 10 to 14
days in UTIs and for 5 days in shigellosis. For simple cystitis or acute urethral syndrome, one to three double-
strength tablets may be given as a single dose. If indicated, I.V. infusion is
given: 8 to 10 mg/kg/day (based on
trimethoprim component) in two to
four divided doses q 6, 8, or 12 hours
for up to 14 days for severe UTIs.
Maximum daily dose is 960 mg trimethoprim.
**Children 2 months and over:** 8 mg/
kg trimethoprim/40 mg/kg sulfamethoxazole P.O. per 24 hours, in two divided doses q 12 hours (10 days for
UTIs; 5 days for shigellosis). If indicated, I.V. infusion is given: 8 to 10
mg/kg/day (based on trimethoprim
component) in two to four divided
doses q 6, 8, or 12 hours. Adult dose
should not be exceeded.

---

*Liquid form contains alcohol.  **May contain tartrazine.  †Canada only.  ‡Australia only.  ◇OTC.

*Otitis media in patients with penicillin allergy or penicillin-resistant infections –*

**Children 2 months and over:** 8 mg/kg trimethoprim/40 mg/kg sulfamethoxazole P.O. per 24 hours, in two divided doses q 12 hours for 10 days.

*Pneumocystis carinii pneumonia –*

**Adults and children 2 months and over:** 15 to 20 mg/kg trimethoprim/100 mg/kg sulfamethoxazole P.O. per 24 hours, in equally divided doses q 6 hours for 14 to 21 days. If indicated, I.V. infusion may be given 15 to 20 mg/kg/day (based on trimethoprim component) in three or four divided doses q 6 to 8 hours for up to 14 days.

*Prophylaxis of P. carinii pneumonia –*

**Adults:** 160 mg trimethoprim/800 mg sulfamethoxazole P.O. daily.

**Children 2 months and over:** 150 mg/m² trimethoprim/750 mg/m² sulfamethoxazole P.O. in equally divided doses b.i.d. on 3 consecutive days per week. Total daily dose should not exceed 320 mg trimethoprim/1,600 mg sulfamethoxazole.

*Chronic bronchitis –*

**Adults:** 160 mg trimethoprim/800 mg sulfamethoxazole P.O. q 12 hours for 10 to 14 days.

*Traveler's diarrhea –*

**Adults:** 160 mg trimethoprim/800 mg sulfamethoxazole P.O. b.i.d. for 3 to 5 days. Some patients may require 2 days of therapy or less.

*UTIs in men with prostatitis –*

**Adults:** 160 mg trimethoprim/800 mg sulfamethoxazole P.O. b.i.d. for 3 to 6 months.

*Chronic UTIs –*

**Adults:** 40 mg trimethoprim/200 mg sulfamethoxazole (½ tablet) or 80 mg trimethoprim/400 mg sulfamethoxazole P.O. daily or three times a week for 3 to 6 months.

## ADVERSE REACTIONS

**CNS:** headache, mental depression, aseptic meningitis, tinnitus, apathy, *seizures,* hallucinations, ataxia, nervousness, fatigue, muscle weakness, vertigo, insomnia.

**GI:** *nausea, vomiting, diarrhea,* abdominal pain, anorexia, stomatitis, pancreatitis, pseudomembranous colitis.

**GU:** *toxic nephrosis with oliguria and anuria,* crystalluria, hematuria, interstitial nephritis.

**Hematologic:** *agranulocytosis, aplastic anemia,* megaloblastic anemia, *thrombocytopenia,* leukopenia, *hemolytic anemia.*

**Hepatic:** jaundice, *hepatic necrosis.*

**Respiratory:** pulmonary infiltrates.

**Skin:** *erythema multiforme (Stevens-Johnson syndrome), generalized skin eruption, epidermal necrolysis, exfoliative dermatitis,* photosensitivity, urticaria, pruritus.

**Other:** hypersensitivity reactions (*serum sickness, drug fever, anaphylaxis*), thrombophlebitis, arthralgia, myalgia.

## INTERACTIONS

*Oral anticoagulants:* increased anticoagulant effect. Monitor for bleeding.

*Oral antidiabetic agents:* increased hypoglycemic effect. Monitor blood glucose levels.

*Oral contraceptives:* decreased contraceptive effectiveness and increased risk of breakthrough bleeding. Suggest a nonhormonal contraceptive.

*Phenytoin:* may inhibit hepatic metabolism of phenytoin. Monitor closely.

*Zidovudine:* may increase serum levels of zidovudine due to decreased renal clearance. Monitor closely.

## CONTRAINDICATIONS

Contraindicated in patients with hypersensitivity to trimethoprim or sulfonamides, severe renal impairment (creatinine clearance less than 15 ml/minute), or porphyria; in megaloblastic anemia caused by folate deficiency; in pregnant women at term; in breast-feeding women; and in children under 2 months.

---

Reactions may be *common,* uncommon, *life-threatening,* or COMMON AND LIFE-THREATENING.

## NURSING CONSIDERATIONS
- Use cautiously and in reduced dosages in patients with impaired hepatic or renal function (creatinine clearance of 15 to 30 ml/minute), severe allergy or bronchial asthma, G6PD deficiency, and blood dyscrasia.
- Obtain specimen for culture and sensitivity tests before first dose. Therapy may begin pending results.
- Note that the "DS" or "DF" product means "double strength."
- **I.V. use:** Dilute I.V. infusion in $D_5W$ before administration. Don't mix with other drugs or solutions. Infuse slowly over 60 to 90 minutes. Don't give by rapid infusion or bolus injection. Don't refrigerate and use within 6 hours.
- Never administer I.M.
- Promptly report complaints of skin rash, sore throat, fever, or mouth sores — early signs of blood dyscrasia.
- Watch for superinfection (fever or other signs of new infection).
- **Alert:** Be aware that adverse reactions, especially hypersensitivity reactions, rash, and fever, occur much more frequently in AIDS patients.

## ☑ PATIENT TEACHING
- Tell the patient to take drug as prescribed, even if he feels better.
- Encourage adequate fluid intake.
- Tell the patient to report adverse reactions promptly.
- Instruct patient receiving drug I.V. to alert nurse if discomfort occurs at I.V. insertion site.

---

# sulfadiazine

*Pregnancy Risk Category: C (contraindicated at term)*

## HOW SUPPLIED
*Tablets:* 500 mg

## ACTION
Inhibits formation of dihydrofolic acid from PABA, decreasing bacterial folic acid synthesis.

## ONSET, PEAK, DURATION
Onset and duration unknown. Serum levels peak within 6 hours of oral dose.

## INDICATIONS & DOSAGE
*Urinary tract infection —*
**Adults:** initially, 2 to 4 g P.O., then 2 to 4 g daily in three to six doses q 24 hours.
**Children 2 months and over:** initially, 75 mg/kg or 2 g/m² P.O., then 150 mg/kg or 4 g/m² P.O. in four to six divided doses daily. Maximum daily dosage is 6 g.
*Rheumatic fever prophylaxis, as an alternative to penicillin —*
**Children over 30 kg:** 1 g P.O. daily.
**Children under 30 kg:** 500 mg P.O. daily.
*Adjunct treatment in toxoplasmosis —*
**Adults:** 2 to 8 g P.O. daily. Usually given with pyrimethamine.
**Children:** 100 to 200 mg/kg P.O. daily. Usually given with pyrimethamine.

## ADVERSE REACTIONS
**CNS:** headache, mental depression, *seizures,* hallucinations.
**GI:** *nausea, vomiting, diarrhea,* abdominal pain, anorexia, stomatitis.
**GU:** *toxic nephrosis* with oliguria and anuria, crystalluria, hematuria.
**Hematologic:** *agranulocytosis, aplastic anemia,* megaloblastic anemia, *thrombocytopenia,* leukopenia, *hemolytic anemia.*
**Skin:** *erythema multiforme (Stevens-Johnson syndrome), generalized skin eruption, epidermal necrolysis, exfoliative dermatitis,* photosensitivity, urticaria, pruritus.
**Other:** hypersensitivity reactions (*serum sickness, drug fever, anaphylaxis*), jaundice, local irritation, extravasation.

---

*Liquid form contains alcohol.   **May contain tartrazine.   †Canada only.   ‡Australia only.   ◇OTC.

## INTERACTIONS

*Oral anticoagulants:* increased anticoagulant effect. Monitor for bleeding.
*Oral antidiabetic agents:* increased hypoglycemic effect. Monitor blood glucose levels.
*Oral contraceptives:* decreased contraceptive effectiveness and increased risk of breakthrough bleeding. Suggest a nonhormonal contraceptive.
*PABA-containing drugs:* inhibited antibacterial action. Don't use together.

## CONTRAINDICATIONS

Contraindicated in patients with hypersensitivity to sulfonamides, in those with porphyria, in infants under age 2 months (except in congenital toxoplasmosis), in pregnant women at term, and during breast-feeding.

## NURSING CONSIDERATIONS

• Use cautiously and in reduced doses in patients with impaired hepatic or renal function, bronchial asthma, history of multiple allergies, G6PD deficiency, and blood dyscrasia.
• Obtain specimen for culture and sensitivity tests before first dose. Therapy may begin pending results.
• Give drug on schedule to maintain constant blood level.
• Monitor for signs of blood dyscrasia (purpura, ecchymoses, sore throat, fever, and pallor). Report them immediately.
• Monitor urine cultures, CBCs, and urinalyses before and during therapy, as ordered.
• Watch for superinfection (fever or other signs of new infection).
• Be aware that folic or folinic acid may be used during rest periods in toxoplasmosis therapy to reverse hematopoietic depression or anemia associated with pyrimethamine and sulfadiazine.
• Monitor fluid intake and output. Intake should be sufficient to produce output of 1,500 ml daily (between 3,000 and 4,000 ml daily for adults). If fluid intake is not adequate enough to prevent crystalluria, sodium bicarbonate may be administered to alkalinize urine, as ordered. Monitor urine pH daily.

## ☑ PATIENT TEACHING

• Tell the patient to take drug as prescribed, even if he feels better.
• Tell him to drink a glass of water with each dose and plenty of water each day to prevent crystalluria.
• Instruct the patient to report adverse reactions promptly.
• Warn the patient to avoid sunlight.

---

# sulfamethoxazole (sulphamethoxazole)
Apo-Sulfamethoxazole†, Gantanol, Gantanol DS

*Pregnancy Risk Category: C (contraindicated at term)*

## HOW SUPPLIED
*Tablets:* 500 mg
*Oral suspension:* 500 mg/5 ml

## ACTION
Inhibits formation of dihydrofolic acid from PABA, decreasing bacterial folic acid synthesis.

## ONSET, PEAK, DURATION
Onset and duration unknown. Serum levels peak within 2 hours of oral dose.

## INDICATIONS & DOSAGE
*Urinary tract and systemic infections –*
**Adults:** initially, 2 g P.O., then 1 g P.O. b.i.d. up to t.i.d. for severe infections.
**Children and infants over 2 months:** initially, 50 to 60 mg/kg P.O., then 25 to 30 mg/kg b.i.d. Maximum dosage should not exceed 75 mg/kg daily.

---

Reactions may be *common,* uncommon, *life-threatening,* or COMMON AND LIFE-THREATENING.

## ADVERSE REACTIONS

**CNS:** headache, mental depression, *seizures*, hallucinations, aseptic meningitis, tinnitus, apathy.

**GI:** *nausea, vomiting, diarrhea*, abdominal pain, anorexia, stomatitis, pancreatitis, pseudomembranous colitis.

**GU:** *toxic nephrosis with oliguria and anuria*, crystalluria, hematuria, interstitial nephritis.

**Hematologic:** *agranulocytosis, aplastic anemia*, megaloblastic anemia, thrombocytopenia, leukopenia, *hemolytic anemia*.

**Skin:** *erythema multiforme (Stevens-Johnson syndrome), generalized skin eruption, epidermal necrolysis, exfoliative dermatitis*, photosensitivity, urticaria, pruritus.

**Other:** hypersensitivity reactions (*serum sickness, drug fever, anaphylaxis*), *jaundice*.

## INTERACTIONS

*Oral anticoagulants:* increased anticoagulant effect. Monitor for bleeding.
*Oral antidiabetic agents:* increased hypoglycemic effect. Monitor blood glucose levels.
*Oral contraceptives:* decreased contraceptive effectiveness and increased risk of breakthrough bleeding. Suggest a nonhormonal contraceptive.
*Phenytoin:* may increase phenytoin effect. Monitor closely.

## CONTRAINDICATIONS

Contraindicated in patients with hypersensitivity to sulfonamides; in those with porphyria, in infants under 2 months (except in congenital toxoplasmosis), in pregnant women at term, and during breast-feeding.

## NURSING CONSIDERATIONS

• Use cautiously and in reduced dosages in patients with impaired hepatic or renal function, severe allergy or bronchial asthma, G6PD deficiency, and blood dyscrasia.

• Obtain specimen for culture and sensitivity tests before first dose. Therapy may begin pending results.
• Monitor urine cultures, CBCs, and urinalyses before and during therapy, as ordered.
• Watch for superinfection (fever or other signs of new infection).
• Monitor fluid intake and output. Intake should be sufficient to produce output of 1,500 ml daily (between 3,000 and 4,000 ml daily for adults). If fluid intake is not adequate enough to prevent crystalluria, sodium bicarbonate may be administered to alkalinize urine, as ordered. Monitor urine pH daily.

## ☑ PATIENT TEACHING

• Tell the patient to take drug as prescribed, even if he feels better.
• Tell him to drink a glass of water with each dose and plenty of water each day to prevent crystalluria.
• **Alert:** Tell the patient to report early signs of blood dyscrasia (sore throat, fever, and pallor) to the doctor.
• Warn the patient to avoid sunlight.

---

# sulfisoxazole (sulfafurazole, sulphafurazole)
Azo-Sulfisoxazole†‡, Gantrisin, Novosoxazole†

# sulfisoxazole acetyl
Gantrisin Pediatric

*Pregnancy Risk Category: C (contraindicated at term)*

## HOW SUPPLIED
**sulfisoxazole**
*Tablets:* 500 mg
**sulfisosoxazole acetyl**
*Liquid:* 500 mg/5 ml

## ACTION
Inhibits formation of dihydrofolic acid from PABA, decreasing bacterial folic acid synthesis.

---

*Liquid form contains alcohol. **May contain tartrazine. †Canada only. ‡Australia only. ◊OTC.

## ONSET, PEAK, DURATION
Onset and duration unknown. Serum levels peak in 2 to 4 hours.

## INDICATIONS & DOSAGE
*Urinary tract and systemic infections –*
**Adults:** initially, 2 to 4 g P.O., then 4 to 8 g in 24 hours divided in four to six doses.

**Children over 2 months:** initially, 75 mg/kg P.O. daily or 2 g/m$^2$ P.O. daily in divided doses q 6 hours, then 150 mg/kg or 4 g/m$^2$ P.O. daily in divided doses q 6 hours. Total daily dose should not exceed 6 gm.

## ADVERSE REACTIONS
**CNS:** headache, mental depression, *seizures,* hallucinations.
**CV:** tachycardia, palpitations, syncope, cyanosis.
**GI:** *nausea, vomiting, diarrhea,* abdominal pain, anorexia, stomatitis, *hepatitis,* pseudomembranous colitis.
**GU:** *toxic nephrosis with oliguria and anuria,* crystalluria, hematuria, *acute renal failure.*
**Hematologic:** *agranulocytosis, aplastic anemia,* megaloblastic anemia, *thrombocytopenia,* leukopenia, *hemolytic anemia.*
**Skin:** *erythema multiforme, generalized skin eruption, epidermal necrolysis, exfoliative dermatitis,* photosensitivity, urticaria, pruritus.
**Other:** hypersensitivity reactions (*serum sickness, drug fever, anaphylaxis*), jaundice.

## INTERACTIONS
*Oral anticoagulants:* increased anticoagulant effect. Monitor for bleeding.
*Oral antidiabetic agents:* increased hypoglycemic effect. Monitor blood glucose levels.
*Oral contraceptives:* decreased contraceptive effectiveness, increased risk of breakthrough bleeding. Suggest a nonhormonal contraceptive.

## CONTRAINDICATIONS
Contraindicated in patients with hypersensitivity to sulfonamines, in infants under 2 months (except in congenital toxoplasmosis), in pregnant women at term, and during breastfeeding.

## NURSING CONSIDERATIONS
• Use cautiously in patients with impaired hepatic or renal function, severe allergy or bronchial asthma, and G6PD deficiency.
• Obtain specimen for culture and sensitivity tests before first dose. Therapy may begin pending results.
• Monitor urine cultures, CBCs, PT, and urinalyses before and during therapy, as ordered.
• When drug is given preoperatively, be aware that the patient should receive a low-residue diet and a minimal number of enemas and cathartics.
• Watch for superinfection (fever or other signs of new infection).
• Monitor fluid intake and output. Maintain intake between 3,000 and 4,000 ml daily for adults to produce output of 1,500 ml daily. If fluid intake is not adequate enough to prevent crystalluria, sodium bicarbonate may be administered to alkalinize urine, as ordered. Monitor urine pH daily.

## ☑ PATIENT TEACHING
• Tell the patient to take drug as prescribed, even if he feels better.
• Tell him to drink a glass of water with each dose and plenty of water each day to prevent crystalluria.
• **Alert:** Tell the patient to report early signs of blood dyscrasia (sore throat, fever, and pallor) to the doctor.
• Warn the patient to avoid sunlight.

---

Reactions may be *common,* uncommon, *life-threatening,* or **COMMON AND LIFE-THREATENING.**

# 16

# Fluoroquinolones

cinoxacin
ciprofloxacin
enoxacin
lomefloxacin hydrochloride
nalidixic acid
norfloxacin
ofloxacin

## COMBINATION PRODUCTS
None.

## cinoxacin
Cinobac

*Pregnancy Risk Category: B*

### HOW SUPPLIED
*Capsules:* 250 mg, 500 mg

### ACTION
Inhibits microbial DNA synthesis.

### ONSET, PEAK, DURATION
Onset unknown. Plasma levels peak within 2 hours of an oral dose; urine levels peak in 2 to 4 hours. Urine levels of the drug remain sufficient for antimicrobial effect for at least 12 hours after a dose.

### INDICATIONS & DOSAGE
*Initial and recurrent urinary tract infections caused by susceptible strains of* Escherichia coli, Klebsiella, Enterobacter, Proteus mirabilis, P. vulgaris, P. Serratia, *and* Citrobacter —
**Adults and children over 12 years:** 1 g P.O. daily, in two to four divided doses for 7 to 14 days.

### ADVERSE REACTIONS
**CNS:** *dizziness, headache,* drowsiness, insomnia.
**EENT:** tinnitus, photophobia.
**GI:** *nausea, vomiting, abdominal pain,* diarrhea, distorted taste.
**Skin:** rash, urticaria, pruritus, photosensitivity, erythema multiforme, toxic epidermal necrolysis.
**Other:** elevated liver enzymes, Stevens-Johnson syndrome, *thrombocytopenia, anaphylaxis.*

### INTERACTIONS
*Oral anticoagulants:* increased anticoagulant effect. Monitor for bleeding.
*Probenecid:* may decrease urine levels of cinoxacin by inhibiting renal tubular secretion. Monitor for increased toxicity and reduced antibacterial effectiveness.
*Theophylline, caffeine:* increased effects of these drugs. Monitor closely.

### CONTRAINDICATIONS
Contraindicated in patients with hypersensitivity to the drug or other fluoroquinolones.

### NURSING CONSIDERATIONS
• Use cautiously in patients with impaired renal and hepatic function.
• Obtain clean-catch urine specimen for culture and sensitivity tests before starting therapy and repeat p.r.n. Therapy may begin pending results.
• Give cinoxacin with meals to help decrease adverse GI reactions.
• *Alert:* Report adverse CNS reactions to the doctor immediately. They indicate serious toxicity and usually mean that drug therapy should be stopped.

### ☑ PATIENT TEACHING
• Tell the patient to take drug as prescribed, even if he feels better.
• Instruct the patient to take drug with meals.
• Tell the patient to report adverse reactions promptly, especially CNS reactions.

---

*Liquid form contains alcohol. **May contain tartrazine. †Canada only. ‡Australia only. ◊OTC.

• Warn the patient about photosensitizing effects of the drug, and advise him to avoid bright sunlight and to wear sunblock.

---

# ciprofloxacin
Cipro, Cipro I.V., Ciproxin‡

*Pregnancy Risk Category: C*

## HOW SUPPLIED
*Tablets:* 250 mg, 500 mg, 750 mg
*Infusion (premixed):* 200 mg in 100 ml $D_5W$, 400 mg in 200 ml $D_5W$
*Injection:* 200 mg, 400 mg

## ACTION
Unknown. Bactericidal effects may result from drug's inhibiting bacterial DNA gyrase and preventing replication in susceptible bacteria.

## ONSET, PEAK, DURATION
Onset immediate after I.V. administration, unknown after oral administration. Serum levels peak 0.5 to 2.3 hours after oral administration, immediately after I.V. administration. Duration unknown.

## INDICATIONS & DOSAGE
*Mild to moderate urinary tract infections* –
**Adults:** 250 mg P.O. or 200 mg I.V. q 12 hours.
*Severe or complicated urinary tract infections; mild to moderate bone and joint infections; mild to moderate respiratory tract infections; mild to moderate skin and skin-structure infections; infectious diarrhea* –
**Adults:** 500 mg P.O. or 400 mg I.V. q 12 hours.
*Severe or complicated bone or joint infections; severe respiratory tract infections; severe skin and skin-structure infections* –
**Adults:** 750 mg P.O. q 12 hours.
*Uncomplicated cervical or urethral gonorrhea due to* Neisseria gonorrhoeae –

**Adults:** 250 mg P.O. as single dose.

## ADVERSE REACTIONS
**CNS:** headache, restlessness, tremor, dizziness, fatigue, drowsiness, insomnia, depression, light-headedness, confusion, hallucinations, *seizures,* paresthesia.
**GI:** *nausea, diarrhea,* vomiting, abdominal pain or discomfort, oral candidiasis, pseudomembranous colitis, dyspepsia, flatulence, constipation.
**GU:** crystalluria, increased serum creatinine and BUN levels, interstitial nephritis.
**Musculoskeletal:** arthralgia, joint or back pain, joint inflammation, joint stiffness, aching, neck or chest pain.
**Skin:** *rash,* photosensitivity, toxic epidermal necrolysis, exfoliative dermatitis.
**Other:** photosensitivity, elevated liver enzymes, Stevens-Johnson syndrome, hypersensitivity; with I.V. administration – thrombophlebitis, burning, pruritus, erythema, edema.

## INTERACTIONS
*Antacids containing magnesium hydroxide or aluminum hydroxide, sucralfate, iron supplements, zinc or iron containing multivitamins:* decreased ciprofloxacin absorption. Separate administration by at least 2 hours.
*Caffeine:* increased effect of caffeine. Monitor closely.
*Probenecid:* may elevate serum level of ciprofloxacin. Monitor for toxicity.
*Theophylline:* increased plasma theophylline concentrations and prolonged theophylline half-life. Monitor blood levels of theophylline and observe for adverse effects.

## CONTRAINDICATIONS
Contraindicated in patients sensitive to fluoroquinolone antibiotics.

---

Reactions may be *common,* uncommon, *life-threatening,* or **COMMON AND LIFE-THREATENING.**

## NURSING CONSIDERATIONS
• Use cautiously in patients with CNS disorders, such as severe cerebral arteriosclerosis or seizure disorders, and in those at an increased risk for seizures. May cause CNS stimulation.
• Obtain specimen for culture and sensitivity tests before first dose. Therapy may begin pending results.
• Administer oral form 2 hours after a meal or 2 hours before or after taking antacids, sucralfate, or products that contain iron (such as vitamins with mineral supplements). Food does not affect absorption but may delay peak serum levels.
• **I.V. use:** Dilute drug using $D_5W$ or 0.9% sodium chloride for injection to a final concentration of 1 to 2 mg/ml before use. Infuse slowly (over 1 hour) into a large vein.
• Be aware that dosage adjustments are necessary in patients with renal dysfunction.
• Know that long-term therapy may result in overgrowth of organisms resistant to ciprofloxacin.

## ☑ PATIENT TEACHING
• Tell the patient to take drug as prescribed, even if he feels better.
• Advise him to drink plenty of fluids to reduce the risk of crystalluria.
• Warn the patient to avoid hazardous tasks that require alertness, such as driving, until CNS effects of the drug are known.
• Advise the patient to avoid caffeine while taking the drug because of potential for cumulative caffeine effects.
• Advise the patient that hypersensitivity reactions may occur even after first dose. If he notices a rash or other allergic reaction, he should stop taking the drug immediately and notify the doctor.
• Tell him to avoid excessive sunlight or artificial ultraviolet light during therapy and to stop drug and call the doctor if phototoxicity occurs.
• Instruct the patient to discontinue breast-feeding during treatment or ask to be treated with another drug. Drug is excreted in breast milk.

---

# enoxacin
Penetrex

*Pregnancy Risk Category: C*

## HOW SUPPLIED
*Tablets:* 200 mg, 400 mg

## ACTION
Inhibits bacterial DNA synthesis, mainly by blocking DNA gyrase. Bactericidal.

## ONSET, PEAK, DURATION
Onset and duration unknown. Serum levels peak in 1 to 3 hours.

## INDICATIONS & DOSAGE
*Uncomplicated urinary tract infections (UTIs)* –
**Adults:** 200 mg P.O. q 12 hours for 7 days.
*Severe or complicated UTIs* –
**Adults:** 400 mg P.O. q 12 hours for 14 days.
*Uncomplicated urethral or endocervical gonorrhea* –
**Adults:** 400 mg P.O. as a single dose.
Doxycycline therapy may follow to treat possible coexisting chlamydial infection.
In patients with renal failure: If creatinine clearance is 30 ml/minute or greater, therapy started with usual initial dose. Subsequent doses are decreased by 50%.

## ADVERSE REACTIONS
**CNS:** headache, restlessness, tremor, light-headedness, confusion, hallucinations, *seizures*.
**GI:** *nausea, diarrhea,* vomiting, abdominal pain or discomfort, oral candidiasis.
**GU:** crystalluria.
**Other:** *rash,* photosensitivity, eosino-

---

*Liquid form contains alcohol.   **May contain tartrazine.   †Canada only.   ‡Australia only.   ◇OTC.

philia, dyspnea, cough, elevated liver enzymes, pruritus, hypersensitivity.

## INTERACTIONS
*Aminophylline, cyclosporine, caffeine, theophylline:* increased levels of these drugs because of decreased metabolism. Use together cautiously.
*Antacids containing magnesium hydroxide or aluminum hydroxide, oral iron supplements, sucralfate:* decreased enoxacin absorption. Separate administration times by at least 2 hours.
*Bismuth subsalicylate:* bioavailability of enoxacin is decreased when given within 60 minutes of bismuth subsalicylate. Avoid concomitant use.
*Digoxin:* may increase digoxin serum levels. Monitor closely for toxicity.
*Oral anticoagulants:* increased anticoagulant effect. Use together cautiously.

## CONTRAINDICATIONS
Contraindicated in patients with hypersensitivity to the drug or other fluoroquinolone antibiotics.

## NURSING CONSIDERATIONS
● Use cautiously in patients with CNS disorders, such as severe cerebral arteriosclerosis or seizure disorders, and in those at increased risk for seizures. May cause CNS stimulation.
● Use cautiously and with dosage adjustments in patients with impaired renal or hepatic function.
● Obtain specimen for culture and sensitivity tests before first dose. Therapy may begin pending results.
● *Alert:* Patients being treated for gonorrhea should have an initial serologic test for syphilis before therapy starts. Drug has not been effective in treating syphilis and may mask signs and symptoms of infection. Have the serologic test repeated in 1 to 3 months.
● Administer 2 hours after a meal or 2 hours before or after antacids containing magnesium hydroxide or aluminum hydroxide, sucralfate, or prod-

ucts that contain iron (such as vitamins with mineral supplements).
● Monitor closely for superinfection.

## ☑ PATIENT TEACHING
● Tell the patient to take drug as prescribed, even if he feels better.
● Instruct the patient to take drug on an empty stomach.
● Advise him to drink plenty of fluids to reduce risk of crystalluria.
● Warn the patient to avoid hazardous tasks until adverse CNS effects of the drug are known.
● Warn the patient not to drink beverages containing caffeine. Enoxacin inhibits the metabolism of caffeine and can result in toxicity.
● Advise the patient to avoid overexposure to direct sunlight and to use a sunblock and wear protective clothing while outdoors.

# lomefloxacin hydrochloride
Maxaquin

*Pregnancy Risk Category: C*

## HOW SUPPLIED
*Tablets (film-coated):* 400 mg

## ACTION
Inhibits bacterial DNA gyrase, an enzyme necessary for bacterial replication (bactericidal).

## ONSET, PEAK, DURATION
Onset and duration unknown. Plasma levels peak 1½ hours after oral dose.

## INDICATIONS & DOSAGE
*Acute bacterial exacerbations of chronic bronchitis caused by* Haemophilus influenzae *or* Moraxella (Branhamella) catarrhalis —
**Adults:** 400 mg P.O. daily for 10 days.
*Uncomplicated urinary tract infections (cystitis) caused by* Escherichia coli, Klebsiella pneumoniae, Proteus mirabilis, *or* Staphylococcus saprophyticus —

---

Reactions may be *common,* uncommon, *life-threatening,* or COMMON AND LIFE-THREATENING.

**Adults:** 400 mg P.O. daily for 10 days.
*Complicated urinary tract infections
caused by* E. coli, K. pneumoniae, P.
mirabilis, *or* Pseudomonas aeruginosa; *possibly effective against infections caused by* Citrobacter diversus
*or* Enterobacter cloacae –
**Adults:** 400 mg P.O. daily for 14 days.
*Prophylaxis of infections after trans-
urethral surgical procedures –*
**Adults:** 400 mg P.O. as a single dose
2 to 6 hours before surgery.

Patients with a creatinine clearance
of 10 to 40 ml/minute should receive a
loading dose of 400 mg P.O. on the first
day, followed by 200 mg daily for the
duration of therapy. Hemodialysis removes negligible amounts of drug.

## ADVERSE REACTIONS

**CNS:** *dizziness, headache,* abnormal
dreams, **fatigue,** malaise, asthenia,
agitation, anorexia, anxiety, confusion, depersonalization, depression,
increased appetite, insomnia, nervousness, somnolence, *seizures,
coma,* hyperkinesia, tremor, vertigo,
paresthesia, arthralgia, myalgia.
**CV:** flushing, hypotension, hypertension, edema, syncope, arrhythmia,
tachycardia, bradycardia, extrasystoles, cyanosis, angina pectoris, *MI,
cardiac failure, pulmonary embolism,* cerebrovascular disorder, cardiomyopathy, phlebitis.
**EENT:** epistaxis, abnormal vision,
conjunctivitis, eye pain, earache, tinnitus, tongue discoloration, taste
perversion.
**GI:** *diarrhea, nausea,* dry mouth,
leukorrhea, pseudomembranous colitis, abdominal pain, dyspepsia, vomiting, flatulence, constipation, inflammation, dysphagia, bleeding.
**GU:** dysuria, hematuria, anuria, epididymitis, orchitis, vaginitis, vaginal
moniliasis, intermenstrual bleeding,
perineal pain.
**Hematologic:** thrombocythemia,
*thrombocytopenia,* lymphadenopathy,
increased fibrinolysis.

**Respiratory:** dyspnea, *bronchospasm,* respiratory disorder or infection, increased sputum, stridor.
**Skin:** pruritus, skin disorder, skin ex-
foliation, eczema, rash, urticaria,
*photosensitivity.*
**Other:** *anaphylaxis,* increased diaphoresis, leg cramps, thirst, chest or
back pain, chills, allergic reaction, facial edema, flulike symptoms, decreased heat tolerance, hypoglycemia,
elevated liver enzymes, gout.

## INTERACTIONS

*Antacids, sucralfate:* impaired absorption after binding with lomefloxacin in GI tract. Give no less than 4
hours before or 2 hours after a dose.
*Cimetidine:* increased half-life of
other fluoroquinolones when administered to patients taking cimetidine; lomefloxacin has not been tested. Monitor for toxicity.
*Probenecid:* decreased excretion of
lomefloxacin. Monitor for toxicity.
*Warfarin, cyclosporine:* increased effects or serum levels when combined
with other fluoroquinolones; lomefloxacin has not been tested. Monitor
for toxicity.

## CONTRAINDICATIONS

Contraindicated in patients with hypersensitivity to lomefloxacin or other
fluoroquinolones.

## NURSING CONSIDERATIONS

● Use cautiously in patients with
known or suspected CNS disorders,
such as seizure disorder or cerebral
arteriosclerosis, that may predispose
the patient to seizures.
● Obtain culture and sensitivity tests
before first dose. Therapy may begin
pending results.
● Be aware that although most fluoroquinolones exhibit photosensitizing
effects, early studies suggest that pho-
tosensitization and phototoxicity are
more common with lomefloxacin.
● Keep in mind that prolonged use

may result in overgrowth of organisms resistant to lomefloxacin.

### ☑ PATIENT TEACHING
• Tell the patient to take drug as prescribed, even if he feels better.
• Advise the patient that hypersensitivity reactions may occur even after first dose. If rash or other allergic reaction occurs, the patient should stop taking the drug and notify the doctor.
• Warn the patient to avoid hazardous tasks until CNS effects of drug are known.
• Advise the patient to wear protective clothing, use a sunblock, and avoid prolonged exposure to sunlight during treatment and for a few days after therapy ends. If sunburn occurs, the patient should call the doctor as soon as possible.

---

## nalidixic acid
NegGram

*Pregnancy Risk Category: B (safe use in first trimester not known)*

### HOW SUPPLIED
*Tablets:* 250 mg, 500 mg, 1 g
*Oral suspension:* 250 mg/5 ml

### ACTION
Inhibits microbial DNA synthesis by bacterial DNA gyrase.

### ONSET, PEAK, DURATION
Onset and duration unknown. Serum levels peak 1 to 2 hours after an oral dose. Urine levels peak 3 to 4 hours after a dose.

### INDICATIONS & DOSAGE
*Acute and chronic urinary tract infections caused by susceptible gram-negative organisms* (Proteus, Klebsiella, Enterobacter, *and* Escherichia coli) —
**Adults:** 1 g P.O. q.i.d. for 7 to 14 days; 2 g daily for long-term use.
**Children over 3 months:** 55 mg/kg

P.O. daily divided q.i.d. for 7 to 14 days; 33 mg/kg daily for long-term use.

### ADVERSE REACTIONS
**CNS:** drowsiness, weakness, headache, dizziness, vertigo, *seizures,* malaise, confusion, hallucinations, psychosis.
**EENT:** sensitivity to light, change in color perception, diplopia, blurred vision.
**GI:** *abdominal pain, nausea, vomiting,* diarrhea.
**Hematologic:** eosinophilia, *leukopenia, thrombocytopenia,* hemolytic anemia.
**Skin:** pruritus, photosensitivity, urticaria, rash.
**Other:** angioedema, *increased intracranial pressure and bulging fontanelles in infants and children,* arthralgia, joint stiffness, anaphylactoid reaction.

### INTERACTIONS
*Nitrofurantoin:* decreased nalidixic acid effectiveness. Avoid concomitant use.
*Oral anticoagulants:* increased anticoagulant effect. Monitor for bleeding.

### CONTRAINDICATIONS
Contraindicated in patients with hypersensitivity to the drug, in those with seizure disorders, and in infants under 3 months.

### NURSING CONSIDERATIONS
• Use with extreme caution in prepubertal children; erosion of cartilage of immature animals has been reported.
• Use cautiously in patients with impaired hepatic or renal function or with severe cerebral arteriosclerosis.
• Use cautiously in patients with pulmonary disease; nalidixic acid may increase respiratory depression in those with respiratory impairment.
• Obtain specimen for culture and sensitivity tests before starting ther-

---

Reactions may be *common,* uncommon, *life-threatening,* or COMMON AND LIFE-THREATENING.

apy and repeat p.r.n. Therapy may begin pending results.

• Monitor CBC, renal, and liver function studies during long-term therapy, as ordered.

• Be aware that resistant bacteria may emerge in the first 48 hours of therapy.

• Know that drug may cause a false-positive Clinitest reaction. Use Clinistix or Tes-Tape to monitor urine glucose. Also may cause false elevations in urine vanilmandelic acid and 17-ketosteroids. Tests should be repeated after therapy is completed.

### ☑ PATIENT TEACHING

• Tell the patient to take drug as prescribed, even if he feels better.

• Instruct the patient to take drug 1 hour before meals.

• Tell the patient to avoid undue exposure to sunlight.

• Tell the patient to report visual disturbances; these usually disappear with reduced dose.

---

## norfloxacin
Noroxin

*Pregnancy Risk Category: C*

### HOW SUPPLIED
*Film-coated tablets:* 400 mg

### ACTION
Inhibits bacterial DNA synthesis, mainly by blocking DNA gyrase. Bactericidal.

### ONSET, PEAK, DURATION
Onset and duration unknown. Plasma levels peak 1 to 2 hours after oral dose.

### INDICATIONS & DOSAGE
*Complicated or uncomplicated urinary tract infections caused by susceptible strains of* Escherichia coli, Klebsiella, Enterobacter, Proteus, Pseudomonas aeruginosa, Citrobacter, Staphylococcus aureus *(and* epi-

dermidis*), and group D strepto-cocci —*
**Adults:** for uncomplicated infections, 400 mg P.O. b.i.d. for 7 to 10 days. For complicated infections, 400 mg b.i.d. for 10 to 21 days.
*Cystitis caused by* E. coli, Klebsiella pneumoniae, *or* P. mirabilis —
**Adults:** 400 mg P.O. b.i.d. for 3 days.
*Acute, uncomplicated gonorrhea —*
**Adults:** 800 mg P.O. as a single dose, followed by doxycycline therapy to treat any coexisting chlamydial infection. Adults with creatinine clearance 30 ml/minute or less should receive 400 mg once daily.

### ADVERSE REACTIONS
**CNS:** fatigue, somnolence, headache, dizziness, *seizures,* depression, insomnia.
**GI:** nausea, constipation, flatulence, heartburn, dry mouth, abdominal pain, diarrhea, vomiting, anorexia.
**GU:** increased serum creatinine and BUN levels, crystalluria.
**Hematologic:** eosinophilia.
**Musculoskeletal:** back pain.
**Skin:** rash, photosensitivity.
**Other:** hypersensitivity reactions (rash, *anaphylactoid reaction*), transient elevations of AST and ALT, fever, hyperhidrosis.

### INTERACTIONS
*Antacids, iron products, sucralfate:* may hinder absorption. Separate administration times by 2 hours.
*Cyclosporine:* increased serum concentrations of cyclosporine. Monitor serum levels.
*Nitrofurantoin:* decreased norfloxacin effectiveness. Don't use together.
*Oral anticoagulants:* increased anticoagulant effect. monitor closely.
*Probenecid:* may increase serum levels of norfloxacin by decreasing its excretion. Monitor for toxicity.
*Theophylline:* possibly impaired theophylline metabolism, resulting in in-

---

creased plasma levels and risk of toxicity. Monitor closely.

**CONTRAINDICATIONS**
Contraindicated in patients with hypersensitivity to fluoroquinolones.

**NURSING CONSIDERATIONS**
• Use cautiously in patients with conditions that may predispose them to seizure disorders, such as cerebral arteriosclerosis. Also use cautiously in those with renal impairment.

☑ **PATIENT TEACHING**
• Tell the patient to take drug as prescribed, even if he feels better.
• Advise the patient to take the drug 1 hour before or 2 hours after meals because food, antacids, iron products, and sucralfate may hinder absorption.
• Warn the patient not to exceed the recommended dosages and to drink several glasses of water throughout the day to maintain hydration and adequate urine output.
• Warn the patient to avoid hazardous tasks that require alertness until CNS effects of the drug are known.

## ofloxacin
Floxin, Floxin I.V.

*Pregnancy Risk Category: C*

**HOW SUPPLIED**
*Tablets:* 200 mg, 300 mg, 400 mg
*Injection:* 20 mg/ml, 40 mg/ml; 4 mg/ml premixed in $D_5W$

**ACTION**
Unknown. Thought to inhibit bacterial DNA gyrase and prevent DNA replication in susceptible bacteria.

**ONSET, PEAK, DURATION**
Onset immediate after I.V. infusion, unknown after oral administration. Plasma levels peak immediately after an I.V. infusion, within 1 to 2 hours after an oral dose.

**INDICATIONS & DOSAGE**
*Lower respiratory tract infections caused by susceptible strains of* Haemophilus influenzae *or* Streptococcus pneumoniae —
**Adults:** 400 mg I.V. or P.O. q 12 hours for 10 days.
*Cervicitis or urethritis caused by* Chlamydia trachomatis *or* Neisseria gonorrhoeae —
**Adults:** 300 mg I.V. or P.O. q 12 hours for 7 days.
*Acute, uncomplicated gonorrhea —*
**Adults:** 400 mg I.V. or P.O. as a single dose.
*Mild to moderate skin and skin-structure infections caused by susceptible strains of* Staphylococcus aureus, S. epidermidis, Streptococcus pyogenes, *or* Proteus mirabilis —
**Adults:** 400 mg I.V. or P.O. q 12 hours for 10 days.
*Cystitis caused by* Escherichia coli *or* Klebsiella pneumoniae —
**Adults:** 200 mg I.V. or P.O. q 12 hours for 3 days.
*Urinary tract infections caused by susceptible strains of* Citrobacter diversus, Enterobacter aerogenes, Escherichia coli, P. mirabilis, *or* Pseudomonas aeruginosa —
**Adults:** 200 mg I.V. or P.O. q 12 hours for 7 days. Complicated infections may require therapy for 10 days.
*Prostatitis caused by* E. coli —
**Adults:** 300 mg I.V. or P.O. q 12 hours for 6 weeks.
   If creatinine clearance is 10 to 50 ml/minute, dosage interval is decreased to once q 24 hours. If creatinine clearance is less than 10 ml/minute, half the recommended dose is given q 24 hours.

**ADVERSE REACTIONS**
**CNS:** headache, dizziness, fatigue, lethargy, malaise, drowsiness, sleep disorders, nervousness, insomnia, visual disturbances, *seizures.*
**CV:** chest pain.
**GI:** *nausea,* anorexia, abdominal pain

Reactions may be *common,* uncommon, *life-threatening,* or COMMON AND LIFE-THREATENING.

or discomfort, diarrhea, vomiting, constipation, dry mouth, flatulence, dysgeusia.
**GU:** vaginitis, vaginal discharge, genital pruritus.
**Musculoskeletal:** trunk pain.
**Skin:** rash, pruritus, photosensitivity.
**Other:** hypersensitivity reactions *(anaphylactoid reaction),* elevated liver enzymes, fever, phlebitis.

## INTERACTIONS
*Antacids containing aluminum or magnesium hydroxide, iron salts, sucralfate, products containing zinc:* may interfere with the GI absorption of ofloxacin. Separate administration by at least 2 hours.
*Antidiabetic agents:* may cause alterations in levels. Monitor concentrations closely.
*Antineoplastic agents:* may lower serum levels of fluoroquinolones. Monitor for lack of effect.
*Oral anticoagulants:* increased effect. Monitor for bleeding and altered PT.
*Theophylline:* decreased clearance of theophylline with some fluoroquinolones. Monitor theophylline levels.

## CONTRAINDICATIONS
Contraindicated in patients with hypersensitivity to the drug or other fluoroquinolones.

## NURSING CONSIDERATIONS
● Use cautiously during pregnancy and only when benefits outweigh risks to the fetus.
● Use cautiously in patients with a history of seizure disorders or other CNS diseases, such as cerebral arteriosclerosis. If patient experiences excessive CNS stimulation (restlessness, tremor, confusion, hallucinations), discontinue medication and notify doctor. Institute seizure precautions.
● Use cautiously and with dosage adjustment in patients with renal failure, as prescribed, because the drug is mainly eliminated by renal excretion.

● **I.V. use:** Dilute concentrate for injection before use. Single-use vials containing 20 or 40 mg/ml must be diluted to a maximum concentration of 4 mg/ml with a compatible I.V. solution, such as $D_5W$, 0.9% sodium chloride for injection, $D_5W$ in 0.9% sodium chloride for injection, or sterile water for injection. Infuse over not less than 60 minutes.
● Because compatibility with other drugs is not known, don't mix ofloxacin with other drugs. If giving infusion at a Y-site, discontinue the flow of the other solution.
● Monitor regular blood studies and hepatic and renal function tests during prolonged therapy, as ordered.
● *Alert:* Know that patients treated for gonorrhea should have a serologic test for syphilis. Drug is not effective against syphilis, and treatment of gonorrhea may mask or delay symptoms of syphilis.

## ☑ PATIENT TEACHING
● Tell the patient to take drug as prescribed, even if he feels better.
● Advise the patient to take the drug with plenty of fluids, but not with meals, and to avoid antacids, sucralfate, and products containing iron or zinc for at least 2 hours before and after each dose.
● Warn the patient to avoid hazardous tasks until adverse CNS effects of drug are known.
● Advise the patient to use sunblock and wear protective clothing.
● Tell the patient to stop drug and notify the doctor if a rash or other signs of hypersensitivity develop.

---

*Liquid form contains alcohol. **May contain tartrazine. †Canada only. ‡Australia only. ◊OTC.

acyclovir sodium
amantadine hydrochloride
didanosine
famciclovir
foscarnet sodium
ganciclovir
lamivudine
ribavirin
rimantadine
saquinavir mesylate
stavudine
valacyclovir hydrochloride
zalcitabine
zidovudine

**COMBINATION PRODUCTS**
None.

---

## acyclovir sodium
Zovirax

*Pregnancy Risk Category: C*

**HOW SUPPLIED**
*Capsules:* 200 mg
*Tablets:* 400 mg, 800 mg
*Suspension:* 200 mg/5 ml
*Injection:* 500 mg/vial, 1 g/vial

**ACTION**
Interferes with DNA synthesis and inhibits viral multiplication.

**ONSET, PEAK, DURATION**
Onset immediate after I.V. infusion, unknown after oral administration. Serum levels peak immediately after I.V. infusion, within 1.7 hours of oral dose. Duration unknown.

**INDICATIONS & DOSAGE**
*Initial and recurrent episodes of mucocutaneous herpes simplex virus (HSV-1 and HSV-2) infections in immunocompromised patients; severe initial episodes of genital herpes in patients who are not immunocompromised –*
**Adults and children over 11 years:** 5 mg/kg, given at a constant rate over a period of 1 hour by I.V. q 8 hours for 7 days (5 days for genital herpes).
**Children under 12 years:** 250 mg/m², given at a constant rate over a period of 1 hour by I.V. q 8 hours for 7 days (5 days for genital herpes).
*Initial genital herpes –*
**Adults:** 200 mg P.O. q 4 hours while awake (a total of 5 capsules daily). Treatment should continue for 10 days.
*Intermittent therapy for recurrent genital herpes –*
**Adults:** 200 mg P.O. q 4 hours while awake (a total of 5 capsules daily). Treatment should continue for 5 days. Initiate therapy at the first sign of recurrence.
*Chronic suppressive therapy for recurrent genital herpes –*
**Adults:** 400 mg P.O. b.i.d. for up to 12 months. Alternatively, 200 mg P.O. three to five times daily for up to 12 months.
*Chicken pox –*
**Adults and children:** 20 mg/kg P.O. q.i.d. for 5 days. Therapy should be started as soon as symptoms appear.
*Varicella zoster infections in immunocompromised patients –*
**Adults and children over 12 years:** 10 mg/kg I.V. infused at a constant rate over 1 hour q 8 hours for 7 days.
**Children under 12 years:** 500 mg/m² I.V. infused at a constant rate over 1 hour q 8 hours for 7 days.

**ADVERSE REACTIONS**
*CNS: malaise, headache, encephalopathic changes (lethargy, obtundation, tremor, confusion, hallucinations, agitation, **seizures, coma**).*

---

**GI:** *nausea, vomiting,* diarrhea.
**GU:** *transient elevations of serum creatinine levels,* hematuria.
**Skin:** rash, itching, urticaria.
**Other:** *inflammation and phlebitis at injection site.*

**INTERACTIONS**
*Probenecid:* increased acyclovir blood levels. Monitor for possible toxicity.
*Zidovudine:* may cause drowsiness or lethargy. Use together cautiously.

**CONTRAINDICATIONS**
Contraindicated in patients with hypersensitivity to the drug.

**NURSING CONSIDERATIONS**
• Use cautiously in patients with underlying neurologic problems, renal disease, or dehydration and in those receiving other nephrotoxic drugs.
• Be aware that it is recommended that acyclovir be administered in a reduced dosage to patients with impaired renal function.
• **I.V. use:** Administer I.V. infusion over at least 1 hour to prevent renal tubular damage. Bolus injection, dehydration (decreased urine output), preexisting renal disease, and the concomitant use of other nephrotoxic drugs increase the risk of renal toxicity.
• **Alert:** Don't give by bolus injection or administer I.M. or S.C.
• Be alert that concentrated solutions (10 mg/ml or more) may be associated with a higher incidence of phlebitis.
• Encourage fluid intake because the patient must be adequately hydrated during acyclovir infusion.
• Know that encephalopathic changes are more likely in patients with neurologic disorders or in those who have had neurologic reactions to cytotoxic drugs.
• Keep in mind that Burroughs-Wellcome, the manufacturer, maintains an ongoing registry of women exposed to the drug during pregnancy. Follow-up

studies to date have not shown an increased risk for birth defects for infants born to patients exposed to the drug during pregnancy. Health care providers are encouraged to report such exposures to the registrar at (800) 722-9292.

☑ **PATIENT TEACHING**
• Tell the patient to take drug as prescribed, even when he feels better.
• Instruct the patient that drug is effective in managing herpes infection but does not eliminate or cure it. Warn the patient that acyclovir will not prevent spread of infection to others.
• Urge the patient to recognize early symptoms of herpes infection (such as tingling, itching, or pain). He can then notify doctor and get a prescription for acyclovir before the infection fully develops.

---

## amantadine hydrochloride
Antadine‡, Symadine, Symmetrel
*Pregnancy Risk Category: C*

**HOW SUPPLIED**
*Capsules:* 100 mg
*Syrup:* 50 mg/5 ml

**ACTION**
Unknown. Appears to interfere with influenza A virus penetration into susceptible cells. In parkinsonism, its action is unknown.

**ONSET, PEAK, DURATION**
Onset for antidyskinetic symptoms usually within 48 hours, unknown for antiviral activity. Peak plasma levels occur 2 to 4 hours after an oral dose. Duration unknown.

**INDICATIONS & DOSAGE**
*Prophylaxis or symptomatic treatment of influenza type A virus, respiratory tract illnesses –*
**Adults up to 64 years and children**

**10 years and over:** 200 mg P.O. daily in a single dose or divided b.i.d.

**Children 1 to 9 years:** 4.4 to 8.8 mg/kg P.O. daily, as a single dose or divided b.i.d. Maximum dose is 150 mg daily.

**Adults over 64 years:** 100 mg P.O. once daily.

Treatment should continue for 24 to 48 hours after symptoms disappear. Prophylaxis should start as soon as possible after initial exposure and continue for at least 10 days after exposure. May continue prophylactic treatment up to 90 days for repeated or suspected exposures if influenza vaccine unavailable. If used with influenza vaccine, dose is continued for 2 to 3 weeks until protection from vaccine develops.

*Drug-induced extrapyramidal reactions –*

**Adults:** 100 mg P.O. b.i.d. Some patients may benefit from as much as 400 mg daily, but dosages over 200 mg must be closely supervised.

*Idiopathic parkinsonism, parkinsonian syndrome –*

**Adults:** 100 mg P.O. b.i.d.; in patients who are seriously ill or receiving other antiparkinsonian drugs, 100 mg daily for at least 1 week, then 100 mg b.i.d., p.r.n.

## ADVERSE REACTIONS

**CNS:** depression, fatigue, confusion, *dizziness,* hallucinations, anxiety, *irritability,* ataxia, *insomnia,* headache, *light-headedness.*

**CV:** peripheral edema, orthostatic hypotension, *CHF.*

**GI:** anorexia, *nausea,* constipation, vomiting, dry mouth.

**Skin:** *livedo reticularis* (with prolonged use).

## INTERACTIONS

*Anticholinergics:* increased adverse anticholinergic effects. Use together cautiously. Dosage of anticholinergic

agent may be reduced prior to initiation of amantadine by some doctors.

*CNS stimulants:* additive CNS stimulation. Use together cautiously.

*Hydrochlorothiazide, triamterene:* increased levels of amantadine. Use together cautiously.

## CONTRAINDICATIONS

Contraindicated in patients with hypersensitivity to the drug.

## NURSING CONSIDERATIONS

● Use cautiously in those with seizure disorders, CHF, peripheral edema, hepatic disease, mental illness, eczematoid rash, renal impairment, orthostatic hypotension, and CV disease and in elderly patients. Dosage may need to be adjusted in patients with renal failure and in patients 65 years and older.

● *Alert:* Be aware that elderly patients are more susceptible to neurologic adverse effects. Taking the drug in two daily doses rather than as a single dose may reduce their incidence.

## ☑ PATIENT TEACHING

● If insomnia occurs, tell the patient to take the drug several hours before bedtime.

● If orthostatic hypotension occurs, instruct the patient not to stand or change positions too quickly.

● Instruct the patient to report adverse reactions to the doctor, especially dizziness, depression, anxiety, nausea, and urine retention.

● In the patient with parkinsonism, warn against discontinuing the drug abruptly to prevent precipitating a parkinsonian crisis.

## didanosine (ddI)
Videx

*Pregnancy Risk Category: B*

---

Reactions may be *common,* uncommon, *life-threatening,* or **COMMON AND LIFE-THREATENING.**

## HOW SUPPLIED
*Tablets (chewable):* 25 mg, 50 mg, 100 mg, 150 mg
*Powder for oral solution (buffered):* 100 mg/packet, 167 mg/packet, 250 mg/packet, 375 mg/packet
*Powder for oral solution (pediatric):* 10 mg/ml in 2- and 4-g bottles

## ACTION
Unknown. Appears to inhibit replication of HIV by preventing DNA replication. In addition, dideoxyadenosine triphosphate inhibits the enzyme HIV-RNA-dependent DNA polymerase (reverse transcriptase).

## ONSET, PEAK, DURATION
Onset and duration unknown. Peak levels occur in ½ to 1 hour.

## INDICATIONS & DOSAGE
*Advanced HIV infection in patients who cannot tolerate or who no longer respond to zidovudine therapy –*
**Adults 60 kg and over:** 200 mg (tablets) P.O. q 12 hours; or 250 mg buffered powder P.O. q 12 hours.
**Adults less than 60 kg:** 125 mg (tablets) P.O. q 12 hours; or 167 mg buffered powder P.O. q 12 hours.
**Children:** 200 mg/m$^2$ P.O. daily in divided doses q 12 hours (average dose).

## ADVERSE REACTIONS
**CNS:** *headache, seizures,* confusion, anxiety, nervousness, abnormal thinking, twitching, depression, *peripheral neuropathy.*
**GI:** *diarrhea, nausea, vomiting, abdominal pain, pancreatitis,* dry mouth, anorexia.
**Hematologic:** *leukopenia,* granulocytosis, *thrombocytopenia,* anemia.
**Hepatic:** *hepatic failure,* elevated liver enzymes.
**Skin:** rash, pruritus.
**Other:** asthenia, pain, pneumonia, infection, sarcoma, dyspnea, allergic reactions, myopathy, increased serum uric acid levels, *chills, fever.*

## INTERACTIONS
*Antacids containing magnesium or aluminum hydroxides:* enhanced adverse effects of the antacid component (including diarrhea or constipation) when administered with didanosine tablets or pediatric suspension. Avoid concomitant use.
*Dapsone, ketoconazole, drugs that require gastric acid for adequate absorption:* decreased absorption from buffering action. Administer these drugs 2 hours before didanosine.
*Fluoroquinolones, tetracyclines:* decreased absorption from buffering agents in didanosine tablets or antacids in pediatric suspension.
*Itraconazole:* decreased serum concentrations of itraconazole. Avoid concomitant use.

## CONTRAINDICATIONS
Contraindicated in patients with a history of hypersensitivity to any component of the formulation.

## NURSING CONSIDERATIONS
● Use cautiously in patients with a history of pancreatitis; fatalities have occurred. Also use cautiously in patients with peripheral neuropathy, renal or hepatic impairment, or hyperuricemia.
● Administer didanosine on an empty stomach, regardless of the dosage form used; administering the drug with meals can decrease absorption by 50%.
● To administer single-dose packets containing buffered powder for oral solution, pour contents into 4 oz (120 ml) of water. Do not use fruit juice or other beverages that may be acidic. Stir for 2 or 3 minutes until the powder dissolves completely. Administer immediately.
● Use care when preparing the powder or crushing tablets to avoid exces-

---

*Liquid form contains alcohol. **May contain tartrazine. †Canada only. ‡Australia only. ◇OTC.

sive dispersal of the powder into the air.

• Keep in mind that in early clinical trials, the powder for oral solution was associated with a high incidence of diarrhea. The manufacturer suggests switching to the tablet formulation if diarrhea is a problem.

• *Alert:* Know that the pediatric powder for oral solution must be prepared by a pharmacist before dispensing. It must be constituted with purified USP water and then diluted with an antacid (either Mylanta Double Strength Liquid or Maalox TC Suspension) to a final concentration of 10 mg/ml. The admixture is stable for 30 days if refrigerated (at 36° to 46° F [2° to 8° C]). Shake the solution well before measuring the dose.

☑ **PATIENT TEACHING**
• Instruct the patient to take drug on an empty stomach.

• Because the tablets contain buffers that raise stomach pH to levels that prevent degradation of the active drug, instruct the patient to chew tablets thoroughly before swallowing and drink at least 1 oz (30 ml) of water with each dose. Teach the patient how to prepare crushed tablets or buffered powder form for ingestion, if appropriate.

• Inform the patient receiving a sodium-restricted diet that each two-tablet dose of didanosine contains 529 mg of sodium; each single packet of buffered powder for oral solution contains 1.38 g of sodium.

# famciclovir
Famvir

*Pregnancy Risk Category: B*

**HOW SUPPLIED**
*Tablets:* 500 mg

**ACTION**
A guanosine nucleoside that is converted to penciclovir, which enters viral cells and inhibits DNA polymerase and viral DNA synthesis.

**ONSET, PEAK, DURATION**
Onset and duration unknown. Serum levels peak within 1 hour.

**INDICATIONS & DOSAGE**
*Acute herpes zoster –*
**Adults:** 500 mg P.O. q 8 hours.
In patients with reduced renal function: If creatinine clearance is greater than or equal to 60 ml/minute, give 500 mg P.O. q 8 hours; if 40 to 59 ml/minute, 500 mg P.O. q 12 hours; if 20 to 39 ml/minute, 500 mg P.O. q 24 hours.

**ADVERSE REACTIONS**
**CNS:** *headache,* fatigue, dizziness, paresthesia, somnolence.
**GI:** diarrhea, *nausea,* vomiting, constipation, anorexia, abdominal pain.
**Musculoskeletal:** back pain, arthralgia.
**Respiratory:** pharyngitis, sinusitis.
**Skin:** pruritus; zoster-related signs, symptoms, and complications.
**Other:** fever, injury, pain, rigors.

**INTERACTIONS**
*Probenecid:* may increase plasma concentrations of famciclovir. Monitor patient for increased adverse effects.

**CONTRAINDICATIONS**
Contraindicated in patients with hypersensitivity to the drug.

**NURSING CONSIDERATIONS**
• Use cautiously in patients with renal or hepatic impairment. Know that dosage adjustment may be needed.
• Famciclovir may be taken without regard to meals.

---

Reactions may be *common,* uncommon, *life-threatening,* or COMMON AND LIFE-THREATENING.

### ☑ PATIENT TEACHING
● Teach the patient how to prevent spread of infection to others.
● Urge the patient to recognize the early symptoms of herpes infection, such as tingling, itching, or pain, and to report them. Treatment is more effective if therapy is started within 48 hours of rash onset.

---

## foscarnet sodium (phosphonoformic acid)
Foscavir

*Pregnancy Risk Category: C*

### HOW SUPPLIED
*Injection:* 24 mg/ml in 250- and 500-ml bottles

### ACTION
Inhibits all known herpesviruses in vitro by blocking the pyrophosphate binding site on DNA polymerases and reverse transcriptases.

### ONSET, PEAK, DURATION
Onset immediate. Peak levels occur immediately after I.V. infusion. Duration unknown.

### INDICATIONS & DOSAGE
*CMV retinitis in patients with AIDS –*
**Adults:** initially, 60 mg/kg I.V. as an induction treatment in patients with normal renal function. Administer I.V. over 1 hour q 8 hours for 2 to 3 weeks, depending on clinical response. Followed with a maintenance infusion of 90 mg/kg daily, administered over 2 hours; this dose may be increased as needed and tolerated to 120 mg/kg daily if the disease shows signs of progression.

### ADVERSE REACTIONS
**CNS:** *headache, seizures, fatigue, malaise, asthenia, paresthesia, dizziness, hypoesthesia, neuropathy,* tremor, ataxia, generalized spasms, dementia, stupor, sensory disturbances, meningitis, aphasia, abnormal coordination, EEG abnormalities, depression, confusion, anxiety, insomnia, somnolence, nervousness, amnesia, agitation, aggressive reaction, hallucinations.
**CV:** *hypertension, palpitations, ECG abnormalities, sinus tachycardia,* cerebrovascular disorder, *first-degree AV block, hypotension, flushing,* edema.
**EENT:** visual disturbances, taste perversion, eye pain, conjunctivitis.
**GI:** *nausea, diarrhea, vomiting, abdominal pain, anorexia,* constipation, dysphagia, rectal hemorrhage, dry mouth, dyspepsia, melena, flatulence, ulcerative stomatitis, *pancreatitis.*
**GU:** *abnormal renal function, decreased creatinine clearance and increased serum creatinine levels, albuminuria, dysuria, polyuria, urethral disorder, urine retention, urinary tract infections, acute renal failure,* moniliasis.
**Hematologic:** *anemia, granulocytopenia, leukopenia, bone marrow suppression, thrombocytopenia,* platelet abnormalities, thrombocytosis, WBC count abnormalities, lymphadenopathy.
**Respiratory:** *cough, dyspnea,* pneumonitis, sinusitis, pharyngitis, rhinitis, respiratory insufficiency, pulmonary infiltration, stridor, pneumothorax, *bronchospasm,* hemoptysis, flulike symptoms.
**Skin:** *rash, increased sweating,* pruritus, skin ulceration, erythematous rash, seborrhea, skin discoloration, facial edema.
**Other:** *death, fever,* pain, infection, sepsis, hypokalemia, hypomagnesemia, hypophosphatemia or hyperphosphatemia, hypocalcemia, leg cramps, rigors, inflammation and pain at infusion site, lymphoma-like disorder, sarcoma, back or chest pain, abnormal hepatic function, bacterial or fungal infections, abscess, in-

---

creased liver enzymes, arthralgia, myalgia.

## INTERACTIONS
*Nephrotoxic drugs such as amphotericin B, aminoglycosides:* increased risk of nephrotoxicity. Avoid concomitant use.

*Pentamidine:* increased risk of nephrotoxicity; severe hypocalcemia has also been reported. Avoid concomitant use.

*Zidovudine:* possible increased incidence or severity of anemia. Monitor blood counts.

## CONTRAINDICATIONS
Contraindicated in patients with hypersensitivity to the drug.

## NURSING CONSIDERATIONS
● Use cautiously and with reduced dosage in patients with abnormal renal function as ordered because it will result in accumulation of the drug and enhanced toxicity. Because foscarnet is nephrotoxic, it has the potential to worsen renal impairment. Some degree of nephrotoxicity occurs in most patients treated with the drug.
● Obtain serum electrolyte levels and creatinine clearance before beginning therapy, as ordered.
● Because the drug is highly toxic and toxicity is probably dose-related, keep in mind that the lowest effective maintenance dose should be used throughout therapy.
● **I.V. use:** Use an infusion pump to administer foscarnet. To minimize renal toxicity, make sure the patient is adequately hydrated before and during the infusion.
● **Alert:** Do not exceed the recommended dosage, infusion rate, or frequency of administration. All doses must be individualized according to the patient's renal function.
● Monitor creatinine clearance frequently during therapy because of the drug's adverse effects on renal func-

tion. A baseline 24-hour creatinine clearance is recommended, followed by regular determinations two to three times weekly during induction and at least once every 1 to 2 weeks during maintenance. If creatinine clearance falls below 0.4 ml/minute/kg, drug should be discontinued.
● Because the drug can adversely affect important serum electrolytes such as potassium, calcium, magnesium, and phosphorus, monitor serum electrolyte levels using a schedule similar to that established for creatinine clearance. Assess the patient for tetany and seizures associated with abnormal electrolyte levels.
● Monitor the patient's hemoglobin and hematocrit levels. Anemia is common (in up to 33% of patients treated with the drug). It may be severe enough to require transfusions.
● Keep in mind that administration of the drug is associated with a dose-related transient decrease in ionized serum calcium, which may not always be reflected in the patient's laboratory values.

### ☑ PATIENT TEACHING
● Explain to the patient the importance of adequate hydration throughout therapy.
● Advise the patient to report perioral tingling, numbness in the extremities, and paresthesia.
● Instruct the patient to alert the nurse if discomfort occurs at I.V. insertion site.

# ganciclovir
Cytovene

*Pregnancy Risk Category: C*

## HOW SUPPLIED
*Capsules:* 250 mg
*Injection:* 500 mg/vial

## ACTION

Unknown. Thought to inhibit viral DNA synthesis of CMV.

## ONSET, PEAK, DURATION

Onset is immediate with I.V. infusion. Peak serum levels occur immediately after I.V. infusion. Duration unknown.

## INDICATIONS & DOSAGE

*CMV retinitis in immunocompromised individuals, including patients with AIDS —*

**Adults:** induction treatment — 5 mg/kg I.V. q 12 hours for 14 to 21 days (normal renal function); maintenance treatment — 5 mg/kg I.V. daily for 7 days each week, or 6 mg/kg daily for 5 days each week. Alternatively, 1,000 mg P.O. t.i.d. with food.

Dosage is adjusted for patients with impaired renal function and is based on creatinine clearance levels.

## ADVERSE REACTIONS

**CNS:** altered dreams, confusion, ataxia, headache, *seizures, coma,* dizziness, somnolence, tremor, abnormal thinking, agitation, amnesia, anxiety, neuropathy, paresthesia, asthenia.

**CV:** phlebitis.

**GI:** *nausea, vomiting, diarrhea, anorexia, abdominal pain,* flatulence, dyspepsia, dry mouth.

**GU:** *increased serum creatinine levels.*

**Hematologic:** *granulocytopenia, thrombocytopenia, leukopenia, anemia.*

**Other:** retinal detachment in CMV retinitis patients; abnormal liver function tests results; *fever;* infection; chills; sepsis; *rash; sweating;* pruritus; pneumonia; at injection site — inflammation, pain, phlebitis.

## INTERACTIONS

*Cytotoxic agents:* increased toxic effects, especially hematologic effects and stomatitis. Monitor closely.
*Imipenem/cilastatin:* heightened seizure activity with concomitant use. Monitor closely.
*Immunosuppressants such as azathioprine, cyclosporine, corticosteroids:* enhanced immune and bone marrow suppression. Use together cautiously.
*Probenecid:* increased ganciclovir blood levels. Monitor closely.
*Zidovudine:* increased incidence of granulocytopenia with concurrent use. Monitor closely.

## CONTRAINDICATIONS

Contraindicated in patients with hypersensitivity to the drug and with an absolute neutrophil count below 500/mm³ or a platelet count below 25,000/mm³.

## NURSING CONSIDERATIONS

• Use cautiously and in reduced dosage in patients with renal dysfunction.
• **I.V. use:** Administer infusion over at least 1 hour. Too-rapid infusions will result in increased toxicity. Use an infusion pump. Do not administer as an I.V. bolus.
• Use caution when preparing ganciclovir solution, which is alkaline.
• *Alert:* Do not administer S.C. or I.M.
• Because of the frequency of granulocytopenia and thrombocytopenia, obtain neutrophil and platelet counts every 2 days during twice-daily ganciclovir dosing and at least weekly thereafter.

## ☑ PATIENT TEACHING

• Explain to patient the importance of adequate hydration throughout therapy.
• Instruct patient to report adverse ractions promptly.
• Tell patient to alert the nurse if discomfort occurs at I.V. insert site.

---

*Liquid form contains alcohol. **May contain tartrazine. †Canada only. ‡Australia only. ◇OTC.

▼ **NEW DRUG**

# lamivudine
Epivir

*Pregnancy Risk Category: C*

## HOW SUPPLIED
*Tablets:* 150 mg
*Oral solution:* 10 mg/ml

## ACTION
A synthetic nucleoside analogue that inhibits HIV reverse transcription via viral DNA chain termination. RNA- and DNA-dependent DNA polymerase activities are also inhibited.

## ONSET, PEAK, DURATION
Unknown.

## INDICATIONS & DOSAGE
*Treatment of HIV infection concomitantly with zidovudine –*
**Adults weighing 50 kg (110 lbs) or more and children 12 years and older:** 150 mg P.O. b.i.d.
**Adults weighing less than 50 kg (110 lbs):** 2 mg/kg P.O. b.i.d.
**Children ages 3 months to 12 years:** 4 mg/kg P.O. b.i.d. Maximum dosage is 150 mg b.i.d.

## ADVERSE REACTIONS
NOTE: Adverse reactions pertain to the combination therapy of lamivudine and zidovudine.
**CNS:** *headache, fatigue, neuropathy, dizziness, insomnia and other sleep disorders,* depressive disorders.
**GI:** *nausea, diarrhea, vomiting, anorexia,* abdominal pain, abdominal cramps, dyspepsia, pancreatitis (in children 3 months to 12 years).
**EENT:** *nasal alterations.*
**Hematologic:** neutropenia, anemia, *thrombocytopenia.*
**Respiratory:** *cough.*
**Skin:** rash.
**Other:** *malaise, fever, chills, musculoskeletal pain,* myalgia, arthralgia, elevated liver enzymes and bilirubin.

## INTERACTIONS
*Trimethoprim/sulfamethoxazole:* may cause increased blood level of lamivudine because of decreased clearance of lamivudine. The clinical significance of this interaction is unknown. Monitor patient closely.

## CONTRAINDICATIONS
Contraindicated in patients with hypersensitivity to the drug.

## NURSING CONSIDERATIONS
● *Alert:* Know that this drug should be used with extreme caution, and only if there's no satisfactory alternative therapy, in pediatric patients with a history of pancreatitis or other significant risk factors for development of pancreatitis. Treatment with lamivudine should be stopped immediately and the doctor notified if clinical signs, symptoms, or laboratory abnormalities suggest pancreatitis.
● Use cautiously in patients with renal impairment. Know that dosage reduction is necessary.
● Breast-feeding should be discontinued if lamivudine is prescribed.
● Drug must be administered concomitantly with zidovudine. It is not intended for use alone.
● Monitor the patient's CBC, platelet count, and liver function studies, as ordered. Report abnormalities.
● Be aware that an Antiretroviral Pregnancy Registry has been established to monitor maternal-fetal outcomes of pregnant women exposed to lamivudine. To register a pregnant patient, the doctor can call 1-800-722-9292, ext. 38465.

## ☑ PATIENT TEACHING
● Inform the patient that long-term effects of lamivudine are unknown.
● Remind the patient that tablets and solutions are for oral ingestion only.
● Stress the importance of taking lamivudine exactly as prescribed.
● For a pediatric patient, teach par-

---

Reactions may be *common*, uncommon, *life-threatening*, or **COMMON AND LIFE-THREATENING**.

ents the signs and symptoms of pancreatitis, and tell them to report such occurrences immediately.

---

## ribavirin
Virazole

*Pregnancy Risk Category: X*

### HOW SUPPLIED
*Powder to be reconstituted for inhalation:* 6 g in 100-ml glass vial

### ACTION
Inhibits viral activity by an unknown mechanism, possibly by inhibiting RNA and DNA synthesis by depleting intracellular nucleotide pools.

### ONSET, PEAK, DURATION
Onset is immediate upon exposure to the drug. Peak levels occur immediately after an aerosol treatment. Duration unknown.

### INDICATIONS & DOSAGE
*Hospitalized infants and young children infected by RSV –*
**Infants and young children:** solution in concentration of 20 mg/ml delivered via the Viratek Small Particle Aerosol Generator (SPAG-2) and mechanical ventilator or oxygen hood, face mask, or oxygen tent at a rate of about 12.5 liters of mist per minute. Treatment is carried out for 12 to 18 hours/day for at least 3 days, and no more than 7 days.

### ADVERSE REACTIONS
**CV:** *cardiac arrest,* hypotension.
**EENT:** conjunctivitis.
**Hematologic:** anemia, reticulocytosis.
**Respiratory:** worsening respiratory state, apnea, bacterial pneumonia, pneumothorax.
**Other:** rash or erythema of eyelids.

### INTERACTIONS
None significant.

### CONTRAINDICATIONS
Contraindicated in patients with hypersensitivity to the drug. Know that although the drug is used in children, manufacturer states that it's also contraindicated in women who are or may become pregnant during treatment.

### NURSING CONSIDERATIONS
● Administer ribavirin aerosol by the Viratek Small Particle Aerosol Generator (SPAG-2) only. Don't use any other aerosol-generating device.
● Use sterile USP water for injection, *not* bacteriostatic water. Water used to reconstitute this drug must not contain any antimicrobial agent.
● Discard solutions placed in the SPAG-2 unit at least every 24 hours before adding newly reconstituted solution.
● Avoid unnecessary occupational exposure to the drug. The most frequent adverse effects reported in health care personnel exposed to aerosolized ribavirin include eye irritation and headache.
● *Alert:* Monitor ventilator function frequently. Ribavirin may precipitate in ventilator apparatus, causing equipment malfunction with serious consequences.
● Monitor patients receiving ribavirin therapy longer than 1 to 2 weeks for the development of anemia.
● Store reconstituted solutions at room temperature for 24 hours.
● Continue providing supportive respiratory and fluid management.
● Keep in mind that ribavirin aerosol is indicated only for severe lower respiratory tract infection caused by RSV. Although treatment may begin while awaiting diagnostic test results, existence of RSV infection must eventually be documented.
● Be aware that most infants and children with RSV infection don't require treatment because the disease is commonly mild and self-limiting. Infants with underlying conditions, such as

---

*Liquid form contains alcohol. **May contain tartrazine. †Canada only. ‡Australia only. ◊OTC.

prematurity or cardiopulmonary disease, get RSV in its severest form and benefit most from treatment with ribavirin aerosol.

☑ **PATIENT TEACHING**
• Inform parents of need for drug and answer any questions.
• Encourage parents to report any subtle change in child immediately to nurse.

---

## rimantadine
Flumadine

*Pregnancy Risk Category: C*

### HOW SUPPLIED
*Tablets:* 100 mg
*Syrup:* 50 mg/5 ml

### ACTION
Unknown. Appears to prevent viral uncoating, an early step in virus reproductive cycle.

### ONSET, PEAK, DURATION
Onset and duration unknown. Peak plasma levels occur in 1 to 4 hours.

### INDICATIONS & DOSAGE
*Prophylaxis of influenza A –*
**Adults and children 10 years and over:** 100 mg P.O. b.i.d.
**Children under 10 years:** 5 mg/kg (not to exceed 150 mg) P.O. once a day.
**Elderly patients, patients with severe hepatic or renal dysfunction:** 100 mg P.O. daily.
*Treatment of influenza A –*
**Adults:** 100 mg P.O. b.i.d.

### ADVERSE REACTIONS
**CNS:** insomnia, headache, dizziness, nervousness, fatigue, asthenia.
**GI:** nausea, vomiting, anorexia, dry mouth, abdominal pain.

### INTERACTIONS
*Acetaminophen, aspirin:* reduced concentration of rimantadine. Monitor for decreased effectiveness of rimantadine.
*Cimetidine:* may decrease clearance of rimantadine. Monitor for adverse reactions.

### CONTRAINDICATIONS
Contraindicated in patients with hypersensitivity to the drug or amantadine.

### NURSING CONSIDERATIONS
• Use cautiously in patients with renal or hepatic impairment and in patients with a history of seizures. Pregnant patients should consider the risks compared to the benefits before taking this drug.
• For influenza infections, begin therapy within 48 hours of onset of symptoms and continue for 7 days after the initial signs and symptoms occurred, as ordered.
• Consider the risk to contacts of treated patients who may be subject to morbidity from influenza A. Influenza A-resistant strains can emerge during therapy. Patients taking the drug may still be able to spread the disease.

☑ **PATIENT TEACHING**
• Instruct the patient to take drug several hours before bedtime to prevent insomnia.
• Inform the patient that he may still be able to infect others with influenza A and to take infection-control precautions.

▼ *NEW DRUG*

---

## saquinavir mesylate
Invirase

*Pregnancy Risk Category: B*

### HOW SUPPLIED
*Capsules:* 200 mg

---

## ACTION
Inhibits the activity of HIV protease and prevents the cleavage of HIV polyproteins, which are essential for HIV maturation.

## ONSET, PEAK, DURATION
Unknown.

## INDICATIONS & DOSAGE
*Adjunct treatment of advanced HIV infection in selected patients –*
**Adults:** 600 mg P.O. t.i.d. taken within 2 hours after a full meal and in combination with a nucleoside analogue, such as zalcitabine at a dosage of 0.75 mg P.O. t.i.d. or zidovudine at a dosage of 200 mg P.O. t.i.d.

## ADVERSE REACTIONS
**CNS:** paresthesia, headache.
**GI:** diarrhea, ulcerated buccal mucosa, abdominal pain, nausea.
**Other:** asthenia, rash, musculoskeletal pain.

## INTERACTIONS
*Rifabutin, rifampin:* reduces the steady state concentration of saquinavir. Use together cautiously.

## CONTRAINDICATIONS
Contraindicated in patients with hypersensitivity to the drug or to any component contained in the capsule.

## NURSING CONSIDERATIONS
• Safety of drug is not established in pregnant or breast-feeding women or in children under age 16.
• CBC, platelets, electrolytes, uric acid, liver enzymes, and bilirubin should be evaluated before therapy begins and at appropriate intervals throughout therapy, as ordered.
• Be aware that if serious toxicity occurs during treatment, saquinavir should be discontinued until the etiology of the event is identified or the toxicity resolves. When drug is re-

sumed, it may be done with no dosage modifications.
• Monitor patient's hydration if adverse GI reactions occur.
• Notify doctor if adverse reactions occur. Obtain an order for a mild analgesic if drug causes headache, an antiemetic if drug causes nausea, or an antidiarrheal agent if drug causes diarrhea.
• Be alert for adverse reactions associated with adjunct therapy (zidovudine or zalcitabine).

## ☑ PATIENT TEACHING
• Advise the patient to take drug within 2 hours after a full meal.
• Tell the patient to notify doctor if adverse reactions occur.
• Inform the patient that drug is usually administered with other AIDS-related antiviral agents.

---

## stavudine (2,3 didehydro-3-deoxythymidine, d4T)
Zerit
*Pregnancy Risk Category: C*

## HOW SUPPLIED
*Capsules:* 15 mg, 20 mg, 30 mg, 40 mg

## ACTION
Unknown. A primidine nucleoside analogue that appears to prevent replication of retroviruses, including HIV, by inhibiting the enzyme reverse transcriptase.

## ONSET, PEAK, DURATION
Onset and duration unknown. Serum levels peak within 1 hour.

## INDICATIONS & DOSAGE
*Patients with advanced HIV infection who cannot tolerate or are unresponsive to other antiviral therapies –*
**Adults weighing 60 kg or more:** 40 mg P.O. q 12 hours.

**Adults weighing less than 60 kg:** 30 mg P.O. q 12 hours.

**ADVERSE REACTIONS**
**CNS:** *peripheral neuropathy, headache, malaise, insomnia, anxiety, depression, nervousness,* dizziness.
**CV:** chest pain.
**GI:** *abdominal pain, diarrhea, nausea, vomiting, anorexia,* dyspepsia, constipation, weight loss.
**Hematologic:** *neutropenia, **thrombocytopenia,*** anemia.
**Skin:** *rash, diaphoresis, pruritus,* maculopapular rash.
**Other:** *myalgia, hepatotoxicity, chills, fever, asthenia, back pain, arthralgia, dyspnea,* conjunctivitis.

**INTERACTIONS**
*Myelosuppressants:* additive myelosuppression. Avoid concomitant use.

**CONTRAINDICATIONS**
Contraindicated in patients with hypersensitivity to the drug.

**NURSING CONSIDERATIONS**
• Use cautiously in patients with renal impairment or history of peripheral neuropathy. Also use cautiously in pregnant women.
• *Alert:* Know that peripheral neuropathy appears to be the major dose-limiting adverse effect of stavudine. It may or may not resolve after drug is discontinued.
• Periodically monitor CBC and serum levels of creatinine, AST, ALT, and alkaline phosphatase, as ordered.

☑ **PATIENT TEACHING**
• Tell the patient that the drug may be taken without regard to meals.
• Warn the patient not to take any other drugs for HIV or AIDS unless the doctor has approved them.
• Teach the patient signs and symptoms of peripheral neuropathy — pain, burning, aching, weakness, or pins

and needles in the extremities — and tell him to report these immediately.

▼ *NEW DRUG*

# valacyclovir hydrochloride
Valtrex
*Pregnancy Risk Category: B*

**HOW SUPPLIED**
*Caplets:* 500 mg

**ACTION**
Rapidly converts to acyclovir, which in turn becomes incorporated into viral DNA and inhibits viral DNA polymerase, thereby inhibiting viral multiplication.

**ONSET, PEAK, DURATION**
Onset occurs about 30 minutes after oral administration. Peak and duration are unknown.

**INDICATIONS & DOSAGE**
*Treatment of herpes zoster (shingles) in immunocompetent patients* —
**Adults:** 1 g P.O. t.i.d. for 7 days. Dosage is adjusted for patients with impaired renal function, based on creatinine clearance level.

**ADVERSE REACTIONS**
**CNS:** *headache,* dizziness.
**GI:** *nausea,* vomiting, diarrhea, constipation, abdominal pain, anorexia.
**Other:** asthenia.

**INTERACTIONS**
*Cimetidine, probenecid:* reduces the rate but not the extent of valacyclovir to acyclovir and reduces the renal clearance of acyclovir, thus increasing acyclovir blood levels. Monitor for possible toxicity.

**CONTRAINDICATIONS**
Contraindicated in patients with hypersensitivity or intolerance to valacyclovir, acyclovir, or any component of the formulation.

Reactions may be *common,* uncommon, *life-threatening,* or **COMMON AND LIFE-THREATENING.**

## NURSING CONSIDERATIONS

• Know that valacyclovir is not recommended for use in immunocompromised patients. Thrombotic thrombocytopenic purpura and hemolytic uremic syndrome have occurred, resulting in death in some patients with advanced HIV disease and in bone marrow transplant and renal transplant recipients participating in clinical trials of valacyclovir.
• Use cautiously in patients with renal impairment and in those receiving other nephrotoxic drugs.
• Safety and efficacy in children have not been established.
• Know that Burroughs-Wellcome, the manufacturer, maintains an ongoing registry of women exposed to the drug during pregnancy. Follow-up studies have not shown an increased risk for birth defects for infants born to patients exposed to the drug during pregnancy. Health care providers are encouraged to report such exposures to the registrar at (800) 722-9292, ext 38465.
• Alert the doctor if the patient is breast-feeding; the drug may need to be discontinued.
• Know that dosage adjustment may be necessary in an elderly patient, depending on the patient's underlying renal status.
• Although there have been no reports of overdosage, precipitation of acyclovir in renal tubules may occur when solubility (2.5 mg/ml) is exceeded in the intratubular fluid. With acute renal failure and anuria, the patient may benefit from hemodialysis until renal function is restored.

## ☑ PATIENT TEACHING
• Inform the patient that valacyclovir may be taken without regard to meals.
• Teach the patient the signs and symptoms of herpes infection (rash, tingling, itching, and pain), and advise him to notify the doctor immediately if they occur. Treatment should be initiated as soon as possible after symptoms appear, preferably within 48 hours of the onset of zoster rash.

---

## zalcitabine (dideoxycytidine, ddC)
HIVID
*Pregnancy Risk Category: C*

### HOW SUPPLIED
*Tablets:* 0.375 mg, 0.75 mg

### ACTION
Inhibits replication of HIV by blocking viral DNA synthesis.

### ONSET, PEAK, DURATION
Onset and duration unknown. Peak plasma levels occur 1 to 2 hours after an oral dose.

### INDICATIONS & DOSAGE
*Monotherapy for treatment of advanced HIV disease in patients who either cannot tolerate zidovudine or who have disease progression while receiving zidovudine –*
**Adults and children 13 years or older:** 0.75 mg P.O. q 8 hours.
*Combination therapy with zidovudine for treatment of advanced HIV disease (CD4+ cell count equal to or less than 300 cells/mm³) –*
**Adults and children 13 years or older:** 0.75 mg P.O. q 8 hours administered concomitantly with zidovudine 200 mg P.O. q 8 hours.

### ADVERSE REACTIONS
**CNS:** *peripheral neuropathy, headache, fatigue,* dizziness, confusion, *seizures,* impaired concentration, amnesia, insomnia, mental depression, tremor, hypertonia, anxiety.
**EENT:** pharyngitis, cough, ocular pain, abnormal vision, ototoxicity, nasal discharge.
**GI:** nausea, vomiting, diarrhea, abdominal pain, anorexia, constipation, stomatitis, esophageal ulcer, glossitis.

---

*Liquid form contains alcohol. **May contain tartrazine. †Canada only. ‡Australia only. ◊OTC.

**Hematologic:** anemia, neutropenia, leukopenia, *thrombocytopenia.*
**Skin:** pruritus; night sweats; *erythematous, maculopapular, or follicular rash;* urticaria.
**Other:** myalgia, arthralgia, *fever,* hypoglycemia, *pancreatitis,* increased liver enzymes.

## INTERACTIONS
*Aminoglycosides, amphotericin B, foscarnet, and other drugs that may impair renal function:* increased risk of nephrotoxicity. Avoid concomitant use, when possible.
*Chloramphenicol, cisplatin, dapsone, disulfiram, ethionamide, glutethimide, gold salts, hydralazine, iodoquinol, isoniazid, metronidazole, nitrofurantoin, phenytoin, ribavirin, and vincristine as well as other drugs that can cause peripheral neuropathy:* increased risk of peripheral neuropathy. Avoid concomitant use.
*Pentamidine:* increased risk of pancreatitis. Avoid concomitant use when possible.

## CONTRAINDICATIONS
Contraindicated in patients with hypersensitivity to the drug or any component of the formulation.

## NURSING CONSIDERATIONS
• Use with extreme caution in patients with preexisting peripheral neuropathy.
• Use cautiously in patients with renal impairment (creatinine clearance below 55 ml/minute) because they may be at increased risk for toxicity to the drug. Dosage adjustments are necessary. Also use cautiously in patients with hepatic failure, history of pancreatitis, and baseline cardiomyopathy or history of CHF.
• Do not administer the drug with food because it decreases the rate and extent of absorption.
• Assess for signs of peripheral neuropathy, characterized by numbness

and burning in the extremities, which are the major toxic effects of the drug. If drug isn't withdrawn, peripheral neuropathy can progress to sharp shooting pain or severe continuous burning pain requiring opioid analgesics. It may or may not be reversible.
• If the patient experiences symptoms that resemble peripheral neuropathy, prepare to withdraw the drug, as ordered. It should be discontinued if symptoms are bilateral and persist beyond 72 hours. If symptoms persist or worsen beyond 1 week, drug should be permanently discontinued. However, if all findings relevant to peripheral neuropathy have resolved to minor symptoms, the drug may be reintroduced at 0.375 mg P.O. q 8 hours.

## ☑ PATIENT TEACHING
• Instruct the patient to take drug on an empty stomach.
• Make sure the patient understands that the drug doesn't cure HIV infection and that opportunistic infections may still occur despite continued use. Review safe sex practices with the patient.
• Inform the patient that peripheral neuropathy is the major toxicity associated with this drug and that pancreatitis is the major life-threatening toxic reaction. Review the signs and symptoms of these adverse reactions, and instruct the patient to call the doctor promptly if any appear.
• Instruct the patient of childbearing age to use an effective contraceptive while taking this drug.

# zidovudine (azidothymidine, AZT)
Apo-Zidovudine†, Novo-AZT†, Retrovir

*Pregnancy Risk Category: C*

## HOW SUPPLIED
*Capsules:* 100 mg
*Syrup:* 50 mg/5 ml

---

Reactions may be *common,* uncommon, *life-threatening,* or COMMON AND LIFE-THREATENING.

*Injection:* 10 mg/ml

## ACTION
Unknown. Appears to prevent replication of HIV by inhibiting the enzyme reverse transcriptase.

## ONSET, PEAK, DURATION
Onset immediate after I.V. infusion, unknown after oral administration. Peak plasma levels occur in ½ to 1½ hours. Duration unknown.

## INDICATIONS & DOSAGE
*Symptomatic HIV infection, including AIDS –*
**Adults and children 12 years and over:** 100 mg P.O. q 4 hours around the clock.
**Children 3 months to 12 years:** 180 mg/m² P.O. q 6 hours (720 mg/m²/day), not to exceed 200 mg q 6 hours.
*Selected patients with AIDS or advanced AIDS-related complex (ARC) who have a history of* Pneumocystis carinii *pneumonia or a CD4+ lymphocyte count below 200 cells/mm³ –*
**Adults:** 1 to 2 mg/kg I.V. infused over 1 hour q 4 hours around the clock, followed by 200 mg P.O. q 4 hours around the clock when oral administration can replace parenteral administration.
*Asymptomatic HIV infection –*
**Adults and children 12 years and over:** 100 mg P.O. q 4 hours while awake (500 mg daily).
**Children 3 months to 12 years:** 180 mg/m² P.O. q 6 hours (720 mg/m²/day), not to exceed 200 mg q 6 hours.
*To reduce risk of transmission of HIV from infected mother with a baseline CD4+ lymphocyte counts greater than 200 cells/mm³ to the newborn –*
**Adults:** 100 mg P.O. given initially between 14 and 34 weeks gestation and continued throughout pregnancy. During labor, administer loading dose of 2 mg/kg I.V. followed by continuous infusion of 1 mg/kg/hour until delivery.

**Infants:** 2 mg/kg P.O. (syrup) q 6 hours for 6 weeks beginning 8 to 12 hours after birth.
*Combination therapy with zalcitabine for treatment of advanced HIV disease (CD4+ cell count equal to or less than 300 cells/mm³) –*
**Adults and children 13 years or older:** 200 mg P.O. q 8 hours administered concomitantly with zalcitabine 0.75 mg P.O. q 8 hours.

## ADVERSE REACTIONS
**CNS:** *headache, seizures,* paresthesia, *malaise,* insomnia, *dizziness,* somnolence.
**GI:** *nausea, anorexia, abdominal pain, vomiting,* constipation, *diarrhea,* dyspepsia.
**Hematologic:** *severe bone marrow suppression (resulting in anemia), agranulocytosis, thrombocytopenia.*
**Skin:** *rash.*
**Other:** myalgia, diaphoresis, *fever, asthenia,* taste perversion.

## INTERACTIONS
*Acetaminophen, aspirin, co-trimoxazole, indomethacin:* may impair hepatic metabolism of zidovudine, increasing the drug's toxicity. Monitor closely.
*Acyclovir:* possible seizures, lethargy, and fatigue. Use together cautiously.
*Amphotericin B, dapsone, flucytosine, pentamidine:* increased risk of nephrotoxicity and bone marrow suppression. Monitor closely.
*Ganciclovir:* increased risk and hematologic toxicity. Monitor closely.
*Other cytotoxic drugs:* additive adverse effects on the bone marrow. Avoid concomitant use.
*Probenecid:* may decrease the renal clearance of zidovudine. Avoid concomitant use.
*Ribavirin:* antagonizes the antiviral activity of zidovudine against HIV. Avoid concomitant use.

---

*Liquid form contains alcohol.   **May contain tartrazine.   †Canada only.   ‡Australia only.   ◊OTC.

## CONTRAINDICATIONS
Contraindicated in patients with hypersensitivity to the drug.

## NURSING CONSIDERATIONS
• Use cautiously and with close monitoring in patients with advanced symptomatic HIV infection and in patients with severe bone marrow depression.
• Use with caution in any patient with hepatomegaly, hepatitis, or other known risk factors for liver disease and in patients with renal insufficiency.
• **I.V. use:** Dilute before administration. Remove the calculated dose from the vial; add to $D_5W$ to achieve a concentration that does not exceed 4 mg/ml. Infuse drug over 1 hour at a constant rate; give every 4 hours around the clock. Avoid rapid infusion or bolus injection. Adding mixture to biological or colloidal fluids (for example, blood products, protein solutions) is not recommended. After drug is diluted, the solution is physically and chemically stable for 24 hours at room temperature and for 48 hours if refrigerated at 35.6° to 46.4° F (2° to 8° C) to minimize the risk of microbial contamination. Store undiluted vials at 59° to 77° F (15° to 25° C) and protect them from light.
• Monitor blood studies every 2 weeks, as ordered, to detect anemia or agranulocytosis. Patients may require dosage reduction or temporary discontinuation of the drug.
• Be aware that zidovudine has been shown to temporarily decrease morbidity and mortality in certain patients with AIDS or ARC.

## ☑ PATIENT TEACHING
• Tell patient to take drug exactly as directed and not to share it with others.
• Instruct patient to take drug on an empty stomach. To avoid esophageal irritation, tell patient to take drug while sitting upright and with adequate amount of fluids.
• Remind patient that he *must* comply with the every-4-hour dosage schedule. Suggest ways to avoid missing doses, perhaps by using an alarm clock.
• Advise patient that blood transfusions may be needed during treatment. Zidovudine frequently causes a low RBC count.
• Warn patient not to take any other drugs for AIDS unless the doctor has approved them.
• Advise pregnant, HIV-infected patient that zidovudine therapy only *reduces* the risk of HIV transmission to her newborn. Long-term risks to infants are unknown.
• Advise health care workers who consider zidovudine prophylaxis after occupational exposure (following needle-stick injury, for example) that animal and human studies have not yet proved the drug's safety or efficacy. Some clinicians do not advocate such use of zidovudine.

# 18

## Macrolide anti-infectives

**azithromycin**
**clarithromycin**
**dirithromycin**
**erythromycin base**
**erythromycin estolate**
**erythromycin ethylsuccinate**
**erythromycin gluceptate**
**erythromycin lactobionate**
**erythromycin stearate**

**COMBINATION PRODUCTS**
None.

---

## azithromycin
Zithromax

*Pregnancy Risk Category: B*

**HOW SUPPLIED**
*Capsules:* 250 mg

**ACTION**
Binds to the 50S subunit of bacterial ribosomes, blocking protein synthesis; bacteriostatic or bactericidal, depending on concentration.

**ONSET, PEAK, DURATION**
Onset and duration unknown. Serum levels peak in young patients in 2.5 to 3.2 hours, in elderly patients in 3.8 to 4.4 hours.

**INDICATIONS & DOSAGE**
*Acute bacterial exacerbations of COPD caused by* Haemophilus influenzae, Moraxella (Branhamella) catarrhalis, *or* Streptococcus pneumoniae; *mild community-acquired pneumonia caused by* H. influenzae *or* S. pneumoniae; *uncomplicated skin and skin-structure infections caused by* Staphylococcus aureus, Streptococcus pyogenes, *or* S. agalactiae; *second-line therapy of pharyngitis or tonsillitis caused by* S. pyogenes —

**Adults and adolescents 16 years and over:** 500 mg P.O. as a single dose on day 1, followed by 250 mg daily on days 2 through 5. Total dose is 1.5 g.
*Nongonococcal urethritis or cervicitis caused by* Chlamydia trachomatis —
**Adults and adolescents 16 years and over:** 1 g P.O. as a single dose.

**ADVERSE REACTIONS**
**CNS:** dizziness, vertigo, headache, fatigue, somnolence.
**CV:** palpitations, chest pain.
**GI:** *nausea, vomiting, diarrhea, abdominal pain,* dyspepsia, flatulence, melena, cholestatic jaundice, pseudomembranous colitis.
**GU:** monilia, vaginitis, nephritis.
**Skin:** rash, photosensitivity.
**Other:** angioedema.

**INTERACTIONS**
*Aluminum- and magnesium-containing antacids:* lowered peak plasma levels of azithromycin. Separate administration times by at least 2 hours.
*Astemizole and terfenadine:* prolongation of QT interval and ventricular tachycardia have been associated with other macrolide anti-infectives. Monitor patient closely.
*Digoxin:* may cause elevated digoxin levels. Monitor closely.
*Theophylline:* may increase plasma theophylline levels with other macrolides; effect of azithromycin is unknown. Monitor theophylline levels carefully.
*Warfarin:* may increase PT with other macrolides; effect of azithromycin is unknown. Monitor PT carefully.

**CONTRAINDICATIONS**
Contraindicated in patients with hypersensitivity to erythromycin or other macrolides.

---

*Liquid form contains alcohol. **May contain tartrazine. †Canada only. ‡Australia only. ◇OTC.

## NURSING CONSIDERATIONS
- Use cautiously in patients with impaired hepatic function.
- Obtain specimen for culture and sensitivity tests before first dose. Therapy may begin pending results.
- Administer 1 hour before or 2 hours after meals; do not administer with antacids.
- Monitor for superinfection. May cause overgrowth of nonsusceptible bacteria or fungi.

☑ **PATIENT TEACHING**
- Tell the patient to take drug as prescribed, even if he feels better.
- Tell the patient to take drug on an empty stomach because food or antacids will decrease absorption.

---

# clarithromycin
Biaxin

*Pregnancy Risk Category: C*

## HOW SUPPLIED
*Tablets:* 250 mg, 500 mg
*Suspension:* 125 mg/5 ml, 250 mg/5 ml

## ACTION
Binds to the 50S subunit of bacterial ribosomes, blocking protein synthesis; bacteriostatic or bactericidal, depending on concentration.

## ONSET, PEAK, DURATION
Onset and duration unknown. Serum levels peak in 2 to 3 hours.

## INDICATIONS & DOSAGE
*Pharyngitis or tonsillitis caused by* Streptococcus pyogenes —
**Adults:** 250 mg P.O. q 12 hours for 10 days.
**Children:** 15 mg/kg/day P.O. in divided doses q 12 hours for 10 days.
*Acute maxillary sinusitis caused by* S. pneumoniae —
**Adults:** 500 mg P.O. q 12 hours for 14 days.
**Children:** 15 mg/kg/day P.O. in divided doses q 12 hours for 10 days.
*Acute exacerbations of chronic bronchitis caused by* Moraxella (Branhamella) catarrhalis *or* S. pneumoniae; *pneumonia caused by* S. pneumoniae *or* Mycoplasma pneumoniae —
**Adults:** 250 mg P.O. q 12 hours for 7 to 14 days.
*Acute exacerbations of chronic bronchitis caused by* Haemophilus influenzae —
**Adults:** 500 mg P.O. q 12 hours for 7 to 14 days.
*Uncomplicated skin and skin-structure infections caused by* Staphylococcus aureus *or* Streptococcus pyogenes —
**Adults:** 250 mg P.O. q 12 hours for 7 to 14 days.
**Children:** 15 mg/kg/day P.O. in divided doses q 12 hours for 10 days.
*Acute otitis media —*
**Children:** 15 mg/kg/day P.O. in divided doses q 12 hours for 10 days.

## ADVERSE REACTIONS
**CNS:** headache.
**GI:** *diarrhea, nausea, abnormal taste,* dyspepsia, abdominal pain or discomfort.

## INTERACTIONS
*Carbamazepine:* may increase serum levels of carbamazepine. Monitor blood levels.
*Digoxin:* may increase serum digoxin levels. Monitor for digitalis toxicity.
*Terfenadine:* altered metabolism of terfenadine, with prolongation of QT interval and ventricular tachycardia. Avoid concurrent use.
*Theophylline:* increased plasma theophylline levels possible with other macrolides; effect of clarithromycin is unknown. Monitor theophylline levels carefully.
*Warfarin:* increased PT possible with other macrolides; effect of clarithromycin is unknown. Monitor PT carefully.

---

Reactions may be *common,* uncommon, *life-threatening,* or COMMON AND LIFE-THREATENING.

*Zidovudine:* decreased zidovudine levels. Monitor effectivenss of zidovudine closely.

## CONTRAINDICATIONS
Contraindicated in patients with hypersensitivity to erythromycin or other macrolides.

## NURSING CONSIDERATIONS
• Use cautiously in patients with hepatic or renal impairment.
• Obtain urine specimen for culture and sensitivity tests before first dose. Therapy may begin pending results.
• Monitor the patient for superinfection. Drug may cause overgrowth of nonsusceptible bacteria or fungi.

☑ **PATIENT TEACHING**
• Tell the patient to take drug as prescribed, even if he feels better.
• Instruct the patient to report persistent adverse reactions.

▼ *NEW DRUG*
━━━━━━━━━━━━━━━━━━━━

# dirithromycin
Dynabac
*Pregnancy Risk Category: C*

## HOW SUPPLIED
*Tablets:* 250 mg

## ACTION
Inhibits bacterial RNA-dependent protein synthesis by binding to the 50S subunit of the ribosome.

## ONSET, PEAK, DURATION
Onset and duration are unknown. Peak level occurs in about 4 hours.

## INDICATIONS & DOSAGE
*Acute bacterial exacerbations of chronic bronchitis due to* Moraxella catarrhalis *or* Streptococcus pneumoniae; *secondary bacterial infection of acute bronchitis due to* M. catarrhalis *or* S. pneumoniae; *uncomplicated skin and skin structure infec-*

*tions due to* Staphylococcus aureus *(methicillin-susceptible) —*
**Adults and children 12 years and older:** 500 mg P.O. daily with food for 7 days.
*Community-acquired pneumonia due to* Legionella pneumophila, Mycoplasma pneumoniae, *or* S. pneumoniae —
**Adults and children 12 years and older:** 500 mg P.O. daily with food for 14 days.
*Pharyngitis or tonsillitis due to* Streptococcus pyogenes —
**Adults and children 12 years and older:** 500 mg P.O. daily with food for 10 days.

## ADVERSE REACTIONS
**CNS:** headache, dizziness, vertigo, insomnia.
**GI:** abdominal pain, nausea, diarrhea, vomiting, dyspepsia, GI disorder, flatulence.
**Hematologic:** increased platelet eosinophil, and neutrophil count.
**Respiratory:** increased cough, dyspnea.
**Skin:** rash, pruritus, urticaria.
**Other:** pain (nonspecific), asthenia, hyperkalemia, decreased bicarbonate levels, increased CPK levels.

## INTERACTIONS
*Antacids and histamine₂ antagonists:* absorption slightly enhanced when dirithromycin is administered immediately after these drugs.
*Terfenadine:* may decrease metabolism, which may lead to increased levels of terfenadine and cardiotoxicity. Monitor terfenadine levels when dirithromycin and terfenadine are administered comcomitantly.
*Theophylline:* may alter steady-state plasma concentration of theophylline. Monitor theophylline plasma concentrations. Dosage adjustments may be needed.
**NOTE:** Alfentanil, anticoagulants, astemizole, bromocriptine, carbamazepine, cyclosporine, digoxin, diso-

pyramide, ergotamine, hexobarbital, lovastatin, phenytoin, triazolam, and valproate have been reported to interact with erythromycin products. It's unknown whether these same drugs interact with dirithromycin. Until further data are available, caution should be used during coadministration.

**CONTRAINDICATIONS**
Contraindicated in patients with hypersensitivity to the drug, erythromycin, or any other macrolide antibiotic.

**NURSING CONSIDERATIONS**
• Use cautiously in patients with hepatic insufficiency and in breast-feeding women.
• Safety of the drug in children under age 12 has not been established.
• Obtain culture and sensitivity tests before first dose. Therapy may begin pending results.
• Be aware that drug should not be used in patients with known, suspected, or potential bacteremias because serum levels are inadequate to provide antibacterial coverage of the bloodstream.
• Administer drug with food or within 1 hour of food intake.
• Monitor the patient for superinfection. Drug may cause overgrowth of nonsusceptible bacteria or fungi.

☑ **PATIENT TEACHING**
• Tell patient to take drug as prescribed, even if he feels better.
• Tell patient to take drug with food or within 1 hour after eating and not to cut, chew, or crush the tablet.

# erythromycin base
Apo-Erythro†, EMU-V‡, E-Mycin, Erybid†, ERYC, ERYC-125†, ERYC-250†, Ery-Tab, Erythromid†, Erythromycin Base Filmtab, Erythromycin Delayed-Release, Novo-rythro†, PCE Disperstab, Robimycin

# erythromycin estolate
Ilosone, Novo-rythro†

# erythromycin ethylsuccinate
Apo-Erythro-ES†, EEG Dulcets‡, E.E.S., EES-400‡, EES granules‡, EryPed, EryPed 200, EryPed 400

# erythromycin gluceptate
Ilotycin

# erythromycin lactobionate
Erythrocin, Erythromycin Lactobionate

# erythromycin stearate
Apo-Erythro-S†, Eramycin, Erythrocin Stearate, Novo-rythro†

*Pregnancy Risk Category: B*

**HOW SUPPLIED**
**erythromycin base**
*Tablets (enteric-coated):* 250 mg, 333 mg, 500 mg
*Tablets (filmtabs):* 250 mg, 500 mg
*Capsules (enteric-coated):* 250 mg
**erythromycin estolate**
*Tablets:* 500 mg
*Capsules:* 250 mg
*Oral suspension:* 125 mg/5 ml, 250 mg/5 ml
**erythromycin ethylsuccinate**
*Tablets:* 400 mg
*Tablets (chewable):* 200 mg
*Oral suspension:* 200 mg/5 ml, 400 mg/5 ml, 100 mg/2.5 ml
**erythromycin gluceptate**
*Injection:* 1-g vials
**erythromycin lactobionate**
*Injection:* 500-mg, 1-g vials
**erythromycin stearate**
*Tablets (film-coated):* 250 mg, 500 mg

**ACTION**
Inhibits bacterial protein synthesis by binding to the 50S subunit of the ribosome.

---

Reactions may be *common,* uncommon, *life-threatening,* or COMMON AND LIFE-THREATENING.

## ONSET, PEAK, DURATION
Onset immediate after I.V. infusion, unknown after oral administration. Peak serum levels occur 1 to 4 hours after an oral dose or immediately after I.V. infusion. Duration unknown.

## INDICATIONS & DOSAGE
*Acute pelvic inflammatory disease caused by* Neisseria gonorrhoeae —
**Adults:** 500 mg I.V. (erythromycin gluceptate, lactobionate) q 6 hours for 3 days, then 250 mg (erythromycin base, estolate, stearate) or 400 mg (erythromycin ethylsuccinate) P.O. q 6 hours for 7 days.
*Endocarditis prophylaxis for dental procedures in patients allergic to penicillin —*
**Adults:** initially, 800 mg (ethylsuccinate) or 1 g (stearate) P.O. 1½ to 2 hours before procedure; then 400 mg (ethylsuccinate) or 500 mg (stearate) P.O. 6 hours later.
**Children:** initially, 20 mg/kg (ethylsuccinate or stearate) P.O. 1½ to 2 hours before procedure; then half the initial dose 6 hours later.
*Intestinal amebiasis —*
**Adults:** 250 mg (base, estolate, stearate) or 400 mg (ethylsuccinate) P.O. q 6 hours for 10 to 14 days.
**Children:** 30 to 50 mg/kg (base, estolate, ethylsuccinate, stearate) P.O. daily, in divided doses q 6 hours for 10 to 14 days.
*Mild to moderately severe respiratory tract, skin, and soft-tissue infections caused by sensitive group A beta-hemolytic streptococci,* Diplococcus pneumoniae, Mycoplasma pneumoniae, Corynebacterium diphtheriae, Bordetella pertussis, *or* Listeria monocytogenes —
**Adults:** 250 to 500 mg (erythromycin base, estolate, stearate) P.O. q 6 hours; or 400 to 800 mg (erythromycin ethylsuccinate) P.O. q 6 hours; or 15 to 20 mg/kg I.V. daily, as continuous infusion or in divided doses q 6 hours.
**Children:** 30 mg/kg to 50 mg/kg (oral erythromycin salts) P.O. daily, in divided doses q 6 hours; or 15 to 20 mg/kg I.V. daily, in divided doses q 4 to 6 hours.
*Syphilis —*
**Adults:** 500 mg (erythromycin base, estolate, stearate) P.O. q.i.d. for 15 days.
*Legionnaire's disease —*
**Adults:** 500 mg to 1 g I.V. or P.O. (base, estolate, stearate) or 800 to 1,600 mg (ethylsuccinate) q 6 hours for 21 days.
*Uncomplicated urethral, endocervical, or rectal infections when tetracyclines are contraindicated —*
**Adults:** 500 mg (base, estolate, stearate) or 800 mg (ethylsuccinate) P.O. q.i.d. for at least 7 days.
*Urogenital* Chlamydia trachomatis *infections during pregnancy —*
**Adults:** 500 mg (base, estolate, stearate) P.O. q.i.d. for at least 7 days or 250 mg (base, estolate, stearate) or 400 mg (ethylsuccinate) P.O. q.i.d. for at least 14 days.
*Conjunctivitis caused by* C. trachomatis *in neonates —*
**Neonates:** 50 mg/kg P.O. daily in four divided doses for at least 2 weeks.
*Pneumonia in infants caused by* C. trachomatis —
**Infants:** 50 mg/kg/day in four divided doses for at least 3 weeks.

## ADVERSE REACTIONS
**EENT:** hearing loss with high I.V. doses.
**GI:** *abdominal pain and cramping, nausea, vomiting, diarrhea.*
**Hepatic:** cholestatic jaundice (with erythromycin estolate).
**Skin:** urticaria, rash, eczema.
**Other:** overgrowth of nonsusceptible bacteria or fungi; *anaphylaxis;* fever; *venous irritation, thrombophlebitis after I.V. injection.*

---

*Liquid form contains alcohol.   **May contain tartrazine.   †Canada only.   ‡Australia only.   ◇OTC.

## INTERACTIONS

*Astemizole, terfenadine:* decreased metabolism, leading to increased levels of these antihistamines and cardiotoxicity. Avoid concomitant use.

*Carbamazepine:* increased carbamazepine blood levels and increased risk of toxicity. Monitor closely.

*Clindamycin, lincomycin:* may be antagonistic. Don't use together.

*Cyclosporine:* increased concentrations of cyclosporine. Monitor closely.

*Digoxin:* increased serum digoxin levels. Monitor for digoxin toxicity.

*Disopyramide:* increased disopyramide plasma levels resulting, in some cases, in arrhythmias and increased QT intervals. Monitor ECG.

*Midazolam and triazolam:* increased effects of these drugs. Monitor closely.

*Oral anticoagulants:* increased anticoagulant effect. Monitor PT closely.

*Theophylline:* decreased erythromycin blood level and increased theophylline toxicity. Use together cautiously.

## CONTRAINDICATIONS

Contraindicated in patients with hypersensitivity to the drug or other macrolides. Erythromycin estolate is contraindicated in patients with hepatic disease.

## NURSING CONSIDERATIONS

● Use erythromycin salts cautiously in patients with impaired hepatic function.

● Obtain urine specimen for culture and sensitivity tests before first dose. Therapy may begin pending results.

● When administering suspension, be sure to note the concentration.

● **I.V. use:** Reconstitute according to manufacturer's directions and dilute each 250 mg in at least 100 ml of 0.9% sodium chloride solution. Infuse over 1 hour.

● *Alert:* Do not administer erythromycin lactobionate with other drugs.

● Monitor the patient for superinfection. May cause overgrowth of non-susceptible bacteria or fungi.

● Monitor hepatic function (increased serum levels of alkaline phosphatase, ALT, AST, and bilirubin may occur). Erythromycin estolate may cause serious hepatotoxicity in adults (reversible cholestatic jaundice). Other erythromycin salts cause hepatotoxicity to a lesser degree.

● Keep in mind that the drug may falsely elevate concentrations of urinary catecholamines, 17-hydroxycorticosteroids, and 17-ketosteroids.

● Be aware that drug may interfere with colorimetric assays, resulting in falsely elevated AST and ALT levels.

● Keep in mind that coated tablets or encapsulated pellets have caused fewer instances of GI upset; they may be better tolerated by patients who cannot tolerate erythromycin.

## ☑ PATIENT TEACHING

● Tell the patient to take drug as prescribed, even if he feels better.

● For best absorption, instruct the patient to take oral form of drug with full glass of water 1 hour before or 2 hours after meals. Coated tablets may be taken with meals. Tell the patient not to drink fruit juice with drug. Chewable erythromycin tablets should not be swallowed whole.

● Instruct the patient to report adverse reactions, especially nausea, abdominal pain, and fever.

---

Reactions may be *common,* uncommon, *life-threatening,* or **COMMON AND LIFE-THREATENING.**

# 19

## Miscellaneous anti-infectives

aztreonam
bacitracin
chloramphenicol
chloramphenicol palmitate
chloramphenicol sodium
   succinate
clindamycin hydrochloride
clindamycin palmitate
   hydrochloride
clindamycin phosphate
imipenem/cilastatin sodium
lincomycin hydrochloride
methenamine hippurate
methenamine mandelate
nitrofurantoin macrocrystals
nitrofurantoin microcrystals
polymyxin B sulfate
rifabutin
spectinomycin hydrochloride
trimethoprim
trimetrexate glucuronate
vancomycin hydrochloride

### COMBINATION PRODUCTS
CYSTEX: methenamine 165 mg, salicylamide 65 mg, sodium salicylate 97 mg, and benzoic acid 32 mg.
HEXALOL: methenamine 40.8 mg, phenyl salicylate 18.1 mg, atropine sulfate 0.03 mg, hyoscyamine 0.03 mg, benzoic acid 4.5 mg, and methylene blue 5.4 mg.
MACRODID: nitrofurantoin macrocrystals 25 mg and nitrofurantoin monohydrate 75 mg.
THIACIDE: methenamine mandelate 500 mg and potassium acid phosphate 250 mg.
TRAC TABS 2X: methenamine 120 mg, methylene blue 6 mg, phenyl salicylate 30 mg, atropine sulfate 0.06 mg, hyoscyamine sulfate 0.03 mg, and benzoic acid 7.5 mg.
URISEDAMINE: methenamine mandelate 500 mg and hyoscyamine 0.15 mg.

URO-PHOSPHATE: methenamine 300 mg and sodium acid phosphate 500 mg. Sugar coated.
UROQUID-ACID: methenamine mandelate 350 mg and sodium acid phosphate 200 mg.
UROQUID-ACID NO. 2: methenamine mandelate 500 mg and sodium acid phosphate 500 mg.

---

## aztreonam
Azactam

*Pregnancy Risk Category: B*

### HOW SUPPLIED
*Injection:* 500-mg, 1-g, 2-g vials

### ACTION
Inhibits bacterial cell-wall synthesis, ultimately causing cell-wall destruction; bactericidal.

### ONSET, PEAK, DURATION
Onset immediate after I.V. administration, unknown after I.M. injection. Serum levels peak in 0.6 to 1.3 hours after I.M. injection, immediately after I.V. infusion. Duration unknown.

### INDICATIONS & DOSAGE
*Urinary tract infections, lower respiratory tract infections, septicemia, skin and skin-structure infections, intra-abdominal infections, surgical infections, and gynecologic infections caused by various gram-negative aerobic organisms—*
**Adults:** 500 mg to 2 g I.V. or I.M. q 8 to 12 hours. For severe systemic or life-threatening infections, 2 g q 6 to 8 hours may be given. Maximum dosage is 8 g daily.

---

## ADVERSE REACTIONS
**CNS:** *seizures,* headache, insomnia, confusion.
**CV:** hypotension.
**GI:** diarrhea, nausea, vomiting.
**Hematologic:** neutropenia, anemia, pancytopenia, *thrombocytopenia,* leukocytosis, thrombocytosis.
**Other:** hypersensitivity reactions (rash, *anaphylaxis*), transient elevation of ALT and AST, thrombophlebitis at I.V. site, discomfort and swelling at I.M. injection site.

## INTERACTIONS
*Aminoglycosides, beta-lactam antibiotics and other anti-infectives:* synergistic effect. Monitor patient closely.
*Cefoxitin, imipenem:* possible antagonistic effect. Do not use together.
*Probenecid:* increased serum aztreonam levels. Avoid concomitant use.

## CONTRAINDICATIONS
Contraindicated in patients with hypersensitivity to the drug.

## NURSING CONSIDERATIONS
• Use cautiously in elderly patients and in those with impaired renal function. Dosage adjustment may be necessary.
• Obtain culture and sensitivity tests before first dose. Therapy may begin pending results.
• **I.V. use:** To administer a bolus of aztreonam, inject drug slowly (over 3 to 5 minutes) directly into a vein or I.V. tubing. Give infusions over 20 minutes to 1 hour.
• Administer I.M. injections deep into a large muscle mass, such as the upper outer quadrant of the gluteus maximus or the lateral aspect of the thigh. Know that doses greater than 1 g should be given I.V.
• Observe the patient for signs of superinfection.
• Because aztreonam is ineffective against gram-positive and anaerobic

organisms, anticipate using it with other antibiotics for immediate treatment of life-threatening illnesses. Aztreonam is a narrow-spectrum antibiotic, effective only against gram-negative organisms.
• Be aware that patients who are allergic to penicillins or cephalosporins may not be allergic to aztreonam. However, close monitoring of those who have had an immediate hypersensitivity reaction to these antibiotics is recommended.

## ☑ PATIENT TEACHING
• Warn patient receiving I.M. drug that pain and swelling at the injection site may occur.
• Tell patient to alert nurse if discomfort occurs at I.V. insertion site.
• Instruct patient to report adverse reactions promptly.

---

# bacitracin
*Pregnancy Risk Category: NR*

## HOW SUPPLIED
*Injection:* 10,000-unit, 50,000-unit vials

## ACTION
Hinders bacterial cell-wall synthesis, damaging the bacterial plasma membrane and making the cell more vulnerable to osmotic pressure.

## ONSET, PEAK, DURATION
Onset and duration unknown. Plasma levels peak within 1 to 2 hours of an I.M. injection.

## INDICATIONS & DOSAGE
*Pneumonia or empyema caused by susceptible staphylococci –*
**Infants over 2.5 kg:** 1,000 units/kg I.M. daily, divided q 8 to 12 hours.
**Infants under 2.5 kg:** 900 units/kg I.M. daily, divided q 8 to 12 hours.

## ADVERSE REACTIONS
**EENT:** ototoxicity.
**GI:** nausea, vomiting.
**GU:** *nephrotoxicity (albuminuria,* cylindruria, oliguria, anuria, increased BUN, *tabular and glomerular necrosis).*
**Skin:** urticaria, rash.
**Other:** pain at injection site.

## INTERACTIONS
*Nephrotoxic drugs (such as aminoglycosides):* increased nephrotoxicity. Use together cautiously.
*Neuromuscular blockers, inhalation anesthetics:* prolonged muscle weakness. Monitor the patient for excessive muscle weakness or respiratory distress.

## CONTRAINDICATIONS
Contraindicated in patients with hypersensitivity to the drug or impaired renal function.

## NURSING CONSIDERATIONS
• Use cautiously in those with myasthenia gravis and neuromuscular disease.
• Obtain culture and sensitivity tests before first dose. Therapy may begin pending results.
• Assess baseline renal function studies before starting therapy.
• Administer by deep I.M. injection only.
• Know that concentration of bacitracin should be between 5,000 and 10,000 units/ml. Store in refrigerator. Drug is inactivated if stored at room temperature.
• Monitor renal function daily during therapy. Notify the doctor of any change.
• Maintain adequate fluid intake, and monitor urine output closely. If fluid intake or output decreases, notify the doctor.
• Provide measures to keep urine pH above 6.0 to reduce the risk of nephrotoxicity.

• Be aware that prolonged therapy may result in overgrowth of nonsusceptible organisms, especially *Candida albicans.*

## ☑ PATIENT TEACHING
• Warn the patient that injection may be painful.
• Instruct the patient to report adverse reactions promptly.

---

## chloramphenicol
Chloromycetin, Novochlorocap†

## chloramphenicol palmitate
Chloromycetin Palmitate

## chloramphenicol sodium succinate
Chloromycetin Sodium Succinate, Pentamycetin†

*Pregnancy Risk Category: NR*

## HOW SUPPLIED
**chloramphenicol**
*Capsules:* 250 mg, 500 mg
**chloramphenicol palmitate**
*Oral suspension:* 150 mg/5 ml
**chloramphenicol sodium succinate**
*Injection:* 1-g vial

## ACTION
Inhibits bacterial protein synthesis by binding to the 50S subunit of the ribosome; bacteriostatic.

## ONSET, PEAK, DURATION
Onset immediate after I.V. administration, unknown after oral administration. Serum levels peak immediately after I.V. administration, 1 to 3 hours after oral dose. Duration unknown.

## INDICATIONS & DOSAGE
Haemophilus influenzae *meningitis, acute* Salmonella typhi *infection, and meningitis, bacteremia, or other severe infections caused by sensitive* Salmonella *species,* Rickettsia, *lympho-*

*granuloma, psittacosis, or various
sensitive gram-negative organisms* —
**Adults:** 50 to 100 mg/kg P.O. or I.V.
daily, divided q 6 hours. Maximum
dosage is 100 mg/kg daily.
**Full-term infants older than 2
weeks with normal metabolic processes:** up to 50 mg/kg P.O. or I.V.
daily, divided q 6 hours.
**Premature infants, neonates 2
weeks or younger, and children and
infants with immature metabolic
processes:** 25 mg/kg P.O. or I.V. once
daily. I.V. route must be used to treat
meningitis.

## ADVERSE REACTIONS
**CNS:** headache, mild depression,
confusion, delirium, peripheral neuropathy with prolonged therapy.
**EENT:** optic neuritis (in patients with
cystic fibrosis), glossitis, decreased
visual acuity.
**GI:** nausea, vomiting, stomatitis,
diarrhea, enterocolitis.
**Hematologic:** *aplastic anemia, hypoplastic anemia, granulocytopenia,
thrombocytopenia.*
**Other:** hypersensitivity reactions (fever, rash, urticaria, *anaphylaxis*),
jaundice, *gray syndrome in neonates,
(abdominal distention, gray cyanosis, vasomotor collapse, respiratory
distress, death within a few hours of
onset of symptoms).*

## INTERACTIONS
*Anticoagulants, barbiturates, hydan-
toins, iron salts, sulfonylureas:* increased blood levels of these agents
possible. Monitor for toxicity.
*Penicillins:* synergistic effects may
develop in the treatment of certain
microorganisms, but antagonism may
also occur. Monitor effectiveness
closely.
*Rifampin:* may reduce chloramphenicol levels. Monitor for changes in effectiveness.
*Vitamin B₁₂:* may decrease response of

vitamin B in patients with pernicious
anemia. Monitor closely.

## CONTRAINDICATIONS
Contraindicated in patients with hypersensitivity to the drug.

## NURSING CONSIDERATIONS
● Use cautiously in patients with impaired hepatic or renal function, acute
intermittent porphyria, and G6PD deficiency and with other drugs that
cause bone marrow suppression or
blood disorders.
● Obtain specimen for culture and
sensitivity tests before first dose.
Therapy may begin pending results.
● **I.V. use:** Give I.V. slowly over at
least 1 minute. Check injection site
daily for phlebitis and irritation.
● Reconstitute 1-g vial of powder for
injection with 10 ml of sterile water
for injection. Concentration will be
100 mg/ml. Stable for 30 days at room
temperature, but refrigeration recommended. Do not use cloudy solutions.
● Obtain plasma concentration levels.
Therapeutic plasma concentrations
are 5 to 25 mcg/ml.
● Monitor CBC, platelets, serum iron,
and reticulocytes before and every 2
days during therapy, as ordered. Stop
drug immediately if anemia, reticulocytopenia, leukopenia, or thrombocytopenia develops, and notify doctor.
● Monitor for evidence of superinfection.

## ☑ PATIENT TEACHING
● Tell the patient to take medication
for as long as prescribed, exactly as
directed, even after he feels better.
● Instruct the patient to report adverse reactions to the doctor, especially nausea, vomiting, diarrhea, fever, confusion, sore throat, or mouth
sores.
● Tell the patient receiving drug I.V.
to alert nurse if discomfort occurs at
I.V. insertion site.

---

Reactions may be *common,* uncommon, *life-threatening,* or **COMMON AND LIFE-THREATENING.**

# clindamycin hydrochloride
Cleocin HCl, Dalacin C†‡

# clindamycin palmitate hydrochloride
Cleocin Pediatric, Dalacin C Palmitate†‡

# clindamycin phosphate
Cleocin Phosphate, Dalacin C†‡, Dalacin C Phosphate

*Pregnancy Risk Category: NR*

## HOW SUPPLIED
**clindamycin hydrochloride**
*Capsules:* 75 mg, 150 mg, 300 mg
**clindamycin palmitate hydrochloride**
*Oral solution:* 75 mg/5 ml
**clindamycin phosphate**
*Injection:* 150 mg base/ml, 300 mg base/2ml, 600 mg base/4ml, 900 mg base/6ml

## ACTION
Inhibits bacterial protein synthesis by binding to the 50S subunit of the ribosome.

## ONSET, PEAK, DURATION
Onset immediate after I.V. administration, unknown after oral and I.M. administration. Serum levels peak immediately after I.V. administration, 3 hours after an I.M. injection, or within 45 minutes to 1 hour after an oral dose. Duration unknown.

## INDICATIONS & DOSAGE
*Infections caused by sensitive staphylococci, streptococci, pneumococci,* Bacteroides, Fusobacterium, Clostridium perfringens, *and other sensitive aerobic and anaerobic organisms* –
**Adults:** 150 to 450 mg P.O. q 6 hours; or 300 mg I.M. or I.V. q 6, 8, or 12 hours.
**Children over 1 month:** 8 to 20 mg/kg P.O. daily, in divided doses q 6 to 8

hours; or 20 to 40 mg/kg I.M. or I.V. daily, in divided doses q 6 or 8 hours.
*Endocarditis prophylaxis for dental procedures in patients allergic to penicillin* –
**Adults:** initially, 300 mg P.O. 1 hour before procedure; then 150 mg 6 hours later.
**Children:** initially, 10 mg/kg P.O. 1 hour before procedure; then half the initial dose 6 hours later.

## ADVERSE REACTIONS
**GI:** *nausea,* vomiting, abdominal pain, *diarrhea, pseudomembranous colitis.*
**Hematologic:** transient leukopenia, eosinophilia, *thrombocytopenia.*
**Skin:** maculopapular rash, urticaria.
**Other:** *anaphylaxis,* jaundice, abnormal liver function tests.

## INTERACTIONS
*Erythromycin:* may block access of clindamycin to its site of action. Don't use together.
*Kaolin:* decreased absorption of oral clindamycin. Separate administration times.
*Neuromuscular blockers:* potentiated neuromuscular blockade possible. Monitor closely.

## CONTRAINDICATIONS
Contraindicated in patients with hypersensitivity to the antibiotic congener lincomycin.

## NURSING CONSIDERATIONS
● Use cautiously in neonates and patients with renal or hepatic disease, asthma, history of GI disease, or significant allergies.
● Know that drug does not penetrate blood-brain barrier.
● Obtain culture and sensitivity tests before first dose. Therapy may begin pending results.
● **I.V. use:** When giving I.V., check site daily for phlebitis and irritation. For I.V. infusion, dilute each 300 mg in 50

---

*Liquid form contains alcohol.   **May contain tartrazine.   †Canada only.   ‡Australia only.   ◇OTC.

ml solution, and give no faster than 30 mg/minute (over 10 to 60 minutes). Never give undiluted as a bolus.
• For I.M. administration, inject deeply. Rotate sites. Doses greater than 600 mg per injection are not recommended.
• Be aware that I.M. injection may raise CK in response to muscle irritation.
• Don't refrigerate reconstituted oral solution because it will thicken. Drug is stable for 2 weeks at room temperature.
• Monitor renal, hepatic, and hematopoietic functions during prolonged therapy, as ordered.
• Observe the patient for signs of superinfection.
• *Alert:* Don't give opioid antidiarrheals to treat drug-induced diarrhea. They may prolong and worsen diarrhea.

### ☑ PATIENT TEACHING
• Advise the patient taking the capsule form to take it with a full glass of water to prevent dysphagia.
• Warn the patient that I.M. injection may be painful.
• Tell the patient to alert nurse if discomfort occurs at I.V. insertion site.
• Instruct the patient to report adverse reactions, especially diarrhea, to the doctor. Warn the patient not to treat such diarrhea himself.

---

## imipenem/cilastatin sodium
Primaxin IM, Primaxin IV

*Pregnancy Risk Category: C*

### HOW SUPPLIED
*Powder for injection:* 250 mg, 500 mg

### ACTION
Imipenem is bactericidal and inhibits bacterial cell-wall synthesis. Cilastatin inhibits the enzymatic breakdown of imipenem in the kidneys, making it effective in the urinary tract.

### ONSET, PEAK, DURATION
Onset unknown. Serum levels peak immediately after I.V. infusion, within 1 hour for cilastatin and within 2 hours for imipenem after I.M. administration. Duration is 4 to 6 hours.

### INDICATIONS & DOSAGE
*Serious infections of the lower respiratory and urinary tracts, intra-abdominal and gynecologic infections, bacterial septicemia, bone and joint infections, skin and soft-tissue infections, and endocarditis. Most known microorganisms are susceptible:* Staphylococcus, Streptococcus, Escherichia coli, Klebsiella, Proteus, Enterobacter, Pseudomonas aeruginosa, *and* Bacteroides, *including* B. fragilis—
**Adults:** 250 mg to 1 g by I.V. infusion q 6 to 8 hours. Maximum daily dosage is 50 mg/kg/day or 4 g/day, whichever is less. Alternatively, 500 to 750 mg I.M. q 12 hours. Maximum daily dosage is 1,500 mg/day.

### ADVERSE REACTIONS
**CNS:** *seizures,* dizziness, somnolence.
**CV:** hypotension.
**GI:** nausea, vomiting, diarrhea, *pseudomembranous colitis.*
**Skin:** rash, urticaria, pruritus.
**Other:** *hypersensitivity reactions (anaphylaxis); thrombophlebitis, pain at injection site,* fever, transient increases in liver enzymes.

### INTERACTIONS
*Beta-lactam antibiotics:* possible in vitro antagonism. Avoid concomitant use.
*Ganciclovir:* may cause seizures. Avoid concomitant use.
*Probenecid:* increased serum concentrations of cilastatin. Avoid concomitant use.

### CONTRAINDICATIONS
Contraindicated in patients with hypersensitivity to the drug.

---

Reactions may be *common,* uncommon, *life-threatening,* or COMMON AND LIFE-THREATENING.

## NURSING CONSIDERATIONS

• Use cautiously in patients allergic to penicillins or cephalosporins because this drug has similar properties.
• Also use cautiously in patients who have a history of seizure disorders, especially if they also have compromised renal function.
• Be aware that patients with impaired renal function may need a lower dose or longer intervals between doses.
• Obtain culture and sensitivity tests before first dose. Therapy may begin pending results.
• **I.V. use:** Don't administer by direct I.V. bolus injection. Each 250- or 500-mg dose should be given by I.V. infusion over 20 to 30 minutes. Each 1-g dose should be infused over 40 to 60 minutes. If nausea occurs, the infusion may be slowed.
• When reconstituting powder, shake until the solution is clear. Solutions may range from colorless to yellow, and variations of color within this range do not affect the drug's potency. After reconstitution, solution is stable for 10 hours at room temperature and for 48 hours when refrigerated.
• **Alert:** If seizures develop and persist, despite anticonvulsant therapy, notify the doctor. The drug should then be discontinued.
• Monitor patients for bacterial or fungal superinfections and resistant infections during and after therapy.

## ☑ PATIENT TEACHING

• Instruct patient to report adverse reactions promptly.
• Tell patient to alert nurse if discomfort occurs at I.V. insertion site.

---

## lincomycin hydrochloride
Lincocin

*Pregnancy Risk Category: NR*

## HOW SUPPLIED
*Capsules:* 500 mg
*Pediatric capsules:* 250 mg

*Injection:* 300 mg/ml in 2-ml and 10-ml vials and 2-ml U-Ject

## ACTION
Unknown. Appears to inhibit bacterial protein synthesis by binding to the 50S subunit of the ribosome.

## ONSET, PEAK, DURATION
Onset immediate after I.V. infusion, unknown after I.M. or oral administration. Peak levels occur immediately after an I.V. infusion, 30 minutes after an I.M. injection, or 2 to 4 hours after an oral dose. Duration unknown.

## INDICATIONS & DOSAGE
*Respiratory tract, skin and soft-tissue, and urinary tract infections; osteomyelitis, septicemia caused by sensitive group A beta-hemolytic streptococci, pneumococci, and staphylococci* —
**Adults:** 500 mg P.O. q 6 to 8 hours (not to exceed 8 g daily); or 600 mg I.M. daily or q 12 hours; or 600 mg to 1 g I.V. q 8 to 12 hours (not to exceed 8 g daily).
**Children over 1 month:** 30 to 60 mg/kg P.O. daily, in divided doses q 6 to 8 hours; or 10 mg/kg I.M. daily or in divided doses q 12 hours; or 10 to 20 mg/kg I.V. daily, in divided doses q 6 to 8 hours.

## ADVERSE REACTIONS
**CNS:** dizziness, headache.
**CV:** hypotension, *cardiopulmonary arrest* (with rapid I.V. infusion).
**EENT:** glossitis, tinnitus.
**GI:** nausea, vomiting, *pseudomembranous colitis, persistent diarrhea,* abdominal cramps, stomatitis, pruritus ani.
**Hematologic:** *neutropenia, leukopenia, thrombocytopenia,* purpura, *agranulocytosis.*
**Skin:** rash, urticaria.
**Other:** hypersensitivity reactions *(anaphylaxis),* cholestatic jaundice, pain at injection site.

---

*Liquid form contains alcohol.  **May contain tartrazine.  †Canada only.  ‡Australia only.  ◊OTC.

### INTERACTIONS
*Antidiarrheals (such as kaolin, pectin, and attapulgite):* reduced oral absorption of lincomycin by as much as 90%. Antidiarrheals should be avoided or given at least 2 hours before lincomycin.
*Neuromuscular blockers:* may potentiate neuromuscular blockade. Monitor for prolonged weakness.

### CONTRAINDICATIONS
Contraindicated in patients with hypersensitivity to lincomycin or clindamycin.

### NURSING CONSIDERATIONS
• Use cautiously in patients with GI disorders (especially colitis), asthma or significant allergies, hepatic or renal disease, and endocrine or metabolic disorders.
• Obtain specimen for culture and sensitivity tests before first dose. Therapy may begin pending results.
• **I.V. use:** For I.V. infusion, dilute to 100 ml; infuse over 1 hour. Rapid I.V. infusion may cause hypotension and syncope. Monitor blood pressure in the patient receiving the drug parenterally.
• When giving I.V., check site daily for phlebitis and irritation and rotate infusion sites regularly.
• For I.M. administration, inject deeply. Rotate injection sites.
• Monitor CBC and platelets. Stop drug immediately if neutropenia, leukopenia, or other blood disorders develop and notify doctor.
• Monitor hepatic function (increased levels of alkaline phosphatase, ALT, AST, or bilirubin may occur).
• Monitor for signs of bacterial and fungal superinfection, especially when therapy exceeds 10 days.

### ☑ PATIENT TEACHING
• Advise the patient to take drug exactly as directed, even after he feels better, and to take entire amount prescribed.

• For best absorption, instruct the patient to take oral form of drug with a full glass of water 1 hour before or 2 hours after meals.
• Warn the patient that I.M. injection may be painful.
• Tell the patient to report adverse reactions to the doctor, especially diarrhea. Warn him not to treat diarrhea himself because it may signal the onset of antibiotic-associated pseudomembranous colitis.

---

## methenamine hippurate
Hiprex**, Hip-Rex†, Urex

## methenamine mandelate
Mandameth, Mandelamine, Sterinet†
*Pregnancy Risk Category: C*

### HOW SUPPLIED
**methenamine hippurate**
*Tablets:* 1 g
**methenamine mandelate**
*Tablets:* 500 mg, 1 g
*Tablets (enteric-coated):* 500 mg, 1 g
*Tablets (film-coated):* 500 mg, 1 g
*Suspension:* 250 mg/5ml, 500 mg/5 ml

### ACTION
Hydrolyzed to ammonia and to formaldehyde, causing antibacterial action against gram-positive and gram-negative organisms. Mandelic and hippuric acids, with which methenamines are combined, are also antibacterial by unknown mechanisms.

### ONSET, PEAK, DURATION
Onset and duration unknown. Plasma levels peak within 1 hour of administration. Urine levels of formaldehyde peak within 2 hours of administration of a film-coated tablet, or 3 to 8 hours after an enteric-coated tablet.

---

Reactions may be *common,* uncommon, *life-threatening,* or **COMMON AND LIFE-THREATENING.**

## INDICATIONS & DOSAGE

*Long-term prophylaxis or suppression of chronic urinary tract infections (UTIs)* –
**Adults and children over 12 years:** 1 g (hippurate) P.O. q 12 hours.
**Children age 6 to 12:** 500 mg to 1 g (hippurate) P.O. q 12 hours.
*UTIs, infected residual urine in patients with neurogenic bladder* –
**Adults:** 1 g (mandelate) P.O. q.i.d. after meals and h.s.
**Children 6 to 12 years:** 500 mg (mandelate) P.O. q.i.d. after meals and h.s.
**Children under 6 years:** 50 mg/kg (mandelate) P.O. divided in four doses after meals and h.s.

## ADVERSE REACTIONS

**GI:** nausea, vomiting, abdominal cramps, anorexia.
**GU:** with high doses, urinary tract irritation, dysuria, frequency, hematuria.
**Skin:** rash, pruritus.
**Other:** elevated liver enzymes, headache, dyspnea.

## INTERACTIONS

*Acetazolamide:* antagonized methenamine effect. Use together cautiously.
*Sulfamethizole:* forms an insoluble precipitate in acid urine. Do not administer together.
*Urine alkalinizing agents:* inhibited methenamine action. Don't use together.

## CONTRAINDICATIONS

Contraindicated in patients with renal insufficiency, severe hepatic disease, or severe dehydration.

## NURSING CONSIDERATIONS

● Administer cautiously to elderly or debilitated patients because aspiration could cause lipid pneumonia. Oral suspension contains vegetable oil.
● Obtain a clean-catch urine specimen for culture and sensitivity tests before starting therapy, and repeat as needed. Therapy may begin pending results.
● Administer after meals to minimize GI upset.
● Monitor fluid intake and output. Fluid intake should be at least 1,500 to 2,000 ml daily.
● For best results, maintain urine pH at 5.5 or below. Use Nitrazine paper to check pH. Large doses of ascorbic acid (12 g/day) may be necessary to effectively acidify urine.
● Monitor liver function studies periodically during long-term therapy.
● **Alert:** If rash appears, withhold dose and contact the doctor.
● Be aware that *Proteus* and *Pseudomonas* tend to raise urine pH; urine acidifiers are usually necessary when treating these infections.
● Keep in mind that drug interferes with fluorometric procedures for determination of urine catecholamines and vanillylmandelic acid, causing false-high results.

## ☑ PATIENT TEACHING

● Instruct the patient to take medication for as long as prescribed, exactly as directed, even after he feels better.
● Tell the patient to take drug after meals.
● Instruct the patient to limit intake of alkaline foods, such as vegetables, milk, and peanuts. Patients may drink cranberry, plum, and prune juices. These juices or ascorbic acid may be used to acidify urine.
● Warn the patient not to take antacids, including Alka-Seltzer and sodium bicarbonate.

---

# nitrofurantoin macrocrystals
Macrodantin

# nitrofurantoin microcrystals

Apo-Nitrofurantoin†, Furadantin, Furanite, Macrodantin, Nephronex†, Nitrofan, Novofuran†

*Pregnancy Risk Category: B*

## HOW SUPPLIED
**nitrofurantoin macrocrystals**
*Capsules:* 25 mg, 50 mg, 100 mg
**nitrofurantoin microcrystals**
*Tablets:* 50 mg, 100 mg
*Capsules:* 50 mg, 100 mg
*Oral suspension:* 25 mg/5 ml

## ACTION
Unknown. Appears to interfere with bacterial enzyme systems and possibly with bacterial cell-wall formation.

## ONSET, PEAK, DURATION
Unknown.

## INDICATIONS & DOSAGE
*Urinary tract infections caused by susceptible* Escherichia coli, Staphylococcus aureus, *enterococci; certain strains of* Klebsiella, Proteus, *and* Enterobacter—
**Adults and children over 12 years:** 50 to 100 mg P.O. q.i.d. with meals and h.s.
**Children 1 month to 12 years:** 5 to 7 mg/kg P.O. daily, divided q.i.d.
*Long-term suppression therapy—*
**Adults:** 50 to 100 mg P.O. daily h.s.
**Children:** 1 to 2 mg/kg P.O. daily in a single dose h.s. or divided into two doses given q 12 hours.

## ADVERSE REACTIONS
**CNS:** *peripheral neuropathy,* headache, dizziness, drowsiness, *ascending polyneuropathy with high doses or renal impairment.*
**GI:** *anorexia, nausea, vomiting,* abdominal pain, *diarrhea.*
**Hematologic:** *hemolysis in patients with G6PD deficiency* (reversed after stopping drug), *agranulocytosis, thrombocytopenia.*

**Hepatic:** *hepatitis, hepatic necrosis.*
**Respiratory:** *pulmonary sensitivity reactions* (cough, chest pain, fever, chills, dyspnea, pulmonary infiltration with consolidation or pleural effusion), *asthmatic attacks in patients with history of asthma.*
**Skin:** maculopapular, erythematous, or eczematous eruption; pruritus; urticaria; *exfoliative dermatitis; Stevens-Johnson syndrome.*
**Other:** hypersensitivity reactions *(anaphylaxis),* transient alopecia, drug fever, overgrowth of nonsusceptible organisms in the urinary tract.

## INTERACTIONS
*Magnesium-containing antacids:* decreased nitrofurantoin absorption. Separate administration times by 1 hour.
*Nalidixic acid, norfloxacin:* possible decreased effectiveness. Avoid using together.
*Probenecid, sulfinpyrazone:* increased blood levels and decreased urine levels. May result in increased toxicity and lack of therapeutic effect. Don't use together.

## CONTRAINDICATIONS
Contraindicated in children 1 month and under and in patients with moderate to severe renal impairment, anuria, oliguria, or creatinine clearance under 60 ml/minute.

## NURSING CONSIDERATIONS
● Use cautiously in patients with renal impairment, anemia, diabetes mellitus, electrolyte abnormalities, vitamin B deficiency, debilitating disease, and G6PD deficiency.
● Obtain urine specimen for culture and sensitivity tests before starting therapy and repeat p.r.n. Therapy may begin pending results.
● Give with food or milk to minimize GI distress.
● Monitor fluid intake and output

---

Reactions may be *common,* uncommon, *life-threatening,* or **COMMON AND LIFE-THREATENING.**

carefully. May turn urine brown or darker.
- Monitor CBC and pulmonary status regularly.
- Monitor the patient for signs of superinfection. Use of nitrofurantoin may result in growth of nonsusceptible organisms, especially *Pseudomonas.*
- *Alert:* Know that hypersensitivity may develop when used for long-term therapy.
- Be aware that some patients may experience fewer adverse GI effects with nitrofurantoin macrocrystals.
- Keep in mind that drug may cause false-positive results with urine glucose test using copper sulfate reduction method (Clinitest) but not with glucose enzymatic tests (Tes-Tape, Diastix, Clinistix).
- Know that dual-release capsules (25 mg nitrofurantoin macrocrystals combined with 75 mg nitrofurantoin monohydrate) enable patients to take drug only twice daily.
- Continue treatment for 3 days after sterile urine specimens have been obtained.
- Store drug in amber container. Keep away from metals other than stainless steel or aluminum to avoid precipitate formation.

### ☑ PATIENT TEACHING
- Instruct patient to take medication for as long as prescribed, exactly as directed, even after he feels better.
- Tell patient to take drug with food or milk to minimize stomach upset.
- Instruct patient to report adverse reactions.
- Alert patient that drug may turn urine a harmless dark yellow or brown color.
- Warn patient not to store drug in container made of metal other than stainless steel or aluminum.

# polymyxin B sulfate
Aerosporin

*Pregnancy Risk Category: NR*

**HOW SUPPLIED**
*Powder for injection:* 500,000-unit vials

**ACTION**
Hinders bacterial cell-wall synthesis, damaging the bacterial plasma membrane and making the cell more vulnerable to osmotic pressure (bactericidal).

**ONSET, PEAK, DURATION**
Onset immediate after I.V. infusion, unknown after I.M. injection. Peak serum levels occur immediately after I.V. infusion, within 2 hours of an I.M. injection. Duration unknown.

**INDICATIONS & DOSAGE**
*Acute urinary tract infections (UTIs) or septicemia caused by sensitive* Pseudomonas aeruginosa, *or when other antibiotics are ineffective or contraindicated; bacteremia caused by sensitive* Enterobacter aerogenes *and* Klebsiella pneumoniae, *or acute UTIs caused by* Escherichia coli—
**Adults and children over 2 years:** 15,000 to 25,000 units/kg daily I.V. infusion, in divided doses q 12 hours; or 25,000 to 30,000 units/kg I.M. daily, in divided doses q 4 to 8 hours.
*Meningitis caused by sensitive* P. aeruginosa *or* Haemophilus influenzae *when other antibiotics are ineffective or contraindicated—*
**Adults and children over 2 years:** 50,000 units intrathecally once daily for 3 to 4 days, then 50,000 units every other day for at least 2 weeks after CSF tests are negative and CSF glucose level is normal.
**Children under 2 years:** 20,000 units intrathecally once daily for 3 to 4 days, then 25,000 units q.o.d. for at

least 2 weeks after CSF tests are negative and CSF glucose level is normal.

## ADVERSE REACTIONS
**CNS:** *neurotoxicity,* irritability, drowsiness, facial flushing, weakness, ataxia, *respiratory paralysis,* headache and meningeal irritation with intrathecal administration, peripheral and perioral paresthesias.
**EENT:** blurred vision.
**GU:** *nephrotoxicity* (albuminuria, cylindruria, hematuria, proteinuria, decreased urine output, increased BUN level).
**Skin:** urticaria.
**Other:** drug fever, pain or thrombophlebitis at injection site.

## INTERACTIONS
*Aminoglycosides, amphotericin B, cisplatin, vancomycin, zidovudine:* increased risk of nephrotoxicity. Avoid concomitant use.
*Neuromuscular blockers:* may potentiate neuromuscular blockade. Monitor closely.

## CONTRAINDICATIONS
Contraindicated in patients with hypersensitivity to the drug.

## NURSING CONSIDERATIONS
• Use cautiously in those with impaired renal function or myasthenia gravis.
• Give only to a hospitalized patient under constant supervision.
• Obtain culture and sensitivity tests before first dose. Therapy may begin pending results.
• **I.V. use:** When giving I.V., check site daily for phlebitis and irritation. Dilute each 500,000 units in 300 to 500 ml of $D_5W$; infuse over 60 to 90 minutes. Rotate I.V. sites regularly.
• Avoid administering by I.M. injection because of severe local pain. If I.M. route must be used, give deeply and check dosage carefully. I.M. dosage differs from I.V. dosage.

• Refrigerate parenteral solutions and use within 72 hours.
• Know that for meningitis, the drug is given intrathecally to achieve adequate CSF levels.
• Don't give solution containing local anesthetics I.V. or intrathecally.
• Monitor renal function (BUN, serum creatinine, creatinine clearance, urine output) before and during therapy, as ordered. Fluid intake should be sufficient to maintain output at 1,500 ml/day (between 3,000 and 4,000 ml/day for adults).
• Notify the doctor immediately if the patient develops fever, adverse CNS effects, rash, or symptoms of nephrotoxicity.
• If the patient is scheduled for surgery, tell the anesthesiologist about preoperative treatment with this drug because it may prolong neuromuscular blockade.

## ☑ PATIENT TEACHING
• Warn patient receiving drug I.M. that it may cause pain at injection site.
• Tell patient receiving drug I.V. to alert nurse if discomfort occurs at I.V. insertion site.
• Instruct patient to drink at least 3,000 to 4,000 ml/day of fluid to maintain adequate output, if not contraindicated.
• Tell patient to report adverse reactions promptly.

---

## rifabutin
Mycobutin

*Pregnancy Risk Category: B*

## HOW SUPPLIED
*Capsules:* 150 mg

## ACTION
Inhibits DNA-dependent RNA polymerase in susceptible bacteria, blocking bacterial protein synthesis.

---

## ONSET, PEAK, DURATION
Onset and duration unknown. Plasma levels peak 1½ to 4 hours after an oral dose.

## INDICATIONS & DOSAGE
*Prevention of disseminated* Mycobacterium avium *complex (MAC) in patients with advanced HIV infection* —
**Adults:** 300 mg P.O. daily as a single dose or divided b.i.d.

## ADVERSE REACTIONS
**GI:** dyspepsia, eructation, flatulence, diarrhea, nausea, vomiting, abdominal pain.
**GU:** *discolored urine.*
**Hematologic:** *neutropenia, leukopenia,* **thrombocytopenia,** eosinophilia.
**Skin:** *rash.*
**Other:** fever, myalgia, headache.

## INTERACTIONS
*Oral contraceptives:* decreased effectiveness. Instruct patient to use nonhormonal forms of birth control.
*Zidovudine, drugs metabolized by the liver:* may alter serum levels of these drugs. Dosage adjustments may be necessary.

## CONTRAINDICATIONS
Contraindicated in patients with hypersensitivity to the drug or other rifamycin derivatives (such as rifampin). Also contraindicated in patients with active tuberculosis because single-agent therapy with rifabutin increases the risk of inducing bacterial resistance to both rifabutin and rifampin.

## NURSING CONSIDERATIONS
• Use cautiously in patients with pre-existing neutropenia and thrombocytopenia. Perform baseline hematologic studies and repeat periodically.
• Know that high-fat meals slow the rate, but not the extent, of absorption.
• Mix with soft foods, such as apple-

sauce, for patients who have difficulty swallowing.
• Know that patients requiring prophylaxis against both *M. tuberculosis* and MAC may require rifampin and rifabutin therapy.

## ☑ PATIENT TEACHING
• Instruct the patient to take drug for as long as prescribed, exactly as directd, even after he feels better.
• Tell the patient that drug or its metabolites may discolor urine, feces, sputum, saliva, tears, and skin brownish orange. Tell him to avoid wearing soft contact lenses because they may be permanently stained.
• Tell the patient to report photophobia, excessive lacrimation, or eye pain immediately. Rarely, the drug has caused uveitis.

# spectinomycin hydrochloride
Trobicin
*Pregnancy Risk Category: NR*

## HOW SUPPLIED
*Powder for injection:* 2 g, 4 g

## ACTION
Inhibits protein synthesis by binding to the 30S subunit of the ribosome.

## ONSET, PEAK, DURATION
Onset and duration unknown. Serum levels peak 1 hour after a single 2-g I.M. dose, 2 hours after a single 4-g I.M. dose.

## INDICATIONS & DOSAGE
*Gonorrhea* —
**Adults:** 2 to 4 g I.M. single dose injected deeply into the upper outer quadrant of the buttock.

## ADVERSE REACTIONS
**CNS:** insomnia, dizziness.
**GI:** nausea.

---

*Liquid form contains alcohol. **May contain tartrazine. †Canada only. ‡Australia only. ◊OTC.

**GU:** decreased urine output and creatinine clearance, increased BUN.
**Hematologic:** decreased hemoglobin and hematocrit levels.
**Skin:** urticaria.
**Other:** fever, chills (may mask or delay symptoms of incubating syphilis), transient increases in liver enzymes, pain at injection site.

**INTERACTIONS**
None significant.

**CONTRAINDICATIONS**
Contraindicated in patients with hypersensitivity to the drug.

**NURSING CONSIDERATIONS**
• Shake vial vigorously after reconstitution and before withdrawing dose. Store at room temperature after reconstitution and use within 24 hours.
• Use 20G needle to administer drug. Divide the 4-g dose (10 ml) into two 5-ml injections—give one in each buttock.

☑ **PATIENT TEACHING**
• Inform patient that drug is not effective in the treatment of syphilis. Tell him that serologic test for syphilis should be done before therapy begins and for 3 months afterward.
• Tell patient to report adverse reactions promptly.

---

# trimethoprim
Aiprin‡, Proloprim, Trimpex, Triprim‡

*Pregnancy Risk Category: C*

**HOW SUPPLIED**
*Tablets:* 100 mg, 200 mg

**ACTION**
Interferes with the action of dihydrofolate reductase, inhibiting bacterial synthesis of folic acid.

**ONSET, PEAK, DURATION**
Onset and duration unknown. Plasma levels peak 1 to 4 hours after an oral dose.

**INDICATIONS & DOSAGE**
*Uncomplicated urinary tract infections caused by susceptible strains of* Escherichia coli, Proteus mirabilis, Klebsiella, *and* Enterobacter—
**Adults:** 200 mg P.O. daily as a single dose or in divided doses q 12 hours for 10 days.
  Not recommended for children under age 12.

**ADVERSE REACTIONS**
**GI:** *epigastric distress, nausea, vomiting,* glossitis.
**Hematologic:** *thrombocytopenia,* leukopenia, megaloblastic anemia, methemoglobinemia.
**Skin:** *rash, pruritus, **exfoliative dermatitis.***
**Other:** fever.

**INTERACTIONS**
*Phenytoin:* may decrease phenytoin metabolism and increase its serum levels. Monitor for toxicity.

**CONTRAINDICATIONS**
Contraindicated in patients with hypersensitivity to the drug and in those with documented megaloblastic anemia caused by folate deficiency.

**NURSING CONSIDERATIONS**
• Use cautiously in patients with impaired hepatic or renal function. Dosage should be decreased in patients with severely impaired renal function. Be aware that the drug is not recommended for use in patients with creatinine clearance less than 15 ml/minute. Also use cautiously in patients with possible folate deficiency.
• Obtain urine specimen for culture and sensitivity tests before first dose. Therapy may begin pending results.
• Monitor CBC routinely. Clinical

---

signs such as sore throat, fever, pallor, or purpura may be early indications of serious blood disorders.
• **Alert:** Prolonged use of trimethoprim at high doses may cause bone marrow suppression.
• Keep in mind that because resistance to trimethoprim develops rapidly when administered alone, it is usually given in combination with other drugs.

☑ **PATIENT TEACHING**
• Instruct the patient to take entire amount of the drug, as prescribed, even if he feels better.
• Tell the patient to report adverse reactions promptly, especially signs of infection or unusual bruising.

---

## trimetrexate glucuronate
NeuTrexin

*Pregnancy Risk Category: D*

**HOW SUPPLIED**
*Injection:* 25-mg vials

**ACTION**
Prevents reduction of folic acid to tetrahydrofolate by binding to dihydrofolate reductase.

**ONSET, PEAK, DURATION**
Unknown.

**INDICATIONS & DOSAGE**
*Alternative treatment of* Pneumocystis carinii *pneumonia in patients with AIDS* –
**Adults:** 45 mg/m² I.V. infusion over 60 to 90 minutes daily for 21 days, administered with 20 mg/m² of leucovorin I.V. or P.O. q 6 hours for 24 days.

**ADVERSE REACTIONS**
**CNS:** peripheral neuropathy.
**GI:** nausea, vomiting, stomatitis.
**Hematologic:** *neutropenia, thrombocytopenia, anemia.*
**Hepatic:** hepatotoxicity.

**Skin:** rash.

**INTERACTIONS**
*Acetaminophen, cimetidine, clotrimazole, erythromycin, fluconazole, ketoconazole, miconazole, rifampin, rifabutin:* may interfere with trimetrexate metabolism and lead to toxicity. Monitor closely.
*Chloride-containing solutions, leucovorin:* precipitate will form if mixed with trimetrexate. Administer separately.
*Hepatotoxic, myelosuppressive, or nephrotoxic drugs:* enhanced toxicity. Use together cautiously and monitor closely.

**CONTRAINDICATIONS**
Contraindicated in patients with hypersensitivity to trimetrexate, methotrexate, or leucovorin.

**NURSING CONSIDERATIONS**
• Use cautiously in patients with impaired hematologic, renal, or hepatic function and in women of childbearing age because the drug may cause fetal harm. Avoid using during pregnancy.
• Follow institutional policy when administering parenteral form of this drug because parenteral form is associated with carcinogenic, mutagenic, and teratogenic risks for personnel.
• **I.V. use:** Reconstitute 25-mg vial with 2 ml of D₅W or sterile water for injection to yield a solution of 12.5 mg/ml. Complete dissolution usually occurs within 30 seconds. Further dilute reconstituted solution with D₅W to yield a final concentration of 0.25 to 2 mg/ml. Infuse over 60 minutes. After reconstitution, the drug is stable at room temperature or refrigerated for 24 hours.
• Use only D₅W for I.V. infusion. Drug is incompatible with chloride-containing solutions (including 0.9% sodium chloride solution) and leucovorin.

- Flush the I.V. line with at least 10 ml of D₅W immediately before and after the trimetrexate infusion.
- Administer leucovorin either before or after trimetrexate. When giving I.V., be sure to flush the I.V. line with D₅W because the two drugs are incompatible. Leucovorin calcium may be infused over 5 to 10 minutes.
- **Alert:** Know that leucovorin therapy must accompany trimetrexate treatments to avoid potentially life-threatening toxicity. Leucovorin therapy must extend for 3 days after trimetrexate therapy.
- When calculating the oral dose of leucovorin, round dosage up to the next increment of 25 mg.
- Monitor patients closely. Many adverse effects may be decreased by adjusting the dosage of leucovorin.
- Avoid I.M. injections in patients with thrombocytopenia.

☑ **PATIENT TEACHING**
- Instruct patient to alert nurse if discomfort occurs at I.V. site.
- Warn patient to watch for signs of infection (fever, sore throat, fatigue) and bleeding (easy bruising, epitaxis, bleeding gums, melena) and instruct how to take infection control and bleeding precautions. Tell patients to take temperature daily.
- Advise women of childbearing age to avoid becoming pregnant during therapy. Also recommend consulting doctor before becoming pregnant.

---

## vancomycin hydrochloride
Vancocin, Vancoled

*Pregnancy Risk Category: C*

**HOW SUPPLIED**
*Capsules:* 125 mg, 250 mg
*Powder for oral solution:* 1-g, 10-g bottles
*Powder for injection:* 500-mg, 1-g vials
*Pharmacy bulk package:* 5 g, 10 g

**ACTION**
Hinders bacterial cell-wall synthesis, damaging the bacterial plasma membrane and making the cell more vulnerable to osmotic pressure.

**ONSET, PEAK, DURATION**
Onset immediate after I.V. infusion, unknown after oral administration. Serum levels peak immediately after I.V. infusion, unknown after oral administration. Duration unknown.

**INDICATIONS & DOSAGE**
*Serious or severe infections when other antibiotics are ineffective or contraindicated –*
**Adults:** 500 mg I.V. q 6 hours, or 1 g q 12 hours.
**Children:** 10 mg/kg I.V. daily q 6 hours.
**Neonates and young infants:** 15 mg/kg I.V. loading dose, followed by 10 mg/kg I.V. q 12 hours if less than 1 week of age or 10 mg/kg I.V. q 8 hours if older than 1 week but less than 1 month.
*Antibiotic-associated pseudomembranous and staphylococcal enterocolitis –*
**Adults:** 125 to 500 mg P.O. q 6 hours for 7 to 10 days.
**Children:** 40 mg/kg P.O. daily, in divided doses q 6 hours for 7 to 10 days. Maximum daily dosage is 2 g.
*Endocarditis prophylaxis for dental procedures –*
**Adults:** 1 g I.V. slowly over 1 hour, starting 1 hour before procedure.
**Children:** 20 mg/kg I.V. over 1 hour, starting 1 hour before procedure.

**ADVERSE REACTIONS**
**EENT:** tinnitus, ototoxicity.
**GI:** nausea.
**GU:** nephrotoxicity.
**Hematologic:** neutropenia.
**Skin:** "red-neck" syndrome with rapid I.V. infusion (maculopapular rash on face, neck, trunk, and extremities).

---

Reactions may be *common,* uncommon, *life-threatening,* or COMMON AND LIFE-THREATENING.

**Other:** chills, fever, *anaphylaxis,* superinfection, pain or thrombophlebitis at injection site, hypotension, wheezing, dyspnea.

## INTERACTIONS
*Aminoglycosides, amphotericin B, cisplatin, pentamidine:* increased risk of nephrotoxicity and ototoxicity. Monitor closely.

## CONTRAINDICATIONS
Contraindicated in patients with hypersensitivity to the drug.

## NURSING CONSIDERATIONS
• Use cautiously in patients receiving other neurotoxic, nephrotoxic, or ototoxic drugs; in patients over 60 years, and in those with impaired hepatic or renal function, preexisting hearing loss, or allergies to other antibiotics. Patients with renal dysfunction require dosage adjustment.
• Obtain culture and sensitivity tests before first dose. Therapy may begin pending results.
• Obtain hearing evaluation and renal function studies before therapy.
• **I.V. use:** For I.V. infusion, dilute in 200 ml 0.9% sodium chloride injection or $D_5W$, and infuse over 60 minutes. Check site daily for phlebitis and irritation. Report pain at infusion site. Avoid extravasation. Severe irritation and necrosis can result.
• Monitor the patient carefully for "red-neck" syndrome, which can occur if drug is infused too rapidly. If this reaction occurs, stop infusion and report to the doctor.
• Refrigerate I.V. solution after reconstitution and use within 96 hours.
• Do not give drug I.M..
• Know that the oral preparation is stable for 2 weeks if refrigerated.
• Monitor renal function (BUN, serum creatinine, urinalysis, creatinine clearance, and urine output) during therapy. Also monitor for signs of superinfection.

• Have the patient's hearing evaluated during prolonged therapy.
• Be aware that when using the drug to treat staphylococcal endocarditis, it will be given for at least 4 weeks.

☑ **PATIENT TEACHING**
• Tell the patient to take entire amount of medication exactly as directed, even after he feels better.
• Tell the patient to stop oral drug immediately and report adverse reactions, especially fullness or ringing in ears.
• Instruct the patient receiving drug I.V. to alert nurse if discomfort occurs at I.V. insertion site.

---

amrinone lactate
digitoxin
digoxin
milrinone lactate

**COMBINATION PRODUCTS**
None.

---

## amrinone lactate
Inocor

*Pregnancy Risk Category: C*

### HOW SUPPLIED
*Injection:* 5 mg/ml

### ACTION
Unknown. Thought to produce inotropic action by increasing cellular levels of cAMP. Produces vasodilation through a direct relaxant effect on vascular smooth muscle.

### ONSET, PEAK, DURATION
Onset begins within 2 to 5 minutes. Serum levels peak in 10 minutes. Effects persist ½ to 2 hours after dose.

### INDICATIONS & DOSAGE
*Short-term management of CHF –*
**Adults:** initially, 0.75 mg/kg I.V. bolus over 2 to 3 minutes. Then begin maintenance infusion of 5 to 10 mcg/kg/minute. Additional bolus of 0.75 mg/kg may be given 30 minutes after start of therapy. Total daily dosage should not exceed 10 mg/kg.

### ADVERSE REACTIONS
**CV:** *arrhythmias,* hypotension.
**GI:** nausea, vomiting, anorexia, abdominal pain.
**Hematologic:** *thrombocytopenia* (depends on dose and duration of therapy).
**Hepatic:** elevated enzymes, hepatotoxicity (rare).

**Other:** burning at injection site, *hypersensitivity reactions* (pericarditis, ascites, myositis vasculitis, pleuritis), fever, chest pain.

### INTERACTIONS
*Digitalis glycosides:* enhanced inotropic effect. Beneficial drug interaction.

### CONTRAINDICATIONS
Contraindicated in patients with hypersensitivity to amrinone or bisulfites.

### NURSING CONSIDERATIONS
● Know that amrinone should not be used in patients with severe aortic or pulmonic valvular disease in place of surgical correction of the obstruction or during acute phase of MI.
● Use cautiously in patients with hypertrophic cardiomyopathy.
● Be aware that amrinone is primarily prescribed for patients who have not responded to digitalis glycosides, diuretics, and vasodilators.
● Dosage depends on clinical response, including assessment of pulmonary artery wedge pressure and cardiac output.
● Anticipate that amrinone may be added to digitalis glycoside therapy in patients with atrial fibrillation and flutter because it slightly enhances AV conduction and increases ventricular response rate.
● **I.V. use:** Administer amrinone with an infusion pump and use as supplied, or dilute in 0.45% or 0.9% sodium chloride solution to a concentration of 1 to 3 mg/ml. Use diluted solution within 24 hours.
● Don't dilute with solutions containing dextrose because a slow chemical reaction occurs over 24 hours. Amrinone can be injected into free-flowing

dextrose infusions through a Y-connector or directly into tubing.
- **Alert:** Don't administer furosemide and amrinone through the same I.V. line because precipitation occurs.
- Monitor blood pressure and heart rate throughout the infusion. If the patient's blood pressure falls, slow or stop infusion and notify the doctor.
- Monitor platelet count. If it falls below 150,000/mm³, decrease dosage as ordered.
- Patients with end-stage cardiac disease may receive home treatment with an amrinone drip while awaiting heart transplantation.

☑ **PATIENT TEACHING**
- Warn patient that burning may occur at the site of injection.
- Instruct home care patient and family on administration; tell them to report adverse reactions promptly.

## digitoxin
Crystodigin, Digitaline†

*Pregnancy Risk Category: C*

**HOW SUPPLIED**
*Tablets:* 0.05 mg, 0.1 mg, 0.15 mg, 0.2 mg

**ACTION**
Inhibits sodium-potassium activated adenosine triphosphatase, promoting movement of calcium from extracellular to intracellular cytoplasm and thereby strengthening myocardial contraction. Also acts on CNS to enhance vagal tone, slowing conduction through the AV node and providing an antiarrhythmic effect.

**ONSET, PEAK, DURATION**
Onset occurs in ½ to 2 hours. Serum levels peak 4 to 12 hours after oral dose. Effects may persist for 3 to 4 weeks after last dose.

**INDICATIONS & DOSAGE**
*CHF, paroxysmal supraventricular tachycardia, atrial fibrillation and flutter –*
**Adults and children 12 years and older:** loading dose is 1.2 to 1.6 mg P.O. in divided doses over 24 hours; average maintenance dosage is 0.15 mg daily (range: 0.05 to 0.3 mg daily).
**Neonates, premature infants, severely ill older infants:** loading dose is 0.022 mg/kg or 0.3 to 0.35 mg/m² P.O. in divided doses over 24 hours; maintenance dosage is 0.0022 mg/kg daily.
**Children 2 weeks to 1 year:** loading dose is 0.045 mg/kg P.O. in divided doses over 24 hours; maintenance dosage is 0.0045 mg/kg daily.
**Children 1 to 2 years:** loading dose is 0.04 mg/kg P.O. in divided doses over 24 hours; maintenance dosage is 0.004 mg/kg daily.
**Children 2 to 12 years:** loading dose is 0.03 mg/kg or 0.75 mg/m² P.O. in divided doses over 24 hours; maintenance dosage is 0.003 mg/kg or 0.075 mg/m² daily.

**ADVERSE REACTIONS**
*The following signs of toxicity may occur with all digitalis glycosides:*
**CNS:** *fatigue, generalized muscle weakness, agitation, hallucinations,* headache, malaise, dizziness, vertigo, stupor, paresthesia.
**CV:** *arrhythmias* (most commonly conduction disturbances with or without AV block, PVCs, and supraventricular arrhythmias); arrhythmias may lead to increased severity of CHF and hypotension. *Toxic effects on heart may be life-threatening and require immediate attention.*
**EENT:** *yellow-green halos around visual images, blurred vision,* light flashes, photophobia, diplopia.
**GI:** *anorexia, nausea,* vomiting, diarrhea.

## INTERACTIONS

*Amiodarone, quinidine, verapamil:* possible increased serum digitoxin levels. Monitor patient closely.

*Amphotericin B, corticosteroids, diuretics (including loop diuretics, chlorthalidone, metolazone, and thiazides), ticarcillin:* hypokalemia or hypomagnesemia, predisposing patient to digitalis toxicity. Monitor serum potassium and serum magnesium levels.

*Antacids, kaolin-pectin, oral neomycin, sulfasalazine:* decreased absorption of digitoxin. Schedule doses as far as possible from digitoxin administration.

*Cholestyramine, colestipol, metoclopramide:* decreased absorption of digitoxin. Monitor for decreased digitoxin effect and low blood levels. Increase dosage as ordered.

*Parenteral calcium, thiazides:* hypercalcemia and hypomagnesemia, predisposing patient to digitalis toxicity. Monitor serum calcium and serum magnesium levels.

*Phenobarbital, phenylbutazone, phenytoin, rifampin:* faster metabolism and shorter duration of digitoxin. Observe for underdigitalization.

## CONTRAINDICATIONS

Contraindicated in patients with hypersensitivity to the drug; digitalis-induced toxicity; ventricular fibrillation; or ventricular tachycardia unless caused by CHF.

## NURSING CONSIDERATIONS

• Use with extreme caution in elderly patients and in those with acute MI, incomplete AV block, sinus bradycardia, PVCs, chronic constrictive pericarditis, hypertrophic cardiomyopathy, severe pulmonary disease, and thyroid disease. Reduce dosage in patients with renal impairment.

• Be aware that hypothyroid patients are sensitive to glycosides; hyperthyroid patients may need larger doses.

• Before administering loading dose, obtain baseline data (heart rate and rhythm, blood pressure, and electrolytes) and question the patient about use of digitalis glycosides within the previous 2 to 3 weeks.

• Be aware that the loading dose is divided over the first 24 hours unless the situation indicates otherwise.

• Before giving, take apical-radial pulse for a full minute. Record and report to the doctor significant changes (sudden increase or decrease in the pulse rate, pulse deficit, irregular beats and, particularly, regularization of a previously irregular rhythm). If any occurs, check blood pressure and obtain a 12-lead ECG.

• Monitor serum digitoxin levels. Therapeutic blood levels of digitoxin range from 25 to 35 ng/ml.

• Because digitoxin is a long-acting drug, watch for cumulative effects and signs of toxicity, especially in children and elderly patients. Ask the patient about nausea, vomiting, anorexia, visual disturbances, and other symptoms of toxicity.

• *Alert:* Excessive slowing of pulse rate (60 beats/minute or less) may be a sign of digitalis toxicity. Withhold drug and notify the doctor.

• For digitalis toxicity, administer agents that bind the drug in the intestine (for example, colestipol or cholestyramine). Treat arrhythmias with phenytoin I.V. or lidocaine I.V. and potentially life-threatening toxicity with specific antigen-binding fragments (such as digoxin immune FAB) as ordered. Correct any electrolyte abnormalities, as ordered.

• Monitor serum potassium level carefully. Take corrective action before hypokalemia occurs.

• Withhold drug for 1 to 2 days before elective cardioversion, as ordered. Adjust dose after cardioversion.

## ☑ PATIENT TEACHING

• Instruct the patient and a responsible family member about drug action,

---

dosage regimen, pulse taking, reportable signs, and follow-up plans.
• Encourage the patient to eat potassium-rich foods.
• Tell the patient not to substitute one brand of digitoxin for another.

## digoxin
Digoxin, Lanoxicaps, Lanoxin*, Novodigoxin†

*Pregnancy Risk Category: C*

### HOW SUPPLIED
*Tablets:* 0.125 mg, 0.25 mg, 0.5 mg
*Capsules:* 0.05 mg, 0.1 mg, 0.2 mg
*Elixir:* 0.05 mg/ml
*Injection:* 0.05 mg/ml†, 0.1 mg/ml (pediatric), 0.25 mg/ml

### ACTION
Inhibits sodium-potassium activated adenosine triphosphatase, thereby promoting movement of calcium from extracellular to intracellular cytoplasm and strengthening myocardial contraction. Also acts on CNS to enhance vagal tone, slowing conduction through the SA and AV nodes and providing an antiarrhythmic effect.

### ONSET, PEAK, DURATION
Onset occurs ½ to 2 hours after oral dose or 5 to 30 minutes after I.V. administration. Serum levels peak 2 to 6 hours after oral dose or 1 to 4 hours after I.V. administration. Effects persist 3 to 4 days after last dose.

### INDICATIONS & DOSAGE
*CHF, paroxysmal supraventricular tachycardia, atrial fibrillation and flutter –*
**Adults:** loading dose is 0.5 to 1 mg I.V. or P.O. in divided doses over 24 hours; maintenance dosage is 0.125 to 0.5 mg I.V. or P.O. daily (average is 0.25 mg). Depending on response, larger doses may be needed for arrhythmias. Smaller loading and maintenance doses are given to patients with impaired renal function.
**Adults over 65 years:** 0.125 mg P.O. daily as maintenance dose. Frail or underweight elderly patients may require only 0.0625 mg daily or 0.125 mg every other day.
**Premature neonates:** loading dose is 0.025 mg/kg I.V. in three divided doses over 24 hours; maintenance dosage is 0.01 mg/kg daily, divided q 12 hours.
**Neonates:** loading dose is 0.035 mg/kg P.O., divided q 8 hours over 24 hours; I.V. loading dose is 0.02 to 0.03 mg/kg; maintenance dosage is 0.01 mg/kg P.O. daily, divided q 12 hours.
**Children 1 month to 2 years:** loading dose is 0.035 to 0.06 mg/kg P.O. in three divided doses over 24 hours; I.V. loading dose is 0.03 to 0.05 mg/kg; maintenance dosage is 0.01 to 0.02 mg/kg P.O. daily, divided q 12 hours.
**Children over 2 years:** loading dose is 0.02 to 0.04 mg/kg P.O. daily, divided q 8 hours over 24 hours; I.V. loading dose is 0.015 to 0.035 mg/kg; maintenance dosage is 0.012 mg/kg P.O. daily, divided q 12 hours.

### ADVERSE REACTIONS
*The following signs of toxicity may occur with all digitalis glycosides:*
**CNS:** *fatigue, generalized muscle weakness, agitation, hallucinations,* headache, malaise, dizziness, vertigo, stupor, paresthesia.
**CV:** *arrhythmias* (most commonly, conduction disturbances with or without AV block, PVCs, and supraventricular arrhythmias); arrhythmias may lead to increased severity of CHF and hypotension. **Toxic effects on the heart may be life-threatening and require immediate attention.**
**EENT:** *yellow-green halos around visual images, blurred vision,* light flashes, photophobia, diplopia.
**GI:** *anorexia, nausea,* vomiting, diarrhea.

---

*Liquid form contains alcohol.  **May contain tartrazine.  †Canada only.  ‡Australia only.  ◊OTC.

## INTERACTIONS

*Amiloride:* inhibited digoxin effect and increased digoxin excretion. Monitor for altered digoxin effect.

*Amiodarone, diltiazem, nifedipine, quinidine, verapamil:* increased digoxin blood levels. Monitor for toxicity.

*Amphotericin B, carbenicillin, corticosteroids, diuretics (including loop diuretics, chlorthalidone, metolazone, and thiazides), ticarcillin:* hypokalemia, predisposing patient to digitalis toxicity. Monitor serum potassium levels.

*Antacids, kaolin-pectin:* decreased absorption of oral digoxin. Schedule doses as far as possible from oral digoxin administration.

*Anticholinergics:* may increase digoxin absorption of oral digoxin tablets. Monitor blood levels and observe for toxicity.

*Cholestyramine, colestipol, metoclopramide:* decreased absorption of oral digoxin. Monitor for decreased digitoxin effect and low blood levels. Increase dosage as ordered.

*Parenteral calcium, thiazides:* hypercalcemia and hypomagnesemia, predisposing patient to digitalis toxicity. Monitor serum calcium and serum magnesium levels.

## CONTRAINDICATIONS

Contraindicated in patients with hypersensitivity to the drug; any digitalis-induced toxicity; ventricular fibrillation; or ventricular tachycardia unless caused by CHF.

## NURSING CONSIDERATIONS

● Use with extreme caution in elderly patients and in those with acute MI, incomplete AV block, sinus bradycardia, PVCs, chronic constrictive pericarditis, hypertrophic cardiomyopathy, renal insufficiency, severe pulmonary disease, or hypothyroidism. Reduce dosage in patients with renal impairment.

● Be aware that hypothyroid patients are extremely sensitive to digitalis

glycosides; hyperthyroid patients may need larger doses.

● Before administering the loading dose, obtain baseline data (heart rate and rhythm, blood pressure, and electrolytes) and question the patient about use of digitalis glycosides within the previous 2 to 3 weeks.

● Be aware that the loading dose is divided over the first 24 hours unless the situation indicates otherwise.

● Before giving, take apical-radial pulse for a full minute. Record and report to the doctor significant changes (sudden increase or decrease in pulse rate, pulse deficit, irregular beats and, particularly, regularization of a previously irregular rhythm). If any occurs, check blood pressure and obtain a 12-lead ECG.

● **I.V. use:** Infuse drug slowly over at least 5 minutes.

● Absorption of digoxin from parenteral route and from liquid-filled capsules is superior to absorption from tablets or elixir. Expect dosage reduction of 20% to 25% when changing from tablets or elixir to liquid-filled capsules or parenteral therapy.

● Monitor serum digoxin levels. Therapeutic levels range from 0.5 to 2.0 ng/ml. Obtain blood for digoxin levels 8 hours after last oral dose.

● *Alert:* Excessive slowing of the pulse rate (60 beats/minute or less) may be a sign of digitalis toxicity. Withhold drug and notify the doctor.

● Monitor serum potassium levels carefully. Take corrective action before hypokalemia occurs.

● Withhold drug for 1 to 2 days before elective cardioversion. Adjust dose after cardioversion.

## ☑ PATIENT TEACHING

● Instruct the patient and a responsible family member about drug action, dosage regimen, how to take pulse, reportable signs, and follow-up care.

● Encourage the patient to eat potassium-rich foods.

Reactions may be *common,* uncommon, *life-threatening,* or COMMON AND LIFE-THREATENING.

• Tell the patient not to substitute one brand of digoxin for another.

---

# milrinone lactate
Primacor

*Pregnancy Risk Category: C*

## HOW SUPPLIED
*Injection:* 1 mg/ml

## ACTION
Produces inotropic action by increasing cellular levels of cAMP. Produces vasodilation by directly relaxing vascular smooth muscle.

## ONSET, PEAK, DURATION
Onset occurs within 5 to 15 minutes. Serum levels peak within 1 to 2 hours. Duration is 3 to 6 hours.

## INDICATIONS & DOSAGE
*Short-term treatment of CHF* —
**Adults:** initial loading dose is 50 mcg/kg I.V., administered slowly over 10 minutes, followed by continuous I.V. infusion of 0.375 to 0.75 mcg/kg/ minute. Adjust infusion dose according to clinical and hemodynamic responses, as ordered.

In patients with renal failure: if creatinine clearance is 50 ml/minute or less, dosage is titrated to maximum clinical effect and not to exceed 1.13 mg/kg/day.

## ADVERSE REACTIONS
**CNS:** headache.
**CV:** VENTRICULAR ARRHYTHMIAS, *ventricular ectopic activity,* nonsustained ventricular tachycardia, SUSTAINED VENTRICULAR TACHYCARDIA, VENTRICULAR FIBRILLATION.

## INTERACTIONS
None significant.

## CONTRAINDICATIONS
Contraindicated in patients with hypersensitivity to the drug.

## NURSING CONSIDERATIONS
• Know that milrinone should not be used in patients with severe aortic or pulmonic valvular disease in place of surgical correction of the obstruction or during acute phase of MI.
• Use cautiously in patients with atrial flutter or fibrillation because drug slightly shortens AV node conduction time and may increase ventricular response rate. Administer a digitalis glycoside, if ordered, before beginning milrinone therapy.
• Be aware that milrinone is typically given with digoxin and diuretics.
• Be aware that inotropic agents may aggravate outflow tract obstruction in hypertrophic subaortic stenosis.
• **I.V. use:** Prepare I.V. infusion solution using 0.45% or 0.9% sodium chloride or $D_5W$. Prepare the 100-mcg/ml solution by adding 180 ml of diluent per 20-mg (20-ml) vial, the 150-mcg/ml solution by adding 113 ml of diluent per 20-mg (20-ml) vial, and the 200-mcg/ ml solution by adding 80 ml of diluent per 20-mg (20-ml) vial.
• Be aware that improved cardiac output may enhance urine output. Expect dosage reduction in patient's diuretic therapy as CHF improves. Potassium loss may predispose patient to digitalis toxicity.
• Monitor fluid and electrolyte status, blood pressure, heart rate, and renal function during therapy. Excessive decrease in blood pressure requires discontinuing or slowing rate of infusion.
• Monitor patient closely. Patients treated with milrinone have exhibited supraventricular and ventricular arrhythmias.

## ☑ PATIENT TEACHING
• Instruct patient to report adverse reactions promptly.
• Tell patient to alert the nurse if discomfort is felt at I.V. insertion site.

---

# Antiarrhythmics

adenosine
amiodarone hydrochloride
atropine sulfate
bretylium tosylate
diltiazem hydrochloride
  (See Chapter 22, ANTIANGINALS.)
disopyramide
disopyramide phosphate
esmolol hydrochloride
flecainide acetate
ibutilide fumarate
lidocaine hydrochloride
mexiletine hydrochloride
moricizine hydrochloride
phenytoin
  (See Chapter 30, ANTICONVULSANTS.)
phenytoin sodium
  (See Chapter 30, ANTICONVULSANTS.)
procainamide hydrochloride
propafenone hydrochloride
propranolol hydrochloride
  (See Chapter 22, ANTIANGINALS.)
quinidine bisulfate
quinidine gluconate
quinidine polygalacturonate
quinidine sulfate
sotalol
tocainide hydrochloride
verapamil hydrochloride
  (See Chapter 22, ANTIANGINALS.)

**COMBINATION PRODUCTS**
None.

---

## adenosine
Adenocard

*Pregnancy Risk Category: C*

**HOW SUPPLIED**
*Injection:* 3 mg/ml in 2-ml vials

**ACTION**
A naturally occurring nucleoside that acts on the AV node to slow conduction and inhibit reentry pathways.

Adenosine is also useful in treating paroxysmal supraventricular tachy-cardia (PSVT) associated with acces-sory bypass tracts (Wolff-Parkinson-White syndrome).

**ONSET, PEAK, DURATION**
Onset and peak serum levels occur immediately. Duration is extremely short; the exact time is unknown.

**INDICATIONS & DOSAGE**
*Conversion of PSVT to sinus rhythm –*
**Adults:** 6 mg I.V. by rapid bolus injec-tion over 1 to 2 seconds. If PSVT is not eliminated in 1 to 2 minutes, 12 mg by rapid I.V. push may be given and re-peated (if necessary). Single doses over 12 mg are not recommended.

**ADVERSE REACTIONS**
**CNS:** apprehension, back pain, blurred vision, burning sensation, dizziness, heaviness in arms, light-headedness, neck pain, numbness, tingling in arms.
**CV:** chest pain, *facial flushing,* head-ache, hypotension, palpitations, dia-phoresis.
**GI:** metallic taste, nausea.
**Respiratory:** *chest pressure, dyspnea, shortness of breath,* hyperventilation.
**Other:** *throat tightness, groin pressure.*

**INTERACTIONS**
*Carbamazepine:* higher degrees of heart block may occur.
*Dipyridamole:* may potentiate adeno-sine's effects. Smaller doses may be necessary.
*Methylxanthines:* antagonism of aden-osine's effects. Patients receiving the-ophylline or caffeine may require higher doses or may not respond to adenosine therapy.

---

Reactions may be *common,* uncommon, *life-threatening,* or **COMMON AND LIFE-THREATENING.**

## CONTRAINDICATIONS

Contraindicated in patients with hypersensitivity to the drug and also in those with second- or third-degree heart block or sick sinus syndrome, unless an artificial pacemaker is present, because adenosine decreases conduction through the AV node and may produce first-, second-, or third-degree heart block. These effects are usually transient; however, patients who develop significant heart block after a dose of adenosine should not receive additional doses.

## NURSING CONSIDERATIONS

• Use cautiously in patients with asthma because bronchoconstriction may occur.
• Crystals may form if solution is cold. If crystals are visible, gently warm solution to room temperature. Don't use solutions that aren't clear.
• Because adenosine contains no preservatives, discard any unused drug.
• **I.V. use:** Rapid I.V. injection is necessary to ensure drug action. Administer directly into a vein if possible; when giving through an I.V. line, use the most proximal port, and flush immediately and rapidly with 0.9% sodium chloride solution to ensure that the drug reaches the systemic circulation quickly.
• Monitor patient's ECG for arrhythmias. In clinical trials, more than half the patients exhibited new arrhythmias, including sinus bradycardia or tachycardia, premature atrial contractions, various degrees of AV block, PVCs, and skipped beats, when adenosine was used to convert to normal sinus rhythm. Such arrhythmias are usually transient.

## ☑ PATIENT TEACHING

• Instruct patient to report adverse reactions promptly.
• Tell patient to alert nurse if discomfort occurs at I.V. site.

## amiodarone hydrochloride

Aratac‡, Cordarone, Cordarone X‡

*Pregnancy Risk Category: D*

### HOW SUPPLIED

*Tablets:* 100 mg†‡, 200 mg
*Injection:* 50 mg/ml

### ACTION

Unknown. Thought to prolong the refractory period and action potential duration and decrease repolarization.

### ONSET, PEAK, DURATION

Onset may occur in 2 to 3 days despite more rapid peak concentration, but more commonly takes 1 to 3 weeks, even with loading doses. Serum levels peak 3 to 7 hours after oral administration. Duration of antiarrhythmic effects may last for weeks or months but rate variable and unpredictable.

### INDICATIONS & DOSAGE

*Recurrent ventricular fibrillation and recurrent hemodynamically unstable ventricular tachycardia refractory to other antiarrhythmics –*
**Adults:** give loading dose of 800 to 1,600 mg P.O. daily for 1 to 3 weeks until initial therapeutic response occurs, then 600 to 800 mg/day P.O. for 1 month, and then, for maintenance, 200 to 600 mg P.O. daily.
  Or, give loading dose of 150 mg I.V. over 10 minutes (15 mg/minute); then 360 mg I.V. over the next 6 hours (1 mg/minute); then 540 mg I.V. over the next 18 hours (0.5 mg/minute). After the first 24 hours, a maintenance I.V. infusion of 720 mg/24 hours (0.5 mg/minute) should be continued.

### ADVERSE REACTIONS

**CNS:** peripheral neuropathy, ataxia, paresthesia, tremor, insomnia, sleep disturbances, headache, *malaise, fatigue.*
**CV:** bradycardia, hypotension, *ar-*

*rhythmias, CHF, heart block, sinus arrest.*
**EENT:** *corneal microdeposits,* visual disturbances.
**GI:** *nausea, vomiting,* constipation, abdominal pain.
**Hepatic:** *altered liver enzymes,* hepatic dysfunction, ***hepatic failure.***
**Respiratory:** SEVERE PULMONARY TOXICITY (PNEUMONITIS, ALVEOLITIS).
**Skin:** *photosensitivity,* blue-gray skin pigmentation, solar dermatitis.
**Other:** hypothyroidism, hyperthyroidism, edema, coagulation abnormalities.

## INTERACTIONS
*Antiarrhythmics:* amiodarone may reduce the hepatic or renal clearance of certain antiarrhythmics (especially flecainide, procainamide, or quinidine); concomitant use of amiodarone with other antiarrhythmics (especially mexilitine, propafenone, quinidine, disopyramide, or procainamide) may induce torsades de pointes.
*Antihypertensives:* increased hypotensive effect. Use together cautiously.
*Beta blockers, calcium channel blockers:* increased cardiac depressant effects; may potentiate slowing of SA node and AV conduction. Use together cautiously.
*Digitalis glycosides:* increased serum digoxin levels (average of 70% to 100%). Monitor digoxin levels closely and adjust dosage as ordered.
*Phenytoin:* may decrease phenytoin metabolism. Monitor serum phenytoin levels and adjust dosage as ordered.
*Theophylline:* increased theophylline levels with toxicity may occur. Monitor serum theophylline levels.
*Warfarin:* increased PT (average of 100% within 1 to 4 weeks of therapy). Decrease warfarin dosage 33% to 50% when amiodarone is initiated. Monitor patient closely.

## CONTRAINDICATIONS
Contraindicated in patients with hypersensitivity to the drug and in those with severe SA node disease resulting in preexisting bradycardia. Unless an artificial pacemaker is present, drug is also contraindicated in patients with second- or third-degree AV block and in those in whom bradycardia has caused syncope.

## NURSING CONSIDERATIONS
● Use with extreme caution in those receiving other antiarrhythmics.
● Use cautiously in patients with pulmonary or thyroid disease.
● Be aware that although amiodarone is often effective for treatment of arrhythmias resistant to other drug therapy, the high incidence of adverse reactions limits its use.
● Obtain baseline pulmonary, liver, and thyroid function tests.
● Administer loading doses in a hospital setting and with continuous ECG monitoring because of the slow onset of antiarrhythmic effect and risk of life-threatening arrhythmias.
● Divide oral loading dose into three equal doses and give with meals to decrease GI intolerance. Maintenance dosage may be given once daily, but may be divided into two doses taken with meals if GI intolerance occurs.
● **I.V. use:** Know that amiodarone may be given I.V. where facilities for close monitoring of cardiac function and resuscitation are available. Initial dosage of 150 mg should be mixed in 100 ml of dextrose 5% solution. Repeat doses should be administered through a central venous catheter.
● Continuously monitor cardiac status of patient receiving drug I.V.
● Monitor blood pressure and heart rate and rhythm frequently. Perform continuous ECG monitoring during initiation and alteration of dosage. Notify doctor of significant change.
● ***Alert:*** Monitor carefully for pulmonary toxicity, which can be fatal. Inci-

dence increases in patients receiving more than 400 mg/day.
• Monitor for symptoms of pneumonitis – exertional dyspnea, nonproductive cough, and pleuritic chest pain. Monitor pulmonary function tests and chest X-ray.
• Monitor liver and thyroid function tests and serum electrolytes, particularly potassium and magnesium levels.
• Instillation of methylcellulose ophthalmic solution is recommended during amiodarone therapy to minimize corneal microdeposits. Within 1 to 4 months after beginning amiodarone therapy, most patients show corneal microdeposits upon slit-lamp ophthalmic examination. However, only 2% to 3% have actual vision disturbances.

☑ **PATIENT TEACHING**
• Advise the patient to use a sunscreen to prevent photosensitivity reaction. Monitor for burning or tingling skin followed by erythema and possible skin blistering.
• Tell the patient to take oral drug with food if GI reactions occur.
• Inform the patient that amiodarone's adverse effects are more prevalent at high doses but are generally reversible when drug therapy is stopped. Resolution of adverse reactions may take up to 4 months.

---

### atropine sulfate

*Pregnancy Risk Category: C*

**HOW SUPPLIED**
*Tablets:* 0.4 mg, 0.6 mg
*Injection:* 0.05 mg/ml, 0.1 mg/ml, 0.3 mg/ml, 0.4 mg/ml, 0.5 mg/ml, 0.6 mg/ml, 0.8 mg/ml, 1 mg/ml, 1.2 mg/ml

**ACTION**
An anticholinergic that inhibits acetylcholine at the parasympathetic neuroeffector junction, blocking vagal effects on the SA node; this enhances

conduction through the AV node and speeds heart rate.

**ONSET, PEAK, DURATION**
Onset occurs 30 minutes to 1 hour after oral administration, 30 minutes after I.M. administration, and immediately after I.V. administration. Serum levels peak 2 hours after oral administration, 1 to 1.6 hours after I.M. administration, and 2 to 4 minutes after I.V. administration. Duration is about 4 hours.

**INDICATIONS & DOSAGE**
*Symptomatic bradycardia, bradyarrhythmia (junctional or escape rhythm)* –
**Adults:** usually 0.5 to 1 mg I.V. push; repeated q 3 to 5 minutes to maximum of 2 mg as needed. Lower doses (less than 0.5 mg) can cause bradycardia.
**Children:** 0.01 mg/kg I.V. up to maximum of 0.4 mg; or 0.3 mg/m²; may repeat q 4 to 6 hours.
*Antidote for anticholinesterase insecticide poisoning* –
**Adults:** 2 to 3 mg I.V. repeated q 5 to 10 minutes until muscarinic symptoms disappear or signs of atropine toxicity appear. Severe poisoning may require up to 6 mg q hour.
**Children:** 1 mg I.V. or I.M., then 0.5 to 1 mg I.V. or I.M. q 5 to 10 minutes until muscarinic signs disappear or signs of atropine toxicity appear.
*Preoperatively to diminish secretions and block cardiac vagal reflexes* –
**Adults and children weighing 20 kg or more:** 0.4 to 0.6 mg I.M. or S.C. 45 to 60 minutes before anesthesia.
**Children weighing less than 20 kg:** 0.01 mg/kg I.M. or S.C. up to maximum dose of 0.4 mg 45 to 60 minutes before anesthesia.
*Adjunct treatment of peptic ulcer disease; treatment of functional GI disorders such as irritable bowel syndrome* –
**Adults:** 0.4 to 0.6 mg P.O. q 4 to 6 hours.

---

**Children:** 0.01 mg/kg or 0.3 mg/m² (not to exceed 0.4 mg) q 4 to 6 hours.

## ADVERSE REACTIONS
**CNS:** *headache, restlessness,* ataxia, disorientation, hallucinations, delirium, *insomnia, dizziness,* excitement, agitation, confusion (especially in elderly patients).
**CV:** palpitations and bradycardia following low dose of atropine, tachycardia after higher doses.
**EENT:** photophobia, *blurred vision, mydriasis,* cycloplegia, increased intraocular pressure.
**GI:** *dry mouth,* thirst, *constipation,* nausea, vomiting.
**GU:** urine retention, impotence.
**Hematologic:** leukocytosis.
**Other:** severe allergic reactions, including ***anaphylaxis*** and urticaria.

## INTERACTIONS
*Antacids:* decreased absorption of anticholinergics. Separate administration times by at least 1 hour.
*Anticholinergics or drugs with anticholinergic effects, such as amantadine, glutethimide, meperidine, antiarrhythmics, antiparkinsonian agents, phenothiazines, and tricyclic antidepressants:* additive anticholinergic effects. Use together cautiously.
*Ketoconazole, levodopa:* decreased absorption. Avoid concomitant use.
*Methotrimeprazine:* may produce extrapyramidal symptoms. Monitor patient carefully.
*Potassium chloride wax-matrix tablets:* increased risk of mucosal lesions. Use cautiously.

## CONTRAINDICATIONS
Contraindicated in patients with hypersensitivity to drug, acute angle-closure glaucoma, obstructive uropathy, obstructive disease of GI tract, paralytic ileus, toxic megacolon, intestinal atony, unstable CV status in acute hemorrhage, asthma, and myasthenia gravis.

## NURSING CONSIDERATIONS
• Use cautiously in patients with Down syndrome because they may be more sensitive to the drug.
• **I.V. use:** Administer via direct I.V. into a large vein or I.V. tubing over at least 1 minute.
• Be aware that many adverse reactions (such as dry mouth and constipation) vary with the dose.
• Monitor patients for paradoxical initial bradycardia, especially those receiving small doses (0.4 to 0.6 mg). This is caused by the drug's effect in the CNS and usually disappears within 2 minutes.
• ***Alert:*** Watch for tachycardia in cardiac patients because it may precipitate ventricular fibrillation.
• Monitor fluid intake and urine output. Drug causes urine retention and urinary hesitancy.

☑ **PATIENT TEACHING**
• Teach patient receiving oral form of drug how to handle distressing anticholinergic effects.
• Instruct patient to report serious or persistent adverse reactions promptly.

---

# bretylium tosylate
Bretylate†‡, Bretylol, Critifib‡
*Pregnancy Risk Category: C*

## HOW SUPPLIED
*Injection:* 50 mg/ml

## ACTION
Unknown but considered a class III antiarrhythmic that initially exerts transient adrenergic stimulation through release of norepinephrine. Subsequent depletion of norepinephrine causes adrenergic blocking actions to predominate, prolonging repolarization and increasing the duration of action potential and an effective refractory period.

---

Reactions may be *common,* uncommon, *life-threatening,* or **COMMON AND LIFE-THREATENING.**

## ONSET, PEAK, DURATION
Onset occurs within a few minutes but suppression of ventricular tachycardia and ventricular fibrillation may not occur for 20 minutes to 6 hours. Serum levels peak within 6 to 9 hours. Effects may persist 6 to 24 hours.

## INDICATIONS & DOSAGE
*Ventricular fibrillation or hemodynamically unstable ventricular tachycardia unresponsive to other antiarrhythmics* —
**Adults:** 5 mg/kg by I.V. push over 1 minute. If necessary, dose increased to 10 mg/kg and repeated q 15 to 30 minutes until 30 to 35 mg/kg have been given. For continuous suppression, diluted solution administered at 1 to 2 mg/minute continuously or 5 to 10 mg/kg diluted over more than 8 minutes q 6 hours.

## ADVERSE REACTIONS
**CNS:** *vertigo, dizziness, light-headedness, syncope* (usually secondary to hypotension).
**CV:** SEVERE HYPOTENSION (especially orthostatic), bradycardia, anginal pain, transient arrhythmias, transient hypertension, increased PVCs.
**GI:** severe nausea, vomiting (with rapid infusion).

## INTERACTIONS
*All antihypertensives:* may potentiate hypotension. Monitor blood pressure.
*Other antiarrhythmics:* additive or antagonistic antiarrhythmic effects. Monitor for additive toxicity.
*Sympathomimetics:* bretylium may potentiate effects of drugs given to correct hypotension.

## CONTRAINDICATIONS
Contraindicated in digitalized patients unless the arrhythmia is life-threatening, not caused by digitalis, and unresponsive to other antiarrhythmics.

## NURSING CONSIDERATIONS
● Use with extreme caution in patients with fixed cardiac output (aortic stenosis and pulmonary hypertension) to avoid severe and sudden drop in blood pressure.
● Bretylium is used with other cardiac life-support measures, such as cardiopulmonary resuscitation, countershock, epinephrine, sodium bicarbonate, and lidocaine.
● **I.V. use:** When used for maintenance therapy, dilute using dextrose or sodium chloride for injection before administration. Follow manufacturer's guidelines for specific dilution guidelines (varies according to dosage). When administering as direct I.V. injection, use a 20G to 22G needle and inject over 1 minute into a vein or I.V. line containing a free-flowing, compatible solution.
● To prevent nausea and vomiting, follow dosage directions carefully.
● Keep the patient supine until tolerance to hypotension develops.
● Monitor the patient closely. The initial release of norepinephrine caused by bretylium may induce transient hypertension and arrhythmias.
● Monitor blood pressure and heart rate and rhythm continuously. Notify doctor immediately of any significant change. If supine systolic blood pressure falls below 75 mm Hg, the doctor may order norepinephrine, dopamine, or volume expanders.
● Observe for increased anginal pain in susceptible patients.

☑ **PATIENT TEACHING**
● Instruct the patient to report adverse reactions immediately.
● Tell the patient to alert nurse if discomfort occurs at I.V. insertion site.
● Tell the patient to avoid sudden postural changes.

---

*Liquid form contains alcohol. **May contain tartrazine. †Canada only. ‡Australia only. ◊OTC.

# disopyramide
Rythmodan†

# disopyramide phosphate
Norpace, Norpace CR,
Rythmodan LA†

*Pregnancy Risk Category: C*

## HOW SUPPLIED
**disopyramide**
*Capsules:* 100 mg†, 150 mg†
**disopyramide phosphate**
*Tablets (sustained-release):* 250 mg†
*Capsules:* 100 mg, 150 mg
*Capsules (controlled-release):* 100 mg, 150 mg
*Injection:* 10 mg/ml‡

## ACTION
Unknown, but the drug is considered a class Ia antiarrhythmic that depresses phase O and prolongs the action potential. All class I drugs have membrane-stabilizing effects.

## ONSET, PEAK, DURATION
Onset occurs within ½ to 3½ hours after an oral dose. Plasma levels peak within 2 to 2½ hours after an oral dose. Effects persist for 1½ to 8½ hours after last dose.

## INDICATIONS & DOSAGE
*Symptomatic PVCs (unifocal, multifocal, or coupled); ventricular tachycardia not severe enough to require cardioversion –*
**Adults weighing more than 50 kg:** 150 mg q 6 hours with conventional capsules or 300 mg q 12 hours with extended-release preparations.
**Adults weighing 50 kg or less:** highly individualized.
**Children under 1 year:** 10 to 30 mg/ kg P.O. daily.
**Children 1 to 4 years:** 10 to 20 mg/ kg P.O. daily.
**Children 4 to 12 years:** 10 to 15 mg/ kg P.O. daily.

**Children 12 to 18 years:** 6 to 15 mg/ kg P.O. daily.
For pediatric dosages, divide into equal amounts and give q 6 hours.
Recommended dosages in advanced renal insufficiency: If creatinine clearance is 30 to 40 ml/minute, 100 mg q 8 hours; if 15 to 30 ml/minute, 100 mg q 12 hours; if less than 15 ml/ minute, 100 mg q 24 hours.
For parenteral use in adults, initially give 2 mg/kg I.V. slowly (over not less than 15 minutes). Administer until arrhythmia is eliminated or patient has received 150 mg. Repeat dosage if conversion is successful but arrhythmia returns. Total I.V. dosage should not exceed 300 mg in the first hour. Follow with an I.V. infusion of 0.4 mg/kg/hour (usually 20 to 30 mg/ hour) to a maximum of 800 mg/day.

## ADVERSE REACTIONS
**CNS:** dizziness, agitation, depression, fatigue, muscle weakness, syncope.
**CV:** *hypotension, CHF, heart block,* edema, weight gain, *arrhythmias,* shortness of breath, chest pain.
**EENT:** *blurred vision, dry eyes or nose.*
**GI:** nausea, vomiting, anorexia, bloating, abdominal pain, diarrhea.
**Hepatic:** cholestatic jaundice.
**Skin:** rash, pruritus, dermatosis.
**Other:** aches, pain, muscle weakness, hypoglycemia (rare).

## INTERACTIONS
*Antiarrhythmics:* possible additive or antagonized antiarrhythmic effects.
*Phenytoin:* increased metabolism of disopyramide. Monitor for decreased antiarrhythmic effect.
*Rifampin:* may decrease disopyramide levels. Monitor closely.

## CONTRAINDICATIONS
Contraindicated in patients with hypersensitivity to the drug, cardiogenic shock, or second- or third-degree

---

Reactions may be *common,* uncommon, *life-threatening,* or COMMON AND LIFE-THREATENING.

heart block in the absence of an artificial pacemaker.

## NURSING CONSIDERATIONS
• Use with extreme caution and avoid, if possible, in patients with CHF. Use cautiously in patients with underlying conduction abnormalities, urinary tract diseases (especially prostatic hyperplasia), hepatic or renal impairment, myasthenia gravis, or acute angle-closure glaucoma.
• Correct electrolyte abnormalities before therapy begins, as ordered.
• Check apical pulse before administering drug. Notify the doctor if pulse rate is slower than 60 beats/minute or faster than 120 beats/minute.
• Know that sustained or controlled-release preparations should not be used for rapid control of ventricular arrhythmias, when therapeutic blood levels must be rapidly attained, in patients with cardiomyopathy or possible cardiac decompensation, or in those with severe renal impairment.
• For administration to young children, pharmacist may prepare disopyramide suspension, using 100 mg capsules and cherry syrup. Suspension should be dispensed in amber glass bottles and protected from light.
• **I.V. use:** Add 200 mg to 200 to 500 ml of a compatible solution, such as 0.9% sodium chloride or D$_5$W. Do not mix with other drugs; switch to oral therapy as soon as possible.
• Watch for recurrence of arrhythmias and check for adverse reactions; notify the doctor if any occur.
• Discontinue drug if heart block develops, if QRS complex widens by more than 25%, or if QT interval lengthens by more than 25% above baseline; also notify the doctor.
• When transferring the patient from immediate-release to sustained-release capsules, advise him to take the first sustained-release capsule 6 hours after taking the last immediate-release capsule.

☑ **PATIENT TEACHING**
• Teach the patient the importance of taking drug on time and exactly as prescribed. This may require use of an alarm clock for overnight doses.
• Advise the patient to chew gum or hard candy to relieve dry mouth and to increase fiber and fluid intake to relieve constipation, if not contraindicated.

## esmolol hydrochloride
Brevibloc

*Pregnancy Risk Category: C*

### HOW SUPPLIED
*Injection:* 10 mg/ml, 250 mg/ml

### ACTION
A class II antiarrhythmic and ultra-short-acting selective beta$_1$-adrenergic blocker that decreases heart rate, contractility, and blood pressure.

### ONSET, PEAK, DURATION
Onset occurs almost immediately. Peak serum levels vary with infusion rate but typically occur in 30 minutes. Effects subside within 30 minutes after infusion ends.

### INDICATIONS & DOSAGE
*Supraventricular tachycardia; to control ventricular rate in patients with atrial fibrillation or flutter in perioperative, postoperative, or other emergent circumstances; noncompensatory sinus tachycardia when heart rate requires specific interventions –*
**Adults:** loading dose is 500 mcg/kg/minute by I.V. infusion over 1 minute, followed by 4-minute maintenance infusion of 50 mcg/kg/minute. If adequate response does not occur within 5 minutes, loading dose is repeated and followed by maintenance infusion of 100 mcg/kg/minute for 4 minutes. Loading dose is repeated and maintenance infusion is increased in a stepwise fashion as needed. Maximum

---

*Liquid form contains alcohol.   **May contain tartrazine.   †Canada only.   ‡Australia only.   ◊OTC.

maintenance infusion for tachycardia is 200 mcg/kg/minute.

*Perioperative and postoperative tachycardia or hypertension –*

**Adults:** for perioperative treatment of tachycardia or hypertension, 80 mg (approximately 1 mg/kg) I.V. bolus over 30 seconds, followed by 150 mcg/kg/minute I.V. infusion, if needed. Adjust the infusion rate as needed up to a maximum of 300 mcg/kg/minute; dosage for postoperative treatment of tachycardia and hypertension is the same as for supraventricular tachycardia.

**ADVERSE REACTIONS**
**CNS:** dizziness, somnolence, headache, agitation, fatigue, confusion.
**CV: HYPOTENSION** (sometimes with diaphoresis), peripheral ischemia.
**GI:** *nausea,* vomiting.
**Respiratory:** *bronchospasm,* wheezing, dyspnea, nasal congestion.
**Other:** inflammation and induration at infusion site.

**INTERACTIONS**
*Digoxin:* serum digoxin levels may be increased by 10% to 20%. Monitor serum digoxin levels.
*Morphine:* may increase esmolol blood levels. Titrate esmolol carefully.
*Reserpine (and other catecholamine-depleting drugs):* may cause additive bradycardia and hypotension. Titrate esmolol carefully.
*Succinylcholine:* esmolol may prolong neuromuscular blockade.

**CONTRAINDICATIONS**
Contraindicated in patients with sinus bradycardia, heart block greater than first-degree, cardiogenic shock, or overt heart failure.

**NURSING CONSIDERATIONS**
● Use cautiously in patients with impaired renal function, diabetes, or bronchospasm.

● **I.V. use:** Don't give esmolol by I.V. push; use an infusion control device. The 10-mg/ml single-dose vials may be used without diluting, but the injection concentrate (250 mg/ml) must be diluted to a maximum concentration of 10 mg/ml before infusion. Remove 20 ml from 500 ml of $D_5W$, lactated Ringer's solution, or 0.45% or 0.9% sodium chloride solution and add two ampules of esmolol (final concentration 10 mg/ml).

● Remember that esmolol solutions are incompatible with diazepam, furosemide, sodium bicarbonate, and thiopental sodium.

● *Alert:* Monitor ECG and blood pressure continuously during infusion. Up to 50% of all patients treated with esmolol develop hypotension. Monitor closely, especially if patient's pretreatment blood pressure was low.

● Hypotension can usually be reversed within 30 minutes by decreasing the dose or, if necessary, by stopping the infusion. Notify doctor if this becomes necessary.

● If a local reaction develops at the infusion site, change to another site. Avoid using butterfly needles.

● Be aware that esmolol is recommended only for short-term use, for no longer than 48 hours.

● When the patient's heart rate becomes stable, esmolol will be replaced by alternative (longer-acting) antiarrhythmics, such as propranolol, digoxin, or verapamil. A half hour after the first dose of the alternative agent is administered, reduce infusion rate by 50%. Monitor patient response and, if heart rate is controlled for 1 hour after administration of the second dose of the alternative drug, discontinue esmolol infusion.

☑ **PATIENT TEACHING**
● Instruct patient to report adverse reactions promptly.
● Tell patient to alert nurse if discomfort occurs at I.V. site.

Reactions may be *common,* uncommon, *life-threatening,* or **COMMON AND LIFE-THREATENING.**

# flecainide acetate
Tambocor

*Pregnancy Risk Category: C*

## HOW SUPPLIED
*Tablets:* 50 mg, 100 mg, 150 mg
*Injection:* 10 mg/ml‡

## ACTION
A class Ic antiarrhythmic that decreases excitability, conduction velocity, and automaticity as a result of slowed atrial, AV node, His-Purkinje system, and intraventricular conduction and causes a slight but significant prolongation of refractory periods in these tissues.

## ONSET, PEAK, DURATION
Onset immediate with I.V. administration, unknown with oral administration. Serum levels peak immediately after I.V. infusion, 2 to 3 hours after oral administration. Duration unknown.

## INDICATIONS & DOSAGE
*Paroxysmal supraventricular tachycardia, paroxysmal atrial fibrillation or flutter in patients without structural heart disease; life-threatening ventricular arrhythmias, such as sustained ventricular tachycardia* —
**Adults:** for paroxysmal supraventricular tachycardia, 50 mg P.O. q 12 hours. Increased in increments of 50 mg b.i.d. q 4 days. Maximum dosage is 300 mg. In patients with renal impairment (creatinine clearance of 35 ml/minute or less), initial dosage is 100 mg once daily or 50 mg b.i.d. For life-threatening ventricular arrhythmias, 100 mg P.O. q 12 hours. Increase in increments of 50 mg b.i.d. q 4 days until efficacy is achieved. Maximum dosage is 400 mg daily for most patients.

Initial dosage for patients with CHF is 50 mg P.O. q 12 hours.

Where available, flecainide may be given by I.V. injection‡ —
**Adults:** 2 mg/kg I.V. push over not less than 10 minutes; or dilute the dose and administer as an infusion.

## ADVERSE REACTIONS
**CNS:** *dizziness, headache,* fatigue, tremor, anxiety, insomnia, depression, malaise, paresthesia, ataxia, vertigo, *light-headedness, syncope,* asthenia.
**CV:** *new or worsened arrhythmias,* chest pain, *CHF, cardiac arrest,* palpitations.
**EENT:** *blurred vision and other visual disturbances.*
**GI:** nausea, constipation, abdominal pain, dyspepsia, vomiting, diarrhea, anorexia.
**Other:** *dyspnea,* edema, skin rash, flushing, fever.

## INTERACTIONS
*Amiodarone, cimetidine:* altered pharmacokinetics. Monitor for toxicity.
*Digitalis glycosides:* flecainide may increase plasma digoxin levels by 15% to 25%. Monitor serum digoxin levels.
*Propranolol, other beta blockers:* both flecainide and propranolol plasma levels increase by 20% to 30%. Monitor for propranolol and flecainide toxicity.
*Urine acidifying and alkalinizing agents:* extremes of urine pH may substantially alter excretion of flecainide. Monitor for flecainide toxicity or decreased effectiveness.

## CONTRAINDICATIONS
Contraindicated in patients with hypersensitivity to the drug; in those with preexisting second- or third-degree AV block or right bundle branch block when associated with a left hemiblock (in the absence of an artificial pacemaker); and in those with cardiogenic shock.

## NURSING CONSIDERATIONS
● Use cautiously in patients with preexisting CHF, cardiomyopathy, severe renal or hepatic disease, prolonged QT interval, sick sinus syndrome, or blood dyscrasia.
● Know that when used to prevent ventricular arrhythmias, flecainide should be reserved for patients with documented life-threatening arrhythmias.
● Check that pacing threshold was determined 1 week before and after initiating therapy in patients with pacemakers because flecainide can alter endocardial pacing thresholds.
● Correct hypokalemia or hyperkalemia as ordered before giving flecainide because these electrolyte disturbances may alter its effect.
● Know that most patients can be adequately maintained on an every-12-hour dosing schedule, but that some need to receive flecainide every 8 hours.
● **I.V. use:** When administering by I.V. push, give over at least 10 minutes. For I.V. infusion, mix only with $D_5W$.
● Be aware that dosage adjustments should be made only once every 3 to 4 days.
● Because of flecainide's long half-life, its full therapeutic effect may take 3 to 5 days. Administer concomitant I.V. lidocaine as ordered for the first several days.
● Monitor serum flecainide levels, especially in patients with renal failure or CHF. Therapeutic serum levels of flecainide range from 0.2 to 1 mcg/ml. Incidence of adverse effects increases when trough blood levels exceed 1 mcg/ml.

### ☑ PATIENT TEACHING
● Stress importance of taking drug exactly as prescribed.
● Instruct patient to report adverse reactions promptly and to limit fluid and sodium intake to minimize fluid retention.
● Tell patient receiving drug I.V. to alert nurse if discomfort occurs at the insertion site.

▼ **NEW DRUG**

## ibutilide fumarate
Corvert

*Pregnancy Risk Category: C*

### HOW SUPPLIED
*Injection:* 0.1 mg/ml

### ACTION
Prolongs action potential in isolated cardiac myocyte and increases atrial and ventricular refractoriness.

### ONSET, PEAK, DURATION
Unknown. May convert arrhythmia 30 to 90 minutes after infusion starts, with most patients in normal sinus rhythm 24 hours later.

### INDICATIONS & DOSAGE
*Rapid conversion of atrial fibrillation or atrial flutter of recent onset to sinus rhythm –*
**Adults weighing 60 kg (132 lb) or more:** 1 mg I.V. over 10 minutes.
**Adults weighing less than 60 kg:** 0.01 mg/kg I.V. over 10 minutes.
● *Alert:* Infusion should be stopped if arrhythmia is terminated or patient develops ventricular tachycardia (VT) or marked prolongation of QT or QTc. If arrhythmia is not terminated 10 minutes after infusion ends, a second 10-minute infusion of equal strength may be given.

### ADVERSE REACTIONS
**CNS:** headache.
**CV:** ventricular extrasystoles, nonsustained VT, hypotension, bundle branch block, *sustained VT,* AV block, hypertension, QT segment prolongation, bradycardia, palpitation, tachycardia.
**GI:** nausea.

---

Reactions may be *common,* uncommon, *life-threatening,* or COMMON AND LIFE-THREATENING.

## INTERACTIONS

*Class Ia antiarrhythmics (disopyramide, quinidine, procainamide) and other class III drugs (amiodarone, sotalol):* increased potential for prolonged refractoriness. Don't give these drugs for at least 5 half-lives before and 4 hours after ibutilide dose.
*Digoxin:* supraventricular arrhythmias may mask cardiotoxicity associated with excessive digoxin levels. Use cautiously.
*Phenothiazines, tricyclic antidepressants, tetracyclic antidepressants, H₁-receptor antagonist antihistamines, and other drugs that prolong QT interval:* increased risk for proarrhythmia. Monitor closely.

## CONTRAINDICATIONS

Contraindicated in patients with hypersensitivity to drug or its components.

## NURSING CONSIDERATIONS

● Drug is not recommended for use in patients with a history of polymorphic VT, such as torsades de pointes, and in breast-feeding women.
● Use cautiously in patients with hepatic or renal dysfunction.
● Safety of drug has not been established in children.
● Drug should be given only by skilled personnel. Cardiac monitor, intracardiac pacing, cardioverter or defibrillator, and medication for sustained VT must be available.
● Before therapy, hypokalemia and hypomagnesemia should be corrected to reduce the potential for proarrhythmia.
● **I.V. use:** Drug may be given undiluted or diluted in 50 ml of diluent; may be added to 0.9% sodium chloride injection or 5% dextrose injection before infusion. Contents of 10-ml vial (0.1 mg/ml) may be added to 50-ml infusion bag to form admixture of about 0.017 mg/ml ibutilide fumarate. Use aseptic technique. Drug

can be used with polyvinyl chloride plastic bags or polyolefin bags.
● Admixtures with approved diluents are stable for 24 hours at room temperature; 48 hours if refrigerated.
● Inspect parenteral products for particulate and discoloration before administration.
● Monitor ECG continuously during administration and for at least 4 hours afterward or until QTc returns to baseline; drug can induce or worsen ventricular arrhythmias. Longer monitoring is required if ECG shows arrhythmia.

### ☑ PATIENT TEACHING

● Tell patient to report adverse reactions promptly.
● Instruct patient to alert nurse of discomfort at injection site.

---

# lidocaine hydrochloride (lignocaine hydrochloride)
LidoPen Auto-Injector, Xylocaine, Xylocard†‡

*Pregnancy Risk Category: B*

## HOW SUPPLIED

*Injection (for I.M. use):* 300 mg/3 ml automatic injection device
*Injection (for direct I.V. use):* 1% (10 mg/ml), 2% (20 mg/ml)
*Injection (for I.V. admixtures):* 4% (40 mg/ml), 10% (100 mg/ml), 20% (200 mg/ml)
*Infusion (premixed):* 0.2% (2 mg/ ml), 0.4% (4 mg/ml), 0.8% (8 mg/ml)

## ACTION

Lidocaine, a class 1B antiarrhythmic, decreases the depolarization, automaticity, and excitability in the ventricles during the diastolic phase by direct action on the tissues, especially the Purkinje network, without involvement of the autonomic nervous system.

---

## ONSET, PEAK, DURATION

Onset is immediate (45 to 90 seconds) with I.V. bolus administration, 5 to 15 minutes with I.M. administration. Without a bolus loading dose, peak serum levels occur within 30 to 60 minutes of starting an I.V. infusion. After an I.M. injection, plasma levels peak in about 10 minutes. Effects of an I.V. bolus dose last for 10 to 20 minutes; effective blood levels persist for about 60 minutes after an I.M. injection.

## INDICATIONS & DOSAGE

*Ventricular arrhythmias resulting from MI, cardiac manipulation, or digitalis glycosides* –

**Adults:** 50 to 100 mg (1 to 1.5 mg/kg) by I.V. bolus at 25 to 50 mg/minute. Half this amount is given to elderly patients or patients under 50 kg and to those with CHF or hepatic disease. Bolus dose is repeated q 3 to 5 minutes until arrhythmias subside or adverse reactions develop. Don't exceed 300-mg total bolus during a 1-hour period. Simultaneously, constant infusion of 20 to 50 mcg/kg/minute (1 to 4 mg/minute) is begun. If single bolus has been given, smaller bolus dose may be repeated 15 to 20 minutes after start of infusion to maintain therapeutic serum level. After 24 hours of continuous infusion, rate may be decreased by half. Alternatively, 200 to 300 mg I.M., followed by second I.M. dose 60 to 90 minutes later, if needed.

**Children:** 1 mg/kg by I.V. bolus, followed by infusion of 30 mcg/kg/minute.

## ADVERSE REACTIONS

**CNS:** *confusion, tremor,* lethargy, somnolence, *stupor, restlessness,* anxiety, hallucinations, nervousness, *light-headedness,* paresthesia, muscle twitching, *seizures*.

**CV:** *hypotension,* bradycardia, *new or worsened arrhythmias, cardiac arrest.*

**EENT:** *tinnitus, blurred or double vision.*

**Other:** *anaphylaxis,* soreness at injection site, sensation of cold.

## INTERACTIONS

*Beta blockers, cimetidine:* decreased metabolism of lidocaine. Monitor for toxicity.

*Phenytoin, procainamide, propranolol, quinidine:* additive cardiac depressant effects. Monitor carefully.

## CONTRAINDICATIONS

Contraindicated in patients with hypersensitivity to the amide-type local anesthetics; Adams-Stokes syndrome; Wolff-Parkinson-White syndrome; and severe degrees of SA, AV, or intraventricular block in absence of artificial pacemaker.

## NURSING CONSIDERATIONS

• Use cautiously in patients with complete or second-degree heart block or sinus bradycardia, in elderly patients, in those with CHF or renal or hepatic disease, and in those who weigh under 50 kg. Reduced dosage in these patients is required.

• **I.V. use:** Patients receiving infusions must be on a cardiac monitor and must be attended *at all times.* Use an infusion control device for administering infusion precisely. Do not exceed rate of 4 mg/minute; faster rate greatly increases risk of toxicity.

• Give I.M. injections in the deltoid muscle only.

• Remind the doctor to monitor isoenzymes when he prescribes I.M. drug for a patient with suspected MI. A patient who has received I.M. lidocaine will show a seven-fold increase in serum CK level. Such an increase originates in the skeletal muscle, not the heart.

• Monitor serum levels as ordered. Therapeutic levels are 2 to 5 mcg/ml.

• *Alert:* Monitor patient for toxicity. In many severely ill patients, seizures

---

may be the first clinical sign of toxicity. However, severe reactions usually are preceded by somnolence, confusion, and paresthesia.
• If signs of toxicity (such as dizziness) occur, stop drug at once and notify the doctor. Continued infusion could lead to seizures and coma. Give oxygen via nasal cannula if not contraindicated. Keep oxygen and cardiopulmonary resuscitation equipment available.
• Monitor the patient's response, especially blood pressure and serum electrolytes, BUN, and creatinine levels, as ordered. Notify the doctor promptly if abnormalities develop.
• Discontinue infusion and notify the doctor if arrhythmias worsen or ECG changes, such as widening QRS complex or substantially prolonged PR interval, are evident.

### ☑ PATIENT TEACHING
• Inform patient receiving drug I.M. that drug may cause soreness at injection site. Instruct patient receiving drug I.V. to alert nurse if discomfort occurs at the insertion site.
• Tell patient to report adverse reactions promptly as toxicity can occur.

---

## mexiletine hydrochloride
Mexitil

*Pregnancy Risk Category: C*

### HOW SUPPLIED
*Capsules:* 50 mg‡, 100 mg†, 150 mg, 200 mg, 250 mg
*Injection:* 250 mg/10 ml‡

### ACTION
A class Ib antiarrhythmic that blocks the fast sodium channel in cardiac tissues, especially the Purkinje network, without involving the autonomic nervous system. Reduces the rate of rise and amplitude of the action potential and decreases automaticity in the Purkinje fibers. Shortens the duration of the action potential and, to a lesser extent, decreases the effective refractory period in the Purkinje fibers.

### ONSET, PEAK, DURATION
Onset occurs ½ to 2 hours after oral administration, immediately after I.V. administration. Serum levels peak 2 to 3 hours after oral administration, immediately after I.V. administration. Duration unknown.

### INDICATIONS & DOSAGE
*Refractory life-threatening ventricular arrhythmias, including ventricular tachycardia and PVCs –*
**Adults:** 200 to 400 mg P.O. followed by 200 mg q 8 hours. Dose increased every 2 to 3 days to 400 mg q 8 hours if satisfactory control is not obtained. Patients who respond well to an every-12-hour schedule may be given up to 450 mg q 12 hours.
    Where available, mexiletine may be given I.V.‡ –
**Adults:** loading dose is 100 to 250 mg I.V. at a rate of 25 mg/minute. Then prepare an infusion solution of 250 mg mexiletine in 500 ml of D₅W, and administer the first 120 ml (60 mg) over 1 hour. If clinical response is inadequate, give another bolus of 200 mg over 10 to 20 minutes. Maintenance dosage is 0.5 mg/minute (1 ml/minute of prepared solution).

### ADVERSE REACTIONS
**CNS:** *tremor, dizziness,* blurred vision, diplopia, confusion, *light-headedness, incoordination,* changes in sleep habits, paresthesia, weakness, fatigue, speech difficulties, tinnitus, depression, *nervousness,* headache.
**CV:** *new or worsened arrhythmias,* palpitations, chest pain, nonspecific edema, angina.
**GI:** *nausea, vomiting, upper GI distress, heartburn,* diarrhea, constipation, dry mouth, changes in appetite, abdominal pain.
**Skin:** rash.

---

## INTERACTIONS

*Antacids, atropine, narcotics:* slowed mexilitine absorption. Monitor patient.
*Cimetidine:* increased or decreased mexiletine blood levels. Monitor carefully.
*Methylxanthines, such as caffeine or theophylline:* reduced clearance of methylxanthines, possibly resulting in toxicity. Monitor carefully.
*Metoclopramide:* mexiletine absorption may be accelerated. Monitor for toxicity.
*Phenobarbital, phenytoin, rifampin, urine acidifiers:* decreased mexiletine blood levels. Monitor carefully.
*Urine alkalinizers:* increased mexiletine blood levels. Monitor carefully.

## CONTRAINDICATIONS

Contraindicated in patients with cardiogenic shock or preexisting second- or third-degree AV block in the absence of an artificial pacemaker.

## NURSING CONSIDERATIONS

• Use cautiously in patients with preexisting first-degree heart block, a ventricular pacemaker, preexisting sinus node dysfunction, intraventricular conduction disturbances, hypotension, severe CHF, or seizure disorder.
• When changing from lidocaine to mexiletine, stop the lidocaine infusion when the first mexiletine dose is given. Keep the infusion line open, however, until the arrhythmia appears to be satisfactorily controlled.
• **I.V. use:** Mexiletine injection is compatible with 0.9% sodium chloride, $D_5W$, 5% sodium bicarbonate, 1/6 M sodium lactate, and 10% fructose (levulose) solutions.
• To lessen GI distress, administer oral dose with meals or antacids.
• If you feel the patient is a good candidate for every-12-hour therapy, notify the doctor. Twice-daily dosage enhances compliance.
• Monitor therapeutic levels, as ordered. Therapeutic levels range from 0.5 to 2 mcg/ml.
• Monitor patient for toxicity. An early sign of mexiletine toxicity is tremor, usually a fine tremor of the hands. This progresses to dizziness and later to ataxia and nystagmus as the drug's blood level increases. Question patients about these symptoms.
• Monitor blood pressure and heart rate and rhythm frequently. Notify the doctor of any significant change.

## ☑ PATIENT TEACHING

• Tell patient to take drug exactly as prescribed and to take with food or antacids if GI reactions occur.
• Instruct patient to report adverse reactions promptly, especially fine hand tremor.
• Tell patient receiving drug I.V. to report discomfort at the insertion site.

# moricizine hydrochloride
Ethmozine

*Pregnancy Risk Category: B*

## HOW SUPPLIED
*Tablets:* 200 mg, 250 mg, 300 mg

## ACTION
A class I antiarrhythmic that reduces the fast inward current carried by sodium ions across myocardial cell membranes. Has potent local anesthetic activity and membrane-stabilizing effect.

## ONSET, PEAK, DURATION
Onset occurs in 2 hours. Serum levels peak in ½ to 2 hours; effects peak in 10 to 14 hours. Effects persist 10 to 24 hours after last dose.

## INDICATIONS & DOSAGE
*Life-threatening ventricular arrhythmias—*
**Adults:** individualized dosage is based on clinical response and patient tolerance. Therapy should begin in

the hospital. Most patients respond to 600 to 900 mg P.O. daily in divided doses q 8 hours. Daily dosage increased q 3 days by 150 mg until the desired clinical effect is seen.

In patients with hepatic or renal impairment, 600 mg or less P.O. daily.

## ADVERSE REACTIONS

**CNS:** *dizziness, headache, fatigue,* hyperesthesias, anxiety, asthenia, nervousness, paresthesia, sleep disorders.
**CV:** *proarrhythmic events (ventricular tachycardia, PVCs, supraventricular arrhythmias), ECG abnormalities (including conduction defects, sinus pause, junctional rhythm, or AV block), CHF,* palpitations, *chest pain, cardiac death,* hypotension, hypertension, vasodilation, cerebrovascular events.
**EENT:** blurred vision.
**GI:** *nausea, vomiting, abdominal pain, dyspepsia, diarrhea, dry mouth.*
**GU:** urine retention, urinary frequency, dysuria.
**Respiratory:** dyspnea.
**Skin:** rash.
**Other:** drug-induced fever, diaphoresis, musculoskeletal pain, thrombophlebitis.

## INTERACTIONS

*Cimetidine:* increased plasma levels and decreased clearance of moricizine. Begin moricizine therapy at low dosage (not more than 600 mg daily), and monitor plasma levels and therapeutic effect closely.
*Digoxin, propranolol:* additive prolongation of PR interval. Monitor closely.
*Theophylline:* increased clearance and reduced plasma levels of theophylline. Monitor plasma levels and therapeutic response; adjust theophylline dosage as needed.

## CONTRAINDICATIONS

Contraindicated in patients with hypersensitivity to the drug; preexisting second- or third-degree AV block or right bundle branch block when associated with left hemiblock (bifascicular block) unless an artificial pacemaker is present; and cardiogenic shock.

## NURSING CONSIDERATIONS

• Know that because drug has been detected in breast milk, a decision should be made to discontinue breast-feeding or discontinue the drug, depending on drug's potential benefit to the mother.
• Use with extreme caution in patients with sick sinus syndrome because drug may cause sinus bradycardia or sinus arrest. Also use with extreme caution in patients with coronary artery disease and left ventricular dysfunction because these patients may be at risk for sudden death when treated with the drug.
• Administer cautiously to patients with liver impairment.
• Patients with hepatic or renal dysfunction will have decreased moricizine clearance. Administer cautiously and monitor effects closely.
• Know that when substituting moricizine for another antiarrhythmic, previous drug should be withdrawn for one to two of the drug's half-lives before moricizine is started. Patients who have shown a tendency to develop life-threatening arrhythmias after withdrawal of previous antiarrhythmic drug therapy should be hospitalized during withdrawal and adjustment to moricizine. Guidelines doctors use for when to start moricizine therapy are as follows:
—disopyramide, 6 to 12 hours after the last dose.
—flecainide, 12 to 24 hours after last dose.
—mexiletine, 8 to 12 hours after the last dose.
—procainamide, 3 to 6 hours after the last dose.
—propafenone, 8 to 12 hours after the last dose.

---

—quinidine, 6 to 12 hours after the last dose.

—tocainide, 8 to 12 hours after the last dose.

• Determine electrolyte status and correct imbalances before therapy as ordered. Hypokalemia, hyperkalemia, and hypomagnesemia may alter the effects of the drug.

## ☑ PATIENT TEACHING
• Instruct patient to take drug exactly as prescribed.
• Tell patient to avoid hazardous activities if adverse CNS reactions or blurred vision occurs.
• Instruct patient to report persistent or serious adverse reactions promptly.

---

## procainamide hydrochloride
Procainamide Durules‡, Procan SR, Promine, Pronestyl**, Pronestyl-SR

*Pregnancy Risk Category: C*

### HOW SUPPLIED
*Tablets:* 250 mg, 375 mg, 500 mg
*Tablets (sustained-release):* 250 mg, 500 mg, 750 mg, 1,000 mg
*Capsules:* 250 mg, 375 mg, 500 mg
*Injection:* 100 mg/ml, 500 mg/ml

### ACTION
A class Ia antiarrhythmic that decreases excitability, conduction velocity, automaticity, and membrane responsiveness with prolonged refractory period. Larger than usual doses may induce AV block.

### ONSET, PEAK, DURATION
Onset occurs immediately with I.V. injection, 10 to 30 minutes after I.M. injection, and 2 hours after oral dose. Peak serum levels occur immediately after I.V. infusion, 15 to 60 minutes after I.M. injection, and 1 to 1½ hours after oral dose. Duration unknown.

### INDICATIONS & DOSAGE
*Life-threatening ventricular arrhythmias—*

**Adults:** 100 mg by slow I.V. push q 5 minutes, no faster than 25 to 50 mg/minute until arrhythmias disappear, adverse reactions develop, or 1 g has been given. Usual effective dose is 500 to 600 mg. When arrhythmias disappear, give continuous infusion of 2 to 6 mg/minute. If arrhythmias recur, repeat bolus as above and increase infusion rate. Alternatively, give 0.5 to 1 g I.M. q 4 to 8 hours until oral therapy begins.

For oral therapy, give 50 mg/kg daily in divided doses q 3 hours (average is 250 to 500 mg q 3 hours); for sustained-release tablets, give 50 mg/kg daily in divided doses q 6 hours.

In patients with renal or hepatic dysfunction, decreased dosages or longer dosing intervals may be needed.

### ADVERSE REACTIONS
**CNS:** hallucinations, confusion, *seizures,* depression, dizziness.
**CV:** *hypotension, bradycardia,* AV block, *ventricular fibrillation* (after parenteral use), *ventricular asystole.*
**GI:** nausea, vomiting, anorexia, diarrhea, bitter taste.
**Hematologic:** *thrombocytopenia, neutropenia* (especially with sustained-release forms), *agranulocytosis, hemolytic anemia.*
**Skin:** *maculopapular rash, urticaria, pruritus, flushing, angioneurotic edema.*
**Other:** *fever, lupuslike syndrome* (especially after prolonged administration).

### INTERACTIONS
*Amiodarone:* increased procainamide levels and toxicity; additive effects on QT interval and QRS complex. Avoid concomitant use.
*Anticholinergics:* additive anticholinergic effects. Monitor closely.
*Anticholinesterase agents:* May decrease effect of anticholinesterase

---

agents. Anticholinesterase dosage may need to be increased.
*Cimetidine:* may increase procainamide blood levels. Monitor for toxicity.
*Neuromuscular blockers:* increased skeletal muscle relaxant effects. Monitor the patient closely.

## CONTRAINDICATIONS
Contraindicated in patients with hypersensitivity to procaine and related drugs; in those with complete, second-, or third-degree heart block in the absence of an artificial pacemaker; and in patients with myasthenia gravis or systemic lupus erythematosus. Also contraindicated in patients with atypical ventricular tachycardia (torsades de pointes) because procainamide may aggravate this condition.

## NURSING CONSIDERATIONS
• Use with extreme caution when treating patients with ventricular tachycardia during coronary occlusion.
• Use cautiously in patients with CHF or other conduction disturbances, such as bundle-branch heart block, sinus bradycardia, or digitalis glycoside intoxication, or with hepatic or renal insufficiency. Also use cautiously in those with preexisting blood dyscrasias or bone marrow suppression.
• **I.V. use:** Patients receiving infusions must be attended *at all times.* Use an infusion control device to administer the infusion precisely.
• Note that the vials for I.V. injection contain 1 g of drug: 100 mg/ml (10 ml) or 500 mg/ml (2 ml).
• Keep patients in the supine position during I.V. administration. If drug is given too rapidly, hypotension can occur. Watch closely for adverse reactions during infusion, and notify the doctor if they occur.
• If procainamide solution becomes discolored, check with pharmacy and expect to discard.
• *Alert:* Monitor blood pressure and

ECG continuously during I.V. administration. Watch for prolonged QT intervals and QRS complexes, heart block, or increased arrhythmias. If these occur, withhold drug, obtain rhythm strip, and notify the doctor immediately.
• Monitor plasma levels of procainamide and its active metabolite NAPA. To suppress ventricular arrhythmias, therapeutic serum concentrations of procainamide are 4 to 8 mcg/ml; therapeutic levels of NAPA are 10 to 30 mcg/ml.
• Monitor QT interval closely in patients with renal failure.
• Hypokalemia predisposes patients to arrhythmias; therefore, monitor serum electrolytes, especially potassium level.
• Elderly patients may be more likely to develop hypotension. Monitor blood pressure carefully.
• Monitor CBC frequently during first 3 months of therapy, particularly in patients taking sustained-release forms.
• Be aware that positive ANA titer is common in about 60% of patients who don't have symptoms of lupuslike syndrome. This response seems to be related to prolonged use, not dosage. May progress to systemic lupus erythematosus if drug is not discontinued.

## ☑ PATIENT TEACHING
• Stress to the patient the importance of taking the drug exactly as prescribed. This may require use of an alarm clock for nighttime doses.
• Instruct the patient to report fever, rash, muscle pain, diarrhea, bleeding, bruises, or pleuritic chest pain.
• Reassure the patient who is taking the extended-release form that a wax-matrix "ghost" from the tablet may be passed in stools. The drug is completely absorbed before this occurs.

# propafenone hydrochloride
Rythmol

*Pregnancy Risk Category: C*

## HOW SUPPLIED
*Tablets:* 150 mg, 300 mg

## ACTION
A class Ic antiarrhythmic that reduces inward sodium current in Purkinje and myocardial cells. Decreases excitability, conduction velocity, and automaticity in AV nodal, His-Purkinje, and intraventricular tissue; causes slight but significant prolongation of refractory period in AV nodal tissue.

## ONSET, PEAK, DURATION
Onset and duration unknown. Plasma levels peak within 3½ hours.

## INDICATIONS & DOSAGE
*Suppression of life-threatening ventricular arrhythmias, such as sustained ventricular tachycardia –*
**Adults:** initially, 150 mg P.O. q 8 hours. Dosage may be increased at 3- to 4-day intervals to 225 mg q 8 hours, if necessary, increase dosage to 300 mg q 8 hours. Maximum daily dosage is 900 mg.

## ADVERSE REACTIONS
**CNS:** anxiety, ataxia, *dizziness,* drowsiness, fatigue, headache, insomnia, syncope, tremor.
**CV:** atrial fibrillation, bradycardia, bundle branch block, *CHF,* angina, chest pain, edema, first-degree AV block, hypotension, increased QRS duration, intraventricular conduction delay, palpitations, *proarrhythmic events (ventricular tachycardia, PVCs, ventricular fibrillation).*
**EENT:** blurred vision.
**GI:** abdominal pain or cramps, constipation, diarrhea, dyspepsia, anorexia, flatulence, *nausea, vomiting,* dry mouth, unusual taste.
**Respiratory:** dyspnea.

**Skin:** rash.
**Other:** diaphoresis, joint pain.

## INTERACTIONS
*Antiarrhythmics:* increased risk of CHF. Monitor closely.
*Cimetidine:* decreased metabolism of propafenone. Monitor closely.
*Digitalis glycosides, oral anticoagulants:* propafenone may increase serum levels of these agents by about 35% to 85%, resulting in toxicity. Monitor closely.
*Local anesthetics:* increased risk of CNS toxicity. Monitor closely.
*Metoprolol, propranolol:* propafenone slows the metabolism of these agents. Adjust dosage as ordered.
*Quinidine:* slowed metabolism of propafenone. Avoid concomitant use.
*Rifampin:* increased clearance of propafenone. Monitor closely.

## CONTRAINDICATIONS
Contraindicated in patients with hypersensitivity to the drug and in those with severe or uncontrolled CHF; cardiogenic shock; SA, AV, or intraventricular disorders of impulse conduction in the absence of a pacemaker; bradycardia; marked hypotension; bronchospastic disorders; and electrolyte imbalance.

## NURSING CONSIDERATIONS
• Use cautiously in patients with CHF because propafenone can exert a negative inotropic effect on the heart. Also use cautiously in patients taking other cardiac depressant drugs and in those with hepatic or renal failure.
• To minimize adverse GI reactions, administer drug with food.
• Continuous cardiac monitoring is recommended during initiation of therapy and during dosage adjustments. If PR interval or QRS complex increases by more than 25%, a reduction in dosage may be necessary.
• During concomitant use with di-

---

Reactions may be *common,* uncommon, *life-threatening,* or **COMMON AND LIFE-THREATENING.**

goxin, frequently monitor ECG and serum digoxin levels.

☑ **PATIENT TEACHING**
• Stress importance of taking drug exactly as prescribed.
• Tell patient to report adverse reactions promptly.

---

## quinidine bisulfate
(66.4% quinidine base)
Biquin Durules†, Kinidin Durules‡

## quinidine gluconate
(62% quinidine base)
Quinaglute Dura-Tabs, Quinalan, Quinate†

## quinidine polygalacturonate
(60.5% quinidine base)
Cardioquin

## quinidine sulfate
(83% quinidine base)
Apo-Quinidine†, Cin-Quin, Novoquinidin†, Quinidex Extentabs, Quinora

*Pregnancy Risk Category: C*

## HOW SUPPLIED
**quinidine bisulfate**
*Tablets (extended-release):* 250 mg†‡
**quinidine gluconate**
*Tablets (extended-release):* 324 mg, 325 mg†, 330 mg
*Injection:* 80 mg/ml
**quinidine polygalacturonate**
*Tablets:* 275 mg
**quinidine sulfate**
*Tablets:* 200 mg, 300 mg
*Tablets (extended-release):* 300 mg
*Capsules:* 200 mg, 300 mg
*Injection:* 200 mg/ml†

## ACTION
A class Ia antiarrhythmic, quinidine has both direct and indirect (anticholinergic) effects on cardiac tissue. Automaticity, conduction velocity, and membrane responsiveness are decreased. The effective refractory period is prolonged. The anticholinergic action reduces vagal tone.

## ONSET, PEAK, DURATION
Onset is immediate after I.V. administration and 1 to 3 hours after oral administration. Peak plasma levels occur immediately after I.V. injection, 1 to 2 hours after oral dose. Effects persist 6 to 8 hours after oral dose.

## INDICATIONS & DOSAGE
*Atrial flutter or fibrillation –*
**Adults:** 200 mg quinidine sulfate or equivalent base P.O. q 2 to 3 hours for five to eight doses, with subsequent daily increases until sinus rhythm is restored or toxic effects develop. Quinidine is administered only after digitalization to avoid increasing AV conduction. Maximum dosage is 3 to 4 g daily.
*Paroxysmal supraventricular tachycardia –*
**Adults:** 400 to 600 mg I.M. or P.O. gluconate q 2 to 3 hours until toxic adverse reactions develop or arrhythmia subsides.
*Premature atrial and ventricular contractions; paroxysmal AV junctional rhythm; paroxysmal atrial tachycardia; paroxysmal ventricular tachycardia; maintenance after cardioversion of atrial fibrillation or flutter –*
**Adults:** test dose is 200 mg P.O. or I.M. Quinidine sulfate or equivalent base 200 to 400 mg P.O. q 4 to 6 hours; or initially, quinidine gluconate 600 mg I.M., then up to 400 mg q 2 hours, p.r.n.; or quinidine gluconate 800 mg (10 ml of the commercially available solution) added to 40 ml of $D_5W$, infused I.V. at 16 mg (1 ml)/minute.
**Children:** test dose is 2 mg/kg; 3 to 6 mg/kg q 2 to 3 hours for five doses P.O. daily.
*Severe Plasmodium falciparum malaria –*

---

**Adults:** 10 mg/kg gluconate I.V. diluted in 250 ml of 0.9% sodium chloride solution and infused over 1 to 2 hours, followed by a continuous maintenance infusion of 0.02 mg/kg/minute for 72 hours or until parasitemia is reduced to less than 1%.

Patients with impaired hepatic function and those with CHF require a reduced dosage.

## ADVERSE REACTIONS
**CNS:** *vertigo, headache, light-headedness,* confusion, ataxia, depression, dementia.
**CV:** *PVCs; ventricular tachycardia; atypical ventricular tachycardia (torsades de pointes); hypotension; complete AV block,* tachycardia; *aggravated CHF; ECG changes (particularly widening of QRS complex, widened QT and PR intervals).*
**EENT:** *tinnitus,* excessive salivation, blurred vision, diplopia, photophobia.
**GI:** *diarrhea, nausea, vomiting,* anorexia, abdominal pain.
**Hematologic:** *hemolytic anemia, thrombocytopenia, agranulocytosis.*
**Hepatic:** *hepatotoxicity.*
**Respiratory:** acute asthmatic attack, *respiratory arrest.*
**Skin:** rash, petechial hemorrhage of buccal mucosa, pruritus, urticaria, lupus erythematosus, photosensitivity.
**Other:** angioedema, *fever, cinchonism.*

## INTERACTIONS
*Acetazolamide, antacids, sodium bicarbonate, thiazide diuretics:* may increase quinidine blood levels because of alkaline urine. Monitor for increased effect.
*Amiodarone, cimetidine:* increased serum quinidine levels. Monitor for increased effect.
*Barbiturates, phenytoin, rifampin:* may lower blood levels of quinidine. Monitor for decreased effect.
*Digoxin:* increased serum digoxin levels after initiating quinidine therapy. Monitor closely.

*Nifedipine:* may decrease quinidine blood levels. Monitor carefully.
*Other antiarrhythmics, such as lidocaine, phenytoin, procainamide, and propranolol:* increased risk of toxicity. Use together cautiously.
*Verapamil:* may result in hypotension, bradycardia, or AV block. Monitor blood pressure and heart rate.
*Warfarin:* increased anticoagulant effect. Monitor closely.

## CONTRAINDICATIONS
Contraindicated in patients with idiosyncrasy or hypersensitivity to quinidine or related cinchona derivatives, intraventricular conduction defects, digitalis toxicity when AV conduction is grossly impaired, and abnormal rhythms due to escape mechanisms.

## NURSING CONSIDERATIONS
• Use cautiously in patients with asthma, muscle weakness, or infection accompanied by fever because hypersensitivity reactions to the drug may be masked.
• Also use cautiously in patients with hepatic or renal impairment because systemic accumulation of quinidine may occur.
• Check apical pulse rate and blood pressure before therapy. If you detect extremes in pulse rate, withhold drug and notify the doctor at once.
• Know that anticoagulant therapy is commonly advised before quinidine therapy in long-standing atrial fibrillation because restoration of normal sinus rhythm may result in thromboembolism caused by dislodgment of thrombi from atrial wall.
• When changing route of administration, be aware that dosage needs to be altered to compensate for variations in quinidine base content.
• Never use discolored (brownish) quinidine solution.
• Do not crush sustained-release tablets.
• *Alert:* When used to treat severe

---

Reactions may be *common,* uncommon, *life-threatening,* or COMMON AND LIFE-THREATENING.

malaria, patients should be hospitalized in an intensive-care setting. Continuous monitoring is necessary. Decrease infusion rate if plasma quinidine level exceeds 6 mcg/ml, uncorrected QT interval exceeds 0.6 second, or QRS complex widening exceeds 25% of baseline.
• Monitor liver function tests during the first 4 to 8 weeks of therapy.
• Monitor serum quinidine levels as ordered. Therapeutic plasma levels for antiarrhythmic effects are 2 to 5 mcg/ml.
• Monitor patient response carefully. Adverse GI reactions, especially diarrhea, are signs of toxicity. Notify the doctor. Check quinidine blood levels, which are toxic when greater than 8 mcg/ml. GI symptoms may be decreased by giving drug with meals.
• Store drug away from heat and direct light.

☑ **PATIENT TEACHING**
• Stress importance of taking drug exactly as prescribed and to take it with food if adverse GI reactions occur.
• Tell patient to report persistent or serious adverse reactions promptly, especially signs and symptoms of quinidine toxicity.

## sotalol
Betapace, Sotacor†‡
*Pregnancy Risk Category: B*

**HOW SUPPLIED**
*Tablets:* 80 mg, 160 mg, 240 mg

**ACTION**
A nonselective beta-adrenergic blocker that depresses sinus heart rate, slows AV conduction, decreases cardiac output, and lowers systolic and diastolic blood pressure.

**ONSET, PEAK, DURATION**
Onset and duration not clearly defined. Peak plasma levels occur within 2½ to 4 hours.

**INDICATIONS & DOSAGE**
*Documented, life-threatening ventricular arrhythmias –*
**Adults:** initially, 80 mg P.O. b.i.d. Dosage is increased q 2 to 3 days as needed and tolerated; most patients respond to daily dosage of 160 to 320 mg. A few patients with refractory arrhythmias have received as much as 640 mg daily.
In patients with renal failure: If creatinine clearance is greater than 60 ml/minute, no adjustment in dosage interval is necessary. If creatinine clearance is 30 to 60 ml/minute, dosage interval is increased to q 24 hours; 10 to 30 ml/minute, q 36 to 48 hours; less than 10 ml/minute, dosage must be individualized.
*Hypertension –*
**Adults:** 80 mg P.O. b.i.d. Dosage is increased at weekly intervals in 80-mg increments b.i.d. as needed and tolerated. Most patients respond to daily dosage of 160 to 320 mg; patients taking 320 mg or less daily may take drug as a single morning dose.
*Angina –*
**Adults:** 80 mg P.O. b.i.d. Dosage is increased at weekly intervals in 80-mg increments b.i.d. as needed and tolerated. Most patients respond to doses of 160 mg b.i.d.; maximum daily dosage is 480 mg.

**ADVERSE REACTIONS**
**CNS:** *asthenia, headache, dizziness, weakness, fatigue,* sleep problems, *light-headedness.*
**CV:** *bradycardia, arrhythmias, CHF, AV block, proarrhythmic events (ventricular tachycardia, PVCs, ventricular fibrillation),* edema, *palpitations, chest pain,* ECG abnormalities, hypotension.
**GI:** *nausea, vomiting,* diarrhea, dyspepsia.
**Respiratory:** *dyspnea, bronchospasm.*

---

## INTERACTIONS

*Antiarrhythmics:* additive effects. Avoid concomitant use.

*Antihypertensives, catecholamine-depleting drugs (such as reserpine and guanethidine):* enhanced hypotensive effects. Monitor closely.

*Calcium channel blockers:* enhanced myocardial depression. Avoid concomitant use.

*Clonidine:* beta blockers may enhance rebound effect after withdrawal of clonidine. Discontinue sotalol several days before withdrawing clonidine.

*General anesthetics:* may cause additional myocardial depression. Monitor closely.

## CONTRAINDICATIONS

Contraindicated in patients with hypersensitivity to the drug, severe sinus node dysfunction, sinus bradycardia, second- and third-degree AV block in the absence of an artificial pacemaker, congenital or acquired long QT syndrome, cardiogenic shock, uncontrolled CHF, and bronchial asthma.

## NURSING CONSIDERATIONS

● Use cautiously in patients with renal impairment or diabetes mellitus. Beta blockers may mask signs and symptoms of hypoglycemia.

● Because proarrhythmic events may occur at start of therapy and during dosage adjustments, patient should be hospitalized. Facilities and personnel should be available for cardiac rhythm monitoring and interpretation of ECG.

● Note that although patients receiving I.V. lidocaine have started sotalol therapy without ill effect, other antiarrhythmic drugs should be withdrawn before therapy with sotalol. Sotalol therapy typically is delayed until two or three half-lives of the withdrawn drug have elapsed. After withdrawal of amiodarone, sotalol shouldn't be administered until the QT interval normalizes.

● Be aware that dosage should be adjusted slowly, allowing 2 to 3 days between dosage increments for adequate monitoring of QT intervals and for plasma levels of drug to reach a steady-state level.

● Monitor serum electrolytes regularly, especially if patient is receiving diuretics. Electrolyte imbalances, such as hypokalemia or hypomagnesemia, may enhance QT-interval prolongation and increase the risk of serious arrhythmias, such as torsades de pointes.

## ☑ PATIENT TEACHING

● Explain to the patient the importance of taking this drug as prescribed, even when he is feeling well. Caution him not to discontinue drug suddenly.

● Because food can interfere with absorption, tell the patient to take this drug on an empty stomach, 1 hour before or 2 hours after meals.

---

## tocainide hydrochloride
Tonocard

*Pregnancy Risk Category: C*

## HOW SUPPLIED
*Tablets:* 400 mg, 600 mg

## ACTION
A class Ib antiarrhythmic that blocks the fast sodium channel in cardiac tissues, especially the Purkinje network, without involvement of the autonomic nervous system. It reduces the rate of rise and amplitude of the action potential and decreases automaticity in the Purkinje fibers. It shortens the duration of action potential and, to a lesser extent, decreases the effective refractory period in the Purkinje fibers.

## ONSET, PEAK, DURATION
Onset unknown. Plasma levels peak ½ to 2 hours after an oral dose. Duration is 8 hours.

## INDICATIONS & DOSAGE
*Suppression of symptomatic life-threatening ventricular arrhythmias, such as sustained ventricular tachycardia –*
**Adults:** initially, 400 mg P.O. q 8 hours. Usual dosage is between 1,200 and 1,800 mg daily in three divided doses.

## ADVERSE REACTIONS
**CNS:** *light-headedness, tremor,* paresthesia, *dizziness, vertigo,* drowsiness, fatigue, confusion, headache.
**CV:** hypotension, *new or worsened arrhythmias, CHF,* bradycardia, palpitations.
**EENT:** blurred vision, tinnitus.
**GI:** *nausea, vomiting,* diarrhea, anorexia.
**Hematologic:** *blood dyscrasias.*
**Hepatic:** hepatitis.
**Respiratory:** *respiratory arrest, pulmonary fibrosis, pneumonitis, pulmonary edema.*
**Skin:** rash, diaphoresis.

## INTERACTIONS
*Beta blockers:* decreased myocardial contractility; increased CNS toxicity. Monitor closely.
*Cimetidine:* may decrease tocainide peak concentration. Monitor closely.
*Rifampin:* increased clearance of tocainide. Monitor efficacy of tocainide.

## CONTRAINDICATIONS
Contraindicated in patients with hypersensitivity to lidocaine or other amide-type local anesthetics and in those with second- or third-degree AV block in the absence of an artificial pacemaker.

## NURSING CONSIDERATIONS
• Use cautiously in patients with CHF or diminished cardiac reserve and in those with hepatic or renal impairment. These patients often may be treated effectively with a lower dose.
• Be aware that drug is considered by cardiologists as "oral lidocaine." May ease transition from I.V. lidocaine to oral antiarrhythmic. Monitor the patient carefully during this transition.
• Correct potassium deficits, if present and as ordered; drug may be ineffective when hypokalemia is present.
• Monitor the patient for tremor, which may indicate that the maximum dosage has been reached.
• Monitor blood levels as ordered. Therapeutic levels range from 4 to 10 mcg/ml. Report deviations.

## ☑ PATIENT TEACHING
• Tell the patient to report immediately any unusual bruising or bleeding or signs of infection. Agranulocytosis and bone marrow suppression have been reported in patients taking usual doses of the drug, typically within the first 12 weeks of therapy.
• Tell the patient to report sudden onset of any pulmonary symptoms, such as coughing, wheezing, or exertional dyspnea. Drug has been associated with serious pulmonary toxicity.
• Tell the patient to take safety precautions, especially if he is elderly because dizziness and falling are more likely to occur in such patients.

amlodipine besylate
amyl nitrate
bepridil hydrochloride
diltiazem hydrochloride
erythrityl tetranitrate
isosorbide dinitrate
isosorbide mononitrate
nadolol
nicardipine
nifedipine
nitroglycerin
pentaerythritol tetranitrate
propranolol hydrochloride
verapamil
verapamil hydrochloride

## COMBINATION PRODUCTS

ANGIJEN NO. 1: pentaerythritol tetranitrate 20 mg and phenobarbital sodium 15 mg.
ARCOTRATE NO. 3: pentaerythritol tetranitrate 20 mg and phenobarbital sodium 8 mg.
BITRATE: pentaerythritol tetranitrate 15 mg and phenobarbital sodium 20 mg.
DIMYCOR: pentaerythritol tetranitrate 10 mg and phenobarbital sodium 15 mg.
NITROTYM-PLUS: nitroglycerin 2.5 mg and butabarbital sodium 48 mg.
PERBUZEM: pentaerythritol tetranitrate 10 mg and butabarbital sodium 15 mg.

---

## amlodipine besylate
Norvasc

*Pregnancy Risk Category: C*

### HOW SUPPLIED
*Tablets:* 2.5 mg, 5 mg, 10 mg

### ACTION
Inhibits calcium ion influx across cardiac and smooth-muscle cells, thus decreasing myocardial contractility and oxygen demand. Also dilates coronary arteries and arterioles.

### ONSET, PEAK, DURATION
Onset unknown. Serum levels peak in 6 to 9 hours. Effects persist for 24 hours.

### INDICATIONS & DOSAGE
*Chronic stable angina; vasospastic angina (Prinzmetal's [variant] angina)* –
**Adults:** initially, 5 to 10 mg P.O. daily. Small, frail, or elderly patients or patients with hepatic insufficiency should begin therapy at 5 mg daily. Most patients require 10 mg daily.
*Hypertension* –
**Adults:** initially, 5 mg P.O. daily. Small, frail, or elderly patients; patients currently receiving other antihypertensives; or patients with hepatic insufficiency should begin therapy at 2.5 mg daily. Dosage adjusted according to patient response and tolerance. Maximum daily dosage is 10 mg.

### ADVERSE REACTIONS
**CNS:** *headache,* somnolence, fatigue, dizziness, light-headedness, paresthesia.
**CV:** *edema,* flushing, palpitations.
**GI:** nausea, abdominal pain.
**Other:** dyspnea, muscle pain, rash, pruritus.

### INTERACTIONS
None significant.

### CONTRAINDICATIONS
Contraindicated in patients with hypersensitivity to the drug.

### NURSING CONSIDERATIONS
• Use cautiously in patients receiving other peripheral vasodilators, especially those with severe aortic stenosis, and in those with CHF. Because drug is

---

Reactions may be *common,* uncommon, *life-threatening,* or COMMON AND LIFE-THREATENING.

metabolized by the liver, use cautiously and in reduced dosage in patients with severe hepatic disease.

• **Alert:** Monitor the patient carefully. Some patients, especially those with severe obstructive coronary artery disease, have developed increased frequency, duration, or severity of angina or even acute MI after initiation of calcium channel blocker therapy or at time of dosage increase.

• Monitor blood pressure frequently during initiation of therapy. Because drug-induced vasodilation has a gradual onset, acute hypotension is rare.

• Notify the doctor if signs of CHF occur, such as swelling of hands and feet or shortness of breath.

☑ **PATIENT TEACHING**
• Caution patient to continue taking the drug, even when feeling better.
• Tell patient sublingual nitroglycerin may be taken as needed when anginal symptoms are acute. If the patient continues nitrate therapy during titration of amlodipine dosage, urge continued compliance.

---

## amyl nitrite

*Pregnancy Risk Category: X*

### HOW SUPPLIED
*Ampules (crushable):* 0.18 ml, 0.3 ml

### ACTION
Antianginal action unknown. Thought to be the result of a reduction in systemic and pulmonary arterial pressure (afterload) and decreased cardiac output caused by peripheral vasodilation, rather than by coronary artery dilation. Converts hemoglobin to methemoglobin (which binds cyanide) to treat cyanide poisoning.

### ONSET, PEAK, DURATION
Onset occurs in 30 seconds. Peak unknown. Effects persist 3 to 5 minutes.

### INDICATIONS & DOSAGE
*Relief of angina pectoris –*
**Adults and children:** 0.18 to 0.3 ml by inhalation (one glass ampule) p.r.n.
*Antidote for cyanide poisoning –*
0.3 ml by inhalation for 30 to 60 seconds q 5 minutes until conscious.

### ADVERSE REACTIONS
**CNS:** *headache, sometimes with throbbing;* dizziness; weakness.
**CV:** *orthostatic hypotension, tachycardia,* flushing, palpitations, fainting.
**GI:** nausea, vomiting.
**Hematologic:** methemoglobinemia.
**Skin:** cutaneous vasodilation, rash.
**Other:** hypersensitivity reactions.

### INTERACTIONS
None significant.

### CONTRAINDICATIONS
Contraindicated in patients with hypersensitivity to nitrites, severe anemia, angle-closure glaucoma, postural hypotension, increased intracranial pressure and in pregnant patients.

### NURSING CONSIDERATIONS
• Use cautiously in patients with glaucoma (except angle-closure type which is a contraindication), volume depletion, or hypotension.
• Extinguish all cigarettes before use, or ampule may ignite.
• Wrap ampule in cloth and crush. Hold near the patient's nose and mouth so vapor is inhaled.
• Watch for orthostatic hypotension.
• Store away from light.
• Be aware that drug is often abused (claimed to have aphrodisiac benefits). Street name is "Amy."

☑ **PATIENT TEACHING**
• Instruct patient how to administer drug. Stress importance of extinguishing all cigarettes before use.
• Tell patient to sit and avoid any position changes while inhaling drug to prevent orthostatic hypotension.

• Instruct patient to take a mild analgesic for drug-induced headache.

# bepridil hydrochloride
Bepadin‡, Vascor

*Pregnancy Risk Category: C*

## HOW SUPPLIED
*Tablets:* 200 mg, 300 mg, 400 mg

## ACTION
A calcium channel blocker that inhibits calcium ion influx across cardiac and smooth-muscle cells. This action dilates coronary arteries as well as peripheral arteries and arterioles; it may reduce heart rate, decrease myocardial contractility, and slow AV node conduction.

## ONSET, PEAK, DURATION
Onset unknown. Plasma levels peak within 2 to 3 hours. Effects persist for 24 hours.

## INDICATIONS & DOSAGE
*Chronic stable angina in patients who cannot tolerate or who fail to respond to other agents –*
**Adults:** initially, 200 mg P.O. daily. After 10 days, dosage increased based on response. Maintenance dosage in most patients is 300 mg/day. Maximum daily dosage is 400 mg.

## ADVERSE REACTIONS
**CNS:** *dizziness,* drowsiness, *nervousness, headache,* insomnia, paresthesia, *asthenia,* tremor.
**CV:** edema, flushing, palpitations, tachycardia, *ventricular arrhythmias, including torsades de pointes, ventricular tachycardia, ventricular fibrillation.*
**EENT:** tinnitus.
**GI:** *nausea, diarrhea,* constipation, abdominal discomfort, dry mouth, anorexia.
**Hematologic:** *agranulocytosis.*

**Respiratory:** dyspnea, shortness of breath.
**Skin:** rash.
**Other:** flu syndrome.

## INTERACTIONS
*Fentanyl anesthesia:* severe hypotension has been reported with concomitant use of a beta blocker and a calcium channel blocker. Inform anesthesiologist that the patient is taking a calcium channel blocker.

## CONTRAINDICATIONS
Contraindicated in patients with hypersensitivity to the drug; uncompensated cardiac insufficiency, sick sinus syndrome or second- or third-degree AV block unless pacemaker is present; hypotension (below 90 mm Hg systolic); congenital QT interval prolongation; or history of serious ventricular arrhythmias. Also contraindicated in those receiving other drugs that prolong the QT interval.

## NURSING CONSIDERATIONS
• Use cautiously in patients with left bundle branch block, sinus bradycardia, impaired renal or hepatic function, or CHF.
• Monitor patient for adverse reactions. Bepridil has been associated with severe ventricular arrhythmias, including torsades de pointes, and with agranulocytosis.

## ☑ PATIENT TEACHING
• Instruct patient to take drug exactly as directed.
• Tell patient to promptly report any unusual bruising or bleeding or signs of persistent infections, including sore throat, fever, or malaise.

---

Reactions may be *common,* uncommon, *life-threatening,* or COMMON AND LIFE-THREATENING.

# diltiazem hydrochloride
Cardizem, Cardizem CD,
Cardizem SR, Dilacor XR,
Vasocardol SR‡

*Pregnancy Risk Category: C*

## HOW SUPPLIED
*Tablets:* 30 mg, 60 mg, 90 mg, 120 mg
*Capsules (extended-release; Cardizem CD):* 120 mg, 180 mg, 240 mg, 300 mg
*Capsules (sustained-release; Cardizem SR, Dilacor XR, Vasocardol SR‡):* 60 mg, 90 mg, 120 mg, 180 mg, 240 mg
*Injection:* 5 mg/ml

## ACTION
A calcium channel blocker that inhibits calcium ion influx across cardiac and smooth-muscle cells, decreasing myocardial contractility and oxygen demand. Also dilates coronary arteries and arterioles.

## ONSET, PEAK, DURATION
Onset is about 3 minutes after I.V. bolus injection, 30 to 60 minutes after oral administration of regular tablets, 2 to 3 hours after extended- or sustained-release preparations. Peak plasma levels occur immediately after I.V. injection, 2 to 3 hours after regular tablet, 6 to 11 hours after sustained-release capsule, or 10 to 14 hours after extended-release capsule. Effects persist 1 to 3 hours after I.V. bolus, up to 10 hours after I.V. infusion, 6 to 8 hours after regular tablet, about 12 hours after sustained-release capsule, about 24 hours after extended-release capsule.

## INDICATIONS & DOSAGE
*Vasospastic angina (Prinzmetal's [variant] angina) and classic chronic stable angina pectoris –*
**Adults:** 30 mg P.O. t.i.d. or q.i.d. before meals and h.s. Dosage increased gradually to maximum of 360 mg/day in divided doses. Alternatively, 120 or 180 mg (extended-release capsule). Titrated as needed and tolerated to a maximum of 480 mg daily.
*Hypertension –*
**Adults:** 60 to 120 mg P.O. b.i.d. (sustained-release). Titrated to effect. Maximum recommended dosage is 360 mg/day. Alternatively, 180 to 240 mg daily (extended-release) initially. Dosage adjusted as necessary.
*Atrial fibrillation or flutter; paroxysmal supraventricular tachycardia –*
**Adults:** 0.25 mg/kg as an I.V. bolus injection over 2 minutes. If response is inadequate, 0.35 mg/kg I.V. after 15 minutes followed with a continuous infusion of 10 mg/hour. Some patients respond well to rates of 5 mg/hour; the maximum dose is 15 mg/hour.

## ADVERSE REACTIONS
**CNS:** *headache,* dizziness, asthenia, somnolence.
**CV:** *edema, **arrhythmias,*** flushing, bradycardia, hypotension, conduction abnormalities, ***CHF,*** AV block, abnormal ECG.
**GI:** *nausea, constipation,* abdominal discomfort.
**Hepatic:** acute hepatic injury.
**Skin:** *rash.*

## INTERACTIONS
*Cimetidine:* may inhibit diltiazem metabolism. Monitor for toxicity.
*Cyclosporine:* diltiazem may increase serum cyclosporine levels, possibly by decreasing its metabolism, leading to increased risk of cyclosporine toxicity. Avoid concomitant use.
*Digoxin:* diltiazem may increase serum levels of digoxin. Monitor for toxicity.
*Furosemide:* forms a precipitate when mixed with diltiazem injection. Administer through separate I.V. lines.
*Propranolol, other beta blockers:* may precipitate CHF or prolong conduction time. Use together cautiously.

## CONTRAINDICATIONS

Contraindicated in patients with sick sinus syndrome or second- or third-degree AV block in the absence of an artificial pacemaker, hypotension (systolic blood pressure below 90 mm Hg), hypersensitivity to the drug, acute MI, and pulmonary congestion (documented by X-ray).

## NURSING CONSIDERATIONS

• Use cautiously in elderly patients and in those with CHF or impaired hepatic or renal function.
• **I.V. use:** Infusions lasting longer than 24 hours are not recommended.
• Monitor blood pressure during initiation of therapy and dosage adjustments.
• If systolic blood pressure is below 90 mm Hg or heart rate is below 60 beats/minute, withhold dose and notify the doctor.

☑ **PATIENT TEACHING**
• Advise patient to avoid hazardous activities during initiation of therapy.
• If nitrate therapy is prescribed during titration of diltiazem dosage, urge patient compliance. Tell patient that sublingual nitroglycerin, especially, may be taken concomitantly as needed when anginal symptoms are acute.
• Tell patient to swallow Dilacor XR whole, not to open, crush, or chew it.

---

# erythrityl tetranitrate
Cardilate

*Pregnancy Risk Category: C*

## HOW SUPPLIED
*Tablets (oral, sublingual):* 10 mg

## ACTION
Unknown. A nitrate that is thought to reduce cardiac oxygen demand by decreasing left ventricular end-diastolic pressure (preload) and, to a lesser extent, systemic vascular resistance (afterload). Drug also may increase

blood flow through the collateral coronary vessels.

## ONSET, PEAK, DURATION
Onset occurs within 5 minutes of S.L. administration, 15 to 30 minutes after oral administration. Peak effects occur within 15 minutes of S.L. administration or 60 minutes of oral administration. Effective for up to 3 hours after S.L. administration, 6 hours after oral administration.

## INDICATIONS & DOSAGE
*Prophylaxis and long-term management of frequent or recurrent anginal pain, reduced exercise tolerance associated with angina pectoris* –
**Adults:** 5 to 10 mg S.L. prior to each anticipated physical or emotional stress and h.s. for patients with history of nocturnal attacks; 10 mg P.O. before each meal, as well as mid-morning and mid-afternoon, if needed, and h.s. for patients with history of nocturnal attacks.

## ADVERSE REACTIONS
**CNS:** *headache* (sometimes with throbbing); *dizziness;* weakness.
**CV:** *orthostatic hypotension, tachycardia, flushing, palpitations,* fainting.
**GI:** nausea, vomiting.
**Skin:** cutaneous vasodilation, rash.
**Other:** hypersensitivity reactions, sublingual burning.

## INTERACTIONS
*Ethanol:* may increase hypotension. Avoid concomitant use.

## CONTRAINDICATIONS
Contraindicated in patients with hypersensitivity or idiosyncratic reactions to nitrates.

## NURSING CONSIDERATIONS
• Use cautiously in those with severe liver or renal disease, acute MI, or CHF.
• To prevent development of toler-

---

Reactions may be *common,* uncommon, **_life-threatening,_** or **COMMON AND LIFE-THREATENING.**

ance, a nitrate-free interval of 8 to 12 hours per day has been recommended.
• Monitor blood pressure and intensity and duration of drug response.
• May cause headaches, especially at beginning of therapy; dosage may be reduced temporarily, but tolerance usually develops. Treat headache with aspirin or acetaminophen.

☑ **PATIENT TEACHING**
• Caution patient to take medication regularly, as prescribed, and to keep it accessible at all times.
• **Alert:** Advise patient that abrupt discontinuation of drug causes coronary vasospasm.
• Tell patient to take S.L. tablet at first sign of attack. The tablet should be wet with saliva and placed under the tongue until absorbed, and the patient should sit down and rest. Dose may be repeated every 10 to 15 minutes for a maximum of three doses. If drug doesn't provide relief, medical help should be obtained promptly.
• Advise patient who complains of tingling sensation with S.L. drug to try holding tablet in buccal pouch.
• Advise patient to take oral tablets on an empty stomach, either ½ hour before or 1 to 2 hours after meals, and to swallow oral tablets whole.
• To minimize orthostatic hypotension, patient should change to upright position slowly. Advise him to go up and down stairs carefully and to lie down at the first sign of dizziness.
• Tell the patient to store drug in a cool place, in a tightly closed container, away from light. To ensure freshness, replace supply every 3 months. Remove cotton from container because it absorbs drug.

# isosorbide dinitrate
Apo-ISDN†, Cedocard-SR†, Coradur†, Coronex†, Dilatrate-SR, Iso-Bid, Isonate, Isorbid, Isordil, Isotrate, Nitro-Spray‡, Novosorbide†, Sorbitrate, Sorbitrate SA

# isosorbide mononitrate
Imdur, ISMO, Monoket

*Pregnancy Risk Category: C*

**HOW SUPPLIED**
**isosorbide dinitrate**
*Tablets:* 5 mg, 10 mg, 20 mg, 30 mg, 40 mg
*Tablets (chewable):* 5 mg, 10 mg
*Tablets (sublingual):* 2.5 mg, 5 mg, 10 mg
*Tablets (sustained-release):* 40 mg
*Capsules:* 40 mg
*Capsules (sustained-release):* 40 mg
*Topical spray:* 10%‡, 12.5 mg metered spray‡
**isosorbide mononitrate**
*Tablets:* 10 mg, 20 mg
*Tablets (extended-release):* 60 mg

**ACTION**
Not completely known. Thought to reduce cardiac oxygen demand by decreasing preload and afterload. Drug also may increase blood flow through the collateral coronary vessels.

**ONSET, PEAK, DURATION**
Onset and peak levels occur as follows: isosorbide dinitrate – 2 to 5 minutes after administration of S.L. or chewable form, 15 to 40 minutes after oral form, 30 minutes after extended-release form. Isosorbide mononitrate – 60 minutes. Duration is as follows: isosorbide dinitrate – effective for 1 to 2 hours after administration of S.L. form, 1 to 2 hours after chewable form, 4 to 6 hours after oral form, 12 hours after extended-release form. Isosorbide mononitrate – not determined.

## INDICATIONS & DOSAGE

*Acute anginal attacks (S.L. and chewable tablets of isosorbide dinitrate only), prophylaxis in situations likely to cause anginal attacks –*

**Adults:** *S.L. form –* 2.5 to 5 mg under the tongue for prompt relief of anginal pain, repeated q 5 to 10 minutes (maximum of three doses for each 30-minute period). For prophylaxis, 2.5 to 10 mg q 2 to 3 hours.

*Chewable form –* 5 to 10 mg p.r.n. for acute attack or q 2 to 3 hours for prophylaxis, but only after initial test dose of 5 mg to determine risk of severe hypotension.

*Oral form (isosorbide dinitrate) –* 5 to 30 mg P.O. t.i.d. or q.i.d. for prophylaxis only (use smallest effective dose); 40 mg P.O. (sustained-release form) q 6 to 12 hours.

*Oral form (isosorbide mononitrate using Imdur) –* 30 to 60 mg P.O. once daily upon arising; increased to 120 mg once daily after several days, if needed.

*Oral form (isosorbide mononitrate using ISMO or Monoket) –* 20 mg b.i.d. with the two doses given 7 hours apart.

*Topical form‡(where available) –* initially, 2 sprays to chest in morning from about 8″ (20 cm). Rub solution in. Increase dosage gradually as needed to 2 to 5 sprays, daily or b.i.d. (in morning and h.s.).

## ADVERSE REACTIONS

**CNS:** *headache* (sometimes with throbbing); dizziness; weakness.
**CV:** *orthostatic hypotension, tachycardia, palpitations, ankle edema,* fainting.
**GI:** nausea, vomiting.
**Skin:** cutaneous vasodilation, *flushing,* rash.
**Other:** hypersensitivity reactions, sublingual burning.

## INTERACTIONS

*Antihypertensives:* may increase hypotensive effects. Monitor closely during initial therapy.

*Ethanol:* may increase hypotension. Avoid concomitant use.

## CONTRAINDICATIONS

Contraindicated in patients with hypersensitivity or idiosyncrasy to nitrates, severe hypotension, shock, or acute MI with low left ventricular filling pressure.

## NURSING CONSIDERATIONS

• Use cautiously in patients with blood volume depletion (such as from diuretic therapy) or mild hypotension.
• To prevent development of tolerance, a nitrate-free interval of 8 to 12 hours per day has been recommended. The regimen for isosorbide mononitrate (one tablet upon awakening with the second dose in 7 hours, or one extended-release tablet daily) is intended to minimize nitrate tolerance by providing a substantial nitrate-free interval.
• Monitor blood pressure and intensity and duration of drug response.
• May cause headaches, especially at beginning of therapy. Dosage may be reduced temporarily, but tolerance usually develops. Treat headache with aspirin or acetaminophen.

## ☑ PATIENT TEACHING

• Caution the patient to take medication regularly, as prescribed, and to keep it accessible at all times.
• ***Alert:*** Advise the patient that abrupt discontinuation of drug causes coronary vasospasm.
• Tell patient to take S.L. tablet at first sign of attack. The tablet should be wet with saliva and placed under the tongue until absorbed, and the patient should sit down and rest. Dose may be repeated every 10 to 15 minutes for a maximum of three doses. If drug doesn't provide relief, medical help should be obtained promptly.
• Advise patient who complains of tingling sensation with S.L. drug to try holding tablet in buccal pouch.

---

Reactions may be *common,* uncommon, *life-threatening,* or **COMMON AND LIFE-THREATENING.**

• Warn the patient not to confuse S.L. with oral form.

• Teach the patient taking oral form of isosorbide dinitrate to take oral tablet on an empty stomach, either ½ before or 1 to 2 hours after meals; to swallow oral tablets whole; and to chew chewable tablets thoroughly before swallowing.

• Tell the patient to minimize orthostatic hypotension by changing to upright position slowly. Advise him to go up and down stairs carefully and to lie down at the first sign of dizziness.

• Tell the patient to store drug in a cool place, in a tightly closed container, away from light.

---

# nadolol
Corgard, Syn-Nadolol†

*Pregnancy Risk Category: C*

## HOW SUPPLIED
*Tablets:* 20 mg, 40 mg, 80 mg, 120 mg, 160 mg

## ACTION
A beta-adrenergic blocker that reduces cardiac oxygen demand by blocking catecholamine-induced increases in heart rate, blood pressure, and force of myocardial contraction. Depresses renin secretion.

## ONSET, PEAK, DURATION
Onset and duration unknown. Plasma levels peak within 2 to 4 hours.

## INDICATIONS & DOSAGE
*Angina pectoris –*
**Adults:** 40 mg P.O. once daily. Dosage increased in 40- to 80-mg increments until optimum response occurs. Usual maintenance dosage is 40 to 240 mg once daily.
*Hypertension –*
**Adults:** 40 mg P.O. once daily. Dosage increased in 40- to 80-mg increments until optimum response occurs. Usual maintenance dosage is 40 to

320 mg once daily. Doses of 640 mg may be necessary in rare cases.

## ADVERSE REACTIONS
**CNS:** fatigue, dizziness.
**CV:** *bradycardia, hypotension, CHF,* peripheral vascular disease, rhythm and conduction disturbances.
**GI:** nausea, vomiting, diarrhea, abdominal pain, constipation, anorexia.
**Respiratory:** *increased airway resistance.*
**Skin:** rash.
**Other:** fever.

## INTERACTIONS
*Antihypertensives:* enhanced antihypertensive effect.
*Digitalis glycosides:* excessive bradycardia and additive effects on AV conduction. Use together cautiously.
*Epinephrine:* severe vasoconstriction and reflex bradycardia. Monitor blood pressure carefully.
*Insulin, oral antidiabetic agents:* can alter dosage requirements in previously stabilized diabetics patients. Observe the patient carefully.
*NSAIDs:* decreased antihypertensive effect. Monitor blood pressure and adjust dosage.

## CONTRAINDICATIONS
Contraindicated in patients with bronchial asthma, sinus bradycardia and greater than first-degree heart block, and cardiogenic shock.

## NURSING CONSIDERATIONS
• Use cautiously in patients with heart failure, chronic bronchitis, emphysema, or renal or hepatic impairment and in patients undergoing major surgery involving general anesthesia. Also use cautiously in diabetic patients because beta-adrenergic blockers may mask certain signs and symptoms of hypoglycemia.
• Check apical pulse before giving drug. If slower than 60 beats/minute, withhold drug and call doctor.

---

*Liquid form contains alcohol. **May contain tartrazine. †Canada only. ‡Australia only. ◊OTC.

• Monitor blood pressure frequently. If the patient develops severe hypotension, administer a vasopressor, as prescribed.

• **Alert:** Know that abrupt discontinuation can exacerbate angina and MI. Dosage should be reduced gradually over 1 to 2 weeks.

• Be aware that nadolol masks signs of shock and hyperthyroidism.

☑ **PATIENT TEACHING**
• Explain to the patient the importance of taking the drug as prescribed, even when he's feeling well.

• Teach the patient how to check pulse rate and to do so before each dose. If pulse rate is below 60 beats/minute, tell the patient to notify the doctor.

• Caution the patient not to discontinue the drug suddenly.

---

# nicardipine
Cardene, Cardene IV, Cardene SR

*Pregnancy Risk Category: C*

## HOW SUPPLIED
*Capsules (immediate-release):* 20 mg, 30 mg
*Capsules (sustained-release):* 30 mg, 45 mg, 60 mg
*Injection:* 2.5 mg/ml

## ACTION
A calcium channel blocker that inhibits calcium ion influx across cardiac and smooth-muscle cells, decreasing myocardial contractility and oxygen demand. Also dilates coronary arteries and arterioles.

## ONSET, PEAK, DURATION
Onset is immediate after I.V. administration, within 20 minutes for both oral formulations. Serum levels peak within minutes after I.V. injection, within ½ to 2 hours after immediate-release capsules, 1 to 4 hours after sustained-release capsule. Effects of immediate-release product persist for 6 to 8 hours, of sustained-release preparation, up to 12 hours; rapid decline after cessation of I.V. infusion.

## INDICATIONS & DOSAGE
*Chronic stable angina (used alone or in combination with other antianginal agents)* –
**Adults:** initially, 20 mg P.O. t.i.d. (immediate-release only). Dosage titrated according to patient response q 3 days. Usual dosage range is 20 to 40 mg t.i.d.
*Hypertension* –
**Adults:** initially, 20 to 40 mg P.O. t.i.d. (immediate-release) or 30 mg b.i.d. (sustained-release). Dosage increased according to patient response. Alternatively, for patients unable to take oral nicardipine, 50 ml/hour (5 mg/hour) I.V. infusion initially; then increased by 25 ml/hour (2.5 mg/hour) every 15 minutes up to a maximum of 150 ml/hour (15 mg/hour).

## ADVERSE REACTIONS
**CNS:** *dizziness, light-headedness, headache, paresthesia, asthenia.*
**CV:** *peripheral edema, palpitations,* angina, tachycardia.
**GI:** nausea, abdominal discomfort, dry mouth.
**Skin:** rash, *flushing.*

## INTERACTIONS
*Antihypertensives:* enhanced antihypertensive effect. Monitor closely.
*Beta blockers:* may increase cardiac depressant effects. Monitor closely.
*Cimetidine:* may decrease metabolism of calcium channel blockers. Monitor for increased pharmacologic effect.
*Cyclosporine:* nicardipine may increase plasma levels of cyclosporine. Monitor for toxicity.
*Theophylline:* pharmacologic effects of theophylline may be enhanced. Monitor for toxicity.

---

Reactions may be *common,* uncommon, *life-threatening,* or COMMON AND LIFE-THREATENING.

## CONTRAINDICATIONS
Contraindicated in patients with hypersensitivity to the drug and in those with advanced aortic stenosis.

## NURSING CONSIDERATIONS
• Use cautiously in patients with cardiac conduction disturbances, hypotension, CHF, and impaired hepatic and renal function.
• **I.V. use:** When switching to oral therapy other than nicardipine, initiate therapy upon discontinuation of the infusion. If oral nicardipine is to be used, administer first dose of t.i.d. regimen 1 hour prior to discontinuation of infusion.
• Adjust infusion rate if hypotension or tachycardia occurs, as ordered.
• Measure blood pressure frequently during initial therapy. Maximum blood pressure response occurs about 1 hour after dosing with the immediate-release form and 2 to 4 hours with the sustained-release form. Check for potential orthostatic hypotension. Because large swings in blood pressure may occur based on blood level of drug, assess adequacy of antihypertensive effect 8 hours after dosing.

## ☑ PATIENT TEACHING
• Tell the patient to take oral form of drug exactly as prescribed.
• Advise the patient to report chest pain immediately. Some patients may experience increased frequency, severity, or duration of chest pain at beginning of therapy or during dosage adjustments.

## nifedipine
Adalat, Adalat CC, Adalat FT†, Adalat P.A.†, Nu-Nifed†, Procardia, Procardia XL

*Pregnancy Risk Category: C*

## HOW SUPPLIED
*Tablets (extended-release):* 30 mg, 60 mg, 90 mg

*Capsules:* 10 mg, 20 mg

## ACTION
Unknown. Thought to inhibit calcium ion influx across cardiac and smooth-muscle cells, decreasing contractility and oxygen demand. Also may dilate coronary arteries and arterioles.

## ONSET, PEAK, DURATION
Onset occurs in 20 minutes. Serum levels peak in about 30 to 60 minutes for capsules, 1 to 2 hours for tablets. Effects persist for 4 to 8 hours for capsules; 12 to 24 hours for extended-release formulations.

## INDICATIONS & DOSAGE
*Vasospastic angina (also called Prinzmetal's [variant] angina) and classic chronic stable angina pectoris –*
**Adults:** starting dose is 10 mg P.O. t.i.d. Usual effective dose range is 10 to 20 mg t.i.d. Some patients may require up to 30 mg q.i.d. Maximum daily dosage is 180 mg.
*Hypertension –*
**Adults:** 30 or 60 mg P.O. (extended-release form) once daily. Titrated over 7 to 14 days. Doses larger than 90 mg are not recommended.

## ADVERSE REACTIONS
**CNS:** *dizziness, light-headedness, flushing, headache, weakness,* syncope, nervousness.
**CV:** *peripheral edema,* hypotension, palpitations, CHF, *MI,* pulmonary edema.
**EENT:** nasal congestion.
**GI:** *nausea,* diarrhea, constipation, abdominal discomfort.
**Respiratory:** dyspnea, cough.
**Skin:** rash, pruritus.
**Other:** muscle cramps, hypokalemia.

## INTERACTIONS
*Cimetidine, ranitidine:* decreased nifedipine metabolism.
*Propranolol, other beta blockers:* may

---

cause hypotension and heart failure. Use together cautiously.

**CONTRAINDICATIONS**
Contraindicated in patients with hypersensitivity to the drug.

**NURSING CONSIDERATIONS**
• Use cautiously in patients with CHF or hypotension and in elderly patients. Use extended-release tablets cautiously in patients with severe GI narrowing.
• When a rapid response to the drug is desired, have the patient bite and swallow the capsule. If he can't chew capsules, the liquid can be withdrawn by puncturing the capsule with a needle and squeezing the contents into the mouth. When these methods are used, continuous blood pressure and ECG monitoring is recommended.
• Despite widespread S.L. use of nifedipine capsules, this route of administration should be avoided. Peak serum levels are lower and take longer to occur than when capsules are bitten and swallowed.
• Monitor blood pressure regularly, especially in patients who are taking beta blockers or antihypertensives.
• Monitor serum potassium level regularly, as ordered.
• Be aware that although rebound effect hasn't been observed when drug is stopped, dosage should be reduced slowly under doctor's supervision.

☑ **PATIENT TEACHING**
• If the patient is kept on nitrate therapy while nifedipine dosage is being titrated, urge continued compliance. S.L. nitroglycerin, especially, may be taken as needed when anginal symptoms are acute.
• Patient may briefly develop anginal exacerbation when beginning drug therapy or when dosage is increased. Reassure him that this is temporary.
• Instruct the patient to swallow extended-release tablets without breaking, crushing, or chewing.

• Reassure the patient who is taking the extended-release form that a wax-matrix "ghost" from the tablet may be passed in the stools. Drug is completely absorbed before this occurs.
• Warn the patient not to switch brands. Procardia XL and Adalat CC are not therapeutically equivalent because of major differences in their pharmacokinetics.
• Tell the patient to protect capsules from direct light and moisture and to store at room temperature.

---

## nitroglycerin (glyceryl trinitrate)
Anginine‡, Deponit, GTN-Pohl‡, Minitran, Nitradisc‡, Nitro-Bid, Nitro-Bid I.V., Nitrocine, Nitrodisc, Nitro-Dur, Nitrogard, Nitroglyn, Nitroject, Nitrol, Nitrolingual, Nitrong, Nitrostat, Transderm-Nitro, Transidem-Nitro‡, Tridil

*Pregnancy Risk Category: C*

**HOW SUPPLIED**
*Tablets (buccal):* 1 mg, 2 mg, 3 mg
*Tablets (sublingual):* 0.15 mg (1/400 gr), 0.3 mg (1/200 gr), 0.4 mg (1/150 gr), 0.6 mg (1/100 gr)
*Tablets (sustained-release):* 2.5 mg, 2.6 mg, 6.5 mg, 9 mg, 13 mg
*Capsules (sustained-release):* 2.5 mg, 6.5 mg, 9 mg, 13 mg
*Aerosol (translingual):* 0.4 mg metered spray
*Topical:* 2% ointment
*Transdermal:* 2.5 mg, 5 mg, 7.5 mg, 10 mg, 15 mg per 24-hour system
*Injection:* 0.5 mg/ml, 0.8 mg/ml, 1 mg/ml, 5 mg/ml, 10 mg/ml

**ACTION**
A nitrate that reduces cardiac oxygen demand by decreasing left ventricular end-diastolic pressure (preload) and, to a lesser extent, systemic vascular resistance (afterload). Also increases blood flow through the collateral coronary vessels.

---

Reactions may be *common,* uncommon, *life-threatening,* or COMMON AND LIFE-THREATENING.

## ONSET, PEAK, DURATION
Onset and peak immediate after I.V. form, 1 to 3 minutes after S.L. form, 2 to 4 minutes after translingual form, 3 minutes after buccal form, 20 to 45 minutes after oral form, 30 minutes after topical ointment, 30 minutes after transdermal system. With I.V. form, effects last 3 to 5 minutes; with S.L. form, 30 to 60 minutes; with translingual form, 30 to 60 minutes; with buccal form, 5 hours; with oral form, 8 to 12 hours; with topical ointment, 4 to 8 hours; with transdermal system, up to 24 hours with system in place (otherwise, effects last several minutes after removal).

## INDICATIONS & DOSAGE
*Prophylaxis against chronic anginal attacks* –
**Adults:** 2.5 mg or 2.6 mg sustained-release capsule q 8 to 12 hours, titrated upward to an effective dose in 2.5- or 2.6-mg increments 2 to 4 times daily. Or, use of 2% ointment: Dosage started with ½" ointment, increasing by ½" increments until headache occurs, then decreasing to previous dose. Range of dosage with ointment is ½" to 5". Usual dose is 1" to 2". Alternatively, transdermal disc or pad (Nitrodisc, Nitro-Dur, or Transderm-Nitro) 0.2 to 0.4 mg/hour once daily.
*Acute angina pectoris, prophylaxis to prevent or minimize anginal attacks before stressful events* –
**Adults:** 1 S.L. tablet (gr ¼400, ½200, ½150, ½100) dissolved under the tongue or in the buccal pouch as soon as angina begins. Repeat q 5 minutes, if needed, for 15 minutes. Or, using Nitrolingual spray, one or two sprays into mouth, preferably onto or under the tongue. Repeat q 3 to 5 minutes, if needed, to a maximum of three doses within a 15-minute period. Or, 1 to 3 mg transmucosally q 3 to 5 hours during waking hours.
*Hypertension associated with surgery; CHF associated with MI; angina pectoris in acute situations; to produce controlled hypotension during surgery (by I.V. infusion)* –
**Adults:** initial infusion rate is 5 mcg/minute, increased as needed by 5 mcg/minute q 3 to 5 minutes until a response is noted. If a 20 mcg/minute rate doesn't produce a response, dosage is increased by as much as 20 mcg/minute q 3 to 5 minutes. Up to 100 mcg/minute may be needed.

## ADVERSE REACTIONS
**CNS:** *headache, sometimes with throbbing; dizziness;* weakness.
**CV:** *orthostatic hypotension, tachycardia, flushing, palpitations,* fainting.
**GI:** nausea, vomiting.
**Skin:** cutaneous vasodilation, contact dermatitis (patch), rash.
**Other:** hypersensitivity reactions, sublingual burning.

## INTERACTIONS
*Antihypertensives:* possible enhanced hypotensive effect. Monitor closely.
*Ethanol:* possible increased hypotension. Advise patient to avoid ethanol.

## CONTRAINDICATIONS
Contraindicated in patients with hypersensitivity to nitrates and in those with early MI (sublingual nitroglycerin), severe anemia, increased intracranial pressure, angle-closure glaucoma, postural hypotension, and allergy to adhesives (transdermal). I.V. nitroglycerin is contraindicated in patients with hypersensitivity to I.V. form, cardiac tamponade, restrictive cardiomyopathy, or constrictive pericarditis.

## NURSING CONSIDERATIONS
• Use cautiously in patients with hypotension or volume depletion.
• **I.V. use:** Dilute with $D_5W$ or 0.9% sodium chloride for injection. Concentration should not exceed 400 mcg/ml. Always administer with an

infusion control device and titrate to desired response. Also, always mix in glass bottles and avoid use of I.V. filters because drug binds to plastic. Regular polyvinyl chloride (PVC) tubing can bind up to 80% of the drug, making it necessary to infuse higher dosages. A special nonabsorbent (non-PVC) tubing is available from the manufacturer; patients receive more drug when these infusion sets are used. Always use the same type of infusion set when changing I.V. lines.

• When changing the concentration of infusion, flush the I.V. administration set with 15 to 20 ml of the new concentration before use. This will clear the line of the old drug solution.

• Closely monitor vital signs during infusion. Be particularly aware of blood pressure, especially in a patient with an MI. Excessive hypotension may worsen the MI.

• To apply ointment, measure the prescribed amount on the application paper; then place the paper on any nonhairy area. Do not rub in. Cover with plastic film to aid absorption and to protect clothing. If using Tape-Surrounded Appli-Ruler (TSAR) system, keep the TSAR on skin to protect patient's clothing and to ensure that ointment remains in place. Remove all excess ointment from previous site before applying the next dose. Avoid getting ointment on fingers.

• Know that transdermal dosage forms can be applied to any nonhairy part of the skin except distal parts of the arms or legs (absorption will not be maximal at from distal sites).

• Remove transdermal patch before defibrillation. Because of its aluminum backing, the electric current may cause the patch to explode.

• When stopping transdermal treatment of angina, gradually reduce the dose and frequency of application over 4 to 6 weeks, as ordered.

• Monitor blood pressure and intensity and duration of drug response.

• May cause headaches, especially at beginning of therapy. Dosage may be reduced temporarily, but tolerance usually develops. Treat headache with aspirin or acetaminophen.

• Tolerance to the drug can be minimized with a 10- to 12-hour nitrate-free interval. To achieve this, remove the transdermal system in the early evening and apply a new system the next morning or omit the last daily dose of a buccal, sustained-release, or ointment form. Check with the doctor for alterations in dosage regimen if tolerance is suspected.

☑ **PATIENT TEACHING**

• Caution the patient to take nitroglycerin regularly, as prescribed, and to have it accessible at all times.

• *Alert:* Advise the patient that abrupt discontinuation of drug causes coronary vasospasms.

• Teach the patient how to administer the prescribed form of nitroglycerin.

• Tell patient to take S.L. tablet at first sign of attack. The tablet should be wet with saliva and placed under the tongue until absorbed, and the patient should sit down and rest. Dose may be repeated every 10 to 15 minutes for a maximum of three doses. If drug doesn't provide relief, medical help should be obtained promptly.

• Advise patient who complains of a tingling sensation with S.L. drug to try holding tablet in buccal pouch.

• Tell the patient to take oral tablets on an empty stomach, either 30 minutes before or 1 to 2 hours after meals; to swallow oral tablets whole; and not to chew tablets.

• Remind the patient using translingual aerosol form that he should *not* inhale the spray, but should release it onto or under the tongue. Also tell him to wait about 10 seconds or so before swallowing.

• Tell the patient to place the buccal tablet between the lip and gum above the incisors or between the cheek and

---

Reactions may be *common,* uncommon, *life-threatening,* or COMMON AND LIFE-THREATENING.

gum. Tablets should not be swallowed or chewed.

• Tell him to take an additional dose before anticipated stress or at bedtime if angina is nocturnal.

• Instruct the patient to use caution when wearing transdermal patch near microwave oven. Leaking radiation may heat patch's metallic backing and cause burns.

• Advise him to avoid alcohol.

• To minimize orthostatic hypotension, tell the patient to change to upright position slowly. Advise him to go up and down stairs carefully and to lie down at the first sign of dizziness.

• Tell the patient to store drug in cool, dark place in a tightly closed container. Remove cotton from container because it absorbs the drug.

• Tell the patient to store S.L. tablets in original container or other container specifically approved for this use and to carry the container in a jacket pocket or purse, not in a pocket close to the body.

---

### pentaerythritol tetranitrate
Dilar, Duotrate, Pentylan, Peritrate, Peritrate Forte†, Peritrate SA, P.E.T.N.

*Pregnancy Risk Category: C*

### HOW SUPPLIED
*Tablets:* 10 mg, 20 mg, 40 mg
*Tablets (sustained-release):* 80 mg
*Capsules (sustained-release):* 30 mg, 45 mg

### ACTION
Reduces cardiac oxygen demand by decreasing preload and afterload. Also increases blood flow through the collateral coronary vessels.

### ONSET, PEAK, DURATION
Onset occurs 30 minutes after oral tablets, 1 hour or more after sustained-release forms. Peak levels unknown. Effects persist for 4 to 5 hours

after oral tablets; 12 hours after sustained-release forms.

### INDICATIONS & DOSAGE
*Prophylaxis against angina pectoris –*
**Adults:** 10 to 20 mg P.O. t.i.d. or q.i.d.; titrated upward as needed to 40 mg P.O. q.i.d. ½ hour before or 1 hour after meals and h.s.; or 30 to 80 mg sustained-release form P.O. b.i.d. on empty stomach.

### ADVERSE REACTIONS
**CNS:** *headache* (sometimes with throbbing); *dizziness;* weakness.
**CV:** *orthostatic hypotension, tachycardia, flushing, palpitations,* fainting.
**GI:** nausea, vomiting.
**Skin:** cutaneous vasodilation, rash.
**Other:** hypersensitivity reactions.

### INTERACTIONS
*Antihypertensives:* possible enhanced hypotensive effect. Monitor closely.
*Ethanol:* may increase hypotension. Avoid concomitant use.

### CONTRAINDICATIONS
Contraindicated in patients with hypersensitivity to nitrates, severe anemia, increased intracranial pressure, angle-closure glaucoma, or postural hypotension.

### NURSING CONSIDERATIONS
• Use cautiously in patients with volume depletion or glaucoma (except angle-closure type).

• Monitor blood pressure and intensity and duration of drug response.

• May cause headaches, especially at beginning of therapy. Dosage may be reduced temporarily, but tolerance usually develops. Treat headache with aspirin or acetaminophen.

### ☑ PATIENT TEACHING
• Caution the patient to take medication regularly, as prescribed, and to have it accessible at all times.

• *Alert:* Advise the patient that abrupt

---

discontinuation of drug causes coronary vasospasm. However, warn the patient that drug is not to be used for relief of acute anginal attacks.
• Tell him additional doses may be taken before anticipated stress or at bedtime for nocturnal angina.
• To minimize orthostatic hypotension, tell the patient to change to upright position slowly. Advise him to go up and down stairs carefully and to lie down at the first sign of dizziness.
• Instruct the patient to store drug in a cool place, in a tightly covered container away from light.

## propranolol hydrochloride
Apo-Propranolol†, Deralin‡, Detensol†, Inderal, Inderal LA, Novopranol†, pms Propranolol†

*Pregnancy Risk Category: C*

### HOW SUPPLIED
*Tablets:* 10 mg, 20 mg, 40 mg, 60 mg, 80 mg, 90 mg
*Capsules (extended-release):* 60 mg, 80 mg, 120 mg, 160 mg
*Oral solution:* 4 mg/ml, 8 mg/ml, 80 mg/ml (concentrate)
*Injection:* 1 mg/ml

### ACTION
Reduces cardiac oxygen demand by blocking catecholamine-induced increases in heart rate, blood pressure, and force of myocardial contraction. Depresses renin secretion and prevents vasodilation of cerebral arteries.

### ONSET, PEAK, DURATION
Onset occurs within 1 minute after I.V. injection, 30 minutes after oral administration. Peak plasma levels occur 60 to 90 minutes after oral administration or immediately after I.V. injection. Effects persist for about 12 hours after oral administration. Drug undetectable in the plasma 5 minutes after I.V. bolus administration.

### INDICATIONS & DOSAGE
*Angina pectoris –*
**Adults:** 10 to 20 mg P.O. t.i.d. or q.i.d. Or one 80-mg extended-release capsule daily. Dosage increased at 7- to 10-day intervals. The average optimum dosage is 160 to 240 mg daily.
*Mortality reduction after MI –*
**Adults:** 180 to 240 mg P.O. daily in divided doses beginning 5 to 21 days after MI has occurred. Usually administered t.i.d. or q.i.d.
*Supraventricular, ventricular, and atrial arrhythmias; tachyarrhythmias caused by excessive catecholamine action during anesthesia, hyperthyroidism, or pheochromocytoma –*
**Adults:** 0.5 to 3 mg by slow I.V. push, not to exceed 1 mg/minute. After 3 mg have been given, another dose may be given in 2 minutes; subsequent doses, no sooner than q 4 hours. May be diluted and infused slowly. Usual maintenance dosage is 10 to 30 mg P.O. t.i.d. or q.i.d.
*Hypertension –*
**Adults:** initially, 80 mg P.O. daily in two to four divided doses or the extended-release form once daily. Increased at 3- to 7-day intervals to maximum daily dosage of 640 mg. Usual maintenance dosage is 160 to 480 mg daily.
*Prevention of frequent, severe, uncontrollable, or disabling migraine or vascular headache –*
**Adults:** initially, 80 mg P.O. daily in divided doses or 1 extended-release capsule daily. Usual maintenance dosage is 160 to 240 mg daily, t.i.d. or q.i.d.
*Essential tremor –*
**Adults:** 40 mg (tablets, oral solution) P.O. b.i.d. Usual maintenance dosage is 120 to 320 mg daily in three divided doses.
*Hypertrophic subaortic stenosis –*
**Adults:** 20 to 40 mg P.O. t.i.d. or q.i.d., or 80 to 160 mg extended-release capsules once daily.

Reactions may be *common*, uncommon, *life-threatening*, or COMMON AND LIFE-THREATENING.

*Adjunct therapy in pheochromocytoma* –
**Adults:** 60 mg P.O. daily in divided doses with an alpha-adrenergic blocker 3 days before surgery.

## ADVERSE REACTIONS
**CNS:** *fatigue, lethargy,* vivid dreams, hallucinations, mental depression, light-headedness, insomnia.
**CV:** *bradycardia, hypotension, CHF,* intermittent claudication, intensification of AV block.
**GI:** nausea, vomiting, diarrhea, abdominal cramping.
**Respiratory:** bronchospasm.
**Skin:** rash.
**Other:** fever, *agranulocytosis.*

## INTERACTIONS
*Aminophylline:* antagonized beta-blocking effects of propranolol. Use together cautiously.
*Cimetidine:* inhibits propranolol's metabolism. Monitor for increased beta-blocking effect.
*Digitalis glycosides, diltiazem, verapamil:* hypotension, bradycardia, and increased depressant effect on myocardium. Use together cautiously.
*Epinephrine:* severe vasoconstriction. Monitor blood pressure and observe the patient carefully.
*Glucagon, isoproterenol:* antagonized propranolol effect. May be used therapeutically and in emergencies.
*Insulin, oral antidiabetic agents:* can alter requirements for these drugs in previously stabilized diabetics. Monitor for hypoglycemia.

## CONTRAINDICATIONS
Contraindicated in patients with bronchial asthma, sinus bradycardia and heart block greater than first-degree, cardiogenic shock, and CHF (unless failure is secondary to a tachyarrhythmia that can be treated with propranolol).

## NURSING CONSIDERATIONS
• Use cautiously in patients with renal impairment, nonallergic bronchospastic diseases, or hepatic disease and in those taking other antihypertensives. Because drug blocks some symptoms of hypoglycemia, use with caution in patients with diabetes mellitus. Also use cautiously in patients with thyrotoxicosis because drug may mask some signs of that disorder. Elderly patients may experience enhanced adverse reactions and may need dosage adjustment.
• Always check patient's apical pulse before giving drug. If you detect extremes in pulse rates, withhold drug and call the doctor immediately.
• Double-check dose and route. I.V. doses are much smaller than oral doses.
• **I.V. use:** Give by direct injection into a large vessel or into the tubing of a free-flowing, compatible I.V. solution; continuous I.V. infusion generally is not recommended. Alternatively, dilute drug with 0.9% sodium chloride and give by intermittent infusion over 10 to 15 minutes in 0.1- to 0.2-mg increments. Drug is compatible with $D_5W$ and 0.45% and 0.9% sodium chloride and lactated Ringer's solutions.
• Give consistently with meals. Food may increase absorption of propranolol.
• Monitor blood pressure, ECG, and heart rate and rhythm frequently, especially during I.V. administration. If the patient develops severe hypotension, notify the doctor; a vasopressor may be prescribed.
• Be aware that drug masks common signs of shock and hypoglycemia.
• *Don't discontinue drug before surgery for pheochromocytoma.* Before any surgical procedure, tell the anesthesiologist that the patient is receiving propranolol.
• For overdose, give I.V. isoproterenol, I.V. atropine, or glucagon; refractory cases may require a pacemaker.
• Compliance may be improved by

---

*Liquid form contains alcohol.   **May contain tartrazine.   †Canada only.   ‡Australia only.   ◊OTC.

administering drug twice daily or as extended-release capsule. Check with the doctor.

### ☑ PATIENT TEACHING
● Caution the patient to continue taking this drug as prescribed, even when he is feeling well.
● Instruct the patient to take drug with food.
● *Alert:* Tell the patient not to discontinue the drug suddenly because this can exacerbate angina and MI.

## verapamil
Apo-Verap†, Calan, Isoptin, Novo-Veramil†, Nu-Verap†

## verapamil hydrochloride
Anpec‡, Calan, Calan SR, Cordilox‡,Cordilox SR‡, Isoptin, Isoptin SR, Veracaps SR‡, Verelan

*Pregnancy Risk Category: C*

### HOW SUPPLIED
**verapamil**
*Tablets:* 40 mg, 80 mg, 120 mg
**verapamil hydrochloride**
*Tablets:* 40 mg‡, 80 mg‡, 120 mg‡, 160 mg‡
*Tablets (extended-release):* 120 mg, 180 mg, 240 mg
*Capsules (extended-release):* 120 mg, 160 mg‡, 180 mg, 240 mg
*Injection:* 2.5 mg/ml

### ACTION
Not clearly defined. Verapamil is a calcium channel blocker that inhibits calcium ion influx across cardiac and smooth-muscle cells, thus decreasing myocardial contractility and oxygen demand; it also dilates coronary arteries and arterioles.

### ONSET, PEAK, DURATION
Onset occurs within 1 to 2 hours with oral administration, within 1 to 5 minutes with I.V. administration. Serum levels peak within 1 to 2 hours (tablets), 7 to 9 hours (extended-release capsules), 5 to 7 hours (extended-release tablets), and immediately after I.V. administration. Effects persist 1 to 6 hours with I.V. form, about 8 to 10 hours with tablets, and about 24 hours with extended-release oral forms.

### INDICATIONS & DOSAGE
*Vasospastic angina (also called Prinzmetal's [variant] angina) and classic chronic, stable angina pectoris; chronic atrial fibrillation –*
**Adults:** starting dose is 80 to 120 mg P.O. t.i.d. Dosage increased at weekly intervals as needed. Some patients may require up to 480 mg daily.
*Supraventricular arrhythmias –*
**Adults:** 0.075 to 0.15 mg/kg (5 to 10 mg) by I.V. push over 2 minutes with ECG and blood pressure monitoring. Repeat dose in 30 minutes if no response occurs.
**Children under 1 year:** 0.1 to 0.2 mg/kg as I.V. bolus over 2 minutes with continuous ECG monitoring. Repeat dose in 30 minutes if no response occurs.
**Children 1 to 15 years:** 0.1 to 0.3 mg/kg as I.V. bolus over 2 minutes.
*Hypertension –*
**Adults:** 240 mg extended-release tablet P.O. once daily in the morning. If response is not adequate, give an additional ½ tablet in the evening or one tablet q 12 hours or an 80 mg immediate-release tablet t.i.d.

### ADVERSE REACTIONS
**CNS:** dizziness, headache, asthenia.
**CV:** *transient hypotension, CHF,* pulmonary edema, bradycardia, AV block, *ventricular asystole, ventricular fibrillation,* peripheral edema.
**GI:** *constipation,* nausea.
**Hepatic:** elevated liver enzymes.
**Skin:** rash.

---

Reactions may be *common,* uncommon, *life-threatening,* or COMMON AND LIFE-THREATENING.

## INTERACTIONS

*Antihypertensives, quinidine:* may result in hypotension. Monitor blood pressure.

*Carbamazepine, digitalis glycosides:* may increase serum levels of these drugs. Monitor for toxicity.

*Cyclosporine:* may increase cyclosporine serum levels. Monitor cyclosporine levels.

*Disopyramide, flecainide, propranolol (and other beta blockers, including ophthalmic timolol):* may cause heart failure. Use together cautiously.

*Lithium:* may decrease serum lithium levels. Monitor closely.

*Rifampin:* may decrease oral bioavailability of verapamil. Monitor the patient for lack of effect.

## CONTRAINDICATIONS

Contraindicated in patients with hypersensitivity to the drug; severe left ventricular dysfunction; cardiogenic shock; second- or third-degree AV block or sick sinus syndrome except in presence of functioning pacemaker; atrial flutter or fibrillation and accessory bypass tract syndrome; severe CHF (unless secondary to verapamil therapy); and severe hypotension. In addition, I.V. verapamil is contraindicated in patients receiving I.V. beta-adrenergic blocking agents and in those with ventricular tachycardia.

## NURSING CONSIDERATIONS

• Use cautiously in elderly patients; in patients with increased intracranial pressure; and in patients with hepatic or renal disease.

• Although the drug should be taken with food, be aware that taking extended-release tablets with food may decrease rate and extent of absorption but allows smaller fluctuations of peak and trough blood levels.

• Patients with severely compromised cardiac function or those receiving beta blockers should receive lower doses of verapamil. Monitor these patients closely.

• **I.V. use:** Give by direct injection into a vein or into the tubing of a free-flowing, compatible I.V. solution. Compatible solutions include $D_5W$ and 0.45%, 0.9% sodium chloride, Ringer's, and lactated Ringer's solutions. Administer I.V. doses over at least 3 minutes to minimize the risk of adverse reactions.

• All patients receiving I.V. verapamil should be on a cardiac monitor. Monitor the R-R interval.

• Be aware that if verapamil is being used to terminate supraventricular tachycardia, the doctor may have the patient perform vagal maneuvers after receiving drug.

• Monitor blood pressure at the start of therapy and during dosage adjustments. Assist the patient with ambulation because dizziness may occur.

• Notify the doctor if signs of CHF, such as swelling of hands and feet or shortness of breath, occur.

• Monitor liver function during prolonged treatment, as ordered.

### ☑ PATIENT TEACHING

• Instruct the patient to take oral form of drug exactly as prescribed.

• Tell the patient to take drug with food.

• If the patient is kept on nitrate therapy during titration of oral verapamil dosage, urge continued compliance. Sublingual nitroglycerin, especially, may be taken as needed when anginal symptoms are acute.

• Encourage the patient to increase fluid and fiber intake to combat constipation. Administer a stool softener as ordered.

# 23
## Antihypertensives

acebutolol
amlodipine besylate
  (See Chapter 22, ANTIANGINALS.)
atenolol
benazepril hydrochloride
betaxolol hydrochloride
bisoprolol fumarate
captopril
carteolol
clonidine
clonidine hydrochloride
diazoxide
diltiazem hydrochloride
  (See Chapter 22, ANTIANGINALS.)
doxazosin mesylate
enalaprilat
enalapril maleate
felodipine
fosinopril sodium
guanabenz acetate
guanadrel sulfate
guanethidine monosulfate
guanfacine hydrochloride
hydralazine hydrochloride
isradipine
labetalol hydrochloride
lisinopril
losartan potassium
methyldopa
methyldopate hydrochloride
metoprolol succinate
metoprolol tartrate
minoxidil
moexipril hydrochloride
nadolol
  (See Chapter 22, ANTIANGINALS.)
nicardipine
  (See Chapter 22, ANTIANGINALS.)
nifedipine
  (See Chapter 22, ANTIANGINALS.)
nisoldipine
nitroprusside sodium
penbutolol sulfate
phentolamine mesylate
pindolol
prazosin hydrochloride

propranolol hydrochloride
  (See Chapter 22, ANTIANGINALS.)
quinapril hydrochloride
ramipril
rauwolfia serpentina
rescinnamine
reserpine
terazosin hydrochloride
timolol maleate
trimethaphan camsylate
verapamil hydrochloride
  (See Chapter 22, ANTIANGINALS.)

**COMBINATION PRODUCTS**
ALDOCLOR-150: chlorothiazide 150 mg and methyldopa 250 mg.
ALDOCLOR-250: chlorothiazide 250 mg and methyldopa 250 mg.
ALDORIL-15: hydrochlorothiazide 15 mg and methyldopa 250 mg.
ALDORIL-25: hydrochlorothiazide 25 mg and methyldopa 250 mg.
ALDORIL D30: hydrochlorothiazide 30 mg and methyldopa 500 mg.
ALDORIL D50: hydrochlorothiazide 50 mg and methyldopa 500 mg.
APRESAZIDE 25/25: hydrochlorothiazide 25 mg and hydralazine hydrochloride 25 mg.
APRESAZIDE 50/50: hydrochlorothiazide 50 mg and hydralazine hydrochloride 50 mg.
APRESAZIDE 100/50: hydrochlorothiazide 50 mg and hydralazine hydrochloride 100 mg.
APRESODEX: hydrochlorothiazide 15 mg and hydralazine hydrochloride 25 mg.
APRESOLINE-ESIDRIX: hydrochlorothiazide 15 mg and hydralazine hydrochloride 25 mg.
CAM-AP-ES: hydrochlorothiazide 15 mg, hydralazine hydrochloride 25 mg, and reserpine 0.1 mg.
CAPOZIDE 25/15: hydrochlorothiazide 15 mg and captopril 25 mg.

Reactions may be *common,* uncommon, *life-threatening,* or COMMON AND LIFE-THREATENING.

CAPOZIDE 25/25: hydrochlorothiazide 25 mg and captopril 25 mg.

CAPOZIDE 50/15: hydrochlorothiazide 15 mg and captopril 50 mg.

CAPOZIDE 50/25: hydrochlorothiazide 25 mg and captopril 50 mg.

CHERAPAS: hydrochlorothiazide 15 mg, hydralazine hydrochloride 25 mg, and reserpine 0.1 mg.

COMBIPRES 0.1: chlorthalidone 15 mg and clonidine hydrochloride 0.1 mg.

COMBIPRES 0.2: chlorthalidone 15 mg and clonidine hydrochloride 0.2 mg.

CORZIDE: nadolol 40 mg or 80 mg and bendroflumethiazide 5 mg.

DEMI-REGROTON: chlorthalidone 25 mg and reserpine 0.125 mg.

DIUPRES-250: chlorothiazide 250 mg and reserpine 0.125 mg.

DIUPRES-500: chlorothiazide 500 mg and reserpine 0.125 mg.

DIURESE-R: trichlormethiazide 4 mg and reserpine 0.1 mg.

DIURIGEN WITH RESERPINE: chlorothiazide 250 mg and reserpine 0.125 mg.

DIUTENSEN-R: methyclothiazide 2.5 mg and reserpine 0.1 mg.

ESIMIL: hydrochlorothiazide 25 mg and guanethidine monosulfate 10 mg.

EXNA-R TABLETS: benzthiazide 50 mg and reserpine 0.125 mg.

H.H.R.: hydrochlorothiazide 15 mg, hydralazine hydrochloride 25 mg, and reserpine 0.1 mg.

HYDROMOX-R: quinethazone 50 mg and reserpine 0.125 mg.

HYDROPINE: hydroflumethiazide 25 mg and reserpine 0.125 mg.

HYDROPINE HP: hydroflumethiazide 50 mg and reserpine 0.125 mg.

HYDROPRES-25: hydrochlorothiazide 25 mg and reserpine 0.125 mg.

HYDRO-RESERP: hydrochlorothiazide 25 or 50 mg and reserpine 0.125 mg.

HYDRO-SERP: hydrochlorothiazide 25 or 50 mg and reserpine 0.125 mg.

HYDROSERPINE: hydrochlorothiazide 25 or 50 mg and reserpine 0.125 mg.

HYDROTENSIN-25 TABLETS: hydrochlorothiazide 25 mg and reserpine 0.125 mg.

HYZAAR: losartan 50 mg and hydrochlorothiazide 12.5 mg.

INDERIDE 40/25: propranolol hydrochloride 40 mg and hydrochlorothiazide 25 mg.

INDERIDE 80/25: propranolol hydrochloride 80 mg and hydrochlorothiazide 25 mg.

INDERIDE LA 80/50: propranolol hydrochloride 80 mg and hydrochlorothiazide 50 mg.

INDERIDE LA 120/50: propranolol hydrochloride 120 mg and hydrochlorothiazide 50 mg.

INDERIDE LA 160/50: propranolol hydrochloride 160 mg and hydrochlorothiazide 50 mg.

LOPRESSOR HCT 50/25: metoprolol tartrate 50 mg and hydrochlorothiazide 25 mg.

LOPRESSOR HCT 100/25: metoprolol tartrate 100 mg and hydrochlorothiazide 25 mg.

LOPRESSOR HCT 100/50: metoprolol tartrate 100 mg and hydrochlorothiazide 50 mg.

MAXZIDE: triamterene 75 mg and hydrochlorothiazide 50 mg.

METATENSIN TABLETS #2 or #4: trichlormethiazide 2 or 4 mg and reserpine 0.1 mg.

MINIZIDE 1: polythiazide 0.5 mg and prazosin hydrochloride 1 mg.

MINIZIDE 2: polythiazide 0.5 mg and prazosin hydrochloride 2 mg.

MINIZIDE 5: polythiazide 0.5 mg and prazosin hydrochloride 5 mg.

NAQUIVAL: trichlormethiazide 4 mg and reserpine 0.1 mg.

NORMOZIDE 100/25: labetalol hydrochloride 100 mg and hydrochlorothiazide 25 mg.

NORMOZIDE 200/25: labetalol hydrochloride 200 mg and hydrochlorothiazide 25 mg.

NORMOZIDE 300/25: labetalol hydrochloride 300 mg and hydrochlorothiazide 25 mg.

PRINZIDE 10-12.5: lisinopril 10 mg and hydrochlorothiazide 12.5 mg.
PRINZIDE 20-12.5: lisinopril 20 mg and hydrochlorothiazide 12.5 mg.
PRINZIDE 20-25: lisinopril 20 mg and hydrochlorothiazide 25 mg.
RAUZIDE**: bendroflumethiazide 4 mg and powdered rauwolfia serpentina 50 mg.
REGROTON: chlorthalidone 50 mg and reserpine 0.25 mg.
RENESE-R: polythiazide 2 mg and reserpine 0.25 mg.
REZIDE: hydrochlorothiazide 15 mg, hydralazine hydrochloride 25 mg, and reserpine 0.1 mg.
R-HCTZ-H: hydrochlorothiazide 15 mg, hydralazine hydrochloride 25 mg, and reserpine 0.1 mg.
SALUTENSIN: hydroflumethiazide 50 mg and reserpine 0.125 mg.
SALUTENSIN DEMI: hydroflumethiazide 25 mg and reserpine 0.125 mg.
SER-A-GEN: hydrochlorothiazide 15 mg, hydralazine hydrochloride 25 mg, and reserpine 0.1 mg.
SERALAZIDE: hydrochlorothiazide 15 mg, hydralazine hydrochloride 25 mg, and reserpine 0.1 mg.
SER-AP-ES: hydrochlorothiazide 15 mg, reserpine 0.1 mg, and hydralazine hydrochloride 25 mg.
SERPASIL-APRESOLINE #1**: reserpine 0.1 mg and hydralazine hydrochloride 25 mg.
SERPASIL-APRESOLINE #2: reserpine 0.2 mg and hydralazine hydrochloride 50 mg.
SERPASIL-ESIDRIX #1: hydrochlorothiazide 25 mg and reserpine 0.1 mg (Serpasil-Esidrix 25 in Canada).
SERPASIL ESIDRIX #2: hydrochlorothiazide 50 mg and reserpine 0.1 mg.
SERPAZIDE: hydrochlorothiazide 15 mg, hydralazine hydrochloride 25 mg, and reserpine 0.1 mg.
TENORETIC 50: atenolol 50 mg and chlorthalidone 25 mg.
TENORETIC 100: atenolol 100 mg and chlorthalidone 25 mg.

TIMOLIDE 10/25: timolol maleate 10 mg and hydrochlorothiazide 25 mg.
TRI-HYDROSERPINE: hydrochlorothiazide 15 mg, hydralazine hydrochloride 25 mg, and reserpine 0.1 mg.
UNIPRES: hydrochlorothiazide 15 mg, reserpine 0.1 mg, and hydralazine hydrochloride 25 mg.
VASERETIC: enalapril maleate 10 mg and hydrochlorothiazide 25 mg.
ZESTORETIC 20-12.5: lisinopril 20 mg and hydrochlorothiazide 12.5 mg
ZESTORETIC 20-25: lisinopril and hydrochlorothiazide 25 mg
ZIAC: bisoprolol fumarate 2.5 mg, 5 mg, or 10 mg and hydrochlorothiazide 6.5 mg.

---

## acebutolol
Monitant, Sectral

*Pregnancy Risk Category: B*

**HOW SUPPLIED**
*Capsules:* 200 mg, 400 mg

**ACTION**
Antihypertensive action is unknown. Possible mechanisms include reduced cardiac output, decreased sympathetic outflow to peripheral vasculature, and inhibition of renin release. Antiarrhythmic action decreases myocardial contractility and decreases heart rate. Drug has mild intrinsic sympathomimetic activity.

**ONSET, PEAK, DURATION**
Onset occurs within 1 to 1½ hours. Peak plasma levels of parent drug occur within 2½ hours; of active metabolite, in about 3½ hours. Effects persist up to 24 hours.

**INDICATIONS & DOSAGE**
*Hypertension –*
**Adults:** 400 mg P.O. either as a single daily dose or in divided doses b.i.d. Patients may receive as much as 1,200 mg daily.
*Suppression of PVCs –*

---

Reactions may be *common,* uncommon, *life-threatening,* or COMMON AND LIFE-THREATENING.

**Adults:** 400 mg P.O. daily divided b.i.d. Dosage increased to provide an adequate clinical response. Usual dosage is 600 to 1,200 mg daily. In patients with impaired renal function, dosage is reduced. Elderly patients may require lower dosage; dosage should not exceed 800 mg daily.

## ADVERSE REACTIONS
**CNS:** *fatigue,* headache, dizziness, insomnia, depression.
**CV:** chest pain, edema, bradycardia, **CHF,** hypotension.
**GI:** nausea, constipation, diarrhea, dyspepsia, flatulence.
**Respiratory:** dyspnea, ***bronchospasm,*** cough.
**Skin:** rash.
**Other:** arthralgia, myalgia.

## INTERACTIONS
*Catecholamine-depleting drugs (such as reserpine):* effects may be additive. Monitor closely.
*Digitalis glycosides, diltiazem, verapamil:* excessive bradycardia and increased depressant effect on myocardium. Use together cautiously.
*Diuretics, other antihypertensive agents:* increased hypotensive effect. Use together cautiously.
*Insulin, oral antidiabetic agents:* can alter dosage requirements in previously stabilized diabetic patients. Observe the patient carefully.
*NSAIDs:* decreased antihypertensive effect. Monitor blood pressure and adjust dosage.
*Sympathomimetic agents:* effects antagonized by acebutolol. Greater than usual dosages of beta-adrenergic agonist bronchodilators may be required.

## CONTRAINDICATIONS
Contraindicated in patients with persistent severe bradycardia, second- and third-degree heart block, overt cardiac failure, and cardiogenic shock.

## NURSING CONSIDERATIONS
• Use cautiously in those with cardiac failure, peripheral vascular disease, bronchospastic disease, and diabetes.
• Check apical pulse before giving drug; if slower than 60 beats/minute, withhold drug and call the doctor. Also monitor blood pressure.
• Before surgery, tell the anesthesiologist that the patient is taking this drug.
• Be aware that acebutolol may mask signs of hyperthyroidism.

## ☑ PATIENT TEACHING
• Instruct patient to take drug exactly as prescribed.
• Warn patient not to discontinue drug suddenly, but to notify the doctor of unpleasant adverse reactions.
• Teach patient how to take his pulse and instruct him to withhold the dose and notify doctor if pulse rate is below 60 beats/minute.

---

# atenolol
Apo-Atenolol†, Noten‡, Nu-Atenol†, Tenormin

*Pregnancy Risk Category: D*

## HOW SUPPLIED
*Tablets:* 25 mg, 50 mg, 100 mg
*Injection:* 5 mg/10 ml

## ACTION
A beta-adrenergic blocker that selectively blocks beta$_1$-adrenergic receptors; decreases cardiac output, peripheral resistance, and cardiac oxygen consumption; and depresses renin secretion.

## ONSET, PEAK, DURATION
Onset occurs 5 minutes after I.V. injection, 1 hour after oral administration. Peak effects occur 2 to 4 hours after oral dose or 5 minutes after direct I.V. injection. Effects persist less than 12 hours after I.V. dose or 24 hours after oral dose.

---

*Liquid form contains alcohol.   **May contain tartrazine.   †Canada only.   ‡Australia only.   ◊OTC.

## INDICATIONS & DOSAGE
*Hypertension –*
**Adults:** initially, 50 mg P.O. daily as a single dose, increased to 100 mg once daily after 7 to 14 days. Dosages over 100 mg are unlikely to produce further benefit. Adjust dosage in patients with creatinine clearance below 35 ml/minute.
*Angina pectoris –*
**Adults:** 50 mg P.O. once daily, increased as needed to 100 mg daily after 7 days for optimal effect. Maximum dosage is 200 mg daily.
*To reduce cardiovascular mortality and risk of reinfarction in patients with acute MI –*
**Adults:** 5 mg I.V. over 5 minutes, followed by another 5 mg 10 minutes later. After an additional 10 minutes, 50 mg P.O., followed by 50 mg P.O. in 12 hours. Thereafter, 100 mg P.O. daily (as a single dose or 50 mg b.i.d.) for at least 7 days.

In patients with renal insufficiency: If creatinine clearance is 15 to 35 ml/minute, a maximum of 50 mg daily; if creatinine clearance is less than 15 ml/minute, maximum dosage is 25 mg daily. Hemodialysis patients require 25 to 50 mg after each dialysis session, but supervise closely because of the risk of hypotension.

## ADVERSE REACTIONS
**CNS:** *fatigue,* lethargy, vertigo, drowsiness, *dizziness.*
**CV:** *bradycardia, hypotension, CHF,* intermittent claudication.
**GI:** nausea, diarrhea.
**Respiratory:** dyspnea, *bronchospasm.*
**Skin:** rash.
**Other:** fever, leg pain.

## INTERACTIONS
*Antihypertensives:* enhanced hypotensive effect. Use together cautiously.
*Digitalis glycosides, diltiazem, verapamil:* excessive bradycardia and increased depressant effect on myocardium. Use together cautiously.

*Insulin, oral antidiabetic agents:* can alter dosage requirements in previously stabilized diabetic patients. Observe the patient carefully.

## CONTRAINDICATIONS
Contraindicated in patients with sinus bradycardia, greater than first-degree heart block, overt cardiac failure, or cardiogenic shock.

## NURSING CONSIDERATIONS
● Use cautiously in patients at risk for CHF and in patients with bronchospastic disease, diabetes, and hyperthyroidism.
● Check apical pulse before giving drug; if slower than 60 beats/minute, withhold drug and call the doctor.
● **I.V. use:** Give by slow I.V. injection, not exceeding 1 mg/minute. I.V. doses may be mixed with $D_5W$, 0.9% sodium chloride, or dextrose and sodium chloride solutions. Solution is stable for 48 hours after mixing.
● Monitor blood pressure.
● ***Alert:*** Know that drug should be withdrawn gradually over 2 weeks to avoid serious adverse reactions.

## ☑ PATIENT TEACHING
● Instruct patient to take drug exactly as prescribed, at the same time every day.
● Caution patient not to stop drug suddenly, but to call the doctor if unpleasant adverse reactions occur.
● Teach patient how to take his pulse. Tell him to withhold drug and call doctor if pulse rate is below 60 beats/minute.
● Tell female patient to notify doctor if pregnancy occurs. Drug will need to be discontinued.

---

## benazepril hydrochloride
Lotensin

*Pregnancy Risk Category: C (D in 2nd and 3rd trimesters)*

---

Reactions may be *common,* uncommon, *life-threatening,* or **COMMON AND LIFE-THREATENING.**

## HOW SUPPLIED
*Tablets:* 5 mg, 10 mg, 20 mg, 40 mg

## ACTION
Benazepril and its active metabolite, benazeprilat, inhibit ACE, preventing conversion of angiotensin I to angiotensin II, a potent vasoconstrictor. Reduced formation of angiotensin II decreases peripheral arterial resistance, thus decreasing aldosterone secretion. This reduces sodium and water retention and lowers blood pressure. Benazepril also has antihypertensive activity in patients with low-renin hypertension.

## ONSET, PEAK, DURATION
Onset occurs within 1 hour. Peak effects occur within 2 to 4 hours. Effects persist for 24 hours.

## INDICATIONS & DOSAGE
*Hypertension –*
**Adults:** In a patient not receiving a diuretic, 10 mg P.O. daily initially. Dosage titrated as needed and tolerated; most patients take 20 to 40 mg daily in one or two doses; a patient receiving a diuretic, 5 mg P.O. daily.

## ADVERSE REACTIONS
**CNS:** headache, dizziness, anxiety, fatigue, insomnia, nervousness, paresthesia.
**CV:** symptomatic hypotension, palpitations.
**EENT:** dysphagia, increased salivation.
**GI:** nausea, vomiting, abdominal pain, constipation.
**Respiratory:** dry, persistent, tickling, nonproductive cough; dyspnea.
**Skin:** hypersensitivity reactions (rash, pruritus).
**Other:** *angioedema,* arthralgia, arthritis, impotence, increased diaphoresis, myalgia, hyperkalemia.

## INTERACTIONS
*Diuretics, other antihypertensives:* risk of excessive hypotension. Discontinue diuretic or lower dose of benazepril as needed.
*Lithium:* increased serum lithium levels and lithium toxicity. Avoid concomitant use.
*Potassium-sparing diuretics, potassium supplements, sodium substitutes containing potassium:* risk of hyperkalemia. Monitor closely.

## CONTRAINDICATIONS
Contraindicated in patients with hypersensitivity to ACE inhibitors.

## NURSING CONSIDERATIONS
• Use cautiously in patients with impaired hepatic or renal function.
• Monitor for hypotension. Excessive hypotension can occur when drug is given with diuretics. If possible, diuretic therapy should be discontinued 2 to 3 days before starting benazepril to decrease potential for excessive hypotensive response. If benazepril does not adequately control blood pressure, diuretic may be reinstituted with care.
• Measure blood pressure when drug levels are at peak (2 to 6 hours after administration) and at trough (just before a dose) to verify adequate blood pressure control.
• Assess renal and hepatic function before and periodically throughout therapy. Monitor serum potassium levels, as ordered.
• Know that other ACE inhibitors have been associated with agranulocytosis and neutropenia. Monitor CBC with differential counts before therapy, every 2 weeks for the first 3 months of therapy, and periodically thereafter.

☑ **PATIENT TEACHING**
• Instruct patient to take this drug on an empty stomach; meals, particularly those high in fat, can impair absorption.

---

*Liquid form contains alcohol.   **May contain tartrazine.   †Canada only.   ‡Australia only.   ◇OTC.

• Tell patient to avoid sodium substitutes; these products may contain potassium, which can cause hyperkalemia in patients taking this drug.
• Light-headedness can occur, especially during the first few days of therapy. Tell patient to rise slowly to minimize this effect and to report symptoms to doctor. Patients who experience syncope should stop taking the drug and call the doctor immediately.
• Tell patient to use caution in hot weather and during exercise. Inadequate fluid intake, vomiting, diarrhea, and excessive perspiration can lead to light-headedness and syncope.
• Advise patient to report signs of infection, such as fever and sore throat. Tell him to call the doctor if the following signs or symptoms occur: easy bruising or bleeding; swelling of tongue, lips, face, eyes, mucous membranes, or extremities; difficulty swallowing or breathing; and hoarseness.
• Tell female patient to notify doctor if pregnancy occurs. Drug will need to be discontinued.

---

## betaxolol hydrochloride
Kerlone

*Pregnancy Risk Category: C*

### HOW SUPPLIED
*Tablets:* 10 mg, 20 mg

### ACTION
Unknown. A selective beta$_1$-adrenergic blocker that decreases blood pressure, possibly by slowing heart rate and decreasing cardiac output.

### ONSET, PEAK, DURATION
Onset occurs within 3 hours. Serum levels peak within 2 to 4 hours after a dose. Peak antihypertensive effects occur after 7 to 14 days of therapy. Effects persist for 24 to 48 hours.

### INDICATIONS & DOSAGE
*Hypertension (used alone or with other antihypertensives) —*
**Adults:** initially, 10 mg P.O. once daily; if necessary, 20 mg P.O. once daily if desired response is not achieved in 7 to 14 days.

### ADVERSE REACTIONS
**CNS:** dizziness, fatigue, headache, insomnia, lethargy, anxiety.
**CV:** bradycardia, chest pain, *CHF,* edema.
**GI:** nausea, diarrhea, dyspepsia.
**Respiratory:** dyspnea, pharyngitis, *bronchospasm.*
**Skin:** rash.
**Other:** impotence, arthralgia.

### INTERACTIONS
*Calcium channel blockers:* increased risk of hypotension, left ventricular failure, and AV conduction disturbances. Use I.V. calcium channel blockers with caution.
*Catecholamine-depleting drugs, reserpine:* may have an additive effect. Monitor closely.
*General anesthetics:* increased hypotensive effects. Observe carefully for excessive hypotension or bradycardia or orthostatic hypotension.
*Lidocaine:* may increase lidocaine's effects.

### CONTRAINDICATIONS
Contraindicated in patients with hypersensitivity to the drug, severe bradycardia, greater than first-degree heart block, cardiogenic shock, or uncontrolled CHF.

### NURSING CONSIDERATIONS
• Use cautiously in patients with CHF controlled by digitalis glycosides and diuretics because these patients may exhibit signs of cardiac decompensation with beta-blocker therapy.
• Monitor blood pressure closely.
• Monitor blood glucose levels regularly in patients with diabetes. Beta

---

Reactions may be *common,* uncommon, *life-threatening,* or COMMON AND LIFE-THREATENING.

blockade may inhibit glycogenolysis as well as the signs and symptoms of hypoglycemia (such as tachycardia and blood pressure changes).
• Know that withdrawal of beta-blocker therapy before surgery is controversial. Some clinicians advocate withdrawal to prevent any impairment of cardiac responsiveness to reflex stimuli and decreased responsiveness to administration of catecholamines. Advise the anesthesiologist that the patient is receiving a beta blocker so that isoproterenol or dobutamine is made readily available for reversal of drug's cardiac effects.
• Beta blockers may mask tachycardia associated with hyperthyroidism. In patients with suspected thyrotoxicosis, withdraw beta blocker gradually, as ordered, to avoid thyroid storm.

☑ **PATIENT TEACHING**
• Instruct patient to take drug exactly as prescribed.
• *Alert:* Advise patient that abrupt discontinuation may precipitate angina pectoris in patients with unrecognized coronary artery disease.
• Emphasize the importance of promptly reporting signs of CHF, including shortness of breath or difficulty breathing, unusually fast heartbeat, cough, or fatigue with exertion.

# bisoprolol fumarate
Zebeta

*Pregnancy Risk Category: C*

**HOW SUPPLIED**
*Tablets:* 5 mg, 10 mg

**ACTION**
Not completely defined. Bisoprolol is a beta$_1$-selective blocker that decreases myocardial contractility, heart rate, and cardiac output; lowers blood pressure; and reduces myocardial oxygen consumption.

**ONSET, PEAK, DURATION**
Onset unknown. Peak effects occur within 2 to 4 hours. Effects last about 24 hours.

**INDICATIONS & DOSAGE**
*Hypertension (used alone or in combination with other antihypertensives)* –
**Adults:** initially, 5 mg P.O. once daily. If response is inadequate, increase to 10 mg once daily or to 20 mg P.O. daily if needed. Maximum recommended dosage is 20 mg daily.
For patients with renal or hepatic impairment, 2.5 mg P.O. daily initially. Subsequent dosage titration is done cautiously.

**ADVERSE REACTIONS**
**CNS:** asthenia, fatigue, dizziness, *headache,* hypoesthesia, vivid dreams, depression, insomnia.
**CV:** bradycardia, peripheral edema, chest pain.
**EENT:** pharyngitis, rhinitis, sinusitis.
**GI:** nausea, vomiting, diarrhea, dry mouth.
**Respiratory:** cough, dyspnea.
**Other:** arthralgia, asthenia.

**INTERACTIONS**
*NSAIDs:* decreased antihypertensive effect. Monitor blood pressure and adjust dosage.

**CONTRAINDICATIONS**
Contraindicated in patients with hypersensitivity to the drug and in those with cardiogenic shock, overt cardiac failure, marked sinus bradycardia, or second- or third-degree AV block.

**NURSING CONSIDERATIONS**
• Use cautiously in patients with bronchospastic disease. In general, these patients should avoid beta-adrenergic blockers because blockade of pulmonary beta$_2$-receptors may result in worsening of symptoms. For patients who cannot tolerate or do not respond to other antihypertensives,

---

bisoprolol is given in low doses, starting with 2.5 mg P.O. daily. Know that bisoprolol blocks beta$_2$-receptors in higher doses (20 mg daily or more).
• Also use cautiously in patients with diabetes, peripheral vascular disease, or thyroid disease and in those with a history of heart failure.
• Monitor blood pressure frequently.
• Monitor blood glucose levels in diabetic patients closely. Beta blockers may mask some manifestations of hypoglycemia, such as tachycardia. Nonselective beta blockers can potentiate insulin-induced hypoglycemia and delay recovery of serum glucose levels. Because bisoprolol is a selective agent, this problem is minimal.
• Know that drug must be withdrawn gradually over 1 to 2 weeks.

☑ **PATIENT TEACHING**
• Explain the importance of taking drug as prescribed, even when he's feeling well.
• Tell the patient not to stop drug suddenly but to call the doctor if unpleasant adverse reactions occur.
• Tell the patient to check with the doctor or pharmacist before taking OTC medications.

---

## captopril
Apo-Capto†, Capoten, Novo-Captopril†, Syn-Captopril†

*Pregnancy Risk Category: C (D in 2nd and 3rd trimesters)*

### HOW SUPPLIED
*Tablets:* 12.5 mg, 25 mg, 50 mg, 100 mg

### ACTION
Not clearly defined. Thought to inhibit ACE, preventing conversion of angiotensin I to angiotensin II, a potent vasoconstrictor. Reduced formation of angiotensin II decreases peripheral arterial resistance, thus decreasing aldosterone secretion. This reduces sodium and water retention and lowers blood pressure.

### ONSET, PEAK, DURATION
Onset occurs in 15 to 60 minutes; peak effects, in 30 to 90 minutes. Effects persist for 6 to 12 hours.

### INDICATIONS & DOSAGE
*Hypertension –*
**Adults:** 25 mg P.O. b.i.d. or t.i.d. initially. If blood pressure isn't satisfactorily controlled in 1 to 2 weeks, dosage increased to 50 mg b.i.d. or t.i.d. If not satisfactorily controlled after another 1 to 2 weeks, expect a diuretic to be added. If further blood pressure reduction is necessary, dosage may be raised to 150 mg t.i.d. while continuing the diuretic. Maximum dosage is 450 mg daily.
*CHF; to reduce risk of death and to slow development of heart failure after MI –*
**Adults:** 6.25 to 12.5 mg P.O. t.i.d. initially. Gradually increased to 50 mg t.i.d. as needed. Maximum daily dosage is 450 mg.
*Diabetic nephropathy –*
**Adults:** 25 mg P.O. t.i.d.

### ADVERSE REACTIONS
**CNS:** dizziness, fainting, headache, malaise, fatigue.
**CV:** *tachycardia, hypotension,* angina pectoris.
**GI:** anorexia, *dysgeusia,* nausea, vomiting, abdominal pain, constipation, dry mouth.
**Hematologic:** *leukopenia, agranulocytosis, pancytopenia,* anemia, *thrombocytopenia.*
**Hepatic:** transient increase in hepatic enzymes.
**Respiratory:** *dry, persistent, tickling, nonproductive cough,* dyspnea.
**Skin:** *urticarial rash, maculopapular rash,* pruritus, alopecia.
**Other:** fever, *angioedema of face and extremities,* hyperkalemia.

---

Reactions may be *common,* uncommon, *life-threatening,* or COMMON AND LIFE-THREATENING.

## INTERACTIONS
*Antacids:* decreased captopril effect. Separate administration times.
*Digitalis glycosides:* may increase serum digoxin concentration by 15% to 30%.
*Diuretics, other antihypertensives:* risk of excessive hypotension. Diuretic may need to be discontinued or captopril dosage lowered.
*Insulin, oral antidiabetic agents:* risk of hypoglycemia when captopril therapy is initiated. Monitor closely.
*Lithium:* increased lithium levels and symptoms of toxicity may occur. Monitor patient closely.
*NSAIDs:* may reduce antihypertensive effect. Monitor blood pressure.
*Potassium supplements, potassium-sparing diuretics:* increased risk of hyperkalemia. Avoid these agents unless hypokalemic blood levels are confirmed.

## CONTRAINDICATIONS
Contraindicated in patients with hypersensitivity to the drug or any other ACE inhibitor.

## NURSING CONSIDERATIONS
• Use cautiously in patients with impaired renal function or serious autoimmune disease (particularly systemic lupus erythematosus) or in patients who have been exposed to other drugs known to affect WBC counts or immune response.
• Monitor the patient's blood pressure and pulse rate frequently.
• **Alert:** Be aware that elderly patients may be more sensitive to the drug's hypotensive effects.
• Monitor WBC and differential counts before starting treatment, every 2 weeks for the first 3 months of therapy, and periodically thereafter, as ordered.

## ☑ PATIENT TEACHING
• Instruct patient to take this medication 1 hour before meals; food in the GI tract may reduce absorption.
• Inform patient that light-headedness can occur, especially during the first few days of therapy. Tell patient to rise slowly to minimize this effect and to report symptoms to the doctor. If he experiences syncope, he should stop taking the drug and call the doctor immediately.
• Tell patient to use caution in hot weather and during exercise. Inadequate fluid intake, vomiting, diarrhea, and excessive perspiration can lead to light-headedness and syncope.
• Advise patient to report signs of infection, such as fever and sore throat.
• Tell female patient to notify doctor if pregnancy occurs. Drug will need to be discontinued.

---

## carteolol
Cartrol

*Pregnancy Risk Category: C*

### HOW SUPPLIED
*Tablets:* 2.5 mg, 5 mg

### ACTION
Unknown. Carteolol is a nonselective beta-adrenergic blocker with intrinsic sympathomimetic activity. Its antihypertensive effects are probably caused by decreased sympathetic outflow from the brain and decreased cardiac output. Carteolol does not have a consistent effect on renin output.

### ONSET, PEAK, DURATION
Onset and duration unknown. Serum levels peak within 1 to 3 hours.

### INDICATIONS & DOSAGE
*Hypertension –*
**Adults:** initially, 2.5 mg P.O. as a single daily dose; gradually increased to 5 or 10 mg as a single daily dose as needed. Dosages that exceed 10 mg

---

*Liquid form contains alcohol. **May contain tartrazine. †Canada only. ‡Australia only. ◇OTC.

daily do not produce a greater response and may actually decrease it.

In patients with substantial renal failure: If creatinine clearance is more than 60 ml/minute, give drug at 24-hour intervals; if 20 to 60 ml/minute, at 48-hour intervals; if less than 20 ml/minute, at 72-hour intervals.

## ADVERSE REACTIONS
**CNS:** lassitude, fatigue, somnolence, *asthenia,* paresthesia.
**CV:** conduction disturbances.
**GI:** diarrhea, nausea, abdominal pain.
**Other:** *muscle cramps,* arthralgia, rash.

## INTERACTIONS
*Calcium channel blockers:* increased risk of hypotension, left ventricular failure, and AV conduction disturbances. Use I.V. calcium antagonists with caution.
*Catecholamine-depleting drugs, reserpine:* may have an additive effect. Monitor closely.
*Digitalis glycosides:* may produce additive effects on slowing AV node conduction. Avoid concomitant use.
*General anesthetics:* increased hypotensive effects. Observe carefully for excessive hypotension or bradycardia or orthostatic hypotension.
*Insulin, oral antidiabetic agents:* may alter hypoglycemic response. Adjust dosage as necessary.

## CONTRAINDICATIONS
Contraindicated in patients with bronchial asthma, severe bradycardia, greater than first-degree heart block, cardiogenic shock, or uncontrolled CHF.

## NURSING CONSIDERATIONS
• Use cautiously in patients with CHF controlled by digitalis glycosides and diuretics because these patients may exhibit signs of cardiac decompensation with beta-blocker therapy.
• Monitor blood pressure frequently.

• Know that beta blockade may inhibit glycogenolysis and the signs and symptoms of hypoglycemia (such as tachycardia and blood pressure changes). It may also attenuate insulin release. Monitor blood glucose levels frequently.
• Know that withdrawal of beta-blocker therapy before surgery is controversial. Some clinicians advocate withdrawal to prevent any impairment of cardiac responsiveness to reflex stimuli and decreased responsiveness to administration of catecholamines. However, the beta-blocking effects of carteolol may persist for weeks, and discontinuing drug before surgery may be impractical. Advise the anesthesiologist that the patient is receiving a beta blocker so that isoproterenol or dobutamine is made readily available for reversal of the drug's cardiac effects.
• Beta blockers may mask tachycardia associated with hyperthyroidism. In patients with suspected thyrotoxicosis, gradually withdraw beta blocker therapy, as ordered, to avoid thyroid storm.
• **Alert:** Be aware that patients with unrecognized coronary artery disease may exhibit signs of angina pectoris on withdrawal of drug. Monitor closely.

## ☑ PATIENT TEACHING
• Instruct patient to take drug exactly as prescribed.
• Tell patient not to stop drug suddenly but to call doctor and discuss unpleasant adverse reactions.
• Emphasize the importance of reporting signs of CHF, including shortness of breath or difficulty breathing, unusually fast heartbeat, cough, or fatigue with exertion.

---

Reactions may be *common,* uncommon, *life-threatening,* or **COMMON AND LIFE-THREATENING.**

# clonidine
Catapres-TTS

## clonidine hydrochloride
Catapres, Dixarit†‡

*Pregnancy Risk Category: C*

## HOW SUPPLIED
**clonidine**
*Transdermal:* TTS-1 (releases 0.1 mg/
24 hours), TTS-2 (releases 0.2 mg/24
hours), TTS-3 (releases 0.3 mg/24
hours)
**clonidine hydrochloride**
*Tablets:* 0.025 mg†‡, 0.1 mg, 0.2 mg,
0.3 mg

## ACTION
Unknown. Thought to inhibit the central vasomotor centers, thereby decreasing sympathetic outflow to the heart, kidneys, and peripheral vasculature; this results in decreased peripheral vascular resistance, decreased systolic and diastolic blood pressure, and decreased heart rate.

## ONSET, PEAK, DURATION
Onset occurs within 15 to 30 minutes after oral administration, 2 to 3 days after transdermal application. Peak effects occur within 1.5 to 2.5 hours after oral dose, about 2 to 3 days after transdermal application. Effects persist for 6 to 8 hours after an oral dose and decline over several days after transdermal system removal.

## INDICATIONS & DOSAGE
*Essential, renal, and malignant hypertension –*
**Adults:** initially, 0.1 mg P.O. b.i.d. Then increased by 0.1 to 0.2 mg daily on a weekly basis. Usual dosage range is 0.2 to 0.8 mg daily in divided doses; infrequently, dosages as high as 2.4 mg daily are used.

Or, a transdermal patch is applied to a nonhairy area of intact skin on the upper arm or torso once every 7 days,
starting with 0.1-mg system and titrated with another 0.1-mg system or larger system.

## ADVERSE REACTIONS
**CNS:** *drowsiness, dizziness,* fatigue, *sedation, weakness,* malaise, agitation, depression.
**CV:** orthostatic hypotension, bradycardia, *severe rebound hypertension.*
**GI:** *constipation, dry mouth,* nausea, vomiting, anorexia.
**GU:** urine retention, impotence, loss of libido.
**Skin:** *pruritus, dermatitis* (with transdermal patch), rash.
**Other:** weight gain.

## INTERACTIONS
*CNS depressants:* enhanced CNS depression. Use together cautiously.
*Diuretics, other antihypertensive agents:* increased hypotensive effect. Monitor closely.
*MAO inhibitors, tricyclic antidepressants:* may decrease antihypertensive effect. Use together cautiously.
*Propranolol, other beta blockers:* paradoxical hypertensive response. Monitor carefully.

## CONTRAINDICATIONS
Contraindicated in patients with hypersensitivity to the drug. Transdermal form is contraindicated in patients with hypersensitivity to any component of the adhesive layer of the transdermal system.

## NURSING CONSIDERATIONS
• Use cautiously in patients with severe coronary insufficiency, recent MI, cerebrovascular disease, chronic renal failure, or impaired liver function.
• Know that clonidine may be given to rapidly lower blood pressure in some hypertensive emergencies.
• Monitor blood pressure and pulse rate frequently. Dosage is usually adjusted to patient's blood pressure and tolerance.

• Elderly patients may be more sensitive to drug's hypotensive effects.
• Observe for patient tolerance to drug's therapeutic effects, which may require increased dosage.
• Antihypertensive effects of transdermal clonidine may take 2 to 3 days to become apparent. Oral antihypertensive therapy may have to be continued in the interim.
• **Alert:** Remove transdermal patch before defibrillation to prevent arcing.
• When stopping therapy in patients receiving both clonidine and a beta blocker, gradually withdraw the beta blocker first to minimize adverse reactions, as ordered.
• Be aware that discontinuation for surgery is not recommended.

☑ **PATIENT TEACHING**
• Instruct the patient to take drug exactly as prescribed.
• Advise the patient that abrupt discontinuation of drug may cause severe rebound hypertension. Tell him dosage must be reduced gradually over 2 to 4 days as instructed by doctor.
• Tell the patient to take the last dose immediately before retiring.
• Reassure the patient that the transdermal patch usually adheres despite showering and other routine daily activities. Instruct him on the use of the adhesive "overlay" to provide additional skin adherence if necessary. Also tell the patient to place the patch at a different site each week.
• Caution the patient that drug may cause drowsiness but that tolerance to this adverse effect will develop.
• Inform the patient that orthostatic hypotension can be minimized by rising slowly and avoiding sudden position changes.

---

**diazoxide**
Hyperstat IV

*Pregnancy Risk Category: C*

**HOW SUPPLIED**
*Injection:* 300 mg/20 ml, 15 mg/ml

**ACTION**
Exact antihypertensive action unknown. Directly relaxes arteriolar smooth muscle and decreases peripheral vascular resistance.

**ONSET, PEAK, DURATION**
Onset occurs within 1 minute after I.V. bolus. Peak effects occur within 2 to 5 minutes after I.V. bolus. Effects persist 2 to 12 hours.

**INDICATIONS & DOSAGE**
*Hypertensive crisis –*
**Adults and children:** 1 to 3 mg/kg by I.V. bolus (up to a maximum of 150 mg) q 5 to 15 minutes until adequate response is seen. Repeat at 4- to 24-hour intervals as needed.

**ADVERSE REACTIONS**
**CNS:** *headache,* dizziness, lightheadedness, weakness, *seizures, paralysis,* euphoria, *cerebral ischemia.*
**CV:** *sodium and water retention, orthostatic hypotension,* diaphoresis, flushing, warmth, angina, myocardial ischemia, *arrhythmias,* ECG changes, *shock, MI.*
**GI:** *nausea, vomiting,* abdominal discomfort, dry mouth, constipation, diarrhea.
**Other:** inflammation and pain resulting from extravasation, *hyperglycemia,* hyperuricemia, optic nerve infarction.

**INTERACTIONS**
*Antihypertensives, such as hydralazine:* may cause severe hypotension. Use together cautiously.
*Thiazide diuretics:* may increase diazoxide's effects. Use together cautiously.

**CONTRAINDICATIONS**
Contraindicated in patients with hypersensitivity to the drug, other thia-

---

Reactions may be *common,* uncommon, ***life-threatening,*** or **COMMON AND LIFE-THREATENING.**

zides, or other sulfonamide-derived drugs. Also contraindicated in the treatment of compensatory hypertension (such as that associated with coarctation of the aorta or arteriovenous shunt).

## NURSING CONSIDERATIONS
• Use cautiously in patients with impaired cerebral or cardiac function or uremia.
• **I.V. use:** Monitor blood pressure and ECG continuously. Place the patient in the supine position or in Trendelenburg's position during and for 1 hour after infusion. Notify the doctor immediately if severe hypotension develops. Keep norepinephrine available.
• Protect I.V. solutions from light. Darkened I.V. solutions of diazoxide are subpotent and should not be used.
• Take care to avoid extravasation.
• Check the patient's standing blood pressure before discontinuing close monitoring for hypotension.
• Monitor the patient's fluid intake and output carefully. If fluid or sodium retention develops, the doctor may order diuretics.
• Weigh the patient daily and notify the doctor of any weight increase.
• Diazoxide may alter requirements for insulin, diet, or oral antidiabetic agents in previously controlled diabetic patients. Monitor blood glucose daily; watch for signs of severe hyperglycemia or hyperosmolar nonketotic syndrome. Insulin may be needed.
• Check uric acid levels frequently and report abnormalities to the doctor.

## ☑ PATIENT TEACHING
• Inform the patient that orthostatic hypotension can be minimized by rising slowly and avoiding sudden position changes. Instruct the patient to remain in the supine position for 30 minutes after injection.
• Tell the patient to alert nurse if discomfort occurs at I.V. insertion site.

## doxazosin mesylate
Cardura
*Pregnancy Risk Category: C*

### HOW SUPPLIED
*Tablets:* 1 mg, 2 mg, 4 mg, 8 mg

### ACTION
An alpha-adrenergic blocker that acts on the peripheral vasculature to produce vasodilation.

### ONSET, PEAK, DURATION
Onset occurs in 1 to 2 hours. Peak antihypertensive effect occurs in 5 to 6 hours. Effects persist about 24 hours.

### INDICATIONS & DOSAGE
*Essential hypertension –*
**Adults:** initially, 1 mg P.O. daily and determine effect on standing and supine blood pressure at 2 to 6 hours and 24 hours after dosing. If necessary, dose is increased to 2 mg daily. To minimize adverse reactions, dosage is titrated slowly (dosage typically increased only q 2 weeks). If necessary, dose increased to 4 mg daily, then 8 mg. Maximum daily dosage is 16 mg, but dosage that exceeds 4 mg daily is associated with a greater incidence of adverse reactions.
*Benign prostatic hyperplasia –*
**Adults:** initially, 1 mg P.O. once daily in the morning or evening; may be increased to 2 mg and, thereafter, 4 mg and 8 mg once daily, as needed. The recommended titration interval is 1 to 2 weeks.

### ADVERSE REACTIONS
**CNS:** *dizziness,* vertigo, somnolence, drowsiness, *asthenia, headache.*
**CV:** *orthostatic hypotension,* hypotension, edema, palpitations, ***arrhythmias,*** tachycardia.
**GI:** nausea, vomiting, diarrhea, constipation.
**Skin:** rash, pruritus.
**Other:** rhinitis, arthralgia, myalgia,

pain, dyspnea, pharyngitis, abnormal vision.

## INTERACTIONS
None significant.

## CONTRAINDICATIONS
Contraindicated in patients with hypersensitivity to the drug and quinazoline derivatives (including prazosin and terazosin).

## NURSING CONSIDERATIONS
• Use cautiously in patients with impaired hepatic function.
• Monitor blood pressure closely.
• If syncope occurs, place the patient in a recumbent position and treat supportively. A transient hypotensive response is not considered a contraindication to continued therapy.

## ☑ PATIENT TEACHING
• Instruct patient to take drug exactly as prescribed.
• **Alert:** Advise patient that he is susceptible to a "first-dose" effect similar to that produced by other alpha-adrenergic blockers — marked orthostatic hypotension accompanied by dizziness or syncope. Orthostatic hypotension is most common after first dose but also can occur during dosage adjustment or interruption of therapy. Warn patient that dizziness or fainting may occur. Advise him to avoid driving and other hazardous activities until drug's CNS effects are known.

---

## enalaprilat
Vasotec I.V.

## enalapril maleate
Amprace‡, Renitec‡, Vasotec

*Pregnancy Risk Category: C (D in 2nd and 3rd trimesters)*

## HOW SUPPLIED
**enalaprilat**
*Injection:* 1.25 mg/ml

## enalapril maleate
*Tablets:* 2.5 mg, 5 mg, 10 mg, 20 mg

## ACTION
Unknown, but does inhibit ACE, preventing conversion of angiotensin I to angiotensin II, a potent vasoconstrictor. Reduced formation of angiotensin II decreases peripheral arterial resistance, thus decreasing aldosterone secretion.

## ONSET, PEAK, DURATION
Onset occurs 15 minutes after I.V. injection, 1 hour after oral dose. Peak effects occur 1 to 4 hours after I.V. injection or 4 to 6 hours after oral dose. Effects persist about 6 hours after I.V. injection or 24 hours after oral dose.

## INDICATIONS & DOSAGE
*Hypertension –*
**Adults:** for patient not receiving diuretics, initially 5 mg P.O. once daily, then adjusted according to response. Usual dosage range is 10 to 40 mg daily as a single dose or two divided doses. Alternatively, 1.25 mg I.V. infusion q 6 hours over 5 minutes. For patient on diuretics, initially 2.5 mg P.O. once daily. Alternatively, 0.625 mg I.V. over 5 minutes, repeated in 1 hour if needed, then followed by 1.25 mg I.V. q 6 hours.
*To convert from I.V. therapy to oral therapy –*
**Adults:** initially, 5 mg P.O. once daily; if patient was receiving 0.625 mg I.V., then 2.5 mg P.O. once daily. Dosage is adjusted to response.
*To convert from oral therapy to I.V. therapy –*
**Adults:** 1.25 mg I.V. over 5 minutes q 6 hours. Higher doses have not demonstrated greater efficacy.
*Renal impairment or hyponatremia –*
If serum creatinine is above 1.6 mg/dl or serum sodium is below 130 mEq/L, dosage is initiated at 2.5 mg P.O. daily and titrated slowly.

---

## ADVERSE REACTIONS

**CNS:** *headache, dizziness, fatigue,* vertigo, asthenia, syncope.
**CV:** *hypotension,* chest pain.
**GI:** diarrhea, nausea, abdominal pain, vomiting.
**GU:** decreased renal·function (in patients with bilateral renal artery stenosis or CHF).
**Hematologic:** *neutropenia, agranulocytosis.*
**Respiratory:** *dry, persistent, tickling, nonproductive cough,* dyspnea.
**Skin:** rash.
**Other:** *angioedema.*

## INTERACTIONS

*Insulin, oral antidiabetic agents:* risk of hypoglycemia, especially at initiation of enalapril therapy. Monitor closely.
*Lithium:* lithium toxicity can occur. Monitor lithium levels.
*NSAIDs:* may reduce antihypertensive effect. Monitor blood pressure.
*Potassium supplements, potassium-sparing diuretics:* increased risk of hyperkalemia. Avoid these drugs unless hypokalemic blood levels are confirmed.

## CONTRAINDICATIONS

Contraindicated in patients with hypersensitivity to the drug or history of angioedema related to previous treatment with an ACE inhibitor.

## NURSING CONSIDERATIONS

● Use cautiously in patients with renal impairment.
● **I.V. use:** Inject drug slowly over at least 5 minutes, or dilute in 50 ml of a compatible solution and infuse over 15 minutes. Compatible solutions include $D_5W$, 0.9% sodium chloride injection, dextrose 5% in lactated Ringer's injection, and dextrose 5% in 0.9% sodium chloride injection.
● Monitor blood pressure response to drug closely.
● Monitor CBC with differential

counts before therapy, every 2 weeks for the first 3 months of therapy, and periodically thereafter.
● Diabetic patients, those with impaired renal function or CHF, and those receiving drugs that can increase serum potassium may develop hyperkalemia. Monitor potassium intake and serum potassium level.

## ☑ PATIENT TEACHING

● Advise the patient to report breathing difficulty or swelling of face, eyes, lips, or tongue. Angioedema (including laryngeal edema) may occur, especially after the first dose.
● Advise him to report signs of infection, such as fever and sore throat.
● Advise the patient that light-headedness can occur, especially during the first few days of therapy. Tell the patient to rise slowly to minimize this effect and to report symptoms to the doctor. Patients who experience syncope should stop taking drug and call the doctor immediately.
● Tell the patient to use caution in hot weather and during exercise. Inadequate fluid intake, vomiting, diarrhea, and excessive perspiration can lead to light-headedness and syncope.
● Advise him to avoid sodium substitutes; these products may contain potassium, which can cause hyperkalemia in patients taking this drug.
● Tell the female patient to notify doctor if pregnancy occurs. Drug will need to be discontinued.

---

## felodipine

Agon‡, Agon SR‡, Plendil, Plendil ER‡, Renedil†

*Pregnancy Risk Category: C*

## HOW SUPPLIED

*Tablets:* 5 mg‡
*Tablets (extended-release):* 2.5 mg, 5 mg, 10 mg

---

## ACTION
Unknown. A dihydropyridine-derivative calcium channel blocker that prevents the entry of calcium ions into vascular smooth-muscle and cardiac cells; shows some selectivity for smooth muscle as compared with cardiac muscle.

## ONSET, PEAK, DURATION
Onset occurs within 2 to 5 hours. Plasma levels peak within 2½ to 5 hours. Effects persist for 24 hours.

## INDICATIONS & DOSAGE
*Hypertension* –
**Adults:** initially, 5 mg P.O. daily. Dosage is adjusted according to patient response, generally at intervals not less than 2 weeks. Usual dose is 5 to 10 mg daily; maximum recommended dosage is 20 mg daily.

In elderly patients and patients with impaired hepatic function, 5 mg P.O. is given daily; dosage is adjusted as for adults. Maximum recommended dosage is 10 mg daily.

## ADVERSE REACTIONS
**CNS:** *headache,* dizziness, paresthesia, asthenia.
**CV:** *peripheral edema,* chest pain, palpitations.
**EENT:** rhinorrhea, pharyngitis.
**GI:** abdominal pain, nausea, constipation, diarrhea.
**Respiratory:** upper respiratory infection, cough.
**Skin:** rash, *flushing.*
**Other:** muscle cramps, back pain, gingival hyperplasia.

## INTERACTIONS
*Anticonvulsants:* decreased plasma concentration of felodipine. Avoid concomitant use.
*Cimetidine:* decreased clearance of felodipine. Use lower doses of felodipine.
*Digoxin:* decreased peak levels of digoxin, but total absorbed drug is unchanged. Clinical significance is unknown.
*Metoprolol:* may alter pharmacokinetics of metoprolol. No dosage adjustment appears necessary; monitor for adverse effects.
*Theophylline:* may slightly decrease theophylline levels. Monitor patient's response closely.

## CONTRAINDICATIONS
Contraindicated in patients with hypersensitivity to the drug.

## NURSING CONSIDERATIONS
● Use cautiously in patients with heart failure, particularly those receiving beta-adrenergic blockers, and in patients with impaired hepatic function.
● Monitor blood pressure for response.
● Monitor patient for peripheral edema. Peripheral edema appears to be both dose- and age-dependent: it's more common in patients taking higher doses, especially those over age 60.

### ☑ PATIENT TEACHING
● Tell the patient to swallow tablets whole and not to crush or chew them.
● Teach the patient to continue taking the drug even when he feels better; to watch his diet; and to check with the doctor or pharmacist before taking any other medications, including OTC drugs.
● Advise the patient to observe good oral hygiene and to see a dentist regularly; use of drug has been associated with mild gingival hyperplasia.

---

# fosinopril sodium
Monopril

*Pregnancy Risk Category: C (D in 2nd and 3rd trimesters)*

## HOW SUPPLIED
Tablets: 10 mg, 20 mg

---

Reactions may be *common,* uncommon, *life-threatening,* or **COMMON AND LIFE-THREATENING.**

## ACTION
Antihypertensive action not clearly defined. Inhibits ACE, preventing conversion of angiotensin I to angiotensin II, a potent vasoconstrictor. Reduced formation of angiotensin II decreases peripheral arterial resistance, thus decreasing aldosterone secretion.

## ONSET, PEAK, DURATION
Onset occurs within 1 hour. Serum levels peak in 2 to 6 hours. Effects persist about 24 hours.

## INDICATIONS & DOSAGE
*Hypertension –*
**Adults:** initially, 10 mg P.O. daily. Dosage is adjusted based on blood pressure response at peak and trough levels. Usual dosage is 20 to 40 mg, up to 80 mg daily. Dosage is divided if needed.
*Heart failure –*
**Adults:** initially, 10 mg P.O. once daily. Dosage increased over several weeks to a maximum dosage of 40 mg P.O. daily, if needed. For patients with moderate to severe renal failure or vigorous diuresis, initially, 5 mg P.O. once daily.

## ADVERSE REACTIONS
**CNS:** headache, dizziness, fatigue, syncope, paresthesia, sleep disturbance, *CVA.*
**CV:** chest pain, angina, *MI, hypertensive crisis,* rhythm disturbances, palpitations, hypotension, orthostatic hypotension.
**EENT:** tinnitus, sinusitis.
**GI:** nausea, vomiting, diarrhea, pancreatitis, hepatitis, dry mouth, abdominal distention, abdominal pain, constipation.
**GU:** sexual dysfunction, decreased libido, renal insufficiency.
**Respiratory:** *dry, persistent, tickling, nonproductive cough; bronchospasm.*
**Skin:** urticaria, rash, photosensitivity, pruritus.

**Other:** *angioedema,* arthralgia, musculoskeletal pain, myalgia, gout, hyperkalemia.

## INTERACTIONS
*Antacids:* may impair absorption. Separate administration times by at least 2 hours.
*Diuretics, other antihypertensives:* risk of excessive hypotension. Diuretic may need to be discontinued or fosinopril dosage lowered.
*Lithium:* increased serum lithium levels and lithium toxicity. Avoid concomitant use.
*Potassium-sparing diuretics, potassium supplements, sodium substitutes containing potassium:* risk of hyperkalemia. Monitor closely during concomitant use.

## CONTRAINDICATIONS
Contraindicated in patients with hypersensitivity to this drug or other ACE inhibitors and in breast-feeding patients.

## NURSING CONSIDERATIONS
• Use cautiously in patients with impaired renal or hepatic function.
• Monitor blood pressure for effect.
• Monitor potassium intake and serum potassium level. Diabetic patients, those with impaired renal function, and those receiving drugs that can increase serum potassium may develop hyperkalemia.
• Other ACE inhibitors have been associated with agranulocytosis and neutropenia. Monitor CBC with differential counts before therapy, every 2 weeks for the first 3 months of therapy, and periodically thereafter, as ordered.
• Assess renal and hepatic function before and periodically throughout therapy.

## ☑ PATIENT TEACHING
• Tell the patient to avoid sodium substitutes; these products may contain

---

*Liquid form contains alcohol. **May contain tartrazine. †Canada only. ‡Australia only. ◇OTC.

potassium, which can cause hyperkalemia in patients taking this drug.
• Advise the patient to report any signs of infection, such as fever and sore throat.
• Also tell the patient to call the doctor if any of the following signs or symptoms occur: easy bruising or bleeding; swelling of tongue, lips, face, eyes, mucous membranes, or extremities; difficulty swallowing or breathing; and hoarseness.
• Tell the patient to use caution in hot weather and during exercise. Inadequate fluid intake, vomiting, diarrhea, and excessive perspiration can lead to light-headedness and syncope.
• Tell the female patient to notify doctor if pregnancy occurs. Drug will need to be discontinued.

---

## guanabenz acetate
Wytensin

*Pregnancy Risk Category: C*

### HOW SUPPLIED
*Tablets:* 4 mg, 8 mg

### ACTION
Unknown. A centrally acting antihypertensive, its action is thought to be due to central alpha-adrenergic stimulation, which results in decreased sympathetic outflow to the heart, kidneys, and peripheral vasculature.

### ONSET, PEAK, DURATION
Onset occurs within 1 hour. Peak effects occur within 2 to 5 hours. Effects for persist about 12 hours.

### INDICATIONS & DOSAGE
*Hypertension* –
**Adults:** initially, 4 mg P.O. b.i.d. Dosage increased in increments of 4 to 8 mg/day q 1 to 2 weeks. Maximum daily dosage is 32 mg b.i.d. To ensure adequate overnight blood pressure control, give last dose h.s.

### ADVERSE REACTIONS
**CNS:** *drowsiness, sedation, dizziness, weakness,* headache.
**CV:** *rebound hypertension.*
**GI:** *dry mouth.*

### INTERACTIONS
*CNS depressants:* may cause increased sedation. Use together cautiously.
*Diuretics, other antihypertensive agents:* increased risk of excessive hypotension.
*Tricyclic antidepressants, MAO inhibitors:* may decrease antihypertensive effect.

### CONTRAINDICATIONS
Contraindicated in patients with hypersensitivity to the drug.

### NURSING CONSIDERATIONS
• Use cautiously in patients with severe coronary insufficiency, recent MI, cerebrovascular disease, or severe hepatic or renal failure. Also use cautiously in elderly patients.
• Monitor blood pressure for effects. Elderly patients may be more sensitive to drug's hypotensive effects.

### ☑ PATIENT TEACHING
• Caution the patient that abrupt discontinuation of drug may cause rebound hypertension.
• Advise him to avoid hazardous tasks that require alertness until drug's CNS effects are known.
• Inform the patient that orthostatic hypotension can be minimized by rising slowly and avoiding sudden position changes. Dry mouth can be relieved with chewing gum, sour hard candy, or ice chips.
• Warn the patient that tolerance to alcohol or other CNS depressants may be diminished.

---

Reactions may be *common,* uncommon, *life-threatening,* or COMMON AND LIFE-THREATENING.

# guanadrel sulfate
Hylorel

*Pregnancy Risk Category: B*

## HOW SUPPLIED
*Tablets:* 10 mg, 25 mg

## ACTION
Acts peripherally, inhibiting norepinephrine release and depleting norepinephrine stores in adrenergic nerve endings.

## ONSET, PEAK, DURATION
Onset occurs in 2 hours. Peak effects occur within 4 to 6 hours. Effects persist for 4 to 14 hours.

## INDICATIONS & DOSAGE
*Hypertension –*
**Adults:** initially, 5 mg P.O. b.i.d. Dosage adjusted until blood pressure is controlled. Most patients require dosages of 20 to 75 mg/day, usually given b.i.d.; however, tolerance to hypotensive effect may necessitate upward titration to 100 to 400 mg daily in three to four divided doses.

In patients with renal impairment, dosage is reduced to 5 mg P.O. once daily if creatinine clearance is 30 to 60 ml/minute; if creatinine clearance is less than 30 ml/minute, increase dosage interval to 48 hours. Dosage is adjusted every 7 to 14 days.

## ADVERSE REACTIONS
**CNS:** *fatigue, drowsiness, faintness, headache, confusion, paresthesia.*
**CV:** *palpitations, chest pain, peripheral edema, orthostatic hypotension.*
**GI:** *diarrhea,* dry mouth, *indigestion, constipation, anorexia,* nausea, vomiting, abdominal pain.
**GU:** impotence, *ejaculation disturbances, nocturia, urination frequency.*
**Respiratory:** *shortness of breath, cough.*

**Other:** *weight gain, aching limbs, leg cramps, visual disturbances,* glossitis.

## INTERACTIONS
*Amphetamines, ephedrine, methylphenidate, norepinephrine, phenothiazines, tricyclic antidepressants:* may inhibit guanadrel's antihypertensive effect. Adjust dose accordingly.
*Diuretics, other antihypertensives:* hypotensive effect of guanadrel increased. Monitor blood pressure closely.
*MAO inhibitors:* antagonized hypotensive effects of guanadrel. Don't give guanadrel concurrently or within 1 week of MAO inhibitor therapy.

## CONTRAINDICATIONS
Contraindicated in patients with hypersensitivity to the drug, known or suspected pheochromocytoma, or frank CHF.

## NURSING CONSIDERATIONS
● Use cautiously in patients with regional vascular disease, bronchial asthma, or history of peptic ulcer disease.
● Monitor both supine and standing blood pressure, especially during dosage adjustment periods.
● Be aware that elderly patients may be more sensitive to drug's hypotensive effects.
● Know that guanadrel should be discontinued 48 to 72 hours before surgery to minimize risk of vascular collapse during anesthesia.

## ☑ PATIENT TEACHING
● Inform the patient that orthostatic hypotension can be minimized by rising slowly from a supine position and by avoiding sudden position changes. Dry mouth can be relieved with chewing gum, sour hard candy, or ice chips.
● Warn the patient to avoid strenuous exercise and hot showers; these may cause a hypotensive reaction. An am-

---

*Liquid form contains alcohol. **May contain tartrazine. †Canada only. ‡Australia only. ◇OTC.

bient temperature that is too hot also may potentiate the hypotensive effects of guanadrel as can alcohol ingestion.

---

# guanethidine monosulfate
Apo-Guanethidine†, Ismelin

*Pregnancy Risk Category: B*

## HOW SUPPLIED
*Tablets:* 10 mg, 25 mg

## ACTION
An adrenergic neuron blocker that acts peripherally, inhibiting norepinephrine release and depleting norepinephrine stores in adrenergic nerve endings. This reduces arteriolar vasoconstriction.

## ONSET, PEAK, DURATION
Onset unknown. Serum levels peak within 8 hours after single dose. Effects persist for 3 to 4 days; blood pressure returns to pretreatment levels in 1 to 3 weeks.

## INDICATIONS & DOSAGE
*Moderate to severe hypertension and renal hypertension –*
**Adults:** initially, 10 mg P.O. daily. Increase by 10 mg at weekly to monthly intervals, p.r.n. Usual dosage is 25 to 50 mg daily. Some patients may require up to 300 mg daily.

## ADVERSE REACTIONS
**CNS:** *syncope, fatigue, headache, drowsiness, paresthesia, confusion.*
**CV:** *palpitations, chest pain, orthostatic hypotension, peripheral edema.*
**EENT:** *visual disturbances,* glossitis.
**GI:** *diarrhea, indigestion, constipation, anorexia,* nausea, vomiting.
**GU:** *nocturia, urination frequency, ejaculation disturbances,* impotence.
**Respiratory:** shortness of breath, cough.
**Other:** *weight gain, aching limbs, leg cramps.*

## INTERACTIONS
*Amphetamines, ephedrine, MAO inhibitors, methylphenidate, norepinephrine, phenothiazines, tricyclic antidepressants:* may inhibit guanethidine's antihypertensive effect. Adjust dose accordingly.
*Ethanol, levodopa:* may increase hypotensive effect of guanethidine. Use together cautiously.

## CONTRAINDICATIONS
Contraindicated in patients with pheochromocytoma, frank CHF, and hypersensitivity to guanethidine.

## NURSING CONSIDERATIONS
• Use cautiously in patients with severe cardiac disease, recent MI, cerebrovascular disease, peptic ulceration, impaired renal function, or bronchial asthma and in those taking other antihypertensives.
• Monitor blood pressure for effects, especially after dosage adjustments.
• Elderly patients may be more sensitive to drug's hypotensive effects.
• Know that drug should be discontinued 2 to 3 weeks before elective surgery to reduce the possibility of vascular collapse and cardiac arrest during anesthesia.
• Know that if the patient develops diarrhea, the doctor may prescribe atropine or paregoric.

## ☑ PATIENT TEACHING
• Inform the patient that orthostatic hypotension can be minimized by rising slowly and avoiding sudden position changes. Dry mouth can be relieved with chewing gum, sour hard candy, or ice chips.
• Patients should receive instruction on a low-sodium diet. Monitor for possible weight gain and edema.
• Warn the patient to avoid strenuous exercise and hot showers; these may cause a hypotensive reaction. An ambient temperature that is too hot also

---

may potentiate the hypotensive effects of guanethidine.

## guanfacine hydrochloride
Tenex

*Pregnancy Risk Category: B*

**HOW SUPPLIED**
*Tablets:* 1 mg, 2 mg

**ACTION**
Unknown. Thought to be due to inhibition of the central vasomotor center, thereby decreasing sympathetic outflow to the heart, kidneys, and peripheral vasculature. This decreases blood pressure.

**ONSET, PEAK, DURATION**
Onset unknown. Serum levels peak in 1 to 4 hours. Effects persist for 24 hours.

**INDICATIONS & DOSAGE**
*Hypertension –*
**Adults:** initially, 1 mg P.O. daily h.s. Dosage may be increased to 2 mg P.O. h.s. after 3 to 4 weeks, as needed. Dosage may be further increased to 3 mg P.O. h.s. after an additional 3 to 4 weeks, as needed. Average dosage is 1 to 3 mg daily.

**ADVERSE REACTIONS**
**CNS:** *dizziness,* fatigue, headache, insomnia, *somnolence,* asthenia.
**CV:** bradycardia.
**GI:** *constipation,* diarrhea, nausea, *dry mouth.*
**Skin:** dermatitis, pruritus.

**INTERACTIONS**
None significant.

**CONTRAINDICATIONS**
Contraindicated in patients with hypersensitivity to the drug.

**NURSING CONSIDERATIONS**
• Use cautiously in patients with severe coronary insufficiency, recent MI, cerebrovascular disease, or chronic renal or hepatic insufficiency.
• Monitor blood pressure frequently.
• Be aware that the incidence and severity of adverse reactions increase with higher dosages.
• Know that guanfacine may be used alone or with a diuretic.

☑ **PATIENT TEACHING**
• Tell the patient not to discontinue therapy abruptly. Rebound hypertension is less common than with similar drugs, such as clonidine, but may occur.
• Because guanfacine causes drowsiness, advise the patient to avoid activities that require alertness until response to drug is established.

## hydralazine hydrochloride
Alphapress‡, Apresoline**, Novo-Hylazin†

*Pregnancy Risk Category: C*

**HOW SUPPLIED**
*Tablets:* 10 mg, 25 mg, 50 mg, 100 mg
*Injection:* 20 mg/ml

**ACTION**
Unknown. A direct-acting vasodilator, its predominant effect relaxes arteriolar smooth muscle.

**ONSET, PEAK, DURATION**
Onset occurs within 5 minutes of I.V. injection, 20 to 30 minutes of oral dose, unknown after I.M. administration. Peak effects occur 15 to 30 minutes after I.V. administration or 1 to 2 hours after oral dose. Unknown after I.M. administration. Effects persist for 3 to 8 hours.

**INDICATIONS & DOSAGE**
*Essential hypertension (orally, alone or in combination with other antihy-*

pertensives); *severe essential hypertension (parenterally, to lower blood pressure quickly)* –

**Adults:** *oral* – initially, 10 mg P.O. q.i.d.; gradually increased to 50 mg q.i.d. as needed. Maximum recommended dosage is 200 mg daily, but some patients may require 300 to 400 mg daily.
*I.V.* – 10 to 20 mg given slowly and repeated as necessary, switching to oral antihypertensives as soon as possible.
*I.M.* – 10 to 50 mg, repeated as necessary, switching to oral form as soon as possible.
**Children:** *oral* – initially, 0.75 mg/kg/day P.O. divided into 4 doses; gradually increased over 3 to 4 weeks to a maximum of 7.5 mg/kg or 200 mg daily.
*I.V.* – 0.1 to 0.2 mg/kg I.V. every 4 to 6 hours as needed.

**ADVERSE REACTIONS**
**CNS:** peripheral neuritis, *headache,* dizziness.
**CV:** orthostatic hypotension, *tachycardia,* edema, *angina, palpitations.*
**GI:** *nausea, vomiting, diarrhea, anorexia,* constipation.
**Hematologic:** neutropenia, leukopenia, *agranulocytopenia.*
**Skin:** rash.
**Other:** *lupuslike syndrome* (especially with high doses).

**INTERACTIONS**
*Diazoxide, MAO inhibitors:* may cause severe hypotension. Use together cautiously.
*Indomethacin:* may decrease effects of hydralazine. Monitor blood pressure.

**CONTRAINDICATIONS**
Contraindicated in patients with hypersensitivity to the drug, coronary artery disease, or mitral valvular rheumatic heart disease.

**NURSING CONSIDERATIONS**
• Use cautiously in patients with suspected cardiac disease, CVA, or severe renal impairment and in those taking other antihypertensives.
• **I.V. use:** Give slowly and repeat as necessary, generally every 4 to 6 hours. Hydralazine will undergo color changes in most infusion solutions; these color changes do not indicate loss of potency. Compatible with 0.9% sodium chloride, Ringer's, and lactated Ringer's solutions, and several other common I.V. solutions. Drug may undergo a reaction with dextrose. The manufacturer does not recommend mixing the drug in infusion solutions. Check with the pharmacist for additional compatibility information.
• Monitor the patient's blood pressure, pulse rate, and body weight frequently. Some clinicians combine hydralazine therapy with diuretics and beta-adrenergic blockers to decrease sodium retention and tachycardia and to prevent anginal attacks.
• Be aware that elderly patients may be more sensitive to drug's hypotensive effects.
• Monitor CBC, lupus erythematosus cell preparation, and antinuclear antibody titer determination before therapy and periodically during long-term therapy, as ordered.
• *Alert:* Watch the patient closely for signs of lupuslike syndrome (sore throat, fever, muscle and joint aches, and rash). Call the doctor immediately if any of these develop.
• Compliance may be improved by administering drug b.i.d. Check with the doctor.

☑ **PATIENT TEACHING**
• Instruct the patient to take oral form with meals to increase absorption.
• Inform the patient that orthostatic hypotension can be minimized by rising slowly and avoiding sudden position changes.

---

Reactions may be *common,* uncommon, *life-threatening,* or COMMON AND LIFE-THREATENING.

## isradipine
DynaCirc

*Pregnancy Risk Category: C*

**HOW SUPPLIED**
*Capsules:* 2.5 mg, 5 mg

**ACTION**
Unknown. A calcium channel blocker that inhibits calcium ion influx across cardiac and smooth-muscle cells and is thought to decrease arteriolar resistance and blood pressure.

**ONSET, PEAK, DURATION**
Onset occurs within 20 minutes. Serum levels peak within 1½ hours. Effects persist more than 12 hours.

**INDICATIONS & DOSAGE**
*Essential hypertension –*
**Adults:** initially, 2.5 mg P.O. b.i.d., alone or with a thiazide diuretic. Dosage increased by gradual titration. If response is inadequate after first 2 to 4 weeks, dosage increased to 5 mg b.i.d., then increased at 5-mg daily intervals q 2 to 4 weeks to a maximum of 20 mg daily.

**ADVERSE REACTIONS**
**CNS:** dizziness, *headache,* fatigue.
**CV:** edema, flushing, syncope, angina, tachycardia.
**GI:** nausea, diarrhea, abdominal discomfort, vomiting.
**Respiratory:** dyspnea.
**Skin:** rash.

**INTERACTIONS**
*Fentanyl anesthesia:* severe hypotension has been reported with concomitant use of a beta blocker and a calcium channel blocker.

**CONTRAINDICATIONS**
Contraindicated in patients with hypersensitivity to the drug.

**NURSING CONSIDERATIONS**
• Use cautiously in patients with CHF, especially if combined with a beta blocker.
• Monitor patient for adverse reactions. Like other calcium channel blockers, isradipine is known to cause symptomatic hypotension; however, syncope and severe dizziness have not been reported. Most adverse reactions are mild and transient and related to vasodilation (dizziness, edema, flushing, palpitations, and tachycardia).
• Monitor blood pressure closely.
• Before surgery, inform the anesthesiologist that the patient is taking a calcium channel blocker.

**☑ PATIENT TEACHING**
• Tell patient that isradipine has some diuretic activity. He may note an increased need to void.
• Advise him to avoid hazardous tasks if adverse CNS reactions occur.

## labetalol hydrochloride
Normodyne, Presolol‡, Trandate

*Pregnancy Risk Category: C*

**HOW SUPPLIED**
*Tablets:* 100 mg, 200 mg, 300 mg
*Injection:* 5 mg/ml

**ACTION**
Unknown. May be related to reduced peripheral vascular resistance mainly as a result of beta-adrenergic blockade.

**ONSET, PEAK, DURATION**
Onset occurs 2 to 5 minutes after I.V. administration, within 20 minutes after oral dose. Peak effects occur within 5 minutes of I.V. administration, 2 to 4 hours of oral dose. Effects persist for 2 to 4 hours after I.V. dose and 12 to 24 hours after oral dose.

**INDICATIONS & DOSAGE**
*Hypertension –*
**Adults:** 100 mg P.O. b.i.d. with or

---

*Liquid form contains alcohol.   **May contain tartrazine.   †Canada only.   ‡Australia only.   ◊OTC.

without a diuretic. If needed, dosage is increased to 200 mg b.i.d. after 2 days. Further increases may be made q 2 to 3 days until optimum response is reached. Usual maintenance dosage is 200 to 400 mg b.i.d.
*Severe hypertension and hypertensive emergencies –*
**Adults:** 200 mg diluted in 160 ml of $D_5W$, infused at 2 mg/minute until satisfactory response is obtained; then infusion is stopped. May be repeated q 6 to 12 hours.

Alternatively, administered by repeated I.V. injection: initially, 20 mg I.V. slowly over 2 minutes. Then repeat injections of 40 to 80 mg q 10 minutes until maximum dosage of 300 mg is reached, as needed.

## ADVERSE REACTIONS
**CNS:** vivid dreams, fatigue, headache, paresthesia, syncope, transient scalp tingling.
**CV:** *orthostatic hypotension and dizziness, ventricular arrhythmias.*
**EENT:** nasal stuffiness.
**GI:** nausea, vomiting, diarrhea.
**GU:** sexual dysfunction, urine retention.
**Respiratory:** dyspnea, bronchospasm.
**Skin:** rash.

## INTERACTIONS
*Beta-adrenergic agonists:* may blunt bronchodilator effect of these drugs in patients with bronchospasm; therefore, greater than normal dose of these agents may be required.
*Cimetidine:* may enhance labetalol's effect. Give together cautiously.
*Halothane:* additive hypotensive effect. Monitor blood pressure closely.
*Insulin, oral antidiabetic agents:* can alter dosage requirements in previously stabilized diabetic patients. Observe the patient carefully.

## CONTRAINDICATIONS
Contraindicated in patients with bronchial asthma, overt cardiac failure, greater than first-degree heart block, cardiogenic shock, severe bradycardia, other conditions associated with severe and prolonged hypotension, and hypersensitivity to the drug.

## NURSING CONSIDERATIONS
● Use cautiously in patients with CHF, hepatic failure, chronic bronchitis, emphysema, preexisting peripheral vascular disease, and pheochromocytoma.
● **I.V. use:** Administer labetalol injection with an infusion control device. Monitor blood pressure closely: every 5 minutes for 30 minutes, then every 30 minutes for 2 hours, then hourly for 6 hours. The patient should remain in a supine position for 3 hours after infusion.
● **Alert:** Be aware that sodium bicarbonate injection is incompatible with I.V. labetalol.
● Monitor blood pressure frequently. Know that drug masks common signs of shock.
● Be aware that when administered I.V. for hypertensive emergencies, labetalol produces a rapid, predictable fall in blood pressure within 5 to 10 minutes.
● If dizziness occurs, ask doctor if patient may take a dose at bedtime or take smaller doses t.i.d. to help minimize this adverse reaction.
● Monitor blood glucose levels in diabetic patients closely because beta blockers may mask certain signs and symptoms of hypoglycemia.

## ☑ PATIENT TEACHING
● Tell the patient that abrupt discontinuation of therapy can exacerbate angina and precipitate MI.
● Dizziness is the most troublesome adverse reaction and tends to occur in early stages of treatment, in patients also receiving diuretics, and in those

---

Reactions may be *common,* uncommon, *life-threatening,* or **COMMON AND LIFE-THREATENING.**

receiving higher dosages. Inform the patient that this can be minimized by rising slowly and avoiding sudden position changes.

• Warn the patient that transient scalp tingling may occur, especially at beginning of therapy, but is harmless.

# lisinopril
Prinivil, Zestril

*Pregnancy Risk Category: C (D in 2nd and 3rd trimesters)*

## HOW SUPPLIED
*Tablets:* 2.5 mg, 5 mg, 10 mg, 20 mg, 40 mg

## ACTION
Unknown. Thought to result primarily from suppression of the renin-angiotensin-aldosterone system.

## ONSET, PEAK, DURATION
Onset occurs within 1 hour. Plasma levels peak within 7 hours. Effects persist for 24 hours.

## INDICATIONS & DOSAGE
*Hypertension –*
**Adults:** initially, 10 mg P.O. daily for the patient not receiving a diuretic; 5 mg P.O. daily for the patient receiving a diuretic. Most patients are well controlled on 20 to 40 mg daily as a single dose.
*Treatment adjunct in heart failure (with diuretics and digitalis) –*
**Adults:** initially, 5 mg P.O. daily; increased as needed to a maximum of 20 mg P.O. daily.

## ADVERSE REACTIONS
**CNS:** *dizziness, headache, fatigue, paresthesia.*
**CV:** hypotension, *orthostatic hypotension,* chest pain.
**EENT:** *nasal congestion.*
**GI:** *diarrhea,* nausea, dyspepsia.
**GU:** impotence.

**Hematologic:** neutropenia, *agranulocytopenia.*
**Respiratory:** *dry, persistent, tickling, nonproductive cough,* dyspnea.
**Skin:** rash.
**Other:** *angioedema,* hyperkalemia.

## INTERACTIONS
*Diuretics:* excessive hypotension. Monitor closely.
*Indomethacin:* attenuated hypotensive effect. Monitor closely.
*Insulin, oral antidiabetic agents:* risk of hypoglycemia, especially at initiation of lisinopril therapy. Monitor closely.
*Potassium-sparing diuretics, potassium supplements, potassium-containing sodium substitutes:* possible hyperkalemia. Monitor closely.
*Thiazide diuretics:* attenuation of potassium loss caused by thiazide diuretics. Discontinue diuretics 2 to 3 days before lisinopril therapy or reduce lisinopril dosage to 5 mg P.O. once daily, as ordered.

## CONTRAINDICATIONS
Contraindicated in patients with hypersensitivity to ACE inhibitors or history of angioedema related to previous treatment with ACE inhibitor.

## NURSING CONSIDERATIONS
• Use cautiously in patients with impaired renal function; dosage adjustment is required. Also use cautiously in patients at risk for hyperkalemia (presence of renal insufficiency, presence of diabetes, or use of drugs that raise potassium levels).
• Monitor blood pressure frequently. Be aware that if drug does not adequately control blood pressure, diuretics may be added.
• Monitor WBC with differential counts before therapy, every 2 weeks for the first 3 months of therapy, and periodically thereafter.

---

## ☑ PATIENT TEACHING

• *Alert:* Angioedema (including laryngeal edema) may occur, especially after first dose. Advise the patient to report signs or symptoms, such as swelling of face, eyes, lips, or tongue or breathing difficulty.

• Light-headedness can occur, especially during the first few days of therapy. Tell the patient to rise slowly to minimize this effect and to report symptoms to the doctor. Patients who experience syncope should stop taking drug and call the doctor immediately.

• Tell the patient not to discontinue drug suddenly, but to call the doctor, if unpleasant adverse reactions occur.

• Advise him to report signs of infection, such as fever and sore throat.

• Tell the female patient to notify doctor if pregnancy occurs. Drug will need to be discontinued.

---

## losartan potassium
Cozaar

*Pregnancy Risk Category: C (D in 2nd and 3rd trimesters)*

---

### HOW SUPPLIED
Tablets: 25 mg, 50 mg

### ACTION
An angiotensin II receptor antagonist that inhibits the vasoconstricting and aldosterone-secreting effects of angiotensin II by selectively blocking the binding of angiotensin II to its receptor sites that are found in many tissues, including vascular smooth muscle and adrenal glands.

### ONSET, PEAK, DURATION
Onset and duration unknown. Serum levels peak in 1 hour for losartan and in 3 to 4 hours for its active metabolite. Although the effect of losartan is substantially present within 1 week, some studies have shown that maximal effect occurs within 3 to 6 weeks.

### INDICATIONS & DOSAGE
*Hypertension –*
**Adults:** initially, 25 to 50 mg P.O. daily. Maximum daily dosage is 100 mg in one or two divided doses.

### ADVERSE REACTIONS
**CNS:** dizziness, insomnia.
**GI:** diarrhea, dyspepsia.
**Musculoskeletal:** muscle cramps, myalgia, back or leg pain.
**Respiratory:** nasal congestion, cough, upper respiratory tract infection, sinus disorder, sinusitis.

### INTERACTIONS
None significant.

### CONTRAINDICATIONS
Contraindicated in patients with hypersensitivity to the drug.

### NURSING CONSIDERATIONS
• Know that breast-feeding is not recommended during losartan therapy.

• Use cautiously in patients with impaired renal or hepatic function.

• Know that drugs that act directly on the renin-angiotensin system (such as losartan) can cause fetal and neonatal morbidity and death when administered to pregnant women. These problems have not been detected when exposure has been limited to the first trimester. If pregnancy is suspected, notify doctor because drug should probably be discontinued.

• Know that the lowest dosage (25 mg) should be used initially in patients with impaired hepatic function and in those who are intravascularly volume-depleted (such as those receiving diuretics).

• Be aware that losartan can be used alone or with other antihypertensives.

• Be aware that if the antihypertensive effect measured by the serum trough level of the drug, using once-daily dosing, is inadequate, a twice-daily regimen using the same total daily dosage or an increase in dosage

---

Reactions may be *common,* uncommon, *life-threatening,* or COMMON AND LIFE-THREATENING.

may give a more satisfactory response.
- Monitor the patient's blood pressure closely to evaluate effectiveness of therapy. Know that when losartan is used alone, the effect on blood pressure is notably less in black patients than in patients of other races.
- Monitor patients who also are taking diuretics for symptomatic hypotension.
- Regularly assess the patient's renal function (via serum creatinine and BUN levels), as ordered.
- Be aware that patients with severe CHF whose renal function depends on the angiotensin-aldosterone system have experienced acute renal failure during ACE inhibitor therapy. Manufacturer of losartan states that drug would be expected to do the same. Closely monitor patient, especially during the first few weeks of therapy.

☑ **PATIENT TEACHING**
- Tell the patient to avoid sodium substitutes; these products may contain potassium, which can cause hyperkalemia in patients taking losartan.
- Inform the female patient of childbearing age about the consequences of second- and third-trimester exposure to losartan, and instruct her to notify the doctor immediately if she suspects that she is pregnant.

---

### methyldopa
Aldomet, Aldomet M‡, Apo-Methyldopa†, Dopamet†, Hydopa‡, Novomedopa†, Nu-Medopa†

### methyldopate hydrochloride
Aldomet, Aldomet Ester Injection‡

*Pregnancy Risk Category: B*

**HOW SUPPLIED**
**methyldopa**
*Tablets:* 125 mg, 250 mg, 500 mg

*Oral suspension:* 250 mg/5 ml
**methyldopate hydrochloride**
*Injection:* 250 mg/5 ml

**ACTION**
Unknown. Thought to involve inhibition of the central vasomotor centers, thereby decreasing sympathetic outflow to the heart, kidneys, and peripheral vasculature.

**ONSET, PEAK, DURATION**
Onset unknown. Serum levels peak within 4 to 6 hours after I.V. or oral administration. Effects persist for 12 to 24 hours after single oral dose, 24 to 48 hours after multiple oral doses, and 10 to 16 hours after I.V. administration.

**INDICATIONS & DOSAGE**
*Hypertension, hypertensive crisis* –
**Adults:** *oral* – initially, 250 mg P.O. b.i.d. to t.i.d. in first 48 hours. Then increased as needed q 2 days. May give entire daily dosage in the evening or h.s. Adjust dosages as needed if other antihypertensives are added to or deleted from therapy. Maintenance dosage is 500 mg to 2 g daily in two to four divided doses. Maximum recommended daily dosage is 3 g.
*I.V.* – 250 to 500 mg q 6 hours, diluted in $D_5W$ and administered over 30 to 60 minutes. Maximum dosage is 1 g q 6 hours. Switch to oral antihypertensives as soon as possible.
**Children:** initially, 10 mg/kg P.O. daily in two to four divided doses; or 20 to 40 mg/kg I.V. daily in four divided doses. Increase dose daily until desired response occurs. Maximum daily dosage is 65 mg/kg or 3 g, whichever is least.

**ADVERSE REACTIONS**
**CNS:** *sedation,* headache, weakness, dizziness, *decreased mental acuity,* paresthesia, parkinsonism, involuntary choreoathetoid movements,

---

psychic disturbances, depression, nightmares.
**CV:** bradycardia, *orthostatic hypotension,* aggravated angina, **myocarditis,** edema.
**EENT:** *nasal congestion.*
**GI:** nausea, vomiting, diarrhea, pancreatitis, *dry mouth,* constipation.
**Hematologic: hemolytic anemia, thrombocytopenia,** leukopenia, bone marrow depression.
**Hepatic: hepatic necrosis,** abnormal liver function tests, hepatitis.
**Skin:** rash.
**Other:** gynecomastia, galactorrhea, drug-induced fever.

## INTERACTIONS
*Amphetamines, norepinephrine, phenothiazines, tricyclic antidepressants:* possible hypertensive effects. Monitor carefully.
*Levodopa:* additive hypotensive effects may increase adverse CNS reactions. Monitor closely.
*Lithium:* may increase lithium levels. Monitor for increased lithium levels.

## CONTRAINDICATIONS
Contraindicated in patients with hypersensitivity to the drug or active hepatic disease (such as acute hepatitis) and active cirrhosis. Also contraindicated if previous methyldopa therapy has been associated with liver disorders.

## NURSING CONSIDERATIONS
• Use cautiously in patients with history of impaired hepatic function and in breast-feeding patients.
• **I.V. use:** Observe for and report any involuntary choreoathetoid movements. The doctor may decide to discontinue drug if this occurs.
• Monitor patient's blood pressure regularly. Be aware that elderly patients are more likely to experience hypotension and sedation.
• After dialysis, monitor the patient for hypertension and notify doctor if

necessary. The patient may need an extra dose of methyldopa.
• Monitor CBC with differential counts before therapy, every 2 weeks for the first 3 months of therapy, and periodically thereafter.
• Patients who require blood transfusions should have direct and indirect Coombs' tests to prevent crossmatching problems.
• Monitor patient's Coombs' test results. In patients who have received this drug for several months, positive reaction to direct Coombs' test indicates hemolytic anemia.

## ☑ PATIENT TEACHING
• Tell the patient not to suddenly stop taking drug, but to contact the doctor, if unpleasant adverse reactions occur.
• Advise him to report signs of infection, such as fever and sore throat.
• Tell the patient to check his weight daily and to notify the doctor of weight gain over 5 lb (about 2 kg). Sodium and water retention may occur but can be relieved with diuretics.
• Warn the patient that drug may impair ability to perform tasks that require mental alertness, particularly at start of therapy. A once-daily dosage at bedtime will minimize daytime drowsiness.
• Inform the patient that orthostatic hypotension can be minimized by rising slowly and avoiding sudden position changes. Dry mouth can be relieved with chewing gum, sour hard candy, or ice chips.
• Tell him that urine may turn dark in toilet bowls treated with bleach.

---

Reactions may be *common,* uncommon, *life-threatening,* or COMMON AND LIFE-THREATENING.

## metoprolol succinate
Toprol XL

## metoprolol tartrate
Apo-Metoprolol†, Apo-Metoprolol
(Type L)†, Betaloc†‡, Betaloc
Durules†, Lopresor†, Lopresor
SR†, Lopressor, Minax‡,
Novometoprol†, Nu-Metop†

*Pregnancy Risk Category: C*

### HOW SUPPLIED
**metoprolol succinate**
*Tablets (extended-release):* 50 mg,
100 mg, 200 mg
**metoprolol tartrate**
*Tablets:* 50 mg, 100 mg
*Tablets (extended-release):* 100 mg†,
200 mg†
*Injection:* 1 mg/ml in 5-ml ampules

### ACTION
Unknown for antihypertensive action.
A beta₁-selective blocking agent that
decreases myocardial contractility,
heart rate, and cardiac output; lowers
blood pressure; and reduces myocardial oxygen consumption. Also depresses renin secretion.

### ONSET, PEAK, DURATION
Onset occurs within 5 minutes of I.V.
dose, 15 minutes of oral dose. Peak
effects occur within 20 minutes of I.V.
dose, 1 hour after regular-release tablet, or 6 to 12 hours after extended-release dosage forms. Effects persist for
5 to 8 hours after I.V. dose, 6 to 12
hours after regular-release oral tablets, up to 24 hours after extended-release forms.

### INDICATIONS & DOSAGE
*Hypertension –*
**Adults:** initially, 50 mg P.O. b.i.d. or
100 mg P.O. once daily, then up to
100 to 450 mg daily in two or three
divided doses. Alternatively, 50 to
100 mg of extended-release tablets
(tartrate) once daily. Dosage is adjusted as needed and tolerated at intervals of not less than 1 week to a
maximum of 450 mg daily.
*Early intervention in acute MI (meto-
prolol tartrate) –*
**Adults:** three 5-mg I.V. boluses q 2
minutes. Then, beginning 15 minutes
after last dose, 25 to 50 mg P.O. q 6
hours for 48 hours. Maintenance dosage is 100 mg P.O. b.i.d. for 3
months to 3 years.
*Angina pectoris –*
**Adults:** initially, 100 mg P.O. daily as
a single dose or in two equally divided
doses; increased at weekly intervals
until an adequate response or a pronounced decrease in heart rate is
seen. Daily dosage beyond 400 mg
has not been studied. Alternatively,
give 100 mg of extended-release tablets (tartrate) once daily. Dosage adjusted as needed and tolerated at intervals of not less than 1 week to a
maximum of 400 mg daily.

### ADVERSE REACTIONS
**CNS:** *fatigue, dizziness,* depression.
**CV:** *bradycardia, hypotension,* **CHF.**
**GI:** nausea, diarrhea.
**Respiratory:** dyspnea, ***broncho-
spasm.***
**Skin:** rash.

### INTERACTIONS
*Barbiturates, rifampin:* increased metabolism of metoprolol. Monitor for
decreased effect.
*Chlorpromazine, cimetidine, verapa-
mil:* decreased hepatic clearance. Monitor for greater beta-blocking effect.
*Digitalis glycosides, diltiazem, verap-
amil:* excessive bradycardia and increased depressant effect on myocardium. Use together cautiously.
*Indomethacin:* decreased antihypertensive effect. Monitor blood pressure
and adjust dosage.
*Insulin, oral antidiabetic agents:* can
alter dosage requirements in previously stabilized diabetic patients. Observe the patient carefully.

## CONTRAINDICATIONS
Contraindicated in patients with hypersensitivity to the drug or other beta blockers. Also contraindicated in patients with sinus bradycardia, heart block greater than first-degree, cardiogenic shock, or overt cardiac failure when used to treat hypertension or angina. When used to treat MI, drug also is contraindicated in patients with heart rate less than 45 beats/minute, second- or third-degree heart block, PR interval of 0.24 seconds or longer with first-degree heart block, systolic blood pressure less than 100 mm Hg, or moderate to severe cardiac failure.

## NURSING CONSIDERATIONS
• Use cautiously in patients with heart failure, diabetes, or respiratory or hepatic disease.
• Always check the patient's apical pulse rate before giving drug. If it's slower than 60 beats/minute, withhold drug and call the doctor immediately.
• **I.V. use:** Give undiluted by direct injection. Although mixing with other drugs should be avoided, studies have shown that metoprolol is compatible when mixed with meperidine hydrochloride or morphine sulfate or when administered with alteplase infusion at a Y-site connection.
• Food may increase drug absorption. Give consistently with meals.
• Monitor blood glucose levels closely in diabetic patients because drug masks common signs of hypoglycemia.
• Monitor blood pressure frequently. Know that metoprolol masks common signs of shock.
• Store drug at room temperature and protect from light. Discard solution if it's discolored or contains particles.

## ☑ PATIENT TEACHING
• Instruct the patient to take drug exactly as prescribed and to take it with meals.

• Tell the patient not to stop drug suddenly but to notify the doctor about unpleasant adverse reactions. Inform him that drug must be withdrawn gradually over 1 to 2 weeks.

---

## minoxidil
Loniten
*Pregnancy Risk Category: C*

### HOW SUPPLIED
*Tablets:* 2.5 mg, 10 mg, 25 mg‡

### ACTION
Unknown. Predominant effect produces direct arteriolar vasodilation.

### ONSET, PEAK, DURATION
Onset occurs in about 30 minutes. Peak effects occur within 1 hour. Effects persist for 2 to 5 days.

### INDICATIONS & DOSAGE
*Severe hypertension* –
**Adults:** initially, 5 mg P.O. as a single dose. Effective dosage range is usually 10 to 40 mg daily. Maximum dosage is 100 mg daily.
**Children under 12 years:** 0.2 mg/kg P.O. (maximum 5 mg) as a single daily dose. Effective dosage range usually is 0.25 to 1 mg/kg daily. Maximum dosage is 50 mg.

### ADVERSE REACTIONS
**CV:** *edema, tachycardia, pericardial effusion and tamponade, CHF,* ECG changes, rebound hypertension.
**GI:** nausea, vomiting.
**Skin:** rash, *Stevens-Johnson syndrome.*
**Other:** *hypertrichosis* (elongation, thickening, and enhanced pigmentation of fine body hair), breast tenderness, weight gain.

### INTERACTIONS
*Guanethidine:* severe orthostatic hypotension. Advise the patient to stand up slowly.

---

Reactions may be *common,* uncommon, *life-threatening,* or **COMMON AND LIFE-THREATENING.**

## CONTRAINDICATIONS
Contraindicated in patients with pheochromocytoma or hypersensitivity to the drug.

## NURSING CONSIDERATIONS
• Use cautiously in those with impaired renal function and after acute MI.
• Closely monitor blood pressure and pulse at beginning of therapy.
• Know that elderly patients may be more sensitive to drug's hypotensive effects.
• Minoxidil is removed by hemodialysis. Be sure to administer dose after dialysis.
• Monitor fluid intake and urine output. Check for weight gain and edema.

## ☑ PATIENT TEACHING
• Make sure the patient receives and reads the manufacturer's package insert that describes in layman's terms the drug and its adverse reactions. Also provide an oral explanation.
• Tell the patient not to suddenly stop taking the drug, but to call the doctor, if unpleasant adverse effects occur.
• Make sure the patient understands the importance of compliance with total treatment regimen. Minoxidil usually is prescribed with a beta blocker to control tachycardia and a diuretic to counteract fluid retention.
• Teach the patient how to take his own pulse and to report increases greater than 20 beats/minute to the doctor.
• Tell the patient to weigh himself at least weekly and to report weight gain of over 5 lb (about 2 kg).
• About 8 out of 10 patients will experience hypertrichosis within 3 to 6 weeks of beginning treatment. Unwanted hair can be controlled with a depilatory or shaving. Assure the patient that extra hair will disappear within 1 to 6 months of stopping minoxidil. Advise the patient, however,

not to discontinue drug without the doctor's approval.

▼ NEW DRUG

# moexipril hydrochloride
Univasc

*Pregnancy Risk Category: C (first trimester), D (second and third trimester)*

## HOW SUPPLIED
*Tablets:* 7.5 mg, 15 mg

## ACTION
Unknown. Thought to result primarily from suppression of renin-angiotensin-aldosterone system.

## ONSET, PEAK, DURATION
Onset occurs in about 1 hour. Plasma levels peak in 3 to 6 hours. Effects persist for 24 hours.

## INDICATIONS & DOSAGE
*Hypertension –*
**Adults:** initially, 7.5 mg (3.75 mg if patient is receiving a diuretic) P.O. once daily 1 hour before meal. If control is inadequate, dose may be increased or divided. Recommended dosage is 7.5 mg to 30 mg daily, in one or two divided doses 1 hour before meal. Subsequent dosage depends on response.

## ADVERSE REACTIONS
**CNS** *dizziness,* headache, fatigue.
**CV:** peripheral edema, hypotension, orthostatic hypotension, chest pain, flushing.
**EENT:** pharyngitis, rhinitis, sinusitis.
**GI:** diarrhea, dyspepsia, nausea.
**GU:** urinary frequency.
**Hematologic:** neutropenia.
**Respiratory:** *dry, persistent, tickling, nonproductive cough.*
**Skin:** rash.
**Other:** myalgia, ***anaphylactoid reactions, angioedema,*** hyperkalemia, flu

---

syndrome, upper respiratory infection, pain.

## INTERACTIONS

*Diuretics:* risk of excessive hypotension. Expect diuretic to be discontinued or moexipril dose lowered.
*Lithium:* increased serum lithium level and lithium toxicity. Avoid concomitant use.
*Potassium-sparing diuretics, potassium supplements, sodium substitutes containing potassium:* risk of hyperkalemia. Monitor serum potassium level closely.

## CONTRAINDICATIONS

Contraindicated in patients with hypersensitivity to drug or history of angioedema related to treatment with ACE inhibitor.

## NURSING CONSIDERATIONS

• Safety of drug is not established in children.
• Use cautiously in patients with impaired renal function, CHF, or renal artery stenosis and in breast-feeding women.
• Monitor for excessive hypotension.
• Measure blood pressure at trough (just before dose) to verify blood pressure control.
• Assess renal function before and during therapy. Monitor serum potassium level, as ordered.
• Know that other ACE inhibitors have been associated with agranulocytosis and neutropenia. Monitor CBC with differential before therapy, especially in patients who have collagen-vascular disease with impaired renal function.
• Because angioedema associated with the tongue, glottis, or larynx can cause a fatal airway obstruction, have appropriate therapy, such as subcutaneous epinephrine 1:1000 (0.3 to 0.5 ml), and equipment to ensure a patent airway is available.

## ☑ PATIENT TEACHING

• Tell patient to take this drug on an empty stomach; meals can impair absorption.
• Advise patient to avoid sodium substitutes, which can cause hyperkalemia in patients taking this drug.
• Tell patient to use caution in hot weather and during exercise. Inadequate fluid intake, vomiting, diarrhea, and excessive perspiration can lead to light-headedness and syncope.
• Urge patient to rise slowly to minimize light-headedness. Tell him to stop taking drug and to call the doctor immediately if he experiences syncope.
• Advise patient to report fever; sore throat; easy bruising or bleeding; swelling of tongue, lips, face, eyes, mucous membranes, or extremities; difficulty swallowing or breathing; or hoarseness.
• Tell female patient to notify doctor if pregnancy occurs. Drug must be discontinued.

▼ *NEW DRUG*

# nisoldipine
Sular

*Pregnancy Risk Category: C*

## HOW SUPPLIED

*Extended-release tablets:* 10 mg, 20 mg, 30 mg, 40 mg

## ACTION

Prevents calcium ions from entering vascular smooth muscle cells, thereby causing dilation of arterioles, which in turn decreases peripheral vascular resistance.

## ONSET, PEAK, DURATION

Onset and duration unknown. Peak plasma levels occur in 6 to 12 hours.

## INDICATIONS & DOSAGE

*Hypertension –*
**Adults:** initially, 20 mg (10 mg if patient is over 65 or has liver dysfunc-

tion) P.O. once daily; increased by 10 mg/week or at longer intervals, as needed. Usual maintenance dosage is 20 to 40 mg/day. Dosages greater than 60 mg/day are not recommended.

**ADVERSE REACTIONS**
**CNS:** *headache,* dizziness.
**CV:** vasodilation, palpitation, chest pain.
**EENT:** sinusitis.
**GI:** nausea.
**Respiratory:** pharyngitis.
**Skin:** rash.
**Other:** *peripheral edema.*

**INTERACTIONS**
*Cimetidine:* increased bioavailability and peak concentration of nisoldipine.
*Quinidine:* decreased bioavailability of nisoldipine.

**CONTRAINDICATIONS**
Contraindicated in patients with hypersensitivity to dihydropyridine calcium channel blockers.

**NURSING CONSIDERATIONS**
• Use cautiously in patients receiving beta-blockers and those with compromised ventricular function, CHF, or hepatic impairment.
• Know that drug should not be used in breast-feeding women.
• Monitor patient carefully. Some patients, especially those with severe obstructive coronary artery disease, have developed increased frequency, duration, or severity of angina or even acute MI after starting calcium channel blocker therapy or at time of dosage increase.
• Monitor blood pressure regularly, especially during the initial administration and titration of drug.

☑ **PATIENT TEACHING**
• Tell the patient to take drug as prescribed, even if he feels better.
• Advise him to swallow tablet whole and not to chew, divide, or crush it.

• Remind him not to take drug with a high-fat meal or with grapefruit products.

---

## nitroprusside sodium
Nipride, Nitropress
*Pregnancy Risk Category: C*

**HOW SUPPLIED**
*Injection:* 50 mg/vial in 2-ml, 5-ml vials

**ACTION**
Relaxes both arteriolar and venous smooth muscle.

**ONSET, PEAK, DURATION**
Onset occurs within 1 minute. Peak effects are evident almost immediately. Effects dissipate within 10 minutes after infusion.

**INDICATIONS & DOSAGE**
*To lower blood pressure quickly in hypertensive emergencies; to produce controlled hypotension during anesthesia; to reduce preload and afterload in cardiac pump failure or cardiogenic shock (may be used with or without dopamine)–*
**Adults:** 50 mg vial diluted with 2 to 3 ml of $D_5W$ and then added to 250, 500, or 1,000 ml of $D_5W$; infused at 0.3 to 10 mcg/kg/minute. Average dose is 3 mcg/kg/minute. Maximum infusion rate is 10 mcg/kg/minute.
Patients taking other antihypertensives along with nitroprusside are extremely sensitive to nitroprusside. Dosage is adjusted accordingly.

**ADVERSE REACTIONS**
**CNS:** *headache, dizziness,* loss of consciousness, apprehension, *restlessness, muscle twitching, diaphoresis.*
**CV:** bradycardia, hypotension, tachycardia, palpitations, ECG changes.
**GI:** *nausea, abdominal pain,* ileus.
**Skin:** pink color, flushing, rash.
**Other:** acidosis, *thiocyanate toxicity,*

---

*Liquid form contains alcohol. **May contain tartrazine. †Canada only. ‡Australia only. ◊OTC.

*methemoglobinemia, cyanide toxicity,* venous streaking, irritation at infusion site, *increased intracranial pressure,* hypothyroidism.

**INTERACTIONS**
*Antihypertensives:* may cause sensitivity to nitroprusside. Adjust dosage as ordered.
*Ganglionic blocking agents, general anesthetics, negative inotropic agents, and other antihypertensives:* additive effects. Monitor blood pressure closely.

**CONTRAINDICATIONS**
Contraindicated in patients with hypersensitivity to the drug, compensatory hypertension (such as in arteriovenous shunt or coarctation of the aorta), inadequate cerebral circulation, congenital optic atrophy, or tobacco-induced amblyopia.

**NURSING CONSIDERATIONS**
• Use with extreme caution in patients with increased intracranial pressure. Use cautiously in patients with hypothyroidism, hepatic or renal disease, hyponatremia, or low vitamin $B_{12}$ concentration.
• Obtain baseline vital signs before giving drug, and find out what parameters the doctor wants to achieve.
• Keep the patient in the supine position when initiating or titrating nitroprusside therapy.
• **I.V. use:** Don't use bacteriostatic water for injection or sterile sodium chloride solution for reconstitution.
• Because the drug is sensitive to light, wrap I.V. solution in foil; it's not necessary to wrap the tubing. Fresh solution should have faint brownish tint. Discard after 24 hours.
• Infuse with an infusion pump. Drug is best given via piggyback through a peripheral line with no other medication. Don't adjust rate of main I.V. line while drug is being infused. Even a small bolus of nitroprusside can cause severe hypotension.

• Check blood pressure every 5 minutes at start of infusion and every 15 minutes thereafter. If severe hypotension occurs, discontinue nitroprusside infusion — effects of drug quickly reverse. Notify the doctor. If possible, start an arterial pressure line. Regulate drug flow to specified level.
• **Alert:** Excessive doses or rapid infusion greater than 10 mcg/kg/minute can cause cyanide toxicity; therefore, check serum thiocyanate levels every 72 hours. Levels above 100 mcg/ml are associated with toxicity. Watch for profound hypotension, metabolic acidosis, dyspnea, headache, loss of consciousness, ataxia, and vomiting. If these occur, discontinue drug immediately and notify the doctor.

☑ **PATIENT TEACHING**
• Instruct patient to report adverse reactions promptly.
• Tell patient to alert nurse if discomfort occurs at I.V. insertion site.

---

## penbutolol sulfate
Levatol

*Pregnancy Risk Category: C*

**HOW SUPPLIED**
*Tablets:* 20 mg

**ACTION**
Unknown.

**ONSET, PEAK, DURATION**
Onset occurs within 1 hour. Peak effects occur within 1½ to 3 hours. Effects persist up to 24 hours.

**INDICATIONS & DOSAGE**
*Mild to moderate hypertension* —
**Adults:** 20 mg P.O. once daily. Usually given with other antihypertensives, such as thiazide diuretics.

**ADVERSE REACTIONS**
**CNS:** *dizziness,* headache, fatigue, insomnia, asthenia.

---

Reactions may be *common,* uncommon, *life-threatening,* or **COMMON AND LIFE-THREATENING.**

**CV:** chest pain, *CHF.*
**GI:** nausea, diarrhea, dyspepsia.
**GU:** impotence.
**Respiratory:** cough, dyspnea.
**Skin:** excessive diaphoresis.

## INTERACTIONS
*Clonidine:* may cause paradoxical hypertension. Also, beta blockers may enhance rebound hypertension when clonidine is withdrawn.
*Digoxin, diltiazem, verapamil:* may produce additive depressant effects on AV node conduction. Monitor closely.
*Insulin, oral antidiabetic agents:* hypoglycemic response to these drugs may be altered. Monitor patient closely.
*NSAIDs:* may decrease antihypertensive effects.
*Prazosin, terazosin:* "first-dose" orthostatic hypotension seen with these drugs may be enhanced.
*Sympathomimetics, including isoproterenol, dopamine, dobutamine, or norepinephrine:* decreased hypotensive response.
*Theophylline:* may decrease bronchodilator effect.

## CONTRAINDICATIONS
Contraindicated in patients with hypersensitivity to the drug or other beta blockers and in those with sinus bradycardia, cardiogenic shock, overt cardiac failure, greater than first-degree heart block, or chronic bronchitis.

## NURSING CONSIDERATIONS
• Use cautiously in patients with CHF controlled by drug therapy and in those with a history of bronchospastic disease. Also use cautiously in diabetic patients because beta-adrenergic blockers may mask certain signs and symptoms of hypoglycemia.
• Always check the patient's apical pulse before giving drug. If you detect extremes in pulse rates, withhold drug and call the doctor immediately.

• Monitor blood pressure, ECG, and heart rate and rhythm frequently.

☑ **PATIENT TEACHING**
• Instruct the patient to take drug exactly as prescribed.
• Tell the patient not to stop drug suddenly but to notify the doctor about unpleasant adverse reactions.
• Teach the patient the signs and symptoms of CHF (edema and pulmonary congestion). Advise him to contact the doctor if these occur.

## phentolamine mesylate
Regitine, Rogitine†
*Pregnancy Risk Category: C*

## HOW SUPPLIED
*Injection:* 5 mg/ml in 1-ml vials, 10 mg/ml‡

## ACTION
An alpha-adrenergic blocker that competitively blocks the effects of catecholamines on alpha-adrenergic receptors.

## ONSET, PEAK, DURATION
Unknown.

## INDICATIONS & DOSAGE
*To aid in diagnosis of pheochromocytoma; to control or prevent hypertension before or during pheochromocytomectomy* –
**Adults:** I.V. diagnostic dose is 5 mg with close monitoring of blood pressure. Before surgical removal of tumor, 5 mg I.M. or I.V. During surgery, the patient may need 5 mg I.V.
**Children:** I.V. diagnostic dose is 1 mg with close monitoring of blood pressure. Before surgical removal of tumor, 1 mg I.V. or I.M. During surgery, the patient may need 1 mg I.V.
*Dermal necrosis and sloughing after I.V. extravasation of norepinephrine* –
**Adults and children:** infiltrate area with 5 to 10 mg phentolamine in 10 ml

of 0.9% sodium chloride solution, or give half the dosage through the infiltrated I.V. and the other half around the site. Must be done within 12 hours.

## ADVERSE REACTIONS
**CNS:** *dizziness, weakness, flushing,* ***cerebrovascular occlusion,*** cerebrovascular spasm.
**CV:** *hypotension,* ***shock,*** *arrhythmias, tachycardia,* ***MI.***
**EENT:** *nasal congestion.*
**GI:** *diarrhea, nausea, vomiting.*

## INTERACTIONS
*Epinephrine:* excessive hypotension. Don't use together.
*Narcotics, sedatives, rauwolfia alkaloids:* false-positive test results for pheochromocytoma. Don't give 24 hours before phentolamine is given as a diagnostic test. Withdraw rauwolfia alkaloids at least 4 weeks before such testing.

## CONTRAINDICATIONS
Contraindicated in patients with angina, coronary artery disease, MI or history of MI, or hypersensitivity to the drug.

## NURSING CONSIDERATIONS
• Use cautiously in patients with gastritis or peptic ulcer.
• When drug is given as a diagnostic test for pheochromocytoma, take the patient's blood pressure first; also monitor blood pressure frequently during administration.
• Know that test is positive for pheochromocytoma if I.V. test dose causes severe hypotension.
• *Alert:* Don't administer epinephrine to treat phentolamine-induced hypotension because it may cause additional fall in blood pressure ("epinephrine reversal"). Use norepinephrine instead, as ordered.

## ☑ PATIENT TEACHING
• Explain to patient why and how drug is administered.
• Tell patient to report adverse reactions promptly.

---

# pindolol
Barbloc‡, Novo-Pindol†, Syn-Pindolol†, Visken

*Pregnancy Risk Category: B*

## HOW SUPPLIED
*Tablets:* 5 mg, 10 mg, 15 mg‡

## ACTION
Unknown. Possible mechanisms include reduced cardiac output, decreased sympathetic outflow to peripheral vasculature, and inhibition of renin release by the kidneys.

## ONSET, PEAK, DURATION
Onset unknown. Peak effects occur in 1 to 2 hours. Effects persist for 24 hours.

## INDICATIONS & DOSAGE
*Hypertension –*
**Adults:** initially, 5 mg P.O. b.i.d. Dosage increased as needed and tolerated to a maximum of 60 mg daily.

## ADVERSE REACTIONS
**CNS:** *insomnia, fatigue, dizziness, nervousness,* vivid dreams, weakness, paresthesia.
**CV:** *edema,* bradycardia, ***CHF,*** chest pain.
**GI:** *nausea,* abdominal discomfort.
**Respiratory:** *increased airway resistance,* dyspnea.
**Skin:** rash, pruritus.
**Other:** *muscle pain, joint pain.*

## INTERACTIONS
*Digitalis glycosides, diltiazem, verapamil:* excessive bradycardia and additive depression of AV node. Use together cautiously.
*Epinephrine:* severe vasoconstriction.

---

Reactions may be *common,* uncommon, ***life-threatening,*** or **COMMON AND LIFE-THREATENING.**

Monitor blood pressure and observe the patient carefully.

*Indomethacin:* decreased antihypertensive effect. Monitor blood pressure and adjust dosage.

*Insulin, oral antidiabetic agents:* can alter requirements for these drugs in previously stabilized diabetic patients. Monitor the patient for hypoglycemia.

## CONTRAINDICATIONS

Contraindicated in patients with hypersensitivity to the drug, bronchial asthma, severe bradycardia, heart block greater than first degree, cardiogenic shock, or overt cardiac failure.

## NURSING CONSIDERATIONS

• Use cautiously in patients with CHF, nonallergic bronchospastic disease, diabetes, hyperthyroidism, and impaired renal or hepatic function.

• Always check the patient's apical pulse rate before giving this drug. If you detect extremes in pulse rates, withhold medication and call the doctor immediately.

• Monitor blood pressure frequently and notify the doctor if severe hypotension occurs. A vasopressor may be required.

• Withdraw drug over 1 to 2 weeks after long-term therapy, as ordered.

• Monitor blood glucose levels in diabetic patients closely because drug masks certain signs and symptoms of hypoglycemia.

## ☑ PATIENT TEACHING

• Tell the patient to take drug exactly as prescribed.

• Tell the patient not to stop drug suddenly but to call doctor to discuss unpleasant adverse drug reactions.

---

## prazosin hydrochloride
Minipress

*Pregnancy Risk Category: C*

## HOW SUPPLIED
*Capsules:* 1 mg, 2 mg, 5 mg

## ACTION
Unknown. Its alpha-adrenergic blocking activity is thought to account primarily for its effects.

## ONSET, PEAK, DURATION
Onset occurs in 30 to 90 minutes. Peak effects occur in 2 to 4 hours, but maximal antihypertensive effect may not occur for 3 to 4 weeks. Effects persist about 7 to 10 hours.

## INDICATIONS & DOSAGE
*Mild to moderate hypertension, alone or in combination with a diuretic or other antihypertensive –*
**Adults:** P.O. test dose is 1 mg h.s. to prevent "first-dose syncope." Initial dose is 1 mg P.O. t.i.d. Dosage increased slowly. Maximum daily dosage is 20 mg. Maintenance dosage is 6 to 15 mg daily in three divided doses. Some patients need dosages larger than this (up to 40 mg daily). If other antihypertensives or diuretics are added to this drug, prazosin is decreased to 1 to 2 mg t.i.d. and retitrated.

## ADVERSE REACTIONS
**CNS:** *dizziness,* headache, drowsiness, nervousness, paresthesia, weakness, *"first-dose syncope,"* depression.
**CV:** orthostatic hypotension, *palpitations.*
**EENT:** blurred vision, tinnitus, conjunctivitis.
**GI:** vomiting, diarrhea, abdominal cramps, *nausea.*
**GU:** priapism, impotence, urinary frequency, incontinence.
**Respiratory:** dyspnea, nasal congestion, epistaxis.
**Other:** arthralgia, myalgia, pruritus, edema, fever.

---

## INTERACTIONS

*Propranolol and other beta blockers:* increased frequency of syncope with loss of consciousness. Advise the patient to sit or lie down if dizziness occurs.

## CONTRAINDICATIONS

None known.

## NURSING CONSIDERATIONS

• Use cautiously in patients receiving other antihypertensives.
• Monitor the patient's blood pressure and pulse rate frequently.
• Know that elderly patients may be more sensitive to drug's hypotensive effects.
• Compliance *might* be improved with twice-daily dosing. Suggest this dosing change with the doctor if you suspect compliance problems.
• *Alert:* Be aware that if initial dose is greater than 1 mg, severe syncope with loss of consciousness may occur ("first-dose syncope").

## ☑ PATIENT TEACHING

• Warn the patient that dizziness may occur with first dose. If he experiences dizziness, tell him to sit or lie down. Reassure him that this effect disappears with continued dosing.
• Tell the patient not to suddenly stop taking this drug but to call the doctor if unpleasant adverse reactions occur.
• Advise the patient to minimize orthostatic hypotension by rising slowly and avoiding sudden position changes. Dry mouth can be relieved with chewing gum, sour hard candy, or ice chips.

---

# quinapril hydrochloride

Accupril, Asig‡

*Pregnancy Risk Category: C (D in 2nd and 3rd trimesters)*

## HOW SUPPLIED

*Tablets:* 5 mg, 10 mg, 20 mg, 40 mg

## ACTION

Unknown, but thought to be related to inhibition of angiotensin I to angiotensin II, a potent vasoconstrictor. Reduced formation of angiotensin II decreases peripheral arterial resistance, thus decreasing aldosterone secretion.

## ONSET, PEAK, DURATION

Onset occurs within 1 hour. Peak serum levels of quinapril are seen in 1 hour; quinaprilat, in 2 hours. Peak effects occur within 2 to 4 hours. Effects persist about 24 hours.

## INDICATIONS & DOSAGE

*Hypertension –*
**Adults:** initially, 10 mg daily. Dosage adjusted based on patient response at intervals of about 2 weeks. Most patients are controlled at 20, 40, or 80 mg daily as a single dose or in two divided doses.
*Heart failure –*
**Adults:** initially, 5 mg P.O. b.i.d. if patient is receiving a diuretic and 10 mg P.O. b.i.d. if patient not receiving a diuretic. Dosage increased at weekly intervals. Usual effective dose is 20 to 40 mg b.i.d. in equally divided doses.

## ADVERSE REACTIONS

**CNS:** somnolence, vertigo, nervousness, headache, dizziness, fatigue, depression.
**CV:** palpitations, tachycardia, angina, hypertensive crisis, orthostatic hypotension, *rhythm disturbances.*
**GI:** dry mouth, abdominal pain, constipation, vomiting, nausea, hemorrhage.
**Hepatic:** elevated liver enzymes.
**Respiratory:** *dry, persistent, tickling, nonproductive cough.*
**Skin:** pruritus, *exfoliative dermatitis, photosensitivity,* diaphoresis.
**Other:** *angioedema,* hyperkalemia.

---

Reactions may be *common,* uncommon, *life-threatening,* or COMMON AND LIFE-THREATENING.

## INTERACTIONS
*Diuretics, other antihypertensives:* risk of excessive hypotension. Discontinue diuretic or lower dose of quinapril as needed.
*Lithium:* increased serum lithium levels and lithium toxicity. Avoid concomitant use.
*Potassium-sparing diuretics, potassium supplements, sodium substitutes containing potassium:* risk of hyperkalemia. Monitor closely during concomitant use.

## CONTRAINDICATIONS
Contraindicated in patients with hypersensitivity to ACE inhibitors or with a history of angioedema related to treatment with an ACE inhibitor.

## NURSING CONSIDERATIONS
• Use cautiously in patients with impaired renal function.
• Assess renal and hepatic function before and periodically throughout therapy. Know that dosage adjustment is necessary for patients with renal impairment.
• Monitor blood pressure for effectiveness of therapy.
• Monitor serum potassium levels as ordered. Be aware that risk factors for the development of hyperkalemia include renal insufficiency, diabetes, and concomitant use of drugs that raise potassium level.
• Other ACE inhibitors have been associated with agranulocytosis and neutropenia. Monitor CBC with differential counts before therapy, every 2 weeks for the first 3 months of therapy, and periodically thereafter, as ordered.

## ☑ PATIENT TEACHING
• Advise the patient to report any signs of infection, such as fever and sore throat.
• *Alert:* Angioedema (including laryngeal edema) may occur, especially after the first dose. Advise the patient to report any signs or symptoms, such as swelling of face, eyes, lips, or tongue or breathing difficulty.
• Light-headedness can occur, especially during the first few days of therapy. Tell the patient to rise slowly to minimize effect and to report symptoms to the doctor. Patients who experience syncope should stop taking drug and call the doctor immediately.
• Inadequate fluid intake, vomiting, diarrhea, and excessive perspiration can lead to light-headedness and syncope. Tell the patient to use caution in hot weather and during exercise.
• Tell the patient to avoid sodium substitutes; these products may contain potassium, which can cause hyperkalemia in patients taking quinapril.
• Tell the female patient to notify doctor if pregnancy occurs. Drug will need to be discontinued.

---

# ramipril
Altace, Ramace‡, Tritace‡
*Pregnancy Risk Category: C (D in 2nd and 3rd trimesters)*

## HOW SUPPLIED
*Capsules:* 1.25 mg, 2.5 mg, 5 mg, 10 mg

## ACTION
Unknown, but thought to be related to inhibition of angiotensin I to angiotensin II, a potent vasoconstrictor. Reduced formation of angiotensin II decreases peripheral arterial resistance, thus decreasing aldosterone secretion.

## ONSET, PEAK, DURATION
Onset occurs within 1 to 2 hours. Peak serum levels of ramipril occur within 1 hour; of ramiprilat, in 3 hours. Peak effects occur in 4 to 6½ hours. Effects persist about 24 hours.

---

## INDICATIONS & DOSAGE

*Hypertension –*

**Adults:** initially, 2.5 mg P.O. once daily for patients not receiving a diuretic, and 1.25 mg P.O. once daily for patients receiving a diuretic. Dosage increased as necessary based on patient response. Maintenance dosage is 2.5 to 20 mg daily as a single dose or in divided doses.

In patients with renal insufficiency: If creatinine clearance is less than 40 ml/minute, 1.25 mg P.O. daily. Dosage is titrated gradually according to response. Maximum daily dosage is 5 mg.

*Heart failure –*

**Adults:** initially, 2.5 mg P.O. b.i.d. If hypotension occurs, dosage should be decreased to 1.25 mg P.O. b.i.d. Dosage may be gradually increased to a maximum of 5 mg P.O. b.i.d. as needed.

In patients with renal insufficiency: If creatinine clearance is less than 40 ml/minute, 1.25 mg P.O. daily. Dosage is titrated gradually according to response. Maximum daily dosage is 2.5 mg b.i.d.

## ADVERSE REACTIONS

**CNS:** headache, dizziness, fatigue, asthenia, malaise, light-headedness, anxiety, amnesia, *seizures,* depression, insomnia, nervousness, neuralgia, neuropathy, paresthesia, somnolence, tremor, vertigo.

**CV:** orthostatic hypotension, syncope, angina, *arrhythmias,* chest pain, palpitations, *MI.*

**EENT:** epistaxis, tinnitus.

**GI:** nausea, vomiting, abdominal pain, anorexia, constipation, diarrhea, dyspepsia, dry mouth, gastroenteritis.

**GU:** impotence.

**Respiratory:** *dry, persistent, tickling, nonproductive cough;* dyspnea.

**Skin:** hypersensitivity reactions, rash, dermatitis, pruritus, photosensitivity.

**Other:** *angioedema,* edema, hyperkalemia, increased diaphoresis, weight gain, arthralgia, arthritis, myalgia.

## INTERACTIONS

*Diuretics:* excessive hypotension, especially at the start of therapy. Discontinue diuretic at least 3 days before therapy begins, increase sodium intake, or reduce starting dose of ramipril.

*Insulin, oral antidiabetic agents:* risk of hypoglycemia, especially at initiation of ramipril therapy. Monitor closely.

*Lithium:* increased serum lithium levels. Use together cautiously and monitor serum lithium levels.

*Potassium-sparing diuretics, potassium supplements, sodium substitutes containing potassium:* increased risk of hyperkalemia because ramipril attenuates potassium loss. Monitor plasma potassium levels closely.

## CONTRAINDICATIONS

Contraindicated in patients with hypersensitivity to ACE inhibitors or a history of angioedema related to treatment with an ACE inhibitor.

## NURSING CONSIDERATIONS

• Use cautiously in patients with renal impairment.

• Monitor blood pressure regularly for drug effectiveness.

• Closely assess renal function in patients during first few weeks of therapy. Regular assessment of renal function (serum creatinine and BUN levels) is advisable. Patients with severe CHF whose renal function depends on the angiotensin-aldosterone system have experienced acute renal failure during ACE inhibitor therapy. Hypertensive patients with renal artery stenosis also may show signs of worsening renal function at start of therapy.

• Monitor CBC with differential counts before therapy, every 2 weeks for the first 3 months of therapy, and periodically thereafter. These effects may occur especially in patients with impaired renal function or collagen vascular diseases (systemic lupus erythematosus or scleroderma).

• Monitor serum potassium levels. Risk factors for the development of hyperkalemia include renal insufficiency, diabetes, and concomitant use of agents that raise potassium levels.

### ☑ PATIENT TEACHING
• Tell the patient to avoid abrupt discontinuation of therapy but to call doctor to discuss any unpleasant adverse reactions.
• *Alert:* Angioedema (including laryngeal edema) may occur, especially after the first dose. Advise the patient to report any signs or symptoms, such as swelling of face, eyes, lips, or tongue or breathing difficulty.
• Light-headedness can occur, especially during the first few days of therapy. Tell the patient to rise slowly to minimize this effect and to report symptoms to the doctor. Patients who experience syncope should stop taking drug and call the doctor immediately.
• Advise him to report signs of infection, such as fever and sore throat.
• Tell the patient to avoid sodium substitutes; these products may contain potassium, which can cause hyperkalemia in patients taking ramipril.
• Tell the female patient to notify doctor if pregnancy occurs. Drug will need to be discontinued.

---

## rauwolfia serpentina
Raudixin**, Rauverid, Wolfina

*Pregnancy Risk Category: C*

### HOW SUPPLIED
*Tablets:* 50 mg, 100 mg

### ACTION
Unknown. Thought to be due to reduced cardiac output and possibly decreased peripheral resistance.

### ONSET, PEAK, DURATION
Onset occurs in several days to 3 weeks. Peak effect is reached in 3 to 6 weeks. Effects persist for 1 to 6 weeks.

### INDICATIONS & DOSAGE
*Mild to moderate hypertension –*
**Adults:** initially and for 1 to 3 weeks thereafter, 200 to 400 mg P.O. daily as a single dose or in two divided doses. Maintenance dosage is 50 to 300 mg daily.

### ADVERSE REACTIONS
**CNS:** dizziness, *depression, drowsiness, nervousness, paradoxical anxiety,* nightmares, headache, extrapyramidal symptoms.
**CV:** bradycardia, syncope, angina, arrhythmias.
**EENT:** glaucoma, *nasal congestion,* epistaxis.
**GI:** *hypersecretion of gastric acid, nausea, vomiting, dry mouth,* bleeding, anorexia, diarrhea.
**GU:** impotence.
**Skin:** pruritus, rash.
**Other:** weight gain, *thrombocytopenic purpura,* dyspnea.

### INTERACTIONS
*CNS depressants:* additive effects. Use together cautiously.
*Digitalis glycosides:* rauwolfia may predispose patients to digitalis-induced arrhythmias. Use together cautiously.
*Diuretics and other antihypertensives:* increased risk of hypotension. Use together cautiously.
*MAO inhibitors:* may cause excitability and hypertension. Use together cautiously.

### CONTRAINDICATIONS
Contraindicated in patients with mental depression, active peptic ulcer disease or ulcerative colitis, hypersensitivity to the drug, and concurrent electroconvulsive therapy.

---

*Liquid form contains alcohol. **May contain tartrazine. †Canada only. ‡Australia only. ◇OTC.

## NURSING CONSIDERATIONS
• Use cautiously in patients with epilepsy, history of peptic ulcer, ulcerative colitis, or gallstones.
• Monitor blood pressure and pulse rate frequently.

### ☑ PATIENT TEACHING
• Tell the patient that drug should be taken with meals.
• Tell the patient not to discontinue drug suddenly, but to call the doctor, if unpleasant adverse reactions occur.
• Warn the patient not to perform tasks that require alertness and good coordination until drug's CNS effects are known.
• Advise the patient to minimize orthostatic hypotension by rising slowly and avoiding sudden position changes. Dry mouth can be relieved with chewing gum, sour hard candy, or ice chips. Tell him to contact the doctor if he needs relief for nasal congestion.
• Tell the patient to weigh himself daily and to notify the doctor of any weight gain over 5 lb (about 2 kg).
• Advise the patient to have periodic eye examinations.
• Tell caregivers to watch the patient closely for signs of mental depression. Warn the patient to notify the doctor promptly if nightmares occur.

---

## rescinnamine
Moderil

*Pregnancy Risk Category: C*

### HOW SUPPLIED
*Tablets:* 0.25 mg, 0.5 mg

### ACTION
Unknown. Thought to be due to reduced cardiac output and possibly decreased peripheral resistance.

### ONSET, PEAK, DURATION
Unknown.

## INDICATIONS & DOSAGE
*Mild hypertension –*
**Adults:** initially, 0.5 mg P.O. b.i.d. Maintenance dosage is 0.25 to 0.5 mg daily.

## ADVERSE REACTIONS
**CNS:** *depression, drowsiness, nervousness, anxiety,* dizziness, *nightmares,* sedation, parkinsonism.
**CV:** *bradycardia, syncope,* angina, arrhythmias.
**EENT:** *nasal congestion,* glaucoma, epistaxis.
**GI:** *hypersecretion of gastric acid, nausea, vomiting, dry mouth,* GI bleeding, anorexia, diarrhea.
**GU:** impotence.
**Skin:** pruritus, rash.
**Other:** *weight gain, **thrombocytopenic purpura,** dyspnea.

## INTERACTIONS
*Digitalis glycosides, quinidine:* arrhythmias may occur. Monitor patient closely.
*MAO inhibitors:* may cause excitability and hypertension. Use together cautiously.

## CONTRAINDICATIONS
Contraindicated in patients with mental depression, active peptic ulcer disease or ulcerative colitis, hypersensitivity to the drug, and concurrent electroconvulsive therapy.

## NURSING CONSIDERATIONS
• Use cautiously in patients with history of peptic ulcer, ulcerative colitis, or gallstones.
• Monitor blood pressure and pulse rate frequently.

### ☑ PATIENT TEACHING
• Tell the patient that drug should be taken with meals.
• Tell the patient not to discontinue drug suddenly, but to call the doctor, if unpleasant adverse reactions occur.
• Warn the patient not to perform

---

tasks that require alertness and coordination until drug's CNS effects are known.

• Advise the patient to minimize orthostatic hypotension by rising slowly and avoiding sudden position changes. Dry mouth can be relieved with chewing gum, sour hard candy, or ice chips. Tell him to contact the doctor if he needs relief for nasal congestion.

• Tell the patient to weigh himself daily and to notify the doctor of any weight gain over 5 lb (about 2 kg).

• Advise the patient to have periodic eye examinations.

• Tell caregivers to watch the patient closely for signs of mental depression. Warn the patient to notify the doctor promptly if nightmares occur.

---

## reserpine
Novoreserpine†, Serpalan, Serpasil*

*Pregnancy Risk Category: C*

### HOW SUPPLIED
*Tablets:* 0.1 mg, 0.25 mg, 1 mg

### ACTION
Unknown. Thought to be due to reduced cardiac output and possibly decreased peripheral resistance.

### ONSET, PEAK, DURATION
Onset occurs in several days to 3 weeks. Peak effect occurs in 3 to 6 weeks. Effects persist for 1 to 6 weeks.

### INDICATIONS & DOSAGE
*Mild to moderate essential hypertension –*
**Adults:** 0.1 to 0.25 mg P.O. daily.
**Children:** 5 to 20 mcg/kg P.O. daily.

### ADVERSE REACTIONS
**CNS:** *drowsiness, sedation, nervousness, paradoxical anxiety,* dizziness, *nightmares, depression,* extrapyramidal symptoms.

**CV:** angina, arrhythmias, *bradycardia, syncope.*
**EENT:** *nasal congestion,* glaucoma, epistaxis.
**GI:** *hyperacidity, nausea, vomiting, dry mouth,* bleeding, anorexia, diarrhea.
**GU:** *impotence.*
**Skin:** pruritus, rash.
**Other:** *weight gain,* **thrombocytopenic purpura,** dyspnea.

### INTERACTIONS
*Digitalis glycosides, quinidine:* arrhythmias may occur. Monitor patient closely.
*Diuretics and other antihypertensives:* increased risk of hypotension. Monitor blood pressure closely.
*MAO inhibitors:* may cause excitability and hypertension. Use together cautiously.

### CONTRAINDICATIONS
Contraindicated in patients with hypersensitivity to the drug, mental depression, ulcerative colitis or peptic ulcer disease and in those receiving electroconvulsive therapy.

### NURSING CONSIDERATIONS
• Use cautiously in patients with history of peptic ulcer, ulcerative colitis, or gallstones.
• Monitor blood pressure and pulse rate frequently.

### ☑ PATIENT TEACHING
• Tell the patient that drug should be taken with meals.
• Tell the patient not to discontinue drug suddenly, but to call the doctor, if unpleasant adverse reactions occur.
• Warn the patient not to perform hazardous tasks that require alertness and coordination until drug's CNS effects are known.
• Advise the patient to minimize orthostatic hypotension by rising slowly and avoiding sudden position changes. Dry mouth can be relieved with chewing gum, sour hard candy, or ice

---

chips. Tell him to contact the doctor if he needs relief for nasal congestion.
• Tell the patient to weigh himself daily and to notify the doctor of any weight gain over 5 lb (about 2 kg).
• Advise the patient to have periodic eye examinations.
• Tell caregivers to watch the patient closely for signs of mental depression. Warn the patient to notify the doctor promptly if nightmares occur.

---

## terazosin hydrochloride
Hytrin
*Pregnancy Risk Category: C*

**HOW SUPPLIED**
*Tablets:* 1 mg, 2 mg, 5 mg, 10 mg

**ACTION**
Decreases blood pressure by vasodilation produced in response to blockade of alpha$_1$-adrenergic receptors. Improves urine flow in patients with benign prostatic hyperplasia (BPH) by blocking alpha$_1$-adrenergic receptors in the smooth muscle of the bladder neck and prostate, thus relieving urethral pressure and reestablishing urine flow.

**ONSET, PEAK, DURATION**
Onset occurs within 15 minutes. Peak effects occur within 2 to 3 hours. Effects persist for 24 hours.

**INDICATIONS & DOSAGE**
*Hypertension* –
**Adults:** initially, 1 mg P.O. h.s. Dosage increased gradually according to patient response. Usual dosage range is 1 to 5 mg daily. Maximum recommended dosage is 20 mg/day.
*Symptomatic BPH* –
**Adults:** initially, 1 mg P.O. h.s. Dosage increased in a stepwise fashion to 2, 5, or 10 mg once daily to achieve optimal response. Most patients require 10 mg daily for optimal response.

**ADVERSE REACTIONS**
**CNS:** *asthenia, dizziness, headache,* nervousness, paresthesia, somnolence.
**CV:** *palpitations,* postural hypotension, tachycardia, *peripheral edema.*
**EENT:** *nasal congestion,* sinusitis, blurred vision.
**GI:** *nausea.*
**GU:** impotence.
**Respiratory:** dyspnea.
**Other:** back pain, muscle pain.

**INTERACTIONS**
*Antihypertensives:* excessive hypotension. Use together cautiously.

**CONTRAINDICATIONS**
Contraindicated in patients with hypersensitivity to the drug.

**NURSING CONSIDERATIONS**
• Monitor blood pressure frequently.
• ***Alert:*** Know that if terazosin is discontinued for several days, the patient will need to be retitrated using initial dosing regimen (1 mg P.O. h.s.).

☑ **PATIENT TEACHING**
• Tell the patient not to discontinue drug suddenly, but to call the doctor, if adverse reactions occur.
• Warn the patient to avoid hazardous activities that require mental alertness, such as driving or operating heavy machinery, for 12 hours after the first dose.

---

## timolol maleate
Apo-Timol†, Blocadren
*Pregnancy Risk Category: C*

**HOW SUPPLIED**
*Tablets:* 5 mg, 10 mg, 20 mg

**ACTION**
Mechanism of antihypertensive action unknown. In MI, may decrease myocardial oxygen requirements. Prevents arterial dilation through beta block-

---

Reactions may be *common,* uncommon, ***life-threatening,*** or **COMMON AND LIFE-THREATENING.**

ade for migraine headache prophylaxis.

## ONSET, PEAK, DURATION
Onset occurs in 15 to 30 minutes. Peak effects occur in 1 to 2 hours. Effects persist for 6 to 12 hours.

## INDICATIONS & DOSAGE
*Hypertension –*
**Adults:** initially, 10 mg P.O. b.i.d. Usual daily maintenance dosage is 20 to 40 mg. Maximum daily dosage is 60 mg. Allow at least 7 days to elapse between increases in dosage.
*MI (long-term prophylaxis in patients who have survived acute phase) –*
**Adults:** 10 mg P.O. b.i.d.
*Migraine headache prophylaxis –*
**Adults:** initially, 20 mg P.O. daily as a single dose or in divided doses b.i.d. Increase dosage as needed and tolerated to maximum of 30 mg daily. Discontinue treatment if no response occurs after 6 to 8 weeks of therapy at maximum dosage.

## ADVERSE REACTIONS
**CNS:** fatigue, lethargy, dizziness.
**CV:** *bradycardia, hypotension, CHF,* peripheral vascular disease, arrhythmias, pulmonary edema.
**GI:** nausea, vomiting, diarrhea.
**Respiratory:** dyspnea, *bronchospasm, increased airway resistance.*
**Skin:** pruritus.

## INTERACTIONS
*Digitalis glycosides, diltiazem, verapamil:* excessive bradycardia and increased depressant effect on myocardium. Use together cautiously.
*Indomethacin:* decreased antihypertensive effect. Monitor blood pressure and adjust dosage.
*Insulin, oral antidiabetic agents:* can alter requirements for these drugs in previously stabilized diabetic patients. Monitor the patient for hypoglycemia.

## CONTRAINDICATIONS
Contraindicated in patients with bronchial asthma, severe COPD, sinus bradycardia and heart block greater than first-degree, cardiogenic shock, overt CHF, or hypersensitivity to the drug.

## NURSING CONSIDERATIONS
• Use cautiously in patients with compensated CHF; hepatic, renal, or respiratory disease; diabetes; and hyperthyroidism.
• Check the patient's apical pulse rate before giving drug. If you detect extremes in pulse rates, withhold drug and call the doctor immediately.
• Monitor blood pressure frequently.
• Monitor blood glucose levels in diabetic patients; drug can mask signs and symptoms of hypoglycemia.

## ☑ PATIENT TEACHING
• Tell the patient to take drug exactly as prescribed.
• Instruct the patient not to discontinue drug suddenly but to call doctor to discuss any unpleasant adverse reactions. Tell him dosage should be reduced gradually over 1 to 2 weeks.

---

# trimethaphan camsylate
Arfonad

*Pregnancy Risk Category: D*

## HOW SUPPLIED
*Injection:* 50 mg/ml in 10-ml ampule, 250 mg/vial‡

## ACTION
A ganglionic blocker that causes vasodilation and increased peripheral blood flow which results in decreased blood pressure.

## ONSET, PEAK, DURATION
Onset and peak are immediate. Effects dissipate within 10 to 15 minutes of discontinuing drug.

---

## INDICATIONS & DOSAGE

*To lower blood pressure quickly in hypertensive emergencies; to control hypotension during surgery –*
**Adults:** 500 mg (10 ml) diluted in 500 ml D₅W, normal saline solution, or Ringer's injection to yield concentration of 1 mg/ml. I.V. drip started at 3 to 4 mg/minute and titrated to achieve desired hypotensive response. Range is 0.3 to 6 mg/minute.

## ADVERSE REACTIONS

**CNS:** *extreme weakness,* restlessness.
**CV:** *severe orthostatic hypotension, tachycardia,* precipitation of angina, syncope.
**EENT:** cycloplegia, mydriasis.
**GI:** anorexia, *nausea, vomiting, dry mouth,* diarrhea, heartburn, abdominal discomfort.
**GU:** urine retention.
**Respiratory:** *respiratory depression.*
**Skin:** urticaria, pruritus.
**Other:** chilliness.

## INTERACTIONS

*Anesthetics, diuretics, procainamide:* increased hypotensive effect. Monitor the patient closely.
*Neuromuscular blockers:* potentiation of neuromuscular blocking action of the nondepolarized agents. Administer together with caution.

## CONTRAINDICATIONS

Contraindicated in patients with uncorrected anemia, hypovolemia, hypovolemic shock, asphyxia, or uncorrected respiratory insufficiency.

## NURSING CONSIDERATIONS

● Use with extreme caution in patients with arteriosclerosis; cardiac, hepatic, or renal disease; degenerative CNS disorders; Addison's disease; or diabetes mellitus. Also use cautiously in those receiving other antihypertensives or glucocorticoids. Also use with extreme caution in elderly or debilitated patients.

● **I.V. use:** Refrigerate before reconstitution, and prepare solution just before use. Solution is stable for 24 hours after reconstitution.
● Use infusion pump to administer drug slowly and precisely.
● Place the patient in the supine position during drug administration. To avoid cerebral anoxia, elevate the head of the bed for maximal effect, if necessary. Do not elevate bed more than 30 degrees.
● Monitor blood pressure and vital signs continuously.
● **Alert:** Watch closely for respiratory distress, especially if large doses are used. Large doses have caused apnea and respiratory arrest.
● If extreme hypotension occurs, discontinue drug and call the doctor. Use phenylephrine or mephentermine to counteract hypotension.
● Discontinue drug before wound closure in surgery as ordered to allow blood pressure to return to normal.

☑ **PATIENT TEACHING**
● Tell patient to report adverse reactions promptly.
● Tell him to alert nurse if he feels discomfort at injection site.

---

Reactions may be *common,* uncommon, *life-threatening,* or **COMMON AND LIFE-THREATENING.**

# 24

# Antilipemics

**cholestyramine**
**clofibrate**
**colestipol hydrochloride**
**dextrothyroxine sodium**
**fluvastatin sodium**
**gemfibrozil**
**lovastatin**
**niacin**
  (See Chapter 90, VITAMINS AND MINERALS.)
**pravastatin sodium**
**simvastatin**

**COMBINATION PRODUCTS**
None.

## cholestyramine
Questran**, Questran Light,
Questran Lite‡
*Pregnancy Risk Category: NR*

### HOW SUPPLIED
*Powder:* 378-g cans, 9-g single-dose packets. Each scoop of powder or single-dose packet contains 4 g of cholestyramine resin.

### ACTION
A bile-acid sequestrant that combines with bile acid to form an insoluble compound that is excreted. The liver must synthesize new bile acid from cholesterol, which reduces low-density-lipoprotein cholesterol levels.

### ONSET, PEAK, DURATION
Reduction of plasma cholesterol concentrations generally reduced within 1 to 2 weeks of therapy. After withdrawal of drug, cholesterol concentrations return to baseline in about 2 to 4 weeks.

### INDICATIONS & DOSAGE
*Primary hyperlipidemia or pruritus caused by partial bile obstruction; adjunct for reduction of elevated serum cholesterol in patients with primary hypercholesterolemia –*
**Adults:** 4 g once or twice daily. Maintenance dosage is 8 to 16 g daily. Maximum daily dosage is 24 g.

### ADVERSE REACTIONS
**CNS:** headache, anxiety, vertigo, dizziness, insomnia, fatigue, syncope, tinnitus.
**GI:** *constipation, fecal impaction,* hemorrhoids, *abdominal discomfort,* flatulence, *nausea,* vomiting, steatorrhea, GI bleeding, diarrhea, anorexia.
**GU:** hematuria, dysuria.
**Skin:** *rash;* irritation of skin, tongue, and perianal area.
**Other:** *vitamin A, D, E, and K deficiencies from decreased absorption,* hyperchloremic acidosis with long-term use or very high dosage, anemia, ecchymoses, backache, muscle and joint pains, bleeding tendencies, osteoporosis.

### INTERACTIONS
*Acetaminophen, beta-adrenergic blockers, corticosteroids, digitalis glycosides, fat-soluble vitamins (A, D, E, and K), iron preparations, thiazide diuretics, thyroid hormones, warfarin and other coumarin derivatives:* absorption may be substantially decreased by cholestyramine. Administer at least 2 hours apart.

### CONTRAINDICATIONS
Contraindicated in patients with hypersensitivity to bile-acid sequestering resins and in those with complete biliary obstruction.

### NURSING CONSIDERATIONS
● Use cautiously in patients predisposed to constipation and in those with conditions aggravated by consti-

pation, such as severe, symptomatic coronary artery disease.
• Monitor serum cholesterol and triglyceride levels regularly during therapy.
• Monitor serum levels of digitalis glycosides in patients receiving digitalis glycosides and cholestyramine concurrently. If cholestyramine therapy is discontinued, adjust dosage of digitalis glycosides as ordered to avoid toxicity.
• Monitor bowel habits. Encourage a diet high in fiber and fluids. If severe constipation develops, decrease dosage, add a stool softener, or discontinue drug, as ordered.
• Be aware that long-term use may be associated with deficiencies of vitamins A, D, E, and K and folic acid.

☑ **PATIENT TEACHING**
• **Alert:** Tell the patient never to take drug in its dry form; esophageal irritation or severe constipation may result.
• Instruct the patient to mix powder as follows: Using a large glass, the patient should sprinkle the powder on the surface of preferred beverage; let the mixture stand a few minutes; then stir thoroughly. The best diluents are water, milk, and juice (especially pulpy fruit juice). Mixing with carbonated beverages may result in excessive foaming. After drinking this preparation, the patient should swirl a small additional amount of liquid in the same glass and then drink it to ensure ingestion of the entire dose.
• Advise the patient to take all other drugs at least 1 hour before or 4 to 6 hours after cholestyramine to avoid blocking their absorption.
• Teach the patient about proper dietary management of serum lipids. When appropriate, recommend weight-control, exercise, and smoking-cessation programs.

# clofibrate
Arterioflexin‡, Atromid-S, Claripex†, Col‡, Novofibrate†

*Pregnancy Risk Category: C*

## HOW SUPPLIED
*Capsules:* 500 mg

## ACTION
Unknown. Seems to inhibit biosynthesis of cholesterol at an early stage.

## ONSET, PEAK, DURATION
Plasma concentrations of very-low-density lipoprotein (VLDL) are reduced within 2 to 5 days. Time to peak effect occurs in 3 weeks with continued use. VLDL concentrations return to pretreatment levels within 3 weeks after drug is withdrawn.

## INDICATIONS & DOSAGE
*Hyperlipidemia –*
**Adults:** 2 g P.O. daily in divided doses. Some patients may respond to lower doses as assessed by serum lipid monitoring.

## ADVERSE REACTIONS
**CNS:** fatigue, weakness, drowsiness, dizziness, headache.
**CV:** *arrhythmias,* angina, ***thromboembolic events,*** intermittent claudication.
**GI:** *nausea, diarrhea, vomiting,* stomatitis, *dyspepsia,* flatulence, ***cholelithiasis, cholecystitis.***
**GU:** impotence and decreased libido, renal dysfunction (dysuria, hematuria, proteinuria, decreased urine output).
**Hematologic:** leukopenia, anemia, eosinophilia.
**Hepatic:** gallstones, *transient and reversible elevations of liver function tests,* hepatomegaly.
**Skin:** rash, urticaria, pruritus, dry skin and hair.
**Other:** myalgia and arthralgia, resembling a flulike syndrome; *weight gain; polyphagia.*

---

Reactions may be *common,* uncommon, *life-threatening,* or **COMMON AND LIFE-THREATENING.**

## INTERACTIONS
*Furosemide, sulfonylureas:* clofibrate may potentiate the clinical effects of these agents. Monitor closely.
*Lovastatin, pravastatin, simvastatin:* risk of myositis, rhabdomyolysis, and renal failure. Avoid concomitant use.
*Oral anticoagulants:* clofibrate may potentiate the anticoagulant effects of warfarin or dicumarol. Decrease the anticoagulant dosage.
*Oral contraceptives, rifampin:* may antagonize clofibrate's lipid-lowering effect. Monitor serum lipids.
*Probenecid:* increased clofibrate effect. Monitor for toxicity.

## CONTRAINDICATIONS
Contraindicated in patients with significant hepatic or renal dysfunction, primary biliary cirrhosis, or hypersensitivity to the drug and in pregnant or breast-feeding women.

## NURSING CONSIDERATIONS
• Use cautiously in patients with peptic ulcer.
• Monitor serum cholesterol and triglyceride levels regularly during therapy.
• Monitor renal and hepatic function, blood counts, and serum electrolyte and blood glucose levels. If liver function tests show steady rise, expect discontinuation of clofibrate.
• Know that drug typically is discontinued if significant lipid lowering is not achieved within 3 months.

### ☑ PATIENT TEACHING
• Teach the patient about proper dietary management of serum lipids. When appropriate, recommend weight-control, exercise, and smoking-cessation programs.
• Advise the patient to report any flu-like symptoms immediately because their occurrence may indicate rhabdomyolysis-induced renal failure.

# colestipol hydrochloride
Colestid

*Pregnancy Risk Category: NR*

## HOW SUPPLIED
*Granules:* 300-g and 500-g bottles, 5-g packets
*Tablets:* 1 g

## ACTION
Combines with bile acid to form an insoluble compound that is excreted in feces. The liver must synthesize new bile acid from cholesterol; this leads to reduced low-density-lipoprotein cholesterol levels.

## ONSET, PEAK, DURATION
Reduced plasma cholesterol levels occur within 1 to 2 days. Antilipemic effects peak after about 1 month of therapy. Lipid levels return to pretreatment values within 1 month of discontinuing treatment.

## INDICATIONS & DOSAGE
*Primary hypercholesterolemia* –
**Adults:** 5 to 30 g P.O. once daily or in divided doses.

## ADVERSE REACTIONS
**CNS:** headache, dizziness, anxiety, vertigo, insomnia, fatigue, syncope, tinnitus.
**GI:** *constipation, **fecal impaction,*** hemorrhoids, abdominal discomfort, flatulence, nausea, vomiting, steatorrhea, GI bleeding, diarrhea, anorexia.
**GU:** dysuria, hematuria.
**Skin:** rash; irritation of tongue and perianal area.
**Other:** vitamin A, D, E, and K deficiencies from decreased absorption; hyperchloremic acidosis with long-term use or high dosage, anemia, ecchymoses, bleeding tendencies, backache, muscle and joint pain, osteoporosis.

## INTERACTIONS

*Oral antidiabetic agents:* may antagonize response to colestipol. Monitor serum lipids.
*Orally administered drugs:* colestipol may decrease absorption. Separate administration times; give other drugs at least 1 hour before or 4 hours after colestipol.

## CONTRAINDICATIONS

Contraindicated in patients with hypersensitivity reactions to bile-acid sequestering resins.

## NURSING CONSIDERATIONS

• Use cautiously in patients predisposed to constipation and in those with conditions aggravated by constipation, such as severe, symptomatic coronary artery disease.
• Monitor serum cholesterol and triglyceride levels regularly during therapy.
• Monitor bowel habits; if severe constipation develops, decrease dosage or add stool softener as ordered. Encourage a diet high in fiber and fluids.
• Monitor serum levels of digitalis glycosides in patients receiving digitalis glycosides and colestipol concurrently. If colestipol therapy is discontinued, adjust dosage of digitalis glycosides to avoid toxicity, as ordered.

☑ **PATIENT TEACHING**
• *Alert:* Tell the patient never to take drug in its dry form; esophageal irritation or severe constipation may result.
• To prepare, instruct the patient to use a large glass containing water, milk, or juice (especially pulpy fruit juice). The patient should sprinkle the powder on the surface of the preferred beverage; let the mixture stand a few minutes; then stir thoroughly to obtain a uniform suspension. After drinking this preparation, the patient should swirl a small additional amount of liquid in the same glass and then drink it to ensure ingestion of the entire dose.
• To enhance palatability, tell the patient to mix and refrigerate the next daily dose the previous evening.
• Instruct the patient taking tablet form to swallow tablets whole and not to crush, cut, or chew them.
• Advise the patient to take all other drugs at least 1 hour before or 4 to 6 hours after colestipol to avoid blocking their absorption.
• Teach the patient about proper dietary management of serum lipids. When appropriate, recommend weight-control, exercise, and smoking-cessation programs.
• Inform the patient that long-term use may be associated with deficiencies of vitamins A, D, E, and K and folic acid. Instruct patient to report any unusual signs and symptoms.

---

# dextrothyroxine sodium (d-thyroxine sodium)
Choloxin**

*Pregnancy Risk Category: NR*

## HOW SUPPLIED
*Tablets:* 1 mg, 2 mg, 4 mg, 6 mg

## ACTION
Unknown. Thought to accelerate hepatic catabolism of cholesterol and increase bile secretion to lower cholesterol levels.

## ONSET, PEAK, DURATION
Onset unknown. Peak effects occur after 1 to 2 months. Effects persist for 1½ to 3 months.

## INDICATIONS & DOSAGE
*Hyperlipidemia in euthyroid patients, especially when cholesterol and triglyceride levels are elevated –*
**Adults:** initially, 1 to 2 mg P.O. daily, increased by 1 to 2 mg daily at monthly intervals to a total of 4 to 8 mg daily.

---

**Children:** initially, 0.05 mg/kg P.O. daily, increased by 0.05 mg/kg daily at monthly intervals to a maximum of 4 mg daily. Alternatively, give 1.5 mg/m² P.O. daily, increased by 1.5 mg/m² daily at monthly intervals. Maximum daily dosage is 4 mg. The usual maintenance dosage is 0.1 mg/kg or 3 mg/m² daily in euthyroid children.

## ADVERSE REACTIONS
**CNS:** insomnia, nervousness, tremor, headache, tinnitus, dizziness, paresthesia.
**CV:** palpitations, angina pectoris, *arrhythmias,* ischemic myocardial changes on ECG, *MI.*
**EENT:** visual disturbances, exophthalmos, retinopathy, ptosis.
**GI:** nausea, vomiting, diarrhea, constipation, decreased appetite, dyspepsia.
**Skin:** *diaphoresis,* flushing, rashes, pruritus.
**Other:** *insomnia, weight loss,* hyperthermia, hyperthyroidism, alopecia, menstrual irregularities.

## INTERACTIONS
*Digitalis glycosides:* dextrothyroxine may decrease clinical effect. Use together cautiously.
*Insulin, sulfonylureas:* increased glucose levels. Monitor closely.
*Oral anticoagulants:* dextrothyroxine may potentiate anticoagulant effect of warfarin or dicumarol. Monitor prothrombin time.
*Sympathomimetics, thyroid hormones:* dextrothyroxine may precipitate arrhythmias or coronary insufficiency in patients with cardiac disease. Monitor closely.

## CONTRAINDICATIONS
Contraindicated in patients with advanced hepatic or renal disease or iodism. Also contraindicated in patients with organic heart disease; history of MI; arrhythmias; rheumatic heart disease; history of CHF or decompensation or borderline compensated cardiac status; and hypertension (other than mild, labile, systolic hypertension).

## NURSING CONSIDERATIONS
● Use cautiously in patients with diabetes mellitus and impaired liver or kidney function.
● Monitor lipid levels, as ordered.
● Observe the patient for signs of hyperthyroidism, such as nervousness, insomnia, and weight loss. If these occur, decrease dosage or discontinue drug as ordered.

## ☑ PATIENT TEACHING
● Instruct the patient to take drug exactly as prescribed.
● Teach the patient about proper dietary management of serum lipids. When appropriate, recommend weight-control, exercise, and smoking-cessation programs.

---

# fluvastatin sodium
Lescol

*Pregnancy Risk Category: X*

## HOW SUPPLIED
*Capsules:* 20 mg, 40 mg

## ACTION
Inhibits 3-hydroxy-3-methylglutaryl coenzyme A reductase. This enzyme is an early (and rate-limiting) step in the synthetic pathway of cholesterol.

## ONSET, PEAK, DURATION
Unknown.

## INDICATIONS & DOSAGE
*Reduction of low-density lipoprotein and total cholesterol levels in patients with primary hypercholesterolemia (types IIa and IIb) –*
**Adults:** initially, 20 mg P.O. h.s. Increase dosage as needed to a maximum of 40 mg daily.

---

## ADVERSE REACTIONS
**CNS:** headache, fatigue, dizziness, insomnia.
**GI:** dyspepsia, diarrhea, nausea, vomiting, abdominal pain, constipation, flatulence, tooth disorder.
**Hematologic:** thrombocytopenia, leukopenia, *hemolytic anemia*.
**Respiratory:** sinusitis, *upper respiratory infection,* rhinitis, cough, pharyngitis, bronchitis.
**Other:** arthropathy, muscle pain, hypersensitivity reactions (rash, pruritus), increased liver enzyme levels.

## INTERACTIONS
*Cholestyramine, colestipol:* may bind with fluvastatin in the GI tract and decrease absorption. Separate administration times by at least 4 hours.
*Cimetidine, omeprazole, ranitidine:* decreased fluvastatin metabolism. Monitor for enhanced effects.
*Cyclosporine and other immunosuppressants, erythromycin, gemfibrozil, niacin:* possible increased risk of polymyositis and rhabdomyolysis. Avoid concomitant use.
*Digoxin:* may alter digoxin pharmacokinetics. Monitor serum digoxin levels carefully.
*Ethanol:* increased risk of hepatotoxicity. Avoid concomitant use.
*Rifampin:* enhanced fluvastatin metabolism and decreased plasma levels. Monitor for lack of effect.

## CONTRAINDICATIONS
Contraindicated in patients with hypersensitivity to the drug; in those with active liver disease or conditions associated with unexplained persistent elevations of serum transaminase levels; in pregnant and breast-feeding women; and in women of childbearing age unless there is no risk of pregnancy.

## NURSING CONSIDERATIONS
• Use cautiously in patients with severe renal impairment and history of liver disease or heavy alcohol use.
• Know that fluvastatin should be initiated only after diet and other non-pharmacologic therapies prove ineffective. The patient should be on a standard low-cholesterol diet during therapy.
• Be aware that liver function tests should be performed at the start of therapy and periodically thereafter.
• Watch for signs of myositis.

## ☑ PATIENT TEACHING
• Tell the patient that drug may be taken without regard to meals; however, efficacy is enhanced if the drug is taken in the evening.
• Teach the patient about proper dietary management, weight control, and exercise. Explain their importance in controlling elevated serum lipids levels.
• Warn the patient to avoid alcohol.
• Tell the patient to inform the doctor of any adverse reactions, particularly muscle aches and pains.
• *Alert:* Inform the female patient that drug is contraindicated during pregnancy. Advise her to notify doctor immediately if pregnancy occurs.

---

# gemfibrozil
Lopid

*Pregnancy Risk Category: C*

## HOW SUPPLIED
*Tablets:* 600 mg
*Capsules:* 300 mg

## ACTION
Inhibits peripheral lipolysis and also reduces triglyceride synthesis in the liver. Lowers serum triglyceride levels and increases high-density-lipoprotein cholesterol levels.

## ONSET, PEAK, DURATION
Onset occurs in 2 to 5 days. Peak effect occurs after 4 weeks of treatment. Duration unknown.

---

Reactions may be *common,* uncommon, *life-threatening,* or **COMMON AND LIFE-THREATENING.**

## INDICATIONS & DOSAGE
*Types IV and V hyperlipidemia unresponsive to diet and other drugs; reduction of risk of coronary heart disease in patients with type IIb hyperlipidemia who cannot tolerate or who are refractory to treatment with bile acid sequestrants or niacin –*
**Adults:** 1,200 mg P.O. daily in two divided doses, 30 minutes before morning and evening meals.

## ADVERSE REACTIONS
**CNS:** headache, fatigue, vertigo.
**CV:** atrial fibrillation.
**GI:** *abdominal and epigastric pain, diarrhea, nausea,* vomiting, *dyspepsia,* constipation, acute appendicitis.
**Hematologic:** anemia, leukopenia, eosinophilia, *thrombocytopenia*.
**Hepatic:** bile duct obstruction, elevated liver enzymes.
**Skin:** rash, dermatitis, pruritus, eczema.

## INTERACTIONS
*Lovastatin:* myopathy with rhabdomyolysis has been reported. Don't use together.
*Oral anticoagulants:* gemfibrozil may enhance the clinical effects of oral anticoagulants. Monitor closely.

## CONTRAINDICATIONS
Contraindicated in patients with hypersensitivity to the drug, or hepatic or severe renal dysfunction (including primary biliary cirrhosis), and preexisting gallbladder disease.

## NURSING CONSIDERATIONS
● Know that periodic CBCs and liver function tests should be performed during the first 12 months of therapy.
● If the drug has no beneficial effects after 3 months of therapy, expect the doctor to discontinue the drug.

## ☑ PATIENT TEACHING
● Instruct the patient to take drug ½ hour before breakfast and dinner.

● Teach the patient about proper dietary management of serum lipids. When appropriate, recommend weight-control, exercise, and smoking-cessation programs.
● Because of possible dizziness and blurred vision, advise the patient to avoid driving or other potentially hazardous activities until drug's CNS effects are known.
● Tell the patient to observe bowel movements and to report any evidence of steatorrhea or other signs of bile duct obstruction.

# lovastatin (mevinolin)
Mevacor
*Pregnancy Risk Category: X*

## HOW SUPPLIED
*Tablets:* 10 mg, 20 mg, 40 mg

## ACTION
Inhibits 3-hydroxy-3-methylglutaryl coenzyme A reductase. This enzyme is an early (and rate-limiting) step in the synthetic pathway of cholesterol.

## ONSET, PEAK, DURATION
Onset unknown. Plasma levels peak within 2 to 6 hours after a dose. After withdrawal of continuous therapy, effects persist for 4 to 6 weeks.

## INDICATIONS & DOSAGE
*Reduction of low-density lipoprotein and total cholesterol levels in patients with primary hypercholesterolemia (types IIa and IIb) –*
**Adults:** initially, 20 mg P.O. once daily with evening meal. For patients with severely elevated cholesterol levels (for example, over 300 mg/dl), initial dose is 40 mg. Recommended daily dosage range is 20 to 80 mg in single or divided doses.

## ADVERSE REACTIONS
**CNS:** headache, dizziness, peripheral neuropathy, insomnia.

**EENT:** blurred vision.

**GI:** constipation, diarrhea, dyspepsia, flatulence, abdominal pain or cramps, heartburn, nausea, vomiting.

**Skin:** rash, pruritus, alopecia.

**Other:** muscle cramps, myalgia, myositis, *rhabdomyolysis*, elevated serum transaminase levels, abnormal liver test results, chest pain.

## INTERACTIONS

*Cyclosporine or other immunosuppressants, erythromycin, gemfibrozil, niacin:* possible increased risk of polymyositis and rhabdomyolysis (maximum recommended lovastatin dosage is 20 mg daily); monitor the patient closely.

*Ethanol:* increased risk of hepatotoxicity. Avoid concomitant use.

*Oral anticoagulants:* lovastatin may enhance the clinical effects of oral anticoagulants. Monitor the patient closely.

## CONTRAINDICATIONS

Contraindicated in patients with hypersensitivity to the drug; in those with active liver disease or conditions associated with unexplained persistent elevations of serum transaminase levels; in pregnant and breast-feeding patients; and in women of childbearing age unless there is no risk of pregnancy.

## NURSING CONSIDERATIONS

• Use cautiously in patients who consume substantial quantities of alcohol or have a past history of liver disease.

• Know that lovastatin should be initiated only after diet and other nonpharmacologic therapies prove ineffective. The patient should be on a standard low-cholesterol diet during therapy.

• Be aware that liver function tests should be performed at the start of therapy and periodically thereafter.

☑ **PATIENT TEACHING**

• Instruct the patient to take lovastatin with the evening meal, when absorption is enhanced and cholesterol biosynthesis is greater.

• Teach the patient about proper dietary management of serum lipids. When appropriate, recommend weight-control, exercise, and smoking-cessation programs.

• Advise him to have periodic eye examinations; related compounds have caused cataracts in laboratory animals.

• Tell him to store tablets at room temperature in a light-resistant container.

• *Alert:* Inform the female patient that drug is contraindicated during pregnancy. Advise her to notify doctor immediately if pregnancy occurs.

## pravastatin sodium (eptastatin)

Pravachol

*Pregnancy Risk Category: X*

## HOW SUPPLIED

*Tablets:* 10 mg, 20 mg, 40 mg

## ACTION

Inhibits 3-hydroxy-3-methylglutaryl coenzyme A reductase. This enzyme is an early (and rate-limiting) step in the synthetic pathway of cholesterol.

## ONSET, PEAK, DURATION

Onset and duration are unknown. Plasma levels peak within 1 hour.

## INDICATIONS & DOSAGE

*Reduction of low-density lipoprotein and total cholesterol levels in patients with primary hypercholesterolemia (types IIa and IIb)* —

**Adults:** initially, 10 or 20 mg P.O. daily h.s. Dosage adjusted q 4 weeks based on patient tolerance and response; maximum daily dosage is 40 mg. Most elderly patients respond to a daily dosage of 20 mg or less.

## ADVERSE REACTIONS
**CNS:** headache, dizziness, fatigue.
**CV:** chest pain.
**EENT:** rhinitis.
**GI:** vomiting, diarrhea, heartburn, abdominal pain, constipation, flatulence, nausea.
**GU:** renal failure secondary to myoglobinuria, urinary abnormality.
**Respiratory:** cough, influenza, common cold.
**Skin:** rash.
**Other:** flulike symptoms, myositis, myopathy, *localized muscle pain,* myalgia, ***rhabdomyolysis.***

## INTERACTIONS
*Cholestyramine, colestipol:* concomitant administration decreases plasma levels of pravastatin. Administer pravastatin 1 hour before or 4 hours after these drugs.
*Drugs that decrease levels or activity of endogenous steroids (such as cimetidine, ketoconazole, spironolactone):* may increase risk of developing endocrine dysfunction. No intervention appears necessary; take complete drug history in patients who develop endocrine dysfunction.
*Erythromycin, fibric acid derivatives (such as clofibrate or gemfibrozil), immunosuppressants (such as cyclosporine), high doses (1 g or more daily) of niacin (nicotinic acid):* may increase the risk of rhabdomyolysis. Monitor the patient closely if concomitant use cannot be avoided.
*Ethanol, hepatotoxic drugs:* increased risk of hepatotoxicity. Avoid concomitant use.
*Gemfibrozil:* decreases protein-binding and urinary clearance of pravastatin. Avoid concomitant use.

## CONTRAINDICATIONS
Contraindicated in patients with hypersensitivity to the drug; in those with active liver disease or conditions that cause unexplained, persistent elevations of serum transaminase levels; in pregnant and breast-feeding patients; and in women of childbearing age unless there is no risk of pregnancy.

## NURSING CONSIDERATIONS
• Use cautiously in patients who consume large quantities of alcohol or have history of liver disease.
• Know that pravastatin should be initiated only after diet and other nonpharmacologic therapies prove ineffective. Patients should be on a standard low-cholesterol diet during therapy.
• Know that liver function tests should be performed at the start of therapy and periodically thereafter. A liver biopsy may be performed if liver enzyme elevations persist.

## ☑ PATIENT TEACHING
• Instruct the patient to take the recommended dosage in the evening, preferably at bedtime.
• Teach the patient about proper dietary management of serum lipids. When appropriate, recommend weight-control, exercise, and smoking-cessation programs.
• **Alert:** Inform the female patient that drug is contraindicated during pregnancy. Advise her to notify doctor immediately if pregnancy occurs.

## simvastatin (syvinolin)
Lipex‡, Zocor
*Pregnancy Risk Category: X*

## HOW SUPPLIED
*Tablets:* 5 mg, 10 mg, 20 mg, 40 mg

## ACTION
Inhibits 3-hydroxy-3-methylglutaryl coenzyme A reductase. This enzyme is an early (and rate-limiting) step in the synthetic pathway of cholesterol.

## ONSET, PEAK, DURATION
Onset and duration unknown. Peak plasma levels occur in 1.3 to 2.4 hours. Peak antilipemic effects occur in 3 to 4 months.

## INDICATIONS & DOSAGE
*Reduction of low-density lipoprotein and total cholesterol levels in patients with primary hypercholesterolemia (types IIa and IIb) —*
**Adults:** initially, 5 to 10 mg P.O. daily in the evening. Dosage adjusted q 4 weeks based on patient tolerance and response; maximum daily dosage is 40 mg.

## ADVERSE REACTIONS
**CNS:** headache, asthenia.
**GI:** abdominal pain, constipation, diarrhea, dyspepsia, flatulence, nausea, vomiting.
**Hepatic:** elevated liver enzymes.
**Respiratory:** upper respiratory tract infection.

## INTERACTIONS
*Digoxin:* simvastatin may elevate digoxin levels slightly. Closely monitor plasma digoxin levels at initiation of simvastatin therapy.
*Drugs that decrease levels or activity of endogenous steroids (such as cimetidine, ketoconazole, spironolactone):* may increase risk of developing endocrine dysfunction. No intervention appears necessary; take complete drug history in patients who develop endocrine dysfunction.
*Erythromycin, fibric acid derivatives (such as clofibrate or gemfibrozil), immunosuppressants (such as cyclosporine), high doses (1 g or more daily) of niacin (nicotinic acid):* may increase risk of rhabdomyolysis. Monitor the patient closely if concomitant use cannot be avoided. Limit daily dosage of simvastatin to 10 mg if the patient must take cyclosporine.
*Ethanol, hepatotoxic drugs:* increased risk of hepatotoxicity. Avoid concomitant use.
*Warfarin:* anticoagulant effect may be slightly enhanced. Monitor the patient's PT at start of therapy and during dosage adjustments.

## CONTRAINDICATIONS
Contraindicated in patients with hypersensitivity to the drug and in those with active liver disease or conditions that cause unexplained persistent elevations of serum transaminase; in pregnant and breast-feeding patients; and in women of childbearing age unless there is no risk of pregnancy.

## NURSING CONSIDERATIONS
• Use cautiously in patients who consume substantial quantities of alcohol or have a history of liver disease.
• Know that simvastatin is initiated only after diet and other nonpharmacologic therapies prove ineffective. The patient should be on a standard low-cholesterol diet during therapy.
• Know that liver function tests should be performed at the start of therapy and periodically thereafter. A liver biopsy may be performed if enzyme elevations persist.

## ☑ PATIENT TEACHING
• Instruct the patient to take simvastatin with the evening meal; absorption is enhanced and cholesterol biosynthesis is greater.
• Teach the patient about proper dietary management of serum lipids. When appropriate, recommend weight-control, exercise, and smoking-cessation programs.
• Tell the patient to inform the doctor of any adverse reactions, particularly muscle aches and pains.
• *Alert:* Inform the female patient that drug is contraindicated during pregnancy. Advise her to notify the doctor immediately if pregnancy occurs.

---

Reactions may be *common*, uncommon, *life-threatening*, or **COMMON AND LIFE-THREATENING**.

# 25

# Miscellaneous cardiovascular drugs

alprostadil
dipyridamole
isoxsuprine hydrochloride
papaverine hydrochloride
pentoxifylline
ticlopidine hydrochloride
tolazoline hydrochloride

## COMBINATION PRODUCTS
None.

## alprostadil
Prostin VR Pediatric
*Pregnancy Risk Category: NR*

## HOW SUPPLIED
*Injection:* 500 mcg/ml

## ACTION
A prostaglandin derivative that relaxes the smooth muscle of the ductus arteriosus.

## ONSET, PEAK, DURATION
Onset occurs in 5 to 10 minutes. Peak levels occur within 20 minutes. Effects persist for 1 to 3 hours.

## INDICATIONS & DOSAGE
*Palliative therapy for temporary maintenance of patency of ductus arteriosus until surgery can be performed –*
**Infants:** 0.05 to 0.1 mcg/kg/minute by I.V. infusion. When therapeutic response is achieved, infusion rate reduced to lowest dosage that will maintain response. Maximum dosage is 0.4 mcg/kg/minute. Alternatively, drug can be administered through umbilical artery catheter placed at ductal opening.

## ADVERSE REACTIONS
**CNS:** *seizures.*
**CV:** bradycardia, hypotension, tachycardia, *cardiac arrest,* edema.
**GI:** diarrhea.
**Hematologic:** *disseminated intravascular coagulation.*
**Other:** APNEA, *flushing, fever, sepsis,* hypokalemia.

## INTERACTIONS
None significant.

## CONTRAINDICATIONS
None known.

## NURSING CONSIDERATIONS
● Know that a differential diagnosis should be made between respiratory distress syndrome and cyanotic heart disease before drug is administered. Drug should not be used in neonates with respiratory distress syndrome.
● Use cautiously in neonates with bleeding tendencies because drug inhibits platelet aggregation.
● Dilute drug before administering. Prepare fresh solution daily; discard solution after 24 hours.
● Do not use diluents that contain benzyl alcohol. Fatal toxic syndrome may occur.
● **I.V. use:** Know that this drug is not recommended for direct injection or intermittent infusion. Administer by continuous infusion using a constant-rate pump. Infuse through a large peripheral or central vein or through an umbilical artery catheter placed at the level of the ductus arteriosus. If flushing occurs from peripheral vasodilation, reposition catheter.
● Reduce infusion rate if fever or significant hypotension occurs.
● Keep respiratory support available.
● In infants with restricted pulmonary

blood flow, measure drug's effectiveness by monitoring blood oxygenation. In infants with restricted systemic blood flow, measure drug's effectiveness by monitoring systemic blood pressure and blood pH.

• Monitor arterial pressure by umbilical artery catheter, auscultation, or Doppler transducer. Slow rate of infusion if arterial pressure falls significantly.

• *Alert:* If apnea and bradycardia (may reflect drug overdose) occur, stop infusion immediately.

• Keep in mind that CV and CNS adverse reactions are more frequent in infants weighing less than 2 kg and in those receiving infusions for longer than 48 hours.

### ☑ PATIENT TEACHING
• Inform parents of the need for alprostadil and explain its use.
• Encourage parents to ask questions and express concerns.

---

## dipyridamole
Apo-Dipyridamole†, Dipridacot, I.V. Persantine, Novodipiradol†, Persantin‡, Persantin 100‡, Persantine**

*Pregnancy Risk Category: B*

### HOW SUPPLIED
*Tablets:* 25 mg, 50 mg, 75 mg
*Injection:* 10 mg/2 ml

### ACTION
Unknown but may involve its ability to increase adenosine, which is a coronary vasodilator and platelet aggregation inhibitor.

### ONSET, PEAK, DURATION
Onset and duration are unknown. Plasma levels peak 45 to 180 minutes after oral dose; within 2 minutes after I.V. administration; unknown after I.M. administration.

### INDICATIONS & DOSAGE
*Inhibition of platelet adhesion in prosthetic heart valves (in combination with warfarin or aspirin)—*
**Adults:** 75 to 100 mg P.O. q.i.d.
*Alternative to exercise in evaluation of coronary artery disease during thallium ($^{201}Tl$) myocardial perfusion scintigraphy—*
**Adults:** 0.57 mg/kg as an I.V. infusion at a constant rate over 4 minutes (0.142 mg/kg/minute).
*Acute coronary insufficiency‡—*
**Adults:** 10 mg I.V. or I.M.

### ADVERSE REACTIONS
**CNS:** *headache, dizziness.*
**CV:** flushing, fainting, *hypotension;* angina, chest pain, *ECG abnormalities, blood pressure lability, hypertension* (with I.V. infusion).
**GI:** *nausea,* vomiting, diarrhea, abdominal distress.
**Skin:** rash, irritation (with undiluted injection), pruritus.

### INTERACTIONS
*Heparin:* may increase risk of bleeding. Monitor closely.

### CONTRAINDICATIONS
None known.

### NURSING CONSIDERATIONS
• Use cautiously in patients with hypotension.
• If the patient develops GI distress, administer 1 hour before meals or with meals.
• **I.V. use:** If administering as a diagnostic agent, dilute in 0.45% or 0.9% sodium chloride solution or $D_5W$ in at least a 1:2 ratio for a total volume of 20 to 50 ml. Inject $^{201}Tl$ within 5 minutes after completing the 4-minute dipyridamole infusion.
• Observe for adverse reactions, especially with large doses. Monitor blood pressure.
• Observe for signs of bleeding; note prolonged bleeding time (especially

---

Reactions may be *common,* uncommon, *life-threatening,* or **COMMON AND LIFE-THREATENING.**

with large doses or long-term therapy).
• Know that dipyridamole's value as part of an antithrombotic regimen is controversial; using it may not provide significantly better results than using aspirin alone.

## ☑ PATIENT TEACHING
• Instruct the patient to take drug exactly as prescribed.
• Tell patient to report adverse reactions promptly.
• Tell patient receiving drug I.V. to alert nurse if discomfort occurs at insertion site.

---

## isoxsuprine hydrochloride
Duvadilan‡, Vasodilan

*Pregnancy Risk Category: NR*

### HOW SUPPLIED
*Tablets:* 10 mg, 20 mg

### ACTION
Produces peripheral vasodilation by a direct effect on vascular smooth muscle.

### ONSET, PEAK, DURATION
Onset and duration unknown. Serum levels peak in 1 hour.

### INDICATIONS & DOSAGE
*Adjunct for relief of symptoms associated with cerebrovascular insufficiency, peripheral vascular diseases (such as arteriosclerosis obliterans, thromboangiitis obliterans, Raynaud's disease)* –
**Adults:** 10 to 20 mg P.O. t.i.d. or q.i.d.

### ADVERSE REACTIONS
**CNS:** trembling, weakness, dizziness.
**CV:** tachycardia, hypotension, chest pain.
**GI:** vomiting, abdominal distress, nausea.
**Skin:** severe rash.

### INTERACTIONS
None significant.

### CONTRAINDICATIONS
Contraindicated in immediate postpartum period and in patients with arterial bleeding.

### NURSING CONSIDERATIONS
• Use cautiously in patients with cardiovascular or cerebrovascular disease.
• Know that safe use during pregnancy and lactation has not been established.
• Discontinue drug if rash develops.

### ☑ PATIENT TEACHING
• Instruct the patient to take drug exactly as prescribed.
• To minimize the risk of orthostasis, instruct the patient to avoid sudden position changes.

---

## papaverine hydrochloride
Cerespan, Genabid, Pavabid, Pavabid HP, Pavabid Plateau, Pavacels, Pavagen, Pavarine, Pavased, Pavatym, Paverolan

*Pregnancy Risk Category: C*

### HOW SUPPLIED
*Tablets:* 30 mg, 60 mg, 100 mg, 150 mg, 200 mg, 300 mg
*Tablets (timed-release):* 200 mg
*Capsules (timed-release):* 150 mg
*Injection:* 30 mg/ml, 32.5 mg/ml†

### ACTION
Has a direct, nonspecific relaxant effect on vascular, cardiac, and other smooth muscle.

### ONSET, PEAK, DURATION
Onset is fairly rapid. Peak unknown. Persists for 12 hours after administration of timed-release form. Unknown for other forms of the drug.

---

*Liquid form contains alcohol. **May contain tartrazine. †Canada only. ‡Australia only. ◇OTC.

## INDICATIONS & DOSAGE
*Relief from vascular spasm associated with acute MI (coronary occlusion), angina pectoris, peripheral and pulmonary embolism, peripheral vascular disease in which there is a vasospastic element or certain cerebral angiostatic states; and visceral spasm, as in ureteral, biliary, or gastrointestinal colic –*
**Adults:** 75 to 300 mg P.O. one to five times daily, or 150- to 300-mg timed-release preparations q 8 to 12 hours; 30 to 120 mg I.M. or I.V. slowly over 1 to 2 minutes q 3 hours, as indicated.

## ADVERSE REACTIONS
**CNS:** *headache,* vertigo, drowsiness, sedation, malaise.
**CV:** *increased heart rate, increased blood pressure* (with parenteral use), depressed AV and intraventricular conduction, ***arrhythmias.***
**GI:** constipation, *nausea,* anorexia, abdominal pain, diarrhea.
**Hepatic:** ***hepatitis*** (jaundice, eosinophilia, abnormal liver function tests), ***cirrhosis.***
**Respiratory:** increased depth and rate of respiration.
**Skin:** *diaphoresis, flushing,* skin rash.

## INTERACTIONS
*Lactated Ringer's solution:* precipitate forms when mixed with papaverine. Don't mix together.
*Levodopa:* papaverine may interfere with levodopa's therapeutic effects in patients with Parkinson's disease. Monitor for decreased effectiveness.

## CONTRAINDICATIONS
I.V. use is contraindicated in patients with Parkinson's disease or complete AV block.

## NURSING CONSIDERATIONS
• Use cautiously in patients with glaucoma.
• **I.V. use:** Give by direct injection over 1 to 2 minutes. Slow administration minimizes the risk of serious adverse reactions. Do not add to Lactated Ringer's Injection because precipitation occurs.
• Be aware that drug is most effective when given early in the course of a disorder.
• Know that the FDA has declared that this drug may not be effective for the disease states indicated.
• Monitor blood pressure and heart rate and rhythm, especially in patients with cardiac disease. Withhold dose and notify the doctor immediately if changes occur.
• *Alert:* Monitor for adverse hepatic reactions in patients receiving long-term therapy.

### ☑ PATIENT TEACHING
• Tell the patient to take medication regularly; long-term therapy is required.
• Advise the patient to avoid tasks that require mental alertness, such as driving or operating heavy machinery, until drug's CNS effects are known.
• To minimize the risk of orthostatic hypotension, instruct the patient to avoid sudden posture changes.

## pentoxifylline
Trental
*Pregnancy Risk Category: C*

## HOW SUPPLIED
*Tablets (extended-release):* 400 mg

## ACTION
Unknown. Improves capillary blood flow probably by increasing RBC flexibility and lowering blood viscosity.

## ONSET, PEAK, DURATION
Onset and duration unknown. Serum levels peak within 2 to 4 hours but are not related to drug effect.

---

Reactions may be *common,* uncommon, *life-threatening,* or COMMON AND LIFE-THREATENING.

## INDICATIONS & DOSAGE
*Intermittent claudication caused by chronic occlusive vascular disease –*
**Adults:** 400 mg P.O. t.i.d. with meals.

## ADVERSE REACTIONS
**CNS:** headache, dizziness.
**GI:** dyspepsia, nausea, vomiting.

## INTERACTIONS
*Anticoagulants:* increased anticoagulant effect. Adjust anticoagulant dosage as ordered.
*Antihypertensives:* increased hypotensive effect. Dosage adjustments may be necessary.

## CONTRAINDICATIONS
Contraindicated in patients who are intolerant to methylxanthines, such as caffeine, theophylline, and theobromine, and in patients with recent cerebral or retinal hemorrhage.

## NURSING CONSIDERATIONS
• Know that drug is useful in patients who are not good surgical candidates.
• Be aware that elderly patients may be more sensitive to drug's effects.

## ☑ PATIENT TEACHING
• Advise the patient to take with meals to minimize GI upset.
• Instruct the patient to swallow medication whole, without breaking, crushing, or chewing.
• Tell the patient to report any GI or CNS adverse reactions; the doctor may reduce the dosage.
• Advise the patient to avoid smoking because nicotine causes vasoconstriction that can worsen his condition.
• Tell the patient not to discontinue drug during the first 8 weeks of therapy unless directed by the doctor.

# ticlopidine hydrochloride
Ticlid
*Pregnancy Risk Category: B*

## HOW SUPPLIED
*Tablets:* 250 mg

## ACTION
Unknown. An antiplatelet agent that probably blocks adenosine diphosphate-induced platelet-to-fibrinogen and platelet-to-platelet binding.

## ONSET, PEAK, DURATION
Onset occurs within 2 days. Serum levels peak in about 2 hours, although time to peak effect takes 8 to 11 days. Effects persist for 1 to 2 weeks.

## INDICATIONS & DOSAGE
*To reduce risk of thrombotic stroke in patients with history of stroke or who have experienced stroke precursors –*
**Adults:** 250 mg P.O. b.i.d. with meals.

## ADVERSE REACTIONS
**CNS:** dizziness, ***intracerebral bleeding,*** peripheral neuropathy.
**CV:** vasculitis.
**EENT:** epistaxis, conjunctival hemorrhage.
**GI:** *diarrhea, nausea, dyspepsia, abdominal pain,* anorexia, vomiting, flatulence, bleeding, light-colored stools.
**GU:** hematuria, ***nephrotic syndrome,*** dark-colored urine.
**Hematologic:** neutropenia, ***pancytopenia, agranulocytosis, immune thrombocytopenia.***
**Hepatic:** hepatitis, cholestatic jaundice, abnormal liver function tests.
**Respiratory:** *allergic pneumonitis.*
**Skin:** *rash,* pruritus, ecchymoses, maculopapular rash, urticaria, ***thrombocytopenic purpura.***
**Other:** hypersensitivity reactions, postoperative bleeding, systemic lupus erythematosus, ***serum sickness,***

arthropathy, myositis, *hyponatremia, increased serum cholesterol levels.*

## INTERACTIONS
*Antacids:* decreased plasma ticlopidine levels. Separate administration times by at least 2 hours.
*Aspirin:* effects of aspirin on platelets potentiated. Avoid concomitant use.
*Cimetidine:* decreased clearance of ticlopidine and increased risk of toxicity. Avoid concomitant use.
*Digoxin:* slight decrease in serum digoxin levels. Monitor serum digoxin levels.
*Theophylline:* decreased theophylline clearance and risk of toxicity. Monitor closely and adjust theophylline dosage as ordered.

## CONTRAINDICATIONS
Contraindicated in patients hypersensitive to the drug; in patients with hematopoietic disorders, such as neutropenia, thrombocytopenia, or disorders of hemostasis; in patients with active pathologic bleeding from peptic ulceration or active intracranial bleeding; and in those with severe hepatic impairment.

## NURSING CONSIDERATIONS
● Use cautiously and with close monitoring of CBC and WBC differentials. Moderate to severe neutropenia and agranulocytosis have occurred in patients taking ticlopidine, usually within the first 3 weeks to 3 months of therapy.
● Monitor baseline liver function tests prior to therapy.
● Determine CBC and WBC differentials at the 2nd week of therapy and repeat every 2 weeks until the end of the 3rd month, as ordered. Frequency of tests is increased in patients who show signs of declining neutrophil count or counts of less than 30% of baseline. After first 3 months of therapy, CBC and WBC differential determinations should be performed only

in patients who show signs of infection.
● Monitor liver function tests and repeat whenever dysfunction is suspected. Monitor closely, especially during first 4 months of treatment.
● Know that thrombocytopenia has occurred rarely. Drug should be discontinued in patients having a platelet count of 80,000/mm$^3$ or less, and doctor should be notified. If necessary, give methylprednisolone 20 mg I.V. to normalize bleeding time within 2 hours, as ordered. Know that platelet transfusions may also be used.
● Know that when used preoperatively, ticlopidine may decrease incidence of graft occlusion in patients receiving coronary artery bypass grafts and reduce severity of drop in platelet count in patients receiving extracorporeal hemoperfusion during open heart surgery.

## ☑ PATIENT TEACHING
● Tell patient to take drug with meals; this substantially increases bioavailability and improves GI tolerance.
● Tell patient to avoid aspirin and aspirin-containing products and to check with the doctor or pharmacist before taking OTC medications.
● Explain to patient that drug will prolong bleeding time and that any unusual or prolonged bleeding should be reported. Advise patient to tell dentists and other doctors that he is taking ticlopidine.
● Stress importance of regular blood tests. Because neutropenia can result from increased risk of infection, tell patient to immediately report signs of infection, such as fever, chills, or sore throat.
● If ticlopidine is being substituted for a fibrinolytic or anticoagulant, tell patient to discontinue those drugs before starting ticlopidine therapy as ordered.
● Advise patient to discontinue drug

---

Reactions may be *common,* uncommon, *life-threatening,* or COMMON AND LIFE-THREATENING.

10 to 14 days before undergoing elective surgery, as ordered.
• Also tell patient to immediately report yellow skin or sclera, severe or persistent diarrhea, rashes, subcutaneous bleeding, light-colored stools, or dark urine.

## tolazoline hydrochloride
Priscoline
*Pregnancy Risk Category: C*

### HOW SUPPLIED
*Injection:* 25 mg/ml

### ACTION
Direct-acting vasodilator. May have some alpha-receptor blocking effects.

### ONSET, PEAK, DURATION
Onset occurs within 30 minutes. Peak and duration unknown.

### INDICATIONS & DOSAGE
*Persistent pulmonary hypertension in neonates —*
**Neonates:** initially, 1 to 2 mg/kg I.V. over 10 minutes, followed by infusion of 1 to 2 mg/kg/hour.

### ADVERSE REACTIONS
**CV:** *arrhythmias,* pain, *hypertension, flushing,* tachycardia, *hypotension.*
**GI:** *nausea, vomiting, diarrhea, GI hemorrhage.*
**GU:** edema, oliguria, hematuria.
**Hematologic:** leukopenia, *thrombocytopenia.*
**Respiratory:** *pulmonary hemorrhage.*
**Skin:** increased pilomotor activity with tingling and chilliness, rash.

### INTERACTIONS
*Vasopressors (epinephrine, norepinephrine):* may cause paradoxical fall in blood pressure.

### CONTRAINDICATIONS
Contraindicated in neonates with hypersensitivity to the drug.

### NURSING CONSIDERATIONS
• Use cautiously in patients with known or suspected mitral stenosis.
• **I.V. use:** Know that response to treatment of persistent pulmonary hypertension of the newborn should be evident within 30 minutes. Little information exists regarding infusions lasting longer than 48 hours.
• Place the patient in the supine position during infusion.
• To increase response, keep the patient warm during parenteral administration.
• *Alert:* Appearance of flushing usually indicates maximum tolerable dose.
• Monitor vital signs. Watch especially for blood pressure changes and arrhythmias.

### ☑ PATIENT TEACHING
• Inform parents of need for drug and explain its use.
• Encourage parents to ask questions and express concerns.

---

*Liquid form contains alcohol.  **May contain tartrazine.  †Canada only.  ‡Australia only.  ◊OTC.

# 26

# Nonnarcotic analgesics and antipyretics

**acetaminophen**
**aspirin**
**choline magnesium trisalicylate**
**choline salicylate**
**diflunisal**
**magnesium salicylate**
**salsalate**
**sodium salicylate**

## COMBINATION PRODUCTS

ALLEREST NO DROWSINESS TABLETS◇, COLDRINE◇, ORNEX NO DROWSINESS CAPLETS◇, SINUS RELIEF TABLETS, SINUTAB MAXIMUM STRENGTH WITHOUT DROWSINESS◇: acetaminophen 325 mg and pseudoephedrine hydrochloride 30 mg.

AMAPHEN, ANOQUAN, BUTACE, ENDOLOR, ESGIC, FEMCET, FIORICET, ISOPAP, MEDIGESIC, REPAN, TENCET, TRIAD, TWO-DYNE: acetaminophen 325 mg, caffeine 40 mg, and butalbital 50 mg.

ASCRIPTIN: aspirin 325 mg, magnesium hydroxide 50 mg, aluminum hydroxide 50 mg, and calcium carbonate 50 mg.◇

ASCRIPTIN A/D: aspirin 325 mg, magnesium hydroxide 75 mg, aluminum hydroxide 75 mg, and calcium carbonate 75 mg.◇

AXOTAL: aspirin 650 mg and butalbital 50 mg.

CAMA ARTHRITIS PAIN RELIEVER: aspirin 500 mg, magnesium oxide 150 mg, and aluminum hydroxide 150 mg.

COPE: aspirin 421 mg, caffeine 32 mg, magnesium hydroxide 50 mg, and aluminum hydroxide 25 mg.

DOAN'S P.M. EXTRA STRENGTH ◇: magnesium salicylate 500 mg and diphenhydramine 25 mg.

EXCEDRIN EXTRA STRENGTH◇: aspirin 250 mg, acetaminophen 250 mg, and caffeine 65 mg.

EXCEDRIN P.M.◇: acetaminophen 500 mg and diphenhydramine citrate 38 mg.

FIORINAL, ISOLLYL IMPROVED, LANORINAL: aspirin 325 mg, caffeine 40 mg, and butalbital 50 mg.

MIDRIN: isometheptene mucate 65 mg, dichloralphenazone 100 mg, and acetaminophen 325 mg.

PAC TABLETS◇: aspirin 400 mg and caffeine 32 mg.

PHRENILIN: acetaminophen 325 mg and butalbital 50 mg.

PHRENILIN FORTE: acetaminophen 650 mg and butalbital 50 mg.

SINUS EXCEDRIN NO DROWSINESS◇: acetaminophen 500 mg and pseudoephedrine hydrochloride 30 mg.

SINUTAB◇: acetaminophen 325 mg, chlorpheniramine 2 mg, and pseudoephedrine hydrochloride 30 mg.

SINUTAB MAXIMUM STRENGTH◇: acetaminophen 500 mg, pseudoephedrine hydrochloride 30 mg, and chlorpheniramine maleate, 2 mg.

TECNAL†: aspirin 330 mg, caffeine 40 mg, and butalbital 50 mg.

VANQUISH◇: aspirin 227 mg, acetaminophen 194 mg, caffeine 33 mg, aluminum hydroxide 25 mg, and magnesium hydroxide 50 mg.

---

# acetaminophen (APAP, paracetamol)

Abenol†◇; Aceta Elixir*◇; Acetaminophen Uniserts◇; Aceta Tablets◇; Actamin◇; Actamin Extra◇; Actimol†◇; Aminofen◇; Aminofen Max◇; Anacin-3◇; Anacin-3 Children's Elixir*◇; Anacin-3 Children's Tablets◇; Anacin-3 Extra Strength◇; Anacin-3 Infants'◇; Anacin-3 Maximum Strength Caplets◇; Apacet Capsules◇; Apacet Elixir*◇; Apacet Extra Strength Caplets◇; Apacet Extra Strength Tablets◇; Apacet Infants'◇; Apacet Regular Strength Tablets◇; Apo-Acetaminophen†◇; Arthritis Pain Formula Aspirin Free◇; Atasol Caplets†◇; Atasol Drops†◇; Atasol Elixir*†◇; Atasol Forte Caplets†◇; Atasol Forte Tablets†◇; Atasol Tablets†◇; Banesin◇; Dapa◇; Dapa X-S◇; Datril Extra-Strength; Dolanex*◇; Dorcol Children's Fever and Pain Reducer◇; Dymadon‡◇; Dymadon P‡◇; Exdol†◇; Exdol Strong†◇; Feverall, Children's‡; Feverall Junior Strength‡; Feverall Sprinkle Caps, Children's‡; Feverall Sprinkle Caps, Junior Strength‡; Genapap Children's Elixir◇; Genapap Children's Tablets◇; Genapap Extra Strength Caplets◇; Genapap Extra Strength Tablets◇; Genapap, Infants'◇; Genapap Regular Strength Tablets◇; Genebs Extra Strength Caplets◇; Genebs Regular Strength Tablets◇; Genebs X-Tra◇; Halenol Children's*◇; Liquiprin Infants' Drops◇; Meda Cap◇; Myapap Elixir*◇; Myapap, Infants'◇; Neopap◇; Oraphen-PD◇; Panadol◇; Panadol, Children's◇; Panadol Extra Strength◇; Panadol, Infants'◇; Panadol Junior Strength Caplets◇; Panadol Maximum Strength Caplets◇; Panadol Maximum Strength Tablets◇; Panamax‡◇; Panex◇; Panex-500◇; Paralgin‡◇; Paraspen‡◇; Redutemp◇; Ridenol Caplets◇; Robigesic†◇; Rounox†◇; Setamol-500‡◇; Snaplets-FR◇; Stanback AF Extra Strength Powder; St. Joseph Aspirin-Free Fever Reducer for Children◇; Suppap-120◇; Suppap-325◇; Suppap-650◇; Tapanol Extra Strength Caplets◇; Tapanol Extra Strength Tablets◇; Tempra◇; Tempra Caplets◇; Tempra Chewable Tablets◇; Tempra Drops◇; Tempra D.S.◇; Tempra, Infants'◇; Tempra Syrup◇; Tenol◇; Tylenol Caplets◇; Tylenol Chewable Tablets◇; Tylenol Children's Elixir◇; Tylenol Children's Tablets◇; Tylenol Drops◇; Tylenol Elixir*◇; Tylenol Extended Relief◇; Tylenol Extra Strength Adult Liquid Pain Reliever◇; Tylenol Extra Strength Caplets◇; Tylenol Extra Strength Gelcaps◇; Tylenol Extra Strength Tablets◇; Tylenol Infants'◇; Tylenol Junior Strength Caplets◇; Tylenol Junior Strength Tablets◇; Tylenol Regular Strength Caplets◇; Tylenol Regular Strength Tablets◇; Tylenol Tablets◇; Ty-Pap◇; Ty-Pap, Infants'◇; Ty-Pap Syrup◇; Ty-Tab Caplets◇; Ty-Tab Capsules◇; Ty-Tab, Children's◇; Ty-Tab Tablets◇; Valorin◇; Valorin Extra◇

*Pregnancy Risk Category: NR*

## HOW SUPPLIED

*Tablets:* 160 mg◇, 325 mg◇, 500 mg◇, 650 mg◇
*Tablets (chewable):* 80 mg◇, 160 mg◇
*Caplets (extended-release):* 650 mg
*Capsules:* 500 mg◇
*Oral liquid:* 160 mg/5 ml◇, 500 mg/15 ml◇
*Oral solution:* 48 mg/ml◇, 100 mg/ml◇
*Oral suspension:* 120 mg/5 ml‡, 100 mg/ml◇, 160 mg/ml◇
*Elixir:* 120 mg/5 ml, 130 mg/5 ml*◇, 160 mg/5 ml*◇, 325 mg/5 ml*◇

---

*Liquid form contains alcohol. **May contain tartrazine. †Canada only. ‡Australia only. ◇OTC.

*Granules:* 80 mg/packet◊, 325 mg/
dosage measure◊
*Powder for solution:* 1 g/packet
*Sprinkles:* 80 mg/capsule, 160 mg/
capsule
*Suppositories:* 80 mg◊, 120 mg◊, 125
mg◊, 300 mg◊, 325 mg◊, 650 mg◊

## ACTION
Unknown. Thought to produce analgesia by blocking generation of pain
impulses, probably by inhibiting prostaglandin synthesis in the CNS or the
synthesis or action of other substances
that sensitize pain receptors to mechanical or chemical stimulation. It is
thought to relieve fever by central action in the hypothalamic heat-regulating center.

## ONSET, PEAK, DURATION
Onset unknown. Peak effects vary;
average peak blood levels occur in 1
to 3 hours. Effects persist about 3 to 4
hours.

## INDICATIONS & DOSAGE
*Mild pain or fever* –
**Adults and children over 11 years:**
325 to 650 mg P.O. q 4 to 6 hours; or
1 g P.O. t.i.d. or q.i.d., p.r.n. Alternatively, 2 extended-release caplets
P.O. q 8 hours. Maximum dosage
should not exceed 4 g daily. Dosage
for long-term therapy should not exceed 2.6 g daily.
**Children 11 years:** 480 mg P.O. or
rectally q 4 to 6 hours.
**Children 9 to 10 years:** 400 mg P.O.
or rectally q 4 to 6 hours.
**Children 6 to 8 years:** 320 mg P.O.
or rectally q 4 to 6 hours.
**Children 4 to 5 years:** 240 mg P.O.
or rectally q 4 to 6 hours.
**Children 2 to 3 years:** 160 mg P.O.
or rectally q 4 to 6 hours.
**Children 12 to 23 months:** 120 mg
P.O. q 4 to 6 hours.
**Children 4 to 11 months:** 80 mg P.O.
q 4 to 6 hours.

**Children up to 3 months:** 40 mg
P.O. q 4 to 6 hours.

## ADVERSE REACTIONS
**Hematologic:** hemolytic anemia,
neutropenia, leukopenia, ***pancyto-
penia, thrombocytopenia*** (rare).
**Hepatic:** *severe liver damage* (with
toxic doses), jaundice.
**Skin:** rash, urticaria.
**Other:** hypoglycemia.

## INTERACTIONS
*Barbiturates, carbamazepine, hydan-
toins, rifampin, sulfinpyrazone:* high
doses or long-term use of these drugs
may reduce the therapeutic effects and
enhance the hepatotoxic effects of acetaminophen. Avoid concomitant use.
*Caffeine:* may enhance analgesic effects of acetaminophen.
*Ethanol:* increased risk of hepatic
damage. Avoid concomitant use.
*Warfarin:* may increase hypoprothrombinemic effects with long-term
use with high doses of acetaminophen. Monitor PTs closely.
*Zidovudine:* may increase the incidence of bone marrow suppression
because of impaired zidovudine metabolism. Monitor patient closely.

## CONTRAINDICATIONS
None known.

## NURSING CONSIDERATIONS
• Use cautiously in patients with history of chronic alcohol abuse because
hepatotoxicity has occurred after
therapeutic doses.
• Many OTC products contain acetaminophen; be aware of this when calculating total daily dosage.
• Liquid form is recommended for
children and for all patients who have
difficulty swallowing.
• Know that acetaminophen may interfere with certain laboratory tests
for urinary 5-hydroxyindoleacetic
acid. It may also produce false-posi-

---

tive decreases in blood glucose levels in home monitoring systems.

### ☑ PATIENT TEACHING
• Tell parents to consult a doctor before giving this drug to child under 2 years.
• Tell patient this drug is only for short-term use. Tell patient to consult a doctor if administering to child for more than 5 days or adults for more than 10 days.
• Tell patient not to use for self-medication of marked fever (over 103.1° F [39.5° C]), fever persisting longer than 3 days, or recurrent fever unless directed by doctor.
• *Alert:* Warn patient that high doses or unsupervised long-term use can cause hepatic damage. Excessive ingestion of alcoholic beverages may increase the risk of hepatotoxicity.
• Tell breast-feeding patient that acetaminophen is found in breast milk in low concentrations (less than 1% of dose). Such patients may use it safely if therapy is short-term and does not exceed recommended doses.

---

## aspirin (acetylsalicylic acid)
Ancasal†◇, Arthrinol†◇, Artria S.R.◇, ASA◇, ASA Enseals◇, Aspergum◇, Aspro‡, Astrint†◇, Bayer Aspirin◇, Bex‡, Coryphen†◇, Easprin◇, Ecotrin◇, Empirin◇, Entrophen†◇, Halfprin, Measurin◇, Norwich Aspirin Extra Strength◇, Novasen†◇, Riphen-10†◇, Sal-Adult†◇, Sal-Infant†◇, Solprin‡, Supasa†◇, Triaphen-10†◇, Vincent's Powders‡, Winsprin Capsules‡, ZORprin◇

*Pregnancy Risk Category: C (D in 3rd trimester)*

### HOW SUPPLIED
*Tablets*◇: 325 mg, 500 mg, 650 mg
*Tablets (chewable):* 81 mg◇
*Tablets (enteric-coated):* 81 mg, 162 mg, 165 mg, 325 mg◇, 500 mg◇, 650 mg◇, 975 mg
*Tablets (extended-release):* 650 mg, 800 mg
*Tablets (timed-release):* 650 mg◇
*Chewing gum:* 227.5 mg◇
*Suppositories*◇: 60 mg, 120 mg, 125 mg, 130 mg, 195 mg, 200 mg, 300 mg, 325 mg, 600 mg, 650 mg, 1.2 g

### ACTION
Produces analgesia by blocking prostaglandin synthesis (peripheral action). Aspirin and other salicylates may prevent the lowering of the pain threshold that occurs when prostaglandins sensitize pain receptors to mechanical and chemical stimulation. Exerts its anti-inflammatory effect by inhibiting prostaglandin synthesis; also may inhibit the synthesis or action of other mediators of the inflammatory response. Relieves fever by acting on the hypothalamic heat-regulating center to cause peripheral vasodilation. This increases peripheral blood supply and promotes sweating, which leads to heat loss and to cooling by evaporation. In low doses, aspirin also appears to impede clotting by blocking prostaglandin synthesis, which prevents formation of the platelet-aggregating substance thromboxane $A_2$.

### ONSET, PEAK, DURATION
Onset occurs 5 to 30 minutes after an oral, rapidly absorbed dose. With oral solution, serum aspirin levels peak in 15 to 40 minutes; peak serum levels of salicylate, its active metabolite, in ½ to 1 hour. With regular tablets, peak serum aspirin levels in 25 to 40 minutes; peak serum salicylate levels, in 1 to 2 hours. With buffered tablets, peak serum aspirin and salicylate levels occur in 1 to 2 hours. With extended-release tablets, peak aspirin levels occur in 1 to 2 hours; peak salicylate levels, in 3 to 4 hours. With enteric-coated tablets, peak aspirin and salicylate

---

*Liquid form contains alcohol.   **May contain tartrazine.   †Canada only.   ‡Australia only.   ◇OTC.

levels occur in 4 to 8 hours. With suppositories, peak aspirin and salicylate levels occur in 3 to 4 hours. Effects persist for 1 to 4 hours.

## INDICATIONS & DOSAGE
*Rheumatoid arthritis, osteoarthritis, or other polyarthritic or inflammatory conditions –*
**Adults:** initially, 2.4 to 3.6 g P.O. daily in divided doses. Maintenance dosage is 3.6 to 5.4 g P.O. daily in divided doses.
*Juvenile rheumatoid arthritis –*
**Children:** weighing 25 kg or less, 60 to 90 mg/kg P.O. daily in divided doses; weighing more than 25 kg, 2.4 to 3.6 g P.O. daily in divided doses.
*Mild pain or fever –*
**Adults and children over 11 years:** 325 to 650 mg P.O. or P.R. q 4 hours, p.r.n.
**Children 2 to 11 years:** 1.5 g/m$^2$ or 65 mg/kg P.O. or P.R. daily in 4 to 6 divided doses.
*Prevention of thrombosis –*
**Adults:** 1.3 g P.O. daily in 2 to 4 divided doses.
*Reduction of risk of heart attack in patients with previous MI or unstable angina –*
**Adults:** 160 to 325 mg P.O. daily.
*Kawasaki syndrome (mucocutaneous lymph node syndrome) –*
**Adults:** 80 to 100 mg/kg P.O. daily in 4 divided doses during the febrile phase. Some patients may need up to 120 mg/kg. When fever subsides, dosage decreased to 3 to 8 mg/kg once daily, adjusted according to serum salicylate concentration.

## ADVERSE REACTIONS
**EENT:** *tinnitus and hearing loss.*
**GI:** *nausea, GI distress, occult bleeding, dyspepsia,* **GI bleeding.**
**Hematologic:** leukopenia, ***thrombocytopenia, prolonged bleeding time.***
**Hepatic:** abnormal liver function studies, hepatitis.

**Skin:** *rash,* bruising, urticaria, angioedema.
**Other:** hypersensitivity reactions, (***anaphylaxis,*** asthma), ***Reye's syndrome.***

## INTERACTIONS
*Ammonium chloride and other urine acidifiers:* increased blood levels of aspirin products. Monitor for aspirin toxicity.
*Angiotensin-converting enzyme inhibitors:* may decrease antihypertensive effects. Monitor blood pressure closely.
*Antacids in high doses (and other urine alkalinizers):* decreased levels of aspirin products. Monitor for decreased aspirin effect.
*Anticoagulants:* increased risk of bleeding. Avoid using together if possible.
*Beta blockers:* decreased antihypertensive effect. Avoid long-term aspirin use if patient is taking antihypertensives.
*Corticosteroids:* enhanced salicylate elimination. Monitor for decreased salicylate effect.
*Ethanol, NSAIDs, steroids:* increased risk of GI bleeding. Avoid concomitant use.
*Methotrexate:* increased risk of methotrexate toxicity. Avoid concomitant use.
*Nizatidine:* may increase risk of salicylate toxicity in patients receiving high doses of aspirin. Monitor closely.
*NSAIDs, including diflunisal, fenoprofen, ibuprofen, indomethacin, piroxicam, meclofenamate, naproxen:* altered pharmacokinetics of these agents, leading to lowered serum levels and decreased effectiveness. Avoid concomitant use.
*Oral antidiabetic agents:* increased hypoglycemic effect. Monitor closely.
*Probenecid, sulfinpyrazone:* decreased uricosuric effect. Avoid aspirin during therapy with these agents.
*Valproic acid:* may increase serum valproic acid concentrations. Avoid concomitant use.

---

Reactions may be *common,* uncommon, *life-threatening,* or COMMON AND LIFE-THREATENING.

## CONTRAINDICATIONS
Contraindicated in patients with hypersensitivity to the drug, G6PD deficiency, bleeding disorders such as hemophilia, von Willebrand's disease, or telangiectasia. Also contraindicated in patients with NSAID-induced sensitivity reactions.

## NURSING CONSIDERATIONS
• Use cautiously in patients with GI lesions, impaired renal function, hypoprothrombinemia, vitamin K deficiency, thrombocytopenia, thrombotic thrombocytopenic purpura, or severe hepatic impairment.
• *Alert:* Because of epidemiologic association with Reye's syndrome, the Centers for Disease Control and Prevention recommends not giving salicylates to children or teenagers with chickenpox or influenza-like illness.
• Be aware that for inflammatory conditions, rheumatic fever, and thrombosis, aspirin is administered on a scheduled, rather than p.r.n., basis.
• Know that because enteric-coated and sustained-release tablets are slowly absorbed, they are not suitable for rapid relief of acute pain, fever, or inflammation. They do cause less GI bleeding and may be more suited for long-term therapy, such as for the treatment of arthritis.
• For patient with swallowing difficulties, crush non-enteric-coated aspirin and dissolve in soft food or liquid. Administer liquid immediately after mixing because drug will break down rapidly.
• For patients who cannot tolerate oral medications, ask doctor about the possibility of using aspirin rectal suppositories. Watch for rectal mucosal irritation or bleeding.
• Be aware that febrile, dehydrated children can develop toxicity rapidly.
• Monitor elderly patients closely because they may be more susceptible to aspirin's toxic effects.
• Monitor blood salicylate levels as

indicated and ordered. Therapeutic blood salicylate level in arthritis is 10 to 30 mg/100 ml. Tinnitus may occur at plasma levels of 30 mg/100 ml and above, but this is not a reliable indicator of toxicity, especially in very young patients and those over age 60. With chronic therapy, mild toxicity may occur at plasma levels of 20 mg/100 ml.
• During prolonged therapy, hematocrit, hemoglobin level, PT, and renal function should be assessed periodically as ordered.
• Know that aspirin irreversibly inhibits platelet aggregation. It should be discontinued 5 to 7 days before elective surgery as ordered to allow time for the production and release of new platelets.

### ☑ PATIENT TEACHING
• Advise patient allergic to tartrazine dye not to take aspirin.
• To reduce adverse GI reactions, advise patient to take with food, milk, antacid, or large glass of water.
• Tell patient that sustained-release or enteric-coated preparations should not be crushed or chewed but swallowed whole.
• Tell patient that aspirin tablets with a strong vinegar-like odor should be discarded.
• Tell patient to consult a doctor if administering to child for more than 5 days or adult for more than 10 days.
• Advise patient receiving prolonged treatment with large doses of aspirin to watch for petechiae, bleeding gums, and signs of GI bleeding, and to maintain adequate fluid intake. Encourage the use of a soft-bristled toothbrush.
• Because of the many possible drug interactions involving aspirin, warn patient taking prescription drugs to check with a doctor or pharmacist before taking aspirin or OTC combination products containing aspirin.
• Inform female patient that she

should not take aspirin during last trimester of pregnancy unless specifically directed to do so by a doctor.
• Caution parents to keep out of reach of children — aspirin is one of the leading causes of poisoning in children. Encourage the use of child-resistant containers.

---

## choline magnesium trisalicylate (choline salicylate and magnesium salicylate)

Tricosal, Trilisate

*Pregnancy Risk Category: C*

### HOW SUPPLIED
*Tablets:* 500 mg, 750 mg, 1,000 mg of salicylate
*Solution:* 500 mg of salicylate/5 ml

### ACTION
Produces analgesia by blocking prostaglandin synthesis (peripheral action). Salicylates may prevent the lowering of the pain threshold that occurs when prostaglandins sensitize pain receptors to mechanical and chemical stimulation. Exerts its anti-inflammatory effect by inhibiting prostaglandin synthesis. Relieves fever by acting on the hypothalamic heat-regulating center to produce peripheral vasodilation. This increases peripheral blood supply and promotes sweating, which leads to heat loss and to cooling by evaporation.

### ONSET, PEAK, DURATION
Onset and duration unknown. Serum levels peak within 1 to 2 hours.

### INDICATIONS & DOSAGE
*Rheumatoid arthritis and osteoarthritis or other polyarthritic or inflammatory conditions —*
**Adults:** initially, 1.5 to 2.5 g P.O. daily as a single dose or in 2 or 3 divided doses. Dosage is adjusted ac-

cording to patient response. Dosage range is 1 to 4.5 g daily.
*Juvenile rheumatoid arthritis —*
**Children:** 60 to 110 mg/kg/day in divided doses (q 6 to 8 hours).
*Mild to moderate pain and fever —*
**Adults:** 2 to 3 g P.O. daily in divided doses q 4 to 6 hours.
**Children:** 10 to 15 mg/kg/day q 4 hours, up to 60 to 80 mg/kg/day.

### ADVERSE REACTIONS
**EENT:** tinnitus and hearing loss.
**GI:** GI distress, nausea, vomiting.
**Skin:** rash.
**Other:** hypersensitivity reactions *(anaphylaxis), Reye's syndrome.*

### INTERACTIONS
*Ammonium chloride and other urine acidifiers:* increased blood levels of salicylates. Monitor for salicylate toxicity.
*Antacids in high doses (and other urine alkalinizers):* decreased levels of salicylates. Monitor for decreased salicylate effect.
*Corticosteroids:* enhanced salicylate elimination. Monitor for decreased salicylate effect.
*Ethanol, steroids, and other NSAIDs:* enhanced risk of adverse GI effects. Avoid concomitant use.
*Methotrexate:* increased risk of methotrexate toxicity. Avoid concomitant use.
*Oral anticoagulants:* increased risk of bleeding. Use together cautiously.
*Uricosuric agents:* decreased uricosuric effect. Avoid concomitant use.

### CONTRAINDICATIONS
Contraindicated in patients hypersensitive to the drug. Also contraindicated in patients with hemophilia, bleeding ulcers, and hemorrhagic states.

### NURSING CONSIDERATIONS
• Use cautiously in patients with renal insufficiency, hepatic impairment, peptic ulcer disease, and gastritis.
• *Alert:* Because of epidemiologic as-

---

Reactions may be *common,* uncommon, *life-threatening,* or COMMON AND LIFE-THREATENING.

sociation with Reye's syndrome, the Centers for Disease Control and Prevention recommends not giving salicylates to children or teenagers with chicken pox or influenza-like illness.
• Be aware that febrile, dehydrated children can develop toxicity rapidly.
• Monitor serum salicylate levels in long-term therapy. Therapeutic blood salicylate level in arthritis is 10 to 30 mg/100 ml. Tinnitus may occur at plasma levels of 30 mg/100 ml and above, but this is not a reliable indicator of toxicity, especially in the very young and those over age 60. In chronic therapy, mild toxicity may occur at plasma levels of 20 mg/100 ml.
• Periodically monitor hemoglobin level and PT in patients receiving long-term treatment with large doses.
• Know that this drug causes less GI distress than aspirin. If an antacid is needed, give it 2 hours after meals and choline magnesium trisalicylate before meals.

☑ **PATIENT TEACHING**
• Tell patient to take tablets with food or a full glass of water. Solution may be mixed with fruit juice, but not antacids.
• Warn patient not to take drug longer than prescribed or to increase dosage without consulting doctor.

---

## choline salicylate
Arthropan, Teejel†*

*Pregnancy Risk Category: NR*

### HOW SUPPLIED
*Liquid:* 870 mg/5 ml◊
*Gel:* 87 mg/g†*

### ACTION
Produces analgesia by blocking prostaglandin synthesis (peripheral action). Salicylates may prevent the lowering of the pain threshold that occurs when prostaglandins sensitize pain receptors to mechanical and chemical stimulation. Exerts its anti-inflammatory effect by inhibiting prostaglandin synthesis. Relieves fever by acting on the hypothalamic heat-regulating center to produce peripheral vasodilation. This increases peripheral blood supply and promotes sweating, which leads to heat loss and to cooling by evaporation.

### ONSET, PEAK, DURATION
Unknown.

### INDICATIONS & DOSAGE
*Rheumatoid arthritis, osteoarthritis, mild to moderate pain or fever –*
**Adults and children over 12 years:** ½ to 1 teaspoonful (435 to 870 mg of choline salicylate) P.O. q 4 hours, p.r.n. If tolerated and needed, dosage may be increased to 2 tsp. Not to exceed 6 tsp daily.
*Relief of pain from inflamed gums –*
**Adults and children over 2 years:** apply 1 cm of gel to affected area q 3 to 4 hours and h.s., p.r.n.

### ADVERSE REACTIONS
**EENT:** *tinnitus* and hearing loss.
**GI:** nausea, vomiting, GI distress.
**Skin:** rash.
**Other:** hypersensitivity reactions *(anaphylaxis), Reye's syndrome.*

### INTERACTIONS
*Ammonium chloride and other urine acidifiers:* increased blood levels of salicylates. Monitor for salicylate toxicity.
*Antacids in high doses and other urine alkalinizers:* decreased levels of salicylates. Monitor for decreased salicylate effect.
*Corticosteroids:* enhanced salicylate elimination. Monitor for decreased salicylate effect.
*Ethanol, other NSAIDs, steroids:* enhanced risk of adverse GI reactions. Avoid concomitant use.
*Methotrexate:* increased risk of methotrexate toxicity. Avoid concomitant use.

---

*Liquid form contains alcohol.   **May contain tartrazine.   †Canada only.   ‡Australia only.   ◊OTC.

## CONTRAINDICATIONS

Contraindicated in patients with hypersensitivity to the drug. Also contraindicated in patients with hemophilia, bleeding ulcers, and hemorrhagic states.

## NURSING CONSIDERATIONS

• Use cautiously in impaired hepatic or renal function, hypoprothrombinemia, vitamin K deficiency, peptic ulcer disease, and gastritis, and in a known allergy to salicylates.
• **Alert:** Because of epidemiologic association with Reye's syndrome, the Centers for Disease Control and Prevention recommends not giving salicylates to children or teenagers with chicken pox or influenza-like illness.
• Know that febrile, dehydrated children can develop toxicity rapidly.
• Monitor serum salicylate levels in prolonged therapy. Therapeutic blood salicylate level in arthritis is 10 to 30 mg/100 ml. Tinnitus may occur at plasma levels of 30 mg/100 ml and above, but this is not a reliable indicator of toxicity, especially in the very young and those over age 60. With chronic therapy, mild toxicity may occur at plasma levels of 20 mg/100 ml.
• Periodically monitor hemoglobin level and PT in patients receiving long-term treatment with large doses.

## ☑ PATIENT TEACHING

• Tell patient that drug should be mixed with water, fruit juice, or carbonated drinks, but not antacids.
• Inform patient that drug causes less GI distress than aspirin. If an antacid is needed, he should take it 2 hours after meals and choline salicylate before meals.

---

### diflunisal
Dolobid
*Pregnancy Risk Category: C*

## HOW SUPPLIED

*Tablets:* 250 mg, 500 mg

## ACTION

Unknown. Probably related to inhibition of prostaglandin synthesis.

## ONSET, PEAK, DURATION

Onset in 1 hour for pain relief; unknown for anti-inflammatory action. Peak plasma levels and analgesic effects in 2 to 3 hours. Effects persist for pain relief 8 to 12 hours; unknown for anti-inflammatory effects.

## INDICATIONS & DOSAGE

*Mild to moderate pain, osteoarthritis, and rheumatoid arthritis –*
**Adults:** 500 to 1,000 mg P.O. daily in two divided doses, usually q 12 hours. Maximum dosage is 1,500 mg daily.
**Adults over 65 years:** one-half the usual adult dose.

## ADVERSE REACTIONS

**CNS:** *dizziness,* somnolence, insomnia, *headache,* fatigue.
**EENT:** *tinnitus, visual disturbances* (rare).
**GI:** *nausea, dyspepsia, GI pain, diarrhea,* vomiting, constipation, flatulence.
**GU:** renal impairment, hematuria, interstitial nephritis.
**Skin:** *rash,* pruritus, sweating, stomatitis, erythema multiforme, ***Stevens-Johnson syndrome.***

## INTERACTIONS

*Acetaminophen, hydrochlorothiazide, indomethacin:* diflunisal may substantially increase blood levels, increasing the risk of toxicity. Avoid concomitant use.
*Antacids, aspirin:* decreased diflunisal blood levels. Monitor for possible decreased therapeutic effect.
*Anticoagulants, thrombolytic agents:* diflunisal may enhance pharmacologic effects of these agents. Use together cautiously.

---

Reactions may be *common*, uncommon, ***life-threatening***, or COMMON AND LIFE-THREATENING.

*Cyclosporine:* diflunisal may enhance the nephrotoxicity of cyclosporine. Avoid concomitant use.
*Methotrexate:* diflunisal may enhance the toxicity of methotrexate. Avoid concomitant use.
*Sulindac:* diflunisal decreases blood levels of sulindac's active metabolite. Monitor for reduced pharmacologic effect.

## CONTRAINDICATIONS
Contraindicated in patients with hypersensitivity to the drug, or for whom acute asthmatic attacks, urticaria, or rhinitis are precipitated by aspirin or other NSAIDs.

## NURSING CONSIDERATIONS
● Use cautiously in GI bleeding, history of peptic ulcer disease, renal impairment, and compromised cardiac function, hypertension, or other conditions predisposing patient to fluid retention.
● *Alert:* Because of the epidemiologic association with Reye's syndrome, the Centers for Disease Control and Prevention recommends not giving salicylates to children and teenagers with chicken pox or influenza-like illness.

## ☑ PATIENT TEACHING
● Advise the patient to take with water, milk, or meals.
● Tell patient that tablets must be swallowed whole; they are not to be crushed or chewed.
● Tell him to avoid aspirin or acetaminophen while using diflunisal unless ordered.

---

## magnesium salicylate
Doan's, Extra-Strength Doan's P.M.◇, Magan◇, Mobidin◇

*Pregnancy Risk Category: NR*

## HOW SUPPLIED
*Tablets:* 545 mg, 600 mg
*Caplets:* 325 mg◇, 500 mg◇

## ACTION
Produces analgesia by blocking prostaglandin synthesis (peripheral action). Salicylates may prevent the lowering of the pain threshold that occurs when prostaglandins sensitize pain receptors to mechanical and chemical stimulation. Exerts its anti-inflammatory effect by inhibiting prostaglandin synthesis. Relieves fever by acting on the hypothalamic heat-regulating center to produce peripheral vasodilation. This increases peripheral blood supply and promotes sweating, which leads to heat loss and to cooling by evaporation.

## ONSET, PEAK, DURATION
Onset and duration unknown. Blood levels peak within 1½ to 2 hours of a dose.

## INDICATIONS & DOSAGE
*Arthritis –*
**Adults:** 545 mg to 1.2 g P.O. t.i.d. or q.i.d.
*Mild pain or fever –*
**Adults and children over 11 years:** 300 to 600 mg P.O. q 4 hours, not to exceed 3.5 g/day.

## ADVERSE REACTIONS
**EENT:** *tinnitus and hearing loss.*
**GI:** *nausea, vomiting, GI distress.*
**Hepatic:** abnormal liver function studies, hepatitis.
**Skin:** *rash,* bruising.
**Other:** hypersensitivity reactions (*anaphylaxis,* asthma), *Reye's syndrome.*

## INTERACTIONS
*Ammonium chloride and other urine acidifiers:* increased blood levels of salicylates. Monitor for salicylate toxicity.
*Antacids in high doses and other urine alkalinizers:* decreased levels of salicylates. Monitor for decreased salicylate effect.

---

*Anticoagulants:* increased risk of bleeding. Avoid using together.

*Corticosteroids:* enhanced salicylate elimination. Monitor for decreased salicylate effect.

*Ethanol, other NSAIDs, steroids:* increased risk of GI bleeding. Avoid concomitant use.

*Methotrexate:* increased risk of methotrexate toxicity. Avoid concomitant use.

## CONTRAINDICATIONS
Contraindicated in patients with hypersensitivity to the drug, or severe chronic renal insufficiency because of risk of magnesium toxicity. Also contraindicated in patients with bleeding disorders, or aspirin hypersensitivity.

## NURSING CONSIDERATIONS
• Use cautiously in hypoprothrombinemia and vitamin K deficiency.

• *Alert:* Because of epidemiologic association with Reye's syndrome, the Centers for Disease Control and Prevention recommends not giving salicylates to children or teenagers with chicken pox or influenza-like illness.

• Know that febrile, dehydrated children can develop toxicity rapidly.

• Monitor serum salicylate levels when drug used long term, as ordered. Therapeutic blood salicylate level in arthritis is 10 to 30 mg/100 ml. Tinnitus may occur at plasma levels of 30 mg/100 ml and above, but this is not a reliable indicator of toxicity, especially in very young patients and those over age 60. With chronic therapy, mild toxicity may occur at plasma levels of 20 mg/100 ml.

• Monitor hemoglobin level and PT in long-term treatment with large doses.

### ☑ PATIENT TEACHING
• Tell patient to take this drug with food, milk, antacid, or large glass of water.

• Tell patient that tablets or caplets must be swallowed whole; they should not be crushed or chewed.

---

# salsalate (disalicylic acid, salicylsalicylic acid)
Amigesic, Argesic-SA, Arthra-G, Disalcid, Mono-Gesic, Salflex, Salgesic, Salsitab

*Pregnancy Risk Category: C*

## HOW SUPPLIED
*Tablets:* 500 mg, 750 mg
*Caplets:* 750 mg
*Capsules:* 500 mg

## ACTION
Salsalate is the salicylic ester of salicylic acid. Each molecule of salsalate is hydrolyzed to two molecules of salicylate in vivo. Produces analgesia by blocking prostaglandin synthesis (peripheral action). Salicylates prevent the lowering of the pain threshold that occurs when prostaglandins sensitize pain receptors to mechanical and chemical stimulation. Drug also has an ill-defined effect on the hypothalamus. Exact mechanism of its anti-inflammatory action is unknown.

## ONSET, PEAK, DURATION
Onset and duration unknown. Plasma levels of salsalate peak within 1½ hours of an oral dose; of salicylate, within 2 to 4 hours.

## INDICATIONS & DOSAGE
*Arthritis —*
**Adults:** 3 g P.O. daily in divided doses b.i.d. or t.i.d.

## ADVERSE REACTIONS
**EENT:** *tinnitus and hearing loss.*
**GI:** *nausea, vomiting, GI distress,* occult bleeding (rare).
**Hepatic:** abnormal liver function studies, hepatitis.
**Skin:** *rash,* bruising.
**Other:** hypersensitivity reactions (**anaphylaxis,** asthma), **Reye's syndrome.**

---

## INTERACTIONS
*Ammonium chloride and other urine acidifiers:* increased blood levels of salicylates. Monitor for salicylate toxicity.
*Antacids in high doses and other urine alkalinizers:* decreased levels of salicylates. Monitor for decreased salicylate effect.
*Corticosteroids:* enhanced salicylate excretion. Monitor for decreased salicylate effect.
*Ethanol, NSAIDs, steroids:* increased risk of GI bleeding. Avoid concomitant use.
*Methotrexate:* increased risk of methotrexate toxicity. Avoid concomitant use.
*Oral anticoagulants:* possible increased risk of bleeding. Avoid using together if possible.
*Uricosuric agents:* decreased uricosuric effect. Avoid concomitant use.

## CONTRAINDICATIONS
Contraindicated in patients with salsalate hypersensitivity.

## NURSING CONSIDERATIONS
● Use cautiously in bleeding disorders, peptic ulcer disease, renal insufficiency, hypoprothrombinemia, vitamin K deficiency, thrombocytopenia, thrombotic thrombocytopenic purpura, or severe hepatic impairment.
● *Alert:* Because of epidemiologic association with Reye's syndrome, the Centers for Disease Control and Prevention recommends not giving salicylates to children or teenagers with chicken pox or influenza-like illness.
● Monitor serum salicylate level as ordered. Therapeutic blood salicylate level in arthritis is 10 to 30 mg/100 ml. Tinnitus may occur at plasma levels of 30 mg/100 ml and above, but this is not a reliable indicator of toxicity, especially in very young patients and those over age 60. With long-term therapy, mild toxicity may occur at plasma levels of 20 mg/100 ml.

● In long-term therapy, obtain hemoglobin and PT tests periodically.

## ☑ PATIENT TEACHING
● Tell patient to take this drug with food, milk, antacid, or large glass of water.
● Advise patient receiving long-term treatment with large doses to watch for petechiae, bleeding gums, and signs of GI bleeding, and to maintain adequate fluid intake. Encourage the use of a soft-bristled toothbrush.

---

# sodium salicylate
*Pregnancy Risk Category: NR*

## HOW SUPPLIED
*Tablets (enteric-coated):* 325 mg◇, 650 mg◇
*Injection:* 100 mg/ml

## ACTION
Produces analgesia by blocking prostaglandin synthesis (peripheral action). Salicylates may prevent the lowering of the pain threshold that occurs when prostaglandins sensitize pain receptors to mechanical and chemical stimulation. Exact anti-inflammatory action unknown although it may exert its anti-inflammatory effect by inhibiting prostaglandin synthesis; also may inhibit the synthesis or action of other mediators of the inflammatory response. Relieves fever by acting on the hypothalamic heat-regulating center to produce peripheral vasodilation. This increases peripheral blood supply and promotes sweating, which leads to heat loss and to cooling by evaporation.

## ONSET, PEAK, DURATION
Onset and duration unknown. Plasma levels peak within 6 hours of oral administration.

## INDICATIONS & DOSAGE
*Minor pain or fever –*
**Adults and children older than 11**

**years:** 325 to 650 mg P.O. q 4 hours, p.r.n. Alternatively, 500 mg I.V., not to exceed 1 g daily except in rheumatic fever in which single daily I.V. infusions of up to 10 g have been given.
**Children 2 to 11 years:** 25 to 50 mg/kg daily or 1.5 g/m$^2$ daily, administered in 4 to 6 divided doses.
*Rheumatoid arthritis, osteoarthritis, and other polyarthritic or inflammatory conditions –*
**Adults:** 3.6 to 5.4 g P.O. daily in divided doses.

## ADVERSE REACTIONS
**EENT:** *tinnitus, hearing loss.*
**GI:** *nausea, vomiting, GI distress.*
**Hepatic:** abnormal liver function studies, hepatitis.
**Skin:** *rash.*
**Other:** hypersensitivity reactions (***anaphylaxis,*** asthma), ***Reye's syndrome.***

## INTERACTIONS
*Ammonium chloride and other urine acidifiers:* increased blood levels of salicylates. Monitor for salicylate toxicity.
*Antacids in large doses and other urine alkalinizers:* decreased levels of salicylates. Monitor for decreased salicylate effect.
*Corticosteroids:* enhanced salicylate elimination. Monitor for decreased salicylate effect.
*Ethanol, other NSAIDs, steroids:* increased risk of GI distress. Avoid concomitant use.
*Methotrexate:* increased risk of methotrexate toxicity. Avoid concomitant use.
*Oral anticoagulants:* increased risk of bleeding. Avoid using together if possible.

## CONTRAINDICATIONS
Contraindicated in patients with GI ulcer, GI bleeding, or aspirin hypersensitivity.

## NURSING CONSIDERATIONS
● Use cautiously in hypoprothrombinemia, vitamin K deficiency, or bleeding disorders and in asthmatic patients with nasal polyps (may cause severe bronchospasm). Also use cautiously in CHF or hypertension because of increased sodium load.
● *Alert:* Because of epidemiologic association with Reye's syndrome, the Centers for Disease Control and Prevention recommends not giving salicylates to children or teenagers with chickenpox or influenza-like illness.
● **I.V. use:** Dilute drug in 1 liter of 0.9% sodium chloride or lactated Ringer's solution, and infuse over 4 to 8 hours. Avoid extravasation because the drug is highly irritating to local tissues. Rapid infusion may cause thrombophlebitis.
● Administer oral drug with food, milk, antacid, or large glass of water.
● Know that febrile, dehydrated children can develop toxicity rapidly.
● Monitor serum salicylate levels as ordered in long-term therapy. Therapeutic salicylate level in arthritis is 10 to 30 mg/100 ml. Tinnitus may occur at plasma levels of 30 mg/100 ml and above (not a reliable indicator of toxicity, especially in very young patients and in those over age 60). With long-term therapy, mild toxicity may occur at plasma levels of 20 mg/100 ml.
● In long-term therapy, monitor hemoglobin level and PT as ordered.

☑ **PATIENT TEACHING**
● Tell patient to take this drug with food, milk, antacid, or large glass of water.
● Advise patient receiving long-term treatment with large doses to watch for petechiae, bleeding gums, and signs of GI bleeding, and to maintain adequate fluid intake.

---

Reactions may be *common,* uncommon, ***life-threatening,*** or **COMMON AND LIFE-THREATENING.**

# 27

## Nonsteroidal anti-inflammatory drugs

diclofenac sodium
diclofenac potassium
etodolac
fenoprofen calcium
flurbiprofen
ibuprofen
indomethacin
indomethacin sodium trihydrate
ketoprofen
ketorolac tromethamine
meclofenamate
mefenamic acid
nabumetone
naproxen
naproxen sodium
oxaprozin
piroxicam
sulindac
tolmetin sodium

### COMBINATION PRODUCTS

ADVIL COLD AND SINUS◇, DRISTAN SINUS CAPLETS◇: pseudoephedrine hydrochloride 30 mg and ibuprofen 200 mg.

---

### diclofenac sodium
Fenac‡, Voltaren, Voltaren SR†

### diclofenac potassium
Cataflam

*Pregnancy Risk Category: B*

### HOW SUPPLIED
*Tablets:* 50 mg
*Tablets (enteric-coated):* 25 mg, 50 mg, 75 mg
*Tablets (slow-release):* 100 mg†
*Suppositories:* 50 mg†, 100 mg†

### ACTION
Unknown. Produces anti-inflammatory, analgesic, and antipyretic effects, possibly by inhibiting prostaglandin synthesis.

### ONSET, PEAK, DURATION
Onset occurs in 30 minutes. Plasma levels peak within 2 to 3 hours of oral administration of enteric-coated tablets; unknown for regular tablets. Analgesic effects persist for up to 8 hours.

### INDICATIONS & DOSAGE
*Ankylosing spondylitis –*
**Adults:** 25 mg P.O. q.i.d. (and h.s., p.r.n.)
*Osteoarthritis –*
**Adults:** 50 mg P.O. b.i.d. or t.i.d., or 75 mg P.O. b.i.d. (diclofenac sodium only).
*Rheumatoid arthritis –*
**Adults:** 50 mg P.O. t.i.d. or q.i.d. Alternatively, 75 mg P.O. b.i.d. (diclofenac sodium only) or 50 to 100 mg P.R. (where available) h.s. as a substitute for the last oral dose of the day. Not to exceed 225 mg daily.
*Analgesia and primary dysmenorrhea –*
**Adults:** 50 mg P.O. t.i.d. (diclofenac potassium only).

### ADVERSE REACTIONS
**CNS:** anxiety, depression, dizziness, drowsiness, insomnia, irritability, headache.
**CV:** *CHF,* hypertension, edema, fluid retention.
**EENT:** *tinnitus,* laryngeal edema, swelling of the lips and tongue, blurred vision, eye pain, night blindness, epistaxis, taste disorder, reversible hearing loss.
**GI:** *abdominal pain or cramps, constipation, diarrhea, indigestion, nausea,* abdominal distention, flatulence, peptic ulceration, **bleeding,** melena, bloody diarrhea, appetite change, colitis.
**GU:** proteinuria, *acute renal failure,*

---

oliguria, interstitial nephritis, papillary necrosis, *nephrotic syndrome, fluid retention.*
**Hepatic:** elevated liver enzymes, jaundice, hepatitis, *hepatotoxicity.*
**Respiratory:** asthma.
**Skin:** rash, pruritus, urticaria, eczema, dermatitis, alopecia, photosensitivity, bullous eruption, *Stevens-Johnson syndrome* (rare), allergic purpura.
**Other:** *anaphylaxis; anaphylactoid reactions;* angioedema; back, leg, or joint pain; hypoglycemia; hyperglycemia.

## INTERACTIONS

*Anticoagulants (including warfarin):* possible increased incidence of bleeding. Monitor patient closely.
*Aspirin:* may decrease effectiveness of diclofenac. Concomitant use not recommended by manufacturer.
*Cyclosporine, digoxin, lithium, methotrexate:* diclofenac may reduce renal clearance of these drugs and increase risk of toxicity. Monitor patient closely.
*Diuretics:* decreased effectiveness of diuretics. Avoid concomitant use.
*Insulin, oral antidiabetic agents:* diclofenac may alter requirements for antidiabetic agents. Monitor patient closely.
*Potassium-sparing diuretics:* enhanced potassium retention and increased serum potassium levels. Monitor serum potassium level.

## CONTRAINDICATIONS

Contraindicated in patients with hypersensitivity to this drug, hepatic porphyria and in patients with a history of asthma, urticaria, or other allergic reactions after taking aspirin or other NSAIDs. Not recommended for use during late pregnancy or while breast-feeding.

## NURSING CONSIDERATIONS

● Use cautiously in patients with a history of peptic ulcer disease, hepatic dysfunction, cardiac disease, hypertension, conditions associated with fluid retention, or impaired renal function.
● Because NSAIDs impair the synthesis of renal prostaglandins, they can decrease renal blood flow and lead to reversible renal impairment, especially in patients with preexisting renal failure, liver dysfunction, or heart failure; in elderly patients; and in those taking diuretics. Monitor these patients closely.
● Elevations of liver tests may occur during therapy. Monitor serum transaminase, especially ALT levels, periodically in patients undergoing long-term therapy as ordered. Know that the first serum transaminase measurement should be no later than 8 weeks after initiation of therapy.
● Be aware that because of their antipyretic and anti-inflammatory actions, NSAIDs may mask the signs and symptoms of infection.

## ☑ PATIENT TEACHING

● To minimize GI distress, tell patient to take diclofenac with milk or meals.
● Instruct patient not to crush, break, or chew enteric-coated tablets.
● Serious GI toxicity, including peptic ulceration and bleeding, can occur in patients taking NSAIDs despite the absence of GI symptoms. Teach patient the signs and symptoms of GI bleeding, and tell him to contact the doctor immediately if any of these occurs.
● Teach patient the signs and symptoms of hepatotoxicity, including nausea, fatigue, lethargy, pruritus, jaundice, right upper quadrant tenderness, and flulike symptoms. Tell him to contact doctor immediately if these symptoms appear.
● Advise patient to avoid consump-

---

Reactions may be *common,* uncommon, *life-threatening,* or **COMMON AND LIFE-THREATENING.**

tion of alcoholic beverages or asprin while taking diclofenac.

• Warn patient to avoid hazardous activities that require alertness until adverse CNS effects of drug are known.

• Tell patient that use during last trimester of pregnancy should be avoided.

---

# etodolac (ultradol)
Lodine

*Pregnancy Risk Category: C*

## HOW SUPPLIED
*Capsules:* 200 mg, 300 mg
*Tablets:* 400 mg

## ACTION
Unknown, but believed related to inhibition of prostaglandin biosynthesis.

## ONSET, PEAK, DURATION
Onset occurs within 30 minutes. Plasma levels peak within 1 to 2 hours. Analgesic effects persist 4 to 12 hours.

## INDICATIONS & DOSAGE
*Acute and chronic management of osteoarthritis and pain –*
**Adults:** 200 to 400 mg P.O. q 6 to 8 hours, p.r.n., not to exceed 1,200 mg daily. For patients weighing 60 kg or less, total daily dose should not exceed 20 mg/kg.

## ADVERSE REACTIONS
**CNS:** *asthenia, malaise, dizziness,* depression, drowsiness, nervousness, insomnia.
**CV:** hypertension, *CHF,* syncope, flushing, palpitations, edema, fluid retention.
**EENT:** blurred vision, tinnitus, photophobia, dry mouth.
**GI:** *dyspepsia, flatulence, abdominal pain, diarrhea, nausea,* constipation, gastritis, melena, vomiting, anorexia, peptic ulceration with or without *GI*

*bleeding* or perforation, ulcerative stomatitis, thirst.
**GU:** dysuria, urinary frequency, *renal failure.*
**Hematologic:** anemia (rare), leukopenia, *thrombocytopenia,* hemolytic anemia, *agranulocytosis.*
**Hepatic:** hepatitis.
**Respiratory:** asthma.
**Skin:** pruritus, rash, *Stevens-Johnson syndrome.*
**Other:** chills, fever, weight gain.

## INTERACTIONS
*Antacids:* may decrease peak levels of the drug. Monitor for decreased effect of etodolac.
*Aspirin:* reduced protein-binding of etodolac without altering its clearance. Clinical significance unknown. Recommend avoiding concomitant use.
*Cyclosporine:* impaired elimination and increased risk of nephrotoxicity. Avoid concomitant use.
*Digoxin, lithium, methotrexate:* etodolac may impair elimination of these drugs, resulting in increased levels and risk of toxicity. Monitor blood levels.
*Warfarin:* etodolac decreases the protein-binding of warfarin but does not change its clearance. Although no dosage adjustment is necessary, monitor PT closely and watch for bleeding.

## CONTRAINDICATIONS
Contraindicated in patients with hypersensitivity to the drug and in those with a history of aspirin- or NSAID-induced asthma, rhinitis, urticaria, or other allergic reactions.

## NURSING CONSIDERATIONS
• Use cautiously in patients with a history of GI bleeding, ulceration, and perforation and renal or hepatic impairment.
• Because NSAIDs impair the synthesis of renal prostaglandins, they can

---

*Liquid form contains alcohol. **May contain tartrazine. †Canada only. ‡Australia only. ◊OTC.

decrease renal blood flow and lead to reversible renal impairment, especially in patients with preexisting renal failure, liver dysfunction, or heart failure; in elderly patients; and in those taking diuretics. Monitor these patients closely during therapy.

• **Alert:** Know that etodolac appears to cause fewer GI problems than most NSAIDs. Minimal GI blood loss has been reported at dosages up to 1,200 mg daily.

• Know that metabolites of etodolac may cause a false-positive test for urinary bilirubin, decreased serum uric acid levels, and borderline elevations of one or more liver function tests.

☑ **PATIENT TEACHING**

• To minimize GI discomfort, tell patient to take etodolac with milk or meals.

• Serious GI toxicity, including peptic ulceration and bleeding, can occur in patient taking NSAIDs despite the absence of GI symptoms. Teach patient the signs and symptoms of GI bleeding, and tell him to contact the doctor immediately if any of these occurs.

• Advise patient to avoid consumption of alcoholic beverages or aspirin while taking drug.

• Warn patient to avoid hazardous activities that require alertness until adverse CNS effects of drug are known.

• This drug has been associated with photosensitivity reactions. Advise patient to use a sunblock, wear protective clothing, and avoid prolonged exposure to sunlight.

• Tell patient that use during last trimester of pregnancy should be avoided.

## fenoprofen calcium
Nalfon, Nalfon 200

*Pregnancy Risk Category: NR*

**HOW SUPPLIED**
*Tablets:* 600 mg
*Capsules:* 200 mg, 300 mg

**ACTION**
Unknown. Produces anti-inflammatory, analgesic, and antipyretic effects, possibly by inhibiting prostaglandin synthesis.

**ONSET, PEAK, DURATION**
Onset occurs within 15 to 30 minutes. Plasma levels peak in about 2 hours. Analgesic effects persist 4 to 6 hours.

**INDICATIONS & DOSAGE**
*Rheumatoid arthritis and osteoarthritis —*
**Adults:** 300 to 600 mg P.O. t.i.d. or q.i.d. Maximum dosage is 3.2 g daily.
*Mild to moderate pain —*
**Adults:** 200 mg P.O. q 4 to 6 hours, p.r.n.

**ADVERSE REACTIONS**
**CNS:** *headache,* dizziness, *somnolence,* fatigue, nervousness, asthenia, tremor, confusion.
**CV:** peripheral edema, palpitations.
**EENT:** tinnitus, blurred vision, decreased hearing.
**GI:** *epigastric distress, nausea, GI bleeding,* vomiting, occult blood loss, peptic ulceration, constipation, anorexia, *dyspepsia,* flatulence.
**GU:** oliguria, interstitial nephritis, proteinuria, reversible renal failure, papillary necrosis, cystitis, hematuria.
**Hematologic:** prolonged bleeding time, anemia, *aplastic anemia, agranulocytosis, thrombocytopenia, hemorrhage,* bruising, hemolytic anemia.
**Hepatic:** elevated enzymes, hepatitis.
**Respiratory:** dyspnea, upper respiratory tract infections, nasopharyngitis.
**Skin:** *pruritus,* rash, urticaria, *anaphylaxis,* increased diaphoresis.
**Other:** angioedema.

---

Reactions may be *common,* uncommon, *life-threatening,* or **COMMON AND LIFE-THREATENING.**

## INTERACTIONS

*Aspirin:* decreased fenoprofen half-life; may increase GI toxicity. Avoid concomitant use.

*Diuretics:* decreased diuretic effectiveness. Monitor patient closely.

*Ethanol, corticosteroids:* increased risk of adverse GI reactions. Avoid concomitant use.

*Oral anticoagulants, sulfonylureas:* fenoprofen enhances pharmacologic effects of these drugs. Use together cautiously.

*Phenobarbital:* enhanced metabolism of fenoprofen. Monitor for lack of fenoprofen effectiveness.

## CONTRAINDICATIONS

Contraindicated in patients with hypersensitivity to this drug, significantly impaired renal function, or history of aspirin- or NSAID-induced asthma, rhinitis, or urticaria. Also contraindicated in pregnancy.

## NURSING CONSIDERATIONS

● Use cautiously in elderly patients; in patients with history of serious GI events or peptic ulcer disease, compromised cardiac function or hypertension.

● Be aware that safety has not been established for pregnancy. Administration to pregnant patients is not recommended.

● Because NSAIDs impair the synthesis of renal prostaglandins, they can decrease renal blood flow and lead to reversible renal impairment, especially in patients with preexisting renal failure, liver dysfunction, or heart failure; in elderly patients; and in those taking diuretics. Monitor these patients closely during therapy.

● Know that because of their antipyretic and anti-inflammatory actions, NSAIDs may mask the signs and symptoms of infection.

● Be aware that renal, hepatic, ocular, and auditory function should be checked periodically in long-term therapy. Drug should be stopped if abnormalities occur.

● Be aware that fenoprofen may cause false elevations in free and total serum $T_3$ levels as measured by the Amerlex-T assay. Fenoprofen or its metabolite may cross-react with the antibody used in the Amerlex-M assay. Limited data suggest that drug may alter free and total $T_3$ concentrations determined by the Corning method.

## ☑ PATIENT TEACHING

● Tell patient that full therapeutic effect for arthritis may be delayed for 2 to 4 weeks.

● Tell patient to take this drug 30 minutes before or 2 hours after meals. If adverse GI reactions occur, drug may be taken with milk or meals.

● Serious GI toxicity, including peptic ulceration and bleeding, can occur in patients taking NSAIDs despite the absence of GI symptoms. Teach patient the signs and symptoms of GI bleeding, and tell him to contact the doctor immediately if any occurs.

● Advise patient to avoid consumption of alcoholic beverages or aspirin while taking drug.

● Warn patient to avoid hazardous activities that require alertness until adverse CNS effects of the drug are known.

● Instruct patient to notify doctor immediately if pregnancy is suspected because drug is not recommended for use during pregnancy.

# flurbiprofen

Ansaid, Apo-Flurbiprofen†, Froben†, Froben SR†

*Pregnancy Risk Category: B*

## HOW SUPPLIED

*Tablets:* 50 mg, 100 mg
*Capsules (extended-release)†:* 200 mg

## ACTION
Unknown. Possibly inhibits prostaglandin synthesis.

## ONSET, PEAK, DURATION
Onset and duration unknown. Serum levels peak about 2 hours after a dose.

## INDICATIONS & DOSAGE
*Rheumatoid arthritis and osteoarthritis* –
**Adults:** 200 to 300 mg P.O. daily, divided b.i.d. to q.i.d. Where available, patients maintained on 200 mg daily may switch to one 200-mg extended-release capsule P.O. daily, taken in the evening after food.

## ADVERSE REACTIONS
**CNS:** *headache,* anxiety, insomnia, dizziness, increased reflexes, tremors, amnesia, asthenia, drowsiness, malaise, depression.
**CV:** *edema,* **CHF,** hypertension, vasodilation.
**EENT:** rhinitis, tinnitus, visual changes, epistaxis.
**GI:** *dyspepsia, diarrhea, abdominal pain, nausea,* constipation, **bleeding,** flatulence, vomiting.
**GU:** *symptoms suggesting urinary tract infection,* hematuria, interstitial nephritis, **renal failure.**
**Hematologic:** **thrombocytopenia,** neutropenia, anemia, **aplastic anemia.**
**Hepatic:** elevated liver enzymes, jaundice.
**Respiratory:** asthma.
**Skin:** rash, photosensitivity, urticaria, angioedema.
**Other:** weight changes.

## INTERACTIONS
*Anticoagulants:* increased risk of bleeding. Monitor patient closely.
*Aspirin:* decreased flurbiprofen levels. Concomitant use is not recommended.
*Beta-adrenergic blockers:* may increase risk of hypotension. Monitor blood pressure.
*Diuretics:* possible decreased diuretic effect. Monitor patient closely.
*Methotrexate:* increased risk of methotrexate toxicity. Monitor patient closely.

## CONTRAINDICATIONS
Contraindicated in patients with hypersensitivity to the drug, or history of aspirin- or NSAID-induced asthma, urticaria, or other allergic-type reactions.

## NURSING CONSIDERATIONS
• Use cautiously in patients with a history of peptic ulcer disease, hepatic dysfunction, cardiac disease, or other conditions associated with fluid retention or impaired renal function.
• Know that use during pregnancy is not recommended in last trimester.
• Be aware that elderly or debilitated patients and those patients with hepatic or renal dysfunction should be closely monitored and probably should receive lower doses. These patients may be at risk for renal toxicity, jaundice, or toxic hepatitis. Periodically monitor renal and hepatic function as ordered.
• Because NSAIDs impair the synthesis of renal prostaglandins, they can decrease renal blood flow and lead to reversible renal impairment, especially in patients with preexisting renal failure, liver dysfunction, or heart failure; in elderly patients; and in those taking diuretics. Monitor these patients closely during therapy.
• Know that patients receiving long-term therapy should have periodic liver function studies, eye examinations, and hematocrit determinations.

## ☑ PATIENT TEACHING
• Tell patient to take drug with food, milk, or antacid if GI upset occurs.
• Tell patient taking extended-release capsules to swallow them whole; do

---

Reactions may be *common,* uncommon, *life-threatening,* or **COMMON AND LIFE-THREATENING.**

not crush, chew, or break open the capsules.

• Serious GI toxicity, including peptic ulceration and bleeding, can occur in patients taking NSAIDs despite the absence of GI symptoms. Teach patient the signs and symptoms of GI bleeding, and tell him to contact the doctor immediately if they occur.

• Advise patients to avoid consumption of alcoholic beverages or aspirin while taking drug.

• Warn patient to avoid hazardous activities that require mental alertness until CNS effects are known.

---

### ibuprofen

Aches-N-Pain◇, ACT-3‡, Advil◇, Amersol†, Apo-Ibuprofen†, Brufen‡, Children's Advil, Children's Motrin◇, Excedrin IB, Caplets◇, Excedrin IB Tablets◇, Genpril Caplets◇,Genpril Tablets◇, Haltran◇, Ibu-Cream‡, Ibuprin◇, Ibuprohm Caplets◇, Ibuprohm Tablets◇, Ibu-Tab◇, Inflam‡, Medipren Caplets◇, Medipren Tablets◇, Midol-200◇, Motrin, Motrin IB Caplets◇, Motrin IB Tablets◇, Novo-Profen†, Nuprin Caplets◇, Nuprin Tablets◇, Nurofen‡, Pamprin-IB, PediaProfen, Rafen‡, Rufen, Saleto-200, Saleto-400, Saleto-600, Saleto-800, Trendar◇

*Pregnancy Risk Category: NR*

### HOW SUPPLIED
*Tablets:* 200 mg◇, 300 mg, 400 mg, 600 mg, 800 mg
*Caplets:* 200 mg◇
*Oral suspension:* 100 mg/5 ml

### ACTION
Unknown. Produces anti-inflammatory, analgesic, and antipyretic effects, possibly by inhibiting prostaglandin synthesis.

### ONSET, PEAK, DURATION
Analgesic and antipyretic effects within 30 minutes; antirheumatic effect within 7 days. Plasma levels peak 2 to 4 hours after oral dose. Effects persist 4 hours or more.

### INDICATIONS & DOSAGE
*Rheumatoid arthritis, osteoarthritis, arthritis –*
**Adults:** 300 to 800 mg P.O. t.i.d. or q.i.d. not to exceed 3.2 g/day.
*Mild to moderate pain, dysmenorrhea –*
**Adults:** 400 mg P.O. q 4 to 6 hours p.r.n.
*Fever –*
**Adults:** 200 to 400 mg P.O. q 4 to 6 hours. Do not exceed 1.2 g daily or give longer than 3 days.
**Children 6 months to 12 years:** if fever is below 102.5° F (39.2° C), the recommended dose is 5 mg/kg P.O. q 6 to 8 hours. Treat higher fevers with 10 mg/kg q 6 to 8 hours. Do not exceed 40 mg/kg daily.
*External treatment of joint pain; swelling of tissues adjacent to joints† –*
**Adults:** apply a 4- to 10-cm strip of cream to the skin and massage briskly. Apply t.i.d.

### ADVERSE REACTIONS
**CNS:** *headache, dizziness,* nervousness, aseptic meningitis.
**CV:** *peripheral edema,* fluid retention, edema.
**EENT:** *tinnitus.*
**GI:** *epigastric distress, nausea, occult blood loss, peptic ulceration,* diarrhea, constipation, dyspepsia, flatulence, heartburn, decreased appetite.
**GU:** *acute renal failure,* azotemia, cystitis, hematuria.
**Hematologic:** prolonged bleeding time, anemia, neutropenia, pancytopenia, *thrombocytopenia, aplastic anemia,* leukopenia, *agranulocytosis.*
**Hepatic:** elevated enzymes.

---

**Respiratory:** *bronchospasm.*
**Skin:** pruritus, *rash,* urticaria, *Stevens-Johnson syndrome.*

### INTERACTIONS

*Antihypertensives, furosemide, thiazide diuretics:* ibuprofen may decrease the effectiveness of diuretics or antihypertensives. Monitor patient closely.

*Aspirin:* may decrease serum levels of ibuprofen. Avoid concomitant use.

*Aspirin, corticosteroids, ethanol:* increased risk of adverse GI reactions. Avoid concomitant use.

*Lithium, oral anticoagulants:* ibuprofen may increase plasma levels or effects of these drug. Monitor for toxicity.

*Methotrexate:* decreased methotrexate clearance and increased toxicity. Use together cautiously.

### CONTRAINDICATIONS

Contraindicated in patients with hypersensitivity to this drug, or who have the syndrome of nasal polyps, angioedema, and bronchospastic reaction to aspirin or other NSAIDs.

### NURSING CONSIDERATIONS

• Use cautiously in patients with GI disorders, history of peptic ulcer disease, hepatic or renal disease, cardiac decompensation, hypertension, known intrinsic coagulation defects.

• Know that use during pregnancy is not recommended.

• Check renal and hepatic function periodically in patients on long-term therapy. Stop drug if abnormalities occur and notify doctor.

• Be aware that because of their antipyretic and anti-inflammatory actions, NSAIDs may mask the signs and symptoms of infection.

### ☑ PATIENT TEACHING

• To reduce adverse GI reactions, tell patient to take with meals or milk.

• *Alert:* Drug is available OTC in several brands (200 mg). Instruct patient not to exceed 1.2 g daily, give to children under age 12, or self-medicate for extended periods without consulting the doctor.

• Tell patient that full therapeutic effect for arthritis may be delayed for 2 to 4 weeks. Although analgesic effect occurs at low dosage levels, anti-inflammatory effect does not occur at dosages below 400 mg q.i.d.

• Caution patient that concomitant use with aspirin, alcohol, or corticosteroids may increase the risk of GI adverse reactions.

• Serious GI toxicity, including peptic ulceration and bleeding, can occur in patients taking NSAIDs despite the absence of GI symptoms. Teach patients the signs and symptoms of GI bleeding, and tell them to contact the doctor immediately if they occur.

• Warn patient to avoid hazardous activities that require mental alertness until CNS effects are known.

---

## indomethacin

Apo-Indomethacin†, Arthrexin‡, Indochron E-R, Indocid†‡, Indocid SR†, Indocin, Indocin SR, Novo-Methacin†, Rheumacin‡

## indomethacin sodium trihydrate

Apo-Indomethacin†, Indocid PDA†, Indocin I.V., Novomethacin†

*Pregnancy Risk Category: NR*

### HOW SUPPLIED

**indomethacin**
*Capsules:* 25 mg, 50 mg
*Capsules (sustained-release):* 75 mg
*Oral suspension:* 25 mg/5 ml
*Suppositories:* 50 mg
**indomethacin sodium trihydrate**
*Injection:* 1-mg vials

### ACTION

Unknown. Produces anti-inflammatory, analgesic, and antipyretic effects, possibly by inhibiting prostaglandin synthesis.

**ONSET, PEAK, DURATION**
Onset occurs within 2 to 4 hours. Serum levels peak within 1 to 2 hours after a dose of immediate-release capsules or oral suspension, within 2 to 4 hours of a sustained-release capsule, or immediately following an I.V. injection. Peak antirheumatic effects occur after 1 to 2 weeks of therapy. Analgesic effects persist 4 to 6 hours.

**INDICATIONS & DOSAGE**
*Moderate to severe rheumatoid arthritis or osteoarthritis, ankylosing spondylitis* –
**Adults:** 25 mg P.O. or P.R. b.i.d. or t.i.d. with food or antacids; increased dosage by 25 or 50 mg daily q 7 days, up to 200 mg daily. Or, sustained-release capsules (75 mg): 75 mg P.O. to start, in the morning or h.s., followed, if necessary, by 75 mg b.i.d.
*Acute gouty arthritis* –
**Adults:** 50 mg P.O. t.i.d. Dose reduced as soon as possible; then discontinued. Sustained-release capsules shouldn't be used for this condition.
*Acute painful shoulders (bursitis or tendinitis)* –
**Adults:** 75 to 150 mg P.O. daily in divided doses t.i.d. or q.i.d. for 7 to 14 days.
*To close a hemodynamically significant patent ductus arteriosus in premature infants (I.V. form only)* –
**Neonates under 48 hours:** 0.2 mg/kg I.V. followed by two doses of 0.1 mg/kg at 12- to 24-hour intervals.
**Neonates 2 to 7 days:** 0.2 mg/kg I.V. followed by two doses of 0.2 mg/kg at 12- to 24-hour intervals.
**Neonates over 7 days:** 0.2 mg/kg I.V. followed by two doses of 0.25 mg/kg at 12- to 24-hour intervals.

**ADVERSE REACTIONS**
*Oral and rectal forms:*
**CNS:** *headache, dizziness,* depression, drowsiness, confusion, somnolence, fatigue, peripheral neuropathy, *seizures,* psychic disturbances, syncope, *vertigo.*
**CV:** hypertension, *edema, CHF.*
**EENT:** blurred vision, corneal and retinal damage, hearing loss, tinnitus.
**GI:** *nausea,* anorexia, *diarrhea, peptic ulceration, GI bleeding,* constipation, dyspepsia, pancreatitis.
**GU:** hematuria, *acute renal failure.*
**Hematologic:** *hemolytic anemia, aplastic anemia, agranulocytosis,* leukopenia, *thrombocytopenic purpura,* iron deficiency anemia.
**Skin:** pruritus, urticaria, *Stevens-Johnson syndrome.*
**Other:** hypersensitivity (rash, respiratory distress, *anaphylaxis, angioedema),* hyperkalemia.
*I.V. form:*
**GU:** *renal failure,* hematuria, proteinuria, interstitial nephritis.

**INTERACTIONS**
*Aminoglycosides, cyclosporine, methotrexate:* indomethacin may enhance the toxicity of these agents. Avoid concomitant use.
*Antihypertensives:* reduced antihypertensive effect. Monitor patient closely.
*Aspirin:* decreased blood levels of indomethacin. Avoid concomitant use.
*Corticosteroids, ethanol:* increased risk of GI toxicity. Don't use together.
*Diflunisal, probenecid:* decreased indomethacin excretion; watch for increased incidence of indomethacin adverse reactions.
*Digoxin:* indomethacin may prolong the half-life of digoxin. Use together cautiously.
*Dipyridamole:* enhanced fluid retention. Avoid concomitant use.
*Furosemide, thiazide diuretics:* impaired response to both drugs. Avoid using together if possible.
*Lithium:* increased plasma lithium levels. Monitor for toxicity.

---

*Liquid form contains alcohol.   **May contain tartrazine.   †Canada only.   ‡Australia only.   ◊OTC.

*Triamterene:* possible nephrotoxicity. Monitor patient closely.

## CONTRAINDICATIONS

Contraindicated in patients with hypersensitivity to this drug, or history of aspirin- or NSAID-induced asthma, rhinitis, or urticaria; in pregnancy or while breast-feeding. Also contraindicated in infants with untreated infection, active bleeding, coagulation defects or thrombocytopenia, congenital heart disease in whom patency of the ductus arteriosus is necessary for satisfactory pulmonary or systemic blood flow, necrotizing enterocolitis, or impaired renal function. Suppositories are contraindicated in patients with a history of proctitis or recent rectal bleeding.

## NURSING CONSIDERATIONS

● Use cautiously in patients with epilepsy, parkinsonism, hepatic or renal disease, cardiovascular disease, infection, and mental illness or depression. Also use cautiously in elderly patients and patients with history of GI disease.
● Be aware that because of its high incidence of adverse effects during chronic use, indomethacin should not be used routinely as an analgesic or antipyretic.
● Know that use during pregnancy is not recommended.
● Administer oral dosage with food, milk, or antacid if GI upset occurs.
● **I.V. use:** Reconstitute powder for injection with sterile water or 0.9% sodium chloride for injection or 0.9% sodium chloride. For each 1-mg vial, add 1 ml of diluent for a solution containing 1 mg/ml; add 2 ml of diluent to yield a solution containing 0.5 mg/ml. Give by direct injection over 5 to 10 seconds.
● **Alert:** Use only preservative-free diluents to prepare I.V. injection. Never use diluents containing benzyl alcohol because this has been associated with a fatal gasping syndrome in neonates. Because the injection contains no preservatives, reconstitute immediately before administration, and discard any unused solution.
● Don't administer second or third scheduled I.V. dose if anuria or marked oliguria is evident; instead, notify doctor.
● Be aware that if ductus arteriosus reopens, a second course of one to three doses may be given. If ineffective, surgery may be necessary.
● Monitor carefully for bleeding and for reduced urine output with I.V. administration. Discontinue drug and notify doctor if either occurs.
● Monitor for bleeding in patients receiving anticoagulants, patients with coagulation defects, and neonates.
● Because NSAIDs impair the synthesis of renal prostaglandins, they can decrease renal blood flow and lead to reversible renal impairment, especially in patients with preexisting renal failure, liver dysfunction, or heart failure; in elderly patients; and in those taking diuretics. Monitor these patients closely during therapy.
● Causes sodium retention; monitor for weight gain (especially in elderly patients) and increased blood pressure in patients with hypertension.
● Be aware that adverse CNS reactions are more common and serious in elderly patients.
● Know that because of their antipyretic and anti-inflammatory actions, NSAIDs may mask the signs and symptoms of infection.
● Indomethacin may enhance the hypothalamic-pituitary-adrenal axis response to the dexamethasone suppression test. Inform clinical laboratory personnel that the patient is taking indomethacin.

☑ **PATIENT TEACHING**
● Tell patient to take oral form of this drug with food, milk, or antacid if GI upset occurs.

---

Reactions may be *common,* uncommon, *life-threatening,* or **COMMON AND LIFE-THREATENING.**

- Alert patient that concomitant use of oral form with aspirin, alcohol, or corticosteroids may increase the risk of adverse GI reactions.
- Serious GI toxicity, including peptic ulceration and bleeding, can occur in patient taking oral NSAIDs despite the absence of GI symptoms. Teach patient the signs and symptoms of GI bleeding, and tell him to contact the doctor immediately if they occur.
- Warn patient to avoid hazardous activities that require mental alertness until CNS effects are known.
- Tell patient to notify the doctor immediately if any visual or hearing changes occurs. Patient on long-term oral therapy should have regular eye examinations, hearing tests, CBC, and renal function tests to monitor for toxicity.

# ketoprofen
Apo-Keto†, Apo-Keto-E†, Novo-Keto-EC†, Orudis, Orudis-E†, Orudis-SR†‡, Oruvail, Rhodis†, Rhodis-E†, Rhodis-EC†

*Pregnancy Risk Category: NR*

## HOW SUPPLIED
*Tablets (extended-release):* 100 mg, 150 mg, 200 mg†
*Tablets (enteric-coated):* 50 mg†, 100 mg†
*Capsules (extended-release):* 200 mg
*Capsules:* 25 mg, 50 mg, 75 mg
*Suppositories:* 100 mg†

## ACTION
Unknown. Produces anti-inflammatory, analgesic, and antipyretic effects, possibly by inhibiting prostaglandin synthesis.

## ONSET, PEAK, DURATION
Analgesic onset occurs in 1 to 2 hours; unknown for arthritis. Serum levels peak ½ to 2 hours. Effects persist for 3 to 4 hours when used for analgesia; unknown for arthritis.

## INDICATIONS & DOSAGE
*Rheumatoid arthritis and osteoarthritis –*
**Adults:** 75 mg t.i.d. or 50 mg q.i.d. or 200 mg as an extended-release tablet once daily. Maximum dosage is 300 mg/day.
Alternatively, where suppository is available, 100 mg P.R. b.i.d.; or 1 suppository h.s. (in conjunction with oral ketoprofen during the day).
*Mild to moderate pain; dysmenorrhea –*
**Adults:** 25 to 50 mg P.O. q 6 to 8 hours p.r.n.

## ADVERSE REACTIONS
**CNS:** *headache,* dizziness, *CNS excitation* or depression.
**EENT:** tinnitus, visual disturbances.
**GI:** *nausea, abdominal pain, diarrhea, constipation, flatulence, peptic ulceration,* dyspepsia, anorexia, vomiting, stomatitis.
**GU:** *nephrotoxicity, elevated BUN.*
**Hematologic:** prolonged bleeding time, *thrombocytopenia, agranulocytosis.*
**Hepatic:** elevated liver enzymes.
**Respiratory:** dyspnea, *bronchospasm, laryngeal edema.*
**Skin:** rash, photosensitivity, *exfoliative dermatitis.*
**Other:** peripheral edema.

## INTERACTIONS
*Aspirin, corticosteroids, ethanol:* increased risk of adverse GI reactions. Avoid concomitant use.
*Aspirin, probenecid:* increased plasma levels of ketoprofen. Avoid concomitant use.
*Hydrochlorothiazide, other diuretics:* decreased diuretic effectiveness. Monitor for lack of effect.
*Lithium, methotrexate:* increased levels of these drugs, leading to toxicity. Monitor patient closely.
*Warfarin:* increased risk of bleeding. Monitor patient closely.

---

*Liquid form contains alcohol.   **May contain tartrazine.   †Canada only.   ‡Australia only.   ◊OTC.

## CONTRAINDICATIONS

Contraindicated in patients with hypersensitivity to this drug, or history of aspirin- or NSAID-induced asthma, urticaria, or other allergic-type reactions.

## NURSING CONSIDERATIONS

• Use cautiously in patients with history of peptic ulcer disease, renal dysfunction, hypertension, heart failure, or fluid retention.
• Know that use during last trimester of pregnancy should be avoided.
• Know that the sustained-release dosage form is not recommended for patients in acute pain.
• Because NSAIDs impair the synthesis of renal prostaglandins, they can decrease renal blood flow and lead to reversible renal impairment, especially in patients with preexisting renal failure, liver dysfunction, or heart failure; in elderly patients; and in those taking diuretics. Monitor these patients closely during therapy.
• Check renal and hepatic function every 6 months or as indicated and ordered during long-term therapy.
• Be aware that NSAIDs may mask the signs and symptoms of infection because of their antipyretic and anti-inflammatory actions.
• Inform laboratory personnel that patient is taking ketoprofen. Ketoprofen may interfere with some laboratory determinations of blood glucose and serum iron levels, depending on the testing method used.

### ☑ PATIENT TEACHING

• Tell patient to take drug 30 minutes before or 2 hours after meals. If adverse GI reactions occur, patient may take the drug with milk or meals.
• Tell patient that full therapeutic effect may be delayed for 2 to 4 weeks.
• Serious GI toxicity, including peptic ulceration and bleeding, can occur in patient taking NSAIDs despite the absence of GI symptoms. Teach patient the signs and symptoms of GI bleeding, and tell him to contact the doctor immediately if they occur.
• Alert patient that concomitant use with aspirin, alcohol, or corticosteroids may increase the risk of adverse GI reactions.
• Warn patient to avoid hazardous activities that require mental alertness until CNS effects are known.
• This drug has been associated with photosensitivity reactions. Advise patient to use a sunblock, wear protective clothing, and avoid prolonged exposure to sunlight.
• Tell patient to report visual or auditory adverse reactions immediately.

---

## ketorolac tromethamine
Toradol

*Pregnancy Risk Category: C*

## HOW SUPPLIED
*Tablets:* 10 mg
*Injection:* 15 mg, 30 mg, 60 mg

## ACTION
Unknown. Thought to inhibit prostaglandin synthesis.

## ONSET, PEAK, DURATION
Onset immediate with I.V. administration; within 10 minutes of an I.M. injection; 30 to 60 minutes after oral dose. Plasma levels peak in 30 minutes to 1 hour after either oral or I.M. administration, immediately after I.V. injection. Analgesic effects persist up to 6 to 8 hours.

## INDICATIONS & DOSAGE
*Short-term management of moderately severe, acute pain for single-dose treatment —*
**Adults under 65 years:** 60 mg I.M. or 30 mg I.V.
**Adults 65 years or older, renally impaired patients, and patients weighing less than 50 kg:** 30 mg I.M. or 15 mg I.V.

---

*Short-term management of moderately severe, acute pain for multiple-dose treatment* —

**Adults under 65 years:** 30 mg I.M. or I.V. q 6 hours. Maximum daily dose should not exceed 120 mg.

**Adults 65 years or older, renally impaired patients, and patients weighing less than 50 kg:** 15 mg I.M. or I.V. q 6 hours. Maximum daily dose should not exceed 60 mg.

*Short-term management of moderately severe, acute pain when switching from parenteral to oral administration (oral therapy is indicated only as continuation of parenterally administered drug and should never be given without the patient first having received parenteral therapy)* —

**Adults under 65 years:** 20 mg P.O. as single dose followed by 10 mg P.O. q 4 to 6 hours, not to exceed 40 mg/day.

**Adults 65 years or older, renally impaired patients, and patients weighing less than 50 kg:** 10 mg P.O. as single dose followed by 10 mg P.O. q 4 to 6 hours, not to exceed 40 mg/day.

## ADVERSE REACTIONS

**CNS:** *drowsiness, sedation,* dizziness, *headache.*

**CV:** edema, hypertension, palpitations, arrhythmias.

**GI:** *nausea, dyspepsia, GI pain,* diarrhea, peptic ulceration, vomiting, constipation, flatulence, stomatitis.

**Hematologic:** decreased platelet adhesion, purpura, ***thrombocytopenia.***

**Other:** pain at injection site, pruritus, rash, diaphoresis.

## INTERACTIONS

*ACE inhibitors:* may increase risk of renal impairment, particularly in volume-depleted patients. Do not use together in volume-depleted patients.

*Antihypertensives, diuretics:* decreased effectiveness. Monitor patient closely.

*Lithium:* increased lithium levels. Monitor patient closely.

*Methotrexate:* decreased methotrexate clearance and increased toxicity. Don't use together.

*Salicylates, anticoagulants:* ketorolac may increase the levels of free (unbound) salicylates or anticoagulants in the blood. Use with extreme caution and monitor patient closely.

## CONTRAINDICATIONS

Contraindicated in patients with hypersensitivity to this drug and in patients with active peptic ulcer disease, recent GI bleeding or perforation, advanced renal impairment, risk for renal impairment due to volume depletion, suspected or confirmed cerebrovascular bleeding, hemorrhagic diathesis, incomplete hemostasis, or high risk of bleeding.

Drug is also contraindicated in patients with a history of peptic ulcer disease or GI bleeding, past allergic manifestations to aspirin or other NSAIDs, and during labor and delivery or breast-feeding. In addition, drug is contraindicated as prophylactic analgesic before major surgery or intraoperatively when hemostasis is critical; in patients currently receiving aspirin, an NSAID, or probenecid; and in patients requiring analgesic to be administered epidurally or intrathecally.

## NURSING CONSIDERATIONS

● Use cautiously in patients with hepatic or renal impairment.

● **Alert:** The maximum combined duration of therapy (parenteral and oral) must be limited to 5 days.

● I.M. administration may cause pain at the injection site. Holding pressure over the site for 15 to 30 seconds after the injection may minimize local effects.

● Carefully observe patients with coagulopathies and those who are taking anticoagulants. Ketorolac inhibits platelet aggregation and can prolong bleeding time. This effect will disappear within 48 hours of discontinuing the drug. It will not alter platelet count, PTT, or PT.

• Be aware that NSAIDs may mask the signs and symptoms of infection because of their antipyretic and anti-inflammatory actions.

### ☑ PATIENT TEACHING

• Warn patient receiving drug I.M. that pain may occur at injection site.
• Serious GI toxicity, including peptic ulceration and bleeding, can occur in patient taking NSAIDs despite the absence of GI symptoms. Teach patient the signs and symptoms of GI bleeding, and tell him to notify the doctor immediately if they occur.

---

## meclofenamate
Meclomen

*Pregnancy Risk Category: NR*

### HOW SUPPLIED
*Capsules:* 50 mg, 100 mg

### ACTION
Unknown. Produces anti-inflammatory, analgesic, and antipyretic effects, possibly by inhibiting prostaglandin synthesis.

### ONSET, PEAK, DURATION
Onset occurs within 30 minutes for analgesic effects; antirheumatic effects, within a few days of therapy. Plasma levels peak in ½ to 1 hour; peak antirheumatic activity occurs after 2 to 3 weeks of therapy. Duration unknown.

### INDICATIONS & DOSAGE
*Rheumatoid arthritis and osteoarthritis –*
**Adults:** 200 to 400 mg/day P.O. in three or four equally divided doses.
*Mild to moderate pain –*
**Adults:** 50 to 100 mg P.O. q 4 to 6

hours. Maximum dosage is 400 mg/day.
*Dysmenorrhea or menorrhagia –*
**Adults:** 100 mg P.O. t.i.d.

### ADVERSE REACTIONS
**CNS:** *dizziness, headache.*
**CV:** edema.
**EENT:** tinnitus.
**GI:** *abdominal pain, flatulence, peptic ulceration, nausea, diarrhea,* constipation, anorexia, stomatitis, *GI bleeding.*
**Hematologic:** leukopenia, *thrombocytopenia, agranulocytosis,* hemolytic anemia.
**Hepatic:** *renal failure,* alterations in liver function tests.
**Skin:** rash, urticaria.

### INTERACTIONS
*Antihypertensives, diuretics:* decreased effectiveness. Monitor patient closely.
*Aspirin:* decreased plasma levels of meclofenamate. Avoid concomitant use.
*Corticosteroids, ethanol, other NSAIDs:* increased risk of GI adverse reactions. Avoid concomitant use.
*Oral anticoagulants:* enhanced anticoagulant effect. Monitor for toxicity.

### CONTRAINDICATIONS
Contraindicated in patients with hypersensitivity to the drug or with a history of aspirin- or NSAID-induced bronchospasm, urticaria, or rhinitis.

### NURSING CONSIDERATIONS
• Use cautiously in patients with hepatic or renal disease, cardiovascular disease, blood dyscrasia, and in those with a history of peptic ulcer disease; and in elderly patients, who are more likely to experience adverse reactions.
• Know that use during pregnancy is not recommended, especially during 1st and 3rd trimesters.
• Because NSAIDs impair the synthesis of renal prostaglandins, they can

---

Reactions may be *common,* uncommon, *life-threatening,* or COMMON AND LIFE-THREATENING.

decrease renal blood flow and lead to reversible renal impairment, especially in patients with preexisting renal failure, liver dysfunction, or heart failure; in elderly patients; and in those taking diuretics. Monitor these patients closely during therapy.
• Know that NSAIDs may mask the signs and symptoms of infection because of their anti-inflammatory and antipyretic actions.
• Be aware that CBC and renal and hepatic function should be assessed every 6 months or as indicated in patients receiving long-term therapy.
• Know that false-positive reactions for urine bilirubin tests using diazo tablets have been reported.

### ☑ PATIENT TEACHING
• Tell patient to take this drug with food to minimize adverse GI reactions.
• Tell patient to stop drug and contact the doctor immediately if rash, visual disturbances, or diarrhea develops.
• Caution patient that concomitant use with other NSAIDs, alcohol, or corticosteroids may increase the risk of GI adverse reactions.
• Serious GI toxicity, including peptic ulceration and bleeding, can occur in patient taking NSAIDs despite the absence of GI symptoms. Teach patient the signs and symptoms of GI bleeding, and tell him to contact the doctor immediately if they occur.
• Advise patient to avoid hazardous activities that require mental alertness until CNS effects are known.

---

## mefenamic acid
Mefic‡, Ponstan†, Ponstel

*Pregnancy Risk Category: C*

### HOW SUPPLIED
*Capsules:* 250 mg

### ACTION
Unknown. Produces anti-inflammatory, analgesic, and antipyretic effects, possibly by inhibiting prostaglandin synthesis.

### ONSET, PEAK, DURATION
Onset and duration unknown. Serum levels peak 2 to 4 hours after a dose.

### INDICATIONS & DOSAGE
*Mild to moderate pain, dysmenorrhea* –
**Adults and children over 14 years:**
Initially, 500 mg P.O.; then 250 mg q 6 hours, p.r.n. Maximum therapy 1 week.

### ADVERSE REACTIONS
**CNS:** drowsiness, dizziness, nervousness, headache, insomnia.
**EENT:** blurred vision.
**GI:** nausea, *diarrhea, peptic ulceration, GI bleeding,* anorexia, flatulence, constipation.
**GU:** dysuria, hematuria, *renal failure.*
**Hematologic:** leukopenia, *thrombocytopenia, agranulocytosis, hemolytic anemia.*
**Hepatic:** *hepatotoxicity.*
**Skin:** rash, urticaria.

### INTERACTIONS
*Antihypertensives, diuretics:* decreased effect. Monitor patient closely.
*Aspirin, corticosteroids, ethanol:* increased risk of GI adverse reactions. Avoid concomitant use.
*Oral anticoagulants, sulfonylureas, and other highly protein-bound drugs:* increased risk of toxicity. Monitor patient closely.

### CONTRAINDICATIONS
Contraindicated in patients with hypersensitivity to the drug; history of aspirin- or NSAID-induced bronchospasm, allergic rhinitis, or urticaria;

---

*Liquid form contains alcohol.   **May contain tartrazine.   †Canada only.   ‡Australia only.   ◊OTC.

GI ulceration or inflammation; or renal disease.

## NURSING CONSIDERATIONS

• Use cautiously in patients with hepatic disease, cardiovascular disease, and in those with a history of peptic ulcer disease.

• Know that use during 3rd trimester of pregnancy is not recommended.

• *Alert:* Be aware that mefenamic acid should not be administered for more than 1 week at a time because of increased risk of toxicity.

• Severe hemolytic anemia may occur with prolonged use. Monitor CBC every 4 to 6 months as ordered or as indicated.

• Because NSAIDs impair the synthesis of renal prostaglandins, they can decrease renal blood flow and lead to reversible renal impairment, especially in patients with preexisting renal failure, liver dysfunction, or heart failure; in elderly patients; and in those taking diuretics. Monitor these patients closely during therapy.

• Know that NSAIDs may mask the signs and symptoms of infection because of their anti-inflammatory and antipyretic actions.

• Note that false-positive reactions for urine bilirubin tests using diazo tablets have been reported.

## ☑ PATIENT TEACHING

• Tell patient to take this drug with food to minimize adverse GI reactions.

• Tell patient to stop drug and contact the doctor immediately if rash, visual disturbances, or diarrhea develops.

• Caution patient that concomitant use with aspirin, alcohol, or corticosteroids may increase the risk of GI adverse reactions.

• Serious GI toxicity, including peptic ulceration and bleeding, can occur in patient taking NSAIDs despite the absence of GI symptoms. Teach patient the signs and symptoms of GI bleeding, and tell him to contact the doctor immediately if they occur.

• Warn patient against hazardous activities that require alertness until CNS effects are known.

---

## nabumetone
Relafen

*Pregnancy Risk Category: C*

### HOW SUPPLIED
*Tablets:* 500 mg, 750 mg

### ACTION
Unknown. Probably acts by inhibiting prostaglandin synthesis.

### ONSET, PEAK, DURATION
Onset and duration unknown. Plasma levels peak 2 to 4 hours after a dose.

### INDICATIONS & DOSAGE
*Rheumatoid arthritis or osteoarthritis —*

**Adults:** initially, 1,000 mg P.O. daily as a single dose or in divided doses b.i.d. Maximum daily dosage is 2,000 mg.

### ADVERSE REACTIONS
**CNS:** *dizziness, headache,* fatigue, insomnia, nervousness, somnolence.
**CV:** vasculitis, edema.
**EENT:** *tinnitus.*
**GI:** *diarrhea, dyspepsia, abdominal pain, constipation, flatulence, nausea,* dry mouth, gastritis, stomatitis, anorexia, vomiting, ***bleeding,*** ulceration.
**Respiratory:** dyspnea, pneumonitis.
**Skin:** *pruritus, rash,* increased diaphoresis.

### INTERACTIONS
*Diuretics:* NSAIDs may decrease diuretic effectiveness. Monitor patients closely during therapy.
*Ethanol:* associated with an increased risk of additive GI toxicity. Concomitant use should be avoided.

---

Reactions may be *common,* uncommon, *life-threatening,* or **COMMON AND LIFE-THREATENING.**

*Warfarin and other highly protein-bound drugs:* increased risk of adverse effects from displacement of drugs by nabumetone. Use cautiously.

## CONTRAINDICATIONS
Contraindicated in patients with hypersensitivity reactions, or history of aspirin- or NSAID-induced asthma, urticaria, or other allergic-type reactions.

## NURSING CONSIDERATIONS
• Use cautiously in patients with renal or hepatic impairment; CHF, hypertension, or other conditions that may predispose the patient to fluid retention; and in patients with a history of peptic ulcer disease.
• Know that use during 3rd trimester of pregnancy is not recommended.
• Because NSAIDs impair the synthesis of renal prostaglandins, they can decrease renal blood flow and lead to reversible renal impairment, especially in patients with preexisting renal failure, liver dysfunction, or heart failure; in elderly patients; and in those taking diuretics. Monitor these patients closely during therapy.
• During long-term therapy, periodically monitor renal and liver function, CBC, and hematocrit as ordered; assess these patients for signs and symptoms of GI bleeding.

## ☑ PATIENT TEACHING
• Instruct patient to take this drug with food, milk, or antacids. Nabumetone is absorbed more rapidly when administered with food or milk.
• Advise patient to limit alcohol intake because of additive GI toxicity risk.
• Serious GI toxicity, including peptic ulceration and bleeding, can occur in patient taking NSAIDs despite the absence of GI symptoms. Teach patient the signs and symptoms of GI bleeding and tell him to contact the doctor immediately if they occur.

• Warn patient against hazardous activities that require mental alertness until CNS effects are known.

# naproxen
Apo-Naproxen†, Inza-250‡, Inza-500‡, Naprosyn, Naprosyn-E†, Naprosyn SR†‡, Naxen†‡, Novo-Naprox†, Nu-Naprox†

# naproxen sodium
Aleve◇, Anaprox, Anaprox DS, Apo-Napro-Na†, Naprogesic‡, Novo-Naprox Sodium†, Synflex†

*Pregnancy Risk Category: NR*

## HOW SUPPLIED
**naproxen**
*Tablets:* 250 mg, 375 mg, 500 mg
*Tablets (extended-release)†:* 750 mg, 1,000 mg
*Oral suspension:* 125 mg/5 ml
*Suppositories:* 500 mg‡
**naproxen sodium**
*Tablets (film-coated):* 220 mg◇, 275 mg, 550 mg
  *Note:* 275 mg of naproxen sodium contains 250 mg of naproxen

## ACTION
Unknown. Produces anti-inflammatory, analgesic, and antipyretic effects, possibly by inhibiting prostaglandin synthesis.

## ONSET, PEAK, DURATION
Onset of analgesic effect within 1 hour, antirheumatic effect within 14 days. Peak serum levels after administration of naproxen sodium occur within 1 to 2 hours; peak levels after naproxen (base) occur in 2 to 4 hours. Analgesic effects persist about 7 hours.

## INDICATIONS & DOSAGE
*Rheumatoid arthritis, osteoarthritis, ankylosing spondylitis –*
**Adults:** 250 to 500 mg P.O. b.i.d. Alternatively, where suppository is

available, give 500 mg P.R. h.s. with oral naproxen during the day. Maximum dosage is 1,500 mg daily.

*Juvenile arthritis –*
**Children:** 10 mg/kg P.O. in two divided doses.

*Acute gout –*
**Adults:** 750 mg P.O., followed by 250 mg q 8 hours until attack subsides.

*Mild to moderate pain, primary dysmenorrhea (naproxen sodium), acute tendinitis and bursitis –*
**Adults:** 500 mg. P.O., followed by 250 mg q 6 to 8 hours p.r.n.

## ADVERSE REACTIONS

**CNS:** *headache, drowsiness, dizziness,* vertigo.
**CV:** *edema,* palpitations.
**EENT:** visual disturbances, *tinnitus,* auditory disturbances.
**GI:** *epigastric distress, occult blood loss, nausea,* **peptic ulceration,** constipation, dyspepsia, heartburn, diarrhea, stomatitis, thirst.
**GU:** nephrotoxicity.
**Hematologic:** *thrombocytopenia,* eosinophilia, **agranulocytosis,** neutropenia.
**Hepatic:** elevated liver enzyme levels.
**Respiratory:** dyspnea.
**Skin:** *pruritus, rash,* urticaria, ecchymosis, diaphoresis, purpura.

## INTERACTIONS

*ACE inhibitors:* may increase risk of renal impairment. Use together cautiously.
*Antihypertensives, diuretics:* decreased effect of these drugs. Monitor patient closely.
*Aspirin, corticosteroids, ethanol:* increased risk of adverse GI reactions. Avoid concomitant use.
*Methotrexate:* increased risk of toxicity. Monitor patient closely.
*Oral anticoagulants, sulfonylureas, and other highly protein-bound drugs:* increased risk of toxicity. Monitor patient closely.

*Probenecid:* decreased elimination of naproxen. Monitor for toxicity.

## CONTRAINDICATIONS

Contraindicated in patients with hypersensitivity to this drug or with the syndrome of asthma, rhinitis, and nasal polyps.

## NURSING CONSIDERATIONS

● Use cautiously in elderly patients and in patients with renal disease, cardiovascular disease, GI disorders, hepatic disease, or a history of peptic ulcer disease.
● Know that use during last trimester of pregnancy should be avoided.
● Because NSAIDs impair the synthesis of renal prostaglandins, they can decrease renal blood flow and lead to reversible renal impairment, especially in patients with preexisting renal failure, liver dysfunction, or heart failure; in elderly patients; and in those taking diuretics. Monitor these patients closely during therapy.
● Monitor CBC and renal and hepatic function every 4 to 6 months or as indicated and ordered during long-term therapy.
● Be aware that because of their antipyretic and anti-inflammatory actions, NSAIDs may mask the signs and symptoms of infection.
● Inform clinical laboratory personnel that patient is taking naproxen. It may interfere with certain urinary assays of 5-hydroxyindoleacetic acid and may cause false elevations of urinary 17-ketosteroid concentrations.

☑ **PATIENT TEACHING**
● Advise patient to take drug with food or milk to minimize GI upset. A full glass of water or other liquid should be taken with each dose.
● Tell patient taking prescription doses of naproxen for arthritis that full therapeutic effect may be delayed 2 to 4 weeks.
● Warn patient against taking both

---

Reactions may be *common,* uncommon, *life-threatening,* or **COMMON AND LIFE-THREATENING.**

naproxen and naproxen sodium at the same time because both circulate in the blood as the naproxen anion.
• Serious GI toxicity, including peptic ulceration and bleeding, can occur in patient taking NSAIDs despite the absence of GI symptoms. Teach patient the signs and symptoms of GI bleeding and tell him to contact the doctor immediately if they occur.
• Caution patient that concomitant use with aspirin, alcohol, or corticosteroids may increase the risk of adverse GI reactions.
• Warn patient against hazardous activities that require mental alertness until CNS effects are known.

# oxaprozin
Daypro
*Pregnancy Risk Category: C*

## HOW SUPPLIED
*Caplets:* 600 mg

## ACTION
Unknown. Produces anti-inflammatory, analgesic, and antipyretic effects, possibly by inhibiting prostaglandin synthesis.

## ONSET, PEAK, DURATION
Onset and duration unknown. Serum levels peak 3 to 5 hours after a dose.

## INDICATIONS & DOSAGE
*Osteoarthritis or rheumatoid arthritis —*
**Adults:** initially, 1,200 mg P.O. daily. Then, individualized to the smallest effective dosage to minimize adverse reactions. Smaller patients or those with mild symptoms may require only 600 mg daily. Maximum is 1,800 mg or 26 mg/kg, whichever is lower, in divided doses.

## ADVERSE REACTIONS
**CNS:** depression, sedation, somnolence, confusion, sleep disturbances.

**EENT:** tinnitus, blurred vision.
**GI:** *nausea, dyspepsia, diarrhea, constipation,* abdominal pain or distress, anorexia, flatulence, vomiting, *hemorrhage,* stomatitis.
**GU:** dysuria, urinary frequency.
**Hepatic:** elevated liver function test results (with chronic use); severe hepatic dysfunction (rare).
**Skin:** *rash,* photosensitivity.

## INTERACTIONS
*Antihypertensives, diuretics:* decreased effect. Monitor patient closely and adjust dosage, as ordered.
*Aspirin:* oxaprozin displaces salicylates from plasma protein-binding sites, increasing risk of salicylate toxicity. Avoid concomitant use.
*Aspirin, corticosteroids, ethanol:* increased risk of adverse GI reactions. Avoid concomitant use.
*Methotrexate:* increased risk of methotrexate toxicity. Avoid concomitant use.
*Oral anticoagulants:* although problems haven't been reported, there is an increased risk of bleeding. Use together cautiously.

## CONTRAINDICATIONS
Contraindicated in patients with hypersensitivity to this drug or with the syndrome of nasal polyps, angioedema, and bronchospastic reaction to aspirin or other NSAIDs.

## NURSING CONSIDERATIONS
• Use cautiously in patients with a history of peptic ulcer disease, hepatic or renal dysfunction, hypertension, cardiovascular disease, or conditions predisposing patient to fluid retention.
• Because renal prostaglandins play a role in the maintenance of renal perfusion, patients with preexisting conditions leading to a reduction in renal blood flow may experience renal toxicity with NSAID therapy. Those at greatest risk are elderly patients, pa-

tients taking diuretics, and those with impaired renal, hepatic, or cardiac function. Closely monitor renal function in these patients, and discontinue NSAID therapy if problems develop.
• Elevations of liver function tests can occur after chronic use. These abnormal findings may persist, worsen, or resolve with continued therapy. Rarely, patients may progress to severe hepatic dysfunction. Periodically monitor liver function tests in patients receiving long-term therapy, and closely monitor patients with abnormal test results.
• Be aware that because of their antipyretic and anti-inflammatory actions, NSAIDs may mask the signs and symptoms of infection.

☑ **PATIENT TEACHING**
• Tell patient to take this drug 30 minutes before or 2 hours after meals. If adverse GI reactions occur, drug may be taken with milk or meals.
• Tell patient that full therapeutic effects may be delayed for 2 to 4 weeks.
• Serious GI toxicity, including peptic ulceration and bleeding, can occur in patient taking NSAIDs despite the absence of GI symptoms. Teach patient the signs and symptoms of GI bleeding and tell him to contact the doctor immediately if they occur.
• Tell patient to report adverse visual or auditory reactions immediately.
• Warn patient against hazardous activities that require mental alertness until CNS effects are known.
• This drug has been associated with photosensitivity reactions. Advise patient to use a sunblock, wear protective clothing, and avoid prolonged exposure to sunlight.

---

## piroxicam
Apo-Piroxicam†, Feldene, Novo-Pirocam†

*Pregnancy Risk Category: NR*

**HOW SUPPLIED**
*Capsules:* 10 mg, 20 mg

**ACTION**
Unknown. Produces anti-inflammatory, analgesic, and antipyretic effects, possibly by inhibiting prostaglandin synthesis.

**ONSET, PEAK, DURATION**
Onset occurs within 15 to 30 minutes for analgesia; antirheumatic action, 7 to 12 days. Serum levels peak in 3 to 5 hours; peak rheumatic action occurs after 2 to 3 weeks of therapy. Analgesic effects persist for about 24 hours.

**INDICATIONS & DOSAGE**
*Osteoarthritis and rheumatoid arthritis—*
**Adults:** 20 mg P.O. daily. If desired, the dosage may be divided b.i.d.

**ADVERSE REACTIONS**
**CNS:** headache, drowsiness, dizziness, somnolence, vertigo.
**CV:** peripheral edema.
**EENT:** auditory disturbances.
**GI:** *epigastric distress, nausea, occult blood loss, peptic ulceration, severe GI bleeding,* diarrhea, constipation, abdominal pain, dyspepsia, flatulence, anorexia, stomatitis.
**GU:** *nephrotoxicity,* elevated BUN level.
**Hematologic:** prolonged bleeding time, anemia, leukopenia, *aplastic anemia, agranulocytosis,* eosinophilia, *thrombocytopenia.*
**Hepatic:** elevated liver enzymes.
**Skin:** pruritus, rash, urticaria, *photosensitivity.*

**INTERACTIONS**
*Aspirin, corticosteroids, ethanol:* increased risk of GI toxicity. Decreased plasma levels of piroxicam. Avoid concomitant use.
*Lithium:* increased plasma lithium levels. Monitor for toxicity.
*Oral anticoagulants and other highly*

---

Reactions may be *common,* uncommon, *life-threatening,* or COMMON AND LIFE-THREATENING.

*protein-bound drugs:* enhanced risk of bleeding. Monitor patient closely.
*Oral antidiabetic agents:* enhanced antidiabetic effects. Monitor patient closely.

## CONTRAINDICATIONS
Contraindicated in patients with hypersensitivity to this drug or with bronchospasm or angioedema precipitated by aspirin or NSAIDs and during pregnancy or while breast-feeding.

## NURSING CONSIDERATIONS
• Use cautiously in elderly patients and in patients with GI disorders, history of renal or peptic ulcer disease, cardiac disease, hypertension, or conditions predisposing to fluid retention.
• Because NSAIDs impair the synthesis of renal prostaglandins, they can decrease renal blood flow and lead to reversible renal impairment, especially in patients with preexisting renal failure, liver dysfunction, or heart failure; in elderly patients; and in those taking diuretics. Monitor these patients closely during therapy.
• Check renal, hepatic, and auditory function and CBC periodically during prolonged therapy. Discontinue drug if abnormalities occur and notify doctor.
• Be aware that NSAIDs may mask the signs and symptoms of infection because of their antipyretic and anti-inflammatory actions.

## ☑ PATIENT TEACHING
• Tell patient to take this drug with milk, antacids, or meals if GI adverse reactions occur.
• Tell patient that full therapeutic effects may be delayed for 2 to 4 weeks.
• Serious GI toxicity, including peptic ulceration and bleeding, can occur in patient taking NSAIDs despite the absence of GI symptoms. Teach patient the signs and symptoms of GI bleeding and tell him to contact the doctor immediately if they occur.

• Warn patient against hazardous activities that require mental alertness until CNS effects are known.
• Advise patient to use a sunblock, wear protective clothing, and avoid prolonged exposure to sunlight. Causes adverse skin reactions more often than other drugs in its class. Photosensitivity reactions are the most common.

# sulindac
Aclin‡, Apo-Sulin†, Clinoril, Novo-Sundac†

*Pregnancy Risk Category: NR*

## HOW SUPPLIED
*Tablets:* 100 mg‡, 150 mg, 200 mg

## ACTION
Unknown. Produces anti-inflammatory, analgesic, and antipyretic effects, possibly by inhibiting prostaglandin synthesis.

## ONSET, PEAK, DURATION
Onset and duration unknown. Plasma levels peak 2 to 4 hours after a dose; peak antirheumatic effects occur in 2 to 3 weeks.

## INDICATIONS & DOSAGE
*Osteoarthritis, rheumatoid arthritis, ankylosing spondylitis –*
**Adults:** initially, 150 mg P.O. b.i.d.; increased to 200 mg b.i.d., p.r.n.
*Acute subacromial bursitis or supraspinatus tendinitis, acute gouty arthritis –*
**Adults:** 200 mg P.O. b.i.d. for 7 to 14 days. Dose reduced as symptoms subside.

## ADVERSE REACTIONS
**CNS:** dizziness, headache, nervousness, psychosis.
**CV:** hypertension, CHF, palpitations.
**EENT:** tinnitus, transient visual disturbances.
**GI:** *epigastric distress,* **peptic ulcera-**

*tion, pancreatitis,* occult blood loss, nausea, constipation, dyspepsia, flatulence, anorexia, *GI bleeding.*
**GU:** interstitial nephritis, *nephrotic syndrome, renal failure.*
**Hematologic:** prolonged bleeding time, *aplastic anemia, thrombocytopenia,* neutropenia, *agranulocytosis,* hemolytic anemia.
**Skin:** *rash,* pruritus.
**Other:** edema, drug fever, *anaphylaxis,* angioedema, *hypersensitivity syndrome.*

## INTERACTIONS
*Anticoagulants:* increased risk of bleeding. Monitor PT closely.
*Aspirin:* decreased sulindac plasma concentration and increased risk of GI adverse reactions. Concomitant use not recommended.
*Cyclosporine:* increased nephrotoxicity of cyclosporine. Avoid concomitant use.
*Diflunisal, dimethyl sulfoxide:* decreased metabolism of sulindac to its active metabolite, reducing its effectiveness. Don't use together.
*Methotrexate:* increased methotrexate toxicity. Avoid concomitant use.
*Probenecid:* increased plasma levels of sulindac and its active metabolite. Monitor for toxicity.
*Sulfonamides, sulfonylureas, other highly protein-bound drugs:* possible displacement of these drugs from plasma protein-binding sites, leading to increased toxicity. Monitor closely.

## CONTRAINDICATIONS
Contraindicated in patients with hypersensitivity to this drug or in whom acute asthmatic attacks, urticaria, or rhinitis is precipitated by aspirin or NSAIDs.

## NURSING CONSIDERATIONS
● Use cautiously in patients with a history of ulcers and GI bleeding, renal dysfunction, compromised cardiac function, hypertension, or conditions predisposing to fluid retention.
● Know that use during pregnancy is not recommended.
● Periodically monitor hepatic and renal function and CBC in patients receiving long-term therapy as ordered.
● Be aware that NSAIDs may mask the signs and symptoms of infection.

### ☑ PATIENT TEACHING
● Tell patient to take this drug with food, milk, or antacids to reduce adverse GI reactions.
● Serious GI toxicity, including peptic ulceration and bleeding, can occur in patient taking NSAIDs despite the absence of GI symptoms. Teach patient the signs and symptoms of GI bleeding and tell him to contact the doctor immediately if they occur.
● *Alert:* Tell patient to notify the doctor immediately if easy bruising or prolonged bleeding occurs.
● Advise patient to avoid hazardous activities that require mental alertness until CNS effects are known.
● Instruct patient to report edema and have blood pressure checked monthly. Drug causes sodium retention but is thought to have less effect on the kidneys than other NSAIDs.
● Patient should notify the doctor and have complete eye examinations if any visual disturbances occur.

## tolmetin sodium
Tolectin 200, Tolectin 400, Tolectin 600, Tolectin DS

*Pregnancy Risk Category: C*

### HOW SUPPLIED
*Tablets:* 200 mg, 600 mg
*Capsules:* 400 mg

### ACTION
Unknown. Produces anti-inflammatory, analgesic, and antipyretic effects, possibly by inhibiting prostaglandin synthesis.

---

Reactions may be *common,* uncommon, *life-threatening,* or COMMON AND LIFE-THREATENING.

## ONSET, PEAK, DURATION
Onset and duration unknown. Serum levels peak in 30 minutes to 1 hour; peak antirheumatic effect occurs after 1 to 2 weeks.

## INDICATIONS & DOSAGE
*Rheumatoid arthritis, osteoarthritis, juvenile rheumatoid arthritis –*
**Adults:** 400 mg P.O. t.i.d. Maximum daily dosage is 1.8 g.
**Children 2 years or over:** initially, 20 mg/kg/day P.O. in divided doses (t.i.d. or q.i.d.), followed by maintenance dosage of 15 to 30 mg/kg P.O. daily in divided doses (t.i.d. or q.i.d.).

## ADVERSE REACTIONS
**CNS:** *headache,* dizziness, drowsiness, asthenia, depression.
**CV:** chest pain, hypertension, edema.
**EENT:** tinnitus, visual disturbances.
**GI:** *epigastric distress,* **peptic ulceration,** occult blood loss, *nausea,* vomiting, diarrhea, constipation, dyspepsia, flatulence, anorexia, *GI bleeding.*
**GU:** hematuria, proteinuria, dysuria, *renal failure.*
**Hematologic:** prolonged bleeding time, granulocytopenia, *thrombocytopenia, agranulocytosis,* hemolytic anemia.
**Skin:** rash, urticaria, pruritus.
**Other:** *anaphylaxis, weight gain,* weight loss.

## INTERACTIONS
*Anticoagulants:* increased risk of bleeding. Monitor patient closely.
*Aspirin:* increased tolmetin levels. Avoid concurrent use.
*Ethanol:* increased risk of GI toxicity. Avoid concomitant use.
*Methotrexate:* increased risk of methotrexate toxicity. Monitor patient closely.

## CONTRAINDICATIONS
Contraindicated in patients with hypersensitivity to this drug or in whom acute asthmatic attacks, urticaria, or rhinitis is precipitated by aspirin or NSAIDs as well as in lactation.

## NURSING CONSIDERATIONS
● Use cautiously in patients with cardiac and renal disease, GI bleeding, history of peptic ulcer disease, hypertension, and conditions predisposing to fluid retention.
● Because NSAIDs impair the synthesis of renal prostaglandins, they can decrease renal blood flow and lead to reversible renal impairment, especially in patients with preexisting renal failure, liver dysfunction, or heart failure; in elderly patients; and in those taking diuretics. Monitor these patients closely during therapy.
● Know that NSAIDs may mask the signs and symptoms of infection because of their antipyretic and anti-inflammatory actions.
● Be aware that tolmetin may interfere with certain tests for urinary proteins; it does not interfere with dye-impregnated reagent strips.

## ☑ PATIENT TEACHING
● Tell patient to take this drug with food, milk, or antacids to reduce adverse GI reactions.
● Tell patient that therapeutic effect begins within 1 week, but full effect may be delayed 2 to 4 weeks.
● Serious GI toxicity, including peptic ulceration and bleeding, can occur in patient taking NSAIDs despite the absence of GI symptoms. Teach patient the signs and symptoms of GI bleeding and tell him to contact the doctor immediately if they occur.
● Tell patient to notify the doctor immediately if any visual or hearing change occurs. During prolonged therapy, patient should have regular eye examinations, hearing tests, CBCs, and renal function tests.
● Advise patient to avoid hazardous activities that require alertness until the CNS effects of the drug are known.

# 28

# Narcotic and opioid analgesics

**alfentanil hydrochloride**
**buprenorphine hydrochloride**
**butorphanol tartrate**
**codeine phosphate**
**codeine sulfate**
**dezocine**
**fentanyl citrate**
**fentanyl transdermal system**
**fentanyl transmucosal**
**hydromorphone hydrochloride**
**meperidine hydrochloride**
**methadone hydrochloride**
**morphine hydrochloride**
**morphine sulfate**
**morphine tartrate**
**nalbuphine hydrochloride**
**oxycodone hydrochloride**
**oxycodone pectinate**
**oxymorphone hydrochloride**
**pentazocine hydrochloride**
**pentazocine hydrochloride and
    naloxone hydrochloride**
**pentazocine lactate**
**propoxyphene hydrochloride**
**propoxyphene napsylate**
**sufentanil citrate**
**tramadol hydrochloride**

## COMBINATION PRODUCTS

222†: aspirin 375 mg, codeine phosphate 8 mg, and caffeine citrate 30 mg.

222 FORTE†: aspirin 500 mg, codeine phosphate 8 mg, and caffeine citrate 30 mg.

282†: aspirin 375 mg, codeine phosphate 15 mg, and caffeine citrate 30 mg.

292†: aspirin 375 mg, codeine phosphate 30 mg, and caffeine citrate 30 mg.

293†: aspirin 375 mg, codeine phosphate 30 mg, codeine phosphate (slow-release) 30 mg, and caffeine citrate 30 mg.

692†: aspirin 375 mg, propoxyphene hydrochloride 65 mg, and caffeine 30 mg.

A.C. & C.†: aspirin 375 mg, codeine phosphate 8 mg, and caffeine 30 mg.

ACETA WITH CODEINE, EMPRACET-30†, EMTEC-30†: acetaminophen 300 mg and codeine phosphate 30 mg.

ANACIN WITH CODEINE†: aspirin 325 mg, codeine phosphate 8 mg, and caffeine 32 mg.

ANCASAL 8†, C2 WITH CODEINE†: aspirin 375 mg, codeine phosphate 8 mg, and caffeine 15 mg.

ANCASAL 15†: aspirin 375 mg, codeine phosphate 15 mg, and caffeine 15 mg.

ANCASAL 30†: aspirin 375 mg, codeine phosphate 30 mg, and caffeine 15 mg.

ANEXSIA 7.5/650: hydrocodone bitartrate 7.5 mg, acetaminophen 650 mg

BUFF-A-COMP NO. 3: aspirin 325 mg, codeine phosphate 30 mg, caffeine 40 mg, and butalbital 50 mg.

CAPITAL WITH CODEINE, MYAPAP WITH CODEINE*, TYLENOL WITH CODEINE ELIXIR*, TY-PAP WITH CODEINE ELIXIR*: acetaminophen 120 mg and codeine phosphate 12 mg/5 ml.

DARVOCET-N 50: acetaminophen 325 mg and propoxyphene napsylate 50 mg.

DARVOCET-N 100, DOXAPAP-N, PROPACET 100: acetaminophen 650 mg and propoxyphene napsylate 100 mg.

DARVON COMPOUND†: aspirin 325 mg, propoxyphene hydrochloride 32 mg, and caffeine 32.4 mg.

DARVON COMPOUND-65†: aspirin 389 mg, propoxyphene hydrochloride 65 mg, and caffeine 32.4 mg.

DARVON-N COMPOUND†: aspirin

---

Reactions may be *common*, uncommon, *life-threatening*, or **COMMON AND LIFE-THREATENING**.

375 mg, propoxyphene napsylate 100 mg, and caffeine 30 mg.

DARVON-N WITH A.S.A.†: aspirin 325 mg and propoxyphene napsylate 100 mg.

DARVON WITH A.S.A.†: aspirin 325 mg and propoxyphene hydrochloride 65 mg.

DOLENE-AP-65, D-REX-65, E-LOR, GENAGESIC, PRO POX WITH APAP, WYGESIC: acetaminophen 650 mg and propoxyphene hydrochloride 65 mg.

EMPIRIN WITH CODEINE NO. 2: aspirin 325 mg and codeine phosphate 15 mg.

EMPIRIN WITH CODEINE NO. 3: aspirin 325 mg and codeine phosphate 30 mg.

EMPIRIN WITH CODEINE NO. 4: aspirin 325 mg and codeine phosphate 60 mg.

EMPRACET-60†: acetaminophen 300 mg and codeine phosphate 60 mg.

ENDOCAN†, OXYCODAN†, PERCODAN†: aspirin 325 mg and oxycodone hydrochloride 5 mg.

ENDOCET†, OXYCOCET†, PERCOCET, ROXICET: acetaminophen 325 mg and oxycodone hydrochloride 5 mg.

FIORICET WITH CODEINE: acetaminophen 325 mg, butalbital 50 mg, caffeine 40 mg, and codeine phosphate 30 mg.

FIORINAL WITH CODEINE: aspirin 325 mg, butalbital 50 mg, caffeine 40 mg, and codeine 30 mg.

INNOVAR INJECTION: droperidol 2.5 mg and fentanyl citrate 0.05 mg/ml.

LENOLTEC WITH CODEINE NO. 1†, NOVOGESIC C8†: acetaminophen 300 mg, codeine phosphate 8 mg, and caffeine 15 mg.

LORCET 10/650: acetaminophen 650 mg and hydrocodone bitartrate 10mg.

LORTAB 2.5/500: acetaminophen 500 mg and hydrocodone bitartrate 2.5 mg.

LORTAB 5/500: acetaminophen 500 mg and hydrocodone bitartrate 5 mg.

LORTAB 7.5/500: acetaminophen 500 mg and hydrocodone bitartrate 7.5 mg.

LORCET PLUS: acetaminophen 650 mg, hydrocodone bitartrate 7.5 mg

PERCODAN-DEMI: aspirin 325 mg, oxycodone hydrochloride 2.25 mg, and oxycodone terephthalate 0.19 mg.

PERCODAN-DEMI†: aspirin 325 mg and oxycodone hydrochloride 2.5 mg.

PERCODAN, ROXIPRIN: aspirin 325 mg, oxycodone hydrochloride 4.5 mg, and oxycodone terephthalate 0.38 mg.

PHENAPHEN-650 WITH CODEINE: acetaminophen 650 mg and codeine phosphate 30 mg.

ROUNOX AND CODEINE 15†: acetaminophen 325 mg and codeine phosphate 15 mg.

ROUNOX AND CODEINE 30†: acetaminophen 325 mg and codeine phosphate 30 mg.

ROUNOX AND CODEINE 60†: acetaminophen 325 mg and codeine phosphate 60 mg.

ROXICET 5/500: acetaminophen 500 mg and oxycodone hydrochloride 5 mg.

ROXICET ORAL SOLUTION*: acetaminophen 325 mg and oxycodone hydrochloride 5 mg/5 ml.

TALACEN: acetaminophen 650 mg and pentazocine hydrochloride 25 mg.

TALWIN COMPOUND: aspirin 325 mg and pentazocine hydrochloride 12.5 mg.

TYLENOL WITH CODEINE NO. 1: acetaminophen 300 mg and codeine phosphate 7.5 mg.

TYLENOL WITH CODEINE NO. 2: acetaminophen 300 mg and codeine phosphate 15 mg.

TYLENOL WITH CODEINE NO. 3: acetaminophen 300 mg and codeine phosphate 30 mg.

TYLENOL WITH CODEINE NO. 4: acetaminophen 300 mg and codeine phosphate 60 mg.

---

*Liquid form contains alcohol.   **May contain tartrazine.   †Canada only.   ‡Australia only.   ◊OTC.

TYLOX: acetaminophen 500 mg and oxycodone hydrochloride 5 mg.
VICODIN: acetaminophen 500 mg and hydrocodone bitartrate 5 mg.
VICODIN ES: acetaminophen 750 mg and hydrocodone bitartrate 7.5 mg.

---

## alfentanil hydrochloride
Alfenta
Controlled Substance Schedule II
*Pregnancy Risk Category: C*

### HOW SUPPLIED
*Injection:* 500 mcg/ml

### ACTION
Binds with opiate receptors in the CNS, altering both perception of and emotional response to pain through an unknown mechanism.

### ONSET, PEAK, DURATION
Onset within 1 minute. Serum levels peak within 1.5 to 2 minutes. Effects persist 5 to 10 minutes.

### INDICATIONS & DOSAGE
*Adjunct to general anesthetic –*
**Adults:** initially, 8 to 50 mcg/kg I.V.; then increments of 3 to 15 mcg/kg I.V. q 5 to 20 minutes.
*As a primary anesthetic –*
**Adults:** initially, 130 to 245 mcg/kg I.V.; then 0.5 to 1.5 mcg/kg/minute I.V.

In elderly and debilitated patients, dosage should be reduced.

### ADVERSE REACTIONS
**CNS:** anxiety, headache, confusion, sleepiness, sedation.
**EENT:** blurred vision.
**CV:** *hypotension, hypertension, bradycardia, tachycardia, **arrhythmias, asystole.***
**GI:** *nausea, vomiting.*
**Respiratory:** *chest wall rigidity, **bronchospasm, respiratory depression,** hypercapnia, **respiratory arrest,** laryngospasm.*

**Skin:** pruritus, urticaria.

### INTERACTIONS
*CNS depressants, ethanol:* additive effects. Use together cautiously.

### CONTRAINDICATIONS
Contraindicated in patients with hypersensitivity to this drug.

### NURSING CONSIDERATIONS
● Use cautiously in patients with head injury, pulmonary disease, decreased respiratory reserve, or hepatic or renal impairment.
● Be aware drug should be administered only by persons specifically trained in the use of I.V. anesthetics.
● **I.V. use:** Compatible with $D_5W$, $D_5W$ in lactated Ringer's solution, and 0.9% sodium chloride solution. Most clinicians use infusions containing 25 to 80 mcg/ml.
● Discontinue infusion at least 10 to 15 minutes before the end of surgery.
● *Alert:* To administer small volumes of alfentanil accurately, use a tuberculin syringe.
● Keep narcotic antagonist (naloxone) and resuscitation equipment available when giving drug I.V.
● Periodically monitor postoperative vital signs and bladder function. Because drug decreases both rate and depth of respirations, monitoring of arterial oxygen saturation may aid in assessing respiratory depression.

### ☑ PATIENT TEACHING
● Explain the anesthetic effect of alfentanil as well as preoperative and postoperative care measures.
● Inform the patient that another analgesic will be available to relieve pain after effects of alfentanil have worn off.

---

Reactions may be *common,* uncommon, *life-threatening,* or COMMON AND LIFE-THREATENING.

# buprenorphine hydrochloride

Buprenex, Temgesic Injection‡
Controlled Substance Schedule V

*Pregnancy Risk Category: C*

## HOW SUPPLIED
*Injection:* 0.324 mg (equivalent to 0.3 mg base/ml)

## ACTION
Binds with opiate receptors in the CNS, altering both perception of and emotional response to pain through an unknown mechanism.

## ONSET, PEAK, DURATION
Onset occurs within 15 minutes after I.M. administration; more rapid after I.V. administration. Analgesic effects peak in 2 to 5 minutes after I.M. administration, 2 minutes after I.V. administration. Effects persist about 6 hours.

## INDICATIONS & DOSAGE
*Moderate to severe pain –*
**Adults and children 13 years and over:** 0.3 mg I.M. or slow I.V. q 6 hours, p.r.n. or around the clock; dosage repeated (up to 0.3 mg) if required, 30 to 60 minutes after initial dose.
**Children 2 to 12 years:** 2 to 6 mcg/ kg I.M. or I.V. q 4 to 6 hours.

## ADVERSE REACTIONS
**CNS:** *dizziness, sedation, headache,* confusion, nervousness, euphoria, *vertigo,* increased intracranial pressure.
**CV:** *hypotension,* bradycardia, tachycardia, hypertension.
**EENT:** *miosis,* blurred vision.
**GI:** *nausea,* vomiting, constipation, dry mouth.
**GU:** urine retention.
**Respiratory:** *respiratory depression,* hypoventilation, dyspnea.
**Skin:** pruritus, *diaporesis.*

## INTERACTIONS
*CNS depressants, ethanol, MAO inhibitors:* additive effects. Use together cautiously.

## CONTRAINDICATIONS
Contraindicated in patients with hypersensitivity to this drug.

## NURSING CONSIDERATIONS
• Use cautiously in elderly or debilitated patients or patients with head injury, intracranial lesions, and increased intracranial pressure; severe respiratory, liver, or kidney impairment; CNS depression or coma; thyroid irregularities; adrenal insufficiency; and prostatic hyperplasia, urethral stricture, acute alcoholism, delirium tremens, or kyphoscoliosis.
• **I.V. use:** Give by direct I.V. injection, slowly into a vein or through the tubing of a free-flowing, compatible I.V. solution over not less than 2 minutes.
• S.C. administration is not recommended.
• Be aware that buprenorphine 0.3 mg is equal to 10 mg of morphine and 75 mg of meperidine in analgesic potency. It has longer duration of action than morphine or meperidine.
• *Alert:* Know that naloxone will not completely reverse the respiratory depression caused by buprenorphine overdose; an overdose may necessitate mechanical ventilation. Larger than customary doses of naloxone (more than 0.4 mg) and doxapram also may be ordered.
• Be aware that drug's narcotic antagonist properties may precipitate withdrawal syndrome in narcotic-dependent patients.
• Know that if dependence occurs, withdrawal symptoms may appear up to 14 days after drug is stopped.

☑ **PATIENT TEACHING**
• Caution ambulatory patient about getting out of bed or walking.

---

*Liquid form contains alcohol. **May contain tartrazine. †Canada only. ‡Australia only. ◇OTC.

• When drug is used postoperatively, encourage patient to turn, cough, and deep breathe to prevent atelectasis.

# butorphanol tartrate
Stadol, Stadol NS

*Pregnancy Risk Category: C*

## HOW SUPPLIED
*Injection:* 1 mg/ml, 2 mg/ml
*Nasal spray:* 10 mg/ml

## ACTION
Binds with opiate receptors in the CNS, altering both perception of and emotional response to pain through an unknown mechanism.

## ONSET, PEAK, DURATION
Onset occurs within 2 to 3 minutes after an I.V. injection; within 10 to 30 minutes after I.M. injection; within 15 minutes of nasal use. Analgesic effects peak within ½ to 1 hour of I.M. or I.V. use, within 1 to 2 hours of nasal use. Analgesic effects persist 3 to 4 hours after I.M. use, 2 to 4 hours after I.V. use, or 4 to 5 hours after nasal administration.

## INDICATIONS & DOSAGE
*Moderate to severe pain –*
**Adults:** 1 to 4 mg I.M. q 3 to 4 hours, p.r.n. or around the clock; or 0.5 to 2 mg I.V. q 3 to 4 hours, p.r.n. or around the clock. Not to exceed 4 mg per dose. Alternatively, 1 mg by nasal spray q 3 to 4 hours (1 spray in one nostril); repeated in 60 to 90 minutes if pain relief is inadequate.
*Labor for patients at full term and in early labor –*
**Adults:** 1 to 2 mg I.V. or I.M., repeated after 4 hours as needed.
*Preoperative anesthesia or preanesthesia –*
**Adults:** 2 mg. I.M. 60 to 90 minutes before surgery.
*Adjunct to balanced anesthesia –*
**Adults:** 2 mg I.V. shortly before induction or 0.5 to 1.0 mg I.V. in increments during anesthesia.

## ADVERSE REACTIONS
**CNS:** *confusion,* nervousness, lethargy, headache, *somnolence, dizziness, insomnia,* anxiety, paresthesia, euphoria, hallucinations, flushing, increased intracranial pressure.
**CV:** palpitations, vasodilation, hypotension.
**EENT:** blurred vision, *nasal congestion* (with nasal spray), tinnitus, unpleasant taste.
**GI:** *nausea, vomiting, constipation,* anorexia.
**Respiratory:** *respiratory depression.*
**Skin:** rash, hives, *clamminess, excessive diaporesis.*
**Other:** sensation of heat.

## INTERACTIONS
*CNS depressants, ethanol:* additive effects. Use together cautiously.

## CONTRAINDICATIONS
Contraindicated in patients with narcotic addiction; may precipitate withdrawal syndrome. Also contraindicated in patient with hypersensitivity to the drug or to the preservative, benzethonium chloride.

## NURSING CONSIDERATIONS
• Use cautiously in patients with head injury, increased intracranial pressure, acute MI, ventricular dysfunction, coronary insufficiency, respiratory disease or depression, and renal or hepatic dysfunction. Also administer cautiously to patients who have recently received repeated doses of narcotic analgesic medication.
• **I.V. use:** Give by direct injection into a vein or the tubing of a free-flowing I.V. solution. Compatible solutions include $D_5W$ and 0.9% sodium chloride.
• S.C. route is not recommended.
• Know that respiratory depression

---

Reactions may be *common,* uncommon, *life-threatening,* or **COMMON AND LIFE-THREATENING.**

apparently does not increase with larger dosage.
• Be aware that psychological and physical addiction may occur.
• Periodically monitor postoperative vital signs and bladder function. Because drug decreases both rate and depth of respirations, monitoring of arterial oxygen saturation may aid in assessing respiratory depression.

### ☑ PATIENT TEACHING
• Caution ambulatory patient about getting out of bed or walking. Warn outpatient to avoid driving and other potentially hazardous activities that require mental alertness until drug's CNS effects are known.
• Instruct patient about administration technique for and storage of nasal spray, if applicable.

## codeine phosphate
Paveral†

## codeine sulfate
Controlled Substance Schedule II
*Pregnancy Risk Category: C*

### HOW SUPPLIED
**codeine phosphate**
*Oral solution:* 15 mg/5 ml, 10 mg/ml†
*Injection:* 30 mg/ml, 60 mg/ml
*Soluble tablets:* 30 mg, 60 mg
**codeine sulfate**
*Tablets:* 15 mg, 30 mg, 60 mg

### ACTION
Binds with opiate receptors in the CNS, altering both perception of and emotional response to pain through an unknown mechanism. Also suppresses the cough reflex by direct action on the cough center in the medulla.

### ONSET, PEAK, DURATION
Onset occurs immediately with I.V. administration, 10 to 30 minutes after I.M. or S.C. injection, 30 to 45 minutes after oral use. Peak effects occur immediately after I.V. administration, within 30 minutes to 1 hour after I.M. injection, unknown after S.C. administration, and 1 to 2 hours after oral administration. Effects persist 4 to 6 hours.

### INDICATIONS & DOSAGE
*Mild to moderate pain –*
**Adults:** 15 to 60 mg P.O. or 15 to 60 mg (phosphate) S.C., I.M., or I.V. q 4 to 6 hours, p.r.n.
**Children over 1 year:** 0.5 mg/kg P.O., S.C., or I.M. q 4 hours, p.r.n.
*Nonproductive cough –*
**Adults:** 10 to 20 mg P.O. q 4 to 6 hours. Maximum dosage is 120 mg/day.
**Children 6 to 12 years:** 5 to 10 mg P.O. q 4 to 6 hours. Maximum dosage is 60 mg/day.
**Children 2 to 6 years:** 2.5 to 5 mg P.O. q 6 hours. Do not exceed 30 mg/day.

### ADVERSE REACTIONS
**CNS:** *sedation, clouded sensorium, euphoria, dizziness, light-headedness.*
**CV:** *hypotension,* bradycardia.
**GI:** *nausea, vomiting, constipation, dry mouth,* ileus.
**GU:** *urine retention.*
**Respiratory:** *respiratory depression.*
**Skin:** pruritus, flushing, *diaphoresis.*
**Other:** physical dependence.

### INTERACTIONS
*CNS depressants, ethanol, general anesthetics, hypnotics, MAO inhibitors, other narcotic analgesics, sedatives, tranquilizers, tricyclic antidepressants:* additive effects. Use together with extreme caution. Monitor patient response.

### CONTRAINDICATIONS
Contraindicated in patients with hypersensitivity to this drug.

---

*Liquid form contains alcohol.  **May contain tartrazine.  †Canada only.  ‡Australia only.  ◇OTC.

## NURSING CONSIDERATIONS

• Use with extreme caution in patients with head injury, increased intracranial pressure, increased CSF pressure, hepatic or renal disease, hypothyroidism, Addison's disease, acute alcoholism, seizures, severe CNS depression, bronchial asthma, COPD, respiratory depression, and shock. Also use with extreme caution in elderly or debilitated patients.

• **I.V. use:** Give by direct injection into a large vein. Administer very slowly.

• *Alert:* Don't mix with other solutions because codeine phosphate is incompatible with many drugs.

• Don't administer discolored injection solution.

• Know that codeine and aspirin or acetaminophen are often prescribed together to provide enhanced pain relief.

• For full analgesic effect, administer drug before patient has intense pain.

• Be aware that drug is an antitussive and should not be used when cough is a valuable diagnostic sign or is beneficial (as after thoracic surgery).

• Monitor cough type and frequency.

• Monitor respiratory and circulatory status.

• Opiates may cause constipation. Assess bowel function and need for stool softeners or laxatives.

## ☑ PATIENT TEACHING

• To minimize GI distress caused by oral administration, advise patient to take this drug with milk or meals.

• Instruct patient to ask for or to take drug before pain is intense.

• Caution ambulatory patient about getting out of bed or walking. Warn outpatient to avoid driving and other potentially hazardous activities that require mental alertness until drug's CNS effects are known.

# dezocine
Dalgan

*Pregnancy Risk Category: C*

## HOW SUPPLIED
*Injection:* 5 mg/ml, 10 mg/ml, 15 mg/ml

## ACTION
Unknown. A synthetic opioid agonist-antagonist that produces postoperative analgesia qualitatively similar to morphine.

## ONSET, PEAK, DURATION
Onset occurs within 15 minutes of I.V. injection, 30 minutes of I.M. injection. Peak effects occur within ½ to 2½ hours. Duration unknown.

## INDICATIONS & DOSAGE
*Management of moderate to severe pain* –
**Adults:** 5 to 20 mg I.M. q 3 to 6 hours or 2.5 to 10 mg I.V. q 2 to 4 hours. Maximum recommended single I.M. dose is 20 mg, with a maximum daily dosage of 120 mg. Maximum dosage for I.V. use has not been determined.

## ADVERSE REACTIONS
**CNS:** *sedation, dizziness, vertigo,* anxiety, sleep disturbances, headache, chills, flushing.
**CV:** edema, hypotension, irregular heartbeat, hypertension, chest pain, thrombophlebitis.
**EENT:** dry mouth.
**GI:** *nausea, vomiting,* constipation, diarrhea, abdominal distress.
**Hematologic:** low hemoglobin.
**Respiratory:** *respiratory depression.*
**Skin:** rash, pruritus, *irritation at injection site,* diaphoresis.

## INTERACTIONS
*CNS depressants, ethanol:* may increase risk of CNS depression. Monitor patient response.

*Opioids:* opioid-dependent patients may experience withdrawal symptoms after receiving dezocine. May increase risk of CNS depression. Avoid concomitant use, if possible.

**CONTRAINDICATIONS**
Contraindicated in patients with hypersensitivity to the drug and in patients physically dependent on narcotics.

**NURSING CONSIDERATIONS**
• Use with extreme caution in patients with head injury because drug's CNS depressant effects may obscure clinical signs. Related drugs have caused elevations of CSF pressure in patients with head injury.
• Use cautiously and in lower doses in patients with chronic respiratory disease and in patients undergoing biliary surgery. Related drugs have caused significant increases in pressure within the common bile duct.
• Like other potent analgesics, dezocine should be administered with caution to elderly patients and patients who have recently received substantial amounts of narcotic medication.
• Use cautiously in patients with renal or hepatic failure. Expect dosages to be lower because of increased elimination half-life in these patients.
• Because it is not known if dezocine is excreted in breast milk, breastfeeding is not recommended.
• Use of dezocine is not recommended in patients who are opioid-dependent because it may precipitate withdrawal syndrome. Also not recommended for patients with chronic pain because of limited clinical experience and because drug can precipitate withdrawal syndrome in patients with substantial tolerance to opiates.
• Dezocine produces a dose-dependent respiratory depression similar to that of morphine. Use only in clinical settings where adequate respiratory support and an opiate antagonist (nal-

oxone) is available to reverse respiratory depression.
• **I.V. use:** Give by direct injection into a large vein. Avoid mixing with other drugs because there is little information regarding drug and solution compatibility. Infuse over at least 5 minutes. The injection contains sulfite preservatives, which may cause allergic reactions in certain sensitive patients.
• *Alert:* Be aware that plasma concentrations higher than 45 ng/ml are associated with an increased incidence of adverse reactions.

☑ **PATIENT TEACHING**
• Instruct patient to ask for drug before pain becomes intense.
• Caution ambulatory patient about getting out of bed or walking. Warn outpatient to avoid driving and other potentially hazardous activities that require mental alertness until drug's CNS effects are known.

## fentanyl citrate
Sublimaze

## fentanyl transdermal system
Duragesic-25, Duragesic-50, Duragesic-75, Duragesic-100

## fentanyl transmucosal
Fentanyl Oralet

Controlled Substance Schedule II
*Pregnancy Risk Category: C*

**HOW SUPPLIED**
*Injection:* 50 mcg/ml
*Transdermal system:* patches designed to release 25 mcg, 50 mcg, 75 mcg, or 100 mcg of fentanyl per hour
*Transmucosal:* 200 mcg, 300 mcg, 400 mcg

**ACTION**
Unknown. Binds with opiate receptors in the CNS, altering both perception

of and emotional response to pain through an unknown mechanism.

## ONSET, PEAK, DURATION
Onset within 1 to 2 minutes with I.V. administration; within 7 to 15 minutes of I.M. injection; within 5 to 15 minutes of transmucosal use; onset after transdermal use may take 12 to 24 hours. Peak effects after I.V. use occur in 3 to 5 minutes; after I.M. or transmucosal use, 20 to 30 minutes; after transdermal use, 1 to 3 days. Effects persist ½ to 1 hour after I.V. use or 1 to 2 hours after I.M. use; variable with transdermal system; not clearly defined with transmucosal use.

## INDICATIONS & DOSAGE
*Adjunct to general anesthetic –*
**Adults:** for low-dose therapy, 2 mcg/kg I.V. For moderate-dose therapy, 2 to 20 mcg I.V.; then 25 to 100 mcg I.V. p.r.n. For high-dose therapy, 20 to 50 mcg I.V.; then 25 mcg to one-half the initial loading dose I.V. p.r.n.
*Adjunct to regional anesthesia –*
**Adults:** 50 to 100 mcg I.M. or slowly I.V. q 1 to 2 hours p.r.n.
*Induction and maintenance of anesthesia –*
**Children 2 to 12 years:** 2 to 3 mcg/kg I.V.
*Postoperatively –*
**Adults:** 50 to 100 mcg I.M. q 1 to 2 hours p.r.n.
*Preoperatively –*
**Adults:** 50 to 100 mcg I.M. 30 to 60 minutes before surgery. Alternatively, 5 mcg/kg dispensed as oralet unit, 20 to 40 minutes prior to need of desired effects.
*Management of chronic pain –*
**Adults:** one transdermal system applied to a portion of the upper torso on an area of skin that is not irritated and has not been irradiated. Therapy initiated with the 25-mcg/hour system; dosage adjusted as needed and tolerated. Each system may be worn for 72 hours although a small number of patients may require systems to be applied q 48 hours.

## ADVERSE REACTIONS
**CNS:** *sedation, somnolence, clouded sensorium, euphoria,* dizziness, headache, *confusion, asthenia,* nervousness, hallucinations, anxiety, depression.
**CV:** *hypotension,* hypertension, arrhythmias, chest pain.
**GI:** *nausea, vomiting, constipation,* ileus, abdominal pain, *dry mouth,* anorexia, diarrhea, dyspepsia.
**GU:** *urine retention.*
**Respiratory:** *respiratory depression,* hypoventilation, dyspnea, apnea.
**Skin:** reaction at application site (erythema, papules, edema), *pruritus, diaphoresis.*
**Other:** physical dependence.

## INTERACTIONS
*CNS depressants, ethanol, general anesthetics, hypnotics, MAO inhibitors, other narcotic analgesics, sedatives, tricyclic antidepressants:* additive effects. Use together with extreme caution. Fentanyl dose should be reduced by one-quarter to one-third. Also give above drugs in reduced dosages.

## CONTRAINDICATIONS
Contraindicated in patients with known intolerance of the drug.

## NURSING CONSIDERATIONS
● Use with caution in patients with head injury, increased CSF pressure, COPD, decreased respiratory reserve, potentially compromised respirations, hepatic or renal disease, and cardiac bradyarrhythmias. Also use with caution in elderly or debilitated patients.
● Keep narcotic antagonist (naloxone) and resuscitation equipment available when giving drug I.V.
● For better analgesic effect, administer drug before patient has intense pain.
● *Alert:* Be aware that high doses can

produce muscle rigidity, which can be reversed with neuromuscular blockers; however, patient must be artificially ventilated.

• Monitor circulatory and respiratory status and urinary function carefully. Drug may cause respiratory depression, hypotension, urine retention, nausea, vomiting, ileus, or altered level of consciousness without regard to route of administration.

• Periodically monitor postoperative vital signs and bladder function. Because drug decreases both rate and depth of respirations, monitoring of arterial oxygen saturation ($SaO_2$) may help assess respiratory depression. Immediately report respiratory rate below 12 breaths/minute, decreased respiratory volume, or decreased $SaO_2$.

*I.V. form:*

• Know that only staff trained in administration of I.V. anesthetics and management of their potential adverse effects should administer I.V. fentanyl.

• Be aware that drug is often used I.V. with droperidol to produce neuroleptanalgesia.

*Transmucosal form:*

• Remove foil overwrap of fentanyl oralet just prior to administration.

• Have patient place the fentanyl oralet in mouth and suck (not chew or swallow) it.

• Remove fentanyl oralet unit using the handle after it has been consumed, patient shows adequate effect, or patient shows signs of respiratory depression. Place any remaining portion in the plastic overwrap provided, and dispose accordingly for Schedule II drugs.

*Transdermal form:*

• Know that transdermal fentanyl is not recommended for postoperative pain.

• Dosage equivalent charts are available to calculate the fentanyl transdermal dose based on the daily morphine intake – for example, for every 90 mg of oral morphine or 15 mg of I.M. morphine per 24 hours, 25 mcg/hour of transdermal fentanyl is required. Some patients will require alternative means of opiate administration when the dosage exceeds 300 mcg/hour.

• Be aware that dosage adjustments in patients using the transdermal system should be made gradually. Reaching steady-state levels of a new dosage may take up to 6 days; delay dosage adjustment until after at least two applications.

• Monitor patients who develop adverse reactions to the transdermal system for at least 12 hours after removal. Serum levels of fentanyl drop gradually and may take as long as 17 hours to decline by 50%.

• Most patients experience good control of pain for 3 days while wearing the transdermal system, but a few may need a new application after 48 hours. Because serum fentanyl concentration rises for the first 24 hours after application, analgesic effect cannot be evaluated on the first day. Be sure the patient has adequate supplemental analgesic to prevent breakthrough pain.

• When reducing opiate therapy or switching to a different analgesic, know the transdermal system should be withdrawn gradually. Because fentanyl's serum level drops gradually after removal, give half of the equianalgesic dose of the new analgesic 12 to 18 hours after removal as ordered.

☑ **PATIENT TEACHING**

• When used for pain control, instruct patient to ask for drug before pain becomes intense.

• When drug is used postoperatively, encourage patient turning, coughing, and deep breathing to prevent atelectasis.

• Instruct patient to avoid performing hazardous activities until CNS effects subside.

• Tell home care patient to avoid drinking alcohol or taking other CNS-type drugs while receiving fentanyl because additive effects can occur.
• Teach patient about the proper application of the prescribed transdermal patch. Tell patient to clip hair at the application site, but not to use a razor, which may irritate the skin. Wash area with clear water if necessary, but not with soaps, oils, lotions, alcohol, or other substances that may irritate the skin or prevent adhesion. Dry the area completely before application.
• Tell patient to remove the transdermal system from the package just before applying. Hold in place for 10 to 20 seconds, and be sure the edges of the patch adhere to the skin.
• Teach patient to dispose of the transdermal patch by folding so the adhesive side adheres to itself and then flushing it down the toilet.
• Tell patient if another patch is needed after 48 to 72 hours, apply to a new site.
• Inform patient that heat from fever or environment may increase transdermal delivery and cause toxicity requiring dosage adjustment. Instruct patient to notify doctor if fever occurs or if he'll be spending time in a hot climate.

## hydromorphone hydrochloride (dihydromorphinone hydrochloride)
Dilaudid, Dilaudid-HP
Controlled Substance Schedule II

*Pregnancy Risk Category: C*

### HOW SUPPLIED
*Tablets:* 1 mg, 2 mg, 3 mg, 4 mg
*Injection:* 1 mg/ml, 2 mg/ml, 3 mg/ml, 4 mg/ml, 10 mg/ml
*Suppositories:* 3 mg
*Syrup:* 1mg/5 ml

### ACTION
Binds with opiate receptors in the CNS, altering both perception of and emotional response to pain through an unknown mechanism. Also suppresses the cough reflex by direct action on the cough center in the medulla.

### ONSET, PEAK, DURATION
Onset occurs 10 to 15 minutes after I.V. injection, about 15 minutes after S.C. or I.M. administration, about 30 minutes after oral dose. Peak effects occur 15 to 30 minutes after I.V. injection, 30 to 60 minutes after I.M. injection, 30 to 90 minutes after S.C. administration, 1½ to 2 hours after oral administration. Effects persist about 2 to 3 hours after I.V. injection, 4 to 5 hours after I.M. injection, 4 hours after S.C. or oral administration.

### INDICATIONS & DOSAGE
*Moderate to severe pain—*
**Adults:** 2 to 4 mg P.O. q 4 to 6 hours, p.r.n.; or 2 to 4 mg I.M., S.C., or I.V. (slowly over at least 2 to 3 minutes) q 4 to 6 hours p.r.n.; or 3 mg rectal suppository q 6 to 8 hours p.r.n.
*Cough—*
**Adults:** 1 teaspoon (5 ml) P.O. q 3 to 4 hours p.r.n.

### ADVERSE REACTIONS
**CNS:** *sedation, somnolence, clouded sensorium,* dizziness, *euphoria.*
**CV:** *hypotension,* bradycardia.
**EENT:** blurred vision, diplopia, nystagmus.
**GI:** *nausea, vomiting, constipation,* ileus.
**GU:** *urine retention.*
**Respiratory:** *respiratory depression, bronchospasm.*
**Other:** induration with repeated S.C. injections, physical dependence.

---

Reactions may be *common,* uncommon, *life-threatening,* or COMMON AND LIFE-THREATENING.

## INTERACTIONS
*CNS depressants, ethanol, general anesthetics, hypnotics, MAO inhibitors, other narcotic analgesics, sedatives, tranquilizers, tricyclic antidepressants:* additive effects. Use together with extreme caution. Reduce hydromorphone dose and monitor patient response.

## CONTRAINDICATIONS
Contraindicated in patients with hypersensitivity to this drug, intracranial lesions associated with increased intracranial pressure, and whenever ventilator function is depressed such as in status asthmaticus, COPD, cor pulmonale, emphysema, and kryphoscoliosis.

## NURSING CONSIDERATIONS
● Use with extreme caution in patients with hepatic or renal disease, hypothyroidism, Addison's disease, prostatic hyperplasia, or urethral stricture. Also use with caution in elderly or debilitated patients.
● For better analgesic effect, give this drug before patient has intense pain.
● Dilaudid-HP, a highly concentrated form (10 mg/ml), may be administered in smaller volumes to prevent the discomfort associated with large-volume I.M. or S.C. injections. Check dosage carefully.
● Rotate injection sites to avoid induration with S.C. injection.
● **I.V. use:** Give by direct injection over no less than 2 minutes. For infusion, drug may be mixed in D₅W, 0.9% sodium chloride, dextrose 5% in 0.9% sodium chloride, dextrose 5% in 0.45% sodium chloride, or Ringer's or lactated Ringer's solutions.
● Respiratory depression and hypotension can occur with I.V. administration. Give very slowly and monitor constantly. Keep resuscitation equipment available.
● Monitor respiratory and circulatory status and bowel function.
● Keep narcotic antagonist (naloxone) available.
● Be aware that drug may worsen or mask gallbladder pain.
● Be aware that drug is a commonly abused narcotic.

☑ **PATIENT TEACHING**
● Instruct patient to ask for or take drug before pain becomes intense.
● Tell patient to store suppositories in refrigerator.
● When drug is used postoperatively, encourage patient to turn, cough, and deep breathe to avoid atelectasis.
● Caution ambulatory patient about getting out of bed or walking. Warn outpatient to avoid hazardous activities that require mental alertness until drug's CNS effects are known.

---

## meperidine hydrochloride (pethidine hydrochloride)
Demerol
Controlled Substance Schedule II
*Pregnancy Risk Category: NR*

### HOW SUPPLIED
*Tablets:* 50 mg, 100 mg
*Syrup:* 50 mg/ml
*Injection:* 10 mg/ml, 25 mg/ml, 50 mg/ml, 75 mg/ml, 100 mg/ml

### ACTION
Binds with opiate receptors in the CNS, altering both perception of and emotional response to pain through an unknown mechanism.

### ONSET, PEAK, DURATION
Onset occurs about 1 minute following I.V. administration, 10 to 15 minutes after S.C. or I.M. injection, about 15 minutes after oral administration. Peak effects occur within 5 to 7 minutes after I.V. injection, 30 to 50 minutes after I.M. or S.C. injection, and 60 to 90 minutes after oral admin-

---

*Liquid form contains alcohol. **May contain tartrazine. †Canada only. ‡Australia only. ◇OTC.

istration. Effects persist 2 to 4 hours for all routes of administration.

## INDICATIONS & DOSAGE
*Moderate to severe pain –*
**Adults:** 50 to 150 mg P.O., I.M., or S.C. q 3 to 4 hours, p.r.n.; or 15 to 35 mg/hour by continuous I.V. infusion.
**Children:** 1.1 to 1.76 mg/kg P.O., I.M., or S.C. q 3 to 4 hours. Maximum dosage is 100 mg q 4 hours, p.r.n.
*Preoperatively –*
**Adults:** 50 to 100 mg I.M. or S.C. 30 to 90 minutes before surgery.
**Children:** 1 to 2.2 mg/kg I.M. or S.C. up to the adult dose 30 to 90 minutes before surgery.
*Adjunct to anesthesia –*
**Adults:** Repeated slow I.V. injections of fractional doses (10 mg/ml); alternatively, continuous I.V. infusion of a more dilute solution (1 mg/ml) titrated to patient's needs.
*Obstetric analgesia –*
**Adults:** 50 to 100 mg I.M. or S.C. when pain becomes regular, repeated at 1- to 3-hour intervals.

## ADVERSE REACTIONS
**CNS:** *sedation, somnolence, clouded sensorium, euphoria,* paradoxical excitement, tremor, *dizziness, seizures* (with large doses), headache, hallucinations, syncope, *light-headedness.*
**CV:** *hypotension,* bradycardia, tachycardia, *cardiac arrest, shock.*
**GI:** *constipation,* ileus, dry mouth, *nausea, vomiting,* biliary tract spasms.
**GU:** *urine retention.*
**Respiratory:** *respiratory depression, respiratory arrest.*
**Skin:** pruritus, urticaria, *diaphoresis.*
**Other:** physical dependence, muscle twitching, phlebitis after I.V. delivery, pain at injection site, local tissue irritation and induration after S.C. injection.

## INTERACTIONS
*Aminophylline, barbiturates, heparin, methicillin, morphine sulfate, phenytoin, sodium bicarbonate, sulfonamides:* incompatible when mixed in the same I.V. container.
*CNS depressants, ethanol, general anesthetics, hypnotics, other narcotic analgesics, phenothiazines, sedatives, tricyclic antidepressants:* possible respiratory depression, hypotension, profound sedation, or coma. Use together with extreme caution. Reduce meperidine dosage.
*MAO inhibitors:* increased CNS excitation or depression that can be severe or fatal. Don't use together.
*Phenytoin:* decreased blood levels of meperidine. Monitor for decreased analgesia.

## CONTRAINDICATIONS
Contraindicated in patients with hypersensitivity to this drug and in patients who have received MAO inhibitors within past 14 days.

## NURSING CONSIDERATIONS
• Use with extreme caution in patients with increased intracranial pressure, head injury, asthma, and other respiratory conditions; in supraventricular tachycardias, seizures, acute abdominal conditions, hepatic or renal disease, hypothyroidism, Addison's disease, urethral stricture, and prostatic hyperplasia; and in elderly or debilitated patients.
• May be used in some patients allergic to morphine.
• **I.V. use:** Give slowly by direct I.V. injection. Meperidine also may be given by slow continuous I.V. infusion. Drug is compatible with most I.V. solutions, including $D_5W$, 0.9% sodium chloride, and Ringer's or lactated Ringer's solutions.
• Keep narcotic antagonist (naloxone) available when giving this drug I.V.
• S.C. injection is not recommended because it is very painful.

---

Reactions may be *common,* uncommon, *life-threatening,* or **COMMON AND LIFE-THREATENING.**

• **Alert:** Oral dose is less than half as effective as parenteral dose. Give I.M. if possible. When changing from parenteral to oral route, know that dosage should be increased.

• Syrup has local anesthetic effect. Give with full glass of water.

• Meperidine and its active metabolite normeperidine accumulate in the body. Monitor for increased toxic effect, especially in patients with impaired renal function.

• Because meperidine toxicity often appears after several days of treatment, this drug is not recommended for treatment of chronic pain.

• Monitor respirations of neonates exposed to drug during labor. Have resuscitation equipment and naloxone available.

• Monitor respiratory and cardiovascular status carefully. Don't give if respirations are below 12 breaths/minute, if respiratory rate or depth is decreased, or if change in pupils is noted.

• Watch for withdrawal symptoms if drug is discontinued abruptly after long-term use.

• Monitor bladder function in postoperative patients.

• Monitor bowel function. Patient may need a laxative or stool softener.

☑ **PATIENT TEACHING**

• When drug is used postoperatively, encourage patient to turn, cough, and deep breathe and to use an incentive spirometer to prevent atelectasis.

• Caution ambulatory patient about getting out of bed or walking. Warn outpatient to avoid driving and other potentially hazardous activities that require mental alertness until drug's CNS effects are known.

# methadone hydrochloride
Dolophine, Methadose, Physeptone‡
Controlled Substance Schedule II

*Pregnancy Risk Category: NR*

## HOW SUPPLIED
*Tablets:* 5 mg, 10 mg
*Dispersible tablets (for methadone maintenance therapy):* 40 mg
*Oral solution:* 5 mg/5 ml, 10 mg/5 ml, 10 mg/ml (concentrate)
*Injection:* 10 mg/ml

## ACTION
Binds with opiate receptors at many sites in the CNS (brain, brain stem, and spinal cord), altering both perception of and emotional response to pain through an unknown mechanism.

## ONSET, PEAK, DURATION
Onset occurs immediately after I.V. administration, 10 to 20 minutes after I.M. injection, 30 to 60 minutes after oral administration. Peak effects occur within 15 to 30 minutes after I.V injection, 1 to 2 hours after I.M. injection, 1½ to 2 hours after oral administration. Effects persist 3 to 4 hours after I.V. use, 4 to 5 hours after I.M. use, 4 to 6 hours after oral use.

## INDICATIONS & DOSAGE
*Severe pain –*
**Adults:** 2.5 to 10 mg P.O., I.M., or S.C. q 3 to 4 hours, p.r.n.
*Narcotic withdrawal syndrome –*
**Adults:** 15 to 40 mg P.O. daily (highly individualized). Maintenance dosage is 20 to 120 mg P.O. daily. Dosage adjusted as needed. Daily dosages greater than 120 mg require special state and federal approval.

## ADVERSE REACTIONS
**CNS:** *sedation, somnolence, clouded sensorium, euphoria, dizziness,* choreic movements, *seizures* (with large

doses), headache, insomnia, agitation, *light-headedness,* syncope.
**CV:** *hypotension,* bradycardia, ***shock, cardiac arrest,*** palpitations.
**EENT:** visual disturbances.
**GI:** *nausea, vomiting, constipation,* ileus, dry mouth, anorexia, biliary tract spasm.
**GU:** *urine retention,* decreased libido.
**Respiratory:** ***respiratory depression, respiratory arrest.***
**Skin:** *diaphoresis,* pruritus, urticaria, edema.
**Other:** physical dependence; pain at injection site; tissue irritation, induration (following S.C. injection).

### INTERACTIONS

*Ammonium chloride and other urine acidifiers, phenytoin:* may reduce methadone effect. Monitor for decreased pain control.
*CNS depressants, ethanol, general anesthetics, hypnotics, MAO inhibitors, sedatives, tranquilizers, tricyclic antidepressants:* possible respiratory depression, hypotension, profound sedation, or coma. Use together with extreme caution. Monitor patient response.
*Rifampin:* withdrawal symptoms; reduced blood levels of methadone. Use together cautiously.

### CONTRAINDICATIONS

Contraindicated in patients with hypersensitivity to this drug.

### NURSING CONSIDERATIONS

• Use with extreme caution in patients with acute abdominal conditions, severe hepatic or renal impairment, hypothyroidism, Addison's disease, prostatic hyperplasia, urethral stricture, head injury, increased intracranial pressure, asthma, and other respiratory conditions. Also use with caution in elderly or debilitated patients.
• Oral liquid form legally required in maintenance programs. Completely

dissolve tablets in 120 ml of orange juice or powdered citrus drink.
• For parenteral use, I.M. injection is preferred. Rotate injection sites.
• **I.V. use:** Dilute to a maximum concentration of 10 mg/ml using 0.9% sodium chloride. Give slowly by direct injection. Alternatively, dilute to 1 mg/ml and give as a slow I.V. infusion (15 to 35 mg/hour).
• Know that oral dose is half as potent as injected dose.
• Know that an around-the-clock regimen is necessary to manage severe, chronic pain.
• Be aware that patient treated for narcotic withdrawal syndrome usually will require an additional analgesic if pain control is necessary.
• Monitor patient closely; has cumulative effect; marked sedation can occur after repeated doses.
• Monitor circulatory and respiratory status and bladder and bowel function. Patient may need a laxative.
• Be aware that when used as an adjunct in the treatment of narcotic addiction (maintenance), withdrawal usually will be delayed and mild.

### ☑ PATIENT TEACHING

• Caution ambulatory patient about getting out of bed or walking. Warn outpatient to avoid hazardous activities that require mental alertness until drug's CNS effects are known.
• Instruct patient to increase fluid and fiber in diet, if not contraindicated, to combat constipation.

---

Reactions may be *common,* uncommon, *life-threatening,* or COMMON AND LIFE-THREATENING.

# morphine hydrochloride
Morphitec†, M.O.S.†, M.O.S.-S.R.†

# morphine sulfate
Astramorph PF, Duramorph, Duramorph PF, Epimorph†, Infumorph 200, Infumorph 500, Morphine H.P.†, MS Contin, MSIR, MS/L, OMS Concentrate, Oramorph SR, RMS Uniserts, Roxanol, Roxanol 100, Roxanol Rescudose, Roxanol SR, Roxanol UD, Statex†

Controlled Substance Schedule II

# morphine tartrate†

*Pregnancy Risk Category: C*

## HOW SUPPLIED
**morphine hydrochloride**
*Tablets:* 10 mg†, 20 mg†, 40 mg†, 60 mg†
*Tablets (extended-release):* 30 mg†, 60 mg†
*Oral solution†:* 1 mg/ml, 5 mg/ml, 10 mg/ml, 20 mg/ml, 50 mg/ml
*Syrup:* 1 mg/ml†, 5 mg/ml†, 10 mg/ml†, 20 mg/ml†, 50 mg/ml†
*Suppositories:* 10 mg†, 20 mg†, 30 mg†
**morphine sulfate**
*Tablets:* 15 mg, 30 mg
*Tablets (extended-release):* 15 mg, 30 mg, 60 mg, 100 mg
*Soluble tablets:* 10 mg, 15 mg, 30 mg
*Oral solution:* 10 mg/5 ml, 20 mg/5 ml, 20 mg/ml (concentrate)
*Syrup:* 1 mg/ml, 5 mg/ml
*Injection (with preservative):* 0.5 mg/ml, 1 mg/ml, 2 mg/ml, 3 mg/ml, 4 mg/ml, 5 mg/ml, 8 mg/ml, 10 mg/ml, 15 mg/ml, 25 mg/ml, 50 mg/ml
*Injection (without preservative):* 0.5 mg/ml, 1 mg/ml, 10 mg/ml, 25 mg/ml
*Suppositories:* 5 mg, 10 mg, 20 mg, 30 mg
**morphine tartrate**
*Injection:* 80 mg/ml‡

## ACTION
Binds with opiate receptors in the CNS, altering both perception of and emotional response to pain through an unknown mechanism.

## ONSET, PEAK, DURATION
Onset occurs within 1 hour after oral dose, 20 to 60 minutes after rectal dose, 10 to 30 minutes after S.C. or I.M. dose, less than 5 minutes after I.V. dose, 15 to 60 minutes after epidural or intrathecal dose. Peak analgesic effect is 1 to 2 hours after oral dose, 20 to 60 minutes after rectal dose, 50 to 90 minutes after S.C. dose, 30 to 60 minutes after I.M. dose, 20 minutes after direct I.V. injection, 15 to 60 minutes after epidural injection. Effects persist 4 to 5 hours after immediate-release oral forms, 8 to 12 hours after extended-release oral forms, 4 to 5 hours after rectal, S.C., I.M., or I.V. dose, up to 24 hours after intrathecal or epidural dose.

## INDICATIONS & DOSAGE
*Severe pain –*
**Adults:** 5 to 20 mg S.C. or I.M. or 2.5 to 15 mg I.V. q 4 hours p.r.n.; or 10 to 30 mg P.O. or 10 to 20 mg rectally q 4 hours, p.r.n. When given by continuous I.V. infusion, a loading dose of 15 mg I.V. may be followed by a continuous infusion of 0.8 to 10 mg/hour. 15 to 30 mg controlled-release tablets P.O. q 12 hours may also be administered. As an epidural injection, 5 mg by epidural catheter; then, if adequate pain relief not obtained within 1 hour, additional doses of 1 to 2 mg given at intervals sufficient to assess efficacy. Maximum total epidural dose should not exceed 10 mg.
**Children:** 0.1 to 0.2 mg/kg S.C. or I.M. q 4 hours. Maximum single dose is 15 mg.

## ADVERSE REACTIONS

**CNS:** *sedation, somnolence, clouded sensorium, euphoria, **seizures** (with large doses), dizziness, nightmares* (with long-acting oral forms), *light-headedness,* hallucinations, nervousness, depression, syncope.

**CV:** *hypotension,* bradycardia, ***shock, cardiac arrest,*** tachycardia, hypertension.

**GI:** *nausea, vomiting, constipation,* ileus, dry mouth, biliary tract spasms, anorexia.

**GU:** *urine retention,* decreased libido.

**Hematologic:** thrombocytopenia.

**Respiratory:** *respiratory depression,* apnea, ***respiratory arrest.***

**Skin:** pruritus and skin flushing (with epidural administration), *diaphoresis,* edema.

**Other:** *physical dependence.*

## INTERACTIONS

*CNS depressants, ethanol, general anesthetics, hypnotics, MAO inhibitors, other narcotic analgesics, sedatives, tranquilizers, tricyclic antidepressants:* possible respiratory depression, hypotension, profound sedation, or coma. Use together with extreme caution. Reduce morphine dosage and monitor patient response.

## CONTRAINDICATIONS

Contraindicated in patients with hypersensitivity to this drug or conditions that would preclude administration of opioids by I.V. route (acute bronchial asthma or upper airway obstruction).

## NURSING CONSIDERATIONS

• Use with extreme caution in patients with head injury, increased intracranial pressure, seizures, chronic pulmonary disease, prostatic hyperplasia, severe hepatic or renal disease, acute abdominal conditions, hypothyroidism, Addison's disease, and urethral stricture. Also use with extreme caution in elderly or debilitated patients.

• Keep narcotic antagonist (naloxone) and resuscitation equipment available.

• **I.V. use:** When given by direct injection, 2.5 to 15 mg may be diluted in 4 or 5 ml of sterile water for injection and given over 4 to 5 minutes. Alternately, the drug may be mixed with $D_5W$ to a concentration of 0.1 to 1 mg/ml and administered by a continuous infusion device. Morphine sulfate is compatible with most common I.V. solutions.

• Oral solutions of various concentrations are available as well as an intensified oral solution (20 mg/ml). Carefully note the strength administered.

• Do not crush or break extended-release tablets.

• S.L. administration may be ordered. Measure oral solution with tuberculin syringe. Administer dose a few drops at a time to allow maximal S.L. absorption and minimize swallowing.

• Refrigeration of rectal suppository is not necessary. In some patients, rectal and oral absorption may not be equivalent.

• Preservative-free preparations are available for epidural and intrathecal administration.

• When given epidurally, monitor closely for respiratory depression up to 24 hours after the injection. Check respiratory rate and depth every 30 to 60 minutes for 24 hours.

• Know that morphine is the drug of choice in relieving pain of MI. May cause transient decrease in blood pressure.

• Be aware that an around-the-clock regimen best manages severe, chronic pain.

• Be aware morphine may worsen or mask gallbladder pain.

• Monitor circulatory, respiratory, bladder, and bowel functions carefully. Drug may cause respiratory depression, hypotension, urine retention, nausea, vomiting, ileus, or altered level of consciousness regard-

less of the route used. Withhold dose and notify doctor if respirations are below 12 breaths/minute.
• Constipation is often severe with maintenance dosage. Ensure that stool softener or other laxative is ordered.

☑ **PATIENT TEACHING**
• When drug is used postoperatively, encourage patient to turn, cough, and deep breathe and to use incentive spirometer to prevent atelectasis.
• Caution ambulatory patient about getting out of bed or walking. Warn outpatient to avoid driving and other potentially hazardous activities that require mental alertness until drug's adverse CNS effects are known.

# nalbuphine hydrochloride
Nubain

*Pregnancy Risk Category: NR*

## HOW SUPPLIED
*Injection:* 10 mg/ml, 20 mg/ml

## ACTION
Binds with opiate receptors in the CNS, altering both perception of and emotional response to pain through an unknown mechanism.

## ONSET, PEAK, DURATION
Onset occurs 2 to 3 minutes after I.V. administration, within 15 minutes of S.C. or I. M. injection. Peak effects occur within 30 minutes of I.V. administration, 60 minutes of I.M. injection. Effects persist 3 to 4 hours after I.V. use, 3 to 6 hours after S.C. or I.M. injection.

## INDICATIONS & DOSAGE
*Moderate to severe pain –*
**Adults:** For an average (70 kg) person, give 10 to 20 mg S.C., I.M., or I.V. q 3 to 6 hours, p.r.n. Maximum daily dosage is 160 mg.
*Adjunct to balanced anesthesia –*
**Adults:** 0.3 mg/kg to 3.0 mg/kg I.V.

over 10 to 15 minutes followed by maintenance doses of 0.25 to 0.50 mg/kg in single I.V. dose, p.r.n.

## ADVERSE REACTIONS
**CNS:** *headache, sedation, dizziness, vertigo,* nervousness, depression, restlessness, crying, euphoria, hostility, unusual dreams, confusion, hallucinations, speech difficulty, delusions.
**CV:** hypertension, hypotension, tachycardia, bradycardia.
**EENT:** blurred vision, *dry mouth.*
**GI:** cramps, dyspepsia, bitter taste, *nausea, vomiting,* constipation, biliary tract spasms.
**GU:** urinary urgency.
**Respiratory:** *respiratory depression,* dyspnea, asthma, *pulmonary edema.*
**Skin:** pruritus, burning, urticaria, *clamminess.*

## INTERACTIONS
*CNS depressants, ethanol, general anesthetics, hypnotics, MAO inhibitors, sedatives, tranquilizers, tricyclic antidepressants:* possible respiratory depression, hypertension, profound sedation, or coma. Use together with extreme caution. Monitor patient response.
*Narcotic analgesics:* possible decreased analgesic effect. Avoid concomitant use.

## CONTRAINDICATIONS
Contraindicated in patients with hypersensitivity to the drug.

## NURSING CONSIDERATIONS
• Use cautiously in patients with history of drug abuse or in patients with emotional instability, head injury, increased intracranial pressure, impaired ventilation, MI accompanied by nausea and vomiting, upcoming biliary surgery, and hepatic or renal disease.
• Respiratory depression can be reversed with naloxone. Keep resuscita-

tion equipment available, particularly when administering I.V.

● Acts as a narcotic antagonist; may precipitate withdrawal syndrome. For patients who have chronically received opiates, administer 25% of the usual dose initially as ordered. Observe for signs of withdrawal.

● **I.V. use:** Inject slowly over at least 2 to 3 minutes into a vein or into an I.V. line containing a compatible, free-flowing I.V. solution, such as $D_5W$, 0.9% sodium chloride, or lactated Ringer's solution.

● *Alert:* Causes respiratory depression, which at 10 mg is equal to the respiratory depression produced by 10 mg of morphine.

● Monitor circulatory and respiratory status and bladder and bowel function. Withhold dose and notify doctor if respirations are shallow or rate is below 12 breaths/minute.

● Constipation is often severe with maintenance therapy. Make sure stool softener or other laxative is ordered.

● Know that psychological and physical dependence may occur with prolonged use.

☑ **PATIENT TEACHING**
● Caution ambulatory patient about getting out of bed or walking. Warn outpatient to avoid driving and other potentially hazardous activities that require mental alertness until drug's CNS effects are known.

● Instruct patient on how to manage troublesome adverse effects such as constipation.

---

## oxycodone hydrochloride
Endone‡, Roxicodone,
Roxicodone Intensol, Supeudol†
Controlled Substance Schedule II

## oxycodone pectinate
Proladone‡

*Pregnancy Risk Category: NR*

---

**HOW SUPPLIED**
**oxycodone hydrochloride**
*Tablets:* 5 mg
*Oral solution:* 5 mg/5 ml, 20 mg/ml (concentrate)
*Suppositories:* 10 mg, 20 mg
**oxycodone pectinate**
*Suppositories:* 30 mg‡

**ACTION**
Binds with opiate receptors in the CNS, altering both perception of and emotional response to pain through an unknown mechanism.

**ONSET, PEAK, DURATION**
Onset occurs in 10 to 15 minutes. Peak effects occur within 1 hour. Effects persist 3 to 6 hours.

**INDICATIONS & DOSAGE**
*Moderate to severe pain—*
**Adults:** 5 mg P.O. q 6 hours, p.r.n. Alternatively, 1 to 3 suppositories P.R. daily, p.r.n.
**Children 6 to 12 years:** 0.61 mg of combined salts P.O. q 6 hours, p.r.n.
**Children 12 years and older:** 1.22 mg of combined salts P.O. q 6 hours, p.r.n.

**ADVERSE REACTIONS**
**CNS:** *sedation, somnolence, clouded sensorium, euphoria, dizziness, lightheadedness.*
**CV:** *hypotension,* bradycardia.
**GI:** *nausea, vomiting, constipation,* ileus.
**GU:** *urine retention.*
**Respiratory:** *respiratory depression.*
**Skin:** *diaphoresis,* pruritus.
**Other:** physical dependence.

**INTERACTIONS**
*Anticoagulants:* oxycodone hydrochloride products containing aspirin may increase anticoagulant effect. Monitor clotting times. Use together cautiously.
*CNS depressants, ethanol, general anesthetics, hypnotics, MAO inhibitors,*

---

Reactions may be *common,* uncommon, *life-threatening,* or COMMON AND LIFE-THREATENING.

*other narcotic analgesics, sedatives, tranquilizers, tricyclic antidepressants:* additive effects. Use together with extreme caution. Reduce oxycodone dose and monitor patient response.

**CONTRAINDICATIONS**
Contraindicated in patients with hypersensitivity to this drug.

**NURSING CONSIDERATIONS**
• Use with extreme caution in patients with head injury, increased intracranial pressure, seizures, asthma, COPD, prostatic hyperplasia, severe hepatic or renal disease, acute abdominal conditions, urethral stricture, hypothyroidism, Addison's disease, and arrhythmias. Also use with extreme caution in elderly or debilitated patients.
• For full analgesic effect, administer drug before patient has intense pain.
• To minimize GI upset, administer drug after meals or with milk.
• Be aware that single-agent oxycodone solution or tablets are especially good for patients who shouldn't take aspirin or acetaminophen.
• Monitor circulatory and respiratory status. Withhold dose and notify doctor if respirations are shallow or if respiratory rate falls below 12 breaths/ minute.
• Monitor patient's bladder and bowel patterns. Patient may require a laxative because drug has a constipating effect.

☑ **PATIENT TEACHING**
• Instruct patient to ask for drug before pain is intense.
• Tell patient to take drug with milk or after eating.
• Caution ambulatory patient about getting out of bed or walking. Warn outpatient to avoid driving and other potentially hazardous activities that require mental alertness until drug's CNS effects are known.

# oxymorphone hydrochloride
Numorphan, Numorphan H.P.
Controlled Substance Schedule II

*Pregnancy Risk Category: NR*

**HOW SUPPLIED**
*Injection:* 1 mg/ml, 1.5 mg/ml
*Suppositories:* 5 mg

**ACTION**
Binds with opiate receptors in the CNS, altering both perception of and emotional response to pain through an unknown mechanism.

**ONSET, PEAK, DURATION**
Onset occurs within 5 to 10 minutes after I.V. use, 10 to 15 minutes after I.M. use, 10 to 20 minutes after S.C. use, 15 to 30 minutes after rectal use. Peak effects occur within 15 to 30 minutes after I.V. use, 30 to 90 minutes after I.M. use, 60 to 90 minutes after S.C. use, 2 hours after rectal use. Effects persist 3 to 4 hours after I.V. use; 3 to 6 hours after I.M., S.C., or rectal use.

**INDICATIONS & DOSAGE**
*Moderate to severe pain –*
**Adults:** 1 to 1.5 mg I.M. or S.C. q 4 to 6 hours, p.r.n.; or 0.5 mg I.V. q 4 to 6 hours, p.r.n.; or 5 mg P.R. q 4 to 6 hours, p.r.n.

**ADVERSE REACTIONS**
**CNS:** *sedation, somnolence, clouded sensorium, euphoria,* dizziness, *seizures* (with large doses), light-headedness, headache.
**CV:** *hypotension,* bradycardia.
**GI:** *nausea, vomiting, constipation,* ileus.
**GU:** *urine retention.*
**Respiratory:** *respiratory depression.*
**Skin:** pruritus.
**Other:** physical dependence.

---

## INTERACTIONS
*CNS depressants, ethanol, general anesthetics, MAO inhibitors, tricyclic antidepressants:* additive effects. Use together with extreme caution.

## CONTRAINDICATIONS
Contraindicated in patients with hypersensitivity to this drug.

## NURSING CONSIDERATIONS
• Use with extreme caution in patients with head injury, increased intracranial pressure, seizures, asthma, COPD, acute abdominal conditions, prostatic hyperplasia, severe hepatic or renal disease, urethral stricture, respiratory depression, hypothyroidism, Addison's disease, and arrhythmias. Also use with extreme caution in elderly or debilitated patients.
• Keep narcotic antagonist (naloxone) and resuscitation equipment available.
• Ddrug is not for mild to moderate pain. May worsen gallbladder pain.
• For better effect, administer drug before patient has intense pain.
• **I.V. use:** Give by direct I.V. injection. If necessary, drug may be diluted in 0.9% sodium chloride solution.
• Monitor cardiovascular and respiratory status. Withhold dose and notify doctor if respirations decrease or rate is below 12 breaths/minute.
• Monitor patient's bladder and bowel function. Patient may need laxative.

## ☑ PATIENT TEACHING
• Instruct patient to ask for drug before pain is intense.
• When drug is used postoperatively, encourage patient to turn, cough, and deep breathe and to use incentive spirometer to avoid atelectasis.
• Caution ambulatory patient about getting out of bed or walking. Warn outpatient to avoid driving and other potentially hazardous activities that require mental alertness until drug's CNS effects are known.

# pentazocine hydrochloride
Fortral†‡, Talwin†

# pentazocine hydrochloride and naloxone hydrochloride
Talwin-Nx
Controlled Substance Schedule IV

# pentazocine lactate
Fortral‡, Talwin
Controlled Substance Schedule IV

*Pregnancy Risk Category: NR*

## HOW SUPPLIED
**pentazocine hydrochloride**
*Tablets:* 25 mg‡, 50 mg†‡
**pentazocine hydrochloride and naloxone hydrochloride**
*Tablets:* 50 mg pentazocine hydrochloride and 500 mcg naloxone hydrochloride
**pentazocine lactate**
*Injection:* 30 mg/ml

## ACTION
Binds with opiate receptors at many sites in the CNS, altering both perception of and emotional response to pain through an unknown mechanism.

## ONSET, PEAK, DURATION
Onset occurs within 2 to 3 minutes after I.V. use, 15 to 20 minutes after I.M. or S.C. use, 15 to 30 minutes after oral use. Peak effects occur within 15 to 30 minutes after I.V. use, 30 to 60 minutes after I.M. or S.C. use, 60 to 90 minutes after oral use. Effects persist 2 to 3 hours after parenteral use, 2 to 3 hours after oral use.

## INDICATIONS & DOSAGE
*Moderate to severe pain –*
**Adults:** 50 to 100 mg P.O. q 3 to 4 hours, p.r.n. Maximum oral dosage is 600 mg/day. Alternatively, 30 mg I.M., I.V., or S.C. q 3 to 4 hours, p.r.n. Maximum parenteral dosage is 360 mg/day. Single doses above 30

---

mg I.V. or 60 mg I.M. or S.C. are not recommended.
*Labor—*
**Adults:** 30 mg I.M. or 20 mg I.V. q 2 to 3 hours when contractions become regular.

## ADVERSE REACTIONS
**CNS:** *sedation,* visual disturbances, hallucinations, drowsiness, *dizziness, light-headedness,* confusion, *euphoria,* headache, psychotomimetic effects.
**CV:** circulatory depression, *shock,* hypertension.
**EENT:** dry mouth.
**GI:** *nausea, vomiting,* constipation.
**GU:** urine retention.
**Respiratory:** *respiratory depression,* dyspnea, apnea.
**Skin:** induration, nodules, sloughing, and sclerosis of injection site; diaphoresis; pruritus.
**Other:** hypersensitivity reactions *(anaphylaxis),* physical and psychological dependence.

## INTERACTIONS
*CNS depressants, ethanol:* additive effects. Use together cautiously.
*Narcotic analgesics:* possible decreased analgesic effect. Avoid concomitant use.

## CONTRAINDICATIONS
Contraindicated in patients with hypersensitivity to the drug or any product component. Not recommended for children under 12 years.

## NURSING CONSIDERATIONS
• Use cautiously in patients with hepatic or renal disease, acute MI, head injury, increased intracranial pressure, and respiratory depression.
• Have naloxone readily available. Respiratory depression can be reversed with naloxone.
• **I.V. use:** Give by direct I.V. injection slowly. Do not mix in syringe with aminophylline, barbiturates, or other alkaline substances.

• *Alert:* When giving by S.C. or I.M. injection, rotate injection sites to minimize tissue irritation. If possible, avoid giving by S.C.route.
• Know that drug possesses narcotic antagonist properties. May precipitate withdrawal syndrome in narcotic-dependent patients.
• Psychological and physical dependence may occur with prolonged use.
• Know that Talwin-Nx, the oral pentazocine available in the U.S., contains the narcotic antagonist naloxone. This prevents illicit I.V. use.
• Know that pentazocine may interfere with certain laboratory tests for urinary 17-hydroxycorticosteroids.

## ☑ PATIENT TEACHING
• Instruct patient to ask for drug before pain is intense.
• Caution ambulatory patient about getting out of bed or walking. Warn outpatient to avoid driving and other potentially hazardous activities that require mental alertness until drug's CNS effects are known.

# propoxyphene hydrochloride (dextropropoxyphene hydrochloride)
Darvon, Dolene, Novopropoxyn†, 642†

# propoxyphene napsylate (dextropropoxyphene napsylate)
Darvon-N, Doloxene‡, Doloxene Co‡

Controlled Substance Schedule IV
*Pregnancy Risk Category: C*

## HOW SUPPLIED
**propoxyphene hydrochloride**
*Capsules:* 32 mg, 65 mg
**propoxyphene napsylate**
*Tablets:* 100 mg
*Oral suspension:* 10 mg/ml

---

## ACTION
Binds with opiate receptors in the CNS, altering both perception of and emotional response to pain through an unknown mechanism.

## ONSET, PEAK, DURATION
Onset occurs within 15 to 60 minutes. Plasma levels peak in 2 to 2½ hours. Effects persist 4 to 6 hours.

## INDICATIONS & DOSAGE
*Mild to moderate pain* –
**Adults:** 65 mg (hydrochloride) P.O. q 4 hours p.r.n. Maximum dosage is 390 mg/day.
*Mild to moderate pain* –
**Adults:** 100 mg (napsylate) P.O. q 4 hours p.r.n. Maximum dosage is 600 mg/day.

## ADVERSE REACTIONS
**CNS:** *dizziness,* headache, *sedation,* euphoria, light-headedness, weakness, hallucinations.
**GI:** *nausea, vomiting,* constipation, abdominal pain.
**Respiratory:** *respiratory depression.*
**Other:** psychological and physical dependence, abnormal liver function tests.

## INTERACTIONS
*Carbamazepine:* may increase carbamazepine levels. Monitor closely.
*CNS depressants, ethanol:* additive effects. Use together cautiously.
*Warfarin:* may increase anticoagulant effect. Monitor PT.

## CONTRAINDICATIONS
Contraindicated in patients with hypersensitivity to this drug.

## NURSING CONSIDERATIONS
• Use cautiously in hepatic or renal disease, emotional instability, or history of drug or alcohol abuse.
• Remember that 65 mg of propoxyphene hydrochloride equals 100 mg of propoxyphene napsylate.

• Drug is considered a mild narcotic analgesic, but pain relief is equivalent to that provided by aspirin. Tolerance and physical dependence may occur. Used with aspirin or acetaminophen to maximize analgesia.
• Know that smokers may need increased dosage because smoking may induce liver enzymes responsible for the metabolism of the drug thereby decreasing its efficacy.
• Drug may cause false decreases in urinary steroid excretion tests.

☑ **PATIENT TEACHING**
• To minimize GI upset, advise patient to take drug with food or milk.
• Warn patient not to exceed recommended dosage. Respiratory depression, hypotension, profound sedation, and coma may result if used in excessive doses or with other CNS depressants. Advise patient to avoid alcohol intake or use of other CNS-type drugs when taking propoxyphene.
• Caution ambulatory patient about getting out of bed or walking. Warn outpatient to avoid driving and other hazardous activities that require mental alertness until drug's CNS effects are known.

---

## sufentanil citrate
Sufenta
Controlled Substance Schedule II
*Pregnancy Risk Category: C*

## HOW SUPPLIED
*Injection:* 50 mcg/ml

## ACTION
Binds with opiate receptors in the CNS, altering both perception of and emotional response to pain through an unknown mechanism.

## ONSET, PEAK, DURATION
Onset and peak for analgesic effects occur within 1 minute . Time to loss of consciousness depends on rate of

---

administration, generally within 1 to 2 minutes. Analgesic effects persist for 5 minutes. Time to awakening is 0.7 to 2.9 hours after average dose.

## INDICATIONS & DOSAGE

*Adjunct to general anesthetic –*
**Adults:** 1 to 8 mcg/kg I.V. administered with nitrous oxide and oxygen; additional 10 to 25 mcg I.V. may be administered, p.r.n., when movement or changes in vital signs indicate surgical stress or lightening of analgesia.
*As a primary anesthetic –*
**Adults:** 8 to 30 mcg/kg I.V. administered with 100% oxygen and a muscle relaxant; additional 10 to 50 mcg I.V. may be administered p.r.n., when movement or changes in vital signs indicate surgical stress or lightening of analgesia.

## ADVERSE REACTIONS

**CNS:** chills, somnolence.
**CV:** *hypotension,* hypertension, arrhythmias, *bradycardia,* tachycardia.
**GI:** nausea, vomiting.
**Respiratory:** *chest wall rigidity,* apnea, bronchospasm.
**Skin:** *pruritus,* erythema.
**Other:** intraoperative muscle movement.

## INTERACTIONS

*CNS depressants, ethanol:* additive effects. Use together cautiously.

## CONTRAINDICATIONS

Contraindicated in patients with hypersensitivity to this drug.

## NURSING CONSIDERATIONS

• Use with extreme caution in head injury; in pulmonary, hepatic, or renal disease; in decreased respiratory reserve; and in elderly or debilitated patients.
• Should be administered only by persons trained in the use of I.V. anesthetics.

• Reduced dosage is required for elderly and debilitated patients.
• For obese patients who exceed 20% of their ideal body weight, dosage calculations should be based upon an estimate of ideal weight.
• When used at doses over 8 mcg/kg, postoperative mechanical ventilation and observation are essential because of prolonged respiratory depression.
• Keep narcotic antagonist (naloxone) and resuscitation equipment available.
• **I.V. use:** Give by direct I.V. injection. Drug has been given by intermittent I.V. infusion, but drug compatibility and stability in I.V. solutions have not been fully investigated.
• Because drug decreases both rate and depth of respirations, monitoring of arterial oxygen saturation may aid in assessing respiratory depression. Notify the doctor if respirations decrease or rate falls below 12 breaths/ minute.
• Monitor respirations of neonates exposed to the drug during labor.
• *Alert:* Know that high doses can produce muscle rigidity reversible by neuromuscular blockers; however, patient must be artificially ventilated.
• Monitor postoperative vital signs frequently, including circulatory and respiratory status and urinary function. Drug may cause respiratory depression, hypotension, urine retention, nausea, vomiting, ileus, or altered level of consciousness.

## ☑ PATIENT TEACHING

• Inform patient and family of need for drug and answer any questions.
• Encourage turning, coughing, and deep breathing postoperatively to prevent atelectasis.

---

# tramadol hydrochloride
Ultram

*Pregnancy Risk Category: C*

## HOW SUPPLIED
*Tablets:* 50 mg

## ACTION
Unknown. A centrally acting synthetic analgesic compound not chemically related to opiates. Thought to bind to opioid receptors and inhibit reuptake of norepinephrine and serotonin.

## ONSET, PEAK, DURATION
Onset and duration unknown. Serum levels peak in about 2 hours.

## INDICATIONS & DOSAGE
*Moderate to moderately severe pain* —
**Adults:** 50 to 100 mg P.O. q 4 to 6 hours, p.r.n. Maximum dosage is 400 mg daily.

## ADVERSE REACTIONS
**CNS:** *dizziness, vertigo, headache, somnolence, CNS stimulation, asthenia,* anxiety, confusion, coordination disturbance, euphoria, nervousness, sleep disorder, *seizures.*
**CV:** *vasodilation.*
**EENT:** *visual disturbances.*
**GI:** *nausea, constipation, vomiting,* dyspepsia, dry mouth, diarrhea, abdominal pain, anorexia, flatulence.
**GU:** urine retention, urinary frequency, menopausal symptoms.
**Respiratory:** *respiratory depression.*
**Skin:** *pruritus,* diaphoresis, rash.
**Other:** malaise, hypertonia.

## INTERACTIONS
*Carbamazepine:* increased tramadol metabolism. Patients receiving chronic carbamazepine therapy at a dosage of up to 800 mg daily may require up to twice the recommended dose of tramadol.
*CNS depressants:* additive effects. Use together with caution. Dosage of tramadol may need to be reduced.
*MAO inhibitors, neuroleptics:* increased risk of seizures. Monitor patient closely.

## CONTRAINDICATIONS
Contraindicated in patients with hypersensitivity to drug or with acute intoxication from alcohol, hypnotics, centrally acting analgesics, opioids, or psychotropic drugs.

## NURSING CONSIDERATIONS
• Use cautiously in risk for seizures or respiratory depression; in increased intracranial pressure or head injury, acute abdominal conditions, or renal or hepatic impairment; and in physical dependence on opioids.
• Monitor CV and respiratory status. Withhold dose and notify doctor if respirations decrease or rate is below 12 breaths/minute.
• Monitor bowel and bladder function. Anticipate the need for a laxative.
• For better analgesic effect, give drug before onset of intense pain.
• Monitor patients at risk for seizures. Drug may reduce seizure threshold.
• Monitor patient for drug dependence. It can produce dependence similar to that of codeine or dextropropoxyphene and thus has potential for abuse.

## ☑ PATIENT TEACHING
• Tell patient to take drug as prescribed and not to increase dosage or dosage interval unless ordered by doctor.
• Caution ambulatory patient to be careful when rising and walking. Warn outpatient to avoid driving and other potentially hazardous activities that require mental alertness until drug's CNS effects are known.
• Advise patient to check with doctor before taking OTC medications; drug interactions can occur.

---

Reactions may be *common,* uncommon, *life-threatening,* or **COMMON AND LIFE-THREATENING.**

amobarbital
amobarbital sodium
aprobarbital
butabarbital sodium
chloral hydrate
estazolam
ethchlorvynol
flurazepam hydrochloride
pentobarbital
pentobarbital sodium
phenobarbital sodium
   (See Chapter 30, ANTICONVULSANTS.)
quazepam
secobarbital sodium
temazepam
triazolam
zolpidem tartrate

## COMBINATION PRODUCTS
TRI-BARBS CAPSULES: phenobarbital 32 mg, butabarbital sodium 32 mg, and secobarbital sodium 32 mg.
TUINAL 50 MG PULVULES: amobarbital sodium 25 mg and secobarbital sodium 25 mg.
TUINAL 100 MG PULVULES: amobarbital sodium 50 mg and secobarbital sodium 50 mg.
TUINAL 200 MG PULVULES: amobarbital sodium 100 mg and secobarbital sodium 100 mg.

---

## amobarbital
Amytal

## amobarbital sodium
Amytal Sodium

Controlled Substance Schedule II
*Pregnancy Risk Category: D*

## HOW SUPPLIED
**amobarbital**
*Tablets:* 30 mg
**amobarbital sodium**
*Capsules:* 200 mg

*Powder for injection:* 250 mg, 500 mg

## ACTION
Unknown. A barbiturate that probably interferes with transmission of impulses from the thalamus to the cortex of the brain.

## ONSET, PEAK, DURATION
Onset occurs in 60 minutes. Peak unknown. Effects persist 10 to 12 hours.

## INDICATIONS & DOSAGE
*Sedation –*
**Adults:** usually 30 to 50 mg P.O. b.i.d. or t.i.d.
**Children:** 2 mg/kg or 70 mg/m² P.O. daily in four equally divided doses.
*Insomnia –*
**Adults:** 65 to 200 mg P.O. or deep I.M. h.s.; I.M. dose not to exceed 500 mg, I.M. injection not to exceed 5 ml in any one site.
**Children:** 2 to 3 mg/kg I.M. h.s.
*Preanesthetic sedation –*
**Adults:** 200 mg P.O. or I.M. 1 to 2 hours before surgery.
*Labor –*
**Adults:** 200 to 400 mg P.O. followed by 200 to 400 mg at 1 to 3 hour intervals up to a maximum dose of 1 g.
*Manic reactions, as an adjunct in psychotherapy, anticonvulsant –*
**Adults and children over 6 years:** 65 to 500 mg slow I.V.; not to exceed 100 mg/minute. Maximum dosage is 1 g.

## ADVERSE REACTIONS
**CNS:** *drowsiness, lethargy, hangover,* paradoxical excitement, somnolence.
**CV:** bradycardia, hypotension, syncope.
**GI:** nausea, vomiting.
**Hematologic:** exacerbation of porphyria.

---

*Liquid form contains alcohol.  **May contain tartrazine.  †Canada only.  ‡Australia only.  ◇OTC.

**Respiratory:** *respiratory depression,* apnea.
**Skin:** rash; urticaria; *Stevens-Johnson syndrome;* pain, irritation, sterile abscess at injection site.
**Other:** angioedema, physical and psychological dependence.

## INTERACTIONS
*Chloramphenicol, MAO inhibitors, valproic acid:* inhibit metabolism of barbiturates; may cause prolonged CNS depression. Reduce barbiturate dosage.
*Corticosteroids, digitoxin, doxycycline, estrogens and oral contraceptives, oral anticoagulants, tricyclic antidepressants:* amobarbital may enhance the metabolism of these drugs. Monitor for decreased effect.
*Ethanol or other CNS depressants, including narcotic analgesics:* excessive CNS and respiratory depression. Use together cautiously.
*Griseofulvin:* decreased absorption of griseofulvin. Monitor effectiveness of griseofulvin.
*Rifampin:* may decrease barbiturate levels. Monitor for decreased effect.

## CONTRAINDICATIONS
Contraindicated in patients with bronchopneumonia or other severe pulmonary insufficiency or hypersensitivity to barbiturates, or porphyria.

## NURSING CONSIDERATIONS
• Use cautiously in patients with acute or chronic pain, suicidal tendencies, depression, history of drug abuse, or hepatic or renal impairment. Use parenteral form cautiously in patients with blood pressure alterations or pulmonary or cardiovascular disease.
• Elderly patients are more sensitive to the drug's adverse CNS effects. Assess mental status before and after initiating therapy.
• To minimize deterioration, use injection solution within 30 minutes after opening container. Don't use cloudy or precipitated solution. Don't shake solution; mix with sterile water only.
• **I.V. use:** Know that I.V. injection is reserved for emergency treatment. Close supervision required. Administer slowly; do not exceed 100 mg/minute.
• I.V. administration of barbiturates may cause severe respiratory depression, laryngospasm, or hypotension. Have emergency resuscitation equipment available.
• Assess patency of I.V. site before and during administration. Local tissue reactions and injection site pain have been noted with I.V. use.
• *Alert:* Administer I.M. injection deeply. Superficial injection may cause pain, sterile abscess, and sloughing.
• Take precautions to prevent hoarding or self-overdosing by patients who are depressed, suicidal, or drug-dependent or who have a history of drug abuse.
• Be aware long-term use not recommended; drug loses its efficacy in promoting sleep after 14 days of continued use.
• Monitor patient for skin changes. Skin eruptions may precede potentially fatal reactions to barbiturate therapy. Discontinue drug when skin reactions occur and notify doctor. In some patients, high fever, stomatitis, headache, or rhinitis may precede skin reactions.
• Watch for signs of barbiturate toxicity: coma, pupillary constriction, cyanosis, clammy skin, and hypotension. Overdose can be fatal.

## ☑ PATIENT TEACHING
• Inform patient that morning "hangover" common after hypnotic dose, which also suppresses REM sleep. Patients may experience increased dreaming after drug is discontinued.

---

Reactions may be *common,* uncommon, *life-threatening,* or **COMMON AND LIFE-THREATENING.**

• Tell patient to avoid alcohol use while taking drug.
• Caution patient about performing activities that require mental alertness or physical coordination.
• Tell patient who uses oral contraceptives that she should consider alternate birth control methods because drug may enhance contraceptive hormone metabolism and decrease its effect.

## aprobarbital
Alurate*
Controlled Substance Schedule III
*Pregnancy Risk Category: D*

**HOW SUPPLIED**
*Elixir:* 40 mg/5 ml

**ACTION**
Unknown. A barbiturate that probably interferes with transmission of impulses from the thalamus to the cortex of the brain.

**ONSET, PEAK, DURATION**
Onset occurs within 45 to 60 minutes. Peak levels occur within 3 hours. Effects persist for 6 to 8 hours.

**INDICATIONS & DOSAGE**
*Sedation –*
**Adults:** 40 mg P.O. t.i.d.
*Insomnia –*
**Adults:** 40 to 160 mg P.O. h.s.

**ADVERSE REACTIONS**
**CNS:** *drowsiness, lethargy, hangover,* paradoxical excitement in elderly patients, somnolence.
**GI:** nausea, vomiting.
**Hematologic:** exacerbation of porphyria.
**Respiratory:** *respiratory depression,* apnea.
**Skin:** rash, urticaria, *Stevens-Johnson syndrome.*
**Other:** *angioedema,* physical and psychological dependence.

**INTERACTIONS**
*Chloramphenicol, MAO inhibitors, valproic acid:* inhibit metabolism of barbiturates; may cause prolonged CNS depression. Reduce barbiturate dosage.
*Corticosteroids, digitoxin, doxycycline, estrogens and oral contraceptives, oral anticoagulants, tricyclic antidepressants:* aprobarbital may enhance the metabolism of these drugs. Monitor for decreased effectiveness.
*Ethanol or other CNS depressants, including narcotic analgesics:* excessive CNS and respiratory depression. Use together cautiously.
*Griseofulvin:* decreased absorption of griseofulvin. Monitor effectiveness of griseofulvin.
*Rifampin:* may decrease barbiturate levels. Monitor for decreased effect.

**CONTRAINDICATIONS**
Contraindicated in patients with hypersensitivity to barbiturates, bronchopneumonia or other severe pulmonary insufficiency, or porphyria.

**NURSING CONSIDERATIONS**
• Use cautiously in patients with acute or chronic pain, suicidal tendencies, depression, history of drug abuse, or hepatic or renal impairment.
• Take precautions to prevent hoarding or self-overdosing by patients who are depressed, suicidal, or drug-dependent or who have a history of drug abuse.
• Be aware that long-term use is not recommended; drug loses its efficacy in promoting sleep after 14 days of continued use.
• Watch for signs of barbiturate toxicity: coma, pupillary constriction, cyanosis, clammy skin, and hypotension. Overdose can be fatal.
• Assess patient's skin. Skin eruptions may precede potentially fatal reactions to barbiturate therapy. Discontinue drug when skin reactions occur.

*Liquid form contains alcohol. **May contain tartrazine. †Canada only. ‡Australia only. ◇OTC.

In some patients, high fever, stomatitis, headache, or rhinitis may precede skin reactions.

### ☑ PATIENT TEACHING
● Tell patient that morning "hangover" common after hypnotic dose, which also suppresses REM sleep. Patients may experience increased dreaming after drug is discontinued.
● Tell patient to avoid alcohol use while taking drug.
● Caution patient about performing activities that require mental alertness or physical coordination.
● Tell patient who uses oral contraceptives that she should consider alternate birth control methods because drug may enhance contraceptive hormone metabolism and decrease its effect.

---

## butabarbital sodium (butabarbitone sodium)
Butalan*, Butisol* **, Saneryl‡, Sarisol No. 2* **
Controlled Substance Schedule III
*Pregnancy Risk Category: D*

### HOW SUPPLIED
*Tablets:* 15 mg, 30 mg, 50 mg, 100 mg
*Elixir:* 30 mg/5 ml, 33.3 mg/5 ml

### ACTION
Unknown. A barbiturate that probably interferes with transmission of impulses from the thalamus to the cortex of the brain.

### ONSET, PEAK, DURATION
Onset occurs in 45 to 60 minutes. Peak levels occur within 3 hours. Effects persist 6 to 8 hours.

### INDICATIONS & DOSAGE
*Sedation –*
**Adults:** 15 to 30 mg P.O. t.i.d. or q.i.d.
**Children:** 6 mg/kg or 180 mg/m² P.O.

divided t.i.d. Dosage range is 7.5 to 30 mg P.O. t.i.d.
*Preoperatively –*
**Adults:** 50 to 100 mg P.O. 60 to 90 minutes before surgery.
**Children:** 2 to 6 mg/kg P.O. (not to exceed 100 mg) 60 to 90 minutes before surgery.
*Insomnia –*
**Adults:** 50 to 100 mg P.O. h.s.

### ADVERSE REACTIONS
**CNS:** *drowsiness, lethargy, hangover,* paradoxical excitement in elderly patients, somnolence.
**GI:** nausea, vomiting.
**Hematologic:** exacerbation of porphyria.
**Respiratory:** *respiratory depression,* apnea.
**Skin:** rash, urticaria, *Stevens-Johnson syndrome.*
**Other:** *angioedema,* physical and psychological dependence.

### INTERACTIONS
*Chloramphenicol, MAO inhibitors, valproic acid:* inhibited metabolism of barbiturates; may cause prolonged CNS depression. Reduce barbiturate dosage.
*Corticosteroids, digitoxin, doxycycline, estrogens and oral contraceptives, oral anticoagulants, tricyclic antidepressants:* barbiturates may enhance the metabolism of these drugs. Monitor for decreased effectiveness.
*Ethanol or other CNS depressants, including narcotic analgesics:* excessive CNS and respiratory depression. Use together cautiously.
*Griseofulvin:* decreased absorption of griseofulvin. Monitor effectiveness of griseofulvin.
*Rifampin:* may decrease barbiturate levels. Monitor for decreased effect.

### CONTRAINDICATIONS
Contraindicated in patients with bronchopneumonia, or other severe pul-

---

Reactions may be *common,* uncommon, *life-threatening,* or COMMON AND LIFE-THREATENING.

monary insufficiency, hypersensitivity to barbiturates, or porphyria.

## NURSING CONSIDERATIONS
• Use cautiously in patients with acute or chronic pain, depression, suicidal tendencies, history of drug abuse, or hepatic or renal impairment.
• Elderly patients are more sensitive to drug's adverse CNS reactions. Assess mental status before and after initiating therapy.
• Take precautions to prevent hoarding or self-overdosing by patients who are depressed, suicidal, or drug-dependent or who have a history of drug abuse.
• Watch for signs of barbiturate toxicity: coma, pupillary constriction, cyanosis, clammy skin, and hypotension. Overdose can be fatal.
• Discontinue drug when skin reactions occur because skin eruptions may precede potentially fatal reactions to barbiturate therapy. In some patients, high fever, stomatitis, headache, or rhinitis may precede skin reactions.
• Long-term use is not recommended; drug loses its efficacy in promoting sleep after 14 days. A drug-free interval of at least 1 week is advised if continued treatment is appropriate. Long-term high dosage may cause drug dependence, and patients may experience withdrawal symptoms if drug is suddenly stopped. Withdraw barbiturates gradually.

## ☑ PATIENT TEACHING
• Tell patient that morning "hangover" common after hypnotic dose. Hypnotic doses suppress REM sleep. Patients may experience increased dreaming after drug is discontinued.
• Tell patient to avoid alcohol use while taking drug.
• Caution patient about performing activities that require mental alertness or physical coordination.

• Tell patient who uses oral contraceptives that she should consider alternate birth control methods because drug may enhance contraceptive hormone metabolism and decrease its effect.

---

# chloral hydrate
Aquachloral Supprettes, Dormel‡, Novo-Chlorhydrate†
Controlled Substance Schedule IV
*Pregnancy Risk Category: C*

## HOW SUPPLIED
*Capsules:* 250 mg, 500 mg
*Syrup:* 250 mg/5 ml, 500 mg/5 ml
*Suppositories:* 324 mg, 500 mg, 648 mg

## ACTION
Unknown. Sedative effects may be caused by its primary metabolite, trichloroethanol.

## ONSET, PEAK, DURATION
Onset occurs within 30 minutes. Peak unknown. Effects persist 4 to 8 hours.

## INDICATIONS & DOSAGE
*Sedation –*
**Adults:** 250 mg P.O. or P.R. t.i.d. after meals.
**Children:** 8.3 mg/kg or 250 mg/m$^2$ P.O. or P.R. t.i.d. Maximum daily dosage is 500 mg t.i.d.
*Insomnia –*
**Adults:** 500 mg to 1 g P.O. or P.R. 15 to 30 minutes before bedtime.
**Children:** 50 mg/kg or 1.5 g/m$^2$ P.O. or P.R. 15 to 30 minutes before bedtime. Maximum single dose is 1 g.
*Preoperatively –*
**Adults:** 500 mg to 1 g P.O. or P.R. 30 minutes before surgery.
*Premedication for EEG –*
**Children:** 20 to 25 mg/kg P.O. or P.R.
*Management of alcohol withdrawal symptoms –*

---

*Liquid form contains alcohol. **May contain tartrazine. †Canada only. ‡Australia only. ◊OTC.

**Adults:** 500 mg to 1 g P.O. or P.R. q 6 hours p.r.n., not to exceed 2 g daily.

## ADVERSE REACTIONS

**CNS:** drowsiness, nightmares, dizziness, ataxia, paradoxical excitement, hangover, somnolence, disorientation, delirium, light-headedness, hallucinations, confusion, vertigo, malaise.
**GI:** *nausea, vomiting, diarrhea,* flatulence.
**Hematologic:** eosinophilia, leukopenia.
**Skin:** hypersensitivity reactions (rash, urticaria).
**Other:** physical and psychological dependence.

## INTERACTIONS

*Alkaline solutions:* incompatible with aqueous solutions of chloral hydrate. Don't mix together.
*Ethanol or other CNS depressants, including narcotic analgesics:* excessive CNS depression or vasodilation reaction. Use together cautiously.
*Furosemide I.V.:* causes sweating, flushes, variable blood pressure, nausea, and uneasiness. Use together cautiously or use a different hypnotic drug.
*Oral anticoagulants:* increased risk of bleeding. Monitor patient closely.
*Phenytoin:* decreased phenytoin levels. Monitor closely.

## CONTRAINDICATIONS

Contraindicated in patients with hepatic or renal impairment, severe cardiac disease, or in those with hypersensitivity to chloral hydrate. Oral administration contraindicated in patients with gastric disorders.

## NURSING CONSIDERATIONS

• Use with extreme caution in patients with severe cardiac disease. Use cautiously in patients with mental depression, suicidal tendencies, or history of drug abuse.
• **Alert:** Note two strengths of oral liquid form. Double-check dose, especially when administering to children. Fatal overdoses have occurred.
• To minimize unpleasant taste and stomach irritation, dilute or administer with liquid. Drug should be taken after meals.
• Take precautions to prevent hoarding or self-overdosing by patients who are depressed, suicidal, or drug-dependent or who have a history of drug abuse.
• Be aware that long-term use is not recommended; drug loses its efficacy in promoting sleep after 14 days of continued use. Long-term use may cause drug dependence, and patient may experience withdrawal symptoms if drug is suddenly stopped.
• Monitor BUN levels as ordered. Large dosage may raise BUN levels.
• May interfere with fluorometric tests for urine catecholamines and Reddy-Jenkins-Thorn test for urine 17-hydroxycorticosteroids. Do not administer drug for 48 hours before fluorometric test as ordered. May also cause false-positive results in urine glucose tests that use copper sulfate. Use glucose enzymatic tests instead.

☑ **PATIENT TEACHING**
• Instruct patient to take capsules with a full glass of water or juice and to swallow the capsule whole.
• Tell patient to avoid alcohol use while taking drug.
• Caution patients about performing activities that require mental alertness or physical coordination.
• Tell patient to store drug in dark container; store suppositories in refrigerator.

## estazolam
ProSom
Controlled Substance Schedule IV
*Pregnancy Risk Category: X*

---

Reactions may be *common,* uncommon, *life-threatening,* or COMMON AND LIFE-THREATENING.

**HOW SUPPLIED**
*Tablets:* 1 mg, 2 mg

**ACTION**
Unknown. Thought to act on the limbic system and thalamus of the CNS by binding to specific benzodiazepine receptors.

**ONSET, PEAK, DURATION**
Onset and duration unknown. Serum levels peak in 1 to 3 hours.

**INDICATIONS & DOSAGE**
*Insomnia –*
**Adults:** 1 mg P.O. h.s. Some patients may require 2 mg.
**Elderly patients:** 1 mg P.O. h.s. Use higher doses with extreme care. Frail elderly or debilitated patients may take 0.5 mg, but this low dose may be only marginally effective.

**ADVERSE REACTIONS**
**CNS:** fatigue, dizziness, *daytime drowsiness, somnolence, asthenia, hypokinesia,* abnormal thinking.
**GI:** dyspepsia, abdominal pain.
**Other:** back pain, stiffness.

**INTERACTIONS**
*Cigarette smoking, rifampin:* may increase metabolism and clearance and decrease plasma half-life. Monitor for decreased effectiveness.
*Cimetidine, disulfiram, isoniazid, oral contraceptives:* may impair the metabolism and clearance of benzodiazepines and prolong their plasma half-life. Monitor for increased CNS depression.
*CNS depressants, including antihistamines, opiate analgesics, and other benzodiazepines; ethanol:* increased CNS depression. Avoid concomitant use.
*Theophylline:* pharmacologic antagonism. Monitor for decreased effectiveness.

**CONTRAINDICATIONS**
Contraindicated in pregnant patients or patients with hypersensitivity to drug.

**NURSING CONSIDERATIONS**
● Use cautiously in patients with hepatic, renal, or pulmonary disease; depression, or suicidal tendencies.
● Liver and renal function and CBC should be checked before and periodically during long-term therapy as ordered.
● Take precautions to prevent hoarding by depressed, suicidal, or drug-dependent patients or those who have a history of drug abuse.
● Be aware that patients who receive prolonged treatment with benzodiazepines may experience withdrawal symptoms if the drug is suddenly discontinued (possibly after 6 weeks of continuous therapy).

☑ **PATIENT TEACHING**
● Tell patient not to increase dosage of the drug but to inform the doctor if he thinks that the drug is no longer effective.
● Caution patient about performing activities that require mental alertness or physical coordination.
● Warn patient that additive depressant effects can occur if alcohol is consumed while taking this drug or within 24 hours after taking drug.
● Tell patient who uses oral contraceptives that she should consider alternate birth control methods when taking this drug because drug may enhance contraceptive hormone metabolism and decrease its effect.

# ethchlorvynol
Placidyl**
Controlled Substance Schedule IV
*Pregnancy Risk Category: C*

**HOW SUPPLIED**
*Capsules:* 200 mg, 500 mg, 750 mg**

---

*Liquid form contains alcohol.  **May contain tartrazine.  †Canada only.  ‡Australia only.  ◊OTC.

## ACTION
Unknown; pharmacologic effects are similar to those produced by barbiturates.

## ONSET, PEAK, DURATION
Onset occurs within 30 minutes to 1 hour. Plasma levels peak within 1 to 2 hours. Effects persist about 5 hours.

## INDICATIONS & DOSAGE
*Insomnia* –
**Adults:** 500 mg to 1 g P.O. h.s. An additional 200 mg dose P.O. if awakened in early morning.

## ADVERSE REACTIONS
**CNS:** facial numbness, dizziness, hangover, ataxia, transient giddiness, syncope, hysteria, muscular weakness.
**CV:** hypotension.
**EENT:** unpleasant aftertaste, blurred vision.
**GI:** nausea, vomiting, gastric upset.
**Hematologic:** *thrombocytopenia,* exacerbation of porphyria.
**Skin:** rashes, urticaria.
**Other:** physical and psychological dependence, cholestatic jaundice.

## INTERACTIONS
*Ethanol or other CNS depressants, including MAO inhibitors, narcotic analgesics, and tricyclic antidepressants:* excessive CNS depression. Use together cautiously.
*Oral anticoagulants:* ethchlorvynol may enhance the metabolism of coumarin derivatives, decreasing their effectiveness. Monitor patient closely.

## CONTRAINDICATIONS
Contraindicated in patients with hypersensitivity to this drug and in those with porphyria.

## NURSING CONSIDERATIONS
• Use cautiously in patients with hepatic or renal impairment, in elderly or debilitated patients, mental depression, and in those with suicidal tendencies.
• Minimize transient dizziness or ataxia, which is caused by rapid absorption, by giving this drug with milk or food.
• Take precautions to prevent hoarding or self-overdosing by patients who are depressed, suicidal, or drug-dependent or who have a history of drug abuse. Overdose is difficult to treat and is associated with high mortality.
• Monitor patient for allergic reactions. The 750-mg strength contains tartrazine dye, which may cause allergic reactions in susceptible patients.
• Watch for signs of toxicity, such as poor muscle coordination, confusion, hypothermia, speech or vision disturbances, tremor, and weakness.
• Be aware that drug is effective for short-term use only; treatment period should not exceed 1 week.
• Know that slight darkening of liquid from exposure to air and light doesn't affect safety or potency, but store in tight, light-resistant container to avoid possible deterioration.

## ☑ PATIENT TEACHING
• Tell patient to take drug with milk or food if dizziness or ataxia occurs.
• Tell patient to avoid alcohol use while taking drug.
• Caution patient about performing activities that require mental alertness or physical coordination.

---

# flurazepam hydrochloride
Apo-Flurazepam†, Dalmane, Novoflupam†
Controlled Substance Schedule IV
*Pregnancy Risk Category: NR*

## HOW SUPPLIED
*Capsules:* 15 mg, 30 mg

## ACTION
Unknown. A benzodiazepine that is thought to act on the limbic system, thalamus, and hypothalamus of the CNS to produce hypnotic effects.

## ONSET, PEAK, DURATION
Onset and duration unknown. Peak effects occur in ½ to 1 hour.

## INDICATIONS & DOSAGE
*Insomnia* –
**Adults:** 15 to 30 mg P.O. h.s. Dose repeated once, p.r.n.

## ADVERSE REACTIONS
**CNS:** *daytime sedation, dizziness, drowsiness, disturbed coordination,* lethargy, confusion, *headache,* lightheadedness, nervousness, hallucinations, staggering, ataxia, disorientation, *coma.*
**GI:** nausea, vomiting, heartburn, diarrhea, abdominal pain.
**Hepatic:** elevated liver enzymes.
**Other:** physical or psychological dependence.

## INTERACTIONS
*Cigarette smoking, rifampin:* enhanced metabolism of benzodiazepines. Monitor for decreased effectiveness.
*Cimetidine:* increased sedation. Monitor carefully.
*Disulfiram, isoniazid, oral contraceptives:* decreased metabolism of benzodiazepines, leading to toxicity. Monitor closely.
*Ethanol or other CNS depressants, including narcotic analgesics:* excessive CNS depression. Use together cautiously.
*Phenytoin:* increased phenytoin levels. Monitor for toxicity.

## CONTRAINDICATIONS
Contraindicated in patients with hypersensitivity to the drug and during pregnancy.

## NURSING CONSIDERATIONS
• Use cautiously in patients with impaired hepatic or renal function, chronic pulmonary insufficiency, mental depression, suicidal tendencies, or history of drug abuse.
• Check hepatic and renal function and CBC before and periodically during long-term therapy. May cause elevations in certain liver function tests (AST, ALT, total and direct bilirubin, and alkaline phosphatase).
• Assess mental status before initiating therapy. Elderly patients are more sensitive to the drug's adverse CNS reactions.
• Take precautions to prevent hoarding or self-overdosing by patients who are depressed, suicidal, or drug-dependent or who have a history of drug abuse.
• Be aware that physical and psychological dependence is possible with long-term use.

## ☑ PATIENT TEACHING
• Advise patient that this drug is more effective on second, third, and fourth nights because active metabolite accumulates. Encourage him to continue drug even if it doesn't relieve insomnia the first night.
• Tell patient to avoid alcohol use while taking this drug.
• Caution patient about performing activities that require mental alertness or physical coordination.
• Tell patient who uses oral contraceptives that she should consider alternate birth control methods when taking this drug.

---

*Liquid form contains alcohol.  **May contain tartrazine.  †Canada only.  ‡Australia only.  ◇OTC.

# pentobarbital
# (pentobarbitone)
Nembutal* **

# pentobarbital sodium
Carbrital‡, Nembutal Sodium*,
Nova Rectal†, Novopentobarb†

Controlled Substance Schedule II
*Pregnancy Risk Category: D*

## HOW SUPPLIED
**pentobarbital**
*Elixir:* 18.2 mg/5 ml
**pentobarbital sodium**
*Capsules:* 50 mg, 100 mg
*Injection:* 50 mg/ml
*Suppositories:* 30 mg, 60 mg, 120 mg,
200 mg

## ACTION
Unknown. Probably interferes with
transmission of impulses from the
thalamus to the cortex of the brain. A
barbiturate.

## ONSET, PEAK, DURATION
Onset occurs immediately after I.V.
administration, within 10 to 25 minutes after I.M. administration, within
15 minutes after oral or rectal administration. Serum levels peak immediately after I.V. administration, 30 to
60 minutes with oral dose, unknown
for I.M. or rectal routes. Effects persist 1 to 4 hours following oral or rectal administration, 15 minutes following I.V. administration, unknown for
I.M. administration.

## INDICATIONS & DOSAGE
*Sedation –*
**Adults:** 20 to 40 mg P.O. b.i.d.,
t.i.d., or q.i.d.
**Children:** 2 to 6 mg/kg daily P.O. in
3 divided doses. Maximum daily dos-
age is 100 mg.
*Insomnia –*
**Adults:** 100 to 200 mg P.O. h.s. or
150 to 200 mg deep I.M.; 100 mg ini-

tially I.V., then additional doses up to
500 mg; 120 or 200 mg P.R.
**Children:** 2 to 6 mg/kg or 125 mg/m2
I.M. Maximum dosage is 100 mg.
P.R. dose for child 2 months to 1 year
is 30 mg; 1 to 4 years, 30 or 60 mg; 5
to 11 years, 60 mg; 12 to 14 years, 60
or 120 mg.
*Preoperative sedation –*
**Adults:** 150 to 200 mg I.M.
**Children:** 5 mg/kg P.O. or I.M. if 10
years or older; 5 mg/kg I.M. or P.R.
if younger than 10 years.

## ADVERSE REACTIONS
**CNS:** *drowsiness, lethargy, hangover,*
paradoxical excitement in elderly pa-
tients, somnolence.
**GI:** nausea, vomiting.
**Hematologic:** exacerbation of por-
phyria.
**Respiratory:** *respiratory depression.*
**Skin:** rash, urticaria, ***Stevens-John-
son syndrome.***
**Other:** *angioedema,* physical and
psychological dependence.

## INTERACTIONS
*Corticosteroids, doxycycline, estro-
gens and oral contraceptives, oral anticoagulants:* pentobarbital may enhance the metabolism of these drugs.
Monitor for decreased effect.
*Ethanol or other CNS depressants, in-
cluding narcotic analgesics:* excessive
CNS and respiratory depression. Use
together cautiously.
*Griseofulvin:* decreased absorption of
griseofulvin. Monitor effectiveness of
griseofulvin.
*MAO inhibitors:* inhibited metabolism
of barbiturates; may cause prolonged
CNS depression. Reduce barbiturate
dosage.
*Rifampin:* may decrease barbiturate
levels. Monitor for decreased effect.

## CONTRAINDICATIONS
Contraindicated in patients with hypersensitivity to barbiturates, or porphyria.

Reactions may be *common,* uncommon, *life-threatening,* or COMMON AND LIFE-THREATENING.

## NURSING CONSIDERATIONS
• Use cautiously in patients with acute or chronic pain, mental depression, suicidal tendencies, history of drug abuse, or hepatic impairment. Also administer cautiously to elderly or debilitated patients.
• Assess mental status before initiating therapy and use reduced doses as ordered. Elderly patients are more sensitive to the drug's adverse CNS effects.
• **I.V. use:** I.V. administration of barbiturates may cause severe respiratory depression, laryngospasm, or hypotension. Have emergency resuscitation equipment available.
• To minimize deterioration, use I.V injection solution within 30 minutes after opening container. Don't use cloudy solution.
• Reserve I.V. injection for emergency treatment, which should be given under close supervision. Administer slowly at a rate not exceeding 50 mg/minute.
• Parenteral solution is alkaline. Local tissue reactions and injection site pain have followed I.V. use. Avoid extravasation. Assess patency of I.V. site before and during administration.
• Do not mix in syringe or in I.V. solutions or lines with other drugs.
• *Alert:* Administer I.M. injection deeply. Superficial injection may cause pain, sterile abscess, and sloughing.
• To ensure accurate dosage, don't divide suppositories.
• Take precautions to prevent hoarding or self-overdosing by patients who are depressed, suicidal, or drug-dependent or who have a history of drug abuse.
• Watch for signs of barbiturate toxicity: coma, pupillary constriction, cyanosis, clammy skin, and hypotension. Overdose can be fatal.
• Inspect patient's skin. Skin eruptions may precede potentially fatal reactions to barbiturate therapy. Dis-

continue drug when skin reactions occur and call doctor. In some patients, high fever, stomatitis, headache, or rhinitis may precede skin reactions.
• Know that pentobarbital has no analgesic effect and may cause restlessness or delirium in patients with pain.
• Be aware that long-term use is not recommended; drug loses its efficacy in promoting sleep after 14 days of continued use. Long-term high dosage may cause drug dependence, and patient may experience withdrawal symptoms if drug is suddenly discontinued. Withdraw barbiturates gradually.

### ☑ PATIENT TEACHING
• Inform patient that morning "hangover" is common after hypnotic dose, which suppresses REM sleep. Patient may experience increased dreaming after drug is discontinued.
• Caution patient about performing activities that require mental alertness or physical coordination.
• Tell patient to avoid alcohol use while taking drug.
• Tell patient who uses oral contraceptives that she should consider alternate birth control methods because drug may enhance contraceptive hormone metabolism and decrease its effect.

## quazepam
Doral
Controlled Substance Schedule IV
*Pregnancy Risk Category: X*

### HOW SUPPLIED
*Tablets:* 7.5 mg, 15 mg

### ACTION
Unknown, although drug acts on the limbic system and thalamus of the CNS by binding to specific benzodiazepine receptors.

**ONSET, PEAK, DURATION**
Onset and duration unknown. Plasma levels peak in about 2 hours.

**INDICATIONS & DOSAGE**
*Insomnia –*
**Adults:** 15 mg P.O. h.s. Some patients may respond to lower dosages. Dosage decreased in elderly patients after 2 days of therapy if possible.

**ADVERSE REACTIONS**
**CNS:** *fatigue, dizziness, daytime drowsiness, headache.*
**GI:** dry mouth, dyspepsia.
**Other:** physical and psychological dependence.

**INTERACTIONS**
*Anticonvulsants, antihistamines, ethanol, psychotropic drugs, and other drugs that produce CNS depression:* additive CNS depressant effects. Avoid concomitant use.

**CONTRAINDICATIONS**
Contraindicated in patients with hypersensitivity to this drug or other benzodiazepines, in pregnant patients, and in patients with suspected or established sleep apnea.

**NURSING CONSIDERATIONS**
● Use cautiously in patients with hepatic, renal, or respiratory disease, depression, and in elderly patients.
● Take precautions to prevent hoarding or self-overdosing by patients who are depressed, suicidal, or drug-dependent or who have a history of drug abuse.
● Be aware that patients on long-term therapy with benzodiazepines may experience withdrawal symptoms if the drug is suddenly withdrawn (possibly after 6 weeks of continuous therapy).

**☑ PATIENT TEACHING**
● Warn patient not to increase the drug dosage but to inform the doctor if he thinks that drug is not effective.

● Caution patient about performing activities that require mental alertness or physical coordination.
● Warn patient about the possible additive depressant effects that can occur if alcohol is consumed within 24 hours of quazepam.

# secobarbital sodium
Novosecobarb†, Seconal Sodium
Controlled Substance Schedule II
*Pregnancy Risk Category: D*

**HOW SUPPLIED**
*Capsules:* 50 mg, 100 mg
*Injection:* 50 mg/ml

**ACTION**
Unknown. Probably interferes with transmission of impulses from the thalamus to the cortex of the brain. A barbiturate.

**ONSET, PEAK, DURATION**
Onset occurs within 15 minutes with oral dose, almost immediate with I.V. dose, unknown for I.M. administration. Serum levels peak 1 to 3 minutes with I.V. administration, 7 to 10 minutes with I.M. administration, and 15 to 30 minutes with oral dose. Effects persist for 1 to 4 hours for oral dose, 15 minutes for I.V. dose, unknown for I.M. dose.

**INDICATIONS & DOSAGE**
*Preoperative sedation –*
**Adults:** 100 to 300 mg P.O. 1 to 2 hours before surgery.
**Children:** 50 to 100 mg P.O. 1 to 2 hours before surgery. Maximum single dose is 100 mg.
*Insomnia –*
**Adults:** 100 to 200 mg P.O. or I.M.
**Children:** 3 to 5 mg/kg I.M. or 125 mg/m$^2$, not to exceed 100 mg, with no more than 5 ml injected in any one site.
*Acute tetanus seizure –*
**Adults and children:** 5.5 mg/kg I.M.

---

Reactions may be *common,* uncommon, *life-threatening,* or **COMMON AND LIFE-THREATENING.**

or slow I.V., repeated q 3 to 4 hours, if needed; I.V. injection rate not to exceed 50 mg/15 seconds.
*Status epilepticus –*
**Children:** 15 to 20 mg/kg I.V. over 15 minutes.

## ADVERSE REACTIONS
**CNS:** *drowsiness, lethargy, hangover,* paradoxical excitement in elderly patients, somnolence.
**CV:** hypotension (with I.V. use).
**GI:** nausea, vomiting.
**Hematologic:** exacerbation of porphyria.
**Respiratory:** *respiratory depression.*
**Skin:** rash, urticaria, *Stevens-Johnson syndrome,* tissue reactions and injection-site pain.
**Other:** *angioedema,* physical and psychological dependence.

## INTERACTIONS
*Chloramphenicol, MAO inhibitors, valproic acid:* inhibited metabolism of barbiturates; may cause prolonged CNS depression. Reduce barbiturate dosage.
*Corticosteroids, digitoxin, doxycycline, estrogens and oral contraceptives, oral anticoagulants, tricyclic antidepressants:* secobarbital may enhance the metabolism of these drugs. Monitor for decreased effect.
*Ethanol or other CNS depressants, including narcotic analgesics:* excessive CNS and respiratory depression. Use together cautiously.
*Griseofulvin:* decreased absorption of griseofulvin. Monitor effectiveness of griseofulvin.
*Lactated Ringer's solution, acidic solutions:* incompatible with I.V. form of drug. Don't mix.
*Rifampin:* may decrease barbiturate levels. Monitor for decreased effect.

## CONTRAINDICATIONS
Contraindicated in patients with marked liver impairment, respiratory disease in which dyspnea or obstruc-tion is evident, hypersensitivity to barbiturates, or porphyria.

## NURSING CONSIDERATIONS
• Use cautiously in patients with acute or chronic pain, depression, suicidal tendencies, history of drug abuse, or hepatic impairment.
• Assess mental status before initiating therapy. Elderly patients are more sensitive to the drug's adverse CNS effects.
• **I.V. use:** Know that I.V. injection is reserved for emergency treatment and given under close supervision by direct injection and administered slowly at a rate not exceeding 50 mg/15 seconds. May be administered as supplied or diluted.
• Local tissue reactions and injection-site pain have been noted with I.V. use. Assess patency of I.V. site before and during administration.
• I.V. administration of barbiturates may cause severe respiratory depression, laryngospasm, or hypotension. Have emergency resuscitation equipment readily available.
• Know that secobarbital sodium injection is not compatible with lactated Ringer's solution, but is compatible with Ringer's solution, sterile water for injection, and 0.9% sodium chloride. Don't mix with acidic solutions.
• Use injection solution within 30 minutes after opening container to minimize deterioration. Don't use cloudy solution.
• *Alert:* Give I.M. injection deeply. Superficial injection may cause pain, sterile abscess, and sloughing.
• Take precautions to prevent hoarding or self-overdosing by patients who are depressed, suicidal, or drug-dependent or who have a history of drug abuse.
• Watch for signs of barbiturate toxicity: coma, pupillary constriction, cyanosis, clammy skin, and hypotension. Overdose can be fatal.
• Inspect patient's skin. Skin erup-

tions may precede potentially fatal reactions to barbiturate therapy. Discontinue drug when skin reactions occur and notify doctor. In some patients, high fever, stomatitis, headache, or rhinitis may precede skin reactions.

• Be aware that long-term use is not recommended; drug loses its efficacy in promoting sleep after 14 days of continued use.

☑ **PATIENT TEACHING**
• Tell patient that morning "hangover" is common after hypnotic dose, which suppresses REM sleep. Patient may experience increased dreaming after drug is discontinued.
• Tell patient to avoid alcohol use while taking drug.
• Caution patient about performing activities that require mental alertness or physical coordination.
• Tell patient who uses oral contraceptives that she should consider alternate birth control methods because drug may enhance contraceptive hormone metabolism and decrease its effect.

---

## temazepam
Euhypnos 10‡, Euhypnos 20‡, Normison‡, Restoril, Temaze‡
Controlled Substance Schedule IV
*Pregnancy Risk Category: X*

### HOW SUPPLIED
*Capsules:* 10 mg‡, 15 mg, 20 mg‡, 30 mg

### ACTION
Unknown. A benzodiazepine that probably acts on the limbic system, thalamus, and hypothalamus of the CNS to produce hypnotic effects.

### ONSET, PEAK, DURATION
Onset and duration unknown. Serum levels peak in 1 to 2 hours.

### INDICATIONS & DOSAGE
*Insomnia* –
**Adults:** 7.5 to 30 mg P.O. h.s.
**Adults over 65 years:** 7.5 mg P.O. h.s.

### ADVERSE REACTIONS
**CNS:** *drowsiness, dizziness, lethargy,* disturbed coordination, daytime sedation, confusion, nightmares, vertigo, euphoria, weakness, headache, fatigue, nervousness, anxiety, depression.
**EENT:** blurred vision.
**GI:** diarrhea, nausea, dry mouth.
**Other:** physical and psychological dependence.

### INTERACTIONS
*Ethanol or other CNS depressants, including narcotic analgesics:* increased CNS depression. Use together cautiously.

### CONTRAINDICATIONS
Contraindicated in patients with hypersensitivity to this drug or other benzodiazepines and during pregnancy.

### NURSING CONSIDERATIONS
• Use cautiously in patients with chronic pulmonary insufficiency, impaired hepatic or renal function, severe or latent mental depression, suicidal tendencies, and history of drug abuse.
• Assess mental status before initiating therapy. Elderly patients are more sensitive to the drug's adverse CNS effects.
• Take precautions to prevent hoarding or self-overdosing by patients who are depressed, suicidal, or drug-dependent or who have a history of drug abuse.

☑ **PATIENT TEACHING**
• Tell patient to avoid alcohol use while taking drug.
• Caution patient about performing

---

Reactions may be *common,* uncommon, *life-threatening,* or **COMMON AND LIFE-THREATENING.**

activities that require mental alertness or physical coordination.
• Tell patient that onset of the drug's effects may take as long as 2 to 2½ hours.

## triazolam
Apo-Triazo†, Halcion, Novo-Triolam†, Nu-Triazo†
Controlled Substance Schedule IV
*Pregnancy Risk Category: X*

### HOW SUPPLIED
*Tablets:* 0.125 mg, 0.25 mg

### ACTION
Unknown. A benzodiazepine that probably acts on the limbic system, thalamus, and hypothalamus of the CNS to produce hypnotic effects.

### ONSET, PEAK, DURATION
Onset and duration unknown. Serum levels peak in 1 to 2 hours.

### INDICATIONS & DOSAGE
*Insomnia –*
**Adults:** 0.125 to 0.5 mg P.O. h.s.
**Adults over 65:** 0.125 mg P.O. h.s.; increased, as needed, to 0.25 mg P.O. h.s.

### ADVERSE REACTIONS
**CNS:** *drowsiness, dizziness, headache,* rebound insomnia, amnesia, light-headedness, lack of coordination, mental confusion, depression, nervousness, ataxia.
**GI:** nausea, vomiting.
**Other:** physical or psychological dependence.

### INTERACTIONS
*Cimetidine, erythromycin:* may cause prolonged triazolam blood levels. Monitor for increased sedation.
*Ethanol or other CNS depressants, including narcotic analgesics:* excessive CNS depression. Use together cautiously.

### CONTRAINDICATIONS
Contraindicated in patients with hypersensitivity to benzodiazepines and during pregnancy.

### NURSING CONSIDERATIONS
• Use cautiously in patients with impaired hepatic or renal function, chronic pulmonary insufficiency, sleep apnea, mental depression, suicidal tendencies, or history of drug abuse.
• Assess mental status before initiating therapy. Elderly patients are more sensitive to the drug's CNS effects.
• Take precautions to prevent hoarding or self-overdosing by patients who are depressed, suicidal, or drug-dependent or who have a history of drug abuse.

### ☑ PATIENT TEACHING
• Warn patient not to take more than the prescribed amount because overdose can occur at a total daily dose of 2 mg (or four times the highest recommended amount).
• Tell patient to avoid alcohol while taking drug.
• Caution patient about performing activities that require mental alertness or physical coordination.
• Inform patient that drug is short-acting and therefore has less tendency to cause morning drowsiness.
• Tell patient that rebound insomnia may develop for one or two nights after stopping therapy.

## zolpidem tartrate
Ambien
Controlled Substance Schedule IV
*Pregnancy Risk Category: B*

### HOW SUPPLIED
*Tablets:* 5 mg, 10 mg

### ACTION
Although zolpidem interacts with one of three identified gamma-aminobu-

tyric acid—benzodiazepine receptor complexes, it's not a benzodiazepine. It exhibits hypnotic activity, but no muscle relaxant or anticonvulsant properties.

## ONSET, PEAK, DURATION
Onset rapid. Serum levels peak within ½ to 2 hours. Duration unknown.

## INDICATIONS & DOSAGE
*Short-term management of insomnia—*
**Adults:** 10 mg P.O. immediately before bedtime.

In elderly or debilitated patients and in patients with hepatic insufficiency, 5 mg P.O. immediately before bedtime. Maximum daily dosage is 10 mg.

## ADVERSE REACTIONS
**CNS:** daytime drowsiness, light-headedness, abnormal dreams, amnesia, dizziness, *headache,* hangover, sleep disorder, lethargy, depression.
**CV:** palpitations.
**EENT:** sinusitis, pharyngitis, dry mouth.
**GI:** nausea, vomiting, diarrhea, dyspepsia, constipation, abdominal pain.
**Skin:** rash.
**Other:** back or chest pain, flulike-symptoms, hypersensitivity reactions, myalgia, arthralgia.

## INTERACTIONS
*Ethanol or other CNS depressants:* enhanced CNS depression. Avoid concomitant use.

## CONTRAINDICATIONS
None known.

## NURSING CONSIDERATIONS
● Use cautiously in patients with diseases or conditions that could affect metabolism or hemodynamic responses and in those with compromised respiratory status because hypnotics may depress respiratory drive. Also use cautiously in patients with depression or a history of alcohol or drug abuse.
● Be aware that hypnotics should be used only for short-term management of insomnia, usually 7 to 10 days. Persistent insomnia may indicate a primary psychiatric or medical disorder.
● Know that because most adverse reactions are dose-related, the smallest effective dose should be used in all patients, especially in elderly and debilitated patients.
● Take precautions to prevent hoarding or self-overdosing by patients who are depressed, suicidal, or drug-dependent or who have a history of drug abuse.

## ☑ PATIENT TEACHING
● For faster sleep onset, instruct patient not to take drug with or immediately after meals. Food decreases drug's absorption.
● Tell patient to avoid alcohol use while taking drug.
● Caution patient about performing activities that require mental alertness or physical coordination.

# 30

## Anticonvulsants

**acetazolamide sodium**
  (See Chapter 62, DIURETICS.)
**carbamazepine**
**clonazepam**
**clorazepate dipotassium**
  (See Chapter 32, ANTIANXIETY DRUGS.)
**diazepam**
  (See Chapter 32, ANTIANXIETY DRUGS.)
**ethosuximide**
**ethotoin**
**gabapentin**
**lamotrigine**
**magnesium sulfate**
**mephenytoin**
**mephobarbital**
**methsuximide**
**phenacemide**
**phenobarbital**
**phenobarbital sodium**
**phensuximide**
**phenytoin**
**phenytoin sodium**
**phenytoin sodium (extended)**
**primidone**
**trimethadione**
**valproate sodium**
**valproic acid**
**divalproex sodium**

**COMBINATION PRODUCTS**
DILANTIN WITH PHENOBARBITAL
KAPSEALS: phenytoin sodium 100
mg and phenobarbital 16 mg; phenytoin sodium 100 mg and phenobarbital
32 mg.

## carbamazepine
Apo-Carbamazepine†, Epitol,
Mazepine†, Novocarbamaz†,
PMS-Carbamazepine†, Tegretol,
Tegretol Chewable Tablets,
Tegretol CR†, Teril‡

*Pregnancy Risk Category: C*

**HOW SUPPLIED**
*Tablets:* 200 mg
*Tablets (chewable):* 100 mg
*Tablets (extended-release)†:* 200 mg,
400 mg
*Oral suspension:* 100 mg/5 ml

**ACTION**
Unknown. Thought to stabilize neuronal membranes and limit seizure activity by either increasing efflux or
decreasing influx of sodium ions
across cell membranes in the motor
cortex during generation of nerve impulses.

**ONSET, PEAK, DURATION**
For trigeminal neuralgia, onset occurs
in 8 to 72 hours; for anticonvulsant effect, in hours to days. Serum levels
peak in 1½ hours after oral suspension, 4 to 12 hours after tablets. Duration unknown.

**INDICATIONS & DOSAGE**
*Generalized tonic-clonic and complex
partial seizures, mixed seizure patterns –*
**Adults and children over 12 years:**
initially, 200 mg P.O. b.i.d. for tablets or 1 tsp of suspension P.O. q.i.d.
May be increased at weekly intervals
by 200 mg P.O. daily, in divided doses
at 6- to 8-hour intervals. Adjusted to
minimum effective level when control
is achieved. Maximum daily dosage is
1 g/day in children ages 12 to 15, or
1.2 g/day in patients over age 15.
**Children under 12 years:** initially, 100
mg P.O. b.i.d. or ½ tsp of suspension
P.O. q.i.d. Increased at weekly intervals by 100 mg P.O. daily. Maximum
daily dosage is1 g/day.
*Trigeminal neuralgia –*
**Adults:** initially, 100 mg P.O. b.i.d.
or ½ tsp of suspension q.i.d. with

*Liquid form contains alcohol. **May contain tartrazine. †Canada only. ‡Australia only. ◊OTC.

meals. Increased by 100 mg q 12 hours for tablets or ½ tsp of suspension q.i.d. until pain is relieved. Maximum daily dosage is 1.2 g/day. Maintenance dosage is 200 to 400 mg P.O. b.i.d.

## ADVERSE REACTIONS

**CNS:** *dizziness, vertigo, drowsiness,* fatigue, *ataxia,* **worsening of seizures** (usually in patients with mixed seizure disorders, including atypical absence seizures), confusion, headache, syncope.
**CV:** *CHF,* hypertension, hypotension, aggravation of coronary artery disease, arrhythmias, AV block.
**EENT:** conjunctivitis, dry mouth and pharynx, blurred vision, diplopia, nystagmus.
**GI:** *nausea, vomiting,* abdominal pain, diarrhea, anorexia, stomatitis, glossitis.
**GU:** urinary frequency, urine retention, impotence, albuminuria, glycosuria, elevated BUN.
**Hematologic:** *aplastic anemia, agranulocytosis,* eosinophilia, leukocytosis, *thrombocytopenia.*
**Hepatic:** abnormal liver function test results, *hepatitis.*
**Respiratory:** pulmonary hypersensitivity.
**Skin:** rash, urticaria, erythema multiforme, *Stevens-Johnson syndrome.*
**Other:** excessive diaphoresis, fever, chills, SIADH.

## INTERACTIONS

*Cimetidine, danazol, diltiazem, macrolides (such as erythromycin), isoniazid, propoxyphene, valproic acid, verapamil:* may increase carbamazepine blood levels. Use cautiously.
*Lithium:* increased CNS toxicity of lithium. Avoid concomitant use.
*MAO inhibitors:* increased depressant and anticholinergic effects. Don't use together.
*Oral contraceptives, doxycycline, haloperidol, phenytoin, theophylline, warfarin:* carbamazepine may decrease blood levels of these drugs. Monitor for decreased effect.
*Phenobarbital, phenytoin, primidone:* may decrease carbamazepine levels. Monitor for decreased effect.

## CONTRAINDICATIONS

Contraindicated in patients with history of previous bone marrow suppression or hypersensitivity to carbamazepine or tricyclic antidepressants and in patients who have taken an MAO inhibitor within 14 days of therapy.

## NURSING CONSIDERATIONS

● Use cautiously in patients with mixed seizure disorders because they may experience an increased incidence of seizures (usually atypical absence or generalized seizures).
● Obtain baseline determinations of urinalysis, BUN level, liver function, CBC, platelet and reticulocyte counts, and serum iron level as ordered. Monitor periodically thereafter.
● Shake oral suspension well before measuring dose.
● When administering by nasogastric tube, mix dose with an equal volume of water, 0.9% sodium chloride solution, or $D_5W$. Flush tube with 100 ml of diluent after administering dose.
● Never discontinue suddenly when treating seizures. Notify doctor immediately if adverse reactions occur.
● Know that adverse reactions may be minimized by increasing dosage gradually.
● Therapeutic carbamazepine blood level is 4 to 12 mcg/ml. Monitor blood levels and effects closely. Ask the patient when last dose of medication was taken to better evaluate blood levels.
● When managing seizures, institute appropriate precautions.
● **Alert:** Observe for signs of anorexia or subtle appetite changes, which may indicate excessive blood levels.

## ☑ PATIENT TEACHING

● Tell patient to take carbamazepine with food to minimize GI distress. Tell patient who takes suspension form to shake container well before measuring dose.

● Tell patient to keep tablets in the original container, tightly closed, and away from moisture. Some formulations may harden when exposed to excessive moisture, resulting in decreased bioavailability and loss of seizure control.

● Inform patient that when used for trigeminal neuralgia, an attempt to decrease dosage or withdraw drug is usually done every 3 months.

● Tell patient to notify the doctor immediately if fever, sore throat, mouth ulcers, or easy bruising or bleeding occurs.

● Tell patient that drug may cause mild to moderate dizziness and drowsiness when first taken. Advise him to avoid hazardous activities until effects disappear. Effect usually disappears within 3 to 4 days.

● Advise patient that periodic eye examinations are recommended.

---

## clonazepam
Klonopin
Controlled Substance Schedule IV
*Pregnancy Risk Category: NR*

### HOW SUPPLIED
*Tablets:* 0.5 mg, 1 mg, 2 mg
*Drops:* 2.5 mg/ml‡
*Injection:* 1 mg/ml‡

### ACTION
Unknown. A benzodiazepine that probably acts by facilitating the effects of the inhibitory neurotransmitter gamma-aminobutyric acid.

### ONSET, PEAK, DURATION
Onset and duration unknown. Serum levels peak in 1 to 2 hours, although peak concentrations may not be achieved for 4 to 8 hours.

### INDICATIONS & DOSAGE
*Lennox-Gastaut syndrome; atypical absence seizures; akinetic and myoclonic seizures –*
**Adults:** initially, not to exceed 1.5 mg P.O. daily in three divided doses. May be increased by 0.5 to 1 mg q 3 days until seizures are controlled. If given in unequal doses, the largest dose given h.s. Maximum recommended daily dosage is 20 mg.
**Children up to 10 years or 30 kg:** initially, 0.01 to 0.03 mg/kg P.O. daily (not to exceed 0.05 mg/kg daily), in 2 or 3 divided doses. Increased by 0.25 to 0.5 mg q third day to a maximum maintenance dosage of 0.1 to 0.2 mg/kg daily as needed.
*Status epilepticus (where parenteral form is available) –*
**Adults:** 1 mg by slow I.V. infusion.
**Children:** 0.5 mg by slow I.V. infusion.

### ADVERSE REACTIONS
**CNS:** *drowsiness, ataxia, behavioral disturbances* (especially in children), slurred speech, tremor, confusion, psychosis, agitation.
**CV:** palpitations.
**EENT:** nystagmus, abnormal eye movements, sore gums.
**GI:** constipation, gastritis, change in appetite, nausea, anorexia, diarrhea.
**GU:** dysuria, enuresis, nocturia, urine retention.
**Hematologic:** leukopenia, *thrombocytopenia,* eosinophilia.
**Respiratory:** *respiratory depression,* chest congestion, shortness of breath.
**Skin:** rash.

### INTERACTIONS
*Ethanol or other CNS depressants:* increased CNS depression. Monitor patient closely.

---

## CONTRAINDICATIONS
Contraindicated in patients with significant hepatic disease; in those with sensitivity to benzodiazepines; or in patients with acute angle-closure glaucoma.

## NURSING CONSIDERATIONS
• Use cautiously in patients with mixed type of seizure because drug may precipitate generalized tonic-clonic seizures. Also use cautiously in children and in patients with chronic respiratory disease, or open-angle glaucoma.
• **I.V. use‡:** Give slowly by direct injection or by slow I.V. infusion. Drug may be diluted with $D_5W$, dextrose 2.5% in water, or 0.9% sodium chloride or 0.45% sodium chloride solution.
• Mix solutions in glass bottles because the drug binds to polyvinyl chloride (PVC) plastic. If PVC infusion bags are used, administer immediately and infuse at a rate of 60 ml/hour or faster.
• Never withdraw suddenly because seizures may worsen. Call the doctor at once if adverse reactions develop.
• Monitor blood levels. Therapeutic blood level is 20 to 80 ng/ml.
• Assess elderly patient's response closely. Elderly patients are more sensitive to the drug's CNS effects.
• Monitor patient for oversedation.
• Monitor CBCs and liver function tests as ordered.
• Know that withdrawal symptoms are similar to those of barbiturates.

## ☑ PATIENT TEACHING
• Advise patient to avoid driving and other potentially hazardous activities that require mental alertness until drug's CNS effects are known.
• Instruct parent to monitor child's school performance because clonazepam may interfere with attentiveness in school.
• Instruct patient and parents never to stop drug abruptly because seizures may occur.

# ethosuximide
Zarontin

*Pregnancy Risk Category: NR*

## HOW SUPPLIED
*Capsules:* 250 mg
*Syrup:* 250 mg/5 ml

## ACTION
Not clearly defined. A succinimide derivative that probably increases seizure threshold. Reduces the paroxysmal spike-and-wave pattern of absence seizures by depressing nerve transmission in the motor cortex.

## ONSET, PEAK, DURATION
Onset and duration unknown. Peak effect occurs in 3 to 7 hours.

## INDICATIONS & DOSAGE
*Absence seizures –*
**Adults and children 6 years and older:** 500 mg P.O. daily. Optimal dose is 20 mg/kg/day.
**Children 3 to 6 years:** 250 mg P.O. daily. Optimal dose is 20 mg/kg/day.
***Alert:*** Dosages exceeding 1.5 g daily (given in divided doses) require administration under the doctor's strict supervision.

## ADVERSE REACTIONS
**CNS:** *drowsiness, headache, fatigue, dizziness, ataxia, irritability, hiccups, euphoria, lethargy, depression, psychosis.*
**EENT:** myopia, tongue swelling, gingival hyperplasia.
**GI:** *nausea, vomiting, diarrhea, weight loss, cramps, anorexia, epigastric and abdominal pain.*
**GU:** vaginal bleeding, urinary frequency.
**Hematologic:** leukopenia, eosinophilia, ***agranulocytosis,*** pancytopenia.

Reactions may be *common,* uncommon, *life-threatening,* or **COMMON AND LIFE-THREATENING.**

**Skin:** urticaria, pruritic and erythematous rashes, hirsutism.

**INTERACTIONS**
None significant.

**CONTRAINDICATIONS**
Contraindicated in patients with hypersensitivity to succinimide derivatives.

**NURSING CONSIDERATIONS**
• Use with extreme caution in patients with hepatic or renal disease.
• Be aware that ethosuximide is currently the drug of choice for treating absence seizures.
• Never withdraw drug suddenly. Abrupt withdrawal may precipitate absence seizures. Call doctor immediately if adverse reactions develop.
• Monitor blood levels. Therapeutic blood levels are 40 to 80 mcg/ml.
• Obtain CBC every 3 to 6 months as ordered.
• Know that drug may increase frequency of generalized tonic-clonic seizures when used alone in patients who have mixed types of seizures.
• Know that drug may cause positive direct Coombs' test.

**☑ PATIENT TEACHING**
• Advise patient to take ethosuximide with food to minimize GI distress.
• Advise patient to avoid driving and other potentially hazardous activities that require mental alertness until drug's CNS effects are known.
• Warn patient and parents not to stop drug abruptly.

---

**ethotoin**
Peganone

*Pregnancy Risk Category: C*

**HOW SUPPLIED**
*Tablets:* 250 mg, 500 mg

**ACTION**
Unknown. A hydantoin derivative that probably stabilizes neuronal membranes and limits seizure activity by either increasing efflux or decreasing influx of sodium ions across cell membranes in the motor cortex during generation of nerve impulses.

**ONSET, PEAK, DURATION**
Unknown.

**INDICATIONS & DOSAGE**
*Tonic-clonic (grand mal) or complex partial (psychomotor) seizures –*
**Adults:** initially, up to 1 g P.O. daily in divided doses. Increased slowly over several days to 3 g daily in divided doses, p.r.n. Usual maintenance dose is 2 to 3 g daily. Daily dose less than 2 g is ineffective in most patients.
**Children:** initially, up to 750 mg P.O. daily in divided doses. Increased up to 1 g daily in divided doses, p.r.n. Rarely, 2 to 3 g daily may be required.

**ADVERSE REACTIONS**
**CNS:** fatigue, insomnia, dizziness, headache, numbness, ataxia.
**CV:** chest pain.
**EENT:** diplopia, nystagmus, gingival hyperplasia (rare).
**GI:** *nausea, vomiting, diarrhea.*
**Hematologic:** blood dyscrasias.
**Skin:** rash.
**Other:** fever, lymphadenopathy, systemic lupus erythematosus.

**INTERACTIONS**
*Antihistamines, chloramphenicol, cimetidine, diazepam, disulfiram, isoniazid, phenylbutazone, salicylates, sulfamethizole, valproate:* increased ethotoin activity and toxicity; monitor patient closely.
*Diazoxide:* decreased ethotoin activity. Monitor closely.
*Ethanol (with chronic use), folic acid:* decreased ethotoin activity; monitor patient closely.

*Phenacemide:* paranoia. Use together cautiously.

## CONTRAINDICATIONS

Contraindicated in patients with hydantoin hypersensitivity and in those with hepatic or hematologic disorders.

## NURSING CONSIDERATIONS

• Know that ethotoin is the hydantoin derivative of choice for young adults prone to gingival hyperplasia caused by phenytoin. Otherwise, it is used infrequently to treat epilepsy.
• Never withdraw drug suddenly because seizures may worsen. Call the doctor at once if adverse reactions develop.
• Monitor CBC and urinalysis when therapy starts and periodically thereafter as ordered. Also, periodically monitor liver function test results during long-term use.
• Monitor blood levels. Therapeutic blood levels are 15 to 50 mcg/ml.
• Notify doctor if lymphadenopathy or lupuslike syndrome (fever, bruising, and sore throat) develops.

☑ **PATIENT TEACHING**
• Tell patient to take drug after meals. Schedule doses as evenly as possible over 24 hours.
• Advise patient to avoid driving and other potentially hazardous activities that require mental alertness until drug's CNS effects are known.
• Caution patient that heavy alcohol use may diminish drug's benefits.
• Warn patient and parents never to stop drug therapy abruptly.

# gabapentin
Neurontin

*Pregnancy Risk Category: C*

## HOW SUPPLIED
*Capsules:* 100 mg, 300 mg, 400 mg

## ACTION
Unknown. Although structurally related to gamma-amino butyric acid (GABA), the drug doesn't interact with GABA receptors and isn't converted metabolically into GABA or a GABA agonist.

## ONSET, PEAK, DURATION
Unknown.

## INDICATIONS & DOSAGE
*Adjunctive treatment of partial seizures with and without secondary generalization in adults with epilepsy –*
**Adults:** initially 300 mg P.O. h.s. on day 1; 300 mg P.O. b.i.d. on day 2; then 300 mg P.O. t.i.d. on day 3. Dosage increased as needed and tolerated to 1,800 mg daily in divided doses. Dosages up to 3,600 mg daily have been well tolerated.

In patients with renal failure: if creatinine clearance is over 60 ml/minute, 400 mg P.O. t.i.d.; if creatinine clearance is 30 to 60 ml/minute, 300 mg P.O. b.i.d.; if creatinine clearance is 15 to 30 ml/minute, 300 mg P.O. daily; if creatinine clearance is under 15 ml/minute, 300 mg P.O. every other day. Patients on dialysis should receive a loading dose of 300 to 400 mg P.O.; then 200 to 300 mg P.O. following every 4 hours of hemodialysis.

## ADVERSE REACTIONS
**CNS:** *fatigue, somnolence, dizziness, ataxia, nystagmus, tremor,* nervousness, dysarthria, amnesia, depression, abnormal thinking, twitching, incoordination.
**CV:** peripheral edema, vasodilation.
**EENT:** *diplopia, rhinitis,* pharyngitis, dry throat, coughing, *amblyopia.*
**GI:** nausea, vomiting, dyspepsia, dry mouth, constipation.
**GU:** impotence.
**Hematologic:** leukopenia, decreased WBC count.
**Skin:** pruritus, abrasion.
**Other:** dental abnormalities, in-

creased appetite, weight gain, back pain, myalgia, fractures.

### INTERACTIONS
*Antacids:* decreased absorption of gabapentin. Separate administration times by at least 2 hours.

### CONTRAINDICATIONS
Contraindicated in patients hypersensitive to the drug.

### NURSING CONSIDERATIONS
• Know that first dose should be given at bedtime to minimize drowsiness, dizziness, fatigue, and ataxia.
• If gabapentin therapy is discontinued or alternative medication is substituted, do so gradually over at least 1 week, as ordered, to minimize risk of precipitating seizures.
• **Alert:** Do not suddenly withdraw other anticonvulsants in patients starting gabapentin therapy.
• Know that routine monitoring of plasma levels of gabapentin is not necessary. The drug does not appear to alter plasma levels of other anticonvulsants.
• Know that it may cause false-positive tests for urine protein when the Ames-N-Multistix SG dipstick test is used.

### ☑ PATIENT TEACHING
• Instruct patient to take first dose at bedtime to minimize adverse CNS reactions.
• Warn patient to avoid driving and operating heavy machinery until drug's CNS effects are known.

---

## lamotrigine
Lamictal
*Pregnancy Risk Category: C*

### HOW SUPPLIED
*Tablets:* 25 mg, 100 mg, 150 mg, 200 mg

### ACTION
Unknown. May cause inhibited release of glutamate and aspartate (excitatory neurotransmitters), in the brain. This may occur by way of an action at voltage-sensitive sodium channels.

### ONSET, PEAK, DURATION
Onset and duration unknown. Serum levels peak in 1.4 to 4.8 hours after administration.

### INDICATIONS & DOSAGE
*Adjunct therapy in treatment of partial seizures caused by epilepsy –*
**Adults:** 50 mg P.O. daily for 2 weeks, followed by 100 mg daily in two divided doses for 2 weeks. Thereafter, usual maintenance dosage is 300 to 500 mg P.O. daily in two divided doses. For patients also taking valproic acid, 25 mg P.O. every other day for 2 weeks, followed by 25 mg P.O. daily for 2 weeks. Thereafter, no more than 150 mg P.O. daily in two divided doses.

### ADVERSE REACTIONS
**CNS:** *dizziness, headache, ataxia, somnolence,* incoordination, insomnia, tremor, depression, anxiety, seizures, irritability, speech disorder, decreased memory, aggravated reaction, concentration disturbance, sleep disorder, emotional lability, vertigo, mind racing.
**CV:** palpitations.
**EENT:** *diplopia, blurred vision,* vision abnormality, nystagmus.
**GI:** *nausea, vomiting,* diarrhea, dyspepsia, abdominal pain, constipation, tooth disorder, anorexia, dry mouth.
**Respiratory:** *rhinitis,* pharyngitis, cough, dyspnea.
**Skin:** *rash,* pruritus, hot flashes, alopecia, acne.
**Other:** dysarthria, muscle spasm, flulike syndrome, fever, infection, neck pain, malaise, chills, dysmenorrhea, vaginitis, amenorrhea.

*Liquid form contains alcohol.   **May contain tartrazine.   †Canada only.   ‡Australia only.   ◊OTC.

## INTERACTIONS
*Carbamazepine, phenobarbital, phenytoin, primidone:* decreased lamotrigine's steady-state concentrations. Monitor patient closely.

*Folate inhibitors (such as cotrimoxazole, methotrexate):* lamotrigine inhibits dihydrofolate reductase, an enzyme involved in folic acid synthesis. May have an additive effect. Monitor patient closely.

*Valproic acid:* decreased clearance of lamotrigine, which increases the drug's steady-state concentrations. Monitor patient closely for toxicity.

## CONTRAINDICATIONS
Contraindicated in patients with hypersensitivity to the drug.

## NURSING CONSIDERATIONS
• Use cautiously in patients with renal, hepatic, or cardiac impairment.
• Know that drug should not be discontinued abruptly because of the possibility of increased seizure frequency. Instead, drug should be tapered over at least 2 weeks.
• Be aware that lamotrigine dose should be lowered if drug is added to a multidrug regimen that includes valproate.
• Know that a lowered maintenance dosage should be used in a patient with severe renal impairment.
• Be aware that patients should be evaluated for reduction in the frequency and duration of seizures. Periodic evaluation of adjunct anticonvulsant's serum levels should be checked, as ordered.

## ☑ PATIENT TEACHING
• Inform patient that lamotrigine may cause a rash, especially in the first 6 weeks of therapy. Combination therapy of valproic acid and lamotrigine appears to be more likely to precipitate a serious rash. Although rash may resolve with continued therapy, tell patient to report it promptly to the doctor because it may warrant drug discontinuation.
• Warn patient not to engage in hazardous activity until drug's CNS effects are known.

---

# magnesium sulfate
*Pregnancy Risk Category: A*

## HOW SUPPLIED
*Injection:* 4%, 8%, 10%, 12.5%, 25%, 50%
*Injection solution:* 1% in 5% dextrose, 2% in 5% dextrose

## ACTION
Unknown. May decrease acetylcholine released by nerve impulses, but its anticonvulsant mechanism is unknown.

## ONSET, PEAK, DURATION
Onset occurs 1 to 2 minutes after I.V. use; 1 hour after I.M. injection. Serum levels peak almost immediately after I.V. administration, unknown after I.M. administration. Effects persist about 30 minutes after I.V. administration, 3 to 4 hours after I.M. injection.

## INDICATIONS & DOSAGE
*Prevention or control of seizures in preeclampsia or eclampsia –*
**Women:** initially, 4 g I.V. in 250 ml $D_5W$ and 4 to 5 g I.M. each buttock; then 4 to 5 g deep I.M. into alternate buttock q 4 hours, p.r.n. Alternatively, 4 g I.V. loading dose, followed by 1 to 2 g hourly as I.V. infusion.

*Hypomagnesemia –*
**Adults:** 1 g I.M. q 6 hours for 4 doses for mild deficiency; up to 250 mg/kg I.M. over 4-hour period for severe deficiency.

*Seizures, hypertension, and encephalopathy associated with acute nephritis in children –*
**Children:** 0.2 ml/kg of 50% solution

---

Reactions may be *common*, uncommon, *life-threatening*, or COMMON AND LIFE-THREATENING.

I.M. q 4 to 6 hours, p.r.n. For severe symptoms, 100 to 200 mg/kg I.V. slowly over 1 hour with one-half of the dose administered in first 15 to 20 minutes. Dosage titrated according to blood magnesium levels and seizure response.

*Management of paroxysmal atrial tachycardia –*
**Adults:** 3 to 4 g I.V. over 30 seconds.
*Management of life-threatening ventricular arrhythmias, such as sustained ventricular tachycardia or torsades de pointes –*
**Adults:** 2 to 6 g I.V. over several minutes, followed by a continuous I.V. infusion of 3 to 20 mg/minute for 5 to 48 hours. Dosage and duration of therapy depend on patient response and serum magnesium levels.

**ADVERSE REACTIONS**
**CNS:** drowsiness, *depressed reflexes,* flaccid paralysis, hypothermia.
**CV:** *hypotension, flushing,* **circulatory collapse,** depressed cardiac function.
**Other:** diaphoresis, *respiratory paralysis,* hypocalcemia.

**INTERACTIONS**
*Anesthetics, CNS depressants:* may cause additive CNS depression. Use cautiously.
*Digitalis:* concomitant use may exacerbate arrhythmias. Use together cautiously.
*Neuromuscular blockers:* may cause increased neuromuscular blockade. Use cautiously.

**CONTRAINDICATIONS**
Parenteral administration of drug contraindicated in patients with heart block or myocardial damage.

**NURSING CONSIDERATIONS**
• Use cautiously in patients with impaired renal function. Also use cautiously in women who are in labor.

• If used to treat seizures, institute appropriate seizure precautions.
• **I.V. use:** If necessary, dilute to a maximum concentration of 20%. Infuse no faster than 150 mg/minute (1.5 ml/minute of a 10% solution or 0.75 ml/minute of a 20% solution). Drug is compatible with $D_5W$.
• Maximum infusion rate is 150 mg/minute. Too-rapid infusion will induce uncomfortable feeling of heat.
• Monitor vital signs every 15 minutes when giving drug I.V.
• *Alert:* Watch for respiratory depression and signs of heart block. Respirations should be approximately 16 breaths/minute before each dose.
• Keep I.V. calcium gluconate available to reverse magnesium intoxication; however, use cautiously in patients undergoing digitalization because of danger of arrhythmias.
• Check blood magnesium levels after repeated doses. Disappearance of knee-jerk and patellar reflexes is a sign of impending magnesium toxicity.
• Signs of hypermagnesemia begin to appear at blood levels of 4 mEq/liter.
• Monitor fluid intake and output. Urine output should be 100 ml or more in 4-hour period before each dose.
• Observe neonates for signs of magnesium toxicity, including neuromuscular or respiratory depression, when giving I.V. form of drug to toxemic mothers within 24 hours before delivery.

☑ **PATIENT TEACHING**
• Inform patient of short-term need for drug, and answer any questions and address concerns.
• Review adverse reactions associated with drug and tell patient to report adverse reactions promptly. Reassure patient that although drug may cause adverse reactions, vital signs, reflexes, and blood levels will be

---

*Liquid form contains alcohol.   **May contain tartrazine.   †Canada only.   ‡Australia only.   ◇OTC.

checked frequently to ensure his safety.

# mephenytoin
Mesantoin

*Pregnancy Risk Category: C*

## HOW SUPPLIED
*Tablets:* 100 mg

## ACTION
Unknown. A hydantoin derivative that probably stabilizes neuronal membranes and limits seizure activity by either increasing efflux or decreasing influx of sodium ions across cell membranes in the motor cortex during generation of nerve impulses.

## ONSET, PEAK, DURATION
Onset and duration unknown. Serum levels peak in 45 minutes to 4 hours.

## INDICATIONS & DOSAGE
*Tonic-clonic, simple partial, and complex partial seizures in patients refractory to less toxic anticonvulsants —*
**Adults:** 50 to 100 mg P.O. daily. Increased by 50 to 100 mg at weekly intervals. Maintenance dosage ranges from 200 to 800 mg daily in three equally divided doses.
**Children:** initially, 50 to 100 mg P.O. daily. Increased by 50 to 100 mg at weekly intervals. Maintenance dosage ranges from 100 to 400 mg or 100 to 450 mg/m² daily in three equally divided doses.

## ADVERSE REACTIONS
**CNS:** ataxia, *drowsiness,* fatigue, irritability, choreiform movements, depression, tremor, insomnia, dizziness (usually transient).
**EENT:** conjunctivitis, diplopia, nystagmus, gingival hyperplasia (with prolonged use).
**GI:** nausea and vomiting (with prolonged use).

**Hematologic:** *leukopenia, neutropenia, agranulocytosis, thrombocytopenia, pancytopenia,* eosinophilia, leukocytosis.
**Skin:** *rash, exfoliative dermatitis,* Stevens-Johnson syndrome, *fatal dermatitides.*
**Other:** edema, lymphadenopathy, polyarthropathy, *pulmonary fibrosis.*

## INTERACTIONS
*Antihistamines, chloramphenicol, cimetidine, diazepam, disulfiram, isoniazid, phenylbutazone, salicylates, sulfamethizole, valproate:* increased mephenytoin activity and toxicity; monitor closely.
*Diazoxide:* decreased mephenytoin activity. Monitor closely.
*Ethanol (with chronic use), folic acid:* decreased mephenytoin activity; monitor closely.

## CONTRAINDICATIONS
Contraindicated in patients with hydantoin hypersensitivity.

## NURSING CONSIDERATIONS
• Use cautiously in patients receiving other hydantoin derivatives.
• Periodically monitor liver function studies with long-term use. Check CBC and platelet count before therapy and periodically thereafter as ordered. Alert doctor if neutrophil count is less than 1,600/mm³.
• *Alert:* Know that risk of potentially life-threatening blood dyscrasias limit this drug's usefulness.
• Never withdraw drug suddenly because seizures may worsen. Call the doctor if adverse reactions develop.
• Monitor blood levels. Therapeutic blood level of mephenytoin and its active metabolite is 25 to 40 mcg/ml.

## ☑ PATIENT TEACHING
• Tell patient to notify the doctor if fever, sore throat, bleeding, or rash occurs.
• Advise patient to avoid driving and

---

Reactions may be *common,* uncommon, *life-threatening,* or **COMMON AND LIFE-THREATENING.**

other hazardous activities that require mental alertness until drug's CNS effects are known.
• Caution patient that heavy alcohol use may diminish drug's benefits.
• This drug has been associated with photosensitivity reactions. Advise patient to use a sunblock, wear protective clothing, and avoid prolonged exposure to sunlight.
• Warn patient and parents never to stop drug abruptly.

## mephobarbital
Mebaral
Controlled Substance Schedule IV
*Pregnancy Risk Category: D*

### HOW SUPPLIED
*Tablets:* 32 mg, 50 mg, 100 mg

### ACTION
Unknown. A barbiturate that probably depresses monosynaptic and polysynaptic transmission in the CNS and increases the threshold for seizure activity in the motor cortex. Some activity comes from phenobarbital, an active metabolite.

### ONSET, PEAK, DURATION
Onset occurs in 60 minutes or longer. Peak unknown. Effects persist for 10 to 12 hours.

### INDICATIONS & DOSAGE
*Generalized tonic-clonic or absence seizures –*
**Adults:** 400 to 600 mg P.O. once daily or in divided doses.
**Children under 5 years:** 16 to 32 mg P.O. t.i.d. or q.i.d.
**Children 5 years and over:** 32 to 64 mg P.O. t.i.d. or q.i.d.
*Relief of anxiety, tension, and apprehension –*
**Adults:** 32 to 100 mg P.O. t.i.d. or q.i.d.
**Children:** 1.6 to 3 mg P.O. t.i.d. or q.i.d.

### ADVERSE REACTIONS
**CNS:** headache, *hangover,* confusion, paradoxical excitation, drowsiness, somnolence, agitation, ataxia, nervousness, hallucinations, insomnia, anxiety, dizziness, nightmares, syncope.
**CV:** hypotension, bradycardia.
**GI:** nausea, vomiting, constipation.
**Respiratory:** *respiratory depression,* apnea.
**Other:** allergic reactions (facial edema, rashes, exfoliative dermatitis), physical and psychological dependence.

### INTERACTIONS
*Chloramphenicol, MAO inhibitors, valproic acid:* potentiated barbiturate effect. Monitor patient for increased CNS and respiratory depression.
*Corticosteroids, digitoxin, doxycycline, estrogens and oral contraceptives, oral anticoagulants, tricyclic antidepressants:* mephobarbital may enhance the metabolism of these drugs. Monitor for decreased effect.
*Ethanol or other CNS depressants, including narcotic analgesics:* excessive CNS depression. Use cautiously.
*Griseofulvin:* decreased absorption of griseofulvin. Monitor effectiveness of griseofulvin.
*Rifampin:* may decrease barbiturate levels. Monitor for decreased effect.

### CONTRAINDICATIONS
Contraindicated in patients with barbiturate hypersensitivity or porphyria.

### NURSING CONSIDERATIONS
• Use cautiously in patients with acute or chronic pain, depression, suicidal tendencies, or history of drug abuse; hepatic, renal, cardiac, or respiratory function impairment; myasthenia gravis; or myxedema. Also use cautiously in elderly or debilitated patients.
• Know that dosage should be reduced in elderly or debilitated pa-

---

*Liquid form contains alcohol.   **May contain tartrazine.   †Canada only.   ‡Australia only.   ◊OTC.

tients because these patients may be more sensitive to barbiturates. Dosage also should be reduced for patients with impaired renal or hepatic disease.
• Never withdraw drug suddenly because seizures may worsen. Call the doctor at once if adverse reactions develop.
• Monitor phenobarbital blood levels. Therapeutic blood levels of phenobarbital are 15 to 40 mcg/ml.
• Periodically monitor CBC and BUN and creatinine levels.

☑ **PATIENT TEACHING**
• Advise patient to avoid driving and drug's other potentially hazardous activities that require mental alertness until drug's CNS effects are known.
• Advise adults with nighttime seizures to take total or largest dose at night after checking with doctor.
• Warn patient and parents never to stop drug abruptly.
• Instruct patient to store in light-resistant container.
• Inform patient who uses oral contraceptives that she should consider another birth-control method because drug may enhance contraceptive hormone metabolism and decrease its effectiveness.
• Tell patient that drug suppresses REM sleep. When drug is discontinued, patient may experience increased dreaming.

# methsuximide (mesuximide)
Celontin

*Pregnancy Risk Category: NR*

## HOW SUPPLIED
*Capsules:* 150 mg, 300 mg

## ACTION
Unknown. A succinimide that probably increases seizure threshold. Reduces the paroxysmal spike-and-wave pattern of absence seizures by depressing nerve transmission in the motor cortex. A succinimide derivative.

## ONSET, PEAK, DURATION
Onset and duration unknown. Serum levels peak in 1 to 4 hours.

## INDICATIONS & DOSAGE
*Refractory absence seizures* –
**Adults and children:** initially, 300 mg P.O. daily. Increased by 300 mg daily at weekly intervals as needed. Maximum daily dosage is 1.2 g in divided doses.

## ADVERSE REACTIONS
**CNS:** *drowsiness, ataxia, dizziness,* irritability, nervousness, headache, insomnia, confusion, depression, aggressiveness.
**EENT:** blurred vision, photophobia, periorbital edema.
**GI:** *nausea, vomiting, anorexia, diarrhea, weight loss, abdominal or epigastric pain, constipation.*
**Hematologic:** eosinophilia, *leukopenia,* monocytosis, *fatal blood dyscrasias, pancytopenia.*
**Skin:** urticaria, pruritic and erythematous rashes.

## INTERACTIONS
None significant.

## CONTRAINDICATIONS
Contraindicated in patients with hypersensitivity to succinimide derivatives.

## NURSING CONSIDERATIONS
• Use with extreme caution in patients with hepatic or renal dysfunction.
• Never change or withdraw drug suddenly. Abrupt withdrawal may precipitate absence seizures. Call the doctor immediately if adverse reactions develop.

---

Reactions may be *common,* uncommon, *life-threatening,* or **COMMON AND LIFE-THREATENING.**

- Check CBC, urinalysis, and liver function tests periodically as ordered.
- Monitor blood levels closely. Therapeutic serum level is 10 to 40 mcg/ml.

☑ **PATIENT TEACHING**
- Advise patient to avoid driving and other hazardous activities that require mental alertness until drug's CNS effects are known.
- Tell patient to call the doctor promptly if lupuslike syndrome develops.
- Warn patient and parents never to stop drug abruptly.
- Caution patient that this drug may color urine pink or brown.

# phenacemide
# (phenacetylcarbamide)
Phenurone

*Pregnancy Risk Category: D*

**HOW SUPPLIED**
*Tablets:* 500 mg

**ACTION**
Unknown. A hydantoin derivative that probably stabilizes neuronal membranes and limits seizure activity by either increasing efflux or decreasing influx of sodium ions across cell membranes in the motor cortex during generation of nerve impulses.

**ONSET, PEAK, DURATION**
Onset unknown. Serum levels peak 1 to 2 hours after a dose. Effects persist for 5 hours.

**INDICATIONS & DOSAGE**
*Severe epilepsy (particularly mixed forms of complex partial seizures) refractory to other drugs –*
**Adults:** 500 mg P.O. t.i.d. Increased by 500 mg P.O. daily at weekly intervals up to a maximum of 5 g daily.
**Children 5 to 10 years:** 250 mg P.O. t.i.d. Increased by 250 mg daily at

weekly intervals, up to a maximum of 2.5 g daily.

**ADVERSE REACTIONS**
**CNS:** *drowsiness,* dizziness, insomnia, headache, paresthesia, *psychic changes,* fatigue.
**GI:** *anorexia,* weight loss.
**GU:** nephritis with marked albuminuria.
**Hematologic:** *aplastic anemia,* leukopenia.
**Hepatic:** *hepatitis.*
**Skin:** rash, Stevens-Johnson syndrome.
**Other:** fever, muscle pain, palpitations.

**INTERACTIONS**
*Ethotoin:* causes paranoia. Use together cautiously.
*Other anticonvulsants:* enhanced risk of toxicity. Monitor patient closely.

**CONTRAINDICATIONS**
Contraindicated in patients with hypersensitivity or severe blood dyscrasias and in patients achieving satisfactory seizure control with other anticonvulsants.

**NURSING CONSIDERATIONS**
- Use cautiously in patients with hepatic dysfunction, history of personality disturbances, or allergies to other anticonvulsants.
- **Alert:** Know that drug is extremely toxic.
- Check liver function tests, CBCs, and urinalyses before and at monthly intervals during therapy as ordered.
- Notify the doctor if the patient develops jaundice or other signs of hepatitis, abnormal urinary findings, or WBC count below 4,000/mm$^3$.
- When phenacemide replaces another anticonvulsant, increase phenacemide dosage slowly while slowly decreasing the dosage of the first drug, as ordered, to maintain adequate seizure control.

---

*Liquid form contains alcohol.   **May contain tartrazine.   †Canada only.   ‡Australia only.   ◊OTC.

● Never withdraw drug suddenly. Call the doctor at once if adverse reactions develop.

● Tell patient to report sore throat, easy bruising, bleeding, or fever to the doctor immediately.
● Warn patient to avoid activities that require alertness or good psychomotor coordination until drug's CNS effects are known.
● Warn patient and parents never to stop drug abruptly.
● Tell the patient's family to watch for personality or psychological changes and report them to the doctor at once.

# phenobarbital (phenobarbitone)
Ancalixir†, Barbita, Solfoton

# phenobarbital sodium (phenobarbitone sodium)
Luminal Sodium

Controlled Substance Schedule IV
*Pregnancy Risk Category: D*

## HOW SUPPLIED
*Tablets:* 15 mg, 16 mg, 30 mg, 32 mg, 60 mg, 65 mg, 100 mg
*Capsules:* 16 mg
*Elixir\*:* 15 mg/5 ml, 20 mg/5 ml
*Injection:* 30 mg/ml, 60 mg/ml, 65 mg/ml, 130 mg/ml

## ACTION
Unknown. A barbiturate that probably depresses monosynaptic and polysynaptic transmission in the CNS and increases the threshold for seizure activity in the motor cortex. As a sedative, probably interferes with transmission of impulses from the thalamus to the cortex of the brain.

## ONSET, PEAK, DURATION
Onset occurs in 60 minutes or longer. Peak concentration levels are reached in 8 to 12 hours. Effects persist for as long as 10 to 12 hours.

## INDICATIONS & DOSAGE
*All forms of epilepsy, febrile seizures in children –*
**Adults:** 60 to 200 mg P.O. daily in divided dose t.i.d. or as single dose h.s.
**Children:** 3 to 6 mg/kg P.O. daily, usually divided q 12 hours. It can, however, be administered once daily, usually h.s.
*Status epilepticus –*
**Adults:** 200 to 600 mg I.V.
**Children:** 100 to 400 mg I.V. Do not exceed 50 mg/minute.
*Sedation –*
**Adults:** 30 to 120 mg P.O. daily in two or three divided doses.
**Children:** 3 to 5 mg/kg P.O. daily in divided doses t.i.d.
*Insomnia –*
**Adults:** 100 to 200 mg P.O. or I.M. h.s.
*Preoperative sedation –*
**Adults:** 100 to 200 mg I.M. 60 to 90 minutes before surgery.
**Children:** 16 to 100 mg I.M. 60 to 90 minutes before surgery.

## ADVERSE REACTIONS
**CNS:** *drowsiness, lethargy, hangover,* paradoxical excitement in elderly patients, somnolence.
**CV:** bradycardia, hypotension.
**GI:** nausea, vomiting.
**Hematologic:** exacerbation of porphyria.
**Respiratory:** *respiratory depression,* apnea.
**Skin:** rash, *erythema multiforme, Stevens-Johnson syndrome,* urticaria; pain, swelling, thrombophlebitis, necrosis, nerve injury at injection site.
**Other:** *angioedema,* physical and psychological dependence.

## INTERACTIONS
*Chloramphenicol, MAO inhibitors, valproic acid:* potentiated barbiturate

---

effect. Monitor patient for increased CNS and respiratory depression.

*Corticosteroids, digitoxin, doxycycline, estrogens and oral contraceptives, oral anticoagulants, tricyclic antidepressants:* phenobarbital may enhance the metabolism of these drugs. Monitor for decreased effect.

*Diazepam:* increased effects of both drugs. Use together cautiously.

*Ethanol or other CNS depressants, including narcotic analgesics:* excessive CNS depression. Use cautiously.

*Griseofulvin:* decreased absorption of griseofulvin. Monitor effectiveness of griseofulvin.

*Mephobarbital, primidone:* excessive phenobarbital blood levels; monitor closely.

*Rifampin:* may decrease barbiturate levels. Monitor for decreased effect.

*Valproic acid:* increased phenobarbital levels. Monitor for toxicity.

**CONTRAINDICATIONS**
Contraindicated in patients with barbiturate hypersensitivity, history of manifest or latent porphyria, hepatic dysfunction, respiratory disease with dyspnea or obstruction, and nephritis.

**NURSING CONSIDERATIONS**
● Use cautiously in patients with acute or chronic pain, depression, suicidal tendencies, history of drug abuse, blood pressure alterations, cardiovascular disease, shock, uremia, and in elderly or debilitated patients.
● **I.V. use:** Know that I.V. injection is reserved for emergency treatment. Give slowly under close supervision. Monitor respirations closely. When administering, do not give more than 60 mg/minute. Have resuscitation equipment available.
● Do not mix parenteral form with acidic solutions; precipitation may result.
● Do not use injectable solution if it contains a precipitate.
● Give I.M. injection deeply. Superfi-

cial injection may cause pain, sterile abscess, and tissue sloughing.
● Know that elderly patients are more sensitive to the drug's effects. Monitor closely.
● **Alert:** Watch for signs of barbiturate toxicity: coma, asthmatic breathing, cyanosis, clammy skin, and hypotension. Overdose can be fatal.
● Monitor blood levels closely. Therapeutic blood levels are 15 to 40 mcg/ml.
● Don't stop drug abruptly because seizures may worsen. Call the doctor immediately if adverse reactions develop.

☑ **PATIENT TEACHING**
● Make sure that patient is aware that phenobarbital is available in different milligram strengths and sizes. Advise him to check prescription and refills closely.
● Inform patient that full therapeutic effects are not seen for 2 to 3 weeks, except when loading dose is used.
● Advise patient to avoid driving and other potentially hazardous activities that require mental alertness until drug's CNS effects are known.
● Warn patient and parents not to discontinue drug abruptly.
● Tell patient who uses oral contraceptives that she should consider another birth-control method because drug may enhance contraceptive hormone metabolism and decrease its effect.

---

## phensuximide
Milontin

*Pregnancy Risk Category: NR*

**HOW SUPPLIED**
*Capsules:* 500 mg

**ACTION**
Unknown. A succinimide that probably increases seizure threshold. Reduces the paroxysmal spike-and-wave

pattern of absence seizures by depressing nerve transmission in the motor cortex. A succinimide derivative.

## ONSET, PEAK, DURATION
Onset and duration unknown. Serum levels peak in 1 to 4 hours.

## INDICATIONS & DOSAGE
*Absence seizures –*
**Adults and children:** 500 mg to 1 g P.O. b.i.d. or t.i.d.

## ADVERSE REACTIONS
**CNS:** muscular weakness, *drowsiness,* dizziness, ataxia, headache, lethargy.
**GI:** *nausea, vomiting,* anorexia.
**GU:** urinary frequency, renal damage, hematuria.
**Hematologic:** transient leukopenia, *pancytopenia, fatal blood dyscrasias.*
**Skin:** pruritus, eruptions, erythema, Stevens-Johnson syndrome, alopecia.
**Other:** lupuslike syndrome.

## INTERACTIONS
None significant.

## CONTRAINDICATIONS
Contraindicated in patients with hypersensitivity to succinimide derivatives.

## NURSING CONSIDERATIONS
● Use with extreme caution in patients with hepatic or renal disease.
● Monitor blood levels, as ordered. Therapeutic blood level is 40 to 80 mcg/ml.
● Check CBC every 3 to 4 months; urinalysis and liver function tests every 6 months, as ordered.
● Never withdraw drug suddenly. Abrupt withdrawal may precipitate absence seizures. Call the doctor immediately if adverse reactions develop.

## ☑ PATIENT TEACHING
● Advise patient to avoid driving and other potentially hazardous activities that require mental alertness until drug's CNS effects are known.
● Warn patient and parents not to stop drug therapy suddenly.
● Tell patient to report lupuslike symptoms immediately.
● Caution patient that this drug may color urine pink, red, or reddish brown.

# phenytoin (diphenylhydantoin)
Dilantin, Dilantin-30 Pediatric, Dilantin-125, Dilantin Infatabs

# phenytoin sodium
Dilantin, Phenytex

# phenytoin sodium (extended)
Dilantin Kapseals

*Pregnancy Risk Category: NR*

## HOW SUPPLIED
**phenytoin**
*Tablets (chewable):* 50 mg
*Oral suspension:* 30 mg/5 ml, 125 mg/5 ml
**phenytoin sodium**
*Capsules:* 30 mg (27.6-mg base), 100 mg (92-mg base)
*Injection:* 50 mg/ml (46-mg base)
**phenytoin sodium (extended)**
*Capsules:* 30 mg (27.6-mg base), 100 mg (92-mg base)

## ACTION
Unknown. A hydantoin derivative that probably stabilizes neuronal membranes and limits seizure activity by either increasing efflux or decreasing influx of sodium ions across cell membranes in the motor cortex during generation of nerve impulses.

---

Reactions may be *common,* uncommon, *life-threatening,* or COMMON AND LIFE-THREATENING.

## ONSET, PEAK, DURATION

Onset immediate with I.V. administration, unknown for other routes. Peak levels occur 1 to 2 hours after I.V. injection, 1½ to 3 hours after tablets or oral solution, 4 to 12 hours after extended-release capsules. Duration unknown.

## INDICATIONS & DOSAGE

*Control of tonic-clonic (grand mal) and complex partial (temporal lobe) seizures –*
**Adults:** highly individualized. Initially, 100 mg P.O. t.i.d., increased in increments of 100 mg P.O. every 2 to 4 weeks until desired response is obtained. Usual range is 300 to 600 mg daily. If patient stabilized with extended-release capsules, once-daily dosing with 300 mg extended-release capsules possible as an alternative.
**Children:** 5 mg/kg or 250 mg/m² P.O. daily b.i.d. or t.i.d. Maximum daily dosage is 300 mg.
*For patient requiring a loading dose –*
**Adults:** initially, 1 g P.O. daily divided into 3 doses and administered at 2-hour intervals. Alternatively, 10 to 15 mg/kg I.V. at a rate not exceeding 50 mg/minute. Normal maintenance dosage instituted 24 hours later.
**Children:** 5 mg/kg/day P.O. in 2 or 3 equally divided doses with subsequent dosage individualized to a maximum of 300 mg daily.
*Prevention and treatment of seizures occurring during neurosurgery –*
**Adults:** 100 to 200 mg I.M. q 4 hours during surgery and continued during the postoperative period.
*Status epilepticus –*
**Adults:** loading dose of 10 to 15 mg/kg I.V. (1 to 1.5 g may be needed) at a rate not exceeding 50 mg/minute, followed by maintenance doses of 100 mg P.O. or I.V. q 6 to 8 hours.
**Children:** loading dose of 15 to 20 mg/kg I.V., at a rate not exceeding 1 to 3 mg/kg/minute, followed by highly individualized maintenance dosages.

## ADVERSE REACTIONS

**CNS:** *ataxia, slurred speech,* dizziness, insomnia, nervousness, twitching, headache, *mental confusion, decreased coordination.*
**CV:** periarteritis nodosa.
**EENT:** *nystagmus, diplopia,* blurred vision, *gingival hyperplasia* (especially in children).
**GI:** *nausea, vomiting,* constipation.
**Hematologic: *thrombocytopenia, leukopenia, agranulocytosis, pancytopenia,*** macrocythemia, megaloblastic anemia.
**Hepatic:** *toxic hepatitis.*
**Skin:** scarlatiniform or morbilliform rash; bullous, *exfoliative,* or purpuric dermatitis; *Stevens-Johnson syndrome;* lupus erythematosus; *hirsutism; toxic epidermal necrolysis;* photosensitivity; pain, necrosis, and inflammation at injection site; discoloration of skin ("purple-glove syndrome") if given by I.V. push in back of hand.
**Other:** lymphadenopathy, hyperglycemia, osteomalacia, hypertrichosis.

## INTERACTIONS

*Amiodarone, antihistamines, chloramphenicol, cimetidine, cycloserine, diazepam, disulfiram, influenza vaccine, isoniazid, phenylbutazone, salicylates, sulfamethizole, valproate:* may increase phenytoin activity and toxicity. Monitor patient closely.
*Dexamethasone, diazoxide, ethanol (with chronic use), folic acid:* decreased phenytoin activity; monitor patient closely.
*Oral tube feedings with Osmolite or Isocal:* may interfere with absorption of oral phenytoin. Schedule feedings as far as possible from drug administration.

## CONTRAINDICATIONS

Contraindicated in patients with hydantoin hypersensitivity, sinus bradycardia, SA block, second- or third-

---

*Liquid form contains alcohol. **May contain tartrazine. †Canada only. ‡Australia only. ◊OTC.

degree AV block, or Adams-Stokes syndrome.

## NURSING CONSIDERATIONS

• Use cautiously in patients with hepatic dysfunction, hypotension, myocardial insufficiency, diabetes, and respiratory depression; in elderly or debilitated patients; and in patients receiving other hydantoin derivatives.

• Be aware that elderly patients tend to metabolize phenytoin slowly and may require lower dosages.

• Know that phenytoin requirements usually increase during pregnancy.

• Suspension available as 30 mg/5 ml or 125 mg/5 ml. Read label carefully. Shake suspension well before each dose.

• Use only clear solution for injection. A slight yellow color is acceptable. Don't refrigerate.

• **I.V. use:** Administer slowly (50 mg/ minute) as I.V. bolus. If giving an infusion, don't mix drug with $D_5W$ because it will precipitate. Clear I.V. tubing first with 0.9% sodium chloride solution. Never use cloudy solution. May mix with 0.9% sodium chloride solution if necessary and give as an infusion over ½ to 1 hour, when possible. Infusion must begin within 1 hour after preparation and should run through an in-line filter. Discard 4 hours after preparation.

• *Alert:* Check patency of I.V. catheter before administering. Extravasation has caused severe local tissue damage.

• Avoid administering phenytoin by I.V. push into veins on the back of the hand to avoid discoloration known as purple-glove syndrome. Inject into larger veins or central venous catheter if available.

• Check vital signs, blood pressure, and ECG during I.V. administration.

• Do not give I.M. unless dosage adjustments are made. Drug may precipitate at injection site, cause pain, and be absorbed erratically.

• Divided doses given with or after meals may decrease adverse GI reactions.

• Be aware that drug should be discontinued if rash appears. If rash is scarlatiniform or morbilliform, drug may be resumed after rash clears. If rash reappears, therapy should be discontinued. If rash is exfoliative, purpuric, or bullous, drug will not be resumed.

• Don't withdraw drug suddenly because seizures may worsen. Call the doctor at once if adverse reactions develop.

• Monitor blood levels as ordered. Therapeutic phenytoin blood level is 10 to 20 mcg/ml.

• Monitor CBC and serum calcium level every 6 months, and periodically monitor hepatic function as ordered. If megaloblastic anemia is evident, the doctor may order folic acid and vitamin $B_{12}$.

• If using to treat seizures, take appropriate safety precautions.

• Mononucleosis may decrease phenytoin levels. Monitor for increased seizure activity.

• Know that therapy with phenytoin may cause altered laboratory test results, including reduced serum protein-bound iodine and free thyroxine levels without clinical signs of hypothyroidism; a slight decrease in urinary 17-hydroxysteroid and 17-ketosteroid levels; increased urine 6-ß hydroxycortisol excretion and serum levels of alkaline phosphatase or gamma-glutamyltransferase; and decreased values for dexamethasone suppression or metyrapone tests.

## ☑ PATIENT TEACHING

• Advise patient to avoid driving and other potentially hazardous activities that require mental alertness until drug's CNS effects are known.

• Advise patient not to change brands or dosage forms once he's stabilized on therapy.

---

Reactions may be *common*, uncommon, *life-threatening*, or COMMON AND LIFE-THREATENING.

- Dilantin capsules are the only oral form that can be given once daily. Toxic levels may result if any other brand or form is given once daily. Dilantin brand tablets and oral suspension should never be taken once daily.
- Warn patient and parents not to stop drug abruptly.
- Stress importance of good oral hygiene and regular dental examinations. Gingivectomy may be necessary periodically if dental hygiene is poor.
- Caution patient that this drug may color urine pink, red, or reddish brown.
- Inform patient that heavy alcohol use may diminish drug's benefits.

---

## primidone
Apo-Primidone†, Mysoline, PMS Primidone†, Sertan†

*Pregnancy Risk Category: NR*

### HOW SUPPLIED
*Tablets:* 50 mg, 250 mg
*Oral suspension:* 250 mg/5 ml

### ACTION
Unknown, but some activity may be caused by phenylethylmalonamide and phenobarbital, which are active metabolites.

### ONSET, PEAK, DURATION
Onset and duration unknown. Serum levels peak in 3 to 4 hours.

### INDICATIONS & DOSAGE
*Tonic-clonic, complex partial, and simple partial seizures –*
**Adults and children 8 years and over:** initially, 100 to 125 mg P.O. h.s. on days 1 to 3; then 100 to 125 mg P.O. b.i.d. on days 4 to 6; then 100 to 125 mg P.O. on days 7 to 9; followed by maintenance dosage of 250 mg P.O. t.i.d. Maintenance dosage increased to 250 mg q.i.d., if needed.

**Children under 8 years:** initially, 50 mg P.O. h.s., then 50 mg P.O. b.i.d., then 100 mg P.O. b.i.d., followed by maintenance dosage of 125 to 250 mg P.O. t.i.d.

### ADVERSE REACTIONS
**CNS:** *drowsiness, ataxia,* emotional disturbances, vertigo, hyperirritability, fatigue, paranoia.
**EENT:** *diplopia,* nystagmus.
**GI:** anorexia, *nausea, vomiting.*
**GU:** impotence, polyuria.
**Hematologic:** megaloblastic anemia, *thrombocytopenia.*
**Skin:** morbilliform rash.

### INTERACTIONS
*Carbamazepine:* increased primidone levels. Observe for toxicity.
*Phenytoin:* stimulated conversion of primidone to phenobarbital. Observe for increased phenobarbital effect.

### CONTRAINDICATIONS
Contraindicated in patients with phenobarbital hypersensitivity or porphyria.

### NURSING CONSIDERATIONS
- Shake liquid suspension well.
- Don't withdraw drug suddenly because seizures may worsen. Call the doctor immediately if adverse reactions develop.
- Monitor blood levels as ordered. Therapeutic blood level of primidone is 5 to 12 mcg/ml. Therapeutic blood level of phenobarbital is 15 to 40 mcg/ml.
- Monitor CBC and routine blood chemistry every 6 months, as ordered.

### ☑ PATIENT TEACHING
- Advise patient to avoid driving and other potentially hazardous activities that require mental alertness until drug's CNS effects are known.
- Warn patient and parents not to stop drug therapy suddenly.

---

*Liquid form contains alcohol. **May contain tartrazine. †Canada only. ‡Australia only. ◊OTC.

• Tell patient that full therapeutic response may take 2 weeks or more.

# trimethadione
Tridione, Tridione Dulcets
*Pregnancy Risk Category: NR*

## HOW SUPPLIED
*Capsules:* 300 mg
*Tablets (chewable):* 150 mg
*Oral solution:* 200 mg/5 ml

## ACTION
Raises the threshold for cortical seizure but does not modify seizure pattern. Decreases projection of focal activity and reduces both repetitive spinal-cord transmission and spike-and-wave patterns of absence (petit mal) seizures. An oxazolidinedione derivative.

## ONSET, PEAK, DURATION
Unknown.

## INDICATIONS & DOSAGE
*Refractory absence seizures –*
**Adults and children over 13 years:** initially, 300 mg P.O. t.i.d. May increase by 300 mg P.O. daily at weekly intervals to a maximum of 600 mg P.O. q.i.d.
**Children:** 13 mg/kg P.O. t.i.d. or 335 mg/m² P.O. t.i.d.; alternatively, give according to age.
**Children under 2 years:** 100 mg P.O. t.i.d.
**Children 2 to 6 years:** 200 mg P.O. t.i.d.
**Children 6 to 13 years:** 300 mg P.O. t.i.d.

## ADVERSE REACTIONS
**CNS:** *drowsiness,* fatigue, *malaise,* insomnia, dizziness, headache, paresthesia, irritability, ***precipitation of tonic-clonic seizures.***
**CV:** hypertension, hypotension.
**EENT:** *day blindness (hemeralopia),* diplopia, photophobia, epistaxis, retinal hemorrhage.
**GI:** nausea, vomiting, anorexia, abdominal pain, bleeding gums.
**GU:** *nephrosis,* vaginal bleeding, proteinuria.
**Hematologic:** *neutropenia, leukopenia,* eosinophilia, *thrombocytopenia, pancytopenia, agranulocytosis, hypoplastic and aplastic anemias.*
**Hepatic:** abnormal liver function test results.
**Skin:** acneiform and morbilliform rash, *exfoliative dermatitis, erythema multiforme,* petechiae, alopecia, photosensitivity.
**Other:** lymphadenopathy, lupuslike syndrome, myasthenic syndrome.

## INTERACTIONS
None significant.

## CONTRAINDICATIONS
Contraindicated in patients with paramethadione and trimethadione hypersensitivity, severe blood dyscrasias, or hepatic dysfunction.

## NURSING CONSIDERATIONS
• Use with extreme caution in patients with retinal and optic nerve diseases.
• Check CBC, hepatic function, and urinalysis before starting therapy and monthly thereafter, as ordered. Notify doctor if neutrophil count falls below 2,500/mm³ because drug should be stopped.
• *Alert:* Watch for impending toxicity; may precipitate tonic-clonic seizure.
• Notify doctor if scotomata or rash develops; drug should be discontinued.
• Don't withdraw drug suddenly. Abrupt withdrawal may precipitate absence seizures. Call doctor immediately if adverse reactions develop.

---

Reactions may be *common,* uncommon, *life-threatening,* or **COMMON AND LIFE-THREATENING.**

## ☑ PATIENT TEACHING
● Warn patient to report skin rash, alopecia, sore throat, fever, bruises, or epistaxis to the doctor immediately.
● Advise patient to avoid driving and other potentially hazardous activities that require mental alertness until drug's CNS effects are known.
● Warn patient and parents not to stop drug therapy abruptly.
● Advise patient to use a sunblock, wear protective clothing, and avoid prolonged exposure to sunlight.
● Suggest sunglasses if bright light blurs the patient's vision. Tell patient to notify the doctor if this occurs.

## valproate sodium
Depakene Syrup, Epilim‡, Myproic Acid Syrup

## valproic acid
Depakene, Myproic Acid

## divalproex sodium
Depakote, Depakote Sprinkle, Epival†, Valcote‡

*Pregnancy Risk Category: D*

## HOW SUPPLIED
**valproate sodium**
*Syrup:* 250 mg/ml
**valproic acid**
*Tablets (enteric-coated):* 200 mg‡, 500 mg‡
*Crushable tablets:* 100 mg‡
*Capsules:* 250 mg
*Syrup:* 200 mg/5 ml‡
**divalproex sodium**
*Capsules (delayed-release):* 125 mg
*Tablets (enteric-coated):* 125 mg, 250 mg, 500 mg

## ACTION
Unknown. Probably increases brain levels of gamma-aminobutyric acid, which transmits inhibitory nerve impulses in the CNS.

## ONSET, PEAK, DURATION
Onset and duration unknown. Serum levels peak within 1 to 4 hours after capsules or syrup; 3 to 4 hours after tablets and delayed-release capsules.

## INDICATIONS & DOSAGE
*Simple and complex absence seizures, mixed seizure types (including absence seizures)* –
**Adults and children:** initially, 15 mg/kg P.O. daily; then increased by 5 to 10 mg/kg daily at weekly intervals up to maximum of 60 mg/kg daily. When dosage exceeds 250 mg daily, drug should be equally divided into two or more divided doses.

## ADVERSE REACTIONS
Because drug usually is used in combination with other anticonvulsants, adverse reactions reported may not be caused by valproic acid alone.
**CNS:** *sedation,* emotional upset, depression, psychosis, aggressiveness, hyperactivity, behavioral deterioration, muscle weakness, tremor, ataxia, headache, dizziness, incoordination.
**EENT:** nystagmus, diplopia.
**GI:** *nausea, vomiting, indigestion,* diarrhea, abdominal cramps, constipation, increased appetite and weight gain, anorexia, *pancreatitis. (Note:* lower incidence of GI effects occur with divalproex sodium.)
**Hematologic:** *thrombocytopenia,* increased bleeding time, petechiae, bruising, eosinophilia, hemorrhage, leukopenia, bone marrow suppression.
**Hepatic:** *elevated liver enzymes,* **toxic hepatitis**.
**Skin:** rash, alopecia, pruritus, photosensitivity, erythema multiforme.

## INTERACTIONS
*Aspirin, chlorpromazine, cimetidine:* May cause valproic acid toxicity. Use together cautiously and monitor blood levels. Monitor patient closely.

*Liquid form contains alcohol.  **May contain tartrazine.  †Canada only.  ‡Australia only.  ◊OTC.

*Ethanol:* excessive CNS depression. Avoid concomitant use.
*Phenobarbital:* increased phenobarbital levels. Monitor patient closely.
*Phenytoin:* increased or decreased phenytoin levels. Monitor patient closely.

## CONTRAINDICATIONS
Contraindicated in patients with hypersensitivity.

## NURSING CONSIDERATIONS
• Use with extreme caution in patients with history of hepatic dysfunction.
• Monitor liver function studies, platelet counts, and PT before starting drug and periodically thereafter as ordered.
• Don't administer syrup to patients who need sodium restriction. Check with the doctor.
• Never withdraw the drug suddenly because sudden withdrawal may worsen seizures. Call the doctor at once if adverse reactions develop.
• *Alert:* Be aware serious or fatal hepatotoxicity may follow nonspecific symptoms, such as malaise, fever, and lethargy. Notify doctor at once as drug will need to be discontinued in the presence of suspected or apparent substantial hepatic dysfunction.
• Know that patients at high risk for hepatotoxicity include those with congenital metabolic disorders, mental retardation or presence of organic brain disease; those taking multiple anticonvulsants; and children under age 2.
• Notify doctor if tremors occur (a dosage reduction may be necessary).
• Monitor blood levels, as ordered. Therapeutic blood level is 50 to 100 mcg/ml.
• Know that drug may produce false-positive test results for ketones in urine.

☑ **PATIENT TEACHING**
• To reduce adverse GI effects, tell patient this drug may be taken with food or milk.
• Advise patient not to chew capsules; irritation of mouth and throat may result.
• Tell patient and parents that syrup shouldn't be mixed with carbonated beverages; may be irritating to mouth and throat.
• Tell patient and parents to keep drug out of children's reach.
• Warn patient and parents not to stop drug therapy abruptly.
• Advise patient to avoid driving and other potentially hazardous activities that require mental alertness until drug's CNS effects are known.

---

Reactions may be *common*, uncommon, *life-threatening*, or COMMON AND LIFE-THREATENING.

# 31

# Antidepressants

amitriptyline hydrochloride
amitriptyline pamoate
amoxapine
bupropion hydrochloride
clomipramine hydrochloride
desipramine hydrochloride
doxepin hydrochloride
fluoxetine hydrochloride
imipramine hydrochloride
imipramine pamoate
isocarboxazid
maprotiline hydrochloride
nefazodone hydrochloride
nortriptyline hydrochloride
paroxetine hydrochloride
phenelzine sulfate
protriptyline hydrochloride
sertraline hydrochloride
tranylcypromine sulfate
trazodone hydrochloride
trimipramine maleate
venlafaxine hydrochloride

## COMBINATION PRODUCTS

ETRAFON: perphenazine 2 mg and amitriptyline hydrochloride 25 mg.
ETRAFON 2-10: perphenazine 2 mg and amitriptyline hydrochloride 10 mg.
ETRAFON-A: perphenazine 4 mg and amitriptyline hydrochloride 10 mg.
ETRAFON-FORTE: perphenazine 4 mg and amitriptyline hydrochloride 25 mg.
LIMBITROL DS: chlordiazepoxide 10 mg and amitriptyline hydrochloride 25 mg.
TRIAVIL 2-10, TRIAVIL 4-10, TRIA-VIL 2-25, TRIAVIL 4-25 are products identical to the Etrafon products listed above. Triavil is also available as TRIAVIL 4-50 (perphenazine 4 mg and amitriptyline hydrochloride 50 mg).

## amitriptyline hydrochloride

Apo-Amitriptyline†, Elavil, Emitrip, Endep, Enovil, Levate†, Novotriptyn†, PMS-Amitriptyline, Tryptanol‡

## amitriptyline pamoate

Elavil†

*Pregnancy Risk Category: NR*

## HOW SUPPLIED

**amitriptyline hydrochloride**
*Tablets:* 10 mg, 25 mg, 50 mg, 75 mg, 100 mg, 150 mg
*Injection:* 10 mg/ml
**amitriptyline pamoate**
*Syrup:* 10 mg/5 ml

## ACTION

Unknown, but a tricyclic antidepressant (TCA) that increases the amount of norepinephrine, serotonin, or both in the CNS by blocking their reuptake by the presynaptic neurons.

## ONSET, PEAK, DURATION

Onset unknown although thought to take several weeks. Serum levels peak in 2 to 12 hours. Duration unknown.

## INDICATIONS & DOSAGE

*Depression –*
**Adults:** 50 to 100 mg P.O. h.s., increasing to 150 mg daily; maximum dosage is 300 mg daily, if needed. Or 20 to 30 mg I.M. q.i.d.
**Elderly patients and adolescents:** 10 mg P.O. t.i.d. and 20 mg h.s. daily.

## ADVERSE REACTIONS

**CNS:** *coma, seizures,* hallucinations, delusions, disorientation, ataxia, tremor, peripheral neuropathy, anxiety, insomnia, restlessness, drowsi-

---

ness, dizziness, weakness, fatigue, headache, extrapyramidal reactions.
**CV:** *MI, stroke, arrhythmias,* heart block, *orthostatic hypotension, tachycardia, ECG changes,* hypertension.
**EENT:** *blurred vision,* tinnitus, mydriasis, increased intraocular pressure.
**GI:** *dry mouth,* nausea, vomiting, anorexia, epigastric distress, diarrhea, constipation, paralytic ileus.
**GU:** urine retention.
**Hematologic:** *agranulocytosis, thrombocytopenia,* leukopenia, eosinophilia.
**Skin:** rash, urticaria, photosensitivity.
**Other:** *diaphoresis,* hypersensitivity reaction, edema.
**After abrupt withdrawal of long-term therapy:** nausea, headache, malaise (does not indicate addiction).

## INTERACTIONS

*Barbiturates, CNS depressants, ethanol:* enhanced CNS depression. Avoid concomitant use.
*Cimetidine, methylphenidate:* increased TCA blood levels. Monitor for enhanced antidepressant effect.
*Epinephrine, norepinephrine:* increased hypertensive effect. Use with caution.
*MAO inhibitors:* may cause severe excitation, hyperpyrexia, or seizures, usually with high dosage. Use with caution.

## CONTRAINDICATIONS

Contraindicated during acute recovery phase of MI, in patients with hypersensitivity, and in patients who have received an MAO inhibitor within the past 14 days.

## NURSING CONSIDERATIONS

● Use cautiously in patients with history of seizures, urine retention, angle-closure glaucoma, or increased intraocular pressure; in those with hyperthyroidism, CV disease, diabetes, or impaired liver function; and in those receiving thyroid medications.
● *Alert:* Know that parenteral form of drug is for I.M. administration only. Drug should not be given I.V.
● Amitriptyline has strong anticholinergic effects and is one of the most sedating TCAs. Be aware that anticholinergic effects have a rapid onset even though therapeutic effect is delayed for weeks.
● If signs of psychosis occur or increase, expect doctor to reduce dosage. Record mood changes. Monitor patients for suicidal tendencies, and allow them only a minimum supply of the drug.
● Because hypertensive episodes have occurred during surgery in patients receiving TCAs, be aware drug should be gradually discontinued several days before surgery.
● Do not withdraw drug abruptly.

### ☑ PATIENT TEACHING

● Advise patient to take full dose at bedtime, but warn him of possible morning orthostatic hypotension.
● Tell patient to avoid alcohol while taking this drug.
● Warn patient to avoid activities that require alertness and good psychomotor coordination until CNS effects of drug are known. Drowsiness and dizziness usually subside after a few weeks.
● Advise patient to consult his doctor before taking any other prescription or OTC medications.
● Tell patient that dry mouth may be relieved with sugarless hard candy or gum. Saliva substitutes may be necessary.
● To prevent photosensitivity reactions, advise patient to use a sunblock, wear protective clothing, and avoid prolonged exposure to strong sunlight.
● Warn patient not to stop drug therapy abruptly.

---

Reactions may be *common,* uncommon, *life-threatening,* or **COMMON AND LIFE-THREATENING.**

## amoxapine
Asendin

*Pregnancy Risk Category: C*

### HOW SUPPLIED
*Tablets:* 25 mg, 50 mg, 100 mg, 150 mg

### ACTION
Unknown, but a tricyclic antidepressant (TCA) that increases the amount of norepinephrine, serotonin, or both in the CNS by blocking their reuptake by the presynaptic neurons.

### ONSET, PEAK, DURATION
Onset thought to occur in 2 to 4 weeks. Serum levels peak in about 90 minutes. Duration unknown.

### INDICATIONS & DOSAGE
*Depression —*
**Adults:** initially, 50 mg P.O. b.i.d. or t.i.d. Increased to 100 mg b.i.d. or t.i.d. on third day of treatment if tolerated. Increases above 300 mg daily are made only if 300 mg daily has been ineffective during a trial period of at least 2 weeks. When effective dosage is established, entire dosage (not to exceed 300 mg) may be given h.s.

### ADVERSE REACTIONS
**CNS:** *drowsiness, dizziness,* excitation, tremor, weakness, confusion, anxiety, insomnia, restlessness, nightmares, ataxia, fatigue, headache, nervousness, *tardive dyskinesia, EEG changes, seizures,* extrapyramidal reactions (rare), **neuroleptic malignant syndrome** (high fever, tachycardia, tachypnea, profuse diaphoresis).
**CV:** *orthostatic hypotension, tachycardia,* hypertension, palpitations.
**EENT:** *blurred vision.*
**GI:** *dry mouth, constipation,* nausea, excessive appetite.
**GU:** *urine retention, acute renal failure* (with overdose).
**Skin:** rash, edema.
**Other:** *diaphoresis.*
**After abrupt withdrawal of long-term therapy:** nausea, headache, malaise (does not indicate addiction).

### INTERACTIONS
*Barbiturates:* decreased TCA blood levels. Monitor for decreased antidepressant effect.
*Cimetidine, methylphenidate, oral contraceptives:* may increase amoxapine serum levels. Monitor for increased adverse effects.
*Clonidine, epinephrine, norepinephrine:* increased hypertensive effect. Use with caution.
*CNS depressants, ethanol:* enhanced CNS depression. Avoid concomitant use.
*MAO inhibitors:* may cause severe excitation, hyperpyrexia, or seizures, usually with high dosage. Use with caution.

### CONTRAINDICATIONS
Contraindicated in patients with hypersensitivity, during acute recovery phase of MI, and in patients who have received an MAO inhibitor within the past 14 days.

### NURSING CONSIDERATIONS
• Use cautiously in patients with history of urine retention, angle-closure glaucoma, or increased intraocular pressure, as well as patients with CV disease. Use with extreme caution in patients with history of seizure disorders or those with overt or latent seizure disorders.
• Be aware that dosage should be reduced in elderly or debilitated persons and adolescents.
• Do not withdraw drug abruptly.
• Because hypertensive episodes have occurred during surgery in patients receiving TCAs, be aware that drug should be gradually discontinued several days before surgery.
• Expect delay of 2 weeks or more be-

fore noticeable effect. Full effect may take 4 weeks or more. However, know that adverse anticholinergic effects can occur rapidly.
• If signs of psychosis occur or increase, expect doctor to reduce dosage. Record mood changes. Monitor patients for suicidal tendencies, and allow them only a minimum supply of the drug.
• Monitor for signs and symptoms of tardive dyskinesia, especially in elderly women.
• Amoxapine therapy has been associated with neuroleptic malignant syndrome, a rare but life-threatening syndrome usually seen with phenothiazines. Discontinue drug immediately and institute appropriate therapy if symptoms occur.
• Relieve dry mouth with sugarless hard candy or gum. Saliva substitutes may be necessary.

☑ **PATIENT TEACHING**
• Whenever possible, tell patient to take full dose at bedtime.
• Warn patient not to stop drug therapy abruptly.
• Warn patient to avoid activities that require alertness and good psychomotor coordination until CNS effects of the drug are known. Drowsiness and dizziness usually subside after first few weeks.
• Some patients may experience photosensitivity reactions. Advise patient to use a sunblock, wear protective clothing, and avoid prolonged exposure to strong sunlight.

---

# bupropion hydrochloride
Wellbutrin

*Pregnancy Risk Category: B*

## HOW SUPPLIED
*Tablets:* 75 mg, 100 mg

## ACTION
Unknown. Bupropion is not a tricyclic antidepressant (TCA), does not inhibit MAO, and is a weak inhibitor of norepinephrine, dopamine, and serotonin reuptake.

## ONSET, PEAK, DURATION
Onset occurs in 1 to 3 weeks. Serum levels peak within 2 hours. Duration unknown.

## INDICATIONS & DOSAGE
*Depression* –
**Adults:** initially, 100 mg P.O. b.i.d., increased after 3 days to 100 mg P.O. t.i.d. if needed. If no response occurs after several weeks of therapy, dosage increased to 150 mg t.i.d.

## ADVERSE REACTIONS
**CNS:** *headache, **seizures,** anxiety, confusion,* delusions, euphoria, hostility, impaired sleep quality, *insomnia, sedation, tremor,* akinesia, akathisia, *agitation, dizziness,* fatigue.
**CV: *arrhythmias,*** hypertension, hypotension, palpitations, syncope, *tachycardia.*
**EENT:** *auditory disturbances,* blurred vision.
**GI:** *dry mouth,* taste disturbance, increased appetite, *constipation,* dyspepsia, *nausea, vomiting, weight loss, anorexia, weight gain,* diarrhea.
**GU:** impotence, menstrual complaints, urinary frequency, decreased libido, urine retention.
**Skin:** pruritus, rash, cutaneous temperature disturbance, *excessive diaphoresis.*
**Other:** arthritis, fever and chills.

## INTERACTIONS
*Ethanol, levodopa, phenothiazines, MAO inhibitors, or TCAs; recent and rapid withdrawal of benzodiazepines:* increased risk of adverse reactions, including seizures. Monitor patient closely.

---

Reactions may be *common,* uncommon, *life-threatening,* or COMMON AND LIFE-THREATENING.

## CONTRAINDICATIONS
Contraindicated in patients who are hypersensitive to the drug, who have taken MAO inhibitors within the previous 14 days, and in patients with seizure disorders. Also contraindicated in patients with a history of bulimia or anorexia nervosa because of a higher incidence of seizures.

## NURSING CONSIDERATIONS
• Use cautiously in patients with recent history of MI or unstable heart disease, as well as impaired renal or hepatic impairment.
• Know that many patients experience a period of increased restlessness, especially at initiation of therapy. This may include agitation, insomnia, and anxiety.
• *Alert:* Risk of seizure may be minimized by not exceeding 450 mg/day and by administering daily dosage in three to four equally divided doses. Be aware that patients who experience seizures often have predisposing factors, including history of head trauma, prior seizures, or CNS tumors, or they may be taking a drug that lowers the seizure threshold.
• Monitor patients with history of bipolar disorders closely. Antidepressants can cause manic episodes during the depressed phase of bipolar disorder.
• From 28% to 30% of patients taking this drug may experience a weight loss of 5 lb (2.3 kg) or more. Consider this if weight loss is a major factor in the patient's depressive illness.

## ☑ PATIENT TEACHING
• Advise patient to take the drug as scheduled and to take each day's dosage in three divided doses to minimize the risk of seizures.
• Tell patient to avoid alcohol while taking this drug because it may contribute to the development of seizures.
• Advise patient to avoid hazardous activities that require alertness and good psychomotor coordination until CNS effects of the drug are known.
• Advise patient to consult his doctor before taking any other prescription or OTC medications.

---

# clomipramine hydrochloride
Anafranil

*Pregnancy Risk Category: C*

## HOW SUPPLIED
*Capsules:* 25 mg, 50 mg, 75 mg

## ACTION
Unknown, but a tricyclic antidepressant (TCA) that selectively inhibits reuptake of serotonin.

## ONSET, PEAK, DURATION
Unknown, although onset is thought to take 2 weeks or longer.

## INDICATIONS & DOSAGE
*Obsessive-compulsive disorder* –
**Adults:** initially, 25 mg P.O. daily in divided doses with meals, gradually increased to 100 mg daily during first 2 weeks. Thereafter, increased to maximum dosage of 250 mg daily in divided doses with meals as needed. After titration, total daily dosage may be given h.s.
**Children and adolescents:** initially, 25 mg P.O. daily in divided doses with meals, gradually increased to daily maximum of 3 mg/kg or 100 mg P.O., whichever is smaller. Maximum daily dosage is 3 mg/kg or 200 mg, whichever is smaller; may be given h.s. after titration. Periodic reassessment and adjustment necessary.

## ADVERSE REACTIONS
**CNS:** *somnolence, tremor, dizziness, headache, insomnia, nervousness, myoclonus, fatigue,* EEG changes, *seizures.*
**CV:** postural hypotension, palpitations, tachycardia.

---

*\*Liquid form contains alcohol.   \*\*May contain tartrazine.   †Canada only.   ‡Australia only.   ◊OTC.*

**EENT:** *pharyngitis, rhinitis, visual changes.*
**GI:** *dry mouth, constipation, nausea, dyspepsia, increased appetite,* diarrhea, *anorexia, abdominal pain.*
**GU:** *urinary hesitancy,* urinary tract infection, *dysmenorrhea, ejaculation failure, impotence.*
**Hematologic:** *purpura.*
**Skin:** *diaphoresis,* rash, pruritus, dry skin.
**Other:** *myalgia, weight gain, altered libido.*

## INTERACTIONS
*Barbiturates:* decreased TCA blood levels. Monitor for decreased antidepressant effect.
*Cimetidine, methylphenidate:* increased TCA blood levels. Monitor for enhanced antidepressant effect.
*Clonidine, epinephrine, norepinephrine:* increased hypertensive effect. Use with caution.
*CNS depressants, ethanol:* enhanced CNS depression. Avoid concomitant use.
*MAO inhibitors:* may cause hyperpyretic crisis, seizures, coma, or death. Don't use together.

## CONTRAINDICATIONS
Contraindicated in patients with hypersensitivity to drug or other TCAs, who have taken MAO inhibitors within the previous 14 days, and in patients during acute recovery period after MI.

## NURSING CONSIDERATIONS
● Use cautiously in patients with history of seizure disorders or with brain damage of varying etiology; in patients receiving other seizure threshold-lowering drugs; in patients at risk for suicide; in patients with history of urine retention or angle-closure glaucoma, increased intraocular pressure, CV disease, impaired hepatic or renal function, or hyperthyroidism; in patients with tumors of the adrenal medulla; in patients receiving thyroid medication or electroconvulsive therapy; and in those undergoing elective surgery.
● Know that total daily dose may be taken at bedtime after titration. During titration, dosage may be divided.
● Do not withdraw drug abruptly.
● Because hypertensive episodes have occurred during surgery in patients receiving TCAs, know that drug should be gradually discontinued several days before surgery.
● Be aware that adverse anticholinergic effects can occur rapidly.
● Relieve dry mouth with sugarless candy or gum. Saliva substitutes may be necessary.

## ☑ PATIENT TEACHING
● Warn patient to avoid hazardous activities requiring alertness and good psychomotor coordination, especially during titration. Daytime sedation and dizziness may occur.
● Tell patient to avoid alcohol while taking this drug.
● Warn patient not to withdraw drug suddenly.
● To prevent photosensitivity reactions, advise patient to use sunblock, wear protective clothing, and avoid prolonged exposure to strong sunlight.

# desipramine hydrochloride
Norpramin**, Pertofran‡, Pertofrane

*Pregnancy Risk Category: NR*

## HOW SUPPLIED
*Tablets:* 10 mg, 25 mg, 50 mg, 75 mg, 100 mg, 150 mg
*Capsules:* 25 mg, 50 mg

## ACTION
Unknown, but a tricyclic antidepressant (TCA) that increases the amount of norepinephrine, serotonin, or both in the CNS by blocking their reuptake by the presynaptic neurons.

Reactions may be *common,* uncommon, *life-threatening,* or **COMMON AND LIFE-THREATENING.**

## ONSET, PEAK, DURATION
Onset unknown but thought to occur in 2 to 4 weeks or longer. Serum levels peak within 4 to 6 hours. Duration unknown.

## INDICATIONS & DOSAGE
*Depression –*
**Adults:** 100 to 200 mg P.O. daily in divided doses, increased to maximum of 300 mg daily. Or entire dosage can be given at h.s.
**Elderly patients and adolescents:** 25 to 100 mg P.O. daily in divided doses, increased gradually to maximum of 150 mg daily if needed.

## ADVERSE REACTIONS
**CNS:** *drowsiness, dizziness,* excitation, tremor, weakness, confusion, anxiety, restlessness, agitation, headache, nervousness, EEG changes, *seizures,* extrapyramidal reactions.
**CV:** orthostatic hypotension, *tachycardia, ECG changes,* hypertension.
**EENT:** *blurred vision,* tinnitus, mydriasis.
**GI:** *dry mouth, constipation,* nausea, vomiting, anorexia, paralytic ileus.
**GU:** *urine retention.*
**Skin:** rash, urticaria, photosensitivity.
**Other:** *diaphoresis,* hypersensitivity reaction, *sudden death* (in children).
**After abrupt withdrawal of long-term therapy:** nausea, headache, malaise (does not indicate addiction).

## INTERACTIONS
*Barbiturates, CNS depressants, ethanol:* enhanced CNS depression. Avoid concomitant use.
*Cimetidine, methylphenidate:* may increase serum desipramine levels. Monitor for adverse reactions.
*Clonidine, epinephrine, norepinephrine:* increased hypertensive effect. Use with caution.
*MAO inhibitors:* may cause severe excitation, hyperpyrexia, or seizures, usually with high dosage. Use with caution.

## CONTRAINDICATIONS
Contraindicated in patients with hypersensitivity to drug, who have taken MAO inhibitors within the previous 14 days, and in patients during acute recovery phase of MI.

## NURSING CONSIDERATIONS
• Use with extreme caution in patients with CV disease, history of urine retention, or glaucoma, thyroid disease, or those taking thyroid medication, and in patients with history of seizure disorders.
• Do not withdraw drug abruptly.
• Because hypertensive episodes have occurred during surgery in patients receiving TCAs, know that drug should be gradually discontinued several days before surgery.
• If signs of psychosis occur or increase, expect the doctor to reduce dosage. Record mood changes. Monitor patients for suicidal tendencies, and allow them only a minimum supply of the drug.
• Know that because desipramine produces fewer anticholinergic effects than other TCAs, it is often prescribed for cardiac patients.
• Be aware that adverse anticholinergic effects can occur rapidly.
• Relieve dry mouth with sugarless hard candy or gum. Saliva substitutes may be necessary.

## ☑ PATIENT TEACHING
• Advise patient to take full dose at bedtime.
• Warn patient to avoid hazardous activities that require alertness and good psychomotor coordination until CNS effects of the drug are known. Drowsiness and dizziness usually subside after a few weeks.
• Tell patient to avoid alcohol while taking this drug because it may antagonize effects of desipramine.

---

*Liquid form contains alcohol. **May contain tartrazine. †Canada only. ‡Australia only. ◇OTC.

• Warn patient not to stop drug therapy suddenly.
• Advise patient to consult his doctor before taking any other prescription or OTC medications.
• To prevent photosensitivity reactions, advise patient to use sunblock, wear protective clothing, and avoid prolonged exposure to strong sunlight.

---

# doxepin hydrochloride
Deptran‡, Novo-Doxepin†, Sinequan, Triadapin†

*Pregnancy Risk Category: NR*

## HOW SUPPLIED
*Capsules:* 10 mg, 25 mg, 50 mg, 75 mg, 100 mg, 150 mg
*Oral concentrate:* 10 mg/ml

## ACTION
Unknown, but a tricyclic antidepressant (TCA) that increases the amount of norepinephrine, serotonin, or both in the CNS by blocking their reuptake by the presynaptic neurons.

## ONSET, PEAK, DURATION
Onset unknown but thought to take 2 to 4 weeks or longer. Serum levels peak within 2 hours. Duration unknown.

## INDICATIONS & DOSAGE
*Depression or anxiety –*
**Adults:** initially, 25 to 75 mg P.O. daily in divided doses to maximum of 300 mg daily. Alternatively, entire maintenance dosage may be given once daily with a maximum dose of 150 mg P.O.

## ADVERSE REACTIONS
**CNS:** *drowsiness, dizziness,* confusion, numbness, hallucinations, paresthesia, ataxia, weakness, headache, *seizures,* extrapyramidal reactions.
**CV:** *orthostatic hypotension, tachycardia.*
**EENT:** *blurred vision,* tinnitus.

**GI:** *dry mouth, constipation,* nausea, vomiting, anorexia.
**GU:** urine retention.
**Skin:** rash, urticaria, photosensitivity.
**Other:** *diaphoresis,* hypersensitivity reaction.
**After abrupt withdrawal of long-term therapy:** nausea, headache, malaise (does not indicate addiction).

## INTERACTIONS
*Barbiturates, CNS depressants, ethanol:* enhanced CNS depression. Avoid concomitant use.
*Cimetidine, methylphenidate:* may increase serum doxepin levels. Monitor for increased adverse reactions.
*Clonidine, epinephrine, norepinephrine:* increased hypertensive effect. Use with caution.
*MAO inhibitors:* may cause severe excitation, hyperpyrexia, or seizures, usually with high dosage. Avoid concomitant use.

## CONTRAINDICATIONS
Contraindicated in patients with hypersensitivity to drugs, glaucoma, or tendency to urine retention.

## NURSING CONSIDERATIONS
• Be aware that dosage should be reduced in elderly or debilitated patients, adolescents, and those receiving other medications (especially anticholinergics).
• Do not withdraw drug abruptly.
• Because hypertensive episodes have occurred during surgery in patients receiving TCAs, be aware that drug should be gradually discontinued several days before surgery.
• If signs of psychosis occur or increase, expect doctor to reduce dosage. Record mood changes. Monitor patients for suicidal tendencies, and allow them only a minimum supply of the drug.
• Doxepin has strong anticholinergic effects; it is one of the most sedating

---

TCAs. Also be aware that adverse anticholinergic effects can occur rapidly.
• Relieve dry mouth with sugarless hard candy or gum. Saliva substitutes may be necessary.

☑ **PATIENT TEACHING**
• Tell patient to dilute oral concentrate with 120 ml (4 oz) of water, milk, or juice (orange, grapefruit, tomato, prune, or pineapple, but not grape juice); preparation is incompatible with carbonated beverages.
• Advise patient to take full dose at bedtime but warn him of possible morning orthostatic hypotension.
• Warn patient to avoid hazardous activities that require alertness and good psychomotor coordination until CNS effects of the drug are known. Drowsiness and dizziness usually subside after a few weeks.
• Tell patient to avoid alcohol while taking this drug.
• Warn patient not to stop drug therapy suddenly.
• Advise patient to consult his doctor before taking any other prescription or OTC medications.
• To prevent photosensitivity reactions, advise patient to use sunblock, wear protective clothing, and avoid prolonged exposure to strong sunlight.

## fluoxetine hydrochloride
Prozac, Prozac-20‡

*Pregnancy Risk Category: B*

**HOW SUPPLIED**
*Pulvules:* 10 mg, 20 mg
*Oral solution:* 20 mg/5 ml

**ACTION**
Unknown, but presumed to be linked to its inhibition of CNS neuronal uptake of serotonin.

**ONSET, PEAK, DURATION**
Onset occurs in 1 to 4 weeks. Serum levels peak in 6 to 8 hours. Duration unknown.

**INDICATIONS & DOSAGE**
*Depression, obsessive-compulsive disorder –*
**Adults:** initially, 20 mg P.O. in the morning; dosage increased according to patient response. May be given b.i.d. in the morning and at noon. Maximum dosage is 80 mg/day.

**ADVERSE REACTIONS**
**CNS:** *nervousness, anxiety, insomnia, headache, drowsiness, tremor, dizziness, asthenia,* fatigue.
**CV:** palpitations, hot flashes.
**EENT:** nasal congestion, pharyngitis, cough, sinusitis.
**GI:** *nausea, diarrhea, dry mouth, anorexia, dyspepsia,* constipation, abdominal pain, vomiting, flatulence, increased appetite.
**GU:** sexual dysfunction.
**Respiratory:** upper respiratory infection, respiratory distress.
**Skin:** *rash, pruritus,* diaphoresis.
**Other:** flulike syndrome, muscle pain, *weight loss,* fever.

**INTERACTIONS**
*Flecainide, carbamazepine, vinblastine:* increased serum levels of these drugs. Monitor serum levels and the patient for adverse effects.
*Insulin, oral antidiabetic agents:* altered blood glucose levels and possible altered requirements for antidiabetic medication. Adjust dosage, as ordered.
*Lithium, tricyclic antidepressants:* risk of increased adverse CNS effects. Avoid concomitant use.
*Phenytoin:* increased plasma phenytoin levels and risk of toxicity. Monitor serum phenytoin levels and adjust dosage, as ordered.
*Tryptophan:* increased toxic reaction

exhibited by agitation, GI distress, and restlessness. Do not use together. *Warfarin, other highly protein-bound agents:* may increase plasma levels of fluoxetine or other highly protein-bound drugs. Monitor patient closely.

**CONTRAINDICATIONS**
Contraindicated in patients hypersensitive to the drug and in patients taking MAO inhibitors within 14 days of starting therapy.

**NURSING CONSIDERATIONS**
• Use cautiously in patients at high risk for suicide and in patients with history of hepatic, renal, or CV disease; diabetes mellitus; or history of seizures.
• Be aware that elderly or debilitated patients and patients with renal or hepatic dysfunction may require lower dosages or less frequent dosing.
• Use antihistamines or topical corticosteroids as ordered to treat rashes or pruritus.

☑ **PATIENT TEACHING**
• Tell patient to avoid taking drug in the afternoon because fluoxetine commonly causes nervousness and insomnia.
• Drug may cause dizziness or drowsiness in some patients. Warn patient to avoid driving and other hazardous activities that require alertness and good psychomotor coordination until CNS effects of the drug are known.
• Advise patient to consult his doctor before taking any other prescription or OTC medications.
• Warn patient to avoid food high in tryptophan, including meats, poultry, fish, liver, kidney, eggs, nuts, peanut butter, broad beans, and wheat germ.

# imipramine hydrochloride
Apo-Imipramine†, Imiprin‡, Impril†, Janimine**, Melipramine‡, Norfranil, Novopramine†, Tipramine, Tofranil**

# imipramine pamoate
Tofranil-PM**

*Pregnancy Risk Category: NR*

**HOW SUPPLIED**
**imipramine hydrochloride**
*Tablets:* 10 mg, 25 mg, 50 mg
*Injection:* 12.5 mg/ml
**imipramine pamoate**
*Capsules:* 75 mg, 100 mg, 125 mg, 150 mg

**ACTION**
Unknown, but a tricyclic antidepressant (TCA) that increases the amount of norepinephrine, serotonin, or both in the CNS by blocking their reuptake by the presynaptic neurons.

**ONSET, PEAK, DURATION**
Onset unknown but thought to take 2 to 4 weeks or longer. Peak plasma concentrations occur within 1 to 2 hours after oral administration and 30 minutes after I.M. administration. Duration unknown.

**INDICATIONS & DOSAGE**
*Depression –*
**Adults:** 75 to 100 mg P.O. or I.M. daily in divided doses, increased in 25- to 50-mg increments up to maximum dosage of 300 mg daily. Or entire dosage may be given h.s. (using pamoate salt).
*Childhood enuresis –*
**Children 6 years and over:**
25 mg P.O. 1 hour before bedtime. If no response within 1 week, increased to 50 mg if child is under 12 years; increased to 75 mg for children 12 years and over. In either case, maximum dosage is 2.5 mg/kg/day.

## ADVERSE REACTIONS

**CNS:** *drowsiness, dizziness,* excitation, tremor, confusion, hallucinations, anxiety, ataxia, paresthesia, nervousness, EEG changes, *seizures,* extrapyramidal reactions.

**CV:** *orthostatic hypotension, tachycardia, ECG changes,* hypertension, *MI, stroke,* arrhythmias, heart block, precipitation of CHF.

**EENT:** *blurred vision,* tinnitus, mydriasis.

**GI:** *dry mouth, constipation,* nausea, vomiting, anorexia, paralytic ileus, abdominal cramps.

**GU:** *urine retention.*

**Skin:** rash, urticaria, photosensitivity, pruritus.

**Other:** *diaphoresis,* hypersensitivity reaction.

**After abrupt withdrawal of long-term therapy:** nausea, headache, malaise (does not indicate addiction).

## INTERACTIONS

*Barbiturates, CNS depressants, ethanol:* enhanced CNS depression. Avoid concomitant use.
*Cimetidine, methylphenidate:* may increase serum imipramine levels. Monitor for adverse reactions.
*Clonidine, epinephrine, norepinephrine:* increased hypertensive effect. Use with caution.
*MAO inhibitors:* may cause hyperpyretic crisis, severe seizures, and death. Avoid concomitant use.

## CONTRAINDICATIONS

Contraindicated during acute recovery phase of MI, in patients with hypersensitivity to drug, and in those receiving MAO inhibitors.

## NURSING CONSIDERATIONS

● Use with extreme caution in patients at risk for suicide; in patients with history of urine retention or angle-closure glaucoma, increased intraocular pressure, CV disease, impaired hepatic function; or hyperthy-roidism, history of seizure disorders, impaired renal function; and in patients receiving thyroid medications. Injectable form contains sulfites, which may cause allergic reactions in hypersensitive patients.

● Be aware that reduced dosage in elderly or debilitated persons, adolescents, and patients with aggravated psychotic symptoms is necessary.

● Do not withdraw drug abruptly.

● Because of hypertensive episodes during surgery in patients receiving TCAs, be aware that drug should be gradually discontinued several days before surgery.

● If signs of psychosis occur or increase, expect doctor to reduce dosage. Record mood changes. Monitor patients for suicidal tendencies, and allow them only a minimum supply of the drug.

● To prevent relapse in children receiving the drug for enuresis, be aware that drug should be withdrawn gradually.

● Relieve dry mouth with sugarless hard candy or gum. Saliva substitutes may be necessary.

## ☑ PATIENT TEACHING

● Advise patient to take full dose at bedtime but warn him of possible morning orthostatic hypotension.

● If the child is an "early night" bed-wetter, tell parents it may be more effective to divide dosage and administer the first dose earlier in the day if approved by doctor.

● Tell patient to avoid alcohol while taking this drug.

● Warn patient to avoid hazardous activities that require alertness and good psychomotor coordination until CNS effects of the drug are known. Drowsiness and dizziness usually subside after a few weeks.

● Warn patient not to stop drug suddenly.

● Advise patient to consult his doctor

---

*Liquid form contains alcohol.  **May contain tartrazine.  †Canada only.  ‡Australia only.  ◇OTC.

before taking any other prescription or OTC medications.
• To prevent photosensitivity reactions, advise patient to use sunblock, wear protective clothing, and avoid prolonged exposure to strong sunlight.

---

## isocarboxazid
Marplan

*Pregnancy Risk Category: NR*

### HOW SUPPLIED
*Tablets:* 10 mg

### ACTION
Unknown, but an MAO inhibitor that probably promotes accumulation of neurotransmitters by inhibiting their metabolism.

### ONSET, PEAK, DURATION
Onset in 7 to 10 days, although up to 4 to 8 weeks may be needed to achieve full therapeutic effect. Peak levels occur within 3 to 5 days. Effects persist for up to 10 days after therapy is stopped.

### INDICATIONS & DOSAGE
*Depression –*
**Adults:** 30 mg P.O. daily as a single dose or in divided doses. Reduced to 10 to 20 mg daily when condition improves.

### ADVERSE REACTIONS
**CNS:** *dizziness,* vertigo, weakness, headache, hyperactivity, hyperreflexia, tremor, muscle twitching, mania, *insomnia,* confusion, memory impairment, fatigue.
**CV:** *orthostatic hypotension,* **arrhythmias.**
**EENT:** blurred vision.
**GI:** dry mouth, *anorexia,* nausea, diarrhea, constipation.
**Skin:** rash.
**Other:** peripheral edema, diaphoresis, weight changes, altered libido.
**After abrupt withdrawal from drug**

**therapy:** restlessness, anxiety, hallucinations, headache, weakness.

### INTERACTIONS
*Amphetamines, antihistamines, ephedrine, levodopa, meperidine, metaraminol, methylphenidate, phenylephrine, phenylpropanolamine, sympathomimetics:* enhanced pressor effects of these drugs. Avoid concomitant use.
*Barbiturates, dextromethorphan, ethanol, methotrimeprazine, narcotics, other sedatives, tricyclic antidepressants:* unpredictable interactions. Use these agents with caution and in reduced dosages.
*Insulin, oral antidiabetic agents:* increased risk of hypoglycemia. Use with caution; may require reduced dosages.
*Foods high in tyramine, tryptophan:* risk of hypertensive crisis. Avoid concomitant use.

### CONTRAINDICATIONS
• Contraindicated in elderly or debilitated patients; in patients with hypersensitivity to the drug, severe hepatic or renal impairment, CHF, pheochromocytoma, hypertension, or CV or cerebrovascular disease; in patients with severe or frequent headaches; and in patients who are currently receiving or have received fluoxetine therapy within the last 5 weeks.
• Also contraindicated with foods containing tryptophan or tyramine; during therapy with other MAO inhibitors (including phenelzine, tranylcypromine) or within 10 days of such therapy; and within 10 days of elective surgery requiring general anesthetic, cocaine use, or local anesthetic containing sympathomimetic vasoconstrictors.

### NURSING CONSIDERATIONS
• Use cautiously in patients at risk for suicide; and in patients with Parkinson's disease, impaired renal function,

---

hyperthyroidism, diabetes, or seizure disorders.
• Obtain baseline blood pressure, heart rate, CBC, and liver function test results before beginning therapy as ordered, and continue to monitor throughout treatment.
• Be aware that dosage is usually reduced to maintenance level as soon as possible.
• Do not withdraw drug abruptly.
• Know that in most patients, MAO inhibitors should be discontinued 14 days before elective surgery to avoid drug interactions that may occur during anesthesia.
• If the patient develops symptoms of overdose (palpitations, frequent headaches, or severe orthostatic hypotension), withhold dose and notify the doctor.
• *Alert:* Have phentolamine available to counteract severe hypertension.
• Monitor patients closely for suicidal tendencies, and allow them only a minimum supply of the drug.
• Continue precautions 10 days after discontinuation of the drug because it has long-lasting effects.

☑ **PATIENT TEACHING**
• Warn patient to avoid foods high in tryptophan (broad beans) or tyramine (aged cheese, Chianti wine, beer, avocados, chicken livers, chocolate, bananas, soy sauce, meat tenderizers, salami, bologna) and large amounts of caffeine.
• Tell patient to avoid alcohol while taking this drug.
• Advise patient to consult doctor before taking any other prescription or OTC medications. Severe adverse effects can occur if MAO inhibitors are taken with OTC cold, hay-fever, or diet preparations.
• Because MAO inhibitors may suppress chest pain in patient with angina, warn such a patient to engage in moderate activities and to avoid overexertion.

• To prevent dizziness from orthostatic hypotension, tell patient to get out of bed slowly, sitting up first for 1 minute. Supervise walking.
• Warn patient not to stop taking the drug suddenly.
• Tell patient to weigh himself biweekly. Teach him how to check for edema and urine retention.

---

# maprotiline hydrochloride
Ludiomil

*Pregnancy Risk Category: B*

**HOW SUPPLIED**
*Tablets:* 25 mg, 50 mg, 75 mg

**ACTION**
Unknown. A tetracyclic antidepressant similar to tricyclic derivatives. Probably increases the amount of norepinephrine, serotonin, or both in the CNS by blocking their reuptake by the presynaptic neurons.

**ONSET, PEAK, DURATION**
Onset usually occurs in 2 to 3 weeks, although sometimes it occurs within 7 days. Serum levels peak in 12 hours. Duration unknown.

**INDICATIONS & DOSAGE**
*Depression* –
**Adults:** initially, 25 to 75 mg P.O. daily for patients with mild to moderate depression, increased gradually in increments of 25 mg to 150 mg daily, if needed. Maximum dosage is 225 mg daily.

**ADVERSE REACTIONS**
**CNS:** *drowsiness, dizziness, seizures,* tremor, confusion, headache, nervousness, extrapyramidal reactions, anxiety, insomnia, agitation, numbness, weakness.
**CV:** *orthostatic hypotension, tachycardia, ECG changes,* hypertension, arrhythmias, heart block, syncope.

---

*Liquid form contains alcohol. **May contain tartrazine. †Canada only. ‡Australia only. ◇OTC.

**EENT:** *blurred vision,* tinnitus, mydriasis.
**GI:** *dry mouth, constipation,* nausea, diarrhea, vomiting.
**GU:** urine retention.
**Skin:** rash, urticaria, photosensitivity.
**Other:** *diaphoresis,* hypersensitivity reaction.
**After abrupt withdrawal of long-term therapy:** nausea, headache, malaise (does not indicate addiction).

## INTERACTIONS
*Barbiturates:* decreased blood maprotiline levels. Monitor for decreased antidepressant effect.
*Cimetidine, methylphenidate:* may increase serum maprotiline levels. Monitor for adverse reactions.
*Clonidine, epinephrine, norepinephrine:* increased hypertensive effect. Use with caution.
*CNS depressants, ethanol:* enhanced CNS depression. Avoid concomitant use.
*MAO inhibitors:* may cause severe excitation, hyperpyrexia, or seizures, usually with high dosage. Use with caution.

## CONTRAINDICATIONS
Contraindicated during acute recovery phase of MI and in patients with hypersensitivity to drug, seizure disorders, or within 14 days of MAO inhibitor therapy.

## NURSING CONSIDERATIONS
• Use with extreme caution in patients with history of MI or CV disease. Use cautiously in patients with suicidal tendency, increased intraocular pressure, or history of urine retention or angle-closure glaucoma.
• Know that dosage needs to be reduced in elderly or debilitated patients and adolescents.
• Do not withdraw drug abruptly.
• Because maprotiline shares toxic potentials with tricyclic antidepres-

sants and may cause hypertensive episodes during surgery, know that dosage should be gradually discontinued several days before surgery.
• If signs of psychosis occur or increase, expect doctor to reduce dosage. Record mood changes. Monitor patients for suicidal tendencies, and allow them only a minimum supply of the drug.
• Relieve dry mouth with sugarless hard candy or gum. Saliva substitutes may be necessary.

☑ **PATIENT TEACHING**
• Warn patient to avoid activities that require alertness and good psychomotor coordination until CNS effects of the drug are known. Drowsiness and dizziness usually subside after a few weeks.
• Advise patient to take full dose at bedtime, but warn him of possible morning orthostatic hypotension.
• Tell patient to avoid alcohol while taking this drug.
• Warn patient not to withdraw drug suddenly.
• Advise patient to consult his doctor before taking any other prescription or OTC medications.
• To prevent photosensitivity reactions, advise patient to use sunblock, wear protective clothing, and avoid prolonged exposure to strong sunlight.

---

# nefazodone hydrochloride
Serzone

*Pregnancy Risk Category: C*

## HOW SUPPLIED
*Tablets:* 100 mg, 150 mg, 200 mg, 250 mg

## ACTION
Not precisely defined. Nefazodone inhibits neuronal uptake of serotonin (5-HT-2) and norepinephrine; it also occupies serotonin and alpha$_1$-adrenergic receptors in the CNS.

## ONSET, PEAK, DURATION
Onset and duration unknown. Serum levels peak in about 1 hour.

## INDICATIONS & DOSAGE
*Depression –*
**Adults:** initially, 200 mg/day P.O. in two divided doses. Dosage increased in increments of 100 to 200 mg/day at intervals of no less than 1 week, p.r.n. Usual dosage range is 300 to 600 mg/day.

## ADVERSE REACTIONS
**CNS:** *headache, somnolence, dizziness, asthenia,* insomnia, *light-headedness, confusion,* memory impairment, paresthesia, vasodilation, abnormal dreams, decreased concentration, ataxia, incoordination, taste perversion, psychomotor retardation, tremor, hypertonia.
**CV:** postural hypotension, hypotension, peripheral edema.
**EENT:** *blurred vision, abnormal vision,* tinnitus, visual field defect.
**GI:** *dry mouth, nausea, constipation,* dyspepsia, diarrhea, increased appetite, vomiting.
**GU:** urinary frequency, urinary tract infection, urine retention, vaginitis.
**Respiratory:** pharyngitis, cough.
**Skin:** pruritus, rash.
**Other:** infection, flulike syndrome, chills, fever, neck rigidity, breast pain, thirst, arthralgia.

## INTERACTIONS
*Alprazolam, triazolam:* coadministration with nefazodone potentiates the effects of these drugs. Do not administer concurrently. However, if necessary, dosage of alprazolam and triazolam may need to be reduced greatly.
*Astemizole, terfenadine:* may cause decreased metabolism, leading to increased levels of these antihistamines and cardiotoxicity. Avoid concomitant use.
*CNS drugs:* may alter CNS activity. Use together cautiously.

*Digoxin:* may increase digoxin level. Use together cautiously and monitor digoxin levels.
*MAO inhibitors:* may cause severe excitation, hyperpyrexia, seizures, delirium, or coma. Avoid concomitant use.
*Other highly protein-bound drugs:* may increase incidence and severity of adverse reactions. Monitor patient closely.

## CONTRAINDICATIONS
Contraindicated in patients with hypersensitivity to the drug or to other phenylpiperazine antidepressants. Also contraindicated within 14 days of MAO inhibitor therapy and in coadministration with terfenadine or astemizole.

## NURSING CONSIDERATIONS
• Use cautiously in patients with CV or cerebrovascular disease that could be exacerbated by hypotension (such as history of MI, angina, or CVA) and conditions that would predispose patients to hypotension (such as dehydration, hypovolemia, and treatment with antihypertensives). Also use cautiously in patients with a history of mania.
• Know that at least 1 week should elapse between stopping nefazodone and starting MAO inhibitor therapy, and that at least 14 days should elapse before a patient begins taking nefazodone after MAO inhibitor therapy has been discontinued.
• Record mood changes. Monitor patients for suicidal tendencies, and allow them only a minimum supply of the drug.

## ☑ PATIENT TEACHING
• Warn patient not to engage in hazardous activity until drug's CNS effects are known.
• *Alert:* Instruct men who experience prolonged or inappropriate erections to stop drug immediately and notify doctor.

---

*Liquid form contains alcohol.   **May contain tartrazine.   †Canada only.   ‡Australia only.   ◇OTC.

• Instruct women to notify doctor if they become pregnant or intend to become pregnant during therapy.
• Instruct patient not to take alcoholic beverages while taking this drug.
• Tell patient who develops a rash, hives, or a related allergic reaction to notify doctor.
• Inform patient that several weeks of therapy may be required to obtain the full antidepressant effect. Once improvement occurs, advise patient not to discontinue drug until directed by doctor.

---

## nortriptyline hydrochloride
Allegron‡, Aventyl*, Nortab‡, Pamelor*

*Pregnancy Risk Category: NR*

### HOW SUPPLIED
*Tablets:* 10 mg‡, 25 mg‡
*Capsules:* 10 mg, 25 mg, 50 mg, 75 mg
*Oral solution:* 10 mg/5 ml (4% alcohol)

### ACTION
Unknown, but a tricyclic antidepressant (TCA) that increases the amount of norepinephrine, serotonin, or both in the CNS by blocking their reuptake by the presynaptic neurons.

### ONSET, PEAK, DURATION
Onset unknown but thought to take at least 2 to 4 weeks or longer. Peak plasma concentrations occur within 7 to 8.5 hours. Duration unknown.

### INDICATIONS & DOSAGE
*Depression* –
**Adults:** 25 mg P.O. t.i.d. or q.i.d., gradually increased to maximum of 150 mg daily. Or, entire dosage may be given h.s.

### ADVERSE REACTIONS
CNS: *drowsiness, dizziness, seizures,* tremor, weakness, confusion, headache, nervousness, EEG changes, extrapyramidal reactions, insomnia, nightmares, hallucinations, paresthesia, ataxia, agitation.
CV: *tachycardia,* hypertension, hypotension, *MI,* heart block, *stroke.*
EENT: *blurred vision,* tinnitus, mydriasis.
GI: dry mouth, *constipation,* nausea, vomiting, anorexia, paralytic ileus.
GU: *urine retention.*
Hematologic: bone marrow depression, *agranulocytosis,* eosinophilia, *thrombocytopenia.*
Skin: rash, urticaria, photosensitivity.
Other: *diaphoresis,* hypersensitivity reaction.
**After abrupt withdrawal of long-term therapy:** nausea, headache, malaise (does not indicate addiction).

### INTERACTIONS
*Barbiturates, CNS depressants, ethanol:* enhanced CNS depression. Avoid concomitant use.
*Cimetidine, methylphenidate:* may increase nortriptyline serum levels. Monitor for adverse reactions.
*Clonidine, epinephrine, norepinephrine:* increased hypertensive effect. Use with caution.
*MAO inhibitors:* may cause severe excitation, hyperpyrexia, or seizures, usually with high dosage. Use with caution.

### CONTRAINDICATIONS
Contraindicated during acute recovery phase of MI and in patients with hypersensitivity to drug or MAO therapy within past 14 days.

### NURSING CONSIDERATIONS
• Use with extreme caution in patients with glaucoma, suicidal tendency, history of urine retention or seizures, CV disease, or hyperthyroidism and in those receiving thyroid medication.
• Know that dosage should be re-

duced in elderly or debilitated patients and adolescents.
• Do not withdraw drug abruptly.
• Because hypertensive episodes have occurred during surgery in patients receiving TCAs, know that dosage should be gradually discontinued several days before surgery.
• If signs of psychosis occur or increase, expect doctor to reduce dosage. Record mood changes. Monitor patients for suicidal tendencies, and allow them only a minimum supply of the drug.
• Be aware that adverse anticholinergic effects can occur rapidly. Drug has anticholinergic effects similar to other TCAs.
• Relieve dry mouth with sugarless hard candy or gum. Saliva substitutes may be necessary.

☑ **PATIENT TEACHING**
• Whenever possible, advise patient to take full dose at bedtime to reduce the risk of orthostatic hypotension.
• Warn patient to avoid activities that require alertness and good psychomotor coordination until CNS effects of the drug are known. Drowsiness and dizziness usually subside after a few weeks.
• Tell patient to avoid alcohol while taking this drug.
• Warn patient not to stop drug suddenly.
• Advise patient to consult his doctor before taking any other prescription or OTC medications.
• To prevent photosensitivity reactions, advise patient to use sunblock, wear protective clothing, and avoid prolonged exposure to strong sunlight.

---

### paroxetine hydrochloride
Paxil
*Pregnancy Risk Category: B*

**HOW SUPPLIED**
*Tablets:* 20 mg, 30 mg

**ACTION**
Unknown, but presumed to be linked to its inhibition of CNS neuronal uptake of serotonin.

**ONSET, PEAK, DURATION**
Onset usually occurs within 1 to 4 weeks. Serum levels peak in 2 to 8 hours. Duration unknown.

**INDICATIONS & DOSAGE**
*Depression –*
**Adults:** initially, 20 mg P.O. daily, preferably in the morning as indicated. If patient does not respond after full antidepressant effect has occurred, dosage may be increased in 10-mg/day increments at weekly intervals, to a maximum of 50 mg daily.
**Elderly or debilitated patients; patients with severe hepatic or renal disease:** initially, 10 mg P.O. daily, preferably in the morning as indicated. If patient does not respond after full antidepressant effect has occurred, dosage may be increased in 10-mg/day increments at weekly intervals, to a maximum of 40 mg daily.

**ADVERSE REACTIONS**
**CNS:** *somnolence, dizziness, insomnia, tremor, nervousness,* anxiety, paresthesia, confusion, *headache,* agitation.
**CV:** palpitations, vasodilation, postural hypotension.
**EENT:** lump or tightness in throat, dysgeusia.
**GI:** *dry mouth, nausea, constipation, diarrhea,* flatulence, vomiting, dyspepsia, increased appetite, abdominal pain.
**GU:** ejaculatory disturbances, male genital disorders (including anorgasmy, erectile difficulties, delayed ejaculation or orgasm, impotence, and sexual dysfunction), urinary frequency, other urinary disorders, female genital disorders (including anorgasmy, difficulty with orgasm).
**Skin:** rash, pruritus.

**Other:** *asthenia, diaphoresis,* myopathy, myalgia, myasthenia, decreased libido, yawning.

## INTERACTIONS
*Cimetidine:* decreased hepatic metabolism of paroxetine, leading to risk of toxicity. Dosage adjustments may be necessary.
*Digoxin:* may decrease digoxin levels. Monitor closely.
*MAO inhibitors:* may increase risk of serious, sometimes fatal, adverse reactions. Avoid concomitant use.
*Phenobarbital, phenytoin:* may alter pharmacokinetics of both drugs. Dosage adjustments may be necessary.
*Procyclidine:* may increase procyclidine levels. Monitor for excessive anticholinergic effects.
*Tryptophan:* may increase incidence of adverse reactions, such as diaphoresis, headache, nausea, and dizziness. Avoid concomitant use.
*Warfarin:* increased risk of bleeding. Use concomitantly with caution.

## CONTRAINDICATIONS
Contraindicated in patients taking MAO inhibitors.

## NURSING CONSIDERATIONS
• Use cautiously in patients with a history of seizure disorders or mania and in those with severe, concomitant systemic illness.
• Use cautiously in patients at risk for volume depletion, and monitor appropriately.
• Don't administer paroxetine with, or within 14 days of discontinuing, MAO inhibitor therapy. Allow at least 2 weeks after discontinuing paroxetine before starting treatment with an MAO inhibitor as ordered.
• If signs of psychosis occur or increase, expect doctor to reduce dosage. Record mood changes. Monitor patients for suicidal tendencies, and allow them only a minimum supply of the drug.

☑ **PATIENT TEACHING**
• Warn patient to avoid activities that require alertness and good psychomotor coordination until CNS effects of the drug are known.
• Advise patient to consult his doctor before taking any other prescription or OTC medications.

---

# phenelzine sulfate
Nardil

*Pregnancy Risk Category: C*

## HOW SUPPLIED
*Tablets:* 15 mg

## ACTION
Unknown. An MAO inhibitor that probably promotes accumulation of neurotransmitters by inhibiting their metabolism.

## ONSET, PEAK, DURATION
Onset occurs in 7 to 10 days, although up to 4 to 8 weeks may be needed to achieve full therapeutic effect. Peak levels occur in 2 to 4 hours. Effects persist for up to 10 days after therapy is stopped.

## INDICATIONS & DOSAGE
*Depression* –
**Adults:** 15 mg P.O. daily t.i.d., increased rapidly to 60 mg daily. Maximum dosage is 90 mg daily. Then dosage can usually be reduced to 15 mg daily.

## ADVERSE REACTIONS
**CNS:** *dizziness,* vertigo, headache, hyperreflexia, tremor, muscle twitching, *insomnia,* drowsiness, weakness, fatigue.
**CV:** postural hypotension, edema.
**GI:** dry mouth, *anorexia,* nausea, constipation.
**Other:** diaphoresis, weight gain.

---

## INTERACTIONS

*Amphetamines, antihistamines, ephedrine, levodopa, meperidine, metaraminol, methylphenidate, phenylephrine, phenylpropanolamine, sympathomimetics:* enhanced pressor effects. Avoid concomitant use.

*Barbiturates, dextromethorphan, ethanol, methotrimeprazine, narcotics, other sedatives, tricyclic antidepressants:* unpredictable interaction. Use these agents with caution and in reduced dosage.

*Insulin, oral antidiabetic agents:* increased risk of hypoglycemia. Use with caution and in reduced dosages.

*Foods high in tryptophan, tyramine:* may precipitate hypertensive crisis. Avoid concomitant use.

## CONTRAINDICATIONS

Contraindicated in patients with hypersensitivity to drug, CHF, pheochromocytoma, hypertension, liver disease, and CV disease. Also contraindicated during therapy with other MAO inhibitors (isocarboxazid, tranylcypromine) or within 10 days of such therapy or within 10 days of elective surgery requiring general anesthesia, cocaine use, or local anesthesia containing sympathomimetic vasoconstrictors.

## NURSING CONSIDERATIONS

• Use cautiously with antihypertensives containing thiazide diuretics, with spinal anesthetics, and in patients at risk for suicide, diabetes, or seizure disorders.

• Obtain baseline blood pressure, heart rate, CBC, and liver function test results before therapy, and continue to monitor throughout treatment.

• Be aware dosage usually is reduced to maintenance level as soon as possible.

• In most patients, discontinue MAO inhibitors 14 days before elective surgery as ordered to avoid drug interactions that may occur during anesthesia.

• Monitor patients closely for suicidal tendencies, and allow them only a minimum supply of the drug.

• If patients develop symptoms of overdose (severe hypotension, palpitations, or frequent headaches), withhold dose and notify the doctor.

• *Alert:* Have phentolamine available to combat severe hypertension.

• Continue precautions 10 days after stopping drug because it has long-lasting effects.

## ☑ PATIENT TEACHING

• Warn patient to avoid foods high in tryptophan (broad beans) or tyramine (aged cheese, Chianti wine, beer, avocados, chicken livers, chocolate, bananas, soy sauce, meat tenderizers, salami, bologna) and large amounts of caffeine.

• Tell patient to avoid alcohol while taking drug.

• Advise patient to consult doctor before taking any other prescription or OTC medications. Severe adverse effects can occur if MAO inhibitors are taken with OTC cold, hay-fever, or diet preparations.

• Warn patient about the probability of orthostatic hypotension. Supervise walking. Tell patient to get out of bed slowly, sitting up first for 1 minute.

• Because MAO inhibitors may suppress chest pain in patient with angina, warn such a patient to engage in moderate activities and to avoid overexertion.

---

# protriptyline hydrochloride
Triptil†, Vivactil

*Pregnancy Risk Category: NR*

## HOW SUPPLIED
*Tablets:* 5 mg, 10 mg

---

## ACTION
Unknown, but a tricyclic antidepressant (TCA) that increases the amount of norepinephrine, serotonin, or both in the CNS by blocking their reuptake by the presynaptic neurons.

## ONSET, PEAK, DURATION
Onset unknown, although therapeutic effect thought to take 2 to 4 weeks or longer. Serum levels peak in 24 to 30 hours. Duration unknown.

## INDICATIONS & DOSAGE
*Depression* –
**Adults:** 15 to 40 mg P.O. daily in divided doses, increasing gradually to maximum of 60 mg daily.

## ADVERSE REACTIONS
**CNS:** *seizures,* tremor, hallucinations, disorientation, anxiety, restlessness, insomnia, ataxia, paresthesia, dizziness, weakness, confusion, headache, nervousness, EEG changes, extrapyramidal reactions.
**CV:** *tachycardia,* orthostatic hypotension, hypertension, *MI, stroke,* heart block, arrhythmias.
**EENT:** *blurred vision,* tinnitus, mydriasis.
**GI:** *dry mouth, constipation,* nausea, vomiting, anorexia, paralytic ileus.
**GU:** *urine retention.*
**Skin:** rash, urticaria, photosensitivity.
**Other:** *diaphoresis,* hypersensitivity reaction.
**After abrupt withdrawal of long-term therapy:** nausea, headache, malaise (does not indicate addiction).

## INTERACTIONS
*Barbiturates:* decreased TCA blood levels. Monitor for decreased antidepressant effect.
*Cimetidine, methylphenidate:* may increase serum protriptyline levels. Monitor for adverse reactions.
*Clonidine, epinephrine, norepineph-*rine: increased hypertensive effect. Use with caution.
*CNS depressants, ethanol:* enhanced CNS depression. Avoid concomitant use.
*MAO inhibitors:* may cause severe excitation, hyperpyrexia, seizures, or death, usually with high dosage. Use with caution.

## CONTRAINDICATIONS
Contraindicated during acute recovery phase of MI, in patients with hypersensitivity to the drug, and within 14 days of MAO inhibitor therapy.

## NURSING CONSIDERATIONS
• Use cautiously in elderly patients; in patients with history of seizures, suicidal tendencies, history of urine retention, increased intraocular pressure, CV disorders, hyperthyroidism, and in those receiving thyroid medications.
• Know that dosage should be reduced in elderly or debilitated patients and adolescents.
• Do not withdraw drug abruptly.
• Because hypertensive episodes have occurred during surgery in patients receiving TCAs, know that drug should be gradually discontinued several days before surgery.
• If signs of psychosis occur or increase, expect doctor to reduce dosage. Record mood changes. Monitor patients for suicidal tendencies, and allow them only a minimum supply of the drug. To prevent insomnia, avoid late-day dosing.
• Know that protriptyline has strong anticholinergic effects.
• Relieve dry mouth with sugarless hard candy or gum. Saliva substitutes may be necessary.

☑ **PATIENT TEACHING**
• Tell patient to avoid alcohol while taking this drug.
• Warn patient not to withdraw drug suddenly.

---

Reactions may be *common,* uncommon, *life-threatening,* or **COMMON AND LIFE-THREATENING.**

• Advise patient to consult doctor before taking any other prescription or OTC medications.
• To prevent photosensitivity reactions, advise patient to use sunblock, wear protective clothing, and avoid prolonged exposure to strong sunlight.

---

## sertraline hydrochloride
Zoloft

*Pregnancy Risk Category: B*

### HOW SUPPLIED
*Tablets:* 50 mg, 100 mg

### ACTION
Unknown, but presumed to be linked to its inhibition of neuronal uptake of serotonin in the CNS.

### ONSET, PEAK, DURATION
Onset occurs in 2 to 4 weeks. Serum levels peak 4½ to 8½ hours after dose. Duration unknown.

### INDICATIONS & DOSAGE
*Depression* –
**Adults:** 50 mg P.O. daily. Dosage adjusted as tolerated and needed; clinical trials involved dosage of 50 to 200 mg daily. Dosage adjustments should be made at intervals of no less than 1 week.

### ADVERSE REACTIONS
**CNS:** *headache, tremor, dizziness, insomnia, somnolence,* paresthesia, hypoesthesia, *fatigue,* nervousness, anxiety, agitation, hypertonia, twitching, confusion.
**CV:** palpitations, chest pain, hot flashes.
**GI:** *dry mouth, nausea, diarrhea, loose stools, dyspepsia,* vomiting, constipation, thirst, flatulence, anorexia, abdominal pain, increased appetite.
**GU:** *male sexual dysfunction.*
**Skin:** rash, pruritus.
**Other:** *diaphoresis,* myalgia.

### INTERACTIONS
*Diazepam, tolbutamide:* decreased clearance of these drugs. Clinical significance unknown; however, monitor patients for increased drug effects.
*MAO inhibitors:* may cause serious, sometimes fatal, reactions including myoclonus rigidity, mental status changes, hyperthermia, autonomic nervous system instability, rapid fluctuations of vital signs, delirium, coma, and death. Avoid concomitant use.
*Warfarin, other highly protein-bound drugs:* may increase plasma levels of sertraline or other highly bound drug. Small (8%) increases in PT have been seen with concomitant use of warfarin. Monitor closely.

### CONTRAINDICATIONS
None known.

### NURSING CONSIDERATIONS
• Use cautiously in patients at risk for suicide, and in those with seizure disorder, major affective disorder, or diseases or conditions that affect metabolism or hemodynamic responses.
• Administer sertraline once daily, either in the morning or evening. May be given with or without food.
• Know that sertraline should not be administered with, or within 14 days of discontinuing, MAO inhibitor therapy. Allow 14 days after discontinuing sertraline before starting treatment with an MAO inhibitor as ordered.
• Record mood changes. Monitor patients for suicidal tendencies, and allow them only a minimum supply of the drug.
• Know that drug may change several laboratory values — increases in serum cholesterol and triglyceride levels, decreases in uric acid concentrations, and elevations in AST and ALT (usually within the first 9 weeks of therapy). AST and ALT values return to normal after discontinuing

---

*Liquid form contains alcohol.   **May contain tartrazine.   †Canada only.   ‡Australia only.   ◇OTC.

drug; clinical significance is unknown.

• Advise patient to use caution when performing hazardous tasks that require alertness and to avoid alcohol while taking this drug. Drugs that influence the CNS may impair judgment.
• Caution patient to check with doctor or pharmacist before taking any OTC medications.

---

### tranylcypromine sulfate
Parnate

*Pregnancy Risk Category: NR*

**HOW SUPPLIED**
*Tablets:* 10 mg

**ACTION**
Unknown. An MAO inhibitor that probably promotes accumulation of neurotransmitters by inhibiting MAO.

**ONSET, PEAK, DURATION**
Onset in 48 hours to 3 weeks may be needed to achieve full therapeutic effect. Peak levels occur in 1 to 3.5 hours. Effects persist for up to 10 days after therapy is stopped.

**INDICATIONS & DOSAGE**
*Depression* –
**Adults:** 10 mg P.O. t.i.d. Increased by 10 mg P.O. daily at 1- to 3-week intervals to maximum of 60 mg daily, if necessary, after 2 weeks of therapy.

**ADVERSE REACTIONS**
**CNS:** *dizziness,* headache, anxiety, agitation, paresthesia, drowsiness, weakness, numbness, tremor, jitters, confusion.
**CV:** *orthostatic hypotension, tachycardia,* paradoxical hypertension, palpitations.
**EENT:** blurred vision, tinnitus.
**GI:** dry mouth, *anorexia,* nausea, diarrhea, constipation, abdominal pain.
**GU:** impotence, SIADH, urine retention, impaired ejaculation.
**Hematologic:** anemia, leukopenia, *agranulocytosis, thrombocytopenia.*
**Skin:** rash.
**Other:** edema, hepatitis, muscle spasm, myoclonic jerks, chills.

**INTERACTIONS**
*Amphetamines, antihistamines, ephedrine, levodopa, meperidine, metaraminol, methylphenidate, phenylephrine, phenylpropanolamine, sympathomimetics:* enhanced pressor effects of these drugs. Avoid concomitant use.
*Barbiturates, dextromethorphan, ethanol, methotrimeprazine, narcotics, other sedatives, tricyclic antidepressants:* enhanced adverse CNS effects. Use with caution and in reduced dosage.
*Buspirone:* may elevate blood pressure. Monitor patient closely.
*Insulin, oral antidiabetic agents:* increased risk of hypoglycemia. Use with caution and in reduced dosages.
*Foods high in tryptophan, tyramine:* may cause hypertensive crisis. Avoid concomitant use.

**CONTRAINDICATIONS**
• Contraindicated in patients receiving MAO inhibitors or dibenzazepine derivatives; sympathomimetics (including amphetamines); some CNS depressants (including narcotics and alcohol); selective serotonin reuptake inhibitors; antihypertensive, diuretic, antihistaminic, sedative or anesthetic drugs; bupropion hydrochloride, buspirone hydrochloride, dextromethorphan, meperidine; cheese or other foods with a high tyramine or tryptophan content; or excessive quantities of caffeine.
• Also contraindicated in patients with a confirmed or suspected cerebrovascular defect, CV disease, hy-

---

pertension, or history of headache and in those undergoing elective surgery.

## NURSING CONSIDERATIONS
• Use cautiously with antiparkinsonian drugs or spinal anesthetics; in patients with renal disease, diabetes, seizure disorder, Parkinson's disease, or hyperthyroidism; and in patients at risk for suicide.
• Obtain baseline blood pressure, heart rate, CBC, and liver function test results before beginning therapy, and continue to monitor throughout treatment.
• Know that dosage usually is reduced to maintenance level as soon as possible.
• Do not withdraw drug abruptly.
• In most patients, discontinue MAO inhibitors 14 days before elective surgery as ordered to avoid drug interactions that may occur during anesthesia.
• Monitor patients for suicidal tendencies, and allow them only a minimum supply of the drug.
• If patients develop symptoms of overdose (palpitations, severe hypotension, or frequent headaches), withhold dose and notify the doctor.
• *Alert:* Have phentolamine available to combat severe hypertension.
• Continue precautions for 10 days after stopping drug because it has long-lasting effects.

## ☑ PATIENT TEACHING
• Warn patient to avoid foods high in tyramine or tryptophan and large amounts of caffeine. Tranylcypromine is the MAO inhibitor most often reported to cause hypertensive crisis with ingestion of foods high in tyramine, including aged cheese, Chianti wine, beer, avocados, chicken livers, chocolate, bananas, soy sauce, meat tenderizers, salami, and bologna.
• Tell patient to avoid alcohol while taking this drug.

• To prevent dizziness resulting from orthostatic hypotension, tell patient to get out of bed slowly, sitting up for 1 minute first.
• Because MAO inhibitors may suppress anginal pain, warn patient to moderate activities and to avoid overexertion.
• Advise patient to consult his doctor before taking any other prescription or OTC medications. Severe adverse effects can occur if MAO inhibitors are taken with OTC cold, hay fever, or diet preparations.
• Warn patient not to stop drug suddenly.

---

## trazodone hydrochloride
Desyrel, Trazon, Trialodine

*Pregnancy Risk Category: C*

### HOW SUPPLIED
*Tablets:* 50 mg, 100 mg, 150 mg, 300 mg

### ACTION
Unknown, although it inhibits serotonin uptake in the brain. Not a tricyclic derivative.

### ONSET, PEAK, DURATION
Onset occurs in 2 to 4 weeks or longer. Plasma levels peak after 1 hour if taken on an empty stomach, 2 hours if taken with food. Duration unknown.

### INDICATIONS & DOSAGE
*Depression* –
**Adults:** initial dosage, 150 mg P.O. daily in divided doses; increased by 50 mg daily q 3 to 4 days, p.r.n. Average dosage ranges from 150 mg to 400 mg daily. Maximum daily dosage is 600 mg.

### ADVERSE REACTIONS
**CNS:** *drowsiness, dizziness,* nervousness, fatigue, confusion, tremor, weakness, hostility, anger, night-

---

*Liquid form contains alcohol.   **May contain tartrazine.   †Canada only.   ‡Australia only.   ◇OTC.

mares, vivid dreams, headache, insomnia.

**CV:** orthostatic hypotension, tachycardia, hypertension, syncope, shortness of breath.

**EENT:** blurred vision, tinnitus, nasal congestion.

**GI:** dry mouth, dysgeusia, constipation, nausea, vomiting, anorexia.

**GU:** urine retention; priapism, possibly leading to impotence; decreased libido; hematuria.

**Hematologic:** anemia.

**Skin:** rash, urticaria.

**Other:** diaphoresis.

### INTERACTIONS
*Antihypertensives:* increased hypotensive effect of trazodone. Antihypertensive dosage may have to be decreased.

*Clonidine, CNS depressants, ethanol:* enhanced CNS depression. Avoid concomitant use.

*Digoxin, phenytoin:* may increase serum levels of these drugs. Monitor for toxicity.

*MAO inhibitors:* effects unknown. Use together with extreme caution.

### CONTRAINDICATIONS
Contraindicated during initial recovery phase of MI or in patients with hypersensitivity to drug.

### NURSING CONSIDERATIONS
• Use cautiously in patients with cardiac disease and in patients at risk for suicide.

• Administer after meals or a light snack for optimal absorption and to decrease incidence of dizziness.

• Record mood changes. Monitor patients for suicidal tendencies, and allow them only minimum supply of the drug.

### ☑ PATIENT TEACHING
• *Alert:* Inform male patient that priapism is a potential problem in men taking trazodone and to report its presence immediately; it may require surgical intervention.

• Warn patient to avoid activities that require alertness and good psychomotor coordination until CNS effects of the drug are known. Drowsiness and dizziness usually subside after the first few weeks.

• Teach caregivers how to recognize signs of suicidal tendency or suicidal ideation.

## trimipramine maleate
Apo-Trimip†, Novo-Tripramine†, Rhotrimine†, Surmontil

*Pregnancy Risk Category: C*

### HOW SUPPLIED
*Tablets:* 25 mg‡
*Capsules:* 25 mg, 50 mg, 100 mg

### ACTION
Unknown, but a tricyclic antidepressant (TCA) that increases the amount of norepinephrine, serotonin, or both in the CNS by blocking their reuptake by the presynaptic neurons.

### ONSET, PEAK, DURATION
Onset unknown, although thought to occur in 2 to 4 weeks or longer. Plasma concentrations peak in 2 hours. Duration unknown.

### INDICATIONS & DOSAGE
*Depression –*
**Adults:** 75 to 100 mg P.O. daily in divided doses, increased to 200 to 300 mg daily. Dosages over 300 mg daily not recommended in hospitalized patients; not over 200 mg in outpatients.

### ADVERSE REACTIONS
**CNS:** *drowsiness, dizziness,* paresthesia, ataxia, hallucinations, delusions, anxiety, agitation, insomnia, tremor, weakness, confusion, headache, EEG changes, *seizures,* extrapyramidal reactions.

**CV:** *orthostatic hypotension, tachy-*

---

Reactions may be *common,* uncommon, *life-threatening,* or COMMON AND LIFE-THREATENING.

*cardia,* hypertension, arrhythmias, heart block, *MI, stroke.*
**EENT:** *blurred vision,* tinnitus, mydriasis.
**GI:** *dry mouth, constipation,* nausea, vomiting, anorexia, paralytic ileus.
**GU:** *urine retention.*
**Skin:** rash, urticaria, photosensitivity.
**Other:** *diaphoresis,* hypersensitivity reaction.
**After abrupt withdrawal of long-term therapy:** nausea, headache, malaise (does not indicate addiction).

## INTERACTIONS
*Barbiturates:* decreased TCA blood levels. Monitor for decreased antidepressant effect.
*Cimetidine, methylphenidate:* may increase serum trimipramine levels. Monitor for increased adverse reactions.
*Clonidine, epinephrine, norepinephrine:* increased hypertensive effect. Use with caution.
*CNS depressants, ethanol:* enhanced CNS depression. Avoid concomitant use.
*MAO inhibitors:* may cause severe excitation, hyperpyrexia, or seizures, usually with high dosage. Use with caution.

## CONTRAINDICATIONS
Contraindicated during acute recovery phase of MI and in patients with hypersensitivity to drug or receiving MAO inhibitor therapy within 14 days.

## NURSING CONSIDERATIONS
• Use with extreme caution in patients with CV disease, history of urine retention or angle-closure glaucoma, increased intraocular pressure, hyperthyroidism, impaired hepatic function, or history of seizures and in those receiving thyroid medications, guanethidine, or similar agents.
• Know that dosage should be reduced in elderly or debilitated persons and adolescents.
• Do not withdraw drug abruptly.
• Because hypertensive episodes have occurred during surgery in patients receiving TCAs, be aware that dosage should be gradually discontinued several days before surgery.
• If signs of psychosis occur or increase, expect doctor to reduce dosage. Record mood changes. Monitor patients for suicidal tendencies, and allow them only a minimum supply of the drug.
• Relieve dry mouth with sugarless hard candy or gum. Saliva substitutes may be necessary.

## ☑ PATIENT TEACHING
• To avoid daytime sedation, tell patient to take full dose at bedtime. Warn him about possible morning orthostatic hypotension.
• Warn patient to avoid hazardous activities that require alertness and good psychomotor coordination until CNS effects of the drug are known. Drowsiness and dizziness usually subside after a few weeks.
• Tell patient to avoid alcohol while taking this drug.
• Warn patient not to stop drug suddenly.
• Advise patient to consult his doctor before taking any other prescription or OTC medications.
• To prevent photosensitivity reactions, advise patient to use sunblock, wear protective clothing, and avoid prolonged exposure to strong sunlight.

# venlafaxine hydrochloride
Effexor

*Pregnancy Risk Category: C*

## HOW SUPPLIED
*Tablets:* 25 mg, 37.5 mg, 50 mg, 75 mg, 100 mg

---

## ACTION
Blocks reuptake of norepinephrine and serotonin into neurons in the CNS.

## ONSET, PEAK, DURATION
Onset unknown but thought to take several weeks. Peak and duration unknown.

## INDICATIONS & DOSAGE
*Depression –*
**Adults:** initially, 75 mg P.O. daily, in two or three divided doses with food. Dosage increased as tolerated and needed in increments of 75 mg/day at intervals of no less than 4 days. For moderately depressed outpatients, usual maximum dosage is 225 mg/day; in certain severely depressed patients, dosage may be as high as 375 mg/day.

## ADVERSE REACTIONS
**CNS:** *headache, somnolence, dizziness, nervousness, insomnia,* anxiety, tremor, abnormal dreams, paresthesia, agitation.
**CV:** hypertension.
**EENT:** blurred vision.
**GI:** *nausea, constipation,* vomiting, *dry mouth, anorexia,* diarrhea, dyspepsia, flatulence.
**GU:** *abnormal ejaculation,* impotence, urinary frequency, impaired urination.
**Other:** *diaphoresis, asthenia,* weight loss, rash, yawning, chills, infection.

## INTERACTIONS
*MAO inhibitors:* may precipitate a syndrome similar to neuroleptic malignant syndrome (myoclonus, hyperthermia, seizures, and death). Do not start venlafaxine within 14 days of discontinuing therapy with an MAO inhibitor, and don't start MAO inhibitor therapy within 7 days of stopping venlafaxine.

## CONTRAINDICATIONS
Contraindicated in patients hypersensitive to the drug. Also contraindicated for use within 14 days of MAO inhibitor therapy.

## NURSING CONSIDERATIONS
• Use cautiously in patients with renal impairment, diseases or conditions that could affect hemodynamic responses or metabolism, and in those with history of mania or seizures.
• Know that total daily dosage should be reduced by 50% in patients with hepatic impairment. In patients with moderate renal impairment (glomerular filtration rate of 10 to 70 ml/minute), total daily dosage should be reduced by 25%. In patients undergoing hemodialysis, know that dose should be withheld until dialysis session is completed and daily dosage is reduced by 50%.
• Carefully monitor blood pressure. Venlafaxine therapy is associated with sustained, dose-dependent increases in blood pressure. Greatest increases (averaging about 7 mm Hg above baseline) occur in patients taking 375 mg daily.

## ☑ PATIENT TEACHING
• Inform patient who has received drug for 6 weeks or more that drug should be gradually discontinued by tapering dosage over a 2-week period as instructed by doctor.
• Warn patient to avoid hazardous activities that require alertness and good psychomotor coordination until CNS effects of the drug are known.

---

# 32

## Antianxiety drugs

alprazolam
buspirone hydrochloride
chlordiazepoxide
chlordiazepoxide hydrochloride
clorazepate dipotassium
diazepam
doxepin hydrochloride
  (See Chapter 31, ANTIDEPRESSANTS.)
hydroxyzine embonate
hydroxyzine hydrochloride
hydroxyzine pamoate
lorazepam
meprobamate
midazolam hydrochloride
oxazepam
prazepam

### COMBINATION PRODUCTS
EQUAGESIC: meprobamate 200 mg and aspirin 325 mg.
LIBRAX: chlordiazepoxide hydrochloride 5 mg and clidinium bromide 2.5 mg.
LIMBITROL DS: chlordiazepoxide 10 mg and amitriptyline hydrochloride 25 mg.

---

### alprazolam
Apo-Alpraz†, Novo-Alprazol†, Nu-Alpraz†, Xanax
Controlled Substance Schedule IV

*Pregnancy Risk Category: D*

#### HOW SUPPLIED
*Tablets:* 0.25 mg, 0.5 mg, 1 mg, 2 mg
*Oral solution:* 0.5 mg/5 ml, 1 mg/ml (concentrate)

#### ACTION
Unknown. A benzodiazepine that probably potentiates the effects of gamma-aminobutyric acid, an inhibitory neurotransmitter, and depresses the CNS at the limbic and subcortical levels of the brain.

#### ONSET, PEAK, DURATION
Onset and duration unknown. Serum levels peak within 1 to 2 hours.

#### INDICATIONS & DOSAGE
*Anxiety –*
**Adults:** usual initial dose, 0.25 to 0.5 mg P.O. t.i.d. Maximum dosage is 4 mg daily in divided doses.
**Elderly or debilitated patients or those with advanced liver disease:** usual initial dose, 0.25 mg P.O. b.i.d. or t.i.d. Maximum dosage is 4 mg daily in divided doses.
*Panic disorders –*
**Adults:** 0.5 mg P.O. t.i.d., increased at intervals of 3 to 4 days in increments of no more than 1 mg. Maximum dosage is 10 mg daily in divided doses.

#### ADVERSE REACTIONS
**CNS:** *drowsiness, light-headedness,* headache, confusion, tremor, dizziness, syncope, *depression,* insomnia, nervousness.
**CV:** hypotension, tachycardia.
**EENT:** blurred vision, nasal congestion.
**GI:** *dry mouth,* nausea, vomiting, *diarrhea, constipation.*
**Skin:** dermatitis.
**Other:** muscle rigidity, weight gain or loss.

#### INTERACTIONS
*Cimetidine:* increased sedation. Monitor patient carefully.
*Digoxin:* may increase serum digoxin levels, increasing toxicity. Monitor patient closely.
*Ethanol, other CNS depressants:* increased CNS depression. Avoid concomitant use.
*Smoking:* increased clearance of benzodiazepines. Monitor for lack of effect.

*Tricyclic antidepressants (TCAs):* increased plasma levels of TCAs. Monitor for toxicity.

## CONTRAINDICATIONS
Contraindicated in patients with hypersensitivity to drug or other benzodiazepines or acute angle-closure glaucoma.

## NURSING CONSIDERATIONS
• Use cautiously in patients with hepatic, renal, or pulmonary disease.
• Also know that drug should not be prescribed for everyday stress or for long-term use (more than 4 months).
• Know that drug should not be withdrawn abruptly after long-term use; withdrawal symptoms may occur. Abuse or addiction is possible.
• Monitor liver, renal, and hematopoietic function studies periodically in patients receiving repeated or prolonged therapy, as ordered.

## ☑ PATIENT TEACHING
• Warn patient to avoid hazardous activities that require alertness and good psychomotor coordination until CNS effects of the drug are known.
• Tell patient to avoid alcohol while taking this drug.

---

## buspirone hydrochloride
BuSpar

*Pregnancy Risk Category: B*

### HOW SUPPLIED
*Tablets:* 5 mg, 10 mg

### ACTION
Unknown. May inhibit neuronal firing and reduce serotonin turnover in cortical, amygdaloid, and septohippocampal tissue.

### ONSET, PEAK, DURATION
Onset unknown but for therapeutic effect, possibly 1 to 2 weeks; optimal results, possibly 3 to 4 weeks. Serum

levels peak within 40 to 90 minutes. Duration unknown.

## INDICATIONS & DOSAGE
*Anxiety disorders; short-term relief of anxiety –*
**Adults:** initially, 5 mg P.O. t.i.d. Dosage increased at 3-day intervals in 5-mg increments. Usual maintenance dosage is 20 to 30 mg daily in divided doses. Do not exceed 60 mg daily.

## ADVERSE REACTIONS
**CNS:** *dizziness, drowsiness,* nervousness, insomnia, headache, light-headedness, fatigue, numbness.
**GI:** dry mouth, nausea, diarrhea, abdominal distress.
**Other:** blurred vision.

## INTERACTIONS
*Ethanol, other CNS depressants:* increased CNS depression. Avoid concomitant use.
*MAO inhibitors:* may elevate blood pressure. Avoid concomitant use.

## CONTRAINDICATIONS
Contraindicated in patients hypersensitive to the drug or within 14 days of therapy with an MAO inhibitor.

## NURSING CONSIDERATIONS
• Use cautiously in patients with hepatic or renal failure.
• Monitor patient closely for adverse CNS reactions. Buspirone is less sedating than other antianxiety agents and does not produce any serious functional impairment. However, CNS effects in individual patients may be unpredictable.
• Be aware that drug has shown no potential for abuse and has not been classified as a controlled substance. However, it is not recommended for relief of everyday stress.

## ☑ PATIENT TEACHING
• *Alert:* Before initiating buspirone therapy in patient already being treated

---

Reactions may be *common,* uncommon, *life-threatening,* or COMMON AND LIFE-THREATENING.

with benzodiazepines, warn him against stopping the benzodiazepine abruptly; withdrawal reaction may occur.

• Warn patient to avoid hazardous activities that require alertness and good psychomotor coordination until CNS effects of the drug are known.

---

## chlordiazepoxide
Libritabs

## chlordiazepoxide hydrochloride
Apo-Chlordiazepoxide†, Librium, Novopoxide†, Sereen, Solium†

Controlled Substance Schedule IV
*Pregnancy Risk Category: NR*

### HOW SUPPLIED
**chlordiazepoxide**
*Tablets:* 5 mg, 10 mg, 25 mg
**chlordiazepoxide hydrochloride**
*Capsules:* 5 mg, 10 mg, 25 mg
*Powder for injection:* 100-mg ampule

### ACTION
Unknown. Thought to depress the CNS at the limbic and subcortical levels of the brain.

### ONSET, PEAK, DURATION
Onset and duration unknown. Plasma levels peak in 30 minutes to 4 hours.

### INDICATIONS & DOSAGE
*Mild to moderate anxiety* –
**Adults:** 5 to 10 mg P.O. t.i.d. or q.i.d.
**Children over 6 years:** 5 mg P.O. b.i.d. to q.i.d. Maximum dosage is 10 mg P.O. b.i.d. or t.i.d.
*Severe anxiety* –
**Adults:** 20 to 25 mg P.O. t.i.d. or q.i.d.
*Withdrawal symptoms of acute alcoholism* –
**Adults:** 50 to 100 mg P.O., I.M., or

I.V. Repeated in 2 to 4 hours, p.r.n. Maximum dosage is 300 mg daily.
*Preoperative apprehension and anxiety* –
**Adults:** 5 to 10 mg P.O. t.i.d. or q.i.d. on day preceding surgery; or 50 to 100 mg I.M. 1 hour before surgery.
*Note:* Parenteral form not recommended in children under 12 years.

### ADVERSE REACTIONS
**CNS:** *drowsiness, lethargy,* ataxia, confusion, extrapyramidal symptoms, EEG changes.
**GI:** nausea, constipation.
**GU:** increased or decreased libido, menstrual irregularities.
**Hematologic:** *agranulocytosis.*
**Hepatic:** jaundice.
**Skin:** *swelling, pain at injection site,* skin eruptions, edema.

### INTERACTIONS
*Cimetidine:* increased sedation. Monitor patient carefully.
*Digoxin:* increased serum digoxin levels and risk of toxicity. Monitor patient closely.
*Ethanol, other CNS depressants:* increased CNS depression. Avoid concomitant use.
*Smoking:* increased clearance of benzodiazepines. Monitor for lack of effect.

### CONTRAINDICATIONS
Contraindicated in patients hypersensitive to the drug.

### NURSING CONSIDERATIONS
• Use cautiously in patients with mental depression, porphyria, or hepatic or renal disease.
• Know that drug should be avoided during pregnancy, especially during first trimester.
• Know that dosage should be reduced in elderly or debilitated patients.
• Also know that drug should not be

---

prescribed regularly for everyday stress.

• Injectable form (as hydrochloride) comes in two types of ampules — as diluent and as powdered drug. Read directions carefully.

• Do not mix injectable form with any other parenteral drug.

• Keep powder away from light and refrigerate; mix just before use and discard remainder.

• For I.M. use, add 2 ml of diluent to powder and agitate gently until clear. Use immediately. I.M. form may be absorbed erratically.

• **Alert:** Recommended for I.M. use only, but may be given I.V..

• **I.V. use:** Use 5 ml of 0.9% sodium chloride solution or sterile water for injection as diluent; do not give packaged diluent I.V. Administer over 1 minute.

• When giving drug I.V., be sure equipment and personnel needed for emergency airway management are available. Monitor respirations every 5 to 15 minutes and before each repeated I.V. dose.

• Monitor liver, renal, and hematopoietic function studies periodically in patients receiving repeated or prolonged therapy, as ordered.

• Possibility of abuse and addiction exists. Drug should not be withdrawn abruptly after long-term administration; withdrawal symptoms may occur.

• May cause false-positive reaction in the Gravindex pregnancy test. May also interfere with certain tests for urine 17-ketosteroids.

☑ **PATIENT TEACHING**
• Warn patient to avoid hazardous activities that require alertness and good psychomotor coordination until CNS effects of the drug are known.

• Tell patient to avoid alcohol while taking this drug.

# clorazepate dipotassium
Apo-Clorazepate†, Gen-XENE, Novoclopate†, Tranxene, Tranxene-SD, Tranxene-T-Tab
Controlled Substance Schedule IV

*Pregnancy Risk Category: NR*

## HOW SUPPLIED
*Tablets:* 3.75 mg, 7.5 mg, 11.25 mg, 15 mg, 22.5 mg
*Capsules:* 3.75 mg, 7.5 mg, 15 mg

## ACTION
Unknown. A benzodiazepine that probably facilitates the action of the inhibitory neurotransmitter gamma-aminobutyric acid. Depresses the CNS at the limbic and subcortical levels of the brain and suppresses the spread of seizure activity produced by epileptogenic foci in the cortex, thalamus, and limbic structures.

## ONSET, PEAK, DURATION
Onset and duration unknown. Plasma levels peak within ½ to 2 hours.

## INDICATIONS & DOSAGE
*Acute alcohol withdrawal –*
**Adults:** day 1 – 30 mg P.O. initially, followed by 30 to 60 mg P.O. in divided doses; day 2 – 45 to 90 mg P.O. in divided doses; day 3 – 22.5 to 45 mg P.O. in divided doses; day 4 – 15 to 30 mg P.O. in divided doses; then gradually reduce dosage to 7.5 to 15 mg daily.
*Anxiety –*
**Adults:** 15 to 60 mg P.O. daily.
*Adjunct in partial seizure disorder –*
**Adults and children over 12 years:** Maximum recommended initial dosage is 7.5 mg P.O. t.i.d. Dosage increases should be no greater than 7.5 mg/week. Maximum dosage should not exceed 90 mg daily.
**Children 9 and 12 years:** Maximum recommended initial dosage is 7.5 mg P.O. b.i.d. Dosage increases should be no greater than 7.5 mg/week.

---

Reactions may be *common*, uncommon, *life-threatening*, or **COMMON AND LIFE-THREATENING**.

Maximum dosage should not exceed 60 mg daily.

### ADVERSE REACTIONS
**CNS:** *drowsiness,* dizziness, nervousness, confusion, headache, insomnia, depression, irritability, tremor.
**CV:** hypotension.
**EENT:** blurred vision, diplopia.
**GI:** nausea, vomiting, abdominal discomfort, dry mouth
**GU:** urine retention, incontinence.
**Skin:** rashes.

### INTERACTIONS
*Cimetidine:* increased sedation. Monitor patient carefully.
*Digoxin:* may increase serum digoxin levels and risk of toxicity. Monitor patient closely.
*Ethanol, other CNS depressants:* increased CNS depression. Avoid concomitant use.
*Smoking:* increased clearance of benzodiazepines. Monitor for lack of effect.

### CONTRAINDICATIONS
Contraindicated in patients with hypersensitivity to the drug and acute angle-closure glaucoma.

### NURSING CONSIDERATIONS
● Know that drug should be avoided during pregnancy, especially the first trimester.
● Use cautiously in patients with suicidal tendencies, renal or hepatic impairment, or history of drug abuse.
● Know that dosage should be reduced in elderly or debilitated patients.
● Monitor liver, renal, and hematopoietic function studies periodically in patients receiving repeated or prolonged therapy as ordered.
● Possibility of abuse and addiction exists. Do not withdraw drug abruptly after prolonged use; withdrawal symptoms may occur.

### ☑ PATIENT TEACHING
● Warn patient to avoid activities that require alertness and good psychomotor coordination until CNS effects of the drug are known.
● Tell patient to avoid alcohol while taking this drug.
● Tell patient that sugarless chewing gum or hard candy can relieve dry mouth.

## diazepam
Apo-Diazepam†, Atenex‡, Diazemuls†‡, Diazepam Intensol, Ducene‡, Novodipam†, PMS-Diazepam†, T-Quil, Valium, Valrelease, Vazepam, Vivol†, Zetran
Controlled Substance Schedule IV
*Pregnancy Risk Category: NR*

### HOW SUPPLIED
*Tablets:* 2 mg, 5 mg, 10 mg
*Capsules (extended-release):* 15 mg
*Oral solution:* 5 mg/5 ml, 5 mg/ml
*Injection:* 5 mg/ml
*Sterile emulsion for injection:* 5 mg/ml†

### ACTION
Unknown. A benzodiazepine that probably depresses the CNS at the limbic and subcortical levels of the brain. Suppresses spread of seizure activity produced by epileptogenic foci in the cortex, thalamus, and limbic structures.

### ONSET, PEAK, DURATION
Onset occurs 30 minutes after oral dose, 1 to 5 minutes after I.V. injection. Plasma levels peak ½ to 2 hours after oral dose, immediately after I.V. injection; peak levels after administration of injectable emulsion occur 15 minutes after I.V. injection, 2 hours after I.M. injection. Effects persist for 3 to 8 hours after oral dose, 15 minutes to 1 hour after I.V. injection.

## INDICATIONS & DOSAGE
*Anxiety –*
**Adults:** depending on severity, 2 to 10 mg P.O. 2 to 4 times daily or 15 to 30 mg extended-release capsules P.O. once daily. Alternatively, 2 to 10 mg I.M. or I.V. q 3 to 4 hours, p.r.n.
**Children 6 months and older:** 1 to 2.5 mg P.O. 3 to 4 times daily, increased gradually, as needed and tolerated.
*Acute alcohol withdrawal –*
**Adults:** 10 mg P.O. 3 or 4 times first 24 hours, reduced to 5 mg P.O. three or four times daily, p.r.n. Alternatively, initially, 10 mg I.M. or I.V., then 5 to 10 mg I.M. or I.V. q 3 to 4 hours, p.r.n..
*Before endoscopic procedures –*
**Adults:** I.V. dose titrated to desired sedative response (up to 20 mg). Alternatively, 5 to 10 mg I.M. 30 minutes before procedure.
*Muscle spasm –*
**Adults:** 2 to 10 mg P.O. two to four times daily or 15 to 30 mg extended-release capsules once daily. Alternatively, 5 to 10 mg I.M. or I.V. initially, then 5 to 10 mg I.M. or I.V. q 3 to 4 hours, p.r.n. For tetanus, larger doses may be required.
**Children over 30 days to 5 years:** 1 to 2 mg I.M. or I.V. slowly, repeated q 3 to 4 hours, p.r.n.
**Children 5 years or older:** 5 to 10 mg I.M. or I.V. q 3 to 4 hours, p.r.n.
*Preoperative sedation –*
**Adults:** 10 mg I.M. (preferred) or I.V. before surgery
*Cardioversion –*
**Adults:** 5 to 15 mg I.V. within 5 to 10 minutes prior to procedure
*Adjunct in seizure disorders –*
**Adults:** 2 to 10 mg P.O. two to four times daily.
**Children 6 months and older:** 1 to 2.5 mg P.O. three or four times daily initially; increased as tolerated and needed.
*Status epilepticus and severe recurrent seizures –*

**Adults:** 5 to 10 mg I.V. (preferred) or I.M. initially. Repeated q 10 to 15 minutes, p.r.n., up to a maximum dose of 30 mg. Repeated q 2 to 4 hours, if necessary.
**Children over 30 days to 5 years:** 0.2 to 0.5 mg I.V. slowly q 2 to 5 minutes up to a maximum of 5 mg. Repeated q 2 to 4 hours, if necessary.
**Children 5 years and older:** 1 mg I.V. q 2 to 5 minutes up to maximum of 10 mg. Repeated q 2 to 4 hours, if necessary.

## ADVERSE REACTIONS
**CNS:** *drowsiness,* slurred speech, tremor, transient amnesia, fatigue, ataxia, headache, insomnia, paradoxical anxiety, hallucinations.
**CV:** hypotension, *cardiovascular collapse,* bradycardia.
**EENT:** diplopia, blurred vision, nystagmus.
**GI:** nausea, constipation.
**GU:** incontinence, urine retention, altered libido.
**Respiratory:** respiratory depression.
**Skin:** rash.
**Other:** physical or psychological dependence, *acute withdrawal syndrome* after sudden discontinuation in physically dependent persons, *pain, phlebitis at injection site, dysarthria, jaundice, neutropenia.*

## INTERACTIONS
*Cimetidine:* increased sedation. Monitor patient carefully.
*Digoxin:* may increase serum digoxin levels and risk of toxicity. Monitor patient closely.
*Ethanol, other CNS depressants:* increased CNS depression. Avoid concomitant use.
*Phenobarbital:* increased effects of both drugs. Use together cautiously.
*Smoking:* increased clearance of benzodiazepines. Monitor for lack of effect.

---

Reactions may be *common,* uncommon, *life-threatening,* or **COMMON AND LIFE-THREATENING.**

## CONTRAINDICATIONS

Contraindicated in patients with hypersensitivity or angle-closure glaucoma; in patients experiencing shock, coma, or acute alcohol intoxication (parenteral form); and in children under 6 months (oral form).

## NURSING CONSIDERATIONS

• Know that drug should be avoided during pregnancy, especially the first trimester.

• Use cautiously in patients with liver or renal impairment, depression, or chronic open-angle glaucoma; and in elderly and debilitated patients.

• Be aware dosage should be reduced in elderly or debilitated patients, who may be more susceptible to the adverse CNS effects of the drug.

• When oral concentrate solution is used, dilute the dose just before administering. Use water, juice, or carbonated beverages, or mix with semisolid food such as applesauce or pudding.

• I.V. route is the most reliable parenteral route; I.M. administration is not recommended because absorption is variable and injection is painful.

• **I.V. use:** Give at rate not exceeding 5 mg/minute. When injecting, administer directly into the vein. If this is impossible, inject slowly through the infusion tubing as near to the vein insertion site as possible. Watch daily for phlebitis at injection site.

• Avoid extravasation. Do not inject into small veins.

• Do not mix injectable form with other drugs because diazepam is incompatible with most drugs.

• **Alert:** Monitor respirations every 5 to 15 minutes and before each repeated I.V. dose. Have emergency resuscitation equipment and oxygen at bedside.

• Do not store parenteral solution in plastic syringes.

• Parenteral emulsion—a stabilized oil-in-water emulsion—should appear milky white and uniform. Avoid mixing with any other drugs or solutions, and avoid infusion sets or containers made from polyvinyl chloride. If dilution is necessary, drug may be mixed with I.V. fat emulsion. Use the admixture within 6 hours.

• Monitor periodic liver, renal, and hematopoietic function studies in patients receiving repeated or prolonged therapy, as ordered.

• Possibility of abuse and addiction exists. Do not withdraw drug abruptly after long-term use; withdrawal symptoms may occur.

### ☑ PATIENT TEACHING

• Warn patient to avoid activities that require alertness and good psychomotor coordination until CNS effects of the drug are known.

• Tell patient to avoid alcohol while taking this drug.

# hydroxyzine embonate‡
Atarax

# hydroxyzine hydrochloride
Anxanil, Apo-Hydroxyzine†, Atarax*, Atozine, Durrax, E-Vista, Hydroxacen, Hyzine-50, Multipax†, Novohydroxyzin†, Quiess, Vistacon-50, Vistaject-25, Vistaject-50, Vistaquel, Vistaril, Vistazine 50

# hydroxyzine pamoate
Hy-Pam, Vamate, Vistaril

*Pregnancy Risk Category: NR*

## HOW SUPPLIED

**hydroxyzine embonate‡**
*Capsules:* 25 mg, 50 mg
**hydroxyzine hydrochloride**
*Tablets:* 10 mg, 25 mg, 50 mg, 100 mg
*Capsules:* 10 mg†‡, 25 mg†‡, 50 mg†‡
*Syrup:* 10 mg/5 ml
*Injection:* 25 mg/ml, 50 mg/ml
**hydroxyzine pamoate**
*Capsules:* 25 mg, 50 mg, 100 mg
*Oral suspension:* 25 mg/5 ml

## ACTION
Unknown. A piperazine antihistamine whose action may be due to a suppression of activity in certain key regions of the subcortical area of the CNS.

## ONSET, PEAK, DURATION
Onset occurs in 15 to 30 minutes with oral administration, unknown after I.M. administration. Serum levels peak about 2 hours after oral dose, unknown after I.M. administration. Effects persist for 4 to 6 hours.

## INDICATIONS & DOSAGE
*Anxiety*–
**Adults:** 50 to 100 mg P.O. q.i.d.
**Children under 6 years:** 50 mg P.O. daily in divided doses.
**Children 6 years and over:** 50 to 100 mg P.O. daily in divided doses.
*Preoperative and postoperative adjunctive therapy*–
**Adults:** 25 to 100 mg I.M. q 4 to 6 hours.
**Children:** 1.1 mg/kg I.M. q 4 to 6 hours.
*Pruritus due to allergies*–
**Adults:** 25 mg P.O. t.i.d. or q.i.d.
**Children under 6 years:** 50 mg P.O. daily in divided doses.
**Children 6 years and over:** 50 to 100 mg P.O. daily in divided doses.
*Psychiatric and emotional emergencies, including acute alcoholism*–
**Adults:** 50 to 100 mg I.M. q 4 to 6 hours, p.r.n.
*Nausea and vomiting (excluding nausea and vomiting of pregnancy)*–
**Adults:** 25 to 100 mg I.M.
**Children:** 1.1 mg/kg I.M.
*Prepartum and postpartum adjunctive therapy*–
**Adults:** 25 to 100 mg I.M.

## ADVERSE REACTIONS
**CNS:** *drowsiness,* involuntary motor activity.
**GI:** *dry mouth.*
**Other:** marked discomfort at I.M. injection site, hypersensitivity reactions (wheezing, dyspnea, chest tightness).

## INTERACTIONS
*Ethanol, other CNS depressants:* increased CNS depression. Avoid concomitant use.

## CONTRAINDICATIONS
Contraindicated in patients hypersensitive to the drug and during early pregnancy.

## NURSING CONSIDERATIONS
● Know that dosage should be reduced in elderly or debilitated patients.
● Parenteral form (hydroxyzine hydrochloride) for I.M. use only; never administer I.V. The Z-track injection method is preferred.
● Aspirate I.M. injection carefully to prevent inadvertent intravascular injection. Inject deeply into a large muscle mass.
● If the patient is taking other CNS drugs, observe for oversedation.
● Be aware that drug may cause false elevations of urine 17-hydroxycorticosteroids, depending on test method used.

## ☑ PATIENT TEACHING
● Warn patient to avoid hazardous activities that require alertness and good psychomotor coordination until CNS effects of the drug are known.
● Tell patient to avoid alcohol while taking this drug.
● To relieve dry mouth, suggest sugarless hard candy or gum.

## lorazepam
Alzapam, Apo-Lorazepam†, Ativan, Lorazepam Intensol, Novo-Lorazem†, Nu-Loraz†
Controlled Substance Schedule IV
*Pregnancy Risk Category: NR*

## HOW SUPPLIED
*Tablets:* 0.5 mg, 1 mg, 2 mg
*Tablets (sublingual):* 0.5 mg†, 1 mg†, 2 mg†
*Oral solution (concentrated):* 2 mg/ml
*Injection:* 2 mg/ml, 4 mg/ml

## ACTION
Unknown. Probably stimulates gamma-aminobutyric receptors in the ascending reticular activating system.

## ONSET, PEAK, DURATION
Onset occurs within 1 to 5 minutes after I.V. administration, 15 to 30 minutes after I.M. injection, 1 to 6 hours after oral administration. Plasma levels peak within 1 to 1½ hours. Effects persist for 12 to 24 hours.

## INDICATIONS & DOSAGE
*Anxiety –*
**Adults:** 2 to 6 mg P.O. daily in divided doses. Maximum dosage is 10 mg daily.
*Insomnia due to anxiety –*
**Adults:** 2 to 4 mg P.O. h.s.
*Preoperative sedation –*
**Adults:** 0.05 mg/kg I.M. 2 hours before procedure. Total dosage should not exceed 4 mg. Alternatively, 2 mg I.V. total or 0.044 mg/kg I.V., whichever is smaller. Larger doses up to 0.05 mg/kg I.V., up to a total of 4 mg, may be required.

## ADVERSE REACTIONS
**CNS:** *drowsiness,* amnesia, insomnia, agitation, *sedation,* dizziness, weakness, unsteadiness, disorientation, depression, headache.
**EENT:** visual disturbances.
**GI:** abdominal discomfort, nausea, change in appetite.
**Other:** *acute withdrawal syndrome* (following sudden discontinuation in physically dependent persons).

## INTERACTIONS
*Digoxin:* may increase serum digoxin levels and risk of toxicity. Monitor patient closely.
*Ethanol, other CNS depressants:* increased CNS depression. Avoid concomitant use.
*Smoking:* increased clearance of benzodiazepines. Monitor for lack of effect.

## CONTRAINDICATIONS
Contraindicated in patients with acute angle-closure glaucoma or hypersensitivity to drug, other benzodiazepines or its vehicle (used in parenteral dosage form).

## NURSING CONSIDERATIONS
• Know that drug should be avoided during pregnancy, especially the first trimester.
• Use cautiously in patients with pulmonary, renal, or hepatic impairment. Also use cautiously in elderly, acutely ill, or debilitated patients.
• Know that dosage should be reduced in elderly or debilitated patients. Preoperative I.V. dose should not exceed 2 mg in patients over age 50.
• For I.M. administration, inject deeply into a muscle mass. Don't dilute.
• **I.V. use:** Give slowly, at rate not exceeding 2 mg/minute. Dilute with an equal volume of sterile water for injection, 0.9% sodium chloride for injection, or dextrose 5% injection.
• ***Alert:*** Monitor respirations every 5 to 15 minutes and before each repeated I.V. dose. Have emergency resuscitation equipment and oxygen available.
• Refrigerate parenteral form to prolong shelf life.
• Monitor liver, renal, and hematopoietic function studies periodically in patients receiving repeated or prolonged therapy, as ordered.
• Possibility of abuse and addiction exists. Do not withdraw drug abruptly

---

*Liquid form contains alcohol.    **May contain tartrazine.    †Canada only.    ‡Australia only.    ◊OTC.

after long-term use; withdrawal symptoms may occur.

### ☑ PATIENT TEACHING
• Warn patient to avoid hazardous activities that require alertness or good psychomotor coordination until CNS effects of the drug are known.
• Tell patient to avoid alcohol while taking this drug.
• As a premedication before surgery, lorazepam provides substantial preoperative amnesia. Patient teaching requires extra care to ensure adequate recall. Provide written materials or inform a family member, if possible.

---

## meprobamate
Apo-Meprobamate†, Equanil**, Meprospan 200, Meprospan-400, Miltown-200, Miltown-400, Miltown-600, Probate, Trancot
Controlled Substance Schedule IV
*Pregnancy Risk Category: NR*

### HOW SUPPLIED
*Tablets:* 200 mg, 400 mg, 600 mg
*Capsules (sustained-release):* 200 mg, 400 mg

### ACTION
Unknown. It appears to act at multiple sites in the CNS.

### ONSET, PEAK, DURATION
Unknown.

### INDICATIONS & DOSAGE
*Anxiety –*
**Adults:** 1.2 to 1.6 g P.O. daily in three or four equally divided doses. Maximum dosage is 2.4 g daily. Alternatively, 400 to 800 mg sustained-release capsule P.O. b.i.d.
**Children 6 to 12 years:** 200 to 600 mg P.O. b.i.d. or t.i.d. Or, 200 mg sustained-release capsule P.O. b.i.d. Not recommended for children under 6 years.

### ADVERSE REACTIONS
**CNS:** *drowsiness,* ataxia, dizziness, slurred speech, headache, vertigo, *seizures.*
**CV:** palpitations, tachycardia, hypotension, arrhythmias, syncope.
**GI:** nausea, vomiting, diarrhea.
**Hematologic:** *aplastic anemia, thrombocytopenia, agranulocytosis.*
**Skin:** pruritus, urticaria, erythematous maculopapular rash, *hypersensitivity reactions.*
• *Alert:* After abrupt withdrawal of long-term therapy, severe generalized tonic-clonic seizures may occur.

### INTERACTIONS
*Ethanol, other CNS depressants:* increased CNS depression. Avoid concomitant use.

### CONTRAINDICATIONS
Contraindicated in patients hypersensitive to meprobamate or related compounds (such as carisoprodol, mebutamate, tybamate, and carbromal) and in patients with porphyria.

### NURSING CONSIDERATIONS
• Know that drug should be avoided during pregnancy, especially the first trimester.
• Use cautiously in patients with impaired hepatic or renal function, seizure disorders, or suicidal tendencies.
• Be aware that dosage should be reduced in elderly or debilitated patients.
• Give drug with meals to reduce GI distress.
• Possibility of abuse and addiction exists with long-term use. Withdraw drug gradually over 2 weeks to avoid withdrawal symptoms.
• Know that drug may interfere with certain laboratory tests for urine 17-ketosteroids and 17-hydroxycorticosteroids.
• Periodically monitor CBC and renal and liver function tests in patients receiving high doses, as ordered.

---

Reactions may be *common,* uncommon, *life-threatening,* or COMMON AND LIFE-THREATENING.

## ☑ PATIENT TEACHING
• Advise patient to take drug with meals and not to crush or chew sustained-release capsules but to swallow them whole.
• Warn patient to avoid hazardous activities that require alertness and good psychomotor coordination until CNS effects of the drug are known.
• Tell patient to avoid alcohol while taking this drug.
• Tell patient to report any unusual bruising or bleeding, fever, or sore throat. These symptoms may indicate serious hematologic toxicity.

---

## midazolam hydrochloride
Hypnovel‡, Versed
Controlled Substance Schedule IV

*Pregnancy Risk Category: D*

### HOW SUPPLIED
*Injection:* 1 mg/ml, 5 mg/ml

### ACTION
Unknown. Thought to depress CNS at the limbic and subcortical levels of the brain by potentiating the effects of gamma-aminobutyric acid.

### ONSET, PEAK, DURATION
Onset occurs 1½ to 5 minutes after I.V. injection, within 15 minutes of I.M. injection. Peak effect occurs rapidly after I.V. administration, within 15 to 60 minutes after I.M. injection. Effects typically persist about 2 hours, but may last up to 6 hours.

### INDICATIONS & DOSAGE
*Preoperative sedation (to induce sleepiness or drowsiness and relieve apprehension) –*
**Adults:** 0.07 mg to 0.08 mg/kg I.M. approximately 1 hour before surgery.
*Conscious sedation before short diagnostic or endoscopic procedures –*
**Adults:** initially, small dose not to exceed 2.5 mg I.V. administered slowly; repeated in 2 minutes, if needed, in small increments of initial dose over at least 2 minutes to achieve desired effect. Total dose of up to 5 mg may be used (3.5 mg for elderly or debilitated patients and patients with decreased pulmonary reserve). For maintenance, additional doses to maintain desired level of sedation may be given by slow titration in increments of 25% of the dose used to first reach the sedative endpoint.
*Induction of general anesthesia –*
**Adults:** 0.3 to 0.35 mg/kg I.V. over 20 to 30 seconds if patient has not received any preanesthesia medication, or 0.2 to 0.25 mg/kg I.V. over 20 to 30 seconds if patient has received preanesthesia medication. Additional increments of 25% of the initial dose may be needed to complete induction.

### ADVERSE REACTIONS
**CNS:** headache, oversedation, drowsiness, amnesia.
**CV:** variations in blood pressure and pulse rate.
**GI:** *nausea,* vomiting, *hiccups.*
**Respiratory:** *decreased respiratory rate,* APNEA.
**Other:** *pain and tenderness at injection site.*

### INTERACTIONS
*Ethanol or other CNS depressants:* may increase the risk of apnea. Avoid concomitant use. Prepare to adjust dosage of midazolam if used with opiates or other CNS depressants.

### CONTRAINDICATIONS
Contraindicated in patients with hypersensitivity to drug, acute angle-closure glaucoma, and those experiencing shock, coma, or acute alcohol intoxication.

### NURSING CONSIDERATIONS
• Use cautiously in patients with uncompensated acute illness and in elderly or debilitated patients.
• *Alert:* Before administering, have

---

oxygen and resuscitation equipment available in case of severe respiratory depression. Excessive dosage or rapid infusion has been associated with respiratory arrest, particularly in elderly or debilitated patients.
• May be mixed in the same syringe with morphine sulfate, meperidine, atropine sulfate, or scopolamine.
• When injecting I.M., give deep into a large muscle mass.
• **I.V. use:** Administer slowly over at least 2 minutes, and wait at least 2 minutes when titrating doses to effect.
• When administering I.V., take care to avoid extravasation.
• Monitor blood pressure, heart rate and rhythm, respirations, airway integrity, and arterial oxygen saturation during procedure, especially in patients premedicated with narcotics.

### ☑ PATIENT TEACHING
• Midazolam's beneficial amnestic effect diminishes a patient's recall of perioperative events. This effect requires extra caution when teaching patients. Written information, family member instruction, and follow-up contact may be required to ensure that the patient has adequate information.
• Warn patient to avoid hazardous activities that require alertness or good psychomotor coordination until CNS effects of the drug are known.

## oxazepam
Alepam‡, Apo-Oxazepam†, Murelax‡, Novoxapam†, Ox-Pam†, Serax**, Serepax‡, Zapex†
Controlled Substance Schedule IV

*Pregnancy Risk Category: NR*

### HOW SUPPLIED
*Tablets:* 10 mg, 15 mg, 30 mg
*Capsules:* 10 mg, 15 mg, 30 mg

### ACTION
Unknown. Believed to stimulate gamma-aminobutyric acid receptors in the ascending reticular activating system.

### ONSET, PEAK, DURATION
Onset and duration unknown. Serum levels peak in about 3 hours.

### INDICATIONS & DOSAGE
*Alcohol withdrawal –*
**Adults:** 15 to 30 mg P.O. t.i.d. or q.i.d.
*Severe anxiety –*
**Adults:** 15 to 30 mg P.O. t.i.d. or q.i.d.
*Mild to moderate anxiety –*
**Adults:** 10 to 15 mg P.O. t.i.d. or q.i.d.

### ADVERSE REACTIONS
**CNS:** *drowsiness, lethargy,* dizziness, vertigo, headache, syncope, tremor, slurred speech.
**CV:** edema.
**GI:** nausea.
**Hematologic:** *leukopenia* (rare).
**Hepatic:** *hepatic dysfunction.*
**Skin:** rash.
**Other:** altered libido.

### INTERACTIONS
*Digoxin:* may increase serum digoxin levels and risk of toxicity. Monitor patient closely.
*Ethanol, cimetidine, other CNS depressants:* increased CNS depression. Avoid concomitant use.
*Smoking:* increased clearance of benzodiazepines. Monitor for lack of effect.

### CONTRAINDICATIONS
Contraindicated in patients hypersensitive to the drug.

### NURSING CONSIDERATIONS
• Know that drug should be avoided during pregnancy, especially the first trimester.
• Use cautiously in elderly patients and in patients with a history of drug abuse

or in whom a drop in blood pressure might lead to cardiac problems.
• Know that dosage should be reduced in elderly or debilitated patients.
• Monitor liver, renal, and hematopoietic function studies periodically in patients receiving repeated or prolonged therapy as ordered.
• Possibility of abuse and addiction exists. Do not stop drug abruptly; withdrawal symptoms may occur.

☑ **PATIENT TEACHING**
• Warn patient to avoid hazardous activities that require alertness or good psychomotor coordination until CNS effects of the drug are known.
• Tell patient to avoid alcohol while taking this drug.

## prazepam
Centrax
Controlled Substance Schedule IV

*Pregnancy Risk Category: NR*

### HOW SUPPLIED
*Tablets:* 5 mg, 10 mg
*Capsules:* 5 mg, 10 mg, 20 mg

### ACTION
Unknown. Believed to potentiate the effects of gamma-aminobutyric acid, an inhibitory neurotransmitter. Depresses the CNS at the limbic and subcortical levels of the brain.

### ONSET, PEAK, DURATION
Unknown.

### INDICATIONS & DOSAGE
*Anxiety* –
**Adults:** 20 to 60 mg P.O. daily in divided doses, or 20 to 40 mg h.s.

### ADVERSE REACTIONS
**CNS:** *drowsiness,* dizziness, ataxia, *fatigue,* weakness, light-headedness, confusion, tremor.
**CV:** transient hypotension, palpitations.

**GI:** dry mouth, nausea, vomiting, abdominal discomfort.
**Skin:** rash, diaphoresis.

### INTERACTIONS
*Cimetidine:* increased sedation. Monitor patient carefully.
*Digoxin:* may increase serum digoxin levels and risk of toxicity. Monitor patient closely.
*Ethanol, other CNS depressants:* increased CNS depression. Avoid concomitant use.
*Smoking:* increased clearance of benzodiazepines. Monitor for lack of effect.

### CONTRAINDICATIONS
Contraindicated in patients with hypersensitivity to drug or acute angle-closure glaucoma.

### NURSING CONSIDERATIONS
• Know that drug should be avoided during pregnancy, especially the first trimester.
• Use cautiously in elderly patients or patients with renal or hepatic impairment.
• Know that dosage should be reduced in elderly or debilitated patients.
• Monitor liver, renal, and hematopoietic function studies periodically in patients receiving repeated or prolonged therapy, as ordered.
• Possibility of abuse and addiction exists. Do not stop drug abruptly; withdrawal symptoms may occur.

☑ **PATIENT TEACHING**
• Warn patient to avoid activities that require alertness or good psychomotor coordination until CNS effects of the drug are known.
• Tell patient to avoid alcohol while taking this drug.

# 33

# Antipsychotics

chlorpromazine hydrochloride
chlorprothixene
clozapine
fluphenazine decanoate
fluphenazine enanthate
fluphenazine hydrochloride
haloperidol
haloperidol decanoate
haloperidol lactate
loxapine hydrochloride
loxapine succinate
mesoridazine besylate
molindone hydrochloride
perphenazine
pimozide
prochlorperazine
  (See Chapter 51, ANTIEMETICS.)
promazine hydrochloride
risperidone
thioridazine hydrochloride
thiothixene
thiothixene hydrochloride
trifluoperazine hydrochloride

## COMBINATION PRODUCTS
ETRAFON 2-10: perphenazine 2 mg
and amitriptyline hydrochloride 10
mg.
ETRAFON-A: perphenazine 2 mg and
amitriptyline hydrochloride 25 mg.
ETRAFON-FORTE: perphenazine 4 mg
and amitriptyline hydrochloride 25
mg.
TRIAVIL 2-10, TRIAVIL 4-10, TRIA-
VIL 2-25 are identical to Etrafon
products above. Triavil also is available as TRIAVIL 4-25 (perphenazine 4
mg and amitriptyline hydrochloride
25 mg) and TRIAVIL 4-50 (perphenazine 4 mg and amitriptyline hydrochloride 50 mg).

## chlorpromazine hydrochloride
Chlorpromanyl-5†, Chlorpromanyl-
20†, Chlorpromanyl-40†,
Largactil†‡, Novo-
Chlorpromazine†, Ormazine,
Thorazine, Thor-Prom

*Pregnancy Risk Category: NR*

### HOW SUPPLIED
*Tablets:* 10 mg, 25 mg, 50 mg, 100
mg, 200 mg
*Capsules (controlled-release):* 30 mg,
75 mg, 150 mg, 200 mg, 300 mg
*Oral concentrate:* 30 mg/ml, 100 mg/
ml
*Syrup:* 10 mg/5ml
*Injection:* 25 mg/ml
*Suppositories:* 25 mg, 100 mg

### ACTION
Unknown. An aliphatic phenothiazine
that probably blocks postsynaptic dopamine receptors in the brain and inhibits the medullary chemoreceptor
trigger zone.

### ONSET, PEAK, DURATION
Onset for full antipsychotic effects, 6
weeks or longer. Onset for other effects, peak, and duration vary.

### INDICATIONS & DOSAGE
*Psychosis –*
**Adults:** 25 to 75 mg P.O. daily in two
to four divided doses. Dosage increased by 20 to 50 mg twice weekly
until symptoms are controlled. Up to
800 mg daily may be required in some
patients. Or, 25 to 50 mg I.M. q 1 to 4
hours, p.r.n. Should progress to oral
therapy as soon as possible.
**Children 6 months and older:** 0.55
mg/kg P.O. q 4 to 6 hours or I.M. q 6
to 8 hours; or 1.1 mg/kg P.R. q 6 to 8

---

Reactions may be *common*, uncommon, *life-threatening*, or COMMON AND LIFE-THREATENING.

hours. Maximum I.M. dose in children under 5 years or weighing less than 22.7 kg is 40 mg. Maximum I.M. dose in children 5 to 12 years or weighing 22.7 to 45.5 kg is 75 mg.

*Nausea and vomiting* –

**Adults:** 10 to 25 mg P.O. q 4 to 6 hours, p.r.n.; or 50 to 100 mg P.R. q 6 to 8 hours, p.r.n., or 25 mg I.M. (if no hypotension occurs), 25 to 50 mg I.M. q 3 to 4 hours, p.r.n., until vomiting stops.

**Children 6 months and older:** 0.55 mg/kg P.O. q 4 to 6 hours or I.M. q 6 to 8 hours; or 1.1 mg/kg P.R. q 6 to 8 hours. Maximum I.M. dose in children under 5 years or weighing less than 22.7 kg is 40 mg. Maximum I.M. dose in children 5 to 12 years or weighing 22.7 to 45.5 kg is 75 mg.

*Intractable hiccups, acute intermittent porphyria* –

**Adults:** 25 to 50 mg P.O. t.i.d. or q.i.d. If symptoms persist for 2 to 3 days, 25 to 50 mg I.M. If symptoms still persist 25 to 50 mg diluted in 500 to 1000 ml of 0.9% sodium chloride solution and infused slowly.

*Tetanus* –

**Adults:** 25 to 50 mg I.V. or I.M. t.i.d. or q.i.d.

**Children 6 months or older:** 0.55 mg/kg I.M. or I.V. q 6 to 8 hours. Maximum parenteral dosage in children weighing less than 22.7 kg. is 40 mg daily; for children weighing 22.7 to 45.5 kg is 75 mg, except in severe cases.

*Surgery* –

**Adults:** preoperatively, 25 to 50 mg P.O. 2 to 3 hours before surgery or 12.5 to 25 mg I.M. 1 to 2 hours before surgery; during surgery, 12.5 mg I.M., repeated in 30 minutes if needed, or fractional 2-mg doses I.V. at 2-minute intervals up to a maximum dose of 25 mg; postoperatively, 10 to 25 mg P.O. q 4 to 6 hours or 12.5 to 25 mg I.M., repeated in 1 hour, if needed.

**Children 6 months and older:** pre-operatively, 0.55 mg/kg P.O. 2 to 3 hours before surgery or I.M. 1 to 2 hours before surgery; during surgery, 0.275 mg/kg I.M., repeated in 30 minutes if needed, or fractional 1 mg doses I.V. at 2-minute intervals up to a total of 0.275 mg/kg; may repeat fractional I.V. regimen in 30 minutes if needed; postoperatively, 0.55 mg/kg P.O. or I.M. q 4 to 6 hours (oral dose) or 1 hour (I.M. dose), if needed, and hypotension does not occur.

## ADVERSE REACTIONS

**CNS:** *extrapyramidal reactions,* drowsiness, *sedation,* **seizures,** *tardive dyskinesia,* pseudoparkinsonism, dizziness.

**CV:** *orthostatic hypotension,* tachycardia, ECG changes.

**EENT:** ocular changes, blurred vision, nasal congestion.

**GI:** *dry mouth, constipation,* nausea.

**GU:** *urine retention,* menstrual irregularities, gynecomastia, inhibited ejaculation, priapism.

**Hematologic:** leukopenia, *agranulocytosis,* eosinophilia, hemolytic anemia, *aplastic anemia, thrombocytopenia.*

**Hepatic:** jaundice, abnormal liver function test results.

**Skin:** *mild photosensitivity,* allergic reactions, *I.M. injection site pain,* sterile abscess, skin pigmentation.

**Other:** *neuroleptic malignant syndrome.*

**After abrupt withdrawal of long-term therapy:** gastritis, nausea, vomiting, dizziness, tremor.

## INTERACTIONS

*Antacids:* inhibited absorption of oral phenothiazines. Separate antacid and phenothiazine doses by at least 2 hours.

*Anticholinergics (including antidepressants and antiparkinsonian agents):* increased anticholinergic ac-

---

*Liquid form contains alcohol. **May contain tartrazine. †Canada only. ‡Australia only. ◊OTC.

tivity, aggravated parkinsonian symptoms. Use with caution.

*Barbiturates, lithium:* may decrease phenothiazine effect. Observe patient.

*Centrally acting antihypertensives:* decreased antihypertensive effect. Monitor blood pressure.

*Ethanol, other CNS depressants:* increased CNS depression. Avoid concomitant use.

*Propranolol:* increased levels of both propranolol and chlorpromazine. Monitor patient closely.

*Warfarin:* decreased effect of oral anticoagulants. Monitor PT.

## CONTRAINDICATIONS

Contraindicated in patients with hypersensitivity or in patients experiencing CNS depression, bone marrow suppression, subcortical damage, and coma.

## NURSING CONSIDERATIONS

• Use cautiously in elderly or debilitated patients and in patients with hepatic or renal disease; severe CV disease (may cause sudden drop in blood pressure); exposure to extreme heat or cold (including antipyretic therapy), to organophosphate insecticides; respiratory disorders; hypocalcemia; seizure disorders (may lower seizure threshold); severe reactions to insulin or electroconvulsive therapy; glaucoma; or prostatic hyperplasia.

• Use cautiously in acutely ill or dehydrated children.

• Obtain baseline measures of blood pressure before starting therapy and monitor regularly. Watch for orthostatic hypotension, especially with parenteral administration. Monitor blood pressure before and after I.M. administration. Keep patient supine for 1 hour afterward and have him get up slowly.

• **I.V. use:** For direct injection, drug may be diluted with 0.9% sodium chloride for injection and adminis-

tered into a large vein or through the tubing of a free-flowing I.V. solution. Do not exceed 1 mg/minute for adults or 0.5 mg/minute for children. Drug also may be given as an intermittent I.V. infusion; dilute with 50 or 100 ml of a compatible solution and infuse over 30 minutes. Chlorpromazine is compatible with most common I.V. solutions, including $D_5W$, Ringer's injection, lactated Ringer's injection, and 0.9% sodium chloride for injection.

• Slight yellowing of injection or concentrate is common and does not affect potency. Discard markedly discolored solutions.

• Give deep I.M. only in upper outer quadrant of buttocks. Massage slowly afterward to prevent sterile abscess. Injection stings.

• Wear gloves when preparing solutions, and prevent any contact with skin and clothing. Oral liquid and parenteral forms can cause contact dermatitis.

• Protect liquid concentrate from light. Dilute with fruit juice, milk, or semisolid food just before administration.

• Monitor patient for tardive dyskinesia, which may occur after prolonged use. It may not appear until months or years later and may disappear spontaneously or persist for life, despite discontinuation of drug.

• Watch for symptoms of neuroleptic malignant syndrome. It is rare, but frequently fatal. It is not necessarily related to length of drug use or type of neuroleptic, but over 60% of affected patients are men.

• Monitor therapy with weekly bilirubin tests during first month; periodic blood tests (CBC and liver function); and ophthalmic tests (long-term use) as ordered.

• Do not withdraw drug abruptly unless required by severe adverse reactions.

• Withhold dose and notify doctor if

patient develops jaundice, symptoms of blood dyscrasia (fever, sore throat, infection, cellulitis, weakness), persistent extrapyramidal reactions (longer than a few hours), or any such reaction in pregnancy or in children.

• Know that acute dystonic reactions may be treated with diphenhydramine.

☑ **PATIENT TEACHING**
• Warn patient to avoid activities that require alertness or good psychomotor coordination until CNS effects of the drug are known. Drowsiness and dizziness usually subside after first few weeks.
• Tell patient to avoid alcohol while taking this drug.
• Have patient report urine retention or constipation.
• Tell patient to use sunblock and to wear protective clothing to avoid photosensitivity reactions. Chlorpromazine causes higher incidence of photosensitivity than any other drug in its class.
• Tell patient to relieve dry mouth with sugarless gum or hard candy.

# chlorprothixene
Taractan**, Tarasan†

*Pregnancy Risk Category: NR*

**HOW SUPPLIED**
*Tablets:* 10 mg, 25 mg, 50 mg, 100 mg
*Oral concentrate:* 100 mg/5 ml (fruit)
*Injection:* 12.5 mg/ml

**ACTION**
Unknown. A thioxanthene that probably blocks postsynaptic dopamine receptors in the brain.

**ONSET, PEAK, DURATION**
Onset unknown but may take several weeks. Peak unknown. Effects persist for up to 12 hours after I.M. administration, unknown for oral form.

**INDICATIONS & DOSAGE**
*Psychotic disorders –*
**Adults and adolescents:** initially, 25 to 50 mg P.O. or I.M. t.i.d. or q.i.d. Increased gradually to maximum of 600 mg daily.
**Children 6 to 12 years:** 10 to 25 mg P.O. t.i.d. or q.i.d.

**ADVERSE REACTIONS**
**CNS:** extrapyramidal reactions (low incidence), tardive dyskinesia, *sedation,* pseudoparkinsonism, EEG changes, dizziness, drowsiness, *seizures,* ataxia, headache, weakness, insomnia.
**CV:** *orthostatic hypotension,* tachycardia, ECG changes.
**EENT:** ocular changes, *blurred vision,* nasal congestion.
**GI:** *dry mouth, constipation,* gastric upset.
**Hematologic:** leukopenia, *agranulocytosis,* hemolytic anemia, eosinophilia, *thrombocytopenia.*
**Hepatic:** jaundice, abnormal liver function test results.
**Skin:** *mild photosensitivity,* allergic reactions, I.M. injection site pain, sterile abscess, dermatitis.
**Other:** weight gain, *neuroleptic malignant syndrome.*
**After abrupt withdrawal of long-term therapy:** gastritis, nausea, vomiting, dizziness, tremor, feeling of warmth or cold, diaphoresis, tachycardia, headache, insomnia.

**INTERACTIONS**
*Anticholinergics:* potentiated central anticholinergic effects. Use together cautiously.
*Centrally acting antihypertensives:* decreased antihypertensive effect. Monitor blood pressure.
*Ethanol:* increased CNS depression. Avoid concomitant use.
*Other CNS depressants:* increased CNS depression. Use together cautiously.

---

*Liquid form contains alcohol.   **May contain tartrazine.   †Canada only.   ‡Australia only.   ◇OTC.

## CONTRAINDICATIONS

Contraindicated in patients with hypersensitivity, blood dyscrasia, CNS depression, bone marrow suppression, or circulatory collapse.

## NURSING CONSIDERATIONS

- Use cautiously in elderly or debilitated patients and in patients with hepatic disease, CV disease (may cause sudden drop in blood pressure), seizure disorders (may lower seizure threshold), glaucoma, or prostatic hyperplasia.
- Also use cautiously in patients with peptic ulcer, respiratory disorders, urine retention, or Parkinson's disease.
- Obtain baseline measures of blood pressure before starting therapy and monitor regularly. Watch for orthostatic hypotension, especially with parenteral administration, because adrenergic blockage is high. Keep patients in a supine position for 1 hour afterward and have them change positions slowly.
- Give deep I.M. only in upper outer quadrant of buttocks or midlateral thigh. Massage slowly afterward to prevent sterile abscess. Injection stings.
- Protect medication from light. Slight yellowing of injection or concentrate is common and does not affect potency. Discard markedly discolored solutions.
- Dilute liquid concentrate with fruit juice, milk, or semisolid food just before administration.
- Oral liquid form can cause contact dermatitis. Wear gloves when preparing solutions, and prevent any contact with skin and clothing.
- Monitor patient for tardive dyskinesia, which may occur after prolonged use. It may not appear until months or years later and may disappear spontaneously or persist for life, despite discontinuation of drug.
- Watch for symptoms related to neuroleptic malignant syndrome. It is rare, but frequently fatal. It is not necessarily related to length of drug use or type of neuroleptic, but over 60% of affected patients are men.
- Monitor therapy with weekly bilirubin tests during first month; periodic blood tests (CBC and liver function) before and during therapy; and ophthalmic tests (long-term therapy) as ordered.
- Do not withdraw drug abruptly unless required by severe adverse reactions.
- Withhold dose and notify doctor if patient develops symptoms of blood dyscrasia (fever, sore throat, infection, cellulitis, weakness), jaundice, or persistent extrapyramidal reactions (longer than a few hours), especially in children.
- Acute dystonic reactions may be treated with diphenhydramine.

☑ **PATIENT TEACHING**

- Warn patient to avoid activities that require alertness or good psychomotor coordination until CNS effects of the drug are known. Drowsiness and dizziness usually subside after first few weeks.
- Tell patient to avoid alcohol while taking this drug.
- Tell patient to relieve dry mouth with sugarless gum or hard candy.
- Tell patient to use sunblock and to wear protective clothing to avoid photosensitivity reactions.

# clozapine
Clozaril

*Pregnancy Risk Category: B*

## HOW SUPPLIED
*Tablets:* 25 mg, 100 mg

## ACTION
Unknown. Binds to dopaminergic receptors (both D-1 and D-2) within the limbic system of the CNS and may in-

---

Reactions may be *common*, uncommon, *life-threatening*, or COMMON AND LIFE-THREATENING.

terfere with adrenergic, cholinergic, histaminergic, and serotoninergic receptors.

## ONSET, PEAK, DURATION
Onset unknown. Serum levels peak in about 2½ hours. Effects persist for 4 to 12 hours.

## INDICATIONS & DOSAGE
*Schizophrenia in severely ill patients unresponsive to other therapies –*
**Adults:** initially, 12.5 mg P.O. once daily or b.i.d., titrated upward at 25 to 50 mg daily (if tolerated) to 300 to 450 mg daily by the end of 2 weeks. Individual dosage is based on clinical response, patient tolerance, and adverse reactions. Subsequent dosage should not be increased more than once or twice weekly, and should not exceed 100 mg. Many patients respond to dosages of 300 to 600 mg daily, but some may require as much as 900 mg daily. Do not exceed 900 mg daily.

## ADVERSE REACTIONS
**CNS:** *drowsiness, sedation, seizures,* dizziness, syncope, vertigo, headache, tremor, disturbed sleep or nightmares, restlessness, hypokinesia or akinesia, agitation, rigidity, akathisia, confusion, fatigue, insomnia, hyperkinesia, weakness, lethargy, ataxia, slurred speech, depression, myoclonus, anxiety.
**CV:** *tachycardia, hypotension,* hypertension, chest pain, ECG changes, orthostatic hypotension.
**GI:** *dry mouth, constipation,* nausea, vomiting, *excessive salivation,* heartburn, constipation, diarrhea.
**GU:** urinary abnormalities (urinary frequency or urgency, urine retention), incontinence, abnormal ejaculation.
**Hematologic:** *leukopenia, agranulocytosis.*
**Skin:** rash.
**Other:** fever, muscle pain or spasm,

muscle weakness, weight gain, visual disturbances, diaphoresis.
**After abrupt withdrawal of long-term therapy:** possible abrupt recurrence of psychotic symptoms. Monitor closely.

## INTERACTIONS
*Anticholinergics:* may potentiate anticholinergic effects of clozapine. Avoid concomitant use. Monitor blood pressure.
*Antihypertensives:* may potentiate hypotensive effects. Monitor blood pressure.
*Bone marrow suppressants:* may increase bone marrow toxicity. Don't use together.
*Psychoactive drugs:* may produce additive effects. Use together cautiously.
*Warfarin, digoxin, and other highly protein-bound drugs:* may increase serum levels of these drugs. Monitor closely for adverse reactions.

## CONTRAINDICATIONS
Contraindicated in patients with uncontrolled epilepsy, a history of clozapine-induced agranulocytosis; in patients with a WBC count below 3,500/mm$^3$; in patients with severe CNS depression or coma; in patients taking other drugs that suppress bone marrow function; and in those with myelosuppressive disorders.

## NURSING CONSIDERATIONS
● Use cautiously in patients with prostatic hyperplasia or angle-closure glaucoma because clozapine has potent anticholinergic effects and also in patients with hepatic, renal, or cardiac disease or those receiving general anesthesia.
● *Alert:* Clozapine carries significant risk of agranulocytosis. If possible, patients should receive at least two trials of drug therapy with a standard antipsychotic before clozapine therapy is initiated. Baseline WBC and differential counts are required before

---

*Liquid form contains alcohol.   **May contain tartrazine.   †Canada only.   ‡Australia only.   ◇OTC.

therapy. Monitor WBC counts weekly for at least 4 weeks after clozapine therapy is discontinued, as ordered.

• When administering clozapine, ensure that WBC counts and blood tests are performed weekly. Also ensure that no more than a 1-week supply of drug is dispensed.

• If WBC count drops below 3,500/mm³ after therapy is initiated or if it exhibits a substantial drop from baseline, monitor patient closely for signs of infection. If WBC count is 3,000 to 3,500/mm³ and granulocyte count is above 1,500/mm³, perform WBC and differential count twice weekly. If WBC count drops below 3,000/mm³ and granulocyte count drops below 1,500/mm³, interrupt therapy, notify doctor, and monitor the patient for signs of infection. Be aware that therapy may be restarted cautiously if WBC count returns to above 3,000/mm³ and granulocyte count returns above 1,500/mm³. Continue monitoring of WBC and differential counts twice weekly until WBC count exceeds 3,500/mm³, as ordered.

• If the WBC count drops below 2,000/mm³ and granulocyte count drops below 1,000/mm³, the patient may require protective isolation. If the patient develops infection, prepare cultures according to institutional policy and administer antibiotics, as ordered. Some clinicians may perform bone marrow aspiration to assess bone marrow function. Know that future clozapine therapy is contraindicated in such patients.

• Be aware that seizures may occur, especially in patients receiving high doses.

• Some patients experience transient fevers (temperature over 100.4° F, [38° C]), especially in the first 3 weeks of therapy. Monitor patients closely.

• If clozapine therapy must be discontinued, the drug usually is withdrawn gradually (over a 1- to 2-week period). However, changes in the patient's medical condition (including the development of leukopenia) may require abrupt discontinuation of the drug. Monitor closely for the recurrence of psychotic symptoms.

• If therapy is reinstated in patients withdrawn from the drug, follow usual guidelines for dosage increase. However, reexposure of the patient to this drug may increase the severity and risk of adverse reactions. If therapy was terminated because WBC counts were below 2,000/mm³ or granulocyte counts below 1,000/mm³, do not expect the drug to be continued.

☑ **PATIENT TEACHING**

• Warn patient about the risk of agranulocytosis. Tell patient that the drug is available only through a special monitoring program that requires weekly blood tests to monitor for agranulocytosis. Advise him to report flulike symptoms, fever, sore throat, lethargy, malaise, or other signs of infection.

• Warn patient to avoid hazardous activities that require alertness and good psychomotor coordination while taking this drug.

• Tell patient to rise slowly to avoid orthostatic hypotension.

• Advise patient to check with the doctor before taking any OTC drugs or alcohol.

• Recommend ice chips or sugarless candy or gum to help relieve dry mouth.

---

Reactions may be *common*, uncommon, *life-threatening*, or COMMON AND LIFE-THREATENING.

## fluphenazine decanoate
Modecate†‡, Modecate
Concentrate†, Prolixin Decanoate

## fluphenazine enanthate
Moditen Enanthate†, Prolixin
Enanthate

## fluphenazine hydrochloride
Anatensol‡*, Apo-Fluphenazine†,
Moditen HCl†, Moditen HCl-H.P.†,
Permitil* **, Permitil Concentrate,
Prolixin* **, Prolixin Concentrate

*Pregnancy Risk Category: NR*

### HOW SUPPLIED
**fluphenazine decanoate**
*Depot injection:* 25 mg/ml
**fluphenazine enanthate**
*Depot injection:* 25 mg/ml
**fluphenazine hydrochloride**
*Tablets:* 1 mg, 2.5 mg, 5 mg, 10 mg
*Oral concentrate:* 5 mg/ml (contains
1% alcohol)
*Elixir:* 2.5 mg/5 ml (with 14% alcohol)
*I.M. injection:* 2.5 mg/ml

### ACTION
Unknown. A piperazine phenothiazine that probably blocks postsynaptic dopamine receptors in the brain.

### ONSET, PEAK, DURATION
Following administration of fluphenazine hydrochloride, onset occurs within 1 hour although full therapeutic effect may take up to several weeks. Serum levels peak within 1½ to 2 hours after I.M. administration; ½ hour after oral administration. Effects persist for 6 to 8 hours. Following I.M. administration of fluphenazine decanoate or enanthate, onset of action occurs within 24 to 72 hours and duration of action is 1 to 6 weeks.

### INDICATIONS & DOSAGE
*Psychotic disorders –*
**Adults:** initially, 2.5 to 10 mg hydro-chloride P.O. daily in divided doses q 6 to 8 hours; may increase cautiously to 20 mg. Higher doses (50 to 100 mg) have been given. Maintenance dosage is 1 to 5 mg P.O. daily. I.M. doses are one-third to one-half of oral doses. Use lower dosages for elderly patients (1 to 2.5 mg daily). Alternatively, 12.5 to 25 mg of long-acting esters (decanoate or enanthate) I.M. or S.C. q 1 to 6 weeks; maintenance dosage is 25 to 100 mg, p.r.n.

### ADVERSE REACTIONS
**CNS:** *extrapyramidal reactions, tardive dyskinesia,* sedation, pseudoparkinsonism, EEG changes, drowsiness, *seizures,* dizziness.
**CV:** *orthostatic hypotension,* tachycardia, ECG changes.
**EENT:** ocular changes, *blurred vision,* nasal congestion.
**GI:** *dry mouth, constipation.*
**GU:** *urine retention,* dark urine, menstrual irregularities, gynecomastia, inhibited ejaculation.
**Hematologic:** leukopenia, *agranulocytosis,* eosinophilia, hemolytic anemia, *aplastic anemia, thrombocytopenia.*
**Hepatic:** cholestatic jaundice, abnormal liver function test results.
**Skin:** *mild photosensitivity,* allergic reactions.
**Other:** weight gain; increased appetite; rarely, *neuroleptic malignant syndrome.*
**After abrupt withdrawal of long-term therapy:** gastritis, nausea, vomiting, dizziness, tremor, feeling of warmth or cold, diaphoresis, tachycardia, headache, insomnia.

### INTERACTIONS
*Antacids:* inhibited absorption of oral phenothiazines. Separate antacid and phenothiazine doses by at least 2 hours.
*Anticholinergics:* increased anticholinergic effects. Avoid concomitant use.

---

*Liquid form contains alcohol. **May contain tartrazine. †Canada only. ‡Australia only. ◇OTC.

*Barbiturates, lithium:* may decrease phenothiazine effect. Observe patient.

*Centrally acting antihypertensives:* decreased antihypertensive effect. Monitor blood pressure.

*Ethanol, other CNS depressants:* increased CNS depression. Avoid concomitant use.

## CONTRAINDICATIONS
Contraindicated in patients with hypersensitivity or in patients experiencing coma, CNS depression, bone marrow suppression or other blood dyscrasia, subcortical damage, or liver damage.

## NURSING CONSIDERATIONS
• Use cautiously in elderly or debilitated patients and in those with pheochromocytoma; severe CV disease (may cause sudden drop in blood pressure); peptic ulcer; exposure to extreme heat or cold (including antipyretic therapy) or phosphorus insecticides; respiratory disorder; hypocalcemia; seizure disorder (may lower seizure threshold); severe reactions to insulin or electroconvulsive therapy; mitral insufficiency; glaucoma; or prostatic hyperplasia. Use parenteral form cautiously in asthmatic patients and patients allergic to sulfites.

• Prolixin Concentrate and Permitil Concentrate are 10 times more concentrated than Prolixin elixir (5 mg/ml versus 0.5 mg/ml). Check dosage order carefully.

• Dilute liquid concentrate with water, fruit juice, milk, or semisolid food just before administration.

• For long-acting forms (decanoate and enanthate), which are oil preparations, use a dry needle of at least 21G. Allow 24 to 96 hours for onset of action. Note and report adverse reactions in patients taking these drug forms.

• Oral liquid and parenteral forms can cause contact dermatitis. Wear gloves when preparing solutions, and prevent contact with skin and clothing.

• Protect medication from light. Slight yellowing of injection or concentrate is common and does not affect potency. Discard markedly discolored solutions.

• Monitor patient for tardive dyskinesia, which may occur after prolonged use. It may not appear until months or years later and disappear spontaneously or persist for life, despite discontinuation of drug.

• Watch patient for neuroleptic malignant syndrome. It is rare, but frequently fatal. It is not necessarily related to length of drug use or type of neuroleptic, but over 60% of affected patients are men.

• Monitor therapy with weekly bilirubin tests during first month; periodic blood tests (CBC and liver function); and periodic renal function and ophthalmic tests (long-term use) as ordered.

• Do not withdraw drug abruptly unless serious adverse reactions occur.

• Withhold dose and notify doctor if patient develops symptoms of blood dyscrasia (fever, sore throat, infection, cellulitis, weakness), persistent extrapyramidal reactions (longer than a few hours) especially in pregnant patients or in children.

• Acute dystonic reactions may be treated with diphenhydramine.

## ☑ PATIENT TEACHING
• Warn patient to avoid activities that require alertness and good psychomotor coordination until CNS effects of the drug are known. Drowsiness and dizziness usually subside after first few weeks.

• Tell patient to avoid alcohol while taking this drug.

• Tell patient to relieve dry mouth with sugarless gum or hard candy.

• Have patient report urine retention or constipation.

---

Reactions may be *common,* uncommon, *life-threatening,* or **COMMON AND LIFE-THREATENING.**

- Tell patient to use sunblock and to wear protective clothing to avoid photosensitivity reactions.
- Tell patient that drug may discolor urine.

## haloperidol
Apo-Haloperidol†, Haldol**, Novo-Peridol†, Peridol†, Serenace‡

## haloperidol decanoate
Haldol Decanoate, Haldol LA†

## haloperidol lactate
Haldol

*Pregnancy Risk Category: C*

### HOW SUPPLIED
**haloperidol**
*Tablets:* 0.5 mg, 1 mg, 2 mg, 5 mg, 10 mg, 20 mg
**haloperidol decanoate**
*Injection:* 50 mg/ml, 100 mg/ml
**haloperidol lactate**
*Oral concentrate:* 2 mg/ml
*Injection:* 5 mg/ml

### ACTION
Unknown. A butyrophenone that probably blocks postsynaptic dopamine receptors in the brain.

### ONSET, PEAK, DURATION
Onset unknown. Serum levels peak in 3 to 6 hours with oral dose, 10 to 20 minutes with I.M. injection (lactate), or 3 to 9 days with long-acting I.M. injection (decanoate). Duration unknown.

### INDICATIONS & DOSAGE
*Psychotic disorders –*
**Adults and children 12 and older:** dosage varies for each patient. Initial range, 0.5 to 5 mg P.O. b.i.d. or t.i.d.; or 2 to 5 mg I.M. q 4 to 8 hours although hourly administration may be needed until control obtained. Maximum dosage is 100 mg P.O. daily.

**Children 3 to 12 years:** 0.05 mg/kg to 0.15 mg/kg P.O. daily. Severely disturbed children may require higher doses.
*Chronic psychotic patients who require prolonged therapy –*
**Adults:** 50 to 100 mg I.M. haloperidol decanoate q 4 weeks.
*Nonpsychotic behavior disorders –*
**Children 3 to 12 years:** 0.05 mg/kg P.O. daily. Maximum daily dosage is 6 mg.
*Tourette syndrome –*
**Adults:** 0.5 to 5 mg P.O. b.i.d. or t.i.d. or p.r.n.
**Children 3 to 12 years:** 0.05 to 0.075 mg/kg P.O. daily in two or three divided doses.

### ADVERSE REACTIONS
**CNS:** *severe extrapyramidal reactions, tardive dyskinesia,* sedation, drowsiness, lethargy, headache, insomnia, confusion, vertigo, *seizures.*
**CV:** tachycardia, hypotension, hypertension, ECG changes.
**EENT:** blurred vision.
**GI:** dry mouth, anorexia, constipation, diarrhea, nausea, vomiting, dyspepsia.
**GU:** urine retention, menstrual irregularities, gynecomastia, priapism.
**Hematologic:** leukopenia and leukocytosis.
**Skin:** rash and other skin reactions, diaphoresis.
**Other:** rarely, *neuroleptic malignant syndrome, altered liver function tests, jaundice.*

### INTERACTIONS
*Ethanol, other CNS depressants:* increased CNS depression. Avoid concomitant use.
*Lithium:* lethargy and confusion after high doses. Monitor the patient.
*Methyldopa:* may cause symptoms of dementia or psychosis. Monitor the patient.

## CONTRAINDICATIONS
Contraindicated in patients with hypersensitivity or in patients experiencing parkinsonism, coma, or CNS depression.

## NURSING CONSIDERATIONS
• Use cautiously in elderly and debilitated patients; in patients with history of seizures or EEG abnormalities, severe CV disorders, allergies, glaucoma, or urine retention; and in conjunction with anticonvulsant, anticoagulant, antiparkinsonian, or lithium medications.
• Know that elderly patients usually require lower initial doses and a more gradual dosage titration.
• **Alert:** Do not administer the decanoate form I.V.
• When changing from tablets to decanoate injection, know that patient should be given 10 to 15 times the oral dose once a month (maximum 100 mg).
• Protect medication from light. Slight yellowing of injection or concentrate is common and does not affect potency. Discard markedly discolored solutions.
• Do not withdraw drug abruptly unless required by severe adverse reactions.
• Monitor patient for tardive dyskinesia, which may occur after prolonged use. It may not appear until months or years later and disappear spontaneously or persist for life, despite discontinuation of drug.
• Watch patient for neuroleptic malignant syndrome. It is rare, but frequently fatal. It is not necessarily related to length of drug use or type of neuroleptic, but over 60% of affected patients are men.
• Know that acute dystonic reactions may be treated with diphenhydramine.

## ☑ PATIENT TEACHING
• Drug is the least sedating of the antipsychotics, but warn the patient to avoid activities that require alertness and good psychomotor coordination until CNS effects of the drug are known. Drowsiness and dizziness usually subside after a few weeks.
• Tell the patient to avoid alcohol while taking this drug.
• Tell the patient to relieve dry mouth with sugarless gum or hard candy.

---

# loxapine hydrochloride
Loxapac†, Loxitane C, Loxitane IM

# loxapine succinate
Loxapac†, Loxitane

*Pregnancy Risk Category: NR*

## HOW SUPPLIED
**loxapine hydrochloride**
*Oral concentrate:* 25 mg/ml
*Injection:* 50 mg/ml
**loxapine succinate**
*Capsules:* 5 mg, 10 mg, 25 mg, 50 mg
*Tablets:* 5 mg†, 10 mg†, 25 mg†, 50 mg†

## ACTION
Unknown. A dibenzoxazepine that probably blocks postsynaptic dopamine receptors in the brain.

## ONSET, PEAK, DURATION
Onset of action occurs in 30 minutes. Serum levels peak in 1.5 to 3 hours. Effects persist up to 12 hours.

## INDICATIONS & DOSAGE
*Psychotic disorders –*
**Adults:** 10 mg P.O. b.i.d. to q.i.d., rapidly increasing to 60 to 100 mg P.O. daily for most patients; dosage varies from patient to patient. If patient is unable to take oral dose, 12.5 to 50 mg I.M. q 4 to 6 hours or longer, both dose and interval depending on patient response. Dosages greater than 250 mg/day are not recommended.

## ADVERSE REACTIONS
**CNS:** *extrapyramidal reactions, sedation,* drowsiness, **seizures**, numbness,

---

Reactions may be *common,* uncommon, *life-threatening,* or **COMMON AND LIFE-THREATENING.**

confusion, syncope, *tardive dyskinesia,* pseudoparkinsonism, EEG changes, dizziness.
**CV:** *orthostatic hypotension,* tachycardia, ECG changes, hypertension.
**EENT:** *blurred vision,* nasal congestion.
**GI:** *dry mouth, constipation,* nausea, vomiting, paralytic ileus.
**GU:** *urine retention,* menstrual irregularities, gynecomastia.
**Hematologic:** leukopenia, *agranulocytosis, thrombocytopenia.*
**Skin:** *mild photosensitivity,* allergic reactions, rash, pruritus.
**Other:** weight gain, *neuroleptic malignant syndrome,* jaundice.

### INTERACTIONS
*Ethanol, other CNS depressants:* increased CNS depression. Avoid concomitant use.

### CONTRAINDICATIONS
Contraindicated in patients with hypersensitivity to dibenzoxazepines and in patients experiencing coma, severe CNS depression, or drug-induced depressed states.

### NURSING CONSIDERATIONS
• Use with extreme caution in patients with seizure disorder, CV disorder, glaucoma, and history of urine retention.
• Obtain baseline measures of blood pressure before starting therapy and monitor regularly.
• Dilute liquid concentrate with orange or grapefruit juice just before giving.
• Monitor patient for tardive dyskinesia, which may occur after prolonged use. It may not appear until months or years later and disappear spontaneously or persist for life, despite discontinuation of drug.
• Monitor patient for neuroleptic malignant syndrome. It is rare, but frequently fatal. It is not necessarily related to length of drug use or type of

neuroleptic, but over 60% of affected patients are men.
• Know that acute dystonic reactions may be treated with diphenhydramine.

### ☑ PATIENT TEACHING
• Warn patient to avoid activities that require alertness and good psychomotor coordination until CNS effects of the drug are known. Drowsiness and dizziness usually subside after first few weeks.
• Tell patient to avoid alcohol while taking this drug.
• Advise patient to get up slowly to avoid orthostatic hypotension.
• Tell patient to relieve dry mouth with sugarless gum or hard candy.
• Tell patient that periodic eye examinations are recommended.

---

## mesoridazine besylate
Serentil* **, Serentil Concentrate
*Pregnancy Risk Category: NR*

### HOW SUPPLIED
*Tablets:* 10 mg, 25 mg, 50 mg, 100 mg
*Oral concentrate:* 25 mg/ml (0.6% alcohol)
*Injection:* 25 mg/ml

### ACTION
Unknown. A piperidine phenothiazine and the major sulfoxide metabolite of thioridazine that probably blocks postsynaptic dopamine receptors in the brain.

### ONSET, PEAK, DURATION
Onset of antipsychotic effect is gradual (up to several weeks) and varies among patients. Peak and duration not clearly defined.

### INDICATIONS & DOSAGE
*Alcoholism—*
**Adults and children over 12 years:**

25 mg P.O. b.i.d. up to maximum of 200 mg daily.
*Behavioral problems associated with chronic organic mental syndrome* –
**Adults and children over 12 years:** 25 mg P.O. t.i.d. up to maximum of 300 mg daily.
*Psychoneurotic manifestations (anxiety)* –
**Adults and children over 12 years:** 10 mg P.O. t.i.d. up to maximum of 150 mg daily.
*Schizophrenia* –
**Adults and children over 12 years:** initially, 50 mg P.O. t.i.d. or 25 mg I.M. repeated in 30 to 60 minutes, p.r.n. Maximum dosage is 400 mg daily.

## ADVERSE REACTIONS
**CNS:** extrapyramidal reactions, *tardive dyskinesia, sedation,* drowsiness, tremor, rigidity, weakness, EEG changes, dizziness.
**CV:** *hypotension,* tachycardia, ECG changes.
**EENT:** *ocular changes, blurred vision,* retinitis pigmentosa, nasal congestion.
**GI:** *dry mouth, constipation,* nausea, vomiting.
**GU:** *urine retention,* menstrual irregularities, gynecomastia, inhibited ejaculation.
**Hematologic:** leukopenia, *agranulocytosis, aplastic anemia,* eosinophilia, *thrombocytopenia.*
**Hepatic:** jaundice, abnormal liver function test results.
**Skin:** *mild photosensitivity,* allergic reactions, pain at I.M. injection site, sterile abscess, rash.
**Other:** weight gain, *neuroleptic malignant syndrome.*
**After abrupt withdrawal of long-term therapy:** gastritis, nausea, vomiting, dizziness, tremor, feeling of warmth or cold, diaphoresis, tachycardia, headache, insomnia.

## INTERACTIONS
*Antacids:* inhibited absorption of oral phenothiazines. Separate antacid and phenothiazine doses by at least 2 hours.
*Anticholinergics:* may increase anticholinergic effects. Use together cautiously.
*Barbiturates:* may decrease phenothiazine effect. Observe patient.
*Ethanol:* increased CNS depression. Avoid concomitant use.
*Other CNS depressants:* increased CNS depression. Use together cautiously.

## CONTRAINDICATIONS
Contraindicated in patients with hypersensitivity to the drug or experiencing severe CNS depression or comatose states.

## NURSING CONSIDERATIONS
● Obtain baseline measures of blood pressure before starting therapy and monitor regularly. Watch for orthostatic hypotension, especially with parenteral administration.
● Oral liquid and parenteral forms may cause contact dermatitis. Wear gloves when preparing solutions, and prevent contact with skin and clothing.
● Give deep I.M. only in upper outer quadrant of buttocks. Massage slowly afterward to prevent sterile abscess. Injection may sting.
● Protect medication from light. Slight yellowing of injection or concentrate is common and does not affect potency. Discard markedly discolored solutions.
● Monitor patient for tardive dyskinesia, which may occur after prolonged use. It may not appear until months or years later and disappear spontaneously or persist for life, despite discontinuation of drug.
● Assess patient for neuroleptic malignant syndrome. It is rare, but frequently fatal. It is not necessarily re-

---

Reactions may be *common,* uncommon, *life-threatening,* or COMMON AND LIFE-THREATENING.

lated to length of drug use or type of neuroleptic, but over 60% of affected patients are men.

• Withhold dose and notify the doctor if patient develops jaundice, symptoms of blood dyscrasia (fever, sore throat, infection, cellulitis, weakness), persistent extrapyramidal reactions (longer than a few hours), especially in pregnant patients or in children.

• Monitor therapy with weekly bilirubin tests during first month; periodic blood tests (CBC and liver function); and ophthalmic tests (long-term use), as ordered.

• Know that acute dystonic reactions may be treated with diphenhydramine.

• Do not withdraw drug abruptly unless required by severe adverse reactions.

### ☑ PATIENT TEACHING

• Warn patient to avoid activities that require alertness and good psychomotor coordination until CNS effects of the drug are known. Drowsiness and dizziness usually subside after a few weeks.

• Advise patient to change position slowly.

• Tell patient to avoid alcohol while taking this drug.

• Have patient report urine retention or constipation.

• Tell patient that drug may discolor urine.

• Instruct patient to relieve dry mouth with sugarless gum or hard candy.

• Tell patient to use sunblock and to wear protective clothing to avoid photosensitivity reactions.

## molindone hydrochloride
Moban

*Pregnancy Risk Category: NR*

### HOW SUPPLIED
*Tablets:* 5 mg, 10 mg, 25 mg, 50 mg, 100 mg
*Oral solution:* 20 mg/ml

### ACTION
Unknown. A dihydroindolone that probably blocks postsynaptic dopamine receptors in the brain.

### ONSET, PEAK, DURATION
Onset unknown but thought to take several weeks. Serum levels peak in 1.5 hours. Effects persist for 24 to 36 hours.

### INDICATIONS & DOSAGE
*Psychotic disorders –*
**Adults:** initially, 50 to 75 mg P.O. daily, then increased to 100 to 225 mg/day in 3 or 4 days. Maintenance dosage as follows: mild severity – 5 to 15 mg P.O. t.i.d. to q.i.d.; moderate severity – 10 to 25 mg P.O. t.i.d. or q.i.d.; or severe severity – 225 mg/day P.O.

### ADVERSE REACTIONS
**CNS:** *extrapyramidal reactions, tardive dyskinesia, sedation,* drowsiness, depression, euphoria, pseudoparkinsonism, EEG changes, dizziness.
**CV:** *orthostatic hypotension,* tachycardia, ECG changes.
**EENT:** *blurred vision.*
**GI:** *dry mouth, constipation,* nausea.
**GU:** *urine retention,* menstrual irregularities, gynecomastia, inhibited ejaculation.
**Hematologic:** leukopenia, leukocytosis.
**Hepatic:** jaundice, abnormal liver function test results.
**Skin:** *mild photosensitivity,* allergic reactions.
**Other:** rarely, ***neuroleptic malignant syndrome.***

## INTERACTIONS
*Ethanol, other CNS depressants:* increased CNS depression. Avoid concomitant use.

## CONTRAINDICATIONS
Contraindicated in patients with hypersensitivity to drug or experiencing coma or severe CNS depression.

## NURSING CONSIDERATIONS
• Use cautiously when increased physical activity would be harmful because this agent increases activity and in patients subject to seizures (may lower seizure threshold).
• Know that drug may be administered in a single daily dose.
• Monitor patient for tardive dyskinesia, which may occur after prolonged use. It may not appear until months or years later and may disappear spontaneously or persist for life, despite discontinuation of drug.
• Assess patient for neuroleptic malignant syndrome. It is rare, but frequently fatal. It is not necessarily related to length of drug use or type of neuroleptic, but over 60% of affected patients are men.
• Know that acute dystonic reactions may be treated with diphenhydramine.

## ☑ PATIENT TEACHING
• Warn patient to avoid activities that require alertness or good psychomotor coordination until CNS effects of the drug are known. Drowsiness and dizziness usually subside after first few weeks.
• Tell patient to avoid alcohol while taking this drug.
• Tell patient to relieve dry mouth with sugarless gum or hard candy.

# perphenazine
Apo-Perphenazine†, PMS Perphenazine†, Trilafon, Trilafon Concentrate

*Pregnancy Risk Category: NR*

## HOW SUPPLIED
*Tablets:* 2 mg, 4 mg, 8 mg, 16 mg
*Oral concentrate:* 16 mg/5ml
*Syrup:* 2 mg/5 ml†
*Injection:* 5 mg/ml

## ACTION
Unknown. Probably blocks postsynaptic dopamine receptors in the brain and inhibits the medullary chemoreceptor trigger zone.

## ONSET, PEAK, DURATION
Onset of antipsychotic effect is gradual (up to several weeks) and varies among patients. Peak and duration not clearly defined.

## INDICATIONS & DOSAGE
*Psychosis in nonhospitalized patients –*
**Adults:** initially, 4 to 8 mg P.O. t.i.d., reduced as soon as possible to minimum effective dosage.
**Children over 12 years:** lowest adult dose.
*Psychosis in hospitalized patients –*
**Adults:** initially, 8 to 16 mg P.O. b.i.d., t.i.d., or q.i.d., increased to 64 mg daily, p.r.n. Alternatively, 5 to 10 mg I.M. q 6 hours, p.r.n. Maximum dosage is 30 mg.
**Children over 12 years:** lowest limit of adult dosage.
*Severe nausea and vomiting –*
**Adults:** 8 to 16 mg P.O. daily in divided doses up to maximum of 24 mg. Alternatively, 5 to 10 mg I.M., p.r.n.

## ADVERSE REACTIONS
**CNS:** *extrapyramidal reactions, tardive dyskinesia,* sedation, pseudoparkinsonism, EEG changes, dizziness, *seizures,* drowsiness.

---

Reactions may be *common,* uncommon, *life-threatening,* or COMMON AND LIFE-THREATENING.

**CV:** *orthostatic hypotension,* tachycardia, ECG changes.
**EENT:** ocular changes, *blurred vision,* nasal congestion.
**GI:** *dry mouth, constipation,* nausea, vomiting, diarrhea.
**GU:** *urine retention,* dark urine, menstrual irregularities, gynecomastia, inhibited ejaculation.
**Hematologic:** leukopenia, *agranulocytosis,* eosinophilia, *hemolytic anemia, thrombocytopenia.*
**Hepatic:** jaundice, abnormal liver function test results.
**Skin:** *mild photosensitivity,* allergic reactions, pain at I.M. injection site, sterile abscess.
**Other:** weight gain, *neuroleptic malignant syndrome.*
**After abrupt withdrawal of long-term therapy:** gastritis, nausea, vomiting, dizziness, tremor, feeling of warmth or cold, diaphoresis, tachycardia, headache, insomnia.

## INTERACTIONS
*Antacids:* inhibited absorption of oral phenothiazines. Separate antacid and phenothiazine doses by at least 2 hours.
*Barbiturates:* may decrease phenothiazine effect. Observe patient.
*Ethanol, other CNS depressants:* increased CNS depression. Avoid concomitant use.

## CONTRAINDICATIONS
Contraindicated in patients with hypersensitivity to the drug; in patients experiencing coma; in those with CNS depression, blood dyscrasia, bone marrow depression, liver damage, or subcortical damage; and in those receiving large doses of CNS depressants.

## NURSING CONSIDERATIONS
• Use cautiously with other CNS depressants or anticholinergics, and in elderly or debilitated patients.
• Also use cautiously in patients with alcohol withdrawal, psychic depression, suicidal tendency, severe adverse reactions to other phenothiazines, impaired renal function, and respiratory disorders.
• Obtain baseline measures of blood pressure before starting therapy and monitor regularly. Watch for orthostatic hypotension, especially with parenteral administration. Keep patient supine for 1 hour afterward; tell him to change positions slowly.
• Prevent contact dermatitis by keeping drug away from skin and clothes. Wear gloves when preparing liquid forms.
• Dilute liquid concentrate with fruit juice, milk, carbonated beverage, or semisolid food just before giving. Exceptions: Oral concentrate causes turbidity or precipitation in colas, black coffee, grape or apple juice, or tea. Do not mix with these liquids.
• Protect drug from light. Slight yellowing of injection or concentrate is common and does not affect potency. Discard markedly discolored solutions.
• Give deep I.M. only in upper outer quadrant of buttocks. Massage slowly afterward to prevent sterile abscess. Injection may sting.
• Monitor patient for tardive dyskinesia, which may occur after prolonged use. It may not appear until months or years later and disappear spontaneously or persist for life, despite discontinuation of drug.
• Assess patient for neuroleptic malignant syndrome. It is rare, but frequently fatal. It is not necessarily related to length of drug use or type of neuroleptic, but over 60% of affected patients are men.
• Know that acute dystonic reactions may be treated with diphenhydramine.
• Monitor therapy with weekly bilirubin tests during first month; periodic blood tests (CBC and liver function); and ophthalmic tests (long-term use), as ordered.
• Do not withdraw drug abruptly un-

---

less required by severe adverse reactions.

• Withhold dose and notify doctor if patient develops jaundice, symptoms of blood dyscrasia (fever, sore throat, infection, cellulitis, weakness), or persistent extrapyramidal reactions (longer than a few hours).

### ☑ PATIENT TEACHING
• Instruct patient what beverages to use to dilute oral concentrate.
• Warn patient to avoid activities that require alertness or good psychomotor coordination until CNS effects of the drug are known. Drowsiness and dizziness usually subside after a few weeks.
• Tell patient to avoid alcohol while taking this drug.
• Advise patient to report urine retention or constipation.
• Tell patient to use sunblock and to wear protective clothing to avoid photosensitivity reactions.
• Tell patient to relieve dry mouth with sugarless gum or hard candy.

---

## pimozide
Orap

*Pregnancy Risk Category: C*

### HOW SUPPLIED
*Tablets:* 2 mg, 4mg†, 10 mg†

### ACTION
Unknown. Although thought to block dopamine nonselectively at both the presynaptic and postsynaptic receptors on neurons in the CNS.

### ONSET, PEAK, DURATION
Onset and duration unknown. Serum levels peak within 4 to 12 hours.

### INDICATIONS & DOSAGE
*Suppression of motor and phonic tics in patients with Tourette syndrome refractory to first-line therapy* –
**Adults and children over 12 years:**
initially, 1 to 2 mg P.O. daily in divided doses, then increased every other day, p.r.n. Maximum dosage is 10 mg daily.

### ADVERSE REACTIONS
**CNS:** *parkinsonian-like symptoms,* drowsiness, headache, insomnia, other extrapyramidal symptoms (dystonia, akathisia, hyperreflexia, opisthotonos, oculogyric crisis), *tardive dyskinesia, sedation.*
**CV:** *ECG changes (prolonged QT interval),* hypotension, hypertension, tachycardia.
**EENT:** visual disturbances.
**GI:** *dry mouth, constipation.*
**GU:** impotence, urinary frequency.
**Skin:** rash, diaphoresis.
**Other:** *neuroleptic malignant syndrome,* muscle rigidity.

### INTERACTIONS
*Ethanol, other CNS depressants:* increased CNS depression. Avoid concomitant use.
*Phenothiazines, tricyclic antidepressants, antiarrhythmics:* increased incidence of ECG abnormalities. Monitor patient closely.

### CONTRAINDICATIONS
Contraindicated in patients with hypersensitivity to drug, in the treatment of simple tics or tics other than those associated with Tourette syndrome, concurrent drug therapy known to cause motor and phonic tics, congenital long QT syndrome or history of arrhythmias, patients with severe toxic CNS depression, and patients experiencing coma.

### NURSING CONSIDERATIONS
• Use cautiously in patients with hepatic or renal dysfunction, glaucoma, prostatic hyperplasia, seizure disorder, or EEG abnormalities.
• *Alert:* Perform an ECG before treatment begins and periodically thereaf-

---

Reactions may be *common*, uncommon, *life-threatening*, or COMMON AND LIFE-THREATENING.

ter as ordered. Monitor for prolonged QT interval.
• Know that concurrent administration of other drugs that prolong the QT interval, such as antiarrhythmics, should be avoided.
• Monitor patient for tardive dyskinesia, which may occur after prolonged use. It may not appear until months or years later and may disappear spontaneously or persist for life, despite discontinuation of drug.
• Assess patient for neuroleptic malignant syndrome. It is rare, but frequently fatal. It is not necessarily related to length of drug use or type of neuroleptic, but over 60% of affected patients are men.
• Know that acute dystonic reactions may be treated with diphenhydramine.
• Monitor patients who also are taking anticonvulsants for increased seizure activity. Pimozide may lower the seizure threshold.

### ☑ PATIENT TEACHING
• Warn patient not to stop taking drug abruptly and not to exceed prescribed dosage.
• Tell patient to avoid alcohol while taking this drug.
• Tell patient to use sugarless hard candy, gum, and liquids to relieve dry mouth.

---

## promazine hydrochloride
Primazine, Prozine-50, Sparine**

*Pregnancy Risk Category: NR*

### HOW SUPPLIED
*Tablets:* 25 mg, 50 mg, 100 mg
*Injection:* 25 mg/ml, 50 mg/ml

### ACTION
Unknown. An aliphatic phenothiazine that probably blocks postsynaptic dopamine receptors in the brain.

### ONSET, PEAK, DURATION
Onset of antipsychotic effect is gradual (up to several weeks) and varies among patients. Peak and duration unknown.

### INDICATIONS & DOSAGE
*Psychosis –*
**Adults:** 10 to 200 mg P.O. or I.M. q 4 to 6 hours, up to 1 g daily, p.r.n. For acutely agitated patients, initial dose is 50 to 150 mg I.M.; repeat within 30 minutes, if necessary, up to a total of 300 mg.
**Children over 12 years:** 10 to 25 mg P.O. or I.M. q 4 to 6 hours.

### ADVERSE REACTIONS
**CNS:** *extrapyramidal reactions, tardive dyskinesia,* drowsiness, **seizures,** *sedation,* pseudoparkinsonism, EEG changes, dizziness.
**CV:** *orthostatic hypotension,* tachycardia, ECG changes.
**EENT:** ocular changes, blurred vision.
**GI:** *dry mouth, constipation.*
**GU:** *urine retention,* menstrual irregularities, gynecomastia, inhibited ejaculation.
**Hematologic:** leukopenia, **hemolytic anemia, thrombocytopenia,** eosinophilia, **agranulocytosis.**
**Hepatic:** jaundice, abnormal liver function test results.
**Skin:** *mild photosensitivity,* allergic reactions, pain at I.M. injection site, sterile abscess.
**Other:** weight gain, **neuroleptic malignant syndrome.**
**After abrupt withdrawal of long-term therapy:** gastritis, nausea, vomiting, dizziness, tremor, feeling of warmth or cold, diaphoresis, tachycardia, headache, insomnia.

### INTERACTIONS
*Antacids:* inhibited absorption of oral phenothiazines. Use together cautiously. Separate antacid and phenothiazine doses by at least 2 hours.

---

*Liquid form contains alcohol.    **May contain tartrazine.    †Canada only.    ‡Australia only.    ◊OTC.

*Anticholinergics (including antidepressants and antiparkinsonian agents):* increased anticholinergic activity, aggravated parkinsonian symptoms. Use together cautiously.
*Barbiturates, lithium:* may decrease phenothiazine effect. Observe patient.
*Centrally acting antihypertensives:* decreased antihypertensive effect. Monitor blood pressure.
*Ethanol:* increased CNS depression. Avoid concomitant use.
*Other CNS depressants:* increased CNS depression. Use together cautiously.

## CONTRAINDICATIONS

Contraindicated in patients with hypersensitivity to the drug or in patients experiencing coma or CNS depression, bone marrow suppression, or subcortical damage.

## NURSING CONSIDERATIONS

• Use cautiously in elderly or debilitated patients and in patients with hepatic or renal disease, severe CV disease (may cause sudden drop in blood pressure); exposure to extreme heat or cold (including antipyretic therapy) or to organophosphate insecticides; respiratory disorder; hypocalcemia; seizure disorder (may lower seizure threshold); severe reactions to insulin or electroconvulsive therapy; glaucoma; or prostatic hyperplasia.
• Monitor blood pressure with patient lying and standing before therapy and routinely throughout treatment.
• Keep drug away from skin and clothes. Wear gloves when preparing liquid forms.
• Dilute liquid concentrate with fruit juice, milk, semisolid food, or chocolate-flavored drinks just before giving. For best taste, use at least 10 ml diluent per 25 mg drug.
• Protect drug from light. Slight yellowing of injection or concentrate

does not affect potency. Discard markedly discolored solutions.
• Give deeply I.M. only in upper outer quadrant of buttocks. Massage slowly afterward to prevent sterile abscess. Injection may sting.
• Watch for orthostatic hypotension, especially with parenteral administration. Keep the patient supine for 1 hour afterward and have patient change positions slowly.
• Monitor patient for tardive dyskinesia, which may occur after prolonged use. It may not appear until months or years later and disappear spontaneously or persist for life, despite discontinuation of drug.
• Assess patient for neuroleptic malignant syndrome. It is rare, but frequently fatal. It is not necessarily related to length of drug use or type of neuroleptic, but over 60% of affected patients are men.
• Monitor therapy with weekly bilirubin tests during first month; periodic blood tests (CBC and liver function); and ophthalmic tests (long-term use).
• Do not withdraw abruptly unless required by severe adverse reactions.
• Withhold dose and notify doctor if patient develops jaundice, blood dyscrasia (fever, sore throat, infection, cellulitis, weakness), or persistent extrapyramidal reactions, especially in pregnant patients or in children.
• Acute dystonic reactions may be treated with diphenhydramine.

☑ **PATIENT TEACHING**
• Warn patient to avoid activities that require alertness until CNS effects of the drug are known.
• Tell patient to avoid alcohol.
• Have patient report urine retention or constipation.
• Tell patient to use sunblock and to wear protective clothing outdoors.
• Tell patient to relieve dry mouth with sugarless gum or hard candy.

# risperidone
Risperdal

*Pregnancy Risk Category: C*

## HOW SUPPLIED
*Tablets:* 1 mg, 2 mg, 3 mg, 4 mg

## ACTION
Blocks dopamine and serotonin receptors; also blocks $alpha_1$, $alpha_2$, and $histamine_1$ receptors in the CNS.

## ONSET, PEAK, DURATION
Onset and duration unknown. Plasma levels peak in about 1 hour.

## INDICATIONS & DOSAGE
*Psychosis –*
**Adults:** initially, 1 mg P.O. b.i.d. Increased in increments of 1 mg b.i.d. on days 2 and 3 of treatment to a target dose of 3 mg b.i.d. At least 1 week must pass before dosage is adjusted further.
**Elderly or debilitated patients, hypotensive patients, or patients with severe renal or hepatic impairment:** initially, 0.5 mg P.O. b.i.d. Increased in increments of 0.5 mg b.i.d. on days 2 and 3 of treatment to a target dosage of 1.5 mg P.O. b.i.d. At least 1 week must pass before dosage increased further.

## ADVERSE REACTIONS
**CNS:** *somnolence, extrapyramidal symptoms, headache, insomnia, agitation, anxiety,* tardive dyskinesia, aggressiveness.
**CV:** tachycardia, chest pain, orthostatic hypotension, prolonged QT interval.
**EENT:** *rhinitis,* coughing, upper respiratory infection, sinusitis, pharyngitis, abnormal vision.
**GI:** *constipation, nausea, vomiting, dyspepsia.*
**Skin:** rash, dry skin, photosensitivity.
**Other:** arthralgia; back pain; fever; rarely, *neuroleptic malignant syndrome.*

## INTERACTIONS
*Carbamazepine:* increased clearance of risperidone, leading to decreased effectiveness. Monitor patient closely.
*Clozapine:* decreased clearance of risperidone, increasing toxicity. Monitor patient closely.
*Ethanol, CNS depressants:* additive CNS depression. Avoid concomitant use.
*Levodopa:* antagonized effects. Don't use together.

## CONTRAINDICATIONS
Contraindicated in patients hypersensitive to the drug. Also contraindicated in breast-feeding patients.

## NURSING CONSIDERATIONS
• Use cautiously in patients with prolonged QT interval, CV disease, cerebrovascular disease, dehydration, hypovolemia, history of seizures, exposure to extreme heat, or conditions that could affect metabolism or hemodynamic responses.
• *Alert:* Obtain baseline measures of blood pressure before starting therapy and monitor regularly. Watch for orthostatic hypotension, especially during initial dosage titration.
• Monitor patient for tardive dyskinesia, which may occur after prolonged use. It may not appear until months or years later and disappear spontaneously or persist for life, despite discontinuation of drug.
• Assess for neuroleptic malignant syndrome. It is rare, but frequently fatal. It is not necessarily related to length of drug use or type of neuroleptic, but over 60% of patients are men.

## ☑ PATIENT TEACHING
• Warn patient to avoid activities that require alertness until CNS effects of the drug are known.
• Warn patient to rise slowly, avoid

hot showers, and use extra caution during the first few days of therapy to avoid fainting.
• Advise patient to use caution in hot weather to prevent heatstroke.
• Tell patient to avoid alcohol.
• Tell patient to use sunblock and to wear protective clothing outdoors.
• Tell female patient to notify her doctor if she is or plans to become pregnant during therapy.

---

# thioridazine hydrochloride
Aldazine‡, Apo-Thioridazine†, Mellaril*, Mellaril Concentrate, Novo-Ridazine†, PMS Thioridazine†

*Pregnancy Risk Category: NR*

## HOW SUPPLIED
*Tablets:* 10 mg, 15 mg, 25 mg, 50 mg, 100 mg, 150 mg, 200 mg
*Oral suspension:* 25 mg/5 ml, 100 mg/5 ml
*Oral concentrate:* 30 mg/ml, 100 mg/ml (3% to 4.2% alcohol)

## ACTION
Unknown. A piperidine phenothiazine that probably blocks postsynaptic dopamine receptors in the brain.

## ONSET, PEAK, DURATION
Onset of antipsychotic effect is gradual (up to several weeks) and variable between patients. Peak and duration unknown.

## INDICATIONS & DOSAGE
*Psychosis –*
**Adults:** initially, 50 to 100 mg P.O. t.i.d., with gradual increments up to 800 mg daily in divided doses, if needed. Dosage varies.
*Short term treatment of moderate to marked depression with variable degrees of anxiety, treatment of multiple symptoms, such as agitation, anxiety, depressed mood, tension, sleep disturbances, and fears in geriatric patients –*

**Adults:** initially, 25 mg P.O. t.i.d. Maximum daily dosage is 200 mg.
**Children 2 to 12 years:** 0.5 to 3 mg/kg P.O. daily in divided doses.

## ADVERSE REACTIONS
**CNS:** extrapyramidal reactions (low incidence), *tardive dyskinesia, sedation* (high incidence), EEG changes, dizziness.
**CV:** *orthostatic hypotension,* tachycardia, ECG changes.
**EENT:** *ocular changes, blurred vision,* retinitis pigmentosa.
**GI:** *dry mouth, constipation.*
**GU:** *urine retention,* dark urine, menstrual irregularities, gynecomastia, inhibited ejaculation.
**Hematologic:** transient leukopenia, *agranulocytosis,* hyperprolactinemia.
**Hepatic:** cholestatic jaundice.
**Skin:** *mild photosensitivity,* allergic reactions.
**Other:** weight gain; increased appetite; rarely, *neuroleptic malignant syndrome.*
**After abrupt withdrawal of long-term therapy:** gastritis, nausea, vomiting, dizziness, tremor, feeling of warmth or cold, diaphoresis, tachycardia, headache, insomnia.

## INTERACTIONS
*Antacids:* inhibited absorption of oral phenothiazines. Separate antacid and phenothiazine doses by at least 2 hours.
*Barbiturates, lithium:* may decrease phenothiazine effect. Observe patient.
*Centrally acting antihypertensives:* decreased antihypertensive effect. Monitor blood pressure.
*Ethanol:* increased CNS depression. Avoid concomitant use.
*Other CNS depressants:* increased CNS depression. Use together cautiously.

## CONTRAINDICATIONS
Contraindicated in patients with hypersensitivity to the drug or in patients experiencing coma or CNS de-

---

Reactions may be *common,* uncommon, *life-threatening,* or COMMON AND LIFE-THREATENING.

pression, or severe hypertensive or hypotensive cardiac disease.

## NURSING CONSIDERATIONS
• Use cautiously in elderly or debilitated patients and in patients with hepatic disease; CV disease; exposure to extreme heat or cold (including antipyretic therapy) or to organophosphate insecticides; respiratory disorder; hypocalcemia; seizure disorder; or severe reactions to insulin or electroconvulsive therapy.
• *Alert:* Remember that different liquid formulations have different concentrations. Check dosage carefully.
• Prevent contact dermatitis by keeping drug away from skin and clothes. Wear gloves when preparing liquid forms.
• Dilute liquid concentrate with water or fruit juice just before giving.
• Shake suspension well before using.
• Monitor patient for tardive dyskinesia, which may occur after prolonged use. It may not appear until months or years later and disappear spontaneously or persist for life, despite discontinuation of drug.
• Assess for neuroleptic malignant syndrome. It is rare, but frequently fatal. Not necessarily related to length of drug use or type of neuroleptic, but over 60% of patients are men.
• Monitor therapy with weekly bilirubin tests during first month; periodic blood tests (CBC and liver function); and ophthalmic tests (long-term use).
• Do not stop drug abruptly unless required by severe adverse reactions.
• Withhold dose and notify doctor if patient develops jaundice, blood dyscrasia (fever, sore throat, infection, cellulitis, weakness), or persistent extrapyramidal reactions, especially in pregnant patients or in children.
• Acute dystonic reactions may be treated with diphenhydramine.

## ☑ PATIENT TEACHING
• Tell patient to shake suspension.
• Warn patient to avoid activities that require alertness until CNS effects of the drug are known.
• Tell patient to watch for orthostatic hypotension, especially with parenteral administration. Advise patient to change positions slowly.
• Tell patient to avoid alcohol.
• Have patient report urine retention, constipation, or blurred vision.
• Tell patient that drug may discolor the urine.
• Advise patient to relieve dry mouth with sugarless gum or hard candy.
• Tell patient to use sunblock and to wear protective clothing outdoors.

---

# thiothixene
Navane

# thiothixene hydrochloride
Navane*

*Pregnancy Risk Category: NR*

## HOW SUPPLIED
**thiothixene**
*Capsules:* 1 mg, 2 mg, 5 mg, 10 mg, 20 mg
**thiothixene hydrochloride**
*Oral concentrate:* 5 mg/ml (7% alcohol)
*Injection:* 2 mg/ml, 5 mg/ml

## ACTION
Unknown. A thioxanthene that probably blocks postsynaptic dopamine receptors in the brain.

## ONSET, PEAK, DURATION
Onset of antipsychotic effect is gradual (up to several weeks). Peak and duration unknown.

## INDICATIONS & DOSAGE
*Mild to moderate psychosis –*
**Adults:** initially, 2 mg P.O. t.i.d. Increased gradually to 15 mg daily, p.r.n.

---

*Severe psychosis* –
**Adults:** initially, 5 mg P.O. b.i.d. Increased gradually to 20 to 30 mg daily, p.r.n. Maximum recommended dosage is 60 mg daily. Alternatively, 4 mg I.M. b.i.d. or q.i.d. Maximum dosage is 30 mg I.M. daily. An oral form should replace the injectable form as soon as possible.

## ADVERSE REACTIONS
**CNS:** *extrapyramidal reactions,* drowsiness, restlessness, agitation, insomnia, *tardive dyskinesia,* sedation, pseudoparkinsonism, EEG changes, dizziness.
**CV:** *hypotension,* tachycardia, ECG changes.
**EENT:** ocular changes, *blurred vision,* nasal congestion.
**GI:** *dry mouth, constipation.*
**GU:** *urine retention,* menstrual irregularities, gynecomastia, inhibited ejaculation.
**Hematologic:** transient leukopenia, leukocytosis, *agranulocytosis.*
**Hepatic:** jaundice.
**Skin:** *mild photosensitivity,* allergic reactions, pain at I.M. injection site, sterile abscess.
**Other:** weight gain, *neuroleptic malignant syndrome.*
**After abrupt withdrawal of long-term therapy:** gastritis, nausea, vomiting, dizziness, tremor, feeling of warmth or cold, diaphoresis, tachycardia, headache, insomnia.

## INTERACTIONS
*Ethanol, other CNS depressants:* increased CNS depression. Avoid concomitant use.

## CONTRAINDICATIONS
Contraindicated in patients with hypersensitivity to the drug or in patients experiencing circulatory collapse, coma, CNS depression, or blood dyscrasia.

## NURSING CONSIDERATIONS
• Use with extreme caution in patients with history of seizure disorder or in a state of alcohol withdrawal.
• Use cautiously in elderly or debilitated patients and in those with CV disease (may cause sudden drop in blood pressure), heat exposure, glaucoma, or prostatic hyperplasia.
• Prevent contact dermatitis by keeping drug off skin and clothes. Wear gloves when preparing liquid forms.
• Dilute liquid concentrate with fruit juice, milk, or semisolid food just before administering.
• Slight yellowing of injection or concentrate is common and does not affect potency. Discard markedly discolored solutions.
• Give I.M. only in upper outer quadrant of buttocks or midlateral thigh. Massage slowly afterward to prevent sterile abscess. Injection may sting.
• Monitor patient for tardive dyskinesia, which may occur after prolonged use; it may not appear until months or years later and disappear spontaneously or persist for life, despite discontinuation of drug.
• Assess for neuroleptic malignant syndrome. It is rare, but frequently fatal. Not necessarily related to length of drug use or type of neuroleptic, but over 60% of patients are men.
• Do not withdraw abruptly unless required by severe adverse reactions.
• Withhold dose and notify doctor if patient develops jaundice, blood dyscrasia (fever, sore throat, infection, cellulitis, weakness), or persistent extrapyramidal reactions, especially in pregnant patients.
• Monitor therapy with weekly bilirubin tests during first month; periodic blood tests (CBC and liver function); and ophthalmic tests (long-term use).
• Acute dystonic reactions may be treated with diphenhydramine.
• Watch for orthostatic hypotension, especially with parenteral administration. Keep the patient in supine posi-

---

Reactions may be *common,* uncommon, *life-threatening,* or **COMMON AND LIFE-THREATENING.**

tion for 1 hour afterward and tell him to change positions slowly.

☑ **PATIENT TEACHING**
• Warn patient to avoid activities that require alertness until CNS effects of the drug are known.
• Tell patient to watch for orthostatic hypotension. Advise him to change positions slowly.
• Tell patient to avoid alcohol.
• Have him report urine retention, constipation, or blurred vision.
• Tell patient to use sunblock and to wear protective clothing outdoors.

---

# trifluoperazine hydrochloride

Apo-Trifluoperazine†, Calmazine‡, Novo-Flurazine†, PMS Trifluoperazine†, Solazine†, Stelazine, Stelazine Concentrate, Terfluzine†, Terfluzine Concentrate†

*Pregnancy Risk Category: NR*

## HOW SUPPLIED
*Tablets (regular and film-coated):*
1 mg, 2 mg, 5 mg, 10 mg
*Oral concentrate:* 10 mg/ml
*Injection:* 2 mg/ml

## ACTION
Unknown. A piperazine phenothiazine that probably blocks postsynaptic dopamine receptors in the brain.

## ONSET, PEAK, DURATION
Onset of antipsychotic effect is gradual (up to several weeks) and variable between patients. Peak and duration unknown.

## INDICATIONS & DOSAGE
*Anxiety states –*
**Adults:** 1 to 2 mg P.O. b.i.d. Maximum dosage is 6 mg/day and drug should not be used longer than 12 weeks for this indication.

*Schizophrenia and other psychotic disorders –*
**Adults:** 2 to 5 mg P.O. b.i.d., gradually increased until therapeutic response. Or 1 to 2 mg deep I.M. q 4 to 6 hours, p.r.n. More than 6 mg I.M. in 24 hours is rarely required.
**Children 6 to 12 years (hospitalized or under close supervision):** 1 mg P.O. daily or b.i.d.; may increase gradually to 15 mg daily, if needed.

## ADVERSE REACTIONS
**CNS:** *extrapyramidal reactions, tardive dyskinesia,* pseudoparkinsonism, dizziness, drowsiness, insomnia, fatigue, headache.
**CV:** *orthostatic hypotension,* tachycardia, ECG changes.
**EENT:** ocular changes, *blurred vision.*
**GI:** *dry mouth, constipation,* nausea.
**GU:** *urine retention.*
**Hematologic:** transient leukopenia, **agranulocytosis.**
**Hepatic:** cholestatic jaundice.
**Skin:** *photosensitivity,* allergic reactions, pain at I.M. injection site, sterile abscess, rash.
**Other:** weight gain; rarely, **neuroleptic malignant syndrome** (fever, tachycardia, tachypnea, profuse diaphoresis), menstrual irregularities, gynecomastia, inhibited lactation.
**After abrupt withdrawal of long-term therapy:** gastritis, nausea, vomiting, dizziness, tremor, feeling of warmth or cold, diaphoresis, tachycardia, headache, insomnia, anorexia, muscle rigidity, altered mental status and evidence of autonomic instability.

## INTERACTIONS
*Antacids:* inhibited absorption of oral phenothiazines. Separate antacid and phenothiazine doses by at least 2 hours.
*Barbiturates, lithium:* may decrease phenothiazine effect. Monitor patient.
*Centrally acting antihypertensives:* decreased antihypertensive effect. Monitor blood pressure.

---

*Liquid form contains alcohol.   **May contain tartrazine.   †Canada only.   ‡Australia only.   ◇OTC.

*Ethanol:* increased CNS depression. Avoid concomitant use.

*Other CNS depressants:* increased CNS depression. Use together cautiously.

*Propranolol:* increased levels of both propranolol and trifluoperazine. Monitor closely.

*Warfarin:* decreased effect of oral anticoagulants. Monitor PT.

## CONTRAINDICATIONS
Contraindicated in patients with hypersensitivity to phenothiazines or in patients experiencing coma, CNS depression, bone marrow suppression, or liver damage.

## NURSING CONSIDERATIONS
● Use cautiously in elderly or debilitated patients and in patients with CV disease (may cause drop in blood pressure), exposure to extreme heat, seizure disorder, glaucoma, or prostatic hyperplasia.
● Wear gloves when preparing liquid forms.
● Dilute liquid concentrate with 60 ml of tomato or fruit juice, carbonated beverages, coffee, tea, milk, water, or semisolid food just before giving.
● Protect drug from light. Slight yellowing of injection or concentrate is common and does not affect potency. Discard markedly discolored solutions.
● Give deeply I.M. only in upper outer quadrant of buttocks. Massage slowly afterward to prevent sterile abscess. Injection may sting.
● Watch for orthostatic hypotension, especially with parenteral administration. Keep patient supine for 1 hour, and tell him to change positions slowly.
● Monitor patient for tardive dyskinesia, which may occur after prolonged use. It may not appear until months or years later and disappear spontaneously or persist for life, despite discontinuation of drug.
● Assess for neuroleptic malignant syndrome. It is rare, but frequently fatal. It is not necessarily related to length of drug use or type of neuroleptic, but over 60% of patients are men.
● Do not withdraw drug abruptly unless severe adverse reactions occur.
● Withhold dose and notify doctor if patient develops jaundice, symptoms of blood dyscrasia (fever, sore throat, infection, cellulitis, weakness), persistent extrapyramidal reactions (longer than a few hours), especially in pregnant patients or in children.
● Monitor therapy with weekly bilirubin tests during first month; periodic blood tests (CBC and liver function); and ophthalmic tests (long-term use).
● Acute dystonic reactions may be treated with diphenhydramine.

## ☑ PATIENT TEACHING
● Warn patient to avoid activities that require alertness until CNS effects of the drug are known.
● Tell patient to avoid alcohol.
● Have him report urine retention or constipation.
● Tell him to use sunblock and to wear protective clothing outdoors.
● Tell patient to relieve dry mouth with sugarless gum or hard candy.

---

amphetamine sulfate
benzphetamine hydrochloride
caffeine
dextroamphetamine sulfate
diethylpropion hydrochloride
doxapram hydrochloride
fenfluramine hydrochloride
mazindol
methamphetamine hydrochloride
methylphenidate hydrochloride
pemoline
phendimetrazine tartrate
phentermine hydrochloride

**COMBINATION PRODUCTS**
None.

## amphetamine sulfate
Controlled Substance Schedule II

*Pregnancy Risk Category: C*

**HOW SUPPLIED**
*Tablets:* 5 mg, 10 mg

**ACTION**
Unknown. Probably promotes nerve impulse transmission by releasing stored norepinephrine from nerve terminals in the brain. Main sites of activity appear to be the cerebral cortex and the reticular activating system.

**ONSET, PEAK, DURATION**
Unknown.

**INDICATIONS & DOSAGE**
*Attention deficit disorder with hyperactivity –*
**Children 3 to 5 years:** 2.5 mg P.O. daily, with 2.5-mg increments weekly, p.r.n.
**Children 6 years and older:** 5 mg P.O. daily, with 5-mg increments weekly, p.r.n. Give first dose on awakening; additional doses (one or two) at intervals of 4 to 6 hours.
*Narcolepsy –*
**Adults and children 12 years and older:** 10 mg P.O. daily. Dosage increased in 10-mg increments weekly, p.r.n. Daily dosage may be divided with first dose given on awakening, additional doses at intervals of 4 to 6 hours.
**Children 6 to 12 years:** 5 mg P.O. daily. Dosage increased in 5-mg increments weekly, p.r.n. Daily dosage may be divided with first dose given on awakening, additional doses at intervals of 4 to 6 hours.
*Short-term adjunct in exogenous obesity –*
**Adults:** 5 to 30 mg P.O. daily in divided doses 30 to 60 minutes before meals.

**ADVERSE REACTIONS**
**CNS:** *restlessness,* tremor, *hyperactivity, talkativeness, insomnia,* irritability, dizziness, headache, chills, dysphoria, euphoria.
**CV:** *tachycardia, palpitations,* hypertension, arrhythmias.
**GI:** dry mouth, metallic taste, diarrhea, constipation, anorexia, weight loss.
**GU:** impotence.
**Skin:** urticaria.
**Other:** altered libido.

**INTERACTIONS**
*Ammonium chloride, ascorbic acid:* decreased serum levels and increased renal excretion of amphetamine. Monitor for decreased amphetamine effect.
*Antacids, sodium bicarbonate, acetazolamide:* increased renal reabsorption. Monitor for enhanced effect.
*Antihypertensives:* reversal of antihy-

---

*Liquid form contains alcohol.   **May contain tartrazine.   †Canada only.   ‡Australia only.   ◇OTC.

pertensive action. Monitor blood pressure.

*Caffeine:* may increase amphetamine and related amine effects. Avoid concomitant use.

*Haloperidol, phenothiazines, tricyclic antidepressants:* altered CNS effect. Avoid concomitant use.

*Insulin, oral antidiabetic agents:* may decrease antidiabetic agent requirements. Monitor blood glucose level.

*MAO inhibitors:* may cause severe hypertension, possibly hypertensive crisis. Don't use together or within 14 days after an MAO inhibitor has been discontinued.

## CONTRAINDICATIONS

Contraindicated in patients with hypersensitivity or idiosyncrasy to the sympathomimetic amines, symptomatic CV disease, hyperthyroidism, moderate to severe hypertension, glaucoma, advanced arteriosclerosis, or history of drug abuse; within 14 days of MAO inhibitor therapy; and in agitated patients.

## NURSING CONSIDERATIONS

- Use cautiously in elderly, debilitated, or hyperexcitable patients; or those with psychopathic personalities or history of suicidal or homicidal tendencies.
- Know that drug is not recommended for first-line treatment of obesity or for treatment of obesity in children under 12 years. Use as an anorexigenic agent is prohibited in some states.
- Be aware that drug should not be used to combat fatigue.
- Make sure obese patient is on a weight-reduction program. Give drug 30 to 60 minutes before meals. Monitor dietary intake and count calories, if necessary.
- If tolerance to anorexigenic effect develops, know that drug should be discontinued. Notify doctor.

## ☑ PATIENT TEACHING

- To avoid sleep interference, tell the patient to take drug at least 6 hours before bedtime.
- Warn the patient to avoid activities that require alertness or good psychomotor coordination until CNS effects of the drug are known.
- Tell the patient to avoid drinks containing caffeine, which increases the effects of amphetamines and related amines.
- Tell the patient to report signs of excessive stimulation.
- Inform patient that fatigue may result as drug effects wear off. The patient will need more rest.

---

# benzphetamine hydrochloride
Didrex**
Controlled Substance Schedule III

*Pregnancy Risk Category: X*

## HOW SUPPLIED
*Tablets:* 25 mg, 50 mg

## ACTION
Unknown. Probably promotes nerve impulse transmission by releasing stored norepinephrine from nerve terminals in the brain. Main sites of activity appear to be the cerebral cortex and the reticular activating system.

## ONSET, PEAK, DURATION
Onset and peak unknown. Effects persist for about 4 hours.

## INDICATIONS & DOSAGE
*Short-term adjunct in exogenous obesity –*
**Adults:** 25 to 50 mg P.O. daily, b.i.d. or t.i.d. Increased as needed in dosage or interval.

## ADVERSE REACTIONS
**CNS:** *restlessness,* tremor, *hyperactivity, talkativeness, insomnia,* irritabil-

---

ity, dizziness, headache, chills, dysphoria, euphoria.
**CV:** *tachycardia, palpitations,* hypertension.
**GI:** dry mouth, metallic taste, diarrhea, constipation, anorexia, weight loss.
**GU:** impotence.
**Skin:** urticaria.
**Other:** altered libido.

## INTERACTIONS
*Ammonium chloride, ascorbic acid:* decreased serum levels and increased renal excretion of benzphetamine. Monitor for decreased amphetamine effects.
*Antacids, sodium bicarbonate, acetazolamide:* increased renal reabsorption. Monitor for enhanced effects.
*Caffeine:* may increase amphetamine and related amine effects. Avoid concomitant use.
*Insulin, oral antidiabetic agents:* may decrease antidiabetic agent requirement. Monitor blood glucose levels.
*MAO inhibitors:* may cause severe hypertension, possibly hypertensive crisis. Don't use together or within 14 days after MAO inhibitor has been discontinued.
*Phenothiazines, haloperidol, tricyclic antidepressants:* increased CNS effects. Avoid concomitant use.

## CONTRAINDICATIONS
Contraindicated in patients with hypersensitivity or idiosyncrasy to sympathomimetic amines; within 14 days of MAO inhibitor therapy; in those with symptomatic CV disease, hyperthyroidism, moderate to severe hypertension, glaucoma, advanced arteriosclerosis, or history of drug abuse; and in agitated patients.

## NURSING CONSIDERATIONS
• Use cautiously in patients with diabetes mellitus and mild hypertension.
• Use in conjunction with a weight-reduction program. Monitor dietary

intake and count calories, if necessary. Give 30 to 60 minutes before meals.
• Give a single daily dose in midmorning or midafternoon, according to patient's eating habits.
• If tolerance to anorexigenic effect develops, know that drug should be discontinued. Notify doctor.

☑ **PATIENT TEACHING**
• Instruct the patient when to take drug.
• To avoid sleep interference, tell the patient to take drug at least 6 hours before bedtime.
• Warn the patient to avoid activities that require alertness or good psychomotor coordination until CNS effects of the drug are known.
• Tell the patient to avoid drinks containing caffeine, which increases the effects of amphetamines and related amines.
• Tell the patient to report signs of excessive stimulation.
• Inform the patient that fatigue may result as drug effects wear off. The patient will need more rest.

---

## caffeine
Caffedrine Caplets◊, Dexitac◊,
NoDoz◊, Quick Pep◊, Vivarin◊

*Pregnancy Risk Category: C*

## HOW SUPPLIED
*Tablets:* 100 mg◊, 150 mg◊, 200 mg◊
*Tablets (timed-release):* 200 mg◊
*Capsules (timed-release):* 200 mg◊
*Injection:* caffeine (250 mg/ml) with sodium benzoate (250 mg/ml)

## ACTION
Inhibits phosphodiesterase, the enzyme that degrades cAMP.

## ONSET, PEAK, DURATION
Onset and duration unknown. Serum levels peak within 50 to 75 minutes after oral administration.

---

## INDICATIONS & DOSAGE
*CNS stimulant* —
**Adults:** 100 to 200 mg anhydrous caffeine P.O. q 3 to 4 hours, p.r.n. Alternatively, 500 mg to 1 g I.M. (or slowly I.V.). Total daily dosage should seldom exceed 2.5 g.

## ADVERSE REACTIONS
**CNS:** *insomnia,* restlessness, nervousness, headache, excitement, agitation, muscle tremor, twitching.
**CV:** *tachycardia, palpitations,* extrasystoles.
**GI:** nausea, vomiting, diarrhea, stomach pain.
**GU:** *diuresis.*
**Other:** abrupt withdrawal symptoms (headache, irritability), tinnitus.

## INTERACTIONS
*Beta-adrenergic agonists, cimetidine, fluoroquinolones, oral contraceptives, phenylpropanolamine, theophylline:* excessive CNS stimulation. Avoid concomitant use.

## CONTRAINDICATIONS
Contraindicated in patients with hypersensitivity to the drug.

## NURSING CONSIDERATIONS
• Use cautiously in patients with history of peptic ulcer, symptomatic arrhythmias, or palpitations, and during the first several days to weeks after an acute MI.
• Know that caffeine does not reverse alcohol intoxication or CNS depressant effects of alcohol. Overvigorous therapy with caffeine may aggravate depression in an already depressed patient.
• **Alert:** Be aware single dose should not exceed 1 g.
• Restrict caffeine-containing beverages in patients who experience palpitations. Caffeine content: cola beverages, 17 to 55 mg/180 ml; tea, 40 to 100 mg/180 ml; instant coffee, 60 to 180 mg/180 ml; brewed coffee, 100 to 150 mg/180 ml; decaffeinated coffee, 1 to 6 mg/180 ml.
• Be alert for signs of overdose: GI pain, mild delirium, insomnia, diuresis, dehydration, and fever. Treat with short-acting barbiturates, gastric emesis, or lavage as ordered.
• Monitor patient for tolerance or psychological dependence.
• Be aware that sudden discontinuation of caffeine may cause headache and irritability.

## ☑ PATIENT TEACHING
• Stress to patient the importance of not exceeding recommended dosage.
• Tell patient to stop taking caffeine if increased or abnormal heart rate, dizziness, or palpitations occur.
• Inform patient that caffeine is not intended for use as a substitute for sleep.

# dextroamphetamine sulfate
Dexedrine* **, Dexedrine
Spansule, Oxydess II, Robese,
Spancap #1
Controlled Substance Schedule II

*Pregnancy Risk Category: C*

## HOW SUPPLIED
*Tablets:* 5 mg, 10 mg
*Capsules (sustained-release):* 5 mg, 10 mg, 15 mg

## ACTION
Unknown. Probably promotes nerve impulse transmission by releasing stored norepinephrine from nerve terminals in the brain. Main sites of activity appear to be the cerebral cortex and the reticular activating system. In children with hyperkinesis, amphetamines have a paradoxical calming effect.

## ONSET, PEAK, DURATION
Unknown.

---

Reactions may be *common,* uncommon, *life-threatening,* or COMMON AND LIFE-THREATENING.

## INDICATIONS & DOSAGE

*Narcolepsy–*
**Adults:** 5 to 60 mg P.O. daily in divided doses.
**Children 6 to 12 years:** 5 mg P.O. daily, with 5-mg increments weekly, p.r.n.
**Children 12 years and older:** 10 mg P.O. daily, with 10-mg increments weekly, p.r.n. Give first dose on awakening; additional doses (one or two) at intervals of 4 to 6 hours.
*Short-term adjunct in exogenous obesity–*
**Adults and children 12 years and older:** 5 to 30 mg P.O. daily 30 to 60 minutes before meals in divided doses of 5 to 10 mg. Alternatively, one 10- or 15-mg sustained-release capsule daily as a single dose in the morning.
*Attention deficit disorder with hyperactivity–*
**Children 3 to 5 years:** 2.5 mg P.O. daily, with 2.5-mg increments weekly, p.r.n.
**Children 6 years and older:** 5 mg P.O. once daily or b.i.d., with 5-mg increments weekly, p.r.n. Only in rare cases will it be necessary to exceed a total dosage of 40 mg/day.

## ADVERSE REACTIONS

**CNS:** *restlessness,* tremor, *insomnia,* dizziness, headache, chills, overstimulation, dysphoria, euphoria.
**CV:** *tachycardia, palpitations,* hypertension, arrhythmias.
**GI:** dry mouth, unpleasant taste, diarrhea, constipation, anorexia, weight loss and other GI disturbances.
**GU:** impotence.
**Skin:** urticaria.
**Other:** altered libido.

## INTERACTIONS

*Acidifying agents, ammonium chloride, ammonium chloride, ascorbic acid:* decreased blood levels and increased renal clearance of dextroamphetamine. Monitor for decreased amphetamine effects.
*Adrenergic blockers:* adrenergic blockers inhibited by amphetamines. Avoid concomitant use.
*Alkalizing agents, antacids, sodium bicarbonate, acetazolamide:* increased renal reabsorption. Monitor for enhanced amphetamine effects.
*Antihistamines:* amphetamines may counteract the sedative effects of antihistamines.
*Caffeine:* may increase amphetamine and related amine effects.
*Chlorpromazine:* inhibits the central stimulant effects of amphetamines. Can be used to treat amphetamine poisoning.
*Insulin, oral antidiabetic agents:* may decrease antidiabetic agent requirements. Monitor blood glucose levels.
*Lithium carbonate:* may inhibit antiobesity and stimulating effects of amphetamines. Monitor patient closely.
*MAO inhibitors:* may cause severe hypertension, possibly hypertensive crisis. Don't use together or within 14 days after MAO inhibitor has been discontinued.
*Meperidine:* amphetamines potentiate analgesic effect. Use together cautiously.
*Methenamine therapy:* increased urinary excretion of amphetamines and efficacy reduced. Monitor effects.
*Norepinephrine:* amphetamines enhance the adrenergic effect of norepinephrine.
*Phenobarbital, phenytoin:* amphetamines may delay absorption. Monitor patient closely.
*Phenothiazines, haloperidol, tricyclic antidepressants:* increased CNS effects. Avoid concomitant use.
*Propoxyphene:* in cases of propoxyphene overdose, amphetamine CNS stimulation is potentiated, and fatal seizures can occur.
*Veratrum alkaloids:* amphetamines inhibit hypotensive effect of veratrum alkaloids. Monitor blood pressure closely.

---

*Liquid form contains alcohol. **May contain tartrazine. †Canada only. ‡Australia only. ◊OTC.

## CONTRAINDICATIONS

Contraindicated in patients with hypersensitivity or idiosyncrasy to the sympathomimetic amines; within 14 days of MAO inhibitor therapy; and in those with hyperthyroidism, moderate to severe hypertension, symptomatic CV disease, glaucoma, advanced arteriosclerosis, and history of drug abuse.

## NURSING CONSIDERATIONS

• Use cautiously in patients with motor and phonic tics, Tourette syndrome, and in agitated states.
• Be aware drug not recommended for first-line treatment of obesity. Use as an anorexigenic agent is prohibited in some states.
• Be aware drug is not to be used to prevent fatigue.
• Make sure the obese patient is on a weight-reduction program.
• If tolerance to anorexigenic effect develops, know that drug should be discontinued. Notify doctor.

## ☑ PATIENT TEACHING

• Tell the patient to take drug 30 to 60 minutes before meals if used for weight reduction and at least 6 hours before bedtime to avoid sleep interference.
• Warn the patient to avoid activities that require alertness or good psychomotor coordination until CNS effects of the drug are known.
• Tell the patient to avoid drinks containing caffeine, which increases the effects of amphetamines and related amines.
• Tell the patient that fatigue may result as drug effects wear off. The patient will need more rest.
• Have the patient report signs of excessive stimulation.

# diethylpropion hydrochloride

M-Orexic, Nobesine†, Nobesine-75†, Propion†, Tenuate, Tenuate Dospan, Tepanil, Tepanil Ten-Tab
Controlled Substance Schedule IV

*Pregnancy Risk Category: B*

## HOW SUPPLIED

*Tablets:* 25 mg
*Tablets (extended-release):* 75 mg
*Capsules (extended-release):* 75 mg†

## ACTION

Unknown. Probably promotes nerve impulse transmission by releasing stored norepinephrine from nerve terminals in the brain. Main sites of activity appear to be the cerebral cortex and the reticular activating system.

## ONSET, PEAK, DURATION

Onset and peak unknown. Effects of regular-release tablets persist for 4 hours; effects of extended-release tablets and capsules, for 12 hours.

## INDICATIONS & DOSAGE

*Short-term adjunct in exogenous obesity—*
**Adults:** 25 mg P.O. before meals t.i.d.; or 75 mg extended-release tablet or capsule P.O. in midmorning.

## ADVERSE REACTIONS

**CNS:** headache, *nervousness,* insomnia, fatigue, anxiety, drowsiness.
**CV:** *tachycardia, palpitations,* elevated blood pressure, ***pulmonary hypertension,*** ECG changes, arrhythmias.
**EENT:** blurred vision, mydriasis.
**GI:** dry mouth, nausea, abdominal cramps, diarrhea, constipation, unpleasant taste, vomiting.
**GU:** impotence.
**Hematologic:** decreased blood glucose levels.
**Skin:** urticaria, rash.

---

Reactions may be *common,* uncommon, *life-threatening,* or COMMON AND LIFE-THREATENING.

**Other:** altered libido, changes in menstruation.

## INTERACTIONS
*Caffeine:* may increase amphetamine and related amine effects. Avoid concomitant use.
*Guanethidine:* decrease antihypertensive effect. Monitor blood pressure.
*Insulin, oral antidiabetic agents:* may decrease antidiabetic agent requirements. Monitor blood glucose levels.
*MAO inhibitors:* may cause hypertension, possibly hypertensive crisis. Don't use together or within 14 days after MAO inhibitor has been discontinued.

## CONTRAINDICATIONS
Contraindicated in patients with hypersensitivity or idiosyncrasy to sympathomimetic amines; within 14 days of MAO inhibitor therapy; in those with hyperthyroidism, severe hypertension, advanced arteriosclerosis, glaucoma, or history of drug abuse; and in agitated patients.

## NURSING CONSIDERATIONS
• Use cautiously in patients with mild to moderate hypertension, symptomatic CV disease (including arrhythmias), or seizure disorders.
• Be sure the patient also is on a weight-reduction program.
• Monitor patient for habituation or psychic dependence.
• If tolerance to anorexigenic effect develops, notify doctor because drug will need to be discontinued.

## ☑ PATIENT TEACHING
• Tell the patient to take drug at least 6 hours before bedtime to avoid sleep interference, although it seldom causes insomnia.
• Tell the patient to avoid drinks containing caffeine, which increases the effects of diethylpropion and related amines.

• Tell the patient to report signs of excessive stimulation.
• Tell the patient that fatigue may result as drug effects wear off. The patient will need more rest.

---

## doxapram hydrochloride
Dopram

*Pregnancy Risk Category: B*

### HOW SUPPLIED
*Injection:* 20 mg/ml (benzyl alcohol 0.9%)

### ACTION
Not clearly defined. Acts either directly on the central respiratory centers in the medulla or indirectly on chemoreceptors.

### ONSET, PEAK, DURATION
Onset occurs in 20 to 40 seconds. Levels peak in 1 to 2 minutes. Effects persist for 5 to 12 minutes.

### INDICATIONS & DOSAGE
*Postanesthesia respiratory stimulation, drug-induced CNS depression, chronic pulmonary disease associated with acute hypercapnia –*
**Adults:** 0.5 to 1 mg/kg of body weight as a single I.V. injection or 2 mg/kg total dosage when given as multiple injections q 5 minutes. Alternatively, 250 mg in 250 ml of 0.9% sodium chloride solution or $D_5W$ infused at 5 mg/minute I.V. Recommended total dosage for infusion should not exceed 4 mg/kg.
*COPD –*
**Adults:** 1 to 2 mg/minute by I.V. infusion. Maximum dosage is 3 mg/minute for a maximum duration of 2 hours.

### ADVERSE REACTIONS
**CNS:** *seizures,* headache, dizziness, apprehension, disorientation, hyperactivity, bilateral Babinski's signs, paresthesia.

---

*Liquid form contains alcohol.   **May contain tartrazine.   †Canada only.   ‡Australia only.   ◊OTC.

**CV:** *chest pain and tightness, variations in heart rate, hypertension,* lowered T waves, arrhythmias.
**EENT:** sneezing, *laryngospasm.*
**GI:** nausea, vomiting, diarrhea.
**GU:** urine retention, bladder stimulation with incontinence.
**Respiratory:** cough, *bronchospasm,* dyspnea.
**Skin:** pruritus.
**Other:** hiccups, rebound hypoventilation, muscle spasms, diaphoresis, flushing.

### INTERACTIONS
*MAO inhibitors, sympathomimetics:* potentiate adverse CV effects. Use together cautiously.

### CONTRAINDICATIONS
Contraindicated in patients with seizure disorders; head injury; CV disorders; frank, uncompensated heart failure; severe hypertension; CVA; respiratory failure or incompetence secondary to neuromuscular disorders, muscle paresis, flail chest, obstructed airway, pulmonary embolism, pneumothorax, restrictive respiratory disease, acute bronchial asthma, or extreme dyspnea; or hypoxia not associated with hypercapnia.

### NURSING CONSIDERATIONS
• Use cautiously in patients with bronchial asthma, severe tachycardia or arrhythmias, cerebral edema or increased CSF pressure, hyperthyroidism, pheochromocytoma, or metabolic disorders.
• Be aware that drug is used only in surgical or emergency department situations.
• *Alert:* Establish an adequate airway before administering drug. Prevent patients from aspirating vomitus by placing them on their side.
• **I.V. use:** Administer slowly; rapid infusion may cause hemolysis. Doxapram is physically incompatible with strongly alkaline drugs, such as thiopental sodium, aminophylline, or sodium bicarbonate.
• Avoid extravasation, which may lead to thrombophlebitis and local skin irritation.
• Monitor blood pressure, heart rate, deep tendon reflexes, and arterial blood gases before giving drug and every 30 minutes afterward.
• Be alert for signs of overdosage: hypertension, tachycardia, arrhythmias, skeletal muscle hyperactivity, and dyspnea. Discontinue drug and notify doctor if patients show signs of increased arterial carbon dioxide or oxygen tension, or if mechanical ventilation is necessary.

### ☑ PATIENT TEACHING
• Inform patient, if alert, and family of need for drug.
• Answer the patient's questions and address his concerns.

---

## fenfluramine hydrochloride
Ponderal†, Ponderal Pacaps†, Ponderax‡, Ponderax Pacaps‡, Pondimin, Pondimin Extentabs
Controlled Substance Schedule IV

*Pregnancy Risk Category: C*

### HOW SUPPLIED
*Tablets:* 20 mg
*Capsules (sustained-release):* 60 mg†‡

### ACTION
Unknown. Stimulates ventromedian nucleus of the hypothalamus. Also may affect serotonin metabolism.

### ONSET, PEAK, DURATION
Onset occurs in 1 to 2 hours. Peak unknown. Effects persist for 4 to 6 hours.

### INDICATIONS & DOSAGE
*Short-term adjunct in exogenous obesity –*
**Adults:** initially, 20 mg P.O. t.i.d. before meals. Maximum dosage is 40

mg t.i.d. Dosage adjusted according to patient response.

### ADVERSE REACTIONS
**CNS:** *drowsiness,* incoordination, headache, euphoria or depression, anxiety, *insomnia,* weakness, fatigue, agitation.
**CV:** *palpitations,* hypotension, hypertension, chest pain.
**EENT:** eye irritation, blurred vision.
**GI:** dry mouth, *diarrhea,* nausea, vomiting, abdominal pain, constipation.
**GU:** dysuria, increased urinary frequency, impotence.
**Skin:** rash, urticaria, burning sensation.
**Other:** diaphoresis, chills, fever, increased libido.

### INTERACTIONS
*Centrally acting antihypertensives:* decreased antihypertensive effect. Monitor blood pressure.
*Ethanol, CNS depressants:* enhanced CNS depression. Don't use together.
*Insulin, oral antidiabetic agents:* may decrease antidiabetic agent requirements. Monitor blood glucose levels.
*MAO inhibitors:* may cause severe hypertension, possibly hypertensive crisis. Don't use together or within 14 days after an MAO inhibitor has been discontinued.

### CONTRAINDICATIONS
Contraindicated in patients with psychotic disorders, severe hypertension, glaucoma, hypersensitivity to sympathomimetic amines, symptomatic CV disease (including arrhythmias), alcoholism, or history of drug abuse.

### NURSING CONSIDERATIONS
● Use cautiously in patients with mild to moderate hypertension and history of mental depression.
● Make sure patient is on a weight-reduction program.

● Monitor patient for tolerance or physical or psychological dependence.
● Monitor blood pressure.

### ☑ PATIENT TEACHING
● Have the patient report signs of excessive sedation, depression, or excessive stimulation.
● Tell patient to avoid alcohol while taking this drug.
● Tell patient not to discontinue abruptly; may precipitate an acute depressive reaction.

---

## mazindol
Mazanor, Sanorex
Controlled Substance Schedule IV
*Pregnancy Risk Category: NR*

### HOW SUPPLIED
*Tablets:* 1 mg, 2 mg

### ACTION
Unknown. Probably inhibits neuronal uptake of norepinephrine and dopamine.

### ONSET, PEAK, DURATION
Onset occurs in 30 to 60 minutes. Peak unknown. Effects persist 10 to 15 hours.

### INDICATIONS & DOSAGE
*Short-term adjunct in exogenous obesity—*
**Adults:** 1 mg P.O. t.i.d. 1 hour before meals, or 2 mg P.O. daily 1 hour before lunch in a single dose. Lowest effective dosage should be used.

### ADVERSE REACTIONS
**CNS:** *nervousness,* restlessness, *insomnia,* dysphoria, headache, depression, drowsiness, weakness, tremor.
**CV:** *palpitations, tachycardia.*
**GI:** dry mouth, dysgeusia, nausea, constipation, diarrhea, vomiting.
**GU:** urinary hesitancy, impotence.
**Hematologic:** decreased blood glucose levels.

---

**Skin:** rash, clamminess, pallor.
**Other:** diaphoresis, altered libido.

## INTERACTIONS
*Caffeine:* may increase amphetamine and related amine effects. Avoid concomitant use.
*Centrally acting antihypertensives:* decreased antihypertensive effect. Monitor blood pressure.
*Insulin, oral antidiabetic agents:* may decrease antidiabetic agent requirements. Monitor blood glucose levels.
*MAO inhibitors:* may cause severe hypertension, possibly hypertensive crisis. Don't use together or within 14 days after stopping MAO inhibitor.

## CONTRAINDICATIONS
Contraindicated in patients with symptomatic glaucoma, hypersensitivity or idiosyncrasy to drug, severe hypertension, CV disease (including arrhythmias) or history of drug abuse; within 14 days of MAO inhibitor therapy; and in agitated patients.

## NURSING CONSIDERATIONS
• Use cautiously in patients with mild to moderate hypertension.
• Make sure the patient also is on a weight-reduction program.
• Monitor patient for tolerance or physical or psychological dependence may develop.

## ☑ PATIENT TEACHING
• Tell the patient to take at least 6 hours before bedtime to avoid sleep interference.
• Warn the patient to avoid activities that require alertness or good psychomotor coordination until CNS effects of the drug are known.
• Tell the patient to avoid drinks containing caffeine, which increases the effects of amphetamines and related amines. Tell him to report signs of excessive stimulation.
• Inform patient that fatigue may result as drug effects wear off. The patient will need more rest.

---

# methamphetamine hydrochloride
Desoxyn, Desoxyn Gradumet
Controlled Substance Schedule II
*Pregnancy Risk Category: C*

## HOW SUPPLIED
*Tablets:* 5 mg
*Tablets (long-acting):* 5 mg, 10 mg, 15 mg**

## ACTION
Unknown. Probably promotes nerve impulse transmission by releasing stored norepinephrine from nerve terminals in the brain. Main sites of activity appear to be the cerebral cortex and the reticular activating system. In children with hyperkinesis, methamphetamine has a paradoxical calming effect.

## ONSET, PEAK, DURATION
Onset and peak unknown. Effects persist up to 24 hours.

## INDICATIONS & DOSAGE
*Attention deficit disorder with hyperactivity –*
**Children 6 years and older:** 2.5 to 5 mg P.O. once daily or b.i.d., with 5-mg increments weekly, p.r.n. Usual effective dosage is 20 to 25 mg daily.
*Short-term adjunct in exogenous obesity –*
**Adults:** 2.5 to 5 mg P.O. b.i.d. to t.i.d., 30 minutes before meals; or 10- to 15-mg long-acting tablet daily before breakfast.

## ADVERSE REACTIONS
**CNS:** *nervousness, insomnia,* irritability, *talkativeness,* dizziness, headache, hyperexcitability, tremor, euphoria.
**CV:** hypertension, *tachycardia, palpitations,* arrhythmias.

---

Reactions may be *common,* uncommon, *life-threatening,* or COMMON AND LIFE-THREATENING.

**EENT:** blurred vision, mydriasis.
**GI:** dry mouth, metallic taste, diarrhea, constipation, anorexia.
**GU:** impotence.
**Skin:** urticaria.
**Other:** altered libido.

## INTERACTIONS
*Ammonium chloride, ascorbic acid:* decreased serum levels and increased renal excretion of methamphetamine. Monitor for decreased methamphetamine effects.
*Antacids, sodium bicarbonate, acetazolamide:* increased renal reabsorption. Monitor for enhanced effects.
*Caffeine:* may increase amphetamine and related amine effects. Avoid concomitant use.
*Insulin, oral antidiabetic agents:* may decrease antidiabetic agent requirements. Monitor blood glucose levels.
*MAO inhibitors:* may cause severe hypertension, possibly hypertensive crisis. Don't use together or within 14 days after stopping MAO inhibitor.
*Phenothiazines, haloperidol, tricyclic antidepressants:* altered CNS effects. Avoid concomitant use.

## CONTRAINDICATIONS
Contraindicated in moderate to severe hypertension, hyperthyroidism, symptomatic CV disease, advanced arteriosclerosis, glaucoma, hypersensitivity or idiosyncrasy to sympathomimetic amines, history of drug abuse; within 14 days of MAO inhibitor therapy; and in agitated patients.

## NURSING CONSIDERATIONS
● Use cautiously in patients who are elderly, debilitated, asthenic, psychopathic, or who have a history of suicidal or homicidal tendencies.
● Be aware that drug is not recommended for first-line treatment of obesity. Use as an anorexigenic agent is prohibited in some states.
● When used for obesity, be sure patient is on a weight-reduction program.

● If tolerance to anorexigenic effect develops, notify doctor because drug will need to be discontinued.

## ☑ PATIENT TEACHING
● Tell the patient to take drug at least 6 hours before bedtime to avoid sleep interference.
● Warn the patient of high potential for abuse. Advise him that drug should not be used to prevent fatigue.
● Tell the patient never to crush sustained-release tablets.
● Warn the patient to avoid activities that require alertness or good psychomotor coordination until CNS effects of the drug are known.
● Tell the patient to avoid drinks containing caffeine, which increases the effects of amphetamines and related amines. Have him report signs of excessive stimulation.

## methylphenidate hydrochloride
PMS-Methylphenidate‡, Ritalin, Ritalin-SR
Controlled Substance Schedule II
*Pregnancy Risk Category: NR*

### HOW SUPPLIED
*Tablets:* 5 mg, 10 mg, 20 mg
*Tablets (sustained-release):* 20 mg

### ACTION
Unknown. Probably promotes nerve impulse transmission by releasing stored norepinephrine from nerve terminals in the brain. Main site of activity appears to be the cerebral cortex and the reticular activating system. In children with hyperkinesis, methylphenidate has a paradoxical calming effect.

### ONSET, PEAK, DURATION
Onset and duration unknown. Peak levels occur about 2 hours after regular-release tablets, 4 or 5 hours after sustained-release tablets.

---

*Liquid form contains alcohol.  **May contain tartrazine.  †Canada only.  ‡Australia only.  ◇OTC.

## INDICATIONS & DOSAGE

*Attention deficit disorder with hyper-activity (ADDH)* –

**Children 6 years and older:** initial dose, 5 to 10 mg P.O. daily before breakfast and lunch, with 5- to 10-mg increments weekly p.r.n., up to 60 mg daily.

*Narcolepsy* –

**Adults:** 10 mg P.O. b.i.d. or t.i.d. 30 to 45 minutes before meals. Dosage varies with patient needs.

## ADVERSE REACTIONS

**CNS:** *nervousness, insomnia,* Tourette syndrome, dizziness, headache, akathisia, dyskinesia, *seizures,* drowsiness.
**CV:** *palpitations,* angina, *tachycardia,* changes in blood pressure and pulse rate, arrhythmias.
**GI:** nausea, abdominal pain, anorexia, weight loss.
**Hematologic:** *thrombocytopenia,* thrombocytopenic purpura, leukopenia, anemia.
**Skin:** rash, urticaria, *exfoliative dermatitis, erythema multiforme.*

## INTERACTIONS

*Caffeine:* may increase amphetamine and related amine effects. Avoid concomitant use.
*Centrally acting antihypertensives:* decreased antihypertensive effect. Monitor blood pressure.
*MAO inhibitors:* may cause severe hypertension, possibly hypertensive crisis. Don't use together or within 14 days after an MAO inhibitor has been discontinued.
*Tricyclic antidepressants:* increased plasma levels of these drugs. Avoid concomitant use.

## CONTRAINDICATIONS

Contraindicated in patients with hypersensitivity to drug, glaucoma, motor tics, family history of or diagnosis of Tourette syndrome, or history of marked anxiety, tension, or agitation.

## NURSING CONSIDERATIONS

● Use cautiously in history of drug abuse, hypertension, history of seizures, or EEG abnormalities.
● Pemoline is the drug of choice for ADDH. It is usually stopped after puberty.
● Drug is not used to prevent fatigue.
● May precipitate Tourette syndrome in children. Monitor especially at start of therapy.
● Observe for signs of excessive stimulation. Monitor blood pressure.
● Monitor results of periodic CBC, differential, and platelet counts with long-term use.
● Monitor height and weight in children on long-term therapy. May delay growth spurt, but children will attain normal height when drug is stopped.
● Monitor patient for tolerance or psychological dependence.

### ☑ PATIENT TEACHING

● Tell the patient to take drug at least 6 hours before bedtime to prevent insomnia and after meals to reduce appetite-suppressant effects.
● Warn the patient against chewing sustained-release tablets.
● Warn the patient to avoid activities that require alertness or good psychomotor coordination until CNS effects of the drug are known.
● Tell the patient to avoid drinks containing caffeine, which increases the effects of amphetamines and related amines.
● Warn patient with seizure disorder that drug may decrease seizure threshold. Instruct him to notify the doctor if seizure occurs.
● Inform the patient that he will need more rest as drug effects wear off.

---

## pemoline
Cylert, Cylert Chewable
Controlled Substance Schedule IV

*Pregnancy Risk Category: B*

---

Reactions may be *common,* uncommon, *life-threatening,* or **COMMON AND LIFE-THREATENING.**

**HOW SUPPLIED**
*Tablets:* 18.75 mg, 37.5 mg, 75 mg
*Tablets (chewable):* 37.5 mg

**ACTION**
Unknown. Probably promotes nerve impulse transmission by releasing stored norepinephrine from nerve terminals in the brain. Main sites of activity appear to be the cerebral cortex and the reticular activating system.

**ONSET, PEAK, DURATION**
Onset and duration unknown. Serum levels peak 2 to 4 hours after dose.

**INDICATIONS & DOSAGE**
*Attention deficit disorder with hyperactivity –*
**Children 6 years and older:** initially, 37.5 mg P.O. in the morning with daily dosage raised by 18.75 mg weekly, p.r.n. Effective dosage range is 56.25 to 75 mg daily; maximum dosage is 112.5 mg daily.

**ADVERSE REACTIONS**
**CNS:** *insomnia,* dyskinetic movements, irritability, fatigue, mild depression, dizziness, headache, drowsiness, hallucinations, *seizures, Tourette syndrome,* abnormal oculomotor function.
**GI:** anorexia, abdominal pain, nausea.
**Hepatic:** elevated liver enzymes.
**Skin:** rash, *aplastic anemia.*

**INTERACTIONS**
*Insulin, oral antidiabetic agents:* may decrease antidiabetic agent requirements. Monitor blood glucose levels.

**CONTRAINDICATIONS**
Contraindicated in patients with hepatic dysfunction and hypersensitivity or idiosyncrasy to the drug.

**NURSING CONSIDERATIONS**
• Use cautiously in patients with impaired renal function.

• Be aware drug is structurally dissimilar to amphetamines or methylphenidate; however, it may produce similar adverse reactions. Drug has greater potential for abuse and dependence than previously thought.
• May precipitate Tourette syndrome in children. Monitor especially at start of therapy.
• Closely monitor patients on longterm therapy for possible blood or hepatic function abnormalities and for growth suppression.

☑ **PATIENT TEACHING**
• Tell patient to take drug at least 6 hours before bedtime to avoid sleep interference.
• Tell patient to avoid activities that require alertness or good psychomotor coordination until CNS effects of the drug are known.
• Warn patient with seizure disorder that drug may decrease seizure threshold. Instruct him to notify doctor if seizure occurs.

---

## phendimetrazine tartrate
Adipost, Anorex SR, Appecon, Bontril PDM, Bontril Slow-Release, Dyrexan OD, Malibar A, Melfiat-105 Unicelles, Metra, Neocurb, Obalan, Obe-Del, Obezine, Panrexin M, Panrexin MTP, Parzine, Phenazine, Phendiet, Phendiet-105, Phendimet, Phentra, Prelu-2, PT 105, Rexigen, Rexigen Forte, Tega-Nil, Trimcaps, Trimstat, Wehless, Weightrol, Wescoid, X-Trozine, X-Trozine LA
Controlled Substance Schedule IV

*Pregnancy Risk Category: NR*

**HOW SUPPLIED**
*Tablets:* 35 mg
*Capsules:* 35 mg
*Capsules (sustained-release):* 105 mg

---

## ACTION
Unknown. Probably promotes nerve impulse transmission by releasing stored norepinephrine from nerve terminals in the brain. Main sites of activity appear to be the cerebral cortex and the reticular activating system.

## ONSET, PEAK, DURATION
Onset and peak unknown. Effects persist about 4 hours.

## INDICATIONS & DOSAGE
*Short-term adjunct in exogenous obesity* –
**Adults:** 35 mg P.O. b.i.d. or t.i.d., 1 hour before meals. Maximum dosage is 70 mg t.i.d. or one (105-mg) sustained-release capsule P.O. once daily in the morning. Lowest effective dosage should be used and adjusted to individual response.

## ADVERSE REACTIONS
**CNS:** *nervousness, insomnia,* tremor, headache.
**CV:** *tachycardia, palpitations,* elevated blood pressure.
**EENT:** blurred vision.
**GI:** dry mouth, nausea, abdominal cramps, diarrhea, constipation.
**GU:** dysuria.

## INTERACTIONS
*Ammonium chloride, ascorbic acid:* decreased serum levels and increased renal excretion of phendimetrazine. Monitor for decreased phendimetrazine effects.
*Antacids, sodium bicarbonate, acetazolamide:* increased renal reabsorption. Monitor for enhanced effects.
*Caffeine:* may increase CNS stimulation. Avoid concomitant use.
*MAO inhibitors:* may cause severe hypertension, possibly hypertensive crisis. Don't use together or within 14 days after MAO inhibitor has been discontinued.
*Phenothiazines, haloperidol, tricyclic antidepressants:* altered CNS effect. Avoid concomitant use.

## CONTRAINDICATIONS
● Contraindicated in patients with hypersensitivity or idiosyncrasy to sympathomimetic amines, advanced arteriosclerosis, hyperthyroidism, moderate to severe hypertension, symptomatic CV disease, or glaucoma.
● Also contraindicated in patients in agitated states or those who are highly nervous, have a history of drug abuse, or have received MAO inhibitors in the last 14 days.

## NURSING CONSIDERATIONS
● Use cautiously in patients with mild hypertension.
● Make sure the patient also is on a weight-reduction program.
● Monitor patient for habituation and tolerance.

## ☑ PATIENT TEACHING
● Tell the patient to take drug at least 6 hours before bedtime to avoid sleep interference.
● Warn the patient to avoid activities that require alertness or good psychomotor coordination until CNS effects of the drug are known.
● Tell the patient to avoid drinks containing caffeine, which increases the effects of amphetamines and related amines. Tell him to report signs of excessive stimulation.
● Inform the patient that fatigue may result as drug effects wear off. The patient will need more rest.

---

Reactions may be *common,* uncommon, *life-threatening,* or COMMON AND LIFE-THREATENING.

# phentermine hydrochloride

Adipex-P, Duromine‡, Fastin, Obe-Mar, Obe-Nix, Obephen, Oby-Trim, Panshape M, Phentercot, Phentride, Phentride Caplets, Phentrol, Phentrol-2, Phentrol-4, Phentrol-5, T-Diet

Controlled Substance Schedule IV

*Pregnancy Risk Category: NR*

## HOW SUPPLIED

*Tablets:* 8 mg, 30 mg, 37.5 mg
*Capsules:* 15 mg, 18.75 mg, 30 mg, 37.5 mg
*Capsules (resin complex, sustained-release):* 15 mg, 30 mg

## ACTION

Unknown. Probably promotes nerve impulse transmission by releasing stored norepinephrine from nerve terminals in the brain. Main sites of activity appear to be the cerebral cortex and the reticular activating system.

## ONSET, PEAK, DURATION

Onset and peak unknown. Effects persist for 12 to 14 hours.

## INDICATIONS & DOSAGE

*Short-term adjunct in exogenous obesity –*
**Adults:** 8 mg P.O. t.i.d. ½ hour before meals. Alternatively, 15 to 30 mg (resin complex) or 15 to 37.5 mg (phentermine hydrochloride) P.O. daily as a single dose in the morning.

## ADVERSE REACTIONS

**CNS:** overstimulation, headache, euphoria, dysphoria, dizziness, *insomnia.*
**CV:** *palpitations, tachycardia,* increased blood pressure.
**GI:** dry mouth, dysgeusia, constipation, diarrhea, other GI disturbances.
**GU:** impotence.
**Skin:** urticaria.
**Other:** altered libido.

## INTERACTIONS

*Ammonium chloride, ascorbic acid:* decreased plasma levels and increased renal excretion of phentermine. Monitor for decreased phentermine effects.
*Antacids, sodium bicarbonate, acetazolamide:* increased renal reabsorption. Monitor for enhanced effects.
*Caffeine:* may increase CNS stimulation.
*Insulin, oral antidiabetic agents:* may alter antidiabetic agent requirements. Monitor blood glucose levels.
*MAO inhibitors:* may cause severe hypertension, possibly hypertensive crisis. Don't use together or within 14 days after MAO inhibitor has been discontinued.
*Phenothiazines, haloperidol, tricyclic antidepressants:* altered CNS effects. Avoid concomitant use.

## CONTRAINDICATIONS

Contraindicated in patients with hyperthyroidism, moderate to severe hypertension, advanced arteriosclerosis, symptomatic CV disease, glaucoma, or hypersensitivity or idiosyncrasy to sympathomimetic amines; within 14 days of MAO inhibitor therapy; and in agitated patients.

## NURSING CONSIDERATIONS

● Use cautiously in patients with mild hypertension.
● Use in conjunction with a weight-reduction program.
● Monitor for tolerance or dependence.

## ☑ PATIENT TEACHING

● Tell the patient to take drug at least 6 hours before bedtime to avoid sleep interference.
● Advise the patient to avoid drinks containing caffeine. Tell him to report signs of excessive stimulation.
● Warn the patient that fatigue may result as drug effects wear off and that the patient will need more rest.

---

*Liquid form contains alcohol.    **May contain tartrazine.    †Canada only.    ‡Australia only.    ◇OTC.

# 35

# Antiparkinsonian drugs

**amantadine hydrochloride**
(See Chapter 17, ANTIVIRALS.)
**benztropine mesylate**
**biperiden hydrochloride**
**biperiden lactate**
**bromocriptine mesylate**
**carbidopa-levodopa**
**levodopa**
**pergolide mesylate**
**procyclidine hydrochloride**
**selegiline hydrochloride**
**trihexyphenidyl hydrochloride**

## COMBINATION PRODUCTS
MADOPAR‡: levodopa 200 mg and
benserazide 50 mg.
MADOPAR HBS‡: levodopa 100 mg
and benserazide 25 mg.
MADOPAR Q‡: levodopa 50 mg and
benserazide 12.5 mg.
SINEMET 10-100: carbidopa 10 mg
and levodopa 100 mg.
SINEMET 25-100: carbidopa 25 mg
and levodopa 100 mg.
SINEMET 25-250: carbidopa 25 mg
and levodopa 250 mg.
SINEMET CR: carbidopa 50 mg and
levodopa 200 mg, in extended-release
tablets.

---

## benztropine mesylate
Apo-Benztropine†, Bensylate†,
Cogentin, PMS Benztropine†

*Pregnancy Risk Category: NR*

### HOW SUPPLIED
*Tablets:* 0.5 mg, 1 mg, 2 mg
*Injection:* 1 mg/ml in 2-ml ampules

### ACTION
Unknown. Thought to block central
cholinergic receptors, helping to balance cholinergic activity in the basal
ganglia.

### ONSET, PEAK, DURATION
Onset occurs within 15 minutes of
parenteral use, or within 1 to 2 hours
of oral use. Peak unknown. Effects
persist for 24 hours.

### INDICATIONS & DOSAGE
*Drug-induced extrapyramidal disor-
ders (except tardive dyskinesia)*
**Adults:** 1 to 4 mg P.O. or I.M. once
or twice daily.
*Acute dystonic reaction –*
**Adults:** 1 to 2 mg I.V. or I.M., followed by 1 to 2 mg P.O. b.i.d. to prevent recurrence.
*Parkinsonism –*
**Adults:** 0.5 to 6 mg P.O. or I.M.
daily. Initial dose is 0.5 mg to 1 mg.,
increased by 0.5 mg q 5 to 6 days.
Dosage adjusted to meet individual
requirements.

### ADVERSE REACTIONS
**CNS:** disorientation, hallucinations,
depression, toxic psychosis, confusion, memory impairment, nervousness.
**CV:** tachycardia.
**EENT:** dilated pupils, blurred vision.
**GI:** dry mouth, *constipation,* nausea,
vomiting, paralytic ileus.
**GU:** urine retention, dysuria.
  Some adverse reactions may result
from atropine-like toxicity and are
dose-related.

### INTERACTIONS
*Amantadine, phenothiazines, tricyclic
antidepressants:* additive anticholinergic adverse reactions, such as confusion and hallucinations. Reduce
dosage before administering.

### CONTRAINDICATIONS
Contraindicated in patients with hypersensitivity to drug or its compo-

---

nents or acute angle-closure glaucoma and in children under age 3.

## NURSING CONSIDERATIONS

• Use cautiously in hot weather, in patients with mental disorders, and in children age 3 and older.
• To help prevent GI distress, administer after meals.
• **I.V. use:** Route is seldom used because of small difference in onset when compared with I.M. route.
• Monitor vital signs carefully. Watch closely for adverse reactions, especially in elderly or debilitated patients. Call the doctor promptly.
• Be aware that drug produces atropine-like adverse reactions and may aggravate tardive dyskinesia.
• Watch for intermittent constipation and abdominal distention and pain; may indicate onset of paralytic ileus.
• *Alert:* Never discontinue this drug abruptly. Reduce dosage gradually.

### ☑ PATIENT TEACHING

• Warn patient to avoid activities that require alertness until CNS effects of the drug are known. If the patient is to receive a single daily dose, tell him to take it at bedtime.
• Advise patient to report signs of urinary hesitancy or urine retention.
• Tell patient to relieve dry mouth with cool drinks, ice chips, or sugarless gum or hard candy.
• Advise limiting activities during hot weather because drug-induced anhydrosis may cause hyperthermia.

---

## biperiden hydrochloride
Akineton

## biperiden lactate
Akineton Lactate

*Pregnancy Risk Category: C*

## HOW SUPPLIED
**biperiden hydrochloride**
*Tablets:* 2 mg

**biperiden lactate**
*Injection:* 5 mg/ml in 1-ml ampules

## ACTION
Unknown. Blocks central cholinergic receptors, helping to balance cholinergic activity in the basal ganglia.

## ONSET, PEAK, DURATION
Onset occurs within 30 minutes of parenteral use, within 1 hour of oral use. Peak unknown. Effects persist for 1 to 8 hours after I.V. use, for 6 to 12 hours after oral use.

## INDICATIONS & DOSAGE
*Drug-induced extrapyramidal disorders –*
**Adults:** 2 mg P.O. once daily b.i.d. or t.i.d., depending on severity. Usual dosage is 2 mg daily, or 2 mg I.M. or I.V. q ½ hour, not to exceed four doses or 8 mg daily.
*Parkinsonism –*
**Adults:** 2 mg P.O. t.i.d. or q.i.d. Some patients may require as much as 16 mg daily.

## ADVERSE REACTIONS
**CNS:** disorientation, euphoria, drowsiness, agitation.
**CV:** transient postural hypotension (with parenteral use).
**EENT:** blurred vision.
**GI:** dry mouth, *constipation*.
**GU:** urine retention.
   Adverse reactions are dose-related and may resemble atropine toxicity.

## INTERACTIONS
*Amantadine, phenothiazines, tricyclic antidepressants:* excessive CNS anticholinergic effects. Avoid concomitant use.

---

*Liquid form contains alcohol.   **May contain tartrazine.   †Canada only.   ‡Australia only.   ◇OTC.

*Antacids:* decreased biperiden absorption. Administer antacids at least 1 hour after biperiden.

## CONTRAINDICATIONS
Contraindicated in patients with hypersensitivity to the drug, angle-closure glaucoma, bowel obstruction, or megacolon.

## NURSING CONSIDERATIONS
• Use cautiously in patients with prostatic hyperplasia, arrhythmias, manifest glaucoma, and seizure disorder.
• To decrease adverse GI effects, give oral doses with or after meals.
• **I.V. use:** Administer very slowly.
• When giving parenterally, keep patient in supine position. Parenteral administration may cause transient postural hypotension and coordination disturbances.
• Monitor vital signs carefully. Watch closely for adverse reactions, especially in elderly or debilitated patients. Call the doctor promptly.
• Monitor patient for tolerance. If it develops, notify doctor because dosage will need to be increased.
• Know that in severe parkinsonism, tremors may increase as spasticity is relieved.

## ☑ PATIENT TEACHING
• Tell the patient to take oral form of drug with or after meals to decrease adverse GI effects.
• Warn the patient to avoid activities that require alertness until CNS effects of the drug are known.
• Because of possible dizziness, help the patient when he gets out of bed.
• Advise the patient to report signs of urinary hesitancy or urine retention.
• Advise the patient to relieve dry mouth with cool drinks, ice chips, sugarless gum, or hard candy.

## bromocriptine mesylate
Parlodel

*Pregnancy Risk Category: NR*

### HOW SUPPLIED
*Tablets:* 2.5 mg
*Capsules:* 5 mg

### ACTION
Inhibits secretion of prolactin and acts as a dopamine-receptor agonist by activating postsynaptic dopamine receptors.

### ONSET, PEAK, DURATION
Antiparkinsonian effects occur in 30 to 90 minutes; effects on serum prolactin, within 2 hours. Antiparkinsonian effects peak in 1 to 3 hours. Peak effects on serum prolactin occur within 8 hours. Antiparkinsonian effects persist for 12 to 18 hours; effects on serum prolactin, about 24 hours.

### INDICATIONS & DOSAGE
*Amenorrhea and galactorrhea associated with hyperprolactinemia; female infertility –*
**Adults:** 1.25 to 2.5 mg P.O. daily, increased by 2.5 mg daily at 3- to 7-day intervals until desired effect is achieved. Therapeutic dosage ranges from 2.5 to 5 mg/day. Safety and efficacy of doses greater than 100 mg daily have not been established.
*Prevention of postpartum lactation –*
**Adults:** 2.5 mg P.O. b.i.d. with meals for 14 days. Treatment may be extended for up to 21 days, if necessary.
*Parkinson's disease –*
**Adults:** 1.25 mg P.O. b.i.d. with meals. Dosage increased q 14 to 28 days, up to 100 mg daily, p.r.n.
*Acromegaly –*
**Adults:** 1.25 to 2.5 mg P.O. with h.s. snack for 3 days. An additional 1.25 to 2.5 mg may be added q 3 to 7 days until patient receives therapeutic benefit. Maximal dosage is 100 mg/day.

---

Reactions may be *common,* uncommon, *life-threatening,* or COMMON AND LIFE-THREATENING.

## ADVERSE REACTIONS

**CNS:** *dizziness, headache,* fatigue, mania, light-headedness, drowsiness, delusions, nervousness, insomnia, depression, *seizures.*
**CV:** *hypotension, stroke, acute MI.*
**EENT:** nasal congestion, blurred vision.
**GI:** *nausea,* vomiting, *abdominal cramps, constipation,* diarrhea, anorexia.
**GU:** urine retention, urinary frequency.
**Skin:** coolness and pallor of fingers and toes.

## INTERACTIONS

*Antihypertensives:* increased hypotensive effects. Adjust dosage of the antihypertensive.
*Haloperidol, loxapine, methyldopa, metoclopramide, MAO inhibitors, phenothiazines, reserpine:* interferes with bromocriptine's effects. Bromocriptine dosage may need to be increased.
*Levodopa:* additive effects. Adjust dosage of levodopa.
*Oral contraceptives, estrogens, progestins:* interfere with effects of bromocriptine. Concurrent use not recommended.

## CONTRAINDICATIONS

Contraindicated in patients with hypersensitivity to ergot derivatives, uncontrolled hypertension, or toxemia of pregnancy.

## NURSING CONSIDERATIONS

• Use cautiously in patients with impaired renal or hepatic function and history of MI with residual arrhythmias.
• Be aware that patients with impaired renal function may require dosage adjustments.
• Know that for Parkinson's disease, bromocriptine usually is given in addition to either levodopa or carbidopalevodopa.

• Give drug with meals.
• *Alert:* Monitor patient for adverse reactions. Incidence of adverse reactions is high (about 68%), particularly at beginning of therapy; however, most are mild to moderate, with nausea being the most common. Minimize adverse reactions by gradually titrating doses to effective levels as ordered. Adverse reactions are more frequent when drug is used for Parkinson's disease.
• Monitor blood pressure closely in patients who receive bromocriptine for suppression of postpartum lactation. In such patients, transient hypotension is common; however, hypertension, seizures, and CVA have also been reported.
• Know that baseline and periodic evaluations of cardiac, hepatic, renal, and hematopoietic function are recommended during prolonged therapy.
• May lead to early postpartum conception. Test for pregnancy every 4 weeks or whenever period is missed after menses resumes.

## ☑ PATIENT TEACHING

• Instruct patient to take drug with meals.
• Advise patient to use contraceptive methods other than oral contraceptives or subdermal implants during treatment.
• Advise patient to avoid dizziness and fainting by rising slowly to an upright position and avoiding sudden position changes.
• Advise patient that it may take 8 weeks or longer for menses to resume and galactorrhea to be suppressed.
• Inform postpartum patient that when therapy is discontinued, she may experience mild to moderate rebound breast secretion, congestion, or engorgement.

---

*Liquid form contains alcohol.   **May contain tartrazine.   †Canada only.   ‡Australia only.   ◊OTC.

## carbidopa-levodopa
Sinemet, Sinemet CR

*Pregnancy Risk Category: NR*

### HOW SUPPLIED
*Tablets:* carbidopa 10 mg with levodopa 100 mg (Sinemet 10-100), carbidopa 25 mg with levodopa 100 mg (Sinemet 25-100), carbidopa 25 mg with levodopa 250 mg (Sinemet 25-250)
*Tablets (extended-release):* carbidopa 50 mg with levodopa 200 mg (Sinemet CR)

### ACTION
Unknown for levodopa. Thought to be decarboxylated to dopamine, countering the depletion of striatal dopamine in extrapyramidal centers. Carbidopa inhibits the peripheral decarboxylation of levodopa without affecting levodopa's metabolism within the CNS. Therefore, more levodopa is available to be decarboxylated to dopamine in the brain.

### ONSET, PEAK, DURATION
Onset and duration unknown. Peak serum levels occur in about 40 minutes for regular-release tablets, or 2½ hours for extended-release tablets.

### INDICATIONS & DOSAGE
*Idiopathic Parkinson's disease, postencephalitic parkinsonism, and symptomatic parkinsonism resulting from carbon monoxide or manganese intoxication —*
**Adults:** one tablet of 25 mg carbidopa/100 mg levodopa P.O. daily t.i.d. followed by an increase of 1 tablet every day or every other day, p.r.n., to a maximum daily dosage of eight tablets. 25 mg carbidopa/250 mg levodopa or 10 mg carbidopa/100 mg levodopa tablets are substituted as required to obtain maximum response. Optimum daily dosage must

be determined by careful titration for each patient.

Patients treated with conventional tablets may receive extended-release tablets; dosage is calculated on current levodopa intake. Initially, the extended-release tablets given should amount to 10% more levodopa per day, increased, as needed and tolerated, to 30% more levodopa per day. Administered in divided doses at intervals of 4 to 8 hours.

### ADVERSE REACTIONS
**CNS:** *choreiform, dystonic, dyskinetic movements; involuntary grimacing, head movements, myoclonic body jerks, ataxia,* tremor, muscle twitching; bradykinetic episodes; psychiatric disturbances, anxiety, disturbing dreams, euphoria, malaise, fatigue; severe depression, suicidal tendencies, dementia, delirium, hallucinations (may necessitate reduction or withdrawal of drug), confusion, insomnia, agitation.
**CV:** *orthostatic hypotension,* **cardiac irregularities,** phlebitis.
**EENT:** blepharospasm, blurred vision, diplopia, mydriasis or miosis, oculogyric crises, excessive salivation.
**GI:** *dry mouth,* bitter taste, *nausea, vomiting, anorexia,* weight loss may occur at start of therapy; constipation; flatulence; diarrhea; abdominal pain.
**GU:** urinary frequency, urine retention, urinary incontinence, darkened urine, priapism.
**Hematologic:** **hemolytic anemia, thrombocytopenia,** leukopenia, **agranulocytosis.**
**Hepatic:** hepatotoxicity.
**Other:** dark perspiration, hyperventilation, hiccups.

### INTERACTIONS
*Antihypertensives:* additive hypotensive effects. Use together cautiously.
*MAO inhibitors:* risk of severe hypertension. Avoid concomitant use.

---

Reactions may be *common,* uncommon, **life-threatening,** or **COMMON AND LIFE-THREATENING.**

*Papaverine, phenytoin:* antagonism of antiparkinsonian actions. Don't use together.

*Phenothiazines and other antipsychotics:* may antagonize antiparkinsonian actions. Use together cautiously.

## CONTRAINDICATIONS

Contraindicated in patients with hypersensitivity to drug, acute angle-closure glaucoma, melanoma, or undiagnosed skin lesions, and within 14 days of MAO inhibitor therapy.

## NURSING CONSIDERATIONS

• Use cautiously in patients with severe CV, renal, hepatic, endocrine, or pulmonary disorders; history of peptic ulcer; psychiatric illness; MI with residual arrhythmias; bronchial asthma; emphysema; and well-controlled, chronic open-angle glaucoma.

• If the patient is being treated with levodopa, the drug should be discontinued at least 8 hours before starting carbidopa-levodopa.

• Know that carbidopa-levodopa typically decreases amount of levodopa needed by 75%, reducing the incidence of adverse reactions.

• Be aware that therapeutic and adverse reactions occur more rapidly with carbidopa-levodopa than with levodopa alone. Observe and monitor vital signs, especially while adjusting dosage. Report significant changes.

• Carefully monitor patients receiving antihypertensives.

• *Alert:* Muscle twitching and blepharospasm may be early signs of drug overdose; report immediately.

• Know that patients receiving long-term therapy should be tested regularly for diabetes and acromegaly and have periodic tests of liver, renal, and hematopoietic function as ordered.

• Depending on reagent and test method used, expect possible false-positive increases in levels of uric acid, urine ketones, urine catecholamines, and urine vanillylmandelic acid.

• False-positive tests for urine glucose can occur if reagents using copper sulfate are used; false-negative results can occur with tests that use glucose enzymatic methods. An accurate measure can be obtained if the paper strip is only partially immersed in the urine sample. Urine will migrate up the strip, as with an ascending chromatographic system. Read only the top of the strip.

## ☑ PATIENT TEACHING

• Tell patient to take the drug with food to minimize GI upset.

• Warn the patient and his caregivers not to increase dosage without doctor's orders.

• Warn the patient of possible dizziness and orthostatic hypotension, especially at start of therapy. Tell him to change position slowly and dangle legs before getting out of bed. Elastic stockings may control this adverse reaction in some patients.

• Instruct the patient to report adverse reactions and therapeutic effects.

• Inform the patient that pyridoxine (vitamin $B_6$) does not reverse the beneficial effects of carbidopa-levodopa. Multivitamins can be taken without losing control of symptoms.

## levodopa
Dopar, Larodopa

*Pregnancy Risk Category: NR*

### HOW SUPPLIED
*Tablets:* 100 mg, 250 mg, 500 mg
*Capsules:* 100 mg, 250 mg, 500 mg

### ACTION
Unknown. Thought to be decarboxylated to dopamine, countering the depletion of striatal dopamine in extrapyramidal centers, which is thought to produce parkinsonism.

## ONSET, PEAK, DURATION
Onset for maximal effects, 3 weeks to 6 months. Plasma levels peak in 1 to 3 hours. Effects vary but usually persist for about 5 hours.

## INDICATIONS & DOSAGE
*Idiopathic parkinsonism, postencephalitic parkinsonism, and symptomatic parkinsonism after carbon monoxide or manganese intoxication or in association with cerebral arteriosclerosis –*
**Adults and children over 12 years:** initially, 0.5 to 1 g P.O. daily, divided in two or more doses with food; increased by no more than 0.75 g daily q 3 to 7 days until usual maximum daily dosage of 8 g is reached. Dosage adjusted to patient requirements, tolerance, and response. Higher dosage requires close supervision.

## ADVERSE REACTIONS
**CNS:** *aggressive behavior; choreiform, dystonic, and dyskinetic movements; involuntary grimacing, head movements, myoclonic body jerks,* **seizures,** *ataxia, tremor, muscle twitching; bradykinetic episodes; psychiatric disturbances; mood changes, nervousness, anxiety, disturbing dreams, euphoria, malaise, fatigue; severe depression, suicidal tendencies, dementia, delirium, hallucinations* (may require reduction or withdrawal of drug).
**CV:** *orthostatic hypotension,* cardiac irregularities, phlebitis.
**EENT:** blepharospasm, blurred vision, diplopia, mydriasis or miosis, activation of latent Horner's syndrome, oculogyric crises, excessive salivation.
**GI:** dry mouth, bitter taste, *nausea, vomiting, anorexia,* weight loss (at start of therapy), constipation, flatulence, diarrhea, abdominal pain.
**GU:** urinary frequency, urine retention, incontinence, darkened urine, priapism.
**Hematologic:** *hemolytic anemia,* leukopenia, *agranulocytosis.*

**Hepatic:** hepatotoxicity.
**Other:** dark perspiration, hyperventilation, hiccups.

## INTERACTIONS
*Antacids:* increased absorption of levodopa. Administer antacids 1 hour after levodopa.
*Cocaine, sympathomimetic agents, inhalation anesthetics:* increased risk of arrhythmias. Monitor closely.
*MAO inhibitors, furazolidone, procarbazine:* risk of severe hypertension. Avoid concomitant use.
*Metoclopramide:* accelerated gastric emptying of levodopa. Give metoclopramide 1 hour after levodopa.
*Papaverine, phenothiazines and other antipsychotics, phenytoin, rauwolfia alkaloids:* decreased levodopa effect. Avoid concomitant use, if possible.
*Pyridoxine:* reversal of antiparkinsonian effects. Check vitamin preparations and nutritional supplements for pyridoxine (vitamin $B_6$) content. Don't give together.
*Foods high in protein:* decreased absorption of levodopa. Don't give levodopa with high-protein foods.

## CONTRAINDICATIONS
Contraindicated in concurrent therapy with MAO inhibitors within 14 days, and in hypersensitivity to the drug, acute angle-closure glaucoma, melanoma, or undiagnosed skin lesions.

## NURSING CONSIDERATIONS
● Use cautiously in severe CV, renal, liver, and pulmonary disorders; peptic ulcer; psychiatric illness; MI with residual arrhythmias; bronchial asthma; emphysema; and endocrine disease.
● Patients who must undergo surgery should continue levodopa therapy as long as oral intake is permitted, generally 6 to 24 hours before surgery. Drug should be resumed as soon as patient is able to take oral medication.
● Carbidopa-levodopa typically decreases amount of levodopa needed by

---

Reactions may be *common,* uncommon, *life-threatening,* or **COMMON AND LIFE-THREATENING.**

75%, reducing the incidence of adverse reactions.
• Monitor vital signs, especially while adjusting dosage. Report changes.
• Muscle twitching and blepharospasm may be early signs of drug overdose; report immediately.
• Coombs' test may become positive during extended use. Expect uric acid elevations with colorimetric method but not with urate oxidase.
• Know that alkaline phosphatase, AST, ALT, lactate dehydrogenase, bilirubin, BUN, and protein-bound iodine show transient elevations in patients receiving levodopa; WBC count, hemoglobin, and hematocrit show occasional reductions.
• Depending on reagent and test method used, expect possible false-positive increases in levels of uric acid, urine ketones, urine catecholamines, and urine vanillylmandelic acid.
• False-positive tests for urine glucose can occur if reagents using copper sulfate are used; false-negative results can occur with tests that use glucose enzymatic methods. An accurate measure can be obtained if the paper strip is only partially immersed in the urine sample. Urine will migrate up the strip, as with an ascending chromatographic system. Read only the top of the strip.
• Know that patients receiving long-term therapy should be tested regularly for diabetes and acromegaly; periodically monitor renal, liver, and hematopoietic function as ordered.
• A doctor-supervised period of drug discontinuance (called a drug holiday) may reestablish the effectiveness of a lower dosage regimen.

☑ **PATIENT TEACHING**
• Tell the patient to take the drug with food to minimize GI upset. However, taking the drug with high-protein meals can impair absorption and reduce effectiveness.
• For the patient who has difficulty swallowing pills, tell him and his caregivers to crush tablets and mix with applesauce or baby food fruits.
• Warn the patient and his caregivers not to increase dosage unless ordered. Daily dosage should not exceed 8 g.
• Tell the patient to protect drug from heat, light, and moisture. If preparation darkens, it has lost potency and should be discarded.
• Warn the patient of possible dizziness and orthostatic hypotension, especially at start of therapy. Tell him to change position slowly and dangle legs before rising. Elastic stockings may control this adverse reaction.
• Advise the patient and his caregivers that multivitamin preparations, fortified cereals, and certain OTC medications may contain pyridoxine (vitamin $B_6$), which can block the effects of levodopa by enhancing its peripheral metabolism.

## pergolide mesylate
Permax

*Pregnancy Risk Category: B*

**HOW SUPPLIED**
*Tablets:* 0.05 mg, 0.25 mg, 1 mg

**ACTION**
A dopamine agonist that directly stimulates dopamine receptors in the nigrostriatal system.

**ONSET, PEAK, DURATION**
Unknown.

**INDICATIONS & DOSAGE**
*Adjunctive treatment with carbidopa-levodopa in the management of the symptoms in Parkinson's disease –*
**Adults:** initially, 0.05 mg P.O. daily for the first 2 days followed by increased dosage of 0.1 to 0.15 mg every third day over 12 days. Subsequent dosage increased by 0.25 mg every third day, if needed, until optimum response is seen. The drug usu-

ally is administered in divided doses t.i.d. Gradual reductions in carbidopa-levodopa dosage could be made during dosage titration.

## ADVERSE REACTIONS
**CNS:** headache, asthenia, *dyskinesia, dizziness, hallucinations, dystonia, confusion, somnolence,* insomnia, anxiety, depression, tremor, abnormal dreams, personality disorder, psychosis, abnormal gait, akathisia, extrapyramidal syndrome, incoordination, akinesia, hypertonia, neuralgia, speech disorder, twitching.
**CV:** *orthostatic hypotension,* vasodilation, palpitations, hypotension, syncope, hypertension, ***arrhythmias, MI.***
**EENT:** *rhinitis,* epistaxis, abnormal vision, diplopia, eye disorder.
**GI:** dry mouth, taste perversion, abdominal pain, *nausea, constipation,* diarrhea, dyspepsia, anorexia, vomiting.
**GU:** urinary frequency, urinary tract infection, hematuria.
**Skin:** rash, diaphoresis, paresthesia.
**Other:** flulike syndrome; chest, neck, and back pain; chills; infection; facial, peripheral, or generalized edema; weight gain; arthralgia; bursitis; myalgia; dyspnea.
   *Note:* The preceding adverse reactions, although not always attributable to the drug, occurred in more than 1% of the study population.

## INTERACTIONS
*Butyrophenones, metoclopramide, other dopamine antagonists, phenothiazines, thioxanthenes:* may antagonize the effects of pergolide. Avoid concomitant use.

## CONTRAINDICATIONS
Contraindicated in patients hypersensitive to the drug or to ergot alkaloids.

## NURSING CONSIDERATIONS
• Use cautiously in patients prone to arrhythmias.

• *Alert:* Monitor blood pressure. Symptomatic orthostatic or sustained hypotension may occur especially at the start of therapy.

## ☑ PATIENT TEACHING
• Inform patient of potential adverse reactions, especially hallucinations and confusion (27% incidence).
• Warn patient to avoid activities that could result in injury from orthostatic hypotension and syncope.

---

# procyclidine hydrochloride
Kemadrin, PMS Procyclidine†, Procyclid†

*Pregnancy Risk Category: NR*

## HOW SUPPLIED
*Tablets:* 5 mg

## ACTION
Unknown. Blocks central cholinergic receptors, helping to balance cholinergic activity in the basal ganglia.

## ONSET, PEAK, DURATION
Onset within 1 hour. Peak in 1 to 3 hours. Effects persist about 4 hours.

## INDICATIONS & DOSAGE
*Parkinsonism, drug-induced extrapyramidal symptoms –*
**Adults:** initially, 2.5 mg P.O. t.i.d. after meals. Increased p.r.n. to 5 mg P.O. t.i.d. after meals and, occasionally, 5 mg P.O. h.s.

## ADVERSE REACTIONS
**CNS:** light-headedness, giddiness.
**EENT:** blurred vision, mydriasis.
**GI:** *dry mouth, constipation,* nausea, vomiting, epigastric distress.
**Skin:** rash.
**Other:** muscle weakness.

## INTERACTIONS
None significant.

---

Reactions may be *common*, uncommon, *life-threatening*, or **COMMON AND LIFE-THREATENING**.

## CONTRAINDICATIONS
Contraindicated in patients with acute angle-closure glaucoma.

## NURSING CONSIDERATIONS
• Use cautiously in patients with tachycardia, hypotension, urine retention, and prostatic hyperplasia.
• Watch for mental confusion, disorientation, agitation, hallucinations, and psychotic symptoms, especially in elderly patients. Call the doctor. In severe parkinsonism, tremors may increase as spasticity is relieved.

## ☑ PATIENT TEACHING
• Tell patient to take drug after meals to minimize GI distress.
• Warn the patient to avoid activities that require alertness until CNS effects of the drug are known.
• Tell the patient to relieve dry mouth with cool drinks, ice chips, or sugarless gum or hard candy.

## selegiline hydrochloride (L-deprenyl hydrochloride)
Eldepryl

*Pregnancy Risk Category: C*

## HOW SUPPLIED
*Tablets:* 5 mg

## ACTION
Unknown. May selectively inhibit MAO type B (found mostly in the brain). At higher-than-recommended doses, it is a nonselective inhibitor of MAO, including MAO type A (found in the GI tract). Also may directly increase dopaminergic activity by decreasing the reuptake of dopamine into nerve cells. Its active metabolites, amphetamine and methamphetamine, may contribute to this effect.

## ONSET, PEAK, DURATION
Onset and duration unknown. Serum levels peak in ½ to 2 hours.

## INDICATIONS & DOSAGE
*Adjunctive treatment with carbidopa-levodopa in the management of the symptoms in Parkinson's disease –*
**Adults:** 10 mg P.O. daily, taken as 5 mg at breakfast and 5 mg at lunch. After 2 or 3 days, gradual decrease of carbidopa-levodopa dosage.

## ADVERSE REACTIONS
**CNS:** *dizziness,* increased tremor, chorea, loss of balance, restlessness, increased bradykinesia, facial grimacing, stiff neck, dyskinesia, involuntary movements, twitching, increased apraxia, behavioral changes, fatigue, headache, confusion, hallucinations, vivid dreams, anxiety, insomnia, lethargy.
**CV:** orthostatic hypotension, hypertension, hypotension, *arrhythmias,* palpitations, new or increased anginal pain, tachycardia, peripheral edema, syncope.
**EENT:** blepharospasm.
**GI:** dry mouth, *nausea,* vomiting, constipation, weight loss, abdominal pain, anorexia or poor appetite, dysphagia, diarrhea, heartburn.
**GU:** slow urination, transient nocturia, prostatic hyperplasia, urinary hesitancy, urinary frequency, urine retention, sexual dysfunction.
**Skin:** rash, hair loss.
**Other:** malaise, diaphoresis.

## INTERACTIONS
*Adrenergic agents:* possible increased pressor response, particularly in patients who have taken an overdose of selegiline. Use together cautiously.
*Meperidine:* may cause stupor, muscle rigidity, severe agitation, and elevated temperature. Avoid concomitant use.
*Foods high in tyramine:* possible hypertensive crisis. Monitor blood pressure.

## CONTRAINDICATIONS
Contraindicated in patients with hypersensitivity to the drug and in patients receiving meperidine.

## NURSING CONSIDERATIONS
● *Alert:* Some patients experience increased adverse reactions with levodopa and require a 10% to 30% reduction of carbidopa-levodopa dosage.

### ☑ PATIENT TEACHING
● Warn patient to move cautiously at the start of therapy because he may experience dizziness.
● Advise patient not to take more than 10 mg daily. A greater amount may increase adverse reactions.

---

# trihexyphenidyl hydrochloride
Aparkane†, Apo-Trihex†, Artane*, Artane Sequels, Novohexidyl†, Trihexane, Trihexy-2, Trihexy-5

*Pregnancy Risk Category: NR*

## HOW SUPPLIED
*Tablets:* 2 mg, 5 mg
*Capsules (sustained-release):* 5 mg
*Elixir:* 2 mg/5 ml

## ACTION
Unknown. Blocks central cholinergic receptors, helping to balance cholinergic activity in the basal ganglia.

## ONSET, PEAK, DURATION
Onset within 1 hour. Peak unknown. Effects persist for 6 to 12 hours.

## INDICATIONS & DOSAGE
*All forms of parkinsonism, drug-induced parkinsonism, and adjunctive treatment to levodopa in the management of parkinsonism –*
**Adults:** 1 mg P.O. first day, 2 mg second day; then increased in 2-mg increments q 3 to 5 days until total of 6 to 10 mg is given daily. Usually given t.i.d. with meals, sometimes given q.i.d. (last dose h.s.) or switched to extended-release form b.i.d. Postencephalitic parkinsonism may require total daily dosage of 12 to 15 mg.

## ADVERSE REACTIONS
**CNS:** nervousness, dizziness, headache, hallucinations, drowsiness, weakness.
**CV:** tachycardia.
**EENT:** blurred vision, mydriasis, increased intraocular pressure.
**GI:** *dry mouth,* constipation, *nausea,* vomiting.
**GU:** urinary hesitancy, urine retention.

## INTERACTIONS
*Amantadine:* additive anticholinergic adverse reactions, such as confusion and hallucinations. Reduce dosage of trihexyphenidyl before administering.

## CONTRAINDICATIONS
Contraindicated in patients hypersensitive to the drug.

## NURSING CONSIDERATIONS
● Use cautiously in glaucoma; cardiac, hepatic, or renal disorders; obstructive disease of the GI and GU tracts; and prostatic hyperplasia.
● Be aware that dosage may need to be gradually increased in patients who develop a tolerance to the drug.
● Monitor patient. Adverse reactions are dose-related and transient.
● Gonioscopic evaluation and monitoring of intraocular pressure are needed, especially in patients over 40 years.

### ☑ PATIENT TEACHING
● Advise the patient that drug may cause nausea if given before meals.
● Tell the patient to avoid activities that require alertness until CNS effects of the drug are known.
● Advise the patient to report signs of urinary hesitancy or urine retention.
● Tell the patient to relieve dry mouth with cool drinks, ice chips, or sugarless gum or hard candy.

---

# 36

## Miscellaneous CNS drugs

fluvoxamine maleate
lithium carbonate
lithium citrate
nicotine polacrilex
nicotine transdermal system
sumatriptan succinate
tacrine hydrochloride

**COMBINATION PRODUCTS**
None.

---

## fluvoxamine maleate
Luvox

*Pregnancy Risk Category: C*

**HOW SUPPLIED**
*Tablets:* 50 mg, 100 mg

**ACTION**
Unknown. Selectively inhibits the neuronal uptake of serotonin, which is thought to improve obsessive-compulsive disorders.

**ONSET, PEAK, DURATION**
Onset and duration unknown. Serum levels peak in 3 to 8 hours.

**INDICATIONS & DOSAGE**
*Obsessive-compulsive disorder –*
**Adults:** initially, 50 mg P.O. daily h.s., increased in 50-mg increments q 4 to 7 days until maximum benefit achieved. Maximum daily dosage is 300 mg. Total daily doses of more than 100 mg should be given in two divided doses.

**ADVERSE REACTIONS**
**CNS:** *headache, asthenia, somnolence, insomnia, nervousness,* dizziness, tremor, anxiety, hypertonia, *agitation,* depression, CNS stimulation, taste perversion.
**CV:** palpitations, vasodilation.

**EENT:** amblyopia.
**GI:** *nausea, diarrhea, constipation, dyspepsia,* anorexia, *vomiting,* flatulence, tooth disorder, dysphagia, *dry mouth.*
**GU:** decreased libido, abnormal ejaculation, urinary frequency, impotence, anorgasmia, urine retention.
**Respiratory:** upper respiratory tract infection, dyspnea, yawning.
**Skin:** sweating.
**Other:** flulike syndrome, chills.

**INTERACTIONS**
*Astemizole, terfenadine:* may cause decreased metabolism, leading to increased levels of these antihistamines and cardiotoxicity. Avoid concomitant use.
*Benzodiazepines, theophylline, warfarin:* reduced clearance of these drugs by fluvoxamine. Use together cautiously (except for diazepam, which should not be administered together with fluvoxamine). Dosage adjustments may be necessary.
*Carbamazepine, clozapine, methadone, metopranolol, propranolol, tricyclic antidepressants:* elevated serum levels of these drugs caused by fluvoxamine. Use together cautiously. Monitor patient closely for adverse reactions. Dosage adjustments may be necessary.
*Diltiazem:* bradycardia may occur. Monitor heart rate.
*Lithium, tryptophan:* may enhance effects of fluvoxamine. Use together cautiously.
*MAO inhibitors:* may cause severe excitation, hyperpyrexia, myoclonus, delirium, and coma. Avoid concomitant use.

---

*Liquid form contains alcohol. **May contain tartrazine. †Canada only. ‡Australia only. ◊OTC.

## CONTRAINDICATIONS
Contraindicated in patients with hypersensitivity to the drug or to other phenylpiperazine antidepressants and within 14 days of MAO inhibitor therapy.

## NURSING CONSIDERATIONS
• Use cautiously in patients with hepatic dysfunction, concomitant conditions that may affect hemodynamic responses or metabolism, or history of mania or seizures.
• Know that at least 14 days should elapse after stopping fluvoxamine before patient is started on an MAO inhibitor and that at least 14 days should elapse before a patient is started on fluvoxamine after MAO inhibitor therapy has been discontinued.
• Record mood changes. Monitor patients for suicidal tendencies, and allow them only a minimum supply of the drug.

## ☑ PATIENT TEACHING
• Warn patient not to engage in hazardous activity until drug's CNS effects are known.
• Advise patient to avoid alcoholic beverages while taking this drug.
• Alert patient that smoking may decrease effectiveness of the drug.
• Instruct female patient who becomes pregnant or intends to become pregnant during therapy to notify doctor.
• Tell patient who develops a rash, hives, or a related allergic reaction to notify doctor.
• Inform patient that several weeks of therapy may be required to obtain the full antidepressant effect. Once improvement is seen, advise patient not to discontinue the drug until directed by doctor.
• Advise patient to check with doctor before taking any OTC medication; drug interactions can occur.

## lithium carbonate
Carbolith†, Duralith†, Eskalith, Eskalith CR, Lithane**, Lithicarb‡, Lithizine†, Lithobid, Lithonate, Lithotabs, Priadel‡

## lithium citrate
Cibalith-S*

*Pregnancy Risk Category: NR*

## HOW SUPPLIED
**lithium carbonate**
*Tablets:* 250 mg‡, 300 mg (300 mg equals 8.12 mEq lithium)
*Tablets (controlled-release):* 300 mg, 400 mg‡, 450 mg
*Capsules:* 150 mg, 300 mg, 600 mg
**lithium citrate**
*Syrup (sugarless):* 8 mEq (of lithium) per 5 ml
   *Note:* 5 ml of lithium citrate (liquid) contains 8 mEq lithium, equal to 300 mg of lithium carbonate.

## ACTION
Unknown. Probably alters chemical transmitters in the CNS, possibly by interfering with ionic pump mechanisms in brain cells, and may compete with or replace sodium ions.

## ONSET, PEAK, DURATION
Onset of clinical effects usually within 1 to 3 weeks. Serum levels peak in $\frac{1}{2}$ to 3 hours depending on dosage form used. Duration unknown.

## INDICATIONS & DOSAGE
*Prevention or control of mania –*
**Adults:** 300 to 600 mg P.O. up to q.i.d., increasing on the basis of blood levels to achieve optimal dosage. Recommended therapeutic lithium blood levels: 1 to 1.5 mEq/L for acute mania; 0.6 to 1.2 mEq/L for maintenance therapy; and 2 mEq/L as maximum dosage.

## ADVERSE REACTIONS

**CNS:** tremors, drowsiness, headache, confusion, restlessness, dizziness, psychomotor retardation, lethargy, *coma,* blackouts, *epileptiform seizures,* EEG changes, worsened organic mental syndrome, impaired speech, ataxia, muscle weakness, incoordination.

**CV:** *reversible ECG changes, arrhythmias,* hypotension, bradycardia, *peripheral vascular collapse* (rare).

**EENT:** tinnitus, blurred vision.

**GI:** dry mouth, metallic taste, nausea, vomiting, anorexia, diarrhea, *thirst,* abdominal pain, flatulence, indigestion.

**GU:** *polyuria,* glycosuria, renal toxicity with long-term use, decreased creatinine clearance, albuminuria.

**Hematologic:** *leukocytosis with leukocyte count of 14,000 to 18,000/mm³* (reversible).

**Skin:** pruritus, rash, diminished or absent sensation, drying and thinning of hair, psoriasis, acne, alopecia.

**Other:** transient hyperglycemia, goiter, hypothyroidism (lowered $T_3$, $T_4$, and protein-bound iodine, but elevated $^{131}I$ uptake), hyponatremia, ankle and wrist edema.

## INTERACTIONS

*Aminophylline, sodium bicarbonate, urine alkalinizers:* increased lithium excretion. Avoid excessive salt and monitor lithium levels.

*Carbamazepine, fluoxetine, indomethacin, methyldopa, piroxicam, probenecid:* increased effect of lithium. Monitor for lithium toxicity.

*Diuretics:* increased reabsorption of lithium by kidneys, with possible toxic effect. Use with extreme caution, and monitor lithium and electrolyte levels (especially sodium).

*Neuroleptics:* may cause encephalopathy. Watch for signs and symptoms (lethargy, tremor, extrapyramidal symptoms), and stop drug if it occurs.

*Neuromuscular blockers:* may cause prolonged paralysis or weakness. Monitor patient closely.

*Thyroid hormones:* may induce hypothyroidism. Monitor thyroid function.

## CONTRAINDICATIONS

Contraindicated if therapy cannot be closely monitored.

## NURSING CONSIDERATIONS

• Know that drug should not be administered during pregnancy.

• Use with extreme caution in patients receiving neuroleptics, neuromuscular blockers, and diuretics; in elderly or debilitated patients; and in patients with thyroid disease, seizure disorder, renal or CV disease, severe debilitation or dehydration, and sodium depletion.

• **Alert:** Be aware that determination of lithium blood concentration is crucial to the safe use of the drug. Drug should not be used in patients who can't have regular lithium blood level checks. Monitor lithium blood levels 8 to 12 hours after first dose, usually before morning dose, two or three times weekly first month, then weekly to monthly during maintenance therapy.

• Know that when blood levels of lithium are below 1.5 mEq/L, adverse reactions are usually mild.

• Monitor baseline ECG, thyroid and renal studies, as well as electrolyte levels, as ordered.

• Check fluid intake and output, especially when surgery is scheduled.

• Weigh the patient daily; check for signs of edema or sudden weight gain.

• Adjust fluid and salt ingestion to compensate if excessive loss occurs as a result of protracted diaphoresis or diarrhea. Under normal conditions, patients should have fluid intake of 2,500 to 3,000 ml daily and a balanced diet with adequate salt intake.

• Check urine specific gravity and report level below 1.005, which may indicate diabetes insipidus.

---

• May alter glucose tolerance in diabetics. Monitor blood glucose closely.
• Perform outpatient follow-up of thyroid and renal functions every 6 to 12 months. Palpate thyroid to check for enlargement.

### ☑ PATIENT TEACHING
• Tell patient to take drug with plenty of water and after meals to minimize GI upset.
• Explain to patient that lithium has a narrow therapeutic margin of safety. A blood level that is even slightly high can be dangerous.
• Warn patient and caregivers to watch for signs of toxicity (diarrhea, vomiting, tremor, drowsiness, muscle weakness, ataxia) and to expect transient nausea, polyuria, thirst, and discomfort during first few days. Patients should withhold one dose and call the doctor if toxic symptoms appear, but not stop drug abruptly.
• Warn ambulatory patient to avoid hazardous activities that require alertness and good psychomotor coordination until CNS effects of the drug are known.
• Tell patient not to switch brands of lithium or take other prescription or OTC drugs without the doctor's guidance.
• Tell patient to carry medical identification at all times.

---

## nicotine polacrilex (nicotine-polacrilin resin complex)
Nicorette, Nicorette DS

*Pregnancy Risk Category: C*

### HOW SUPPLIED
*Chewing gum:* 2 mg/square, 4 mg/square

### ACTION
Provides nicotine, which stimulates nicotinic acetylcholine receptors in the CNS, neuromuscular junction, autonomic ganglia, and adrenal medulla.

### ONSET, PEAK, DURATION
Onset and duration unknown. Serum levels peak within 15 to 30 minutes after the patient begins to chew the gum.

### INDICATIONS & DOSAGE
*Relief of nicotine withdrawal symptoms in patients undergoing smoking cessation –*
**Adults:** initially, one 2-mg square; highly dependent patients should start treatment with 4-mg squares. Patients should chew 1 piece of gum slowly and intermittently for 30 minutes whenever the urge to smoke occurs. Most patients require 9 to 12 pieces of gum daily during the first month. For patients using 4-mg squares, maximum dosage is 20 pieces daily. For patients using 2-mg squares, maximum dosage is 30 pieces daily.

### ADVERSE REACTIONS
**CNS:** dizziness, light-headedness, irritability, insomnia, headache.
**CV:** atrial fibrillation.
**EENT:** *throat soreness, jaw muscle ache* (from chewing).
**GI:** *nausea, vomiting,* indigestion, eructation, anorexia, excessive salivation.
**Other:** *hiccups.*

### INTERACTIONS
*Beta blockers, methylxanthines, propoxyphene, propranolol:* decreased metabolism of these agents, increasing therapeutic effects. Dosage adjustments of these agents may be necessary.

### CONTRAINDICATIONS
Contraindicated in nonsmokers; in patients with recent MI, life-threatening arrhythmias, severe or worsening angina pectoris, or active temporoman-

---

Reactions may be *common,* uncommon, *life-threatening,* or **COMMON AND LIFE-THREATENING.**

dibular joint disease; and during pregnancy.

## NURSING CONSIDERATIONS
• Use cautiously in patients with hyperthyroidism, pheochromocytoma, insulin-dependent diabetes, peptic ulcer disease, history of esophagitis, oral or pharyngeal inflammation, or dental conditions that might be exacerbated by chewing gum.
• Know that smokers most likely to benefit from nicotine gum are those with high "physical" nicotine dependence – those who smoke more than 15 cigarettes daily, prefer brands of cigarettes with high nicotine levels, usually inhale the smoke, smoke the first cigarette within 30 minutes of rising, find the first morning cigarette the hardest to give up, smoke most frequently during the morning, find it difficult to refrain from smoking in places where it's forbidden, or smoke even when ill and confined to bed during the day.

## ☑ PATIENT TEACHING
• Instruct patient to chew gum slowly and intermittently (chew several times; then place between cheek and gum) for about 30 minutes to promote slow and even buccal absorption of nicotine. Fast chewing tends to produce more adverse reactions.
• Be sure that patient reads and understands the instruction sheet included in the package.
• Emphasize the importance of withdrawing the gum gradually.
• Tell patient that successful abstainers will begin to gradually withdraw gum usage after 3 months. Use of the gum for longer than 6 months is not recommended. For gradual withdrawal, cut gum in halves or quarters and mix with other sugarless gum.
• Warn patient that smoking while taking drug will reduce the drug's effectiveness.

## nicotine transdermal system
Habitrol, Nicoderm, Nicotrol, ProStep
*Pregnancy Risk Category: D*

### HOW SUPPLIED
*Transdermal system:* designed to release nicotine at a fixed rate
Habitrol — 21 mg/day, 14 mg/day, 7 mg/day
Nicoderm — 21 mg/day, 14 mg/day, 7 mg/day
ProStep — 22 mg/day, 11 mg/day

### ACTION
Provides nicotine, which stimulates nicotinic acetylcholine receptors in the CNS, neuromuscular junction, autonomic ganglia, and adrenal medulla.

### ONSET, PEAK, DURATION
Users of Habitrol exhibit peak serum levels 5 to 6 hours after application; Nicoderm, 4 hours after application; Nicotrol, 3 to 6 hours; ProStep, 9 hours after application. Duration varies.

### INDICATIONS & DOSAGE
*Relief of nicotine withdrawal symptoms in patients undergoing smoking cessation –*
**Adults:** initially, one transdermal system, delivering the largest available dosage of nicotine in its dosage series, applied once daily to a nonhairy part of body. For Habitrol, Nicoderm, and ProStep, patch should be kept on for 24 hours, then removed and a new system applied to an alternate skin site. For Nicotrol, the patch should be applied upon awakening and removed at bedtime. After 4 to 12 weeks (depending on the brand used), dosage tapered to next largest available dosage of nicotine in its dosage series, followed in 2 to 4 weeks by lowest nicotine dosage system in series being

used. Drug is then stopped in 2 to 4 weeks.

## ADVERSE REACTIONS

**CNS:** somnolence, dizziness, *headache, insomnia,* paresthesia, abnormal dreams, nervousness.
**EENT:** pharyngitis, sinusitis.
**GI:** abdominal pain, constipation, dyspepsia, nausea, diarrhea, vomiting, dry mouth.
**GU:** dysmenorrhea.
**Respiratory:** increased cough, pharyngitis, sinusitis.
**Skin:** *local or systemic erythema, pruritus, burning at application site,* cutaneous hypersensitivity, rash.
**Other:** back pain, myalgia, diaphoresis, hypertension.

## INTERACTIONS

*Acetaminophen, caffeine, imipramine, oxazepam, pentazocine, propranolol, theophylline:* may decrease induction of hepatic enzymes that help metabolize certain drugs. Dosage reductions may be necessary.
*Adrenergic agonists, such as isoproterenol or phenylephrine:* may decrease circulating catecholamines. Dosage increases may be necessary.
*Adrenergic antagonists, such as prazosin or labetalol:* may decrease circulating catecholamines. Dosage reductions may be necessary.
*Insulin:* may increase amount of S.C. insulin absorbed. Dosage reduction of insulin may be necessary.

## CONTRAINDICATIONS

Contraindicated in patients with hypersensitivity to nicotine or any component of the transdermal system. Also contraindicated in nonsmokers; in patients with recent MI, life-threatening arrhythmias, and severe or worsening angina pectoris.

## NURSING CONSIDERATIONS

● Use cautiously in patients with hyperthyroidism, pheochromocytoma, hypertension, insulin-dependent diabetes, or peptic ulcer disease.
● Health care workers' exposure to nicotine within transdermal systems probably is minimal; however, avoid unnecessary contact with the system. Wash hands with water alone because soap may enhance absorption.

## ☑ PATIENT TEACHING

● Inform patient that use of the transdermal system for more than 3 months is not recommended. Warn patient that chronic nicotine consumption by any route can be dangerous and habit-forming.
● Patient should also be warned not to smoke. If he continues to smoke while using the system, he may experience serious adverse effects because peak serum nicotine levels will be substantially higher than those achieved by smoking alone.
● Be sure that patient reads and understands the information that's dispensed with the drug.
● Advise patient to apply the patch promptly because the nicotine can evaporate from the transdermal system once it's removed from its protective packaging. Patch should not be altered in any way (folded or cut) before application. Do not store at temperatures above 86° F (30° C).
● Teach patient proper disposal of the transdermal system. After removal, fold the patch in half, bringing the adhesive sides together. If it comes in a protective pouch, place the used patch in the pouch that contained the system. Careful disposal is necessary to prevent accidental poisoning of children or pets.
● Tell patient who experiences persistent or severe local skin reactions or generalized rash to immediately discontinue use of the patch and contact the doctor.
● Inform patient that patients who cannot stop cigarette smoking during the initial 4 weeks of therapy probably

---

Reactions may be *common,* uncommon, *life-threatening,* or COMMON AND LIFE-THREATENING.

will not benefit from the continued use of the drug. Such patients may benefit from counseling to identify factors that led to treatment failure. Encourage patient to minimize or eliminate factors contributing to treatment failure and to try again, possibly after some time has passed.

---

## sumatriptan succinate
Imitrex

*Pregnancy Risk Category: C*

### HOW SUPPLIED
*Tablets:* 25 mg, 50 mg, 100 mg (base)†
*Injection:* 6 mg/0.5 ml (12 mg/ml) in 0.5-ml prefilled syringes and vials

### ACTION
Unknown. Thought to selectively activate vascular serotonin (5-hydroxytryptamine, 5-HT) receptors. Stimulation of the specific receptor subtype 5-HT$_1$, present on cranial arteries and the dura mater, causes vasoconstriction of cerebral vessels but has minimal effects on systemic vessels, tissue perfusion, and blood pressure.

### ONSET, PEAK, DURATION
Onset occurs within 10 to 20 minutes after S.C. injection, or 30 minutes after oral administration. Serum levels peak about 12 minutes after S.C. injection, within 1½ hours after oral administration. Peak effect occurs within 1 to 2 hours after S.C. administration, within 2 to 4 hours after oral administration. Duration unknown.

### INDICATIONS & DOSAGE
*Acute migraine attacks (with or without aura) –*
**Adults:** 6 mg S.C. Maximum recommended dosage is two 6-mg injections daily, with at least 1 hour allowed between injections. Alternatively, an initial dose of 25 to 100 mg P.O. and a second dose of up to 100 mg in 2

hours, if needed. Additional doses may be given q 2 hours, p.r.n., up to a daily maximum dosage of 300 mg.

### ADVERSE REACTIONS
**CNS:** *dizziness, vertigo,* drowsiness, headache, anxiety, malaise, fatigue.
**CV:** *atrial fibrillation, ventricular fibrillation, ventricular tachycardia, MI, ECG changes such as ischemic ST-segment elevation* (rare).
**EENT:** discomfort of throat, nasal cavity or sinus, mouth, jaw, or tongue; altered vision.
**GI:** abdominal discomfort, dysphagia.
**Skin:** flushing.
**Other:** *tingling; warm or hot sensation; burning sensation; heaviness, pressure or tightness;* feeling of strangeness; tight feeling in head; cold sensation; pressure or tightness in chest; myalgia; muscle cramps; diaphoresis; neck pain; *injection site reaction.*

### INTERACTIONS
*Ergot and ergot derivatives:* prolonged vasospastic effects. Don't use these drugs and sumatriptan within the same 24-hour period.
*MAO inhibitors:* increases sumatriptan's effects. Avoid concomitant use or within 2 weeks of discontinuing MAO inhibitor therapy.

### CONTRAINDICATIONS
Contraindicated in patients with hypersensitivity to the drug; in patients with uncontrolled hypertension or ischemic heart disease (such as angina pectoris, Prinzmetal's angina, history of MI, or documented silent ischemia); in patients with hemiplegic or basilar migraine; in patients taking ergotamine; and within 14 days of MAO therapy.

### NURSING CONSIDERATIONS
• Use cautiously in patients who are or intend to become pregnant.

---

*Liquid form contains alcohol. **May contain tartrazine. †Canada only. ‡Australia only. ◇OTC.

- Also use cautiously in patients who may have unrecognized coronary artery disease (CAD), such as postmenopausal women; male patients over age 40; or patients with risk factors such as hypertension, hypercholesterolemia, obesity, diabetes, smoking, or family history of CAD.
- When giving the drug to patients at risk for unrecognized CAD, consider administering the first dose in the doctor's office. Serious adverse cardiac effects can follow S.C. administration of this drug, but such events are rare.
- After S.C. injection, most patients experience relief within 1 to 2 hours.
- Redness or pain at the injection site should subside within 1 hour after the injection.

☑ **PATIENT TEACHING**
- Tell the patient that the drug is intended only to treat migraine attacks, not to prevent or reduce their occurrence.
- Tell the patient who is pregnant or intends to become pregnant not to use this drug. Advise her to discuss with the doctor the risks and benefits of using the drug during pregnancy.
- Tell the patient that the drug may be given any time during a migraine attack, but should be given as soon as symptoms appear.
- Review information about the drug's injectable form, which is available in a spring-loaded injector system that facilitates self-administration. Be sure the patient understands how to load the injector, administer the injection, and dispose of the used syringes.
- **Alert:** Tell the patient to notify the doctor immediately of persistent or severe chest pain. Tell the patient to stop using the drug and call the doctor if he experiences pain or tightness in the throat, wheezing, heart throbbing, rash, lumps, hives, or swollen eyelids, face, or lips.

## tacrine hydrochloride
Cognex

*Pregnancy Risk Category: C*

### HOW SUPPLIED
*Capsules:* 10 mg, 20 mg, 30 mg, 40 mg

### ACTION
Reversibly inhibits the enzyme cholinesterase in the CNS, allowing the buildup of acetylcholine and thereby temporarily improving cognitive function in patients with Alzheimer's disease.

### ONSET, PEAK, DURATION
Onset and duration unknown. Serum levels peak in ½ to 3 hours.

### INDICATIONS & DOSAGE
*Mild to moderate dementia of the Alzheimer's type –*
**Adults:** initially, 10 mg P.O. q.i.d. After 6 weeks and if the patient tolerates treatment and there are no transaminase elevations, dosage increased to 20 mg q.i.d. After 6 weeks, dosage titrated upward to 30 mg q.i.d. If still tolerated, dosage increased to 40 mg q.i.d. after another 6 weeks.

### ADVERSE REACTIONS
**CNS:** agitation, ataxia, insomnia, abnormal thinking, somnolence, depression, anxiety, *headache,* fatigue, *dizziness,* confusion.
**GI:** *nausea, vomiting, diarrhea,* dyspepsia, loose stools, changes in stool color, anorexia, abdominal pian, flatulence, constipation.
**Respiratory:** rhinitis, upper respiratory tract infection, cough.
**Skin:** rash, jaundice, facial flushing.
**Other:** *elevations in transaminases* (especially *ALT*), myalgia, chest pain, weight loss.

---

Reactions may be *common,* uncommon, **life-threatening,** or **COMMON AND LIFE-THREATENING.**

## INTERACTIONS
*Anticholinergics:* may decrease the effectiveness of anticholinergics. Monitor patient closely.

*Cholinesterase inhibitors, cholinergics (such as bethanechol):* additive effects. Monitor for toxicity.

*Succinylcholine:* enhanced neuromuscular blockade and prolonged duration of action. Monitor patient closely.

*Theophylline:* increased serum theophylline levels and prolonged theophylline half-life. Carefully monitor theophylline plasma levels, and adjust dosage, as ordered.

*Food:* decreased absorption of tacrine if taken concomitantly. Give drug 1 hour before meals.

## CONTRAINDICATIONS
Contraindicated in patients hypersensitive to the drug or acridine derivatives. Also contraindicated in patients who have previously developed tacrine-related jaundice, which has been confirmed with an elevated total bilirubin level of more than 3 mg/dl.

## NURSING CONSIDERATIONS
• Use cautiously in patients with sick sinus syndrome or bradycardia; in patients at risk for peptic ulceration (including patients taking NSAIDs or those with history of peptic ulcer); and in patients with history of hepatic disease. Also use cautiously in patients with renal disease, asthma, prostatic hyperplasia, or other urinary outflow impairment.

• Know that if the drug is discontinued for 4 weeks or more, the full dosage titration and monitoring schedule must be restarted.

• Monitor serum ALT levels weekly during the first 18 weeks of therapy as ordered. If ALT is modestly elevated after the first 18 weeks of monitoring (twice the upper limit of normal range), continue weekly monitoring. If no problems are detected, frequency of serum determinations is decreased to once every 3 months. On each occasion that dosage is increased, resume weekly monitoring for at least 6 weeks as ordered.

## ☑ PATIENT TEACHING
• Patient and caregivers should understand that this drug does not alter the underlying degenerative disease, but can alleviate symptoms. Effect of therapy depends upon drug administration at regular intervals.

• Remind caregivers that dosage titration is an integral part of the safe use of this drug. Abrupt discontinuation or a large reduction in daily dosage (80 mg or more per day) may precipitate behavioral disturbances and a decline in cognitive function.

• Tell caregiver to give the patient the drug between meals whenever possible. If GI upset becomes a problem, the drug may be taken with meals, although doing so may reduce plasma levels by 30% to 40%.

• Advise the patient and caregivers to immediately report any significant adverse effects or changes in status.

# 37

# Cholinergics (parasympathomimetics)

ambenonium chloride
bethanechol chloride
edrophonium chloride
neostigmine bromide
neostigmine methylsulfate
physostigmine salicylate
pyridostigmine bromide

**COMBINATION PRODUCTS**
None.

## ambenonium chloride
Mytelase Caplets

*Pregnancy Risk Category: NR*

**HOW SUPPLIED**
*Tablets:* 10 mg

**ACTION**
Inhibits the destruction of acetylcholine released from the parasympathetic and somatic efferent nerves. Acetylcholine accumulates, promoting increased stimulation of the receptors.

**ONSET, PEAK, DURATION**
Onset ranges from 20 to 30 minutes. Peak unknown. Effects persist for 4 to 8 hours.

**INDICATIONS & DOSAGE**
*Symptomatic treatment of myasthenia gravis in patients who cannot take neostigmine bromide or pyridostigmine bromide –*
**Adults:** dosage individualized for each patient, but usually ranges from 5 to 25 mg P.O. t.i.d. or q.i.d. Starting dose usually is 5 mg P.O. t.i.d. or q.i.d. Increased and adjusted at 1- to 2-day intervals to avoid drug accumulation and overdosage. Usual dosage range is 5 to 25 mg P.O. t.i.d. or q.i.d., but some patients may require as much as 75 mg b.i.d. to q.i.d.

**ADVERSE REACTIONS**
**CNS:** headache, dizziness, muscle weakness, *seizures,* mental confusion, drowsiness.
**CV:** bradycardia, hypotension, tachycardia, *cardiac arrest,* syncope, AV block.
**EENT:** miosis, lacrimation, diplopia.
**GI:** *nausea, vomiting, diarrhea, abdominal cramps,* increased salivation, dysphagia.
**GU:** urinary frequency, incontinence.
**Respiratory:** bronchospasm, *bronchoconstriction,* increased bronchial secretions, *respiratory paralysis,* dyspnea.
**Skin:** rash, flushing, urticaria.
**Other:** muscle cramps, diaphoresis.

**INTERACTIONS**
*Aminoglycosides, anesthetics, atropine, corticosteroids, magnesium, procainamide, quinidine:* prolonged or enhanced muscle weakness. Monitor closely.
*Mecamylamine, other ganglionic blockers:* increased toxicity. Avoid concomitant use.

**CONTRAINDICATIONS**
Contraindicated in patients with mechanical obstruction of intestine or urinary tract and in patients receiving ganglionic blockers.

**NURSING CONSIDERATIONS**
• Use with extreme caution in patients with bronchial asthma. Use cautiously in patients with seizure disorders, bradycardia, recent coronary occlusion, vagotonia, peptic ulcer, hyperthyroidism, arrhythmias, postoperative atelectasis, and pneumonia.
• Discontinue all other cholinergics,

---

Reactions may be *common,* uncommon, *life-threatening,* or COMMON AND LIFE-THREATENING.

as ordered, before administering this drug.

• Know that large doses should be avoided in patients with decreased GI motility or megacolon.

• Administer each dose exactly as ordered, on time. Amount and frequency of dose should vary with the patient's activity level. The doctor probably will order larger doses when the patient is fatigued, for example, in the afternoon and at mealtime.

• Give with milk or food to produce fewer adverse muscarinic reactions.

• Monitor vital signs frequently, especially respirations, and document. Always have atropine injection available and be prepared to give 0.5 to 1 mg S.C. or by slow I.V. push as ordered. Provide respiratory support as needed.

• *Alert:* Watch the patient very closely for adverse reactions, particularly if total dosage is greater than 200 mg daily. When adverse reactions indicate drug toxicity, such as weakness that occurs within 30 to 60 minutes of drug administration, notify the doctor immediately.

• If muscle weakness is severe, know that the doctor must determine if it is caused by drug toxicity or exacerbation of myasthenia gravis. A test dose of edrophonium I.V. will aggravate drug-induced weakness but will temporarily relieve weakness resulting from the disease.

• Seek approval, when indicated, for hospitalized patients to have bedside supply of tablets. Patients with longstanding disease often insist on taking pills themselves.

• Record the patient's variations in muscle strength.

• Be aware that patients may develop resistance to drug.

### ☑ PATIENT TEACHING
• Instruct the patient to take drug with milk or food.
• Show the patient how to monitor

variations in his muscle strength and to keep a record of this information.

• When given for myasthenia gravis, explain that this drug will relieve symptoms of ptosis, double vision, difficulty in chewing and swallowing, and trunk and limb weakness. Stress the importance of taking this drug exactly as ordered.

• Explain to the patient and his family that ambenonium chloride is a long-term drug. Teach them about the disease and the drug's effect on symptoms.

• Advise the patient to wear medical identification bracelet indicating myasthenia gravis.

---

## bethanechol chloride
Duvoid, Myotonachol, Urabeth, Urecholine, Urocarb Liquid‡, Urocarb Tablets‡

*Pregnancy Risk Category: C*

### HOW SUPPLIED
*Tablets:* 5 mg, 10 mg, 25 mg, 50 mg
*Injection:* 5 mg/ml

### ACTION
Directly stimulates cholinergic receptors, mimicking the action of acetylcholine.

### ONSET, PEAK, DURATION
Onset occurs within 5 to 15 minutes of S.C. dose, within 30 to 90 minutes of oral dose. Serum levels peak 15 to 30 minutes after S.C. administration, about 1 hour after oral dose. Effects persist for about 2 hours after S.C. administration, up to 6 hours after oral administration, depending on dose.

### INDICATIONS & DOSAGE
*Acute postoperative and postpartum nonobstructive (functional) urine retention, neurogenic atony of urinary bladder with urine retention—*
**Adults:** 10 to 50 mg P.O. t.i.d. to

q.i.d. Or, 2.5 to 5 mg S.C. Never give I.M. or I.V. When used for urine retention, some patients may require 50 to 100 mg P.O. per dose. Use such doses with extreme caution.

Test dose is 2.5 mg S.C., repeated at 15- to 30-minute intervals to total of four doses to determine the minimal effective dose; then minimal effective dose used q 6 to 8 hours. All doses must be adjusted individually.

## ADVERSE REACTIONS
**CNS:** headache, malaise.
**CV:** hypotension, reflex tachycardia.
**EENT:** lacrimation, miosis.
**GI:** *abdominal cramps, diarrhea,* excessive salivation, nausea, belching, borborygmus.
**GU:** urinary urgency.
**Respiratory:** *bronchoconstriction,* increased bronchial secretions.
**Skin:** flushing, diaphoresis.

## INTERACTIONS
*Atropine, anticholinergic agents, procainamide, quinidine:* may reverse cholinergic effects. Observe for lack of drug effect.
*Cholinergic agonists, anticholinesterase agents:* may cause additive effects, or increase toxicity. Avoid concomitant use.
*Ganglionic blockers:* may cause hypotension. Avoid concomitant use.

## CONTRAINDICATIONS
Contraindicated for I.M. or I.V. use and in patients with hypersensitivity to drug or any of its components; in patients with uncertain strength or integrity of bladder wall; when increased muscular activity of GI or urinary tract is harmful; in patients with mechanical obstructions of GI or urinary tract; in patients with hyperthyroidism, peptic ulceration, latent or active bronchial asthma, pronounced bradycardia or hypotension, vasomotor instability, cardiac or coronary artery disease, seizure disorder, Parkinson's disease, spastic GI disturbances, acute inflammatory lesions of the GI tract, peritonitis, or marked vagotonia.

## NURSING CONSIDERATIONS
● Use cautiously in pregnant patients.
● Give on empty stomach; otherwise, may cause nausea and vomiting.
● **Alert:** *Never* give I.M. or I.V.; could cause circulatory collapse, hypotension, severe abdominal cramping, bloody diarrhea, shock, or cardiac arrest.
● Monitor vital signs frequently, especially respirations. Always have atropine injection available and be prepared to give 0.5 mg S.C. or by slow I.V. push as ordered. Provide respiratory support if needed.
● Watch for toxicity, especially with S.C. administration. Edrophonium is not effective against muscle relaxation caused by bethanechol.
● Watch closely for adverse reactions that may indicate drug toxicity.
● Know that oral drug absorption is poor and variable, requiring larger oral doses. Oral and S.C. doses are not interchangeable.

## ☑ PATIENT TEACHING
● Instruct patient to take oral form on an empty stomach.
● Inform patient that drug is usually effective within 30 to 90 minutes after oral administration and 5 to 15 minutes after S.C. administration.

# edrophonium chloride
Enlon, Reversol, Tensilon

*Pregnancy Risk Category: NR*

## HOW SUPPLIED
*Injection:* 10 mg/ml in 1-ml ampules or in 10-ml or 15-ml vials

## ACTION
Inhibits the destruction of acetylcholine released from the parasympa-

thetic and somatic efferent nerves. Acetylcholine accumulates, promoting increased stimulation of the receptors.

## ONSET, PEAK, DURATION
Onset occurs within 30 to 60 seconds of I.V. administration, within 2 to 10 minutes of I.M. injection. Peak unknown. Effects persist for 5 to 10 minutes after I.V. administration, 5 to 30 minutes after I.M. injection. Duration of action is extremely short.

## INDICATIONS & DOSAGE
*As a curare antagonist (to reverse nondepolarizing neuromuscular blocking action)* –
**Adults:** 10 mg I.V. given over 30 to 45 seconds. Dose may be repeated as necessary to 40 mg maximum dosage. Larger dosages may potentiate effect of curare.
*Diagnostic aid in myasthenia gravis (Tensilon test)* –
**Adults:** 1 to 2 mg I.V. over 15 to 30 seconds, then 8 mg if no response (increase in muscular strength) occurs. Alternatively, 10 mg I.M. If cholinergic reaction occurs, 2 mg I.M. 30 minutes later is given to rule out false-negative response.
**Children over 34 kg:** 2 mg I.V. If no response within 45 seconds, 1 mg q 45 seconds to maximum of 10 mg. Alternatively, 5 mg I.M.
**Children up to 34 kg:** 1 mg I.V. If no response within 45 seconds, 1 mg q 45 seconds to maximum of 5 mg. Alternatively, 2 mg I.M.
   I.M. route may be used in children because of difficulty with I.V. route: for children under 34 kg, 2 mg I.M.; for children over 34 kg, 5 mg I.M. Expect same reactions as with I.V. test, but these appear after 2- to 10-minute delay.
**Infants:** 0.5 mg to 1 mg I.M. or S.C.
*To differentiate myasthenic crisis from cholinergic crisis* –
**Adults:** 1 mg I.V. If no response in 1

minute, dose repeated once. Increased muscular strength confirms myasthenic crisis; no increase or exaggerated weakness confirms cholinergic crisis.

## ADVERSE REACTIONS
**CNS:** *seizures,* weakness, dysarthria, dysphagia.
**CV:** hypotension, bradycardia, AV block.
**EENT:** excessive lacrimation, diplopia, miosis, conjunctival hyperemia.
**GI:** nausea, vomiting, *diarrhea, abdominal cramps,* excessive salivation.
**GU:** urinary frequency, incontinence.
**Respiratory:** *paralysis of muscles of respiration, central respiratory paralysis, bronchospasm, laryngospasm,* increased bronchial secretions.
**Other:** muscle cramps, muscle fasciculation, diaphoresis.

## INTERACTIONS
*Aminoglycosides, anesthetics:* prolonged or enhanced muscle weakness. Monitor closely.
*Corticosteroids, magnesium, procainamide, quinidine:* may antagonize cholinergic effects. Observe for lack of drug effect.
*Digitalis glycosides:* may increase the heart's sensitivity to edrophonium. Use together cautiously.

## CONTRAINDICATIONS
Contraindicated in patients with hypersensitivity to anticholinesterase agents and in those with mechanical obstruction of the intestine or urinary tract.

## NURSING CONSIDERATIONS
• Use cautiously in patients with bronchial asthma or cardiac arrhythmias.
• Stop all other cholinergics before giving this drug, as ordered.
• **I.V. use:** For easier parenteral administration, use tuberculin syringe

---

*Liquid form contains alcohol.  **May contain tartrazine.  †Canada only.  ‡Australia only.  ◇OTC.

with an I.V. needle. When giving drug to differentiate myasthenic crisis from cholinergic crisis, observe patient's muscle strength closely.

• Monitor vital signs frequently, especially respirations. Always have atropine injection available and be prepared to give 0.5 to 1 mg S.C. or by slow I.V. push as ordered. Provide respiratory support as needed.

• Watch closely for adverse reactions; they may indicate toxicity.

• Keep in mind that the drug is effective against muscle relaxation induced by decamethonium bromide and succinylcholine chloride.

• Be aware that this cholinergic has the most rapid onset but shortest duration; therefore, it is not used to treat myasthenia gravis.

☑ **PATIENT TEACHING**
• Teach patient to report adverse reactions promptly.
• Tell patient to alert nurse if discomfort occurs at I.V. site.

---

### neostigmine bromide
Prostigmin

### neostigmine methylsulfate
Prostigmin

*Pregnancy Risk Category: C*

## HOW SUPPLIED
**neostigmine bromide**
*Tablets:* 15 mg
**neostigmine methylsulfate**
*Injection:* 0.25 mg/ml, 0.5 mg/ml, 1 mg/ml

## ACTION
Inhibits the destruction of acetylcholine released from the parasympathetic and somatic efferent nerves. Acetylcholine accumulates, promoting increased stimulation of the receptors.

## ONSET, PEAK, DURATION
Onset occurs 4 to 8 minutes after I.V. administration, 20 to 30 minutes after I.M. injection, or 45 to 75 minutes after oral administration. Peak levels occur within 1 to 2 hours, with considerable individual variations. Effects persist for 2 to 4 hours.

## INDICATIONS & DOSAGE
*Treatment of myasthenia gravis –*
**Adults:** 15 to 30 mg P.O. t.i.d. (range is 15 to 375 mg daily); or 0.5 to 2 mg S.C., I.M., or I.V. q 1 to 3 hours.
**Children:** 7.5 to 15 mg P.O. t.i.d. or q.i.d.

Dosage must be highly individualized, depending on response and tolerance of adverse effects. Therapy may be required day and night.
*Diagnosis of myasthenia gravis –*
**Adults:** 0.022 mg/kg I.M. 30 minutes after 0.4 to 0.6 mg of atropine sulfate.
**Children:** 0.025 to 0.04 mg/kg. I.M. after 0.11 mg/kg atropine sulfate S.C.
*Postoperative abdominal distention and bladder atony –*
**Adults:** 0.5 to 1 mg I.M. or S.C. q 4 to 6 hours.
*Antidote for nondepolarizing neuromuscular blocking agents –*
**Adults:** 0.5 to 2.5 mg I.V. slowly. Repeat p.r.n. to a total of 5 mg. Before antidote dose, 0.6 to 1.2 mg atropine sulfate is given I.V.

*Note:* 1:1,000 solution of injectable solution contains 1 mg/ml; 1:2,000 solution contains 0.5 mg/ml.

## ADVERSE REACTIONS
**CNS:** dizziness, headache, muscle weakness, loss of consciousness, drowsiness.
**CV:** bradycardia, hypotension, tachycardia, AV block, syncope, *cardiac arrest.*
**EENT:** blurred vision, lacrimation, miosis.
**GI:** *nausea, vomiting, diarrhea, abdominal cramps,* excessive salivation, flatulence, increased peristalsis.

---

Reactions may be *common,* uncommon, *life-threatening,* or **COMMON AND LIFE-THREATENING.**

**GU:** urinary frequency.
**Respiratory:** *bronchospasm,* dyspnea, respiratory depression, *respiratory arrest,* increased secretions.
**Skin:** rash, urticaria, diaphoresis, flushing.
**Other:** *muscle cramps,* muscle fasciculations, arthralgia, hypersensitivity reactions *(anaphylaxis).*

## INTERACTIONS
*Atropine, anticholinergic agents, corticosteroids, magnesium sulfate, procainamide, aminoglycosides, quinidine:* may reverse cholinergic effects. Observe for lack of drug effect.

## CONTRAINDICATIONS
Contraindicated in patients with hypersensitivity to cholinergics or to bromide and in those with peritonitis or mechanical obstruction of the intestine or urinary tract.

## NURSING CONSIDERATIONS
• Use cautiously in patients with bronchial asthma, bradycardia, seizure disorders, recent coronary occlusion, vagotonia, hyperthyroidism, arrhythmias, and peptic ulcer.
• Stop all other cholinergics before giving this drug, as ordered.
• In myasthenia gravis, schedule doses before periods of fatigue. For example, if the patient has dysphagia, schedule dose 30 minutes before each meal.
• **I.V. use:** Give at a slow, controlled rate, not exceeding 1 mg/minute in adults and 0.5 mg/minute in children.
• Monitor vital signs frequently, especially respirations. Have atropine injection available and be prepared to give as ordered; provide respiratory support, as needed.
• Monitor and document the patient's response after each dose. Optimum dosage is difficult to judge. Observe closely for improvement in strength, vision, and ptosis 45 to 60 minutes after each dose.

• Although drug is frequently used to reverse the effects of nondepolarizing neuromuscular blockers in patients who have undergone surgery, be aware that it may actually worsen the blockade produced by succinylcholine.
• If patient's muscle weakness is severe, keep in mind that the doctor determines if it is caused by drug-induced toxicity or exacerbation of myasthenia gravis. Test dose of edrophonium I.V. will aggravate drug-induced weakness but will temporarily relieve weakness caused by disease.
• Be aware that I.M. neostigmine may be used instead of edrophonium to diagnose myasthenia gravis. May be preferable to edrophonium when limb weakness is the only symptom.
• When drug is used to prevent abdominal distention and GI distress, be aware that the doctor may order a rectal tube inserted to help passage of gas.
• Know that patients sometimes develop a resistance to neostigmine.
• If appropriate, obtain a doctor's order for a hospitalized patient to have bedside supply of tablets. Patients with long-standing disease often insist on self-administration.

## ☑ PATIENT TEACHING
• Tell the patient to take the drug with food or milk to reduce adverse GI reactions.
• When using for myasthenia gravis, explain that this drug will relieve ptosis, double vision, difficulty in chewing and swallowing, and trunk and limb weakness. Stress importance of taking drug exactly as ordered. Explain that drug may have to be taken for life.
• Show the patient how to observe and record variations in muscle strength.
• Advise the patient to wear medical identification bracelet indicating myasthenia gravis.

*Liquid form contains alcohol.   **May contain tartrazine.   †Canada only.   ‡Australia only.   ◇OTC.

# physostigmine salicylate (eserine salicylate)
Antilirium

*Pregnancy Risk Category: NR*

## HOW SUPPLIED
*Injection:* 1 mg/ml

## ACTION
Inhibits the destruction of acetylcholine released from the parasympathetic and somatic efferent nerves. Acetylcholine accumulates, promoting increased stimulation of the receptor.

## ONSET, PEAK, DURATION
Onset occurs within 3 to 5 minutes of injection. Peak levels occur within 5 minutes of I.V. injection, 20 to 30 minutes after I.M. injection. Effects persist for 30 to 60 minutes after parenteral use.

## INDICATIONS & DOSAGE
*To reverse the CNS toxicity associated with clinical or toxic dosages of drugs capable of producing anticholinergic syndrome—*
**Adults:** 0.5 to 2 mg I.M. or I.V. (1 mg/minute I.V.) repeated q 20 minutes as necessary if life-threatening signs recur (coma, seizures, arrhythmias). Additional doses of 1 to 4 mg I.M. or I.V. q 30 to 60 minutes may be given.
**Children:** reserved for life-threatening situations only. Requires dose of 0.02 mg/kg I.M. or slow I.V., repeated q 5 to 10 minutes until response occurs. Maximum dosage is 2 mg.

## ADVERSE REACTIONS
**CNS:** *seizures,* muscle weakness, *restlessness, excitability.*
**CV:** bradycardia, hypotension.
**EENT:** miosis.
**GI:** nausea, vomiting, epigastric pain, *diarrhea, excessive salivation.*
**GU:** urinary urgency.
**Respiratory:** *bronchospasm,* bronchial constriction, dyspnea.
**Other:** diaphoresis.

## INTERACTIONS
*Atropine, anticholinergic agents, procainamide, quinidine:* may reverse cholinergic effects. Observe for lack of drug effect.
*Ganglionic blockers:* may decrease blood pressure. Avoid concomitant use.

## CONTRAINDICATIONS
Contraindicated in patients with mechanical obstruction of the intestine or urogenital tract, asthma, gangrene, diabetes, CV disease, or vagotonia and in those receiving choline esters or depolarizing neuromuscular blockers.

## NURSING CONSIDERATIONS
• Use cautiously in pregnant patients.
• **I.V. use:** Give I.V. at controlled rate; use direct injection at no more than 1 mg/minute.
• Use only clear solution. Darkening may indicate loss of potency.
• Monitor vital signs frequently, especially respirations. Position the patient to ease breathing. Have atropine injection available and be prepared to give 0.5 mg S.C. or by slow I.V. push as ordered. Provide respiratory support as needed. Best administered in presence of a doctor.
• Watch closely for adverse reactions, particularly CNS disturbances. Raise side rails if the patient becomes restless or hallucinates. Adverse reactions may indicate drug toxicity.
• Know that effectiveness is often immediate and dramatic but may be transient and may require repeated doses.

## ☑ PATIENT TEACHING
- Inform patient of need for drug, explain its use and adverse reactions, and answer any questions or concerns.
- Tell patient to report adverse reactions promptly.
- Instruct patient to alert nurse if discomfort occurs at I.V. site.

---

## pyridostigmine bromide
Mestinon*, Mestinon†, Mestinon Timespans, Regonol

*Pregnancy Risk Category: NR*

### HOW SUPPLIED
*Tablets:* 60 mg
*Tablets (extended-release):* 180 mg
*Syrup:* 60 mg/5 ml
*Injection:* 5 mg/ml in 2-ml ampules or 5-ml vials

### ACTION
Inhibits the destruction of acetylcholine released from the parasympathetic and somatic efferent nerves. Acetylcholine accumulates, promoting increased stimulation of the receptors.

### ONSET, PEAK, DURATION
Onset occurs within 2 to 5 minutes of I.V. injection, 15 minutes after I.M. injection, 30 to 45 minutes after oral ingestion of regular-release tablets or syrup, 30 to 60 minutes after ingestion of extended-release tablets. Levels peak within 1 to 2 hours of oral administration. Effects persist for 2 to 4 hours after parenteral use, 3 to 6 hours after regular-release tablets or syrup, 6 to 12 hours after extended-release tablets.

### INDICATIONS & DOSAGE
*Antidote for nondepolarizing neuromuscular blockers –*
**Adults:** 10 to 20 mg I.V. preceded by atropine sulfate 0.6 to 1.2 mg I.V.
*Myasthenia gravis –*
**Adults:** 60 to 120 mg P.O. q 3 or 4 hours. Usual dosage is 600 mg daily but higher dosage may be needed (up to 1,500 mg daily). For I.M. or I.V. use, ⅓ of oral dosage is given. Dosage must be adjusted for each patient, depending on response and tolerance. Alternatively, 180 to 540 mg extended-release tablets (1 to 3 tablets) P.O. b.i.d., with at least 6 hours between doses.
**Children:** 7 mg/kg or 200 mg/m² daily in five or six divided doses.
*Supportive treatment of neonates born to myasthenic mothers –*
**Neonates:** 0.05 to 0.15 mg/kg I.M. q 4 to 6 hours. Dosage decreased daily until drug can be withdrawn.

### ADVERSE REACTIONS
**CNS:** headache (with high doses), weakness.
**CV:** bradycardia, hypotension.
**EENT:** miosis.
**GI:** abdominal cramps, nausea, vomiting, diarrhea, excessive salivation, increased peristalsis.
**Respiratory:** *bronchospasm, bronchoconstriction,* increased bronchial secretions.
**Skin:** rash, diaphoresis.
**Other:** muscle cramps, muscle fasciculations, thrombophlebitis.

### INTERACTIONS
*Aminoglycosides, anesthetics:* may decrease response to pyridostigmine. Use together cautiously.
*Atropine, anticholinergic agents, corticosteroids, magnesium, procainamide, quinidine:* may antagonize cholinergic effects. Observe for lack of drug effect.
*Ganglionic blockers:* increased risk of hypotension. Monitor closely.

### CONTRAINDICATIONS
Contraindicated in patients with hypersensitivity to anticholinesterase agents and in those with mechanical obstruction of the intestine or urinary tract.

---

*Liquid form contains alcohol. **May contain tartrazine. †Canada only. ‡Australia only. ◇OTC.

## NURSING CONSIDERATIONS

- Use cautiously in patients with bronchial asthma, bradycardia, and arrhythmias.
- Stop all other cholinergics before giving this drug, as ordered.
- **I.V. use:** Administer I.V. injection no faster than 1 mg/minute. With too-rapid I.V. infusion, bradycardia and seizures may result. Monitor vital signs frequently, especially respirations. Position patient to ease breathing. Have atropine injection available and be prepared to give as ordered; provide respiratory support as needed.
- Don't crush the extended-release (Timespans) tablets.
- When using sweet syrup for patients who have difficulty swallowing, give over ice chips if the patient can't tolerate flavor.
- Monitor and document patient's response after each dose. Optimum dosage is difficult to judge.
- If patient's muscle weakness is severe, keep in mind that the doctor determines if it is caused by drug-induced toxicity or exacerbation of myasthenia gravis. Test dose of edrophonium I.V. will aggravate drug-induced weakness, but will temporarily relieve weakness caused by disease.
- **Alert:** In the United States, be aware that Regonol contains benzyl ethanol preservative that may cause toxicity in neonates if administered in high doses. The Canadian formulation of this drug does not contain benzyl ethanol.
- If appropriate, obtain a doctor's order for a hospitalized patient to have bedside supply of tablets. Patients with long-standing disease often insist on self-administration.

## ☑ PATIENT TEACHING

- When using for myasthenia gravis, stress importance of taking drug exactly as ordered, on time, in evenly spaced doses. If the doctor has ordered extended-release tablets, explain that patients must take tablets at the same time each day, at least 6 hours apart. Explain that patients may have to take drug for life.
- Advise patient to wear medical identification indicating he has myasthenia gravis.

---

# 38

# Anticholinergics

**atropine sulfate**
(See Chapter 21, ANTIARRHYTHMICS.)
**belladonna leaf**
**clidinium bromide**
**dicyclomine hydrochloride**
**glycopyrrolate**
**hyoscyamine**
**hyoscyamine sulfate**
**mepenzolate bromide**
**propantheline bromide**
**scopolamine**
**scopolamine butylbromide**
**scopolamine hydrobromide**

## COMBINATION PRODUCTS

BARBIDONNA ELIXIR*: atropine sulfate 0.034 mg/5 ml, phenobarbital 21.6 mg/5 ml, hyoscyamine hydrobromide or sulfate 0.174 mg/5 ml, scopolamine hydrobromide 0.01 mg/5 ml, and ethanol 15%.
BARBIDONNA NO. 2 TABLETS: atropine sulfate 0.025 mg, scopolamine hydrobromide 0.0074 mg, hyoscyamine hydrobromide or sulfate 0.1286 mg, and phenobarbital 32 mg.
BARBIDONNA TABLETS: atropine sulfate 0.025 mg, scopolamine hydrobromide 0.0074 mg, hyoscyamine hydrobromide or sulfate 0.1286 mg, and phenobarbital 16 mg.
CHARDONNA-2: belladonna extract 15 mg and phenobarbital 15 mg.
DONNATAL ELIXIR*: atropine sulfate 0.0194 mg/5 ml, scopolamine hydrobromide 0.0065 mg/5 ml, ethanol 23%, hyoscyamine hydrobromide or sulfate 0.1037 mg/5 ml, and phenobarbital 16 mg/5 ml.
DONNATAL EXTENTABS: atropine sulfate 0.0582 mg, scopolamine hydrobromide 0.0195 mg, hyoscyamine sulfate 0.3111 mg, and phenobarbital 48.6 mg.
DONNATAL NO. 2 TABLETS: atropine sulfate 0.0194 mg, scopolamine hydrobromide 0.0065 mg, hyoscyamine hydrobromide or sulfate 0.1037 mg, and phenobarbital 32.4 mg.
DONNATAL TABLETS AND CAPSULES: atropine sulfate 0.0194 mg, scopolamine hydrobromide 0.0065 mg, hyoscyamine hydrobromide or sulfate 0.1037 mg, and phenobarbital 16 mg.
KINESED TABLETS: atropine sulfate 0.02 mg, scopolamine hydrobromide 0.007 mg, hyoscyamine hydrobromide or sulfate 0.1 mg, and phenobarbital 16 mg.
LIBRAX CAPSULES: clidinium bromide 2.5 mg and chlordiazepoxide hydrochloride 5 mg.

---

# belladonna leaf

(used to prepare extract and tincture)
Belladonna Tincture USP*

*Pregnancy Risk Category: NR*

## HOW SUPPLIED
*Oral solution:* 27 to 33 mg belladonna alkaloids/100 ml in 67% alcohol solution

## ACTION
Blocks acetylcholine, which decreases GI motility and inhibits gastric acid secretion.

## ONSET, PEAK, DURATION
Unknown.

## INDICATIONS & DOSAGE
*Adjunctive therapy for peptic ulceration, irritable bowel syndrome, functional GI disorders, and neurogenic bowel disturbances —*
**Adults:** 0.6 to 1 ml P.O. t.i.d. or q.i.d.
**Children:** 0.1 ml/kg or 2.5 ml/m²

tincture P.O. t.i.d. or q.i.d. Total dosage should not exceed 3.5 ml/day.

## ADVERSE REACTIONS
**CNS:** headache, insomnia, drowsiness, dizziness, *confusion or excitement* (in elderly patients), nervousness, weakness.
**CV:** *palpitations,* tachycardia.
**EENT:** *blurred vision,* mydriasis, increased intraocular pressure, cycloplegia, photophobia.
**GI:** *dry mouth,* dysphagia, heartburn, loss of taste, *constipation,* nausea, vomiting.
**GU:** *urinary hesitancy, urine retention,* impotence.
**Skin:** urticaria, decreased sweating or possible anhidrosis, other dermal manifestations.
**Other:** fever, allergic reactions.
*Note:* Overdose may cause curare-like effects, such as respiratory paralysis.

## INTERACTIONS
*Amantadine, antihistamines, antiparkinsonian agents, disopyramide, glutethimide, meperidine, phenothiazines, procainamide, quinidine, tricyclic antidepressants:* additive adverse effects. Avoid concomitant use.
*Antacids:* decreased absorption of oral anticholinergics. Separate administration times by 2 to 3 hours.
*Ketoconazole:* anticholinergics may interfere with ketoconazole absorption. Avoid concomitant use.
*Methotrimeprazine:* anticholinergics may enhance risk of extrapyramidal reactions. Avoid concomitant use.

## CONTRAINDICATIONS
Contraindicated in patients with angle-closure glaucoma, obstructive uropathy, obstructive disease of the GI tract, severe ulcerative colitis, myasthenia gravis, hypersensitivity to anticholinergics, paralytic ileus, intestinal atony, unstable cardiovascular status in acute hemorrhage, or toxic megacolon.

## NURSING CONSIDERATIONS
● Use cautiously in patients with autonomic neuropathy, hyperthyroidism, coronary artery disease, arrhythmias, CHF, hypertension, hiatal hernia associated with reflux esophagitis, GI infections, hepatic or renal disease, partial obstructive uropathy, and ulcerative colitis and in patients over 40 years because of increased incidence of glaucoma. Also use cautiously in patients in hot or humid environment. Drug-induced heatstroke can develop.
● Give 30 minutes to 1 hour before meals and h.s. Bedtime dose can be larger; give at least 2 hours after last meal of the day.
● Administer smaller doses to elderly patients.
● Monitor the patient's vital signs and urine output carefully.

## ☑ PATIENT TEACHING
● Instruct the patient when to take drug.
● Advise the patient to avoid driving and other hazardous activities if he is drowsy, dizzy, or has blurred vision; to drink plenty of fluids to help prevent constipation; and to report any rash or other skin eruption.

---

# clidinium bromide
Quarzan
*Pregnancy Risk Category: NR*

## HOW SUPPLIED
*Capsules:* 2.5 mg, 5 mg

## ACTION
Blocks acetylcholine, which decreases GI motility and inhibits gastric acid secretion.

---

## ONSET, PEAK, DURATION
Onset occurs within 1 hour of administration. Peak unknown. Effects persist up to 3 hours.

## INDICATIONS & DOSAGE
*Adjunctive therapy for peptic ulcerations –*
**Adults:** 2.5 to 5 mg P.O. t.i.d. or q.i.d. before meals and h.s.
**Elderly or debilitated patients:** 2.5 mg P.O. t.i.d.

## ADVERSE REACTIONS
**CNS:** headache, insomnia, drowsiness, dizziness, *confusion or excitement* (in elderly patients), nervousness, weakness.
**CV:** *palpitations,* tachycardia.
**EENT:** *blurred vision,* mydriasis, increased intraocular pressure, cycloplegia, photophobia.
**GI:** *dry mouth,* dysphagia, heartburn, loss of taste, nausea, vomiting, *paralytic ileus, constipation.*
**GU:** *urinary hesitancy, urine retention,* impotence.
**Skin:** urticaria, decreased sweating or possible anhidrosis, other dermal manifestations.
**Other:** fever, allergic reactions.
*Note:* Overdose may cause curare-like effects, such as respiratory paralysis.

## INTERACTIONS
*Amantadine, antihistamines, antiparkinsonian agents, disopyramide, glutethimide, meperidine, phenothiazines, procainamide, quinidine, tricyclic antidepressants:* additive adverse effects. Avoid concomitant use.
*Antacids:* decreased absorption of oral anticholinergics. Separate administration times by 2 to 3 hours.
*Ketoconazole:* anticholinergics may interfere with ketoconazole absorption. Avoid concomitant use.
*Methotrimeprazine:* anticholinergics may enhance risk of extrapyramidal reactions. Avoid concomitant use.

## CONTRAINDICATIONS
Contraindicated in patients with angle-closure glaucoma, obstructive uropathy, obstructive disease of the GI tract, severe ulcerative colitis, myasthenia gravis, hypersensitivity to anticholinergics, paralytic ileus, intestinal atony, unstable cardiovascular status in acute hemorrhage, or toxic megacolon.

## NURSING CONSIDERATIONS
• Use cautiously in patients with autonomic neuropathy, hyperthyroidism, coronary artery disease, arrhythmias, CHF, hypertension, hiatal hernia associated with reflux esophagitis, GI infections, hepatic or renal disease, partial obstructive uropathy, and ulcerative colitis and in patients over 40 years because of increased incidence of glaucoma. Also use cautiously in patients in hot or humid environment. Drug-induced heatstroke may develop.
• Give 30 minutes to 1 hour before meals and h.s. Bedtime dose can be larger; give at least 2 hours after last meal of the day.
• Monitor the patient's vital signs and urine output carefully.
• Assess the patient for dysphagia, which may cause aspiration.
• Keep in mind that dosage should be individualized according to severity of symptoms and occurrence of adverse reactions.

## ☑ PATIENT TEACHING
• Instruct the patient when to take drug.
• Advise the patient to avoid driving and other hazardous activities if he is drowsy, dizzy, or has blurred vision; to drink plenty of fluids to help prevent constipation; and to report any rash or other skin eruption.

---

# dicyclomine hydrochloride
Antispas, A-Spas, Bemote, Bentyl, Bentylol†, Byclomine, Dibent, Dilomine, Di-Spaz, Formulex†, Lomine†, Merbentyl‡, Neoquess, Or-Tyl, Spasmoban†, Spasmoject

*Pregnancy Risk Category: B*

## HOW SUPPLIED
*Tablets:* 10 mg‡, 20 mg
*Capsules:* 10 mg, 20 mg
*Syrup:* 5 mg/5 ml‡, 10 mg/5 ml
*Injection:* 10 mg/ml

## ACTION
Unknown. Appears to exert a nonspecific, nondirect spasmolytic action on smooth muscle. Also possesses local anesthetic properties that may be partly responsible for spasmolysis.

## ONSET, PEAK, DURATION
Onset and duration unknown. Peak effects occur 1 to 1½ hours after administration.

## INDICATIONS & DOSAGE
*Irritable bowel syndrome and other functional GI disorders –*
**Adults:** initially, 20 mg P.O. q.i.d., increased to 40 mg q.i.d., or 20 mg I.M. q 4 to 6 hours.
**Children 2 years and older:** 10 mg P.O. t.i.d. or q.i.d.
**Children 6 months to 2 years:** 5 to 10 mg P.O. t.i.d. to q.i.d.

## ADVERSE REACTIONS
**CNS:** *headache; dizziness;* insomnia; light-headedness; drowsiness; nervousness, confusion, excitement (in elderly patients).
**CV:** *palpitations,* tachycardia.
**EENT:** blurred vision, increased intraocular pressure, mydriasis.
**GI:** nausea, vomiting, *constipation, dry mouth,* abdominal distention, heartburn, paralytic ileus.
**GU:** *urinary hesitancy, urine retention,* impotence.

**Skin:** urticaria, decreased sweating or possible anhidrosis, other dermal manifestations, local irritation.
**Other:** fever, allergic reactions. Dicyclomine is a synthetic tertiary derivative that may have atropine-like adverse reactions.
   *Note:* Overdose may cause curare-like effects, such as respiratory paralysis.

## INTERACTIONS
*Amantadine, antihistamines, antiparkinsonian agents, disopyramide, glutethimide, meperidine, phenothiazines, procainamide, quinidine, tricyclic antidepressants:* additive adverse effects. Avoid concomitant use.
*Antacids:* decreased absorption of oral anticholinergics. Separate administration times by 2 to 3 hours.
*Ketoconazole:* anticholinergics may interfere with ketoconazole absorption. Avoid concomitant use.
*Methotrimeprazine:* anticholinergics may enhance risk of extrapyramidal reactions. Avoid concomitant use.

## CONTRAINDICATIONS
Contraindicated in patients with obstructive uropathy, obstructive disease of the GI tract, reflux esophagitis, severe ulcerative colitis, myasthenia gravis, hypersensitivity to anticholinergics, unstable cardiovascular status in acute hemorrhage, or glaucoma. Also contraindicated in breast-feeding patients and in children under 6 months.

## NURSING CONSIDERATIONS
• Use cautiously in patients with autonomic neuropathy, hyperthyroidism, coronary artery disease, arrhythmias, CHF, hypertension, hiatal hernia, hepatic or renal disease, prostatic hyperplasia, and ulcerative colitis.
• Give 30 minutes to 1 hour before meals and h.s. Bedtime dose can be larger; give at least 2 hours after last meal of the day.

---

Reactions may be *common,* uncommon, *life-threatening,* or **COMMON AND LIFE-THREATENING.**

- **Alert:** Do not give S.C. or I.V.
- Be prepared to adjust dosage according to patient's needs and response, as ordered. Doses up to 40 mg P.O. q.i.d. have been used in adults, but safety and efficacy for more than 2 weeks has not been established.
- Monitor patient's vital signs and urine output carefully.

☑ **PATIENT TEACHING**
- Instruct the patient when to take drug.
- Advise the patient to avoid driving and other hazardous activities if he is drowsy, dizzy, or has blurred vision; to drink plenty of fluids to help prevent constipation; and to report any rash or other skin eruption.

# glycopyrrolate
Robinul, Robinul Forte

*Pregnancy Risk Category: B*

## HOW SUPPLIED
*Tablets:* 1 mg, 2 mg
*Injection:* 0.2 mg/ml

## ACTION
Inhibits cholinergic (muscarinic) actions of acetylcholine on autonomic effectors innervated by postganglionic cholinergic nerves.

## ONSET, PEAK, DURATION
Onset occurs in 1 minute after I.V. administration, 15 to 30 minutes after S.C. or I.M. injection. Serum levels peak in 30 to 45 minutes after I.M. injection. Vagal blocking effects persist about 3 hours; effect on secretions, up to 7 hours.

## INDICATIONS & DOSAGE
*Blockade of adverse cholinergic effects caused by anticholinesterase agents used to reverse neuromuscular blockade –*
**Adults and children:** 0.2 mg I.V. for

each 1 mg neostigmine or 5 mg of pyridostigmine. May be given I.V. without dilution or may be added to dextrose injection and given by infusion.
*Preoperatively to diminish secretions and block cardiac vagal reflexes –*
**Adults:** 0.0044 mg/kg of body weight I.M. 30 to 60 minutes before anesthesia.
**Children 2 years and older:** 0.0044 mg/kg I.M. 30 to 60 minutes before anesthesia.
**Children under 2 years:** 0.0088 mg/kg I.M. 30 minutes before anesthesia.
*Adjunctive therapy in peptic ulcerations and other GI disorders –*
**Adults:** 1 to 2 mg P.O. t.i.d. or 0.1 mg I.M. t.i.d. or q.i.d. Dosage must be individualized. Maximum P.O. dosage is 8 mg/day.

## ADVERSE REACTIONS
**CNS:** weakness, nervousness, insomnia, drowsiness, dizziness, headache, confusion or excitement (in elderly patients).
**CV:** palpitations, tachycardia.
**EENT:** *dilated pupils, blurred vision,* photophobia, increased intraocular pressure.
**GI:** *constipation, dry mouth,* nausea, loss of taste, abdominal distension, vomiting, epigastric distress.
**GU:** *urinary hesitancy, urine retention,* impotence.
**Skin:** urticaria, decreased sweating or anhidrosis, other dermal manifestations.
**Other:** allergic reactions *(anaphylaxis),* fever.

## INTERACTIONS
*Amantadine, antihistamines, antiparkinsonian agents, disopyramide, glutethimide, meperidine, phenothiazines, procainamide, quinidine, tricyclic antidepressants:* additive adverse effects. Avoid concomitant use.
*Antacids:* decreased absorption of

oral anticholinergics. Separate administration times by 2 to 3 hours.
*Ketoconazole:* anticholinergics may interfere with ketoconazole absorption. Avoid concomitant use.
*Methotrimeprazine:* anticholinergics may enhance risk of extrapyramidal reactions. Avoid concomitant use.

**CONTRAINDICATIONS**
Contraindicated in patients with hypersensitivity to drug and in those with glaucoma, obstructive uropathy, obstructive disease of the GI tract, myasthenia gravis, paralytic ileus, intestinal atony, unstable cardiovascular status in acute hemorrhage, severe ulcerative colitis, or toxic megacolon.

**NURSING CONSIDERATIONS**
● Use cautiously in patients with autonomic neuropathy, hyperthyroidism, coronary artery disease, arrhythmias, CHF, hypertension, hiatal hernia, hepatic or renal disease, and ulcerative colitis. Also use cautiously in patients in hot or humid environment. Drug-induced heatstroke is possible.
● Administer oral form 30 minutes to 1 hour before meals.
● **I.V. use:** Administer by direct injection without dilution. Alternatively, inject into the tubing of a free-flowing I.V. solution.
● Don't mix with I.V. solution containing sodium bicarbonate or alkaline solutions with a pH higher than 6. Alkaline drugs, such as barbiturates (thiopental, methohexital, secobarbital, pentobarbital), chloramphenicol, dexamethasone, dimenhydrinate, diazepam, methylprednisolone, and pentazocine, are incompatible with glycopyrrolate.
● ***Alert:*** Check all dosages carefully; slight overdose can lead to toxicity.
● Monitor vital signs carefully. Watch closely for adverse reactions, especially in elderly or debilitated patients. Call the doctor promptly if they occur.

● Be aware that elderly patients typically receive smaller dosages.

☑ **PATIENT TEACHING**
● Instruct patient to take oral drug 30 to 60 minutes before meals.
● Warn patient to avoid activities that require alertness until drug's CNS effects are known.
● Advise patient to report signs of urinary hesitancy or urine retention.

# hyoscyamine
Cystospaz

## hyoscyamine sulfate
Anaspaz, Bellaspaz, Cystospaz, Cystospaz-M, Gastrosed, Levsin\*, Levsin Drops, Levsinex Timecaps, Levsin S/L, Neoquess

*Pregnancy Risk Category: C*

**HOW SUPPLIED**
**hyoscyamine**
*Tablets:* 0.15 mg
**hyoscyamine sulfate**
*Tablets:* 0.125 mg, 0.13 mg, 0.15 mg
*Capsules (extended-release):* 0.375 mg
*Elixir:* 125 mcg/5 ml
*Oral solution:* 0.125 mg/ml
*Injection:* 0.5 mg/ml

**ACTION**
Competitively blocks acetylcholine, which decreases GI motility and inhibits gastric acid secretion.

**ONSET, PEAK, DURATION**
Onset occurs within 2 minutes after I.V. injection, 5 to 20 minutes after oral elixir, 20 to 30 minutes after oral tablets. Serum levels peak within 15 to 30 minutes after parenteral use, 30 to 60 minutes after oral use. Effects persist for 4 to 12 hours.

---

Reactions may be *common,* uncommon, ***life-threatening,*** or **COMMON AND LIFE-THREATENING.**

## INDICATIONS & DOSAGE
*GI tract disorders caused by spasm; adjunctive therapy for peptic ulcerations –*
**Adults and children 12 years or older:** 0.125 to 0.25 mg P.O. or S.L. t.i.d. or q.i.d. before meals and h.s.; 0.375-mg extended-release form P.O. q 8 to 12 hours; or 0.25 to 0.5 mg (1 or 2 ml) I.M., I.V., or S.C. b.i.d. to q.i.d. (Oral medication substituted when symptoms are controlled.) Maximum daily dosage is 1.5 mg.
**Children 2 to 12 years:** one-half of adult dose P.O., not to exceed 0.75 mg daily.
**Children under 2 years:** one-quarter of adult dose P.O., not to exceed 0.075 mg daily.

## ADVERSE REACTIONS
**CNS:** headache, insomnia, drowsiness, dizziness, *confusion or excitement* (in elderly patients), nervousness, weakness.
**CV:** *palpitations,* tachycardia.
**EENT:** *blurred vision,* mydriasis, increased intraocular pressure, cycloplegia, photophobia.
**GI:** *dry mouth,* dysphagia, *constipation,* heartburn, loss of taste, nausea, vomiting, *paralytic ileus.*
**GU:** *urinary hesitancy, urine retention,* impotence.
**Skin:** urticaria, decreased sweating or possible anhidrosis, other dermal manifestations.
**Other:** fever, allergic reactions.
*Note:* Overdose may cause curare-like effects, such as respiratory paralysis.

## INTERACTIONS
*Amantadine, antihistamines, antiparkinsonian agents, disopyramide, glutethimide, meperidine, phenothiazines, procainamide, quinidine, tricyclic antidepressants:* additive adverse effects. Avoid concomitant use.
*Antacids:* decreased absorption of oral anticholinergics. Separate administration times by 2 to 3 hours.
*Ketoconazole:* anticholinergics may interfere with ketoconazole absorption. Avoid concomitant use.
*Methotrimeprazine:* anticholinergics may enhance risk of extrapyramidal reactions. Avoid concomitant use.

## CONTRAINDICATIONS
Contraindicated in patients with glaucoma, obstructive uropathy, obstructive disease of the GI tract, severe ulcerative colitis, myasthenia gravis, hypersensitivity to anticholinergics, paralytic ileus, intestinal atony, unstable cardiovascular status in acute hemorrhage, or toxic megacolon.

## NURSING CONSIDERATIONS
• Use cautiously in patients with autonomic neuropathy, hyperthyroidism, coronary artery disease, arrhythmias, CHF, hypertension, hiatal hernia associated with reflux esophagitis, hepatic or renal disease, and ulcerative colitis. Also use cautiously in patients in hot or humid environment. Drug-induced heatstroke can develop.
• Give 30 minutes to 1 hour before meals and h.s. Bedtime dose can be larger; give at least 2 hours after the last meal of the day.
• Monitor the patient's vital signs and urine output carefully.
• Be aware that injection contains sodium metabisulfite, which may cause allergic reaction in certain individuals.

## ☑ PATIENT TEACHING
• Instruct the patient when to take drug.
• Advise the patient to avoid driving and other hazardous activities if he is drowsy, dizzy, or has blurred vision; to drink plenty of fluids to help prevent constipation; and to report any rash or other skin eruption.

---

*Liquid form contains alcohol.  **May contain tartrazine.  †Canada only.  ‡Australia only.  ◊OTC.

# mepenzolate bromide
Cantil**

*Pregnancy Risk Category: NR*

## HOW SUPPLIED
*Tablets:* 25 mg

## ACTION
Blocks acetylcholine, which decreases GI motility and inhibits gastric acid secretion.

## ONSET, PEAK, DURATION
Unknown.

## INDICATIONS & DOSAGE
*Adjunctive therapy in treating peptic ulceration, irritable bowel syndrome, and neurogenic bowel disturbances –*
**Adults:** 25 to 50 mg P.O. t.i.d. to q.i.d. with meals and h.s. Dosage adjusted to individual patient's needs.

## ADVERSE REACTIONS
**CNS:** headache, insomnia, drowsiness, dizziness, *confusion or excitement* (in elderly patients), nervousness, weakness.
**CV:** *palpitations,* tachycardia.
**EENT:** *blurred vision,* mydriasis, increased intraocular pressure, cycloplegia, photophobia.
**GI:** *dry mouth,* dysphagia, heartburn, loss of taste, nausea, *constipation,* vomiting, *paralytic ileus.*
**GU:** *urinary hesitancy, urine retention,* impotence.
**Skin:** urticaria, decreased sweating or possible anhidrosis, other dermal manifestations.
**Other:** fever, allergic reactions.
*Note:* Overdose may cause curare-like effects, such as respiratory paralysis.

## INTERACTIONS
*Amantadine, antihistamines, antiparkinsonian agents, disopyramide, glutethimide, meperidine, phenothiazines, procainamide, quinidine, tricyclic antidepressants:* additive adverse effects. Avoid concomitant use.
*Antacids:* decreased absorption of oral anticholinergics. Separate administration times by 2 to 3 hours.
*Ketoconazole:* anticholinergics may interfere with ketoconazole absorption. Avoid concomitant use.
*Methotrimeprazine:* anticholinergics may enhance risk of extrapyramidal reactions. Avoid concomitant use.

## CONTRAINDICATIONS
Contraindicated in patients with angle-closure glaucoma, obstructive uropathy, obstructive disease of the GI tract, severe ulcerative colitis, myasthenia gravis, hypersensitivity to anticholinergics, paralytic ileus, intestinal atony, unstable cardiovascular status in acute hemorrhage, or toxic megacolon. Contains tartrazine, which may precipitate an allergic reaction in certain individuals, especially those with hypersensitivity to aspirin.

## NURSING CONSIDERATIONS
• Use cautiously in patients with autonomic neuropathy, hyperthyroidism, coronary artery disease, arrhythmias, CHF, hypertension, hiatal hernia associated with reflux esophagitis, hepatic or renal disease, and ulcerative colitis. Also use cautiously in patients in hot or humid environment. Drug-induced heatstroke can develop.
• Monitor the patient's vital signs and urine output carefully.

## ☑ PATIENT TEACHING
• Instruct the patient to take drug with meals and h.s.
• Advise the patient to avoid driving and other hazardous activities if he is drowsy, dizzy, or has blurred vision; to drink plenty of fluids to help prevent constipation; and to report any rash or other skin eruption.

---

Reactions may be *common,* uncommon, *life-threatening,* or COMMON AND LIFE-THREATENING.

## propantheline bromide
Pantheline‡, Pro-Banthine,
Propanthel†

*Pregnancy Risk Category: C*

### HOW SUPPLIED
*Tablets:* 7.5 mg, 15 mg

### ACTION
Blocks acetylcholine, which decreases GI motility and inhibits gastric acid secretion.

### ONSET, PEAK, DURATION
Onset unknown. Serum levels may peak in 2 hours. Effects persist for 6 hours.

### INDICATIONS & DOSAGE
*Adjunctive treatment of peptic ulceration—*
**Adults:** 15 mg P.O. t.i.d. before meals and 30 mg h.s.
**Elderly patients:** 7.5 mg P.O. t.i.d. before meals.

### ADVERSE REACTIONS
**CNS:** headache, insomnia, drowsiness, dizziness, *confusion or excitement in elderly patients,* nervousness, weakness.
**CV:** *palpitations,* tachycardia.
**EENT:** *blurred vision,* mydriasis, increased intraocular pressure, cycloplegia, drying of salivary secretions.
**GI:** *dry mouth,* constipation, loss of taste, nausea, vomiting, paralytic ileus, bloated feeling.
**GU:** *urinary hesitancy, urine retention,* impotence.
**Skin:** urticaria, decreased sweating or possible anhidrosis, other dermal manifestations.
**Other:** allergic reactions *(anaphylaxis).*
*Note:* Overdose may cause curarelike effects, such as respiratory paralysis.

### INTERACTIONS
*Amantadine, antihistamines, antiparkinsonian agents, disopyramide, glutethimide, meperidine, phenothiazines, procainamide, quinidine, tricyclic antidepressants:* additive adverse effects. Avoid concomitant use.
*Antacids:* decreased absorption of oral anticholinergics. Separate administration times by 2 to 3 hours.
*Digoxin:* increased serum digoxin levels. Monitor closely for digitalis toxicity.
*Ketoconazole:* anticholinergics may interfere with ketoconazole absorption. Avoid concomitant use.
*Methotrimeprazine:* anticholinergics may enhance risk of extrapyramidal reactions. Avoid concomitant use.

### CONTRAINDICATIONS
Contraindicated in patients with angle-closure glaucoma, obstructive uropathy, obstructive disease of the GI tract, severe ulcerative colitis, myasthenia gravis, hypersensitivity to anticholinergics, paralytic ileus, intestinal atony, unstable cardiovascular status in acute hemorrhage, or toxic megacolon.

### NURSING CONSIDERATIONS
● Use cautiously in patients with autonomic neuropathy, hyperthyroidism, coronary artery disease, arrhythmias, CHF, hypertension, hiatal hernia associated with reflux esophagitis, hepatic or renal disease, and ulcerative colitis. Also use cautiously in patients in hot or humid environment. Drug-induced heatstroke can develop.
● Give 30 minutes to 1 hour before meals and h.s. Bedtime doses can be larger; give at least 2 hours after last meal of the day.
● Monitor the patient's vital signs and urine output carefully.

### ☑ PATIENT TEACHING
● Instruct the patient when to take drug.

- Advise the patient to avoid driving and other hazardous activities if he is drowsy, dizzy, or has blurred vision; to drink plenty of fluids to help prevent constipation; and to report any rash or other skin eruption.

---

# scopolamine (hyoscine)
Scop‡, Transderm-Scōp, Transderm-V†

# scopolamine butylbromide (hyoscine butylbromide)
Buscopan†‡

# scopolamine hydrobromide (hyoscine hydrobromide)

*Pregnancy Risk Category: C*

---

## HOW SUPPLIED
**scopolamine**
*Transdermal patch:* 1.5 mg
**scopolamine butylbromide**
*Capsules:* 0.25 mg
*Suppositories:* 10 mg†
*Tablets:* 10 mg†
**scopolamine hydrobromide**
*Injection:* 0.3 mg, 0.4 mg, 0.5 mg, 0.6 mg, and 1 mg/ml in 1-ml vials and ampules; 0.86 mg/ml in 0.5-ml ampules

## ACTION
Inhibits muscarinic actions of acetylcholine on autonomic effectors innervated by postganglionic cholinergic neurons. Also may affect neural pathways originating in the labyrinth (inner ear) to inhibit nausea and vomiting.

## ONSET, PEAK, DURATION
Onset occurs within 30 minutes after parenteral administration, 30 to 60 minutes after oral administration, unknown after transdermal patch application. Peak unknown. Effects persist about 4 hours after parenteral administration, 4 to 6 hours after oral administration, and up to 72 hours after applying transdermal patch.

## INDICATIONS & DOSAGE
*Spastic states –*
**Adults:** 10 to 20 mg P.O. t.i.d. or q.i.d. Dosage adjusted as needed. Or 10 to 20 mg (butylbromide) S.C., I.M., or I.V. t.i.d. or q.i.d.
*Preoperatively to reduce secretions and block cardiac vagal reflexes –*
**Adults:** 0.2 to 0.6 mg (hydrobromide) I.M. 30 to 60 minutes before induction of anesthesia.
**Children 8 to 12 years:** 300 mcg (hydrobromide) I.M. 45 minutes before induction of anesthesia.
**Children 3 to 8 years:** 200 mcg (hydrobromide) I.M. 45 minutes before induction of anesthesia.
**Children 7 months to 3 years:** 150 mcg (hydrobromide) I.M. 45 minutes before induction of anesthesia.
**Infants 4 to 7 months:** 100 mcg (hydrobromide) I.M. or I.V. 45 minutes before induction of anesthesia.
*Prevention of nausea and vomiting associated with motion sickness –*
**Adults:** one Transderm-Scōp or Transderm-V patch (a circular flat unit) programmed to deliver 0.5 mg scopolamine daily over 3 days (72 hours), applied to the skin behind the ear several hours before the antiemetic is required. Or 300 to 600 mcg (hydrobromide) S.C., I.M., or I.V.
**Children:** 6 mcg/kg or 200 mcg/m² of body surface (hydrobromide) S.C., I.M., or I.V.

## ADVERSE REACTIONS
**CNS:** disorientation, restlessness, irritability, dizziness, drowsiness, headache, confusion, hallucinations, delirium.
**CV:** palpitations, tachycardia, paradoxical bradycardia.
**EENT:** dilated pupils, blurred vision, photophobia, increased intraocular pressure, difficulty swallowing.
**GI:** *constipation, dry mouth, nausea, vomiting, epigastric distress.*
**GU:** urinary hesitancy, urine retention.

**Respiratory:** bronchial plugging, depressed respirations.
**Skin:** rash, flushing, dryness, contact dermatitis (with transdermal patch).
**Other:** fever.

Adverse reactions may be caused by pending atropine-like toxicity and are dose-related. Individual tolerance varies greatly.

Many adverse reactions (such as dry mouth, constipation) are an expected extension of the drug's pharmacologic activity.

### INTERACTIONS

*Centrally acting anticholinergics (tricyclic antidepressants, antihistamines, phenothiazines):* increased incidence of adverse CNS reactions. Avoid concomitant use.
*Digoxin:* increased digoxin levels. Monitor for digitalis toxicity.
*Ethanol, CNS depressants:* increased incidence of CNS depression. Monitor patient closely.

### CONTRAINDICATIONS

Contraindicated in patients with angle-closure glaucoma, obstructive uropathy, obstructive disease of the GI tract, asthma, chronic pulmonary disease, myasthenia gravis, paralytic ileus, intestinal atony, unstable cardiovascular status in acute hemorrhage, or toxic megacolon.

### NURSING CONSIDERATIONS

● Use cautiously in patients with autonomic neuropathy, hyperthyroidism, coronary artery disease, arrhythmias, CHF, hypertension, hiatal hernia associated with reflux esophagitis, hepatic or renal disease, and ulcerative colitis and in children under 6 years. Also use cautiously in patients in hot or humid environment. Drug-induced heatstroke possible.

● **I.V. use:** Keep in mind that intermittent and continuous infusions are not recommended. For direct injection, dilute with sterile water and inject diluted drug at ordered rate through patent I.V. line.
● Protect I.V. solutions from freezing and light, and store at room temperature.
● Raise the bed's side rails as a precaution because some patients become temporarily excited, disoriented, or they develop amnesia or drowsiness. Reorient the patient as needed.
● Be aware that tolerance may develop when given over a long time.

### ☑ PATIENT TEACHING

● Advise the patient to apply patch the night before a planned trip. Transdermal method releases a controlled therapeutic amount of scopolamine. Transderm-Scōp is effective if applied 2 to 3 hours before experiencing motion, but more effective if applied 12 hours before.
● Advise the patient to wash and dry hands thoroughly before and after applying the transdermal patch on dry skin behind the ear and before touching the eye, as pupil may dilate. After removing the system, discard it. Wash hands and application site thoroughly.
● Tell patient that if patch becomes displaced, he should remove it and apply another patch on a fresh skin site behind the ear.
● Alert the patient to possible withdrawal symptoms (nausea, vomiting, headache, dizziness) when the transdermal system is used longer than 72 hours.
● Warn the patient to avoid activities that require alertness until drug's CNS effects are known.
● Have the patient ask the pharmacist for the brochure that comes with the transdermal product.
● Advise the patient to report signs of urinary hesitancy or urine retention.

---

*Liquid form contains alcohol.   **May contain tartrazine.   †Canada only.   ‡Australia only.   ◇OTC.

# 39

# Adrenergics (sympathomimetics)

**dobutamine hydrochloride**
**dopamine hydrochloride**
**mephentermine sulfate**
**metaraminol bitartrate**
**norepinephrine bitartrate**
**phenylephrine hydrochloride**
**pseudoephedrine hydrochloride**
**pseudoephedrine sulfate**

## COMBINATION PRODUCTS

ENTEX: phenylephrine hydrochloride 5 mg, phenylpropanolamine hydrochloride 45 mg, and guaifenesin 400 mg.
ENTEX LIQUID: phenylephrine hydrochloride 5 mg/5 ml, phenylpropanolamine hydrochloride 20 mg/5 ml, and guaifenesin 100 mg/5 ml (alcohol 5%).
ENTEX PSE: pseudophedrine 120 mg and guaifenesin 600 mg.
SEMPREX-D: acrivastine 8 mg and pseudoephedrine hydrochloride 60 mg.

---

# dobutamine hydrochloride

Dobutrex

*Pregnancy Risk Category: NR*

## HOW SUPPLIED

*Injection:* 12.5 mg/ml in 20-ml vials (parenteral)

## ACTION

Directly stimulates beta$_1$ receptors of the heart to increase myocardial contractility and stroke volume. At therapeutic dosages, decreases peripheral vascular resistance (afterload), reduces ventricular filling pressure (preload), and may facilitate AV node conduction. Net result is increased cardiac output.

## ONSET, PEAK, DURATION

Onset occurs in 1 to 2 minutes, up to 10 minutes if I.V. infusion rate is slow. Peak effects usually occur within 10 minutes of starting I.V. infusion. Effects persist for less than 5 minutes after infusion is stopped.

## INDICATIONS & DOSAGE

*To increase cardiac output in the short-term treatment of cardiac decompensation caused by depressed contractility, such as during refractory heart failure, and as adjunct in cardiac surgery—*
**Adults:** 2.5 to 10 mcg/kg/minute I.V. infusion. Infusion rates up to 40 mcg/kg/minute may be needed (rare).

## ADVERSE REACTIONS

**CNS:** headache.
**CV:** *increased heart rate,* **hypertension, PVCs,** angina, nonspecific chest pain, palpitations, hypotension.
**GI:** nausea, vomiting.
**Respiratory:** shortness of breath, *asthmatic episodes.*
**Other:** phlebitis, hypersensitivity reactions *(anaphylaxis).*

## INTERACTIONS

*Beta blockers:* may antagonize dobutamine effects. Don't use together.
*General anesthetics:* greater incidence of ventricular arrhythmias. Monitor ECG closely.

## CONTRAINDICATIONS

Contraindicated in patients with hypersensitivity to the drug or any component of the formulation and in those with idiopathic hypertrophic subaortic stenosis.

---

## NURSING CONSIDERATIONS

• Use cautiously in patients with a history of hypertension. Drug may precipitate an exaggerated pressor response.

• Do not mix with sodium bicarbonate injection because the drug is incompatible with alkaline solutions. Infusions for up to 72 hours produce no more adverse effects than shorter infusions.

• Before initiating therapy with dobutamine, correct hypovolemia with plasma volume expanders, as ordered.

• Administer a digitalis glycoside before dobutamine as ordered. Because drug increases AV node conduction, patients with atrial fibrillation may develop a rapid ventricular rate.

• **I.V. use:** Administer through a central venous catheter or large peripheral vein. Titrate infusion according to the doctor's orders and the patient's condition. Use an infusion pump.

• Dilute concentrate for injection before administration. Compatible solutions include $D_5W$, 0.45% sodium chloride or 0.9% sodium chloride for injection and lactated Ringer's injection. The contents of one vial (250 mg) diluted with 1,000 ml of solution yields a concentration of 250 mcg/ml; diluted with 500 ml, a concentration of 500 mcg/ml; diluted with 250 ml, a concentration of 1,000 mcg/ml. Maximum concentration should not exceed 5 mg/ml.

• Avoid extravasation; may cause an inflammatory response. Change I.V. sites regularly to avoid phlebitis.

• Do not administer through the same I.V. line with other drugs. Drug is incompatible with heparin, hydrocortisone sodium succinate, cefazolin, cefamandole, neutral cephalothin, penicillin, and ethacrynate sodium.

• Keep in mind that I.V. solutions remain stable for 24 hours.

• Be aware that oxidation of drug may slightly discolor admixtures containing dobutamine. This does not indicate a significant loss of potency provided drug is used within 24 hours of reconstitution.

• Continuously monitor ECG, blood pressure, pulmonary capillary wedge pressure, cardiac condition, and urine output.

• Monitor serum electrolytes, as ordered. Drug may lower serum potassium levels.

## ☑ PATIENT TEACHING

• Tell patient to report adverse reactions promptly, especially dyspnea and drug-induced headache.

• Instruct patient to report discomfort at I.V. insertion site.

---

# dopamine hydrochloride
Intropin, Revimine†‡

*Pregnancy Risk Category: C*

## HOW SUPPLIED
*Injection:* 40 mg/ml, 80 mg/ml, 160 mg/ml parenteral concentrate for injection for I.V. infusion; 0.8 mg/ml (200 or 400 mg) in dextrose 5%; 1.6 mg/ml (400 or 800 mg) in dextrose 5%, 3.2 mg/ml (800 mg) in dextrose 5% parenteral injection for I.V. infusion.

## ACTION
Stimulates dopaminergic, beta-adrenergic, and alpha-adrenergic receptors of the sympathetic nervous system.

## ONSET, PEAK, DURATION
Onset occurs within 5 minutes of starting I.V. infusion. Peak unknown. Effects subside within 10 minutes of discontinuing infusion.

## INDICATIONS & DOSAGE
*To treat shock and correct hemodynamic imbalances; to improve perfusion to vital organs; to increase cardiac output; to correct hypotension* –
**Adults:** initially, 1 to 5 mcg/kg/minute by I.V. infusion. Dosage titrated to

desired hemodynamic or renal response; infusion may be increased by 1 to 4 mcg/kg/minute at 10- to 30-minute intervals.

**ADVERSE REACTIONS**
**CNS:** headache.
**CV:** ectopic beats, tachycardia, anginal pain, palpitations, *hypotension.* Less frequently, bradycardia, widening of QRS complex, conduction disturbances, vasoconstriction, hypertension.
**GI:** nausea, vomiting.
**Other:** necrosis and tissue sloughing with extravasation, piloerection, dyspnea, *anaphylactic reactions, asthmatic episodes,* azotemia.

**INTERACTIONS**
*Alpha blockers, beta blockers:* may antagonize dopamine's effects. Don't use together.
*Ergot alkaloids:* extreme elevations in blood pressure. Don't use together.
*Inhalation anesthetics:* increased risk of arrhythmias or hypertension. Monitor closely.
*MAO inhibitors:* may cause hypertensive crisis. Avoid if possible.
*Phenytoin:* may lower blood pressure of dopamine-stabilized patients. Monitor carefully.

**CONTRAINDICATIONS**
Contraindicated in patients with uncorrected tachyarrhythmias, pheochromocytoma, or ventricular fibrillation.

**NURSING CONSIDERATIONS**
• Use cautiously in patients with occlusive vascular disease, cold injuries, diabetic endarteritis, and arterial embolism; in pregnant patients; and in those taking MAO inhibitors.
• Remember that drug is not a substitute for blood or fluid volume deficit. If deficit exists, replace fluid before administering vasopressors, as ordered.

• **I.V. use:** Use a central line or large vein, such as in the antecubital fossa, to minimize risk of extravasation. Watch infusion site carefully for signs of extravasation; if it occurs, stop infusion immediately and call doctor. Extravasation may require treatment by infiltration of the area with 5 to 10 mg phentolamine and 10 to 15 ml 0.9% sodium chloride solution. Don't mix with alkaline solutions. Use $D_5W$, 0.9% sodium chloride solution, or a combination of $D_5W$ and 0.9% sodium chloride solution. Mix just before use.
• Use a continuous infusion pump to regulate flow rate. Keep in mind that patient response depends on dosage and pharmacologic effects. Dosages of 0.5 to 2 mcg/kg/minute predominantly stimulate dopamine receptors and produce vasodilation of the renal vasculature. Dosages of 2 to 10 mcg/kg/minute stimulate beta-adrenergic receptors for a positive inotropic effect. Higher dosages also stimulate alpha-adrenergic receptors, causing vasoconstriction and increased blood pressure. Know that most patients are satisfactorily maintained on dosage less than 20 mcg/kg/minute.
• Do not mix other drugs in I.V. container with dopamine. Do not give alkaline drugs (for example, sodium bicarbonate or phenytoin sodium) through I.V. line containing dopamine.
• Discard after 24 hours (dopamine solutions deteriorate after 24 hours) or earlier if solution is discolored.
• During infusion, frequently monitor ECG, blood pressure, cardiac output, central venous pressure, pulmonary capillary wedge pressure, pulse rate, urine output, and color and temperature of extremities.
• If a disproportionate rise in diastolic pressure (a marked decrease in pulse pressure) is observed in patients receiving dopamine, decrease infusion rate as ordered and observe care-

fully for further evidence of predominant vasoconstrictor activity, unless such an effect is desired.

• Observe patients closely for adverse effects. If they develop, the doctor will adjust dosage or discontinue the drug.

• Check urine output often. If urine flow decreases without hypotension, notify doctor because dosage may need to be reduced.

• *Alert:* After drug is stopped, watch closely for sudden drop in blood pressure. Taper dosage slowly to evaluate stability of blood pressure, as ordered.

• Be aware that acidosis decreases effectiveness of dopamine.

### ☑ PATIENT TEACHING

• Tell patient to report adverse reactions promptly.

• Instruct patient to alert nurse if discomfort occurs at I.V. insertion site.

## mephentermine sulfate
Wyamine

*Pregnancy Risk Category: NR*

### HOW SUPPLIED
*Injection:* 15 mg/ml, 30 mg/ml

### ACTION
Unknown. Appears to indirectly stimulate beta- and alpha-adrenergic receptors by releasing norepinephrine.

### ONSET, PEAK, DURATION
Onset occurs immediately after I.V. administration, within 5 to 15 minutes after I.M. injection. Peak unknown. Effects persist for 15 to 30 minutes after I.V. administration, 1 to 4 hours after I.M. injection.

### INDICATIONS & DOSAGE
*Hypotension after spinal anesthesia –*
**Adults:** 30 to 45 mg I.V. as a single injection, then 30 mg I.V. repeated p.r.n. for maintenance of blood pressure, continuous I.V. infusion of 0.1% solution of mephentermine in D₅W.
**Children:** 0.4 mg/kg I.M. or I.V.
*Hypotension after spinal anesthesia during obstetric procedures –*
**Adults:** initially, 15 mg I.V., then repeated p.r.n.
*Prevention of hypotension during spinal anesthesia –*
**Adults:** 30 to 45 mg I.M. 10 to 20 minutes before anesthesia.

### ADVERSE REACTIONS
**CNS:** nervousness, anxiety, headache, dizziness, tremor, weakness.
**CV: *arrhythmias, marked elevation of blood pressure*** (with large doses), AV block, tachycardia.

### INTERACTIONS
*Antihypertensives, guanethidine, nitrates phenothiazines, reserpine:* decreased effects of these adrenergic blockers. Monitor patient closely.
*Beta-adrenergic blockers, rauwolfia alkaloids:* mutual inhibition of therapeutic effects. Avoid concomitant use.
*CNS stimulants, mazindol, methylphenidate, sympathomimetics:* increased CNS stimulation. Monitor patient closely.
*Digitalis glycosides, levodopa, inhalation anesthetics:* increased risk of arrhythmias. Monitor ECG.
*Ergot alkaloids, oxytocin:* enhanced vasoconstriction. Use together cautiously.
*Inhalation anesthetics:* increased risk of hypertension. Monitor closely.
*MAO inhibitors:* may precipitate hypertension, headache, and related symptoms. Don't use together.
*Maprotiline, tricyclic antidepressants:* decreased pressure response of mephentermine. Monitor for decreased effectiveness.
*Thyroid hormones:* enhanced risk of coronary insufficiency. Monitor patient closely.

---

\*Liquid form contains alcohol.   \*\*May contain tartrazine.   †Canada only.   ‡Australia only.   ◊OTC.

## CONTRAINDICATIONS

Contraindicated in patients with hypersensitivity to the drug and in those with hypotension resulting from hemorrhage, except in emergencies.

## NURSING CONSIDERATIONS

● Use cautiously in patients with CV disease, hyperthyroidism, hypertension, and chronic illness.
● Remember that the drug is not a substitute for blood or fluid volume deficit. If deficit exists, replace fluid before administering vasopressors, as ordered.
● Keep in mind that hypercapnia, hypoxia, or acidosis may reduce effectiveness or increase adverse effects. Identify and correct before and during administration, as ordered.
● **I.V. use:** Administer at 1 to 5 mg/minute. Can be given undiluted; I.V. drug is not irritating to tissue and extravasation has no serious effects. To prepare 0.1% I.V. solution, add 16.6 ml of mephentermine (30 mg/ml) to 500 ml of $D_5W$.
● Don't mix with I.V. hydralazine or epinephrine, which are physically incompatible with mephentermine.
● During infusion, frequently monitor ECG, blood pressure, cardiac output, central venous pressure, pulmonary capillary wedge pressure, pulse rate, urine output, and color and temperature of extremities. Titrate infusion rate according to findings and the doctor's guidelines. Use a continuous infusion pump to regulate flow rate.
● *Alert:* During infusion, check blood pressure every 2 minutes until stabilized; then check every 10 to 15 minutes.
● Know that the I.M. route may be used because drug is not irritating to tissue.
● Monitor blood pressure until stable, even after discontinuing drug.
● Observe patients closely for adverse effects. If they develop, the doctor

will adjust dosage or discontinue the drug.
● Be aware that the drug may increase uterine contractions during third trimester of pregnancy.

## ☑ PATIENT TEACHING

● Tell patient to report adverse reactions promptly.
● Instruct patient to alert nurse if discomfort occurs at I.V. insertion site.

---

## metaraminol bitartrate
Aramine

*Pregnancy Risk Category: C*

## HOW SUPPLIED
*Injection:* 10 mg/ml

## ACTION
Stimulates alpha- and beta$_1$-adrenergic receptors within the sympathetic nervous system.

## ONSET, PEAK, DURATION
Onset occurs in 1 to 2 minutes after I.V. administration, 10 minutes after I.M. administration, 5 to 20 minutes after S.C administration. Peak unknown. Effects last 20 minutes after I.V. administration, up to 90 minutes after S.C. or I.M. administration.

## INDICATIONS & DOSAGE
*Prevention of hypotension associated with spinal anesthesia –*
**Adults:** 2 to 10 mg I.M. or S.C.
*Treatment of hypotension associated with spinal anesthesia –*
**Adults:** 0.5 to 5 mg by direct I.V. injection, followed by I.V. infusion titrated to maintain blood pressure.
**Children:** 0.01 mg/kg as single I.V. injection; 1 mg/25 ml of $D_5W$ as I.V. infusion. Rate adjusted to maintain blood pressure in normal range. Alternatively, 0.1 mg/kg I.M. as single dose, p.r.n. At least 10 minutes should elapse before dosage increased

---

because maximum effect is not immediately apparent.

## ADVERSE REACTIONS

**CNS:** apprehension, dizziness, headache, tremor.
**CV:** hypertension; hypotension; palpitations; *arrhythmias,* including sinus or *ventricular tachycardia; cardiac arrest.*
**GI:** nausea.
**Skin:** flushing, diaphoresis.
**Other:** abscess, necrosis, sloughing upon extravasation.

## INTERACTIONS

*Beta-adrenergic blockers:* mutual inhibition of drug effects, with possible hypertension, bradycardia, and heart block. Avoid concomitant use.
*Cocaine, digitalis glycosides, doxapram, ergot alkaloids, general anesthetics, levodopa, maprotiline, other sympathomimetics, thyroid hormones, tricyclic antidepressants:* increased risk of adverse cardiac effects. Monitor closely.
*Furazolidone, MAO inhibitors, procarbazine:* may cause severe hypertension (hypertensive crisis) and increase action of metaraminol. Avoid this combination.
*Guanadrel, guanethidine:* metaraminol may decrease the hypotensive effect of these drugs; guanadrel and guanethidine may enhance the pressor effect of metaraminol. Avoid concomitant use.

## CONTRAINDICATIONS

Contraindicated in patients with hypersensitivity to the drug and in patients receiving anesthesia with cyclopropane and halogenated hydrocarbon anesthetics.

## NURSING CONSIDERATIONS

● Use cautiously in patients with heart disease, hypertension, peripheral vascular disease, thyroid disease, diabetes, cirrhosis, history of malaria, or sulfite sensitivity and in patients receiving digitalis glycosides.
● Know that drug is not a substitute for blood or fluid volume deficit. If deficit exists, replace fluid before administering vasopressors, as ordered.
● Do not mix metaraminol with other drugs.
● **I.V. use:** To prepare an I.V. infusion, mix 15 to 100 mg in 500 ml of 0.9% sodium chloride solution or $D_5W$. Adjust rate to maintain blood pressure.
● During infusion, check blood pressure every 5 minutes until stabilized; then check every 15 minutes. Frequently monitor ECG, blood pressure, cardiac output, central venous pressure, pulmonary capillary wedge pressure, pulse rate, urine output, and color and temperature of extremities. Titrate infusion rate according to findings and the doctor's guidelines.
● Use a central venous catheter or large vein, such as in the antecubital fossa, to minimize risk of extravasation. Use a continuous infusion pump to regulate infusion flow rate and a piggyback setup so I.V. line remains open if drug is stopped. Watch infusion site carefully for signs of extravasation. If it occurs, stop infusion immediately and call the doctor.
● To treat extravasation, infiltrate site promptly with 10 to 15 ml of 0.9% sodium chloride for injection containing 5 to 10 mg phentolamine. Use a fine needle.
● ***Alert:*** Keep in mind that blood pressure should be raised to slightly less than the patient's normal level. Be careful to avoid excessive blood pressure response. Headache may be a symptom of hypertension. Rapidly induced hypertensive response can cause acute pulmonary edema, arrhythmias, and cardiac arrest.
● Allow at least 10 minutes between doses. Drug effects are not always immediately apparent.
● Be aware that because of prolonged

---

*Liquid form contains alcohol.   **May contain tartrazine.   †Canada only.   ‡Australia only.   ◇OTC.

action, a cumulative effect is possible. With an excessive vasopressor response, elevated blood pressure may persist after drug is stopped.

• Observe patients closely for adverse effects. If they develop, notify the doctor, who will adjust or discontinue dosage.

• Keep emergency drugs on hand to reverse effects of metaraminol: atropine for reflex bradycardia; phentolamine to decrease vasopressor, effects; and propranolol for arrhythmias.

• Report persistent decreased urine output. Urine output may decrease initially, then increase as blood pressure returns to normal level.

• Closely monitor patients with diabetes; insulin dosage may need to be adjusted.

• When discontinuing drug, gradually slow infusion rate, as ordered. Continue monitoring vital signs, watching for possible severe drop in blood pressure. Keep equipment nearby to resume drug, if necessary. Do not reinstate vasopressor therapy until the systolic blood pressure falls below 70 to 80 mm Hg, as ordered.

• Keep solution in light-resistant container, away from heat.

☑ **PATIENT TEACHING**
• Tell patient to report adverse reactions promptly.
• Instruct patient to alert nurse if discomfort occurs at I.V. site.

---

## norepinephrine bitartrate (levarterenol bitartrate, noradrenaline acid tartrate)
Levophed
*Pregnancy Risk Category: C*

**HOW SUPPLIED**
*Injection:* 1 mg/ml

## ACTION
Stimulates alpha- and beta$_1$-adrenergic receptors within the sympathetic nervous system.

## ONSET, PEAK, DURATION
Onset and peak immediately after I.V. infusion begins. Effects persist for 1 to 2 minutes after I.V. infusion ends.

## INDICATIONS & DOSAGE
*To restore blood pressure in acute hypotensive states –*
**Adults:** initially, 8 to 12 mcg/minute I.V. infusion, then adjusted to maintain normal blood pressure. Average maintenance dosage is 2 to 4 mcg/minute.
**Children:** 2 mcg/m$^2$/minute I.V. infusion; dosage adjusted based on patient response.
*Severe hypotension during cardiac arrest –*
**Children:** initial I.V. infusion rate is 0.1 mcg/kg/minute. Rate adjusted according to patient response.

## ADVERSE REACTIONS
**CNS:** *headache,* anxiety, weakness, dizziness, tremor, restlessness, insomnia.
**CV:** bradycardia, *severe hypertension, arrhythmias.*
**Respiratory:** respiratory difficulties, *asthmatic episodes.*
**Other:** *anaphylaxis,* irritation with extravasation.

## INTERACTIONS
*Alpha-adrenergic blockers:* may antagonize drug effects. Avoid concomitant use.
*Antihistamines, ergot alkaloids, guanethidine, methyldopa, tricyclic antidepressants:* when given with sympathomimetics, may cause severe hypertension (hypertensive crisis). Don't give together.
*Inhalation anesthetics:* increased risk of arrhythmias. Monitor closely.

---

Reactions may be *common,* uncommon, *life-threatening,* or COMMON AND LIFE-THREATENING.

*MAO inhibitors:* increased risk of hypertensive crisis. Don't use together.

## CONTRAINDICATIONS

Contraindicated in patients with mesenteric or peripheral vascular thrombosis, profound hypoxia, hypercapnia, or hypotension resulting from blood volume deficit and during cyclopropane and halothane anesthesia.

## NURSING CONSIDERATIONS

• Use with extreme caution in patients receiving MAO inhibitors or triptyline- or imipramine-type antidepressants. Use cautiously in patients with sulfite sensitivity.

• Know that drug is not a substitute for blood or fluid volume deficit. If deficit exists, replace fluid before administering vasopressors.

• **I.V. use:** Use a central venous catheter or a large vein, such as in the antecubital fossa, to minimize risk of extravasation. Administer in dextrose 5% in 0.9% sodium chloride for injection; 0.9% sodium chloride for injection alone is not recommended. Use continuous infusion pump to regulate infusion flow rate and a piggyback setup so I.V. line remains open if norepinephrine is stopped.

• *Alert:* Never leave patients unattended during infusion. Also, check blood pressure every 2 minutes until stabilized; then check every 5 minutes. In previously hypertensive patients, blood pressure should be raised no higher than 40 mm Hg below pre-existing systolic pressure.

• Also during infusion, frequently monitor ECG, cardiac output, central venous pressure, pulmonary capillary wedge pressure, pulse rate, urine output, and color and temperature of extremities. Titrate infusion rate according to findings and the doctor's guidelines.

• Check site frequently for signs of extravasation. If it occurs, stop infusion immediately and call the doctor.

He may counteract effect by infiltrating area with 5 to 10 mg phentolamine and 10 to 15 ml of 0.9% sodium chloride solution. Also check for blanching along course of infused vein; may progress to superficial sloughing.

• If prolonged I.V. therapy is necessary, change injection site frequently.

• Keep emergency drugs on hand to reverse effects of norepinephrine: atropine for reflex bradycardia; phentolamine for increased vasopressor effects; and propranolol for arrhythmias.

• Report decreased urine output to the doctor immediately.

• When discontinuing drug, gradually slow infusion rate, as ordered. Continue monitoring vital signs, watching for possible severe drop in blood pressure.

• Be aware that norepinephrine solutions deteriorate after 24 hours.

• Protect drug from light. Discard discolored solutions or solutions that contain a precipitate.

## ☑ PATIENT TEACHING

• Tell patient to report adverse reactions promptly.

• Advise patient to alert nurse if discomfort occurs at I.V. insertion site.

---

# phenylephrine hydrochloride
Neo-Synephrine

*Pregnancy Risk Category: C*

## HOW SUPPLIED
*Injection:* 10 mg/ml

## ACTION
Predominantly stimulates alpha-adrenergic receptors in the sympathetic nervous system.

## ONSET, PEAK, DURATION
Onset occurs immediately after I.V. administration, within 10 to 15 min-

---

utes after S.C. or I.M. injection. Peak unknown. Effects persist for 15 to 20 minutes after I.V. administration, ½ to 2 hours after I.M. injection, 50 minutes to 1 hour after S.C. injection.

## INDICATIONS & DOSAGE
*Hypotensive emergencies during spinal anesthesia –*
**Adults:** initially, 0.1 to 0.2 mg I.V., then subsequent doses of 0.1 to 0.2 mg, p.r.n.
*Maintenance of blood pressure during spinal or inhalation anesthesia –*
**Adults:** 2 to 3 mg S.C. or I.M. 3 or 4 minutes before anesthesia.
**Children:** 0.044 mg to 0.088 mg/kg S.C. or I.M.
*Prolongation of spinal anesthesia –*
**Adults:** 2 to 5 mg added to anesthetic solution.
*Vasoconstrictor for regional anesthesia –*
**Adults:** 1 mg phenylephrine added to 20 ml local anesthetic.
*Mild to moderate hypotension –*
**Adults:** 2 to 5 mg S.C. or I.M.; repeated in 1 to 2 hours as needed and tolerated. Initial dose should not exceed 5 mg. Alternatively, 0.1 to 0.5 mg slow I.V., not to be repeated more often than 10 to 15 minutes.
**Children:** 0.1 mg/kg I.M. or S.C.; repeated in 1 to 2 hours as needed and tolerated.
*Severe hypotension and shock (including drug-induced) –*
**Adults:** 10 mg in 250 to 500 ml of $D_5W$ or 0.9% sodium chloride for injection. I.V. infusion started at 100 to 180 mcg/minute, then decreased to a maintenance infusion of 40 to 60 mcg/minute when blood pressure stabilizes.
*Paroxysmal supraventricular tachycardia –*
**Adults:** initially, 0.5 mg rapid I.V.; subsequent doses should not exceed the preceding dose by more than 0.1 to 0.2 mg and should not exceed 1 mg.

## ADVERSE REACTIONS
**CNS:** *headache,* excitability.
**CV:** bradycardia, *arrhythmias,* hypertension.
**Other:** tachyphylaxis (may occur with continued use), *anaphylaxis, asthmatic episodes,* decreased organ perfusion (with prolonged use), tissue sloughing with extravasation.

## INTERACTIONS
*Alpha-adrenergic blockers, phenothiazines:* decreased vasopressor response. Monitor closely.
*Beta-adrenergic blockers:* blocked cardiostimulatory effects. Monitor closely.
*Bretylium, halogenated hydrocarbon anesthetics:* may cause serious arrhythmias. Use with extreme caution.
*Guanethidine, oxytocics, tricyclic antidepressants:* increased pressor response. Observe patient.
*MAO inhibitors:* may cause severe hypertension (hypertensive crisis). Don't use together.

## CONTRAINDICATIONS
Contraindicated in patients with hypersensitivity to the drug and in those with severe hypertension or ventricular tachycardia.

## NURSING CONSIDERATIONS
● Use with extreme caution in patients with heart disease, hyperthyroidism, severe atherosclerosis, bradycardia, partial heart block, myocardial disease, or sulfite sensitivity and in elderly patients.
● **I.V. use:** For direct injection, dilute 10 mg (1 ml) with 9 ml sterile water for injection to provide a solution containing 1 mg/ml. I.V. infusions are usually prepared by adding 10 mg of drug to 500 ml of $D_5W$ or 0.9% sodium chloride for injection. The initial infusion rate is usually 100 to 180 mcg/minute; the maintenance infusion rate is usually 40 to 60 mcg/minute.

---

Reactions may be *common,* uncommon, *life-threatening,* or **COMMON AND LIFE-THREATENING.**

• Use a central venous catheter or a large vein, as in the antecubital fossa, to minimize risk of extravasation. Use a continuous infusion pump to regulate infusion flow rate.

• With prolonged I.V. infusions, avoid abrupt withdrawal. During infusion, frequently monitor ECG, blood pressure, cardiac output, central venous pressure, pulmonary capillary wedge pressure, pulse rate, urine output, and color and temperature of extremities. Titrate infusion rate according to findings and the doctor's guidelines. Use a continuous infusion pump to regulate flow rate and avoid severe increase. Maintain blood pressure slightly below the patient's normal level, as ordered. In previously normotensive patients, maintain systolic blood pressure at 80 to 100 mm Hg; in previously hypertensive patients, maintain systolic blood pressure at 30 to 40 mm Hg below usual level.

• To treat extravasation, infiltrate site promptly with 10 to 15 ml of 0.9% sodium chloride for injection containing 5 to 10 mg phentolamine, as ordered. Use a fine needle.

• Remember that drug causes little or no CNS stimulation.

• Keep in mind that drug is incompatible with butacaine sulfate, alkalis, ferric salts, and oxidizing agents.

☑ **PATIENT TEACHING**

• Tell patient to report adverse reactions promptly.

• Instruct patient to alert nurse if discomfort occurs at I.V. insertion site.

## pseudoephedrine hydrochloride

Afrinol Repetabs◊, Allerid◊, Allermed◊, Cenafed◊, Children's Congestion Relief◊, Children's Sudafed Liquid◊, Congestac N.D. Caplets†◊, Congestion Relief◊, Decofed◊, De-Fed-60◊, Dorcol Children's Decongestant Liquid◊, Drixoral Non-Drowsy Formula◊, Efidac/24◊, Eltor 120†◊, Genaphed◊, Halofed◊, Halofed Adult Strength◊, Maxenal†◊, Myfedrine◊, NeoFed◊, Novafed◊, Ornex Cold†◊, PediaCare Infant's Decongestant◊, PediaCare Infants' Oral Decongestant Drops◊, Pseudo◊, Pseudofrin†◊, Pseudo-gest◊, Robidrine◊, Seudotabs◊, Sinufed◊, Sinustat◊, Sinustop Pro◊, Sudafed◊, Sudafed 12 Hour◊, Sudafed-60◊, Sudrin◊, Sufedrin◊

## pseudoephedrine sulfate

Afrin◊, Drixoral Non-Drowsy Formula◊, Drixoral‡

*Pregnancy Risk Category: C*

**HOW SUPPLIED**
**pseudoephedrine hydrochloride**
*Tablets:* 30 mg◊, 60 mg◊
*Tablets (extended-release):* 120 mg◊, 240 mg◊
*Capsules:* 60 mg
*Capsules (extended-release):* 120 mg
*Oral solution:* 15 mg/5 ml◊, 30 mg/5 ml◊, 7.5 mg/0.8 ml◊
*Syrup:* 30 mg/5 ml
**pseudoephedrine sulfate**
*Tablets (extended-release):* 120 mg (60 mg immediate-release, 60 mg delayed-release)◊

**ACTION**
Stimulates alpha-adrenergic receptors in the respiratory tract, producing vasoconstriction.

## ONSET, PEAK, DURATION

Onset occurs in 15 to 30 minutes. Serum levels peak within 30 to 60 minutes. Effects persist for 3 to 4 hours after administration of tablets, oral solution, and syrup, 8 to 12 hours after administration of extended-release capsules and tablets.

## INDICATIONS & DOSAGE

*Nasal and eustachian tube decongestion* –

**Adults:** 60 mg P.O. q 4 hours. Maximum dosage is 240 mg daily. Or, 120 mg extended-release tablet P.O. q 12 hours or 240 mg extended-release (Efidac/24) once daily.

**Children over 12 years:** 120 mg P.O. q 12 hours, or 240 mg P.O. (Efidac/24) once daily.

**Children 6 to 12 years:** 30 mg P.O. regular-release form q 4 to 6 hours. Maximum dosage is 120 mg daily.

**Children 2 to 6 years:** 15 mg P.O. regular-release form q 4 to 6 hours. Maximum dosage is 60 mg/day.

**Children 1 to 2 years:** 7 drops (0.2 ml)/kg q 4 to 6 hours up to 4 doses/day.

**Children 3 to 12 months:** 3 drops/kg q 4 to 6 hours up to 4 doses/day.

*Relief of nasal congestion* –

**Adults:** 120 mg q 12 hours.

## ADVERSE REACTIONS

**CNS:** *anxiety,* transient stimulation, tremor, dizziness, headache, insomnia, *nervousness.*
**CV:** arrhythmias, *palpitations,* tachycardia.
**GI:** anorexia, nausea, vomiting, dry mouth.
**GU:** difficulty urinating.
**Respiratory:** respiratory difficulties.
**Skin:** pallor.

## INTERACTIONS

*Antihypertensives:* may attenuate hypotensive effect. Monitor blood pressure closely.
*MAO inhibitors:* may cause severe hypertension (hypertensive crisis). Don't use together.

## CONTRAINDICATIONS

Contraindicated in patients with severe hypertension or severe coronary artery disease, in patients receiving MAO inhibitors, and in breast-feeding patients. Extended-release preparations are contraindicated in children under age 12.

## NURSING CONSIDERATIONS

• Use cautiously in patients with hypertension, cardiac disease, diabetes, glaucoma, hyperthyroidism, and prostatic hyperplasia.
• Be aware that elderly patients are more sensitive to the drug's effects.

## ☑ PATIENT TEACHING

• Tell the patient not to crush or break extended-release forms.
• Warn against using OTC products containing other sympathomimetics.
• Tell the patient not to take drug within 2 hours of bedtime because it can cause insomnia.
• Tell the patient to stop drug if he becomes unusually restless and to notify the doctor promptly.

**dihydroergotamine mesylate
ergotamine tartrate
methysergide maleate
propranolol hydrochloride**
(See Chapter 22, ANTIANGINALS.)

## COMBINATION PRODUCTS

BELLERGAL-S\*\*, BEL-PHEN-ERGOT
S, PHENERBEL-S: ergotamine tartrate
0.6 mg, levorotatory belladonna alkaloids 0.2 mg, and phenobarbital 40
mg.
CAFERGOT, ERCAF, WIGRAINE: ergotamine tartrate 1 mg and caffeine
100 mg.
CAFERGOT SUPPOSITORIES: ergotamine tartrate 2 mg and caffeine 100
mg.
HYDERGINE: dihydroergocornine
mesylate 0.167 mg, dihydroergocris-
tine mesylate 0.167 mg, and dihy-
droergocryptine mesylate 0.167 mg.
WIGRAINE SUPPOSITORIES: ergotamine tartrate 2 mg and caffeine 100
mg.

---

## dihydroergotamine mesylate

D.H.E. 45, Dihydergot‡,
Dihydroergotamine-Sandoz†

*Pregnancy Risk Category: X*

### HOW SUPPLIED
*Injection:* 1 mg/ml

### ACTION
Causes peripheral vasoconstriction
primarily by stimulating alpha-adrenergic receptors; may abort vascular
headaches by direct vasoconstriction
of dilated carotid artery bed with a
decline in amplitude of pulsations.

### ONSET, PEAK, DURATION
Onset occurs within 5 minutes of I.V.
administration, within 15 to 30 minutes of I.M. injection. Serum levels
peak within 15 minutes of I.V. administration, 30 minutes after I.M. injection, 15 to 45 minutes after S.C. injection. Effects persist for about 8
hours after parenteral use.

### INDICATIONS & DOSAGE
*To prevent or abort vascular or mi-
graine headache—*
**Adults:** 1 mg I.M. or I.V. Repeated
q 1 to 2 hours, p.r.n., up to total of
2 mg I.V. or 3 mg I.M. per attack.
Maximum weekly dosage is 6 mg.

### ADVERSE REACTIONS
**CV:** numbness and tingling in fingers
and toes, transient tachycardia or bradycardia, precordial distress and
pain, increased arterial pressure.
**GI:** *nausea, vomiting.*
**Skin:** itching.
**Other:** weakness in legs, muscle pain
in extremities, localized edema.

### INTERACTIONS
*Erythromycin, other macrolides:* may
cause symptoms of ergot toxicity. Vasodilators (nitroprusside, nifedipine,
or prazosin) may be ordered to treat
such an attack. Monitor closely.
*Propranolol, other beta blockers:*
blocked natural pathway for vasodilation in patients receiving ergot alkaloids; may result in excessive vasoconstriction and cold extremities.
Watch closely if drugs are used together.

### CONTRAINDICATIONS
Contraindicated in patients with hypersensitivity to the drug, during
pregnancy or breast-feeding, and in

---

\*Liquid form contains alcohol.   \*\*May contain tartrazine.   †Canada only.   ‡Australia only.   ◇OTC.

patients with peripheral and occlusive vascular disease, coronary artery disease, uncontrolled hypertension, severe hepatic or renal dysfunction, and sepsis.

## NURSING CONSIDERATIONS
• Know that the drug is most effective when used at first sign of migraine or soon after onset.
• **I.V. use:** Directly inject solution into the vein over 3 minutes. Continuous and intermittent infusion are not recommended.
• Avoid prolonged administration; don't exceed recommended dosage, as ordered. Adjust to most effective minimal dosage, as ordered, for best results.
• Be alert for ergotamine rebound, or an increase in frequency and duration of headache, which may occur when drug is stopped.
• Protect ampules from heat and light. Discard if solution is discolored.

## ☑ PATIENT TEACHING
• Instruct patient to lie down and relax in a quiet, low-light environment after administration of drug.
• Tell patient to report any feeling of coldness in extremities or of tingling in fingers and toes. Severe vasoconstriction may result in tissue damage. Keep extremities warm and administer vasodilators as ordered.
• Help patient evaluate underlying causes of stress, which may precipitate attacks.

---

## ergotamine tartrate
Ergodryl Mono‡, Ergomar, Ergostat, Gynergen†, Medihaler Ergotamine

*Pregnancy Risk Category: X*

## HOW SUPPLIED
*Capsules:* 1 mg‡
*Tablets:* 1 mg†
*Tablets (sublingual):* 2 mg
*Aerosol inhaler:* 360 mcg/metered spray
*Suppositories:* 2 mg

## ACTION
Stimulates alpha-adrenergic receptors, causing peripheral vasoconstriction. Also inhibits reuptake of norepinephrine, increasing vasoconstrictor activity.

## ONSET, PEAK, DURATION
Onset and duration variable. Serum levels peak in ½ to 3 hours or longer after oral dose, unknown for other routes of administration.

## INDICATIONS & DOSAGE
*Vascular or migraine headache* –
**Adults:** initially, 2 mg P.O. or S.L., then 1 to 2 mg P.O. q hour or S.L. q ½ hour, to maximum of 6 mg daily and 10 mg weekly. Alternatively, use aerosol inhaler: 1 spray (360 mcg) initially, repeated q 5 minutes p.r.n. to a maximum of 6 sprays (2.16 mg) per 24 hours or 15 sprays (5.4 mg) per week.

Patient also may use rectal suppositories. Initially, 2 mg P.R. at onset of the attack, repeated in 1 hour p.r.n. Maximum dosage is 2 suppositories per attack or 5 suppositories per week.

## ADVERSE REACTIONS
**CV:** numbness and tingling in fingers and toes, transient tachycardia or bradycardia, precordial distress and pain, increased arterial pressure, angina pectoris, peripheral vasoconstriction.
**GI:** nausea, vomiting.
**Skin:** pruritus, localized edema.
**Other:** weakness in legs, muscle pain in extremities.

## INTERACTIONS
*Erythromycin, other macrolides:* may cause symptoms of ergot toxicity. Va-

---

Reactions may be *common,* uncommon, *life-threatening,* or **COMMON AND LIFE-THREATENING.**

sodilators (nitroprusside, nifedipine, or prazosin) may be ordered to treat such an attack. Monitor closely.
*Propranolol, other beta blockers:* blocked natural pathway for vasodilation in patients receiving ergot alkaloids; may result in excessive vasoconstriction. Watch closely if drugs are used together.

## CONTRAINDICATIONS
Contraindicated in patients with hypersensitivity to ergot alkaloids, during pregnancy, and in patients with peripheral and occlusive vascular diseases, coronary artery disease, hypertension, hepatic or renal dysfunction, severe pruritus, or sepsis.

## NURSING CONSIDERATIONS
• Obtain an accurate dietary history from the patient to determine if a relationship exists between certain foods and onset of headache.
• Be aware that drug is most effective when used during prodromal stage of headache or as soon as possible after onset.
• Avoid prolonged administration; don't exceed recommended dosage.
• Provide a quiet, low-light environment to help patients relax.
• Be alert for ergotamine rebound, or an increase in frequency and duration of headache, which may occur if drug is suddenly discontinued.

## ☑ PATIENT TEACHING
• Tell patient not to eat, drink, or smoke while the tablet is dissolving. S.L. tablet is preferred during early stage of attack because of its rapid absorption.
• Warn patient not to increase dosage without first consulting the doctor.
• Advise patient to avoid prolonged exposure to cold weather whenever possible. Cold may increase many of the adverse reactions to the drug.
• Instruct patient on long-term therapy to check for and report feeling of

coldness in extremities or of tingling in fingers and toes. Severe vasoconstriction may result in tissue damage. Keep extremities warm and administer vasodilators as ordered.
• Instruct patient how to use inhaler correctly.
• Help patient evaluate underlying causes of stress, which may precipitate attacks.

---

## methysergide maleate
Deseril‡, Sansert**

*Pregnancy Risk Category: X*

## HOW SUPPLIED
*Tablets:* 1 mg‡, 2 mg

## ACTION
Unknown. Specifically blocks serotonin (a neurotransmitter) in the peripheral nervous system. In CNS, drug may act as a serotonin agonist.

## ONSET, PEAK, DURATION
Onset occurs within 1 to 2 days after therapy initiated. Peak unknown. Effects persist for 1 to 2 days.

## INDICATIONS & DOSAGE
*Prevention of frequent, severe, uncontrollable, or disabling migraine or vascular headaches —*
**Adults:** 4 to 8 mg P.O. daily with meals.

## ADVERSE REACTIONS
**CNS:** insomnia, drowsiness, *euphoria, vertigo,* ataxia, *light-headedness,* hyperesthesia, weakness, hallucinations or feelings of disassociation, rapid speech, lethargy.
**CV:** *fibrotic thickening of cardiac valves and aorta, inferior vena cava, and common iliac branches (retroperitoneal fibrosis);* vasoconstriction, causing chest pain, abdominal pain, vascular insufficiency of lower limbs; cold, numb, painful extremities with or without paresthesia and diminished

---

*Liquid form contains alcohol. **May contain tartrazine. †Canada only. ‡Australia only. ◊OTC.

or absent pulses; postural hypotension; tachycardia; peripheral edema; murmurs; bruits.
**GI:** nausea, vomiting, diarrhea, constipation, heartburn.
**Hematologic:** neutropenia, eosinophilia.
**Respiratory:** *pulmonary fibrosis* (causing dyspnea, tightness and pain in chest, pleural friction rubs, and effusion).
**Skin:** hair loss, flushing, rash.
**Other:** arthralgia, myalgia.

## INTERACTIONS
*Beta blockers:* may result in peripheral ischemia by cold extremities and possible gangrene. Monitor closely.

## CONTRAINDICATIONS
Contraindicated in patients with severe hypertension or arteriosclerosis, peripheral vascular insufficiency, renal or hepatic disease, coronary artery disease (CAD), phlebitis or cellulitis of lower limbs, collagen diseases, fibrotic processes, or valvular heart disease; in debilitated patients; and during pregnancy.

## NURSING CONSIDERATIONS
● Use cautiously in patients with peptic ulcerations or suspected CAD. ECG and cardiac status evaluation advisable before giving to patients over age 40. Also use cautiously in patients sensitive to aspirin or tartrazine.
● *Alert:* Know that the drug is indicated only for patients who are unresponsive to other drugs and who can be kept under close medical supervision.
● Gradually introduce medication, as ordered, and administer with meals to prevent GI effects.
● Give drug, as ordered, for 3 weeks before evaluating effectiveness.
● Monitor laboratory studies of cardiac and renal function, CBC, and erythrocyte sedimentation rate before and during therapy.
● Know that drug should not be used for treatment of migraine or vascular headache or tension (muscle contraction) headaches.
● Be aware that drug may be withdrawn gradually every 6 months; then restarted after at least 3 weeks.

## ☑ PATIENT TEACHING
● Instruct patient to take drug with meals.
● Instruct patient to keep daily weight record and report unusually rapid weight gain. Teach patient to check for peripheral edema. Explain and suggest low-salt diet if necessary.
● Tell patient not to stop drug abruptly; may cause rebound headaches. Stop gradually over 2 to 3 weeks.
● Tell patient to promptly report any of the following symptoms to the doctor: cold, numb, or painful hands and feet; leg cramps when walking; and pelvic, chest, or flank pain.

---

Reactions may be *common,* uncommon, *life-threatening,* or **COMMON AND LIFE-THREATENING.**

# 41

# Skeletal muscle relaxants

**baclofen**
**carisoprodol**
**chlorphenesin carbamate**
**chlorzoxazone**
**cyclobenzaprine hydrochloride**
**dantrolene sodium**
**methocarbamol**
**orphenadrine citrate**

## COMBINATION PRODUCTS
NORGESIC: orphenadrine citrate 25 mg, aspirin 385 mg, and caffeine 30 mg.
NORGESIC FORTE: orphenadrine citrate 50 mg, aspirin 770 mg, and caffeine 60 mg.
ROBAXISAL: methocarbamol 400 mg and aspirin 325 mg.
SOMA COMPOUND: carisoprodol 200 mg and aspirin 325 mg.
SOMA COMPOUND WITH CODEINE: carisoprodol 200 mg, aspirin 325 mg, caffeine 32 mg, and codeine phosphate 16 mg.

---

## baclofen
Clofen‡, Lioresal, Lioresal Intrathecal

*Pregnancy Risk Category: NR*

### HOW SUPPLIED
*Tablets:* 10 mg, 20 mg, 25 mg‡
*Intrathecal injection:* 500 mcg/ml, 2,000 mcg/ml

### ACTION
Unknown. Appears to reduce transmission of impulses from the spinal cord to skeletal muscle.

### ONSET, PEAK, DURATION
Onset occurs hours to weeks after oral administration, ½ to 1 hour after intrathecal administration. Serum levels peak 2 to 3 hours after an oral dose; peak effects occur about 4 hours after intrathecal administration. Effects of intrathecal injection persist for about 4 to 8 hours, unknown for oral administration.

### INDICATIONS & DOSAGE
*Spasticity in multiple sclerosis, spinal cord injury –*
**Adults:** initially, 5 mg P.O. t.i.d. for 3 days, then 10 mg t.i.d. for 3 days, 15 mg t.i.d. for 3 days, 20 mg t.i.d. for 3 days. Increased according to response up to maximum of 80 mg daily.
*Management of severe spasticity in patients who do not respond to or cannot tolerate oral baclofen therapy –*
**Adults:** *Screening phase –* After a test dose to check responsiveness, drug is given by an implantable infusion pump. The test dose is 1 ml of a 50-mcg/ml dilution administered into the intrathecal space by barbotage over 1 minute or more. Significantly decreased severity or frequency of muscle spasm or reduced muscle tone should appear within 4 to 8 hours. If the response is inadequate, a second test dose of 75 mcg/1.5 ml is given 24 hours after the first. If response is still inadequate, a final test dose of 100 mcg/2 ml is given 24 hours later. Patients unresponsive to the 100-mcg dose shouldn't be considered candidates for the implantable pump.
*Maintenance therapy –* Initial dose is titrated based on the screening dose that elicited an adequate response. This effective dose is doubled and administered over 24 hours. However, if the screening dose efficacy was maintained for 12 hours or more, the dose is not doubled. After the first 24 hours, the dose is increased slowly as needed and tolerated by 10% to 30% daily. During prolonged maintenance

---

therapy, daily dose may be increased by 10% to 40% if needed; if the patient experiences adverse effects, dosage may be decreased by 10% to 20%. Maintenance dosages have ranged from 12 mcg to 1,500 mcg daily; however, experience with dosages over 1,000 mcg daily is limited. Most patients need 300 to 800 mcg daily.

## ADVERSE REACTIONS

**CNS:** *drowsiness, dizziness,* headache, *weakness, fatigue,* hypotonia, *confusion,* insomnia, dysarthria, **SEIZURES.**
**CV:** hypotension, hypertension.
**EENT:** blurred vision, nasal congestion, slurred speech.
**GI:** *nausea,* constipation, *vomiting.*
**GU:** urinary frequency.
**Hepatic:** increased AST and alkaline phosphatase levels.
**Skin:** rash, pruritus.
**Other:** excessive perspiration, hyperglycemia, weight gain, dyspnea.

## INTERACTIONS

*Ethanol, CNS depressants:* increased CNS depression. Avoid concomitant use.

## CONTRAINDICATIONS

Contraindicated in patients with hypersensitivity to the drug.

## NURSING CONSIDERATIONS

• Use cautiously in patients with impaired renal function or seizure disorder or when spasticity is used to maintain motor function.
• Give oral form with meals or with milk to prevent GI distress.
• Know that orally administered drug should not be used to treat muscle spasm caused by rheumatic disorders, cerebral palsy, Parkinson's disease, or CVA because efficacy hasn't been established. Do not administer intrathecal injection by I.V., I.M., S.C., or epidural route.
• Watch for sensitivity reactions, such as fever, skin eruptions, and respiratory distress.
• Watch for increased incidence of seizures in patients with seizure disorder.
• Be aware that amount of relief determines if dosage (and drowsiness) can be reduced.
• Do not withdraw drug abruptly after long-term use unless required by severe adverse reactions; may precipitate hallucinations or rebound spasticity.
• Know that experience with long-term intrathecal use suggests that about 10% of patients may develop tolerance to the drug. In some cases, this may be treated by hospitalizing the patient and slowly withdrawing the drug over a 2-week period.

## ☑ PATIENT TEACHING

• Instruct patient to take oral form with meals or milk.
• Tell patients to avoid activities that require alertness until drug's CNS effects are known. Drowsiness usually is transient.
• Tell patients to avoid alcohol while taking this drug.
• Advise the patient to follow the doctor's orders regarding rest and physical therapy.

---

# carisoprodol

Rela, Sodol, Soma, Soprodol, Soridol

*Pregnancy Risk Category: NR*

## HOW SUPPLIED

*Tablets:* 350 mg

## ACTION

Unknown. Drug appears to modify central perception of pain without modifying pain reflexes. Blocks interneuronal activity in descending reticular activating system and spinal cord.

---

## ONSET, PEAK, DURATION
Onset occurs within 30 minutes. Serum levels peak within 4 hours. Effects persist for 4 to 6 hours.

## INDICATIONS & DOSAGE
*As an adjunct in acute, painful musculoskeletal conditions –*
**Adults:** 350 mg P.O. t.i.d. and h.s.

## ADVERSE REACTIONS
**CNS:** *drowsiness, dizziness,* vertigo, ataxia, tremor, agitation, irritability, headache, depressive reactions, insomnia.
**CV:** orthostatic hypotension, tachycardia, facial flushing.
**GI:** nausea, vomiting, hiccups, epigastric distress.
**Hematologic:** eosinophilia.
**Respiratory:** asthmatic episodes.
**Skin:** rash, *erythema multiforme,* pruritus.
**Other:** fever, angioedema, *anaphylaxis.*

## INTERACTIONS
*Ethanol, CNS depressants:* increased CNS depression. Avoid concomitant use.

## CONTRAINDICATIONS
Contraindicated in patients with hypersensitivity to related compounds (for example, meprobamate or tybamate) or intermittent porphyria.

## NURSING CONSIDERATIONS
• Use cautiously in patients with impaired hepatic or renal function.
• **Alert:** Watch for idiosyncratic reactions after first to fourth dose (weakness, ataxia, visual and speech difficulties, fever, skin eruptions, and mental changes) and for severe reactions, including bronchospasm, hypotension, and anaphylactic shock. Withhold dose and notify the doctor immediately of any unusual reactions.
• Record amount of relief to help the doctor determine whether dosage can be reduced.
• Do not stop drug abruptly; mild withdrawal effects, such as insomnia, headache, nausea, and abdominal cramps, may result.

## ☑ PATIENT TEACHING
• Warn patient to avoid activities that require alertness until drug's CNS effects are known. Drowsiness is transient.
• Advise patient to avoid combining drug with alcohol or other CNS depressants.
• Advise patient to follow doctor's orders regarding rest and physical therapy.

# chlorphenesin carbamate
Maolate**

*Pregnancy Risk Category: NR*

## HOW SUPPLIED
*Tablets:* 400 mg

## ACTION
Unknown. Probably modifies central perception of pain without modifying pain reflexes. Blocks interneuronal activity in descending reticular activating system and in spinal cord.

## ONSET, PEAK, DURATION
Onset and duration unknown. Serum levels peak within 1 to 3 hours.

## INDICATIONS & DOSAGE
*As an adjunct to rest, physical therapy, and other measures for relief in short-term, acute, painful musculoskeletal conditions –*
**Adults:** initial dose is 800 mg P.O. t.i.d. Maintenance dosage is 400 mg P.O. q.i.d. for maximum of 8 weeks.

## ADVERSE REACTIONS
**CNS:** *drowsiness, dizziness,* confusion, headache, paradoxical stimulation, insomnia, nervousness.

---

*Liquid form contains alcohol. **May contain tartrazine. †Canada only. ‡Australia only. ◊OTC.

**GI:** *nausea, GI distress.*
**Hematologic:** *thrombocytopenia,* leukopenia, *agranulocytosis.*
**Other:** *anaphylaxis.*

### INTERACTIONS
*Ethanol, CNS depressants:* increased CNS depression. Avoid concomitant use.

### CONTRAINDICATIONS
Contraindicated in patients with hypersensitivity to the drug.

### NURSING CONSIDERATIONS
• Use cautiously in patients with hepatic disease or impaired renal function and in patients with hypersensitivity to aspirin because tablets contain tartrazine.
• Know that amount of relief determines if dosage (and drowsiness) can be reduced.
• Watch for sensitivity reactions, such as fever, skin eruptions, and respiratory distress. Withhold dose and notify doctor of unusual reactions.
• Monitor CBC and platelet studies in patients on long-term therapy. Watch for unusual bleeding and infections that may indicate blood dyscrasia.
• Be aware that safe use for periods over 8 weeks has not been established.

### ☑ PATIENT TEACHING
• Tell patient to take with meals or milk.
• Tell patient to avoid activities that require mental alertness, such as driving, until drug's adverse CNS effects are known.
• Advise patient to avoid combining drug with alcohol or other CNS depressants.

## chlorzoxazone
Paraflex, Parafon Forte DSC, Remular-S, Strifon Forte DSC

*Pregnancy Risk Category: NR*

### HOW SUPPLIED
*Tablets:* 250 mg, 500 mg
*Caplets:* 250 mg, 500 mg

### ACTION
Unknown. Appears to modify central perception of pain without modifying pain reflexes. Blocks interneuronal activity in descending reticular activating system and in spinal cord.

### ONSET, PEAK, DURATION
Onset occurs within 1 hour. Serum levels peak within 1 to 2 hours. Effects persist for 3 to 4 hours.

### INDICATIONS & DOSAGE
*As an adjunct in acute, painful musculoskeletal conditions –*
**Adults:** 250 to 750 mg P.O. t.i.d. or q.i.d.
**Children:** 20 mg/kg P.O. or 600 mg/$m^2$ daily in divided doses t.i.d. or q.i.d.

### ADVERSE REACTIONS
**CNS:** *drowsiness, dizziness, lightheadedness,* malaise, headache, overstimulation, tremor.
**GI:** anorexia, nausea, vomiting, heartburn, abdominal distress, constipation, diarrhea.
**GU:** urine discoloration (orange or purple-red).
**Hepatic:** hepatic dysfunction.
**Skin:** urticaria, redness, pruritus, petechiae, bruising, angioneurotic edema, *anaphylaxis.*

### INTERACTIONS
*Ethanol, CNS depressants:* increased CNS depression. Avoid concomitant use.

### CONTRAINDICATIONS
Contraindicated in patients with hypersensitivity to the drug or impaired hepatic function.

## NURSING CONSIDERATIONS
• Use cautiously in patients with history of drug allergies.
• Know that the amount of relief determines if dosage (and drowsiness) can be reduced.
• Monitor patient's liver enzyme levels, as ordered. Watch for early signs of hepatic dysfunction or abnormal liver enzyme levels. If they occur, withhold dose and notify the doctor. Serious (including fatal) hepatocellular toxicity has been reported in patients receiving this drug.

## ☑ PATIENT TEACHING
• Tell patient to take drug with meals or milk.
• Warn patient to avoid activities that require alertness until drug's CNS effects are known.
• Instruct patient to report to doctor fever, rash, anorexia, nausea, vomiting, fatigue, right upper quadrant pain, dark urine, or jaundice immediately because these may be signs of heptocellular toxicity, which warrants immediate discontinuation of drug.
• Warn patient to avoid alcohol or other CNS depressants; concomitant use with drug may increase risk of hepatocellular toxicity.
• Tell patient that the drug may discolor urine orange or purple-red.
• Advise patient to follow the doctor's orders regarding physical activity.

---

## cyclobenzaprine hydrochloride
Flexeril

*Pregnancy Risk Category: B*

## HOW SUPPLIED
*Tablets:* 10 mg

## ACTION
Unknown.

## ONSET, PEAK, DURATION
Onset occurs within 1 hour. Serum levels peak in 3 to 8 hours. Effects persist for 12 to 24 hours.

## INDICATIONS & DOSAGE
*Short-term treatment of muscle spasm —*
**Adults:** 10 mg P.O. t.i.d. for 7 days. Maximum dosage is 60 mg daily; maximum duration of treatment is 2 to 3 weeks.

## ADVERSE REACTIONS
**CNS:** *drowsiness,* headache, insomnia, fatigue, asthenia, nervousness, confusion, paresthesia, *dizziness,* depression, visual disturbances, *seizures.*
**CV:** tachycardia, syncope, arrhythmias, palpitations, hypotension, vasodilation.
**EENT:** blurred vision, *dry mouth.*
**GI:** dyspepsia, abnormal taste, constipation, nausea.
**GU:** urine retention, urinary frequency.
**Skin:** rash, urticaria, pruritus.
**Other:** with high doses, watch for adverse reactions similar to those of other tricyclic antidepressants.

## INTERACTIONS
*Anticholinergics:* additive anticholinergic effects. Avoid concomitant use.
*Ethanol, CNS depressants:* may cause additive CNS depression. Avoid concomitant use.
*MAO inhibitors:* may exacerbate CNS depression or anticholinergic effects. Don't give within 14 days after discontinuing MAO inhibitors.

## CONTRAINDICATIONS
Contraindicated in patients who have received MAO inhibitors within 14 days; during acute recovery phase of MI; and in patients with hyperthyroidism, hypersensitivity to the drug, heart block, arrhythmias, conduction disturbances, or CHF.

---

*Liquid form contains alcohol.   **May contain tartrazine.   †Canada only.   ‡Australia only.   ◇OTC.

## NURSING CONSIDERATIONS

• Use cautiously in patients with history of urine retention, acute angle-closure glaucoma, and increased intraocular pressure and in elderly or debilitated patients.
• Be alert for nausea, headache, and malaise, which may occur if drug is stopped abruptly after long-term use.
• Watch for symptoms of overdose, including possible cardiac toxicity. Notify the doctor immediately and have physostigmine available.

## ☑ PATIENT TEACHING

• Advise patient to report urinary hesitancy or urine retention. If constipation is a problem, increase fluid intake and suggest a stool softener.
• Warn patient to avoid activities that require alertness until drug's CNS effects are known.
• Warn patient not to combine with alcohol or other CNS depressants.

---

## dantrolene sodium

Dantrium, Dantrium Intravenous

*Pregnancy Risk Category: NR*

### HOW SUPPLIED

*Capsules:* 25 mg, 50 mg, 100 mg
*Injection:* 20 mg/vial

### ACTION

Acts directly on skeletal muscle to interfere with intracellular calcium movement.

### ONSET, PEAK, DURATION

Onset and duration unknown. Peak levels occur 5 hours after oral administration.

### INDICATIONS & DOSAGE

*Spasticity and sequelae secondary to severe chronic disorders (such as multiple sclerosis, cerebral palsy, spinal cord injury, CVA) –*
**Adults:** 25 mg P.O. daily. Increased gradually in 25-mg increments, up to 100 mg b.i.d. to q.i.d., to maximum of 400 mg daily.
**Children:** initially, 0.5 mg/kg P.O. b.i.d.; increased to t.i.d. then q.i.d. Dosage increased as needed by 0.5 mg/kg daily to 3 mg/kg b.i.d. to q.i.d. Maximum dosage is 100 mg q.i.d.
*Management of malignant hyperthermia crisis –*
**Adults and children:** 1 mg/kg I.V. initially; dose repeated as needed up to cumulative dosage of 10 mg/kg.
*Prevention or attenuation of malignant hyperthermia crisis in susceptible patients who require surgery –*
**Adults:** 4 to 8 mg/kg P.O. daily in three to four divided doses for 1 to 2 days before procedure. Final dose administered 3 to 4 hours before procedure.
*Prevention of recurrence of malignant hyperthermia crisis –*
**Adults:** 4 to 8 mg/kg/day P.O. in four divided doses for up to 3 days after hyperthermic crisis.

### ADVERSE REACTIONS

**CNS:** *muscle weakness, drowsiness,* dizziness, light-headedness, malaise, fatigue, headache, confusion, nervousness, insomnia, *seizures*.
**CV:** tachycardia, blood pressure changes.
**EENT:** excessive lacrimation, speech disturbance, altered taste, diplopia, visual disturbances.
**GI:** anorexia, constipation, cramping, dysphagia, metallic taste, severe diarrhea, GI bleeding.
**GU:** urinary frequency, hematuria, incontinence, nocturia, dysuria, crystalluria, difficult erection, urine retention.
**Hepatic:** *hepatitis*.
**Respiratory:** pleural effusion with pericarditis.
**Skin:** eczematous eruption, pruritus, urticaria.
**Other:** abnormal hair growth, diaphoresis, myalgia, chills, fever, back pain.

---

Reactions may be *common,* uncommon, *life-threatening,* or COMMON AND LIFE-THREATENING.

## INTERACTIONS

*Estrogens:* may increase risk of hepatotoxicity. Use together cautiously.
*Ethanol, CNS depressants:* increased CNS depression. Avoid concomitant use.
*I.V. verapamil:* may result in CV collapse. Stop verapamil before administering I.V. dantrolene.

## CONTRAINDICATIONS

Contraindicated in patients when spasticity is used to maintain motor function, in those with upper motor neuron disorders, for spasms in rheumatic disorders, in patients with active hepatic disease, and in breastfeeding patients.

## NURSING CONSIDERATIONS

• Use cautiously in patients with severely impaired cardiac or pulmonary function or preexisting hepatic disease, in women, and in patients over age 35.
• Obtain liver function tests at the beginning of therapy.
• Prepare oral suspension for single dose by dissolving capsule contents in juice or other suitable liquid. For multiple doses, use acid vehicle, such as citric acid in USP syrup; refrigerate. Use within several days.
• **I.V. use:** Give as soon as malignant hyperthermia reaction is recognized, as ordered. Reconstitute each vial by adding 60 ml of sterile water for injection and shaking vial until clear. Don't use a diluent that contains a bacteriostatic agent. Protect contents from light, and use within 6 hours. Avoid extravasation.
• Watch for hepatitis (fever and jaundice), severe diarrhea, severe weakness, or sensitivity reactions (fever and skin eruptions). Withhold dose and notify the doctor.
• Know that amount of relief in patient determines if dosage (and drowsiness) can be reduced.

## ☑ PATIENT TEACHING

• Instruct patient to take drug with meals or milk in four divided doses.
• Tell patient to use caution when eating to avoid choking. Some patients may experience difficulty swallowing during therapy.
• Warn patient to avoid driving and other hazardous activities until drug's CNS effects are known.
• Advise patient to avoid combining drug with alcohol and other CNS depressants.
• Tell patient to avoid photosensitivity reactions by using sunblock and wearing protective clothing, to report abdominal discomfort or GI problems immediately, and to follow the doctor's orders regarding rest and physical therapy.

## methocarbamol

Delaxin, Marbaxin-750, Robaxin, Robaxin-750, Robomol-500, Robomol-750

*Pregnancy Risk Category: NR*

## HOW SUPPLIED

*Tablets:* 500 mg, 750 mg
*Injection:* 100 mg/ml

## ACTION

Unknown. Probably modifies central perception of pain without modifying pain reflexes.

## ONSET, PEAK, DURATION

Onset is immediate after I.V. administration; within ½ hour after oral administration. Peak levels occur immediately after I.V. administration, or within 2 hours of an oral dose. Duration unknown.

## INDICATIONS & DOSAGE

*As an adjunct in acute, painful musculoskeletal conditions –*
**Adults:** 1.5 g P.O. q.i.d. for 2 to 3 days, then 1 g P.O. q.i.d., or not more than 500 mg (5 ml) I.M. into each glu-

teal region. Repeated q 8 hours p.r.n. Or 1 to 3 g daily (10 to 30 ml) I.V. directly into vein at 3 ml/minute, or 10 ml may be added to no more than 250 ml of D₅W or 0.9% sodium chloride solution. Maximum dosage is 3 g daily.

*Supportive therapy in tetanus management —*
**Adults:** 1 to 2 g by direct I.V. or 1 to 3 g as infusion q 6 hours.
**Children:** 15 mg/kg I.V. q 6 hours.

## ADVERSE REACTIONS
**CNS:** drowsiness, dizziness, lightheadedness, headache, syncope, mild muscular incoordination (with I.M. or I.V. use ), *seizures* (with I.V. use only), vertigo.
**CV:** hypotension, bradycardia (with I.M. or I.V. use).
**EENT:** blurred vision, conjunctivitis, nystagmus, diplopia.
**GI:** nausea, GI upset, metallic taste.
**GU:** hematuria (with I.V. use only), discoloration of urine.
**Skin:** urticaria, pruritus, rash.
**Respiratory:** thrombophlebitis.
**Other:** extravasation (with I.V. use only), fever, flushing, *anaphylactic reactions* (with I.M. or I.V. use).

## INTERACTIONS
*Ethanol, CNS depressants:* increased CNS depression. Avoid concomitant use.

## CONTRAINDICATIONS
Contraindicated in patients with hypersensitivity to the drug, impaired renal function (injectable form), or seizure disorder (injectable form).

## NURSING CONSIDERATIONS
● For nasogastric tube administration, prepare liquid by crushing tablets into water or sodium chloride solution.
● In tetanus management, be aware methocarbamol is used with tetanus antitoxin, penicillin; tracheotomy, and aggressive supportive care. Long

course of I.V. methocarbamol therapy is required.
● **I.V. use:** Dilute 10 ml of drug in not more than 250 ml of solution. Use D₅W or 0.9% sodium chloride for injection. Infuse slowly; maximum rate is 300 mg(3 ml)/minute.
● Know that drug irritates veins; may cause phlebitis, aggravate seizures, and cause fainting if injected rapidly. Make sure the patient remains in a supine position during infusion. Drug is an irritant; avoid extravasation.
● Give I.M. deeply, only into upper outer quadrant of buttocks, with maximum of 5 ml in each buttock.
● Do not give S.C.
● Watch for orthostatic hypotension, especially with parenteral administration. Keep the patient in a supine position for 15 minutes afterward, and supervise ambulation. Have patient get up slowly.
● Watch for sensitivity reactions, such as fever and skin eruptions.
● Have epinephrine, antihistamines, and corticosteroids available.
● Monitor CBC periodically during prolonged therapy.
● Know that drug may interfere with urine tests for 5-hydroxyindoleacetic acid and vanillylmandelic acid.

## ☑ PATIENT TEACHING
● Instruct patient to take drug with food or milk.
● Tell patient that urine may turn green, black, or brown.
● Advise patient to follow the doctor's orders regarding physical activity.
● Warn patient to avoid activities that require alertness until drug's CNS effects are known.
● Advise patient to avoid combining drug with alcohol or other CNS depressants.

---

Reactions may be *common,* uncommon, *life-threatening,* or **COMMON AND LIFE-THREATENING.**

## orphenadrine citrate
Banflex, Flexoject, Flexon, K-Flex, Marflex, Myolin, Neocyten, Noradex, Norflex, O-Flex, Orflagen, Orphenate

*Pregnancy Risk Category: NR*

### HOW SUPPLIED
*Tablets:* 100 mg
*Tablets (extended-release):* 100 mg
*Injection:* 30 mg/ml

### ACTION
Unknown. Appears to modify central perception of pain without modifying pain reflexes. Blocks interneuronal activity in descending reticular activating system and in spinal cord.

### ONSET, PEAK, DURATION
Onset occurs immediately with I.V. use, within 5 minutes of I.M. injection, or within 1 hour of oral administration. Peak levels occur immediately after I.V. infusion, within 30 minutes of I.M. injection, within 2 hours of tablet ingestion, or within 6 to 8 hours of extended-release tablet ingestion. Duration unknown.

### INDICATIONS & DOSAGE
*Adjunctive treatment in painful, acute musculoskeletal conditions –*
**Adults:** 100 mg P.O. b.i.d., or 60 mg I.V. or I.M. q 12 hours, p.r.n. For maintenance therapy, patient switched to oral therapy beginning 12 hours after last parenteral dose.

### ADVERSE REACTIONS
**CNS:** weakness, *drowsiness,* lightheadedness, confusion, agitation, tremor, headache, dizziness, hallucinations.
**CV:** palpitations, tachycardia, syncope.
**EENT:** dilated pupils, blurred vision, difficulty swallowing, increased intraocular pressure.
**GI:** constipation, *dry mouth,* nausea, vomiting, epigastric distress.
**GU:** urinary hesitancy or retention.
**Hematologic:** *aplastic anemia.*
**Skin:** urticaria, pruritus.
**Other:** *anaphylaxis.*

### INTERACTIONS
*Ethanol, CNS depressants, propoxyphene:* increased CNS depression. Avoid concomitant use.

### CONTRAINDICATIONS
Contraindicated in those with hypersensitivity to drug; glaucoma; prostatic hyperplasia; pyloric, duodenal, or bladder-neck obstruction; myasthenia gravis; and peptic ulceration.

### NURSING CONSIDERATIONS
• Use cautiously in elderly or debilitated patients or in those with tachycardia, cardiac disease, arrhythmias, or sulfite sensitivity.
• *Alert:* Check all dosages carefully; a slight overdose can lead to toxicity. Early signs are excessive dry mouth, dilated pupils, blurred vision, skin flushing, and fever.
• **I.V. use:** Inject drug over approximately 5 minutes while the patient is supine. Wait 5 to 10 minutes and then help the patient to sit up.
• When given I.V., assess for paradoxical initial bradycardia; usually disappears in 2 minutes.
• Monitor CBC, hepatic function, and urinalysis in patients receiving long-term therapy as ordered.
• Monitor vital signs carefully.

### ☑ PATIENT TEACHING
• Have patient report urinary hesitancy and urine retention. Tell patient to void before taking the drug.
• Tell him to relieve dry mouth with cool drinks, sugarless gum or hard candy.
• Warn patient to avoid tasks that require alertness until drug's CNS effects are known.
• Advise patient not to combine with alcohol or other CNS depressants.

---

*Liquid form contains alcohol.  **May contain tartrazine.  †Canada only.  ‡Australia only.  ◇OTC.

# 42

## Neuromuscular blockers

atracurium besylate
cisatracurium besylate
doxacurium chloride
metocurine iodide
mivacurium chloride
pancuronium bromide
pipecuronium bromide
rocuronium bromide
succinylcholine chloride
tubocurarine chloride
vecuronium bromide

**COMBINATION PRODUCTS**
None.

---

## atracurium besylate
Tracrium

*Pregnancy Risk Category: C*

### HOW SUPPLIED
*Injection:* 10 mg/ml

### ACTION
Prevents acetylcholine from binding to receptors on muscle end plate, thus blocking depolarization.

### ONSET, PEAK, DURATION
Onset occurs in 2 minutes. Peak occurs in 3 to 5 minutes. About 25% of muscle twitch strength returns in 35 to 45 minutes; 95% in 60 to 70 minutes.

### INDICATIONS & DOSAGE
*Adjunct to general anesthesia to facilitate endotracheal intubation and to provide skeletal muscle relaxation during surgery or mechanical ventilation* –
Dosage depends on anesthetic used, individual needs, and response. Dosages given here are representative only.
**Adults and children over 2 years:**
0.4 to 0.5 mg/kg by I.V. bolus. Maintenance dosage of 0.08 to 0.10 mg/kg within 20 to 45 minutes should be

given during prolonged surgery. Maintenance dosages may be given q 12 to 25 minutes in patients receiving balanced anesthesia. For prolonged procedures, a constant infusion of 5 to 9 mcg/kg/minute may be used.
**Children 1 month to 2 years:** initial dose, 0.3 to 0.4 mg/kg. Frequent maintenance doses may be needed.

### ADVERSE REACTIONS
**CV:** bradycardia, hypotension, tachycardia.
**Respiratory:** *prolonged dose-related apnea,* wheezing, increased bronchial secretions, dyspnea, bronchospasm, laryngospasm.
**Skin:** *skin flushing,* erythema, pruritus, urticaria, rash.
**Other:** *anaphylaxis.*

### INTERACTIONS
*Aminoglycoside antibiotics (amikacin, gentamicin, kanamycin, neomycin, streptomycin); polymyxin antibiotics (polymyxin B sulfate, colistin); clindamycin; quinidine; general anesthetics (halothane, enflurane, isoflurane):* potentiated neuromuscular blockade, leading to increased skeletal muscle relaxation and prolonged effect. Use cautiously during and after surgery.
*Lithium, magnesium salts, opioid analgesics:* potentiated neuromuscular blockade, leading to increased skeletal muscle relaxation and possible respiratory paralysis. Reduce dose of atracurium.

### CONTRAINDICATIONS
Contraindicated in patients with hypersensitivity to the drug.

---

Reactions may be *common,* uncommon, *life-threatening,* or COMMON AND LIFE-THREATENING.

## NURSING CONSIDERATIONS

• Use cautiously in those with CV disease; severe electrolyte disorder; bronchogenic carcinoma; hepatic, renal, or pulmonary impairment; neuromuscular disease; or myasthenia gravis and in elderly or debilitated patients.

• Administer sedatives or general anesthetics before neuromuscular blockers, which don't obtund consciousness or alter pain threshold.

• Administer analgesics, as ordered, for pain. Remember that patient may have pain but not be able to express it.

• Use this drug only under direct medical supervision by personnel skilled in the use of neuromuscular blockers and techniques for maintaining a patent airway. Have emergency respiratory support equipment (endotracheal equipment, ventilator, oxygen, atropine, edrophonium, neostigmine, and epinephrine) available.

• **I.V. use:** Drug usually is administered by rapid I.V. bolus injection but may be given by intermittent infusion or continuous infusion. At concentrations of 0.2 mg/ml to 0.5 mg/ml, atracurium is compatible for 24 hours in $D_5W$, 0.9% sodium chloride for injection, or dextrose 5% in 0.9% sodium chloride for injection.

• Do not use lactated Ringer's solution. In lactated Ringer's injection, atracurium is stable for 8 hours at a concentration of 0.5 mg/ml. However, because of increased degradation in this solution, it is not recommended.

• Do not give by I.M. injection.

• Do not mix with acidic or alkaline solutions (precipitate may form).

• Once spontaneous recovery starts, be prepared to reverse atracurium-induced neuromuscular blockade with an anticholinesterase agent (such as neostigmine or edrophonium), as ordered. Usually given together with an anticholinergic (such as atropine).

• Monitor respirations closely until patient is fully recovered from neuromuscular blockade, as evidenced by tests of muscle strength (hand grip, head lift, and ability to cough).

• A nerve stimulator and train-of-four monitoring are recommended to confirm antagonism of neuromuscular blockade and recovery of muscle strength. Evidence of spontaneous recovery should be seen before attempting reversal with neostigmine.

• Know that prior administration of succinylcholine doesn't prolong duration of action but quickens onset and may deepen neuromuscular blockade.

## ☑ PATIENT TEACHING

• Explain all events and procedures to the patient because he can still hear.

• Answer the family's questions.

▼ *NEW DRUG*

## cisatracurium besylate
Nimbex

*Pregnancy Risk Category: B*

### HOW SUPPLIED
*Injection:* 2 mg/ml, 10 mg/ml

### ACTION
A nondepolarizing agent that binds to cholinergic receptors on the motor end plate, antagonizing acetylcholine and blocking neuromuscular transmission.

### ONSET, PEAK, DURATION
Onset occurs in 1 to 3.3 minutes. Peak levels occur in 2 to 5 minutes. About 95% of muscle twitch strength returns in 46 to 121 minutes.

### INDICATIONS & DOSAGE
*Adjunct to general anesthesia, to facilitate tracheal intubation, and to provide skeletal muscle relaxation during surgery or mechanical ventilation in ICU –*
**Adults:** 0.15 mg/kg I.V., followed by 0.03 mg/kg I.V. q 40 to 50 minutes (or 0.20 mg/kg I.V., followed by 0.03 mg/kg I.V. q 50 to 60 minutes). Alterna-

tively, after initial dose, a maintenance infusion may be given at 3 mcg/kg/minute, reduced to 1 to 2 mcg/kg/minute as needed.

**Children 2 to 12 years:** 0.1 mg/kg I.V. over 5 to 10 seconds. After initial dose, a maintenance infusion may be given at 3 mcg/kg/minute, reduced to 1 to 2 mcg/kg/minute as needed.

*Maintenance of neuromuscular blockade in ICU –*

**Adults and children 2 to 12 years:** 3 mcg/kg/minute (range: 0.5 to 10.2 mcg/kg/minute) I.V. infusion.

**Note:** Dosage requirements vary widely among patients.

## ADVERSE REACTIONS

**CV:** bradycardia, hypotension.
**Respiratory:** bronchospasm.
**Skin:** flushing, rash.

## INTERACTIONS

*Aminoglycosides, bacitracin, clindamycin, colistin, lincomycin, lithium, local anesthetics, magnesium salts, polymyxins, procainamide, quinidine, tetracyclines, sodium colistemethate:* may enhance neuromuscular blocking action of cisatracurium. Use together cautiously.

*Carbamazepine, phenytoin:* may cause slightly shorter duration of neuromuscular block, requiring higher infusion rate. Monitor closely.

*Isoflurane or enflurane administered with nitrous oxide/oxygen:* may prolong duration of action of cisatracurium. Be aware that patient may require less frequent maintenance dosing, lower maintenance doses, or reduced infusion rate of cisatracurium.

## CONTRAINDICATIONS

Contraindicated in patients with hypersensitivity to drug, other bis-benzylisoquinolinium agents, or benzyl alcohol.

## NURSING CONSIDERATIONS

• Drug is not recommended for rapid-sequence endotracheal intubation because of its intermediate onset.

• Use cautiously in pregnant or breast-feeding women.

• Cisatracurium has no known effect on consciousness, pain threshold, or cerebration. To avoid patient distress, neuromuscular block should not be induced before unconsciousness.

• **I.V. use:** 20-ml vial is intended for ICU use only. Drug is not compatible with propofol injection or ketorolac injection for Y-site administration. Drug is acidic and may not be compatible with an alkaline solution having a pH greater than 8.5 (such as barbiturate solutions for Y-site administration). Drug should not be diluted in lactated Ringer's injection because of chemical instability.

• Drug is colorless to slightly yellow or green-yellow. Inspect vials for particulate and discoloration before administration. Unclear solutions or those with visible particulate should not be used.

• Neuromuscular function should be monitored with a nerve stimulator during administration. If nerve stimulation does not elicit a definite response, infusion should be discontinued until a response returns.

• To avoid inaccurate dosing, neuromuscular monitoring should be performed on a nonparetic limb in patients with hemiparesis or paraparesis.

• In patients with neuromuscular disease (myasthenia gravis and myasthenic syndrome), prolonged neuromuscular block is possible. Use of a peripheral nerve stimulator and a dose of not more than 0.02 mg/kg is recommended to assess the level of neuromuscular block and to monitor dosage requirements.

• Because patients with burns have been shown to develop resistance to nondepolarizing neuromuscular blocking agents, they may require increased dosing. Monitor closely.

---

Reactions may be *common,* uncommon, *life-threatening,* or COMMON AND LIFE-THREATENING.

• Monitor acid-base balance and electrolyte levels, as ordered. Abnormalities may potentiate or antagonize the action of cisatracurium.
• Monitor patient for malignant hyperthermia.
• Administer analgesics, if appropriate. Although the patient can feel pain, he cannot indicate its presence.

☑ **PATIENT TEACHING**
• Explain the drug's purpose.
• Assure the patient that he will be monitored continuously.
• Explain all procedures and events; the drug does not interfere with the patient's ability to hear.

---

## doxacurium chloride
Nuromax

*Pregnancy Risk Category: C*

### HOW SUPPLIED
*Injection:* 1 mg/ml

### ACTION
A nondepolarizing neuromuscular blocking agent that competes with acetylcholine for receptor sites at the motor end plate; because this action may be antagonized by cholinesterase inhibitors, doxacurium is considered a competitive antagonist.

### ONSET, PEAK, DURATION
Onset occurs within 5 minutes. Peak effects are dose-dependent and occur within 3 to 9 minutes. Effects persist for 1 to 4 hours.

### INDICATIONS & DOSAGE
*To provide skeletal muscle relaxation during surgery as an adjunct to general anesthesia –*
Dosage is highly individualized. All times of onset and duration are averages; considerable individual variation is normal.
**Adults:** 0.05 mg/kg rapid I.V. produces adequate conditions for endotracheal intubation in 5 minutes in about 90% of patients when used as part of a thiopental-narcotic induction technique. Lower doses may require longer delay before intubation is possible. Neuromuscular blockade at this dose lasts for an average of 100 minutes.
**Children over 2 years:** an initial dose of 0.03 mg/kg I.V. given during halothane anesthesia produces effective blockade in 7 minutes with duration of 30 minutes. Under the same conditions, 0.05 mg/kg produces blockade in 4 minutes with duration of 45 minutes.
*Maintenance of neuromuscular blockade during long procedures –*
**Adults and children:** after initial dose of 0.5 mg/kg I.V., maintenance doses of 0.005 to 0.01 mg/kg will prolong neuromuscular blockade for an average of 30 minutes. Children usually require more frequent administration of maintenance doses.

### ADVERSE REACTIONS
**Respiratory:** dyspnea, respiratory depression, *respiratory insufficiency or apnea.*
**Other:** prolonged muscle weakness.

### INTERACTIONS
*Alkaline solutions (such as barbiturate solutions):* physically incompatible; precipitate may form. Do not administer through same I.V. line.
*Aminoglycosides (gentamicin, kanamycin, neomycin, and streptomycin), bacitracin, colistimethate, colistin, polymyxin B, tetracyclines:* potentiated neuromuscular blockade leading to increased skeletal muscle relaxation and prolonged effect. Use together cautiously.
*Carbamazepine, phenytoin:* may prolong the time to maximal block or shorten the duration of block with neuromuscular blockers.
*Inhalation anesthetics, quinidine:* may enhance or prolong action of nondepolarizing neuromuscular blockers.
*Magnesium salts:* may enhance neuro-

---

*Liquid form contains alcohol.   **May contain tartrazine.   †Canada only.   ‡Australia only.   ◊OTC.

muscular blockade. Monitor for excessive weakness.

## CONTRAINDICATIONS

Contraindicated in patients with hypersensitivity to the drug and in neonates. The drug contains benzyl ethanol, which has been associated with fatalities in newborns.

## NURSING CONSIDERATIONS

• Use cautiously, possibly at reduced dosage, in debilitated patients; in patients with metastatic cancer, severe electrolyte disturbances, or neuromuscular diseases; and in those in whom potentiation or difficulty in reversal of neuromuscular blockade is anticipated. Patients with myasthenia gravis or myasthenic syndrome (Eaton-Lambert syndrome) are particularly sensitive to the effects of nondepolarizing relaxants. Shorter-acting agents are recommended for use in such patients.

• Because of the lack of data supporting the drug's safety, be aware that it is not recommended for use in patients requiring prolonged mechanical ventilation in the intensive care unit, before or after administration of nondepolarizing neuromuscular blocking agents, or during cesarean section.

• Use drug only under direct medical supervision by personnel skilled in the use of neuromuscular blockers and techniques for maintaining a patent airway. Do not use unless facilities and equipment for mechanical ventilation, oxygen therapy, and intubation and an antagonist are within reach.

• To avoid distress to the patient, do not give the drug until the patient's consciousness is obtunded by general anesthetic. Doxacurium has no effect on consciousness or pain threshold.

• Drug is not metabolized; it is excreted in urine and bile. Patients with renal or hepatic insufficiency may require dosage adjustment.

• Keep in mind that the dosage should be adjusted to ideal body weight in obese patients (patients 30% or more above their ideal weight) to avoid prolonged neuromuscular blockade.

• Know that higher initial doses may be required in patients with severe burns and in some patients with severe liver disease. Higher doses (0.8 mg/kg) will produce intubating conditions more rapidly (4 minutes), with neuromuscular blockade for 160 minutes or more. Consequently, these higher doses should be reserved for long procedures. Administration during steady-state anesthesia with enflurane, halothane, or isoflurane may allow 33% reduction of dose.

• **I.V. use:** Prepare drug for I.V. use with $D_5W$, 0.9% sodium chloride for injection, dextrose 5% in 0.9% sodium chloride for injection, lactated Ringer's injection, and dextrose 5% in lactated Ringer's injection.

• When diluted as directed, remember that doxacurium is compatible with alfentanil, fentanyl, and sufentanil.

• Recommend that the product be administered immediately after reconstitution. Diluted solutions are stable for 24 hours at room temperature; however, because reconstitution dilutes the preservative, risk of contamination increases. Unused solutions should be discarded after 8 hours.

• Be aware that a nerve stimulator and train-of-four monitoring are recommended to document antagonism of neuromuscular blockade and recovery of muscle strength. Before attempting pharmacologic reversal with neostigmine, some evidence of spontaneous recovery should be present.

• Because the drug has minimal vagolytic action, monitor for bradycardia, which may occur during anesthesia.

• Monitor respirations until the patient is fully recovered from neuromuscular blockade, as evidenced by tests of muscle strength (hand grip, head lift, and ability to cough).

• Know that experimental evidence suggests that acid-base and electrolyte

---

balance may influence the actions of nondepolarizing neuromuscular blockers. Alkalosis may counteract paralysis; acidosis may enhance it.

☑ **PATIENT TEACHING**
• Inform the patient of need for drug.
• Reassure the patient and family that he'll be monitored at all times.

## metocurine iodide
Metubine Iodide
*Pregnancy Risk Category: C*

### HOW SUPPLIED
*Injection:* 2 mg/ml

### ACTION
Prevents acetylcholine from binding to receptors on the muscle end plate, thus blocking depolarization.

### ONSET, PEAK, DURATION
Onset occurs in 1 to 4 minutes. Peak effects occur in 3 to 5 minutes. Effects persist for 35 to 60 minutes; may take more than 6 hours for more than 50% of muscle twitch strength to return.

### INDICATIONS & DOSAGE
*Adjunct to anesthesia to induce skeletal muscle relaxation; to facilitate intubation, reduction of fractures and dislocations –*
**Adults:** 0.2 to 0.4 mg/kg for endotracheal intubation; supplemented with 0.5 to 1 mg for further relaxation.
*To lessen muscle contractions in pharmacologically or electrically induced seizures –*
**Adults:** 1.75 to 5.5 mg I.V.

### ADVERSE REACTIONS
**CV:** hypotension secondary to histamine release, ganglionic blockade and histamine release, arrhythmias, *cardiac arrest,* bradycardia.
**Respiratory:** *dose-related prolonged apnea, bronchospasm.*
**Other:** residual muscle weakness, in-

creased oropharyngeal secretions, allergic or idiosyncratic hypersensitivity reactions.

### INTERACTIONS
*Alkaline solutions, such as barbiturates, meperidine, or morphine:* instability when combined in same syringe. Do not administer in same syringe.
*Aminoglycoside antibiotics (including amikacin, gentamicin, kanamycin, neomycin, streptomycin); polymyxin antibiotics (polymyxin B sulfate, colistin); clindamycin; quinidine; general anesthetics (such as halothane, enflurane, isoflurane); furosemide; thiazide diuretics; beta-adrenergic blockers:* potentiated neuromuscular blockade, leading to increased skeletal muscle relaxation and possible respiratory paralysis. Use cautiously during and after surgery.
*Opioid analgesics:* potentiated neuromuscular blockade, leading to increased skeletal muscle relaxation and possible respiratory paralysis. Use with extreme caution, and reduce dose of metocurine iodide.

### CONTRAINDICATIONS
Contraindicated in patients with hypersensitivity to iodides or in whom histamine release is a hazard (asthmatic or atopic patients).

### NURSING CONSIDERATIONS
• Use cautiously in elderly or debilitated patients. Also use cautiously in patients with cardiac, renal, hepatic, or pulmonary impairment; respiratory depression; myasthenia gravis; myasthenic syndrome of lung cancer or bronchogenic cancer; dehydration; thyroid disorders; collagen diseases; porphyria; electrolyte disturbances; hyperthermia; hypotension; or shock. Also use large doses cautiously in patients undergoing cesarean section.
• Know that metocurine should only be used by personnel skilled in airway management.
• Administer sedatives or general an-

esthetics before neuromuscular blockers, as ordered. Neuromuscular blockers do not obtund consciousness or alter pain threshold.
• Keep airway clear. Have emergency respiratory support equipment (endotracheal equipment, ventilator, oxygen, atropine, edrophonium, epinephrine, and neostigmine) available.
• I.V. use: Give by direct I.V. injection over 30 to 90 seconds. Dosage depends on anesthetic used, individual needs, and response. Dosages given are representative and must be adjusted. Administer as sustained injection over 30 to 60 seconds. Adults given cyclopropane, 2 to 4 mg I.V. (2.68 mg average); ether, 1.5 to 3 mg I.V. (2.1 mg average); nitrous oxide, 4 to 7 mg I.V. (4.79 mg average) with supplemental injections of 0.5 to 1 mg in 25 to 90 minutes, repeated p.r.n.
• Do not administer I.M.
• Store solution away from heat and sunlight. Do not mix with barbiturates (precipitate will form). Use fresh solutions only.
• Know that a nerve stimulator and train-of-four monitoring are recommended to document antagonism of neuromuscular blockade and recovery of muscle strength. Before attempting pharmacologic reversal with neostigmine, some evidence of spontaneous recovery should be seen.
• Monitor baseline electrolyte determinations (electrolyte imbalance, especially potassium, calcium, and magnesium levels as ordered, can potentiate neuromuscular effects) and vital signs, especially respirations.
• Monitor respirations closely until patient is fully recovered from neuromuscular blockade, as evidenced by tests of muscle strength (hand grip, head lift, and ability to cough).
• Measure fluid intake and output; renal dysfunction prolongs duration of action because drug is mainly unchanged before excretion.
• Give analgesics, as ordered, for pain.

☑ **PATIENT TEACHING**
• Explain all events and procedures to the patient because he can still hear.
• Answer the family's questions.

# mivacurium chloride
Mivacron

*Pregnancy Risk Category: C*

## HOW SUPPLIED
*Injection:* 2 mg/ml in 5-ml and 10-ml vials
*Infusion:* 0.5 mg/ml in 50 ml of $D_5W$

## ACTION
Competes with acetylcholine for receptor sites at the motor end plate. Because this action may be antagonized by cholinesterase inhibitors, mivacurium is considered a competitive antagonist. The drug is a mixture of three stereoisomers, each possessing neuromuscular blocking activity.

## ONSET, PEAK, DURATION
Onset occurs within 1 to 2 minutes. Peak effects occur in 2 to 5 minutes. 95% muscle twitch strength recovery within 20 to 35 minutes.

## INDICATIONS & DOSAGE
*Adjunct to general anesthesia, to facilitate endotracheal intubation, and to relax skeletal muscles during surgery or mechanical ventilation –*
**Adults:** dosage is highly individualized. Usually, 0.15 mg/kg I.V. push over 5 to 15 seconds provides adequate muscle relaxation within 2½ minutes for endotracheal intubation. Supplemental doses of 0.1 mg/kg I.V. q 15 minutes are usually sufficient to maintain muscle relaxation.
    Alternatively, maintain neuromuscular blockade with a continuous infusion of 4 mcg/kg/minute begun simultaneously with the initial dose, or 9 to 10 mcg/kg/minute started after spontaneous recovery caused by the initial dose is evident. When used with iso-

---

Reactions may be *common,* uncommon, *life-threatening,* or COMMON AND LIFE-THREATENING.

flurane or enflurane anesthesia, dosage usually is reduced about 25%.

**Children 2 to 12 years:** 0.20 mg/kg I.V. push administered over 5 to 15 seconds. Neuromuscular blockade is usually evident in less than 2 minutes. Maintenance doses are generally required more frequently in children.

Alternatively, neuromuscular blockade can be maintained with a continuous I.V. infusion titrated to effect. Most children respond to 5 to 31 mcg/kg/minute (average 14 mcg/kg/minute).

## ADVERSE REACTIONS
**CNS:** dizziness.
**CV:** *flushing,* tachycardia, bradycardia, arrhythmias, hypotension.
**Respiratory:** *bronchospasm,* wheezing, *respiratory insufficiency or apnea.*
**Skin:** rash, urticaria, erythema.
**Other:** prolonged muscle weakness, phlebitis, muscle spasms.

## INTERACTIONS
*Alkaline solutions (such as barbiturate solutions):* physically incompatible; precipitate may form. Do not administer through the same I.V. line.
*Aminoglycosides (gentamicin, kanamycin, neomycin, and streptomycin), bacitracin, colistin, colistimethate, polymyxin B sulfate, tetracyclines:* potentiated neuromuscular blockade, leading to increased skeletal muscle relaxation and prolonged effect. Use together cautiously.
*Carbamazepine, phenytoin:* may prolong the time to maximal blockade or shorten the duration of blockade with neuromuscular blockers.
*Inhalation anesthetics (especially isoflurane or enflurane), quinidine:* may enhance or prolong action of nondepolarizing neuromuscular blockers. Monitor for excessive weakness.
*Magnesium salts:* may enhance neuromuscular blockade. Monitor for excessive weakness.

## CONTRAINDICATIONS
Contraindicated in patients with hypersensitivity to the drug.

## NURSING CONSIDERATIONS
● Use cautiously in patients with significant CV disease and in patients who may be adversely affected by release of histamine (such as asthmatic patients). To avoid hypotension, initial dose of the drug should be lower or drug should be given over longer period (60 seconds).
● Also use cautiously, possibly at reduced dosage, in debilitated patients; in patients with metastatic cancer, severe electrolyte disturbances, or neuromuscular diseases; and in those in whom potentiation or difficulty in reversal of neuromuscular blockade is anticipated. Patients with myasthenia gravis or myasthenic syndrome (Eaton-Lambert syndrome) are particularly sensitive to effects of nondepolarizing relaxants. Test dose of 0.015 to 0.020 mg/kg may be used to assess the patient's sensitivity to the drug.
● *Alert:* Use very cautiously, if at all, in patients who are homozygous for the atypical plasma pseudocholinesterase gene. Drug is metabolized to inactive compound by plasma pseudocholinesterase.
● Use only under direct medical supervision by personnel skilled in the use of neuromuscular blockers and techniques for maintaining a patent airway. Do not use unless facilities and equipment for artificial respiration, mechanical ventilation, oxygen therapy, and intubation and an antagonist are within reach.
● To avoid patient distress, do not administer until the patient's consciousness is obtunded by the general anesthetic because drug has no effect on consciousness or pain threshold.
● Administer a test dose to assess the patient's sensitivity to the drug. Patients with severe burns are known to develop resistance to nondepolarizing

---

neuromuscular blockers; however, they also may have reduced plasma pseudocholinesterase activity.
- Keep in mind that dosage should be adjusted to ideal body weight in obese patients (patients 30% or more above their ideal weight) to avoid prolonged neuromuscular blockade.
- Be aware that like other neuromuscular blockers, dosage requirements for children are higher on a mg/kg basis than those for adults. Onset and recovery of neuromuscular blockade occur more rapidly in children.
- **I.V. use:** Prepare drug for I.V. use with D$_5$W, 0.9% sodium chloride for injection, dextrose 5% in 0.9% sodium chloride for injection, lactated Ringer's injection, and dextrose 5% in lactated Ringer's injection. Diluted solutions are stable for 24 hours at room temperature.
- Remember that when diluted as directed, mivacurium is compatible with alfentanil, fentanyl, sufentanil, droperidol, and midazolam.
- For drug available as premixed infusion in D$_5$W, remove the protective outer wrap, then check container for minor leaks by squeezing the bag before administering. Do not add any other drugs to the container, and do not use the container in series connections.
- A nerve stimulator and train-of-four monitoring are recommended to document antagonism of neuromuscular blockade and recovery of muscle strength. Before attempting pharmacologic reversal with neostigmine or edrophonium, some signs of spontaneous recovery should be evident.
- Monitor respirations closely until patient is fully recovered from neuromuscular blockade, as evidenced by tests of muscle strength (hand grip, head lift, and ability to cough).
- Know that experimental evidence suggests that acid-base and electrolyte balances may influence the actions of nondepolarizing neuromuscular

blockers. Alkalosis may counteract the paralysis; acidosis may enhance it.
- Know that duration of drug effect is increased about 150% in patients with end-stage renal disease and 300% in patients with hepatic dysfunction.

☑ **PATIENT TEACHING**
- Explain the drug's purpose.
- Reassure the patient and family that he'll be monitored at all times.

---

## pancuronium bromide
Pavulon

*Pregnancy Risk Category: C*

**HOW SUPPLIED**
*Injection:* 1 mg/ml, 2 mg/ml

**ACTION**
Prevents acetylcholine from binding to receptors on the muscle end plate, thus blocking depolarization.

**ONSET, PEAK, DURATION**
Onset occurs in 30 to 45 seconds. Peak effects occur in 3 to 4½ minutes. Effects persist for 35 to 45 minutes; 90% of muscle twitch strength returns within 1 hour.

**INDICATIONS & DOSAGE**
*Adjunct to anesthesia to induce skeletal muscle relaxation; to facilitate intubation; to lessen muscle contractions in pharmacologically or electrically induced seizures; to assist with mechanical ventilation —*
Dosage depends on anesthetic used, individual needs, and response. Dosages are representative only.
**Adults and children 1 month and over:** initially, 0.04 to 0.1 mg/kg I.V.; then 0.01 mg/kg q 30 to 60 minutes.
**Neonates:** individualized.

**ADVERSE REACTIONS**
**CV:** tachycardia, increased blood pressure.

**Respiratory:** *prolonged, dose-related respiratory insufficiency or apnea.*
**Skin:** transient rashes.
**Other:** excessive salivation, residual muscle weakness, allergic or idiosyncratic hypersensitivity reactions.

## INTERACTIONS
*Aminoglycoside antibiotics (including amikacin, gentamicin, kanamycin, neomycin, streptomycin); polymyxin antibiotics (polymyxin B sulfate, colistin); clindamycin; lincomycin; quinidine; general anesthetics (such as halothane, enflurane, isoflurane):* potentiated neuromuscular blockade, leading to increased skeletal muscle relaxation and prolonged effect. Use cautiously during surgical and postoperative periods.
*Lithium, opioid analgesics:* potentiated neuromuscular blockade, leading to increased skeletal muscle relaxation and possible respiratory paralysis. Use with extreme caution, and reduce dose of pancuronium.
*Succinylcholine:* increased intensity and duration of neuromuscular blockade. Allow effects of succinylcholine to subside before administering pancuronium.

## CONTRAINDICATIONS
Contraindicated in patients with hypersensitivity to bromides or preexisting tachycardia and in patients for whom even a minor increase in heart rate is undesirable.

## NURSING CONSIDERATIONS
• Use cautiously in elderly or debilitated patients; in patients with renal, hepatic, or pulmonary impairment; and in those with respiratory depression, myasthenia gravis, myasthenic syndrome of lung cancer or bronchogenic carcinoma, dehydration, thyroid disorders, collagen diseases, porphyria, electrolyte disturbances, hyperthermia, and toxemic states. Also use large doses cautiously in patients undergoing cesarean section.

• Administer sedatives or general anesthetics before neuromuscular blockers, as ordered. Neuromuscular blockers do not obtund consciousness or alter the pain threshold.
• Know that pancuronium should be used only by personnel skilled in airway management.
• Have emergency respiratory support equipment (endotracheal equipment, ventilator, oxygen, atropine, edrophonium, epinephrine, and neostigmine) immediately available.
• **I.V. use:** Do not mix with alkaline solutions, such as barbiturate solutions, because precipitate will form; use only fresh solutions.
• Allow succinylcholine effects to subside before giving pancuronium.
• Store in refrigerator. Do not store in plastic containers or syringes, although plastic syringes may be used for administration.
• Monitor baseline electrolyte determinations (electrolyte imbalance can potentiate neuromuscular effects) and vital signs, especially respirations and heart rate.
• Measure fluid intake and output; renal dysfunction may prolong duration of action because 25% of the drug is unchanged before excretion.
• Keep in mind that a nerve stimulator and train-of-four monitoring are recommended to confirm antagonism of neuromuscular blockade and recovery of muscle strength. Before attempting pharmacologic reversal with neostigmine, some evidence of spontaneous recovery should be seen.
• Monitor respirations closely until patient is fully recovered from neuromuscular blockade, as evidenced by tests of muscle strength (hand grip, head lift, and ability to cough).
• Once spontaneous recovery starts, pancuronium-induced neuromuscular blockade may be reversed with an anticholinesterase agent (such as neostigmine or edrophonium), which is

usually administered with an anticholinergic (such as atropine).
● Know that drug does not cause histamine release or hypotension but may raise heart rate and blood pressure.
● Give analgesics, as ordered, for pain.

☑ **PATIENT TEACHING**
● Explain all events and procedures to the patient because he can still hear.
● Answer the family's questions.

## pipecuronium bromide
Arduan

*Pregnancy Risk Category: C*

### HOW SUPPLIED
*Powder for injection:* 10-mg vial

### ACTION
A nondepolarizing neuromuscular blocking agent that competes with acetylcholine for receptor sites at the motor end plate. Because this action may be antagonized by cholinesterase inhibitors, pipecuronium is considered a competitive antagonist.

### ONSET, PEAK, DURATION
Onset occurs in 1 to 2 minutes. Peak effects occur within 5 minutes; 25% to 50% of muscle twitch strength returns within 24 minutes.

### INDICATIONS & DOSAGE
*To provide skeletal muscle relaxation during surgery as adjunct to general anesthesia —*
Dosage is highly individualized. The following doses may serve as a guide for use in nonobese patients with normal renal function.
**Adults and children:** initially, 70 to 85 mcg/kg I.V. provides conditions considered ideal for endotracheal intubation and maintains paralysis for 1 to 2 hours. If succinylcholine is used for endotracheal intubation, initial dose of 50 mcg/kg I.V. provides good relaxation for 45 minutes or more. Maintenance dose of 10 to 15 mcg/kg provides relaxation for about 50 minutes.

### ADVERSE REACTIONS
**CV:** hypotension, bradycardia, hypertension, myocardial ischemia, *CVA,* thrombosis, atrial fibrillation, *ventricular extrasystole.*
**GU:** anuria.
**Respiratory:** dyspnea, respiratory depression, *respiratory insufficiency or apnea.*
**Skin:** rash, urticaria.
**Other:** prolonged muscle weakness, increased creatinine levels.

### INTERACTIONS
*Aminoglycosides (gentamicin, kanamycin, neomycin, and streptomycin), bacitracin, colistimethate, colistin, polymyxin B sulfate, tetracyclines:* potentiated neuromuscular blockade, leading to increased skeletal muscle relaxation and prolonged effect. Use together cautiously.
*Inhalation anesthetics, quinidine:* enhances or prolongs action of nondepolarizing neuromuscular blockers.
*Magnesium salts:* may enhance neuromuscular blockade. Monitor for excessive weakness.

### CONTRAINDICATIONS
Contraindicated in patients with hypersensitivity to the drug.

### NURSING CONSIDERATIONS
● Use cautiously and with dosage adjustments in patients with renal failure because the drug is excreted by the kidneys. No information is available regarding use of the drug in patients with hepatic disease.
● Because of the lack of data supporting the drug's safety, know that it is not recommended for use in patients requiring prolonged mechanical ventilation in the intensive care unit, before or after administration of other nondepolarizing neuromuscular blockers, or during cesarean section.

---

Reactions may be *common*, uncommon, *life-threatening*, or COMMON AND LIFE-THREATENING.

• Be aware that patients with myasthenia gravis or myasthenic syndrome (Eaton-Lambert syndrome) are particularly sensitive to the effects of nondepolarizing relaxants. Shorter-acting agents are recommended.

• Keep in mind that the drug is not recommended for use in neonates and infants younger than 3 months. Limited evidence suggests that infants and children (ages 1 to 14) under balanced anesthesia or halothane anesthesia may be less sensitive than adults.

• Know that dosage should be adjusted to ideal body weight in obese patients (30% or more over their ideal weight) to avoid prolonged neuromuscular blockade.

• Use drug under direct medical supervision by personnel skilled in use of neuromuscular blockers and techniques for maintaining a patent airway. Do not use drug unless facilities and equipment for artificial respiration, mechanical ventilation, oxygen therapy, and intubation and an antagonist are within reach.

• *Alert:* Because of its prolonged duration of action, keep in mind that pipecuronium is recommended only for procedures that take 90 minutes or longer.

• Administer pipecuronium after succinylcholine when the latter is used to facilitate intubation.

• Give patients sedatives or general anesthetics before neuromuscular blockers are administered, as ordered. Neuromuscular blockers do not obtund consciousness or alter pain threshold.

• **I.V. use:** Reconstitute with 10 ml solution before use to yield a solution of 1 mg/ml. Using a large volume of diluent or adding the drug to a hanging I.V. solution is not recommended.

• After reconstitution with sterile water for injection or other compatible I.V. solutions (such as 0.9% sodium chloride for injection, $D_5W$, lactated Ringer's injection, dextrose 5% in 0.9% sodium chloride for injection), drug is stable for 24 hours if refrigerated.

• After reconstitution with any solution other than bacteriostatic water for injection, discard unused drug.

• After reconstitution with bacteriostatic water for injection, know that the drug is stable for 5 days at room temperature or in the refrigerator. Note that bacteriostatic water contains benzyl alcohol and is not intended for use in neonates.

• Store the powder at room temperature or in the refrigerator (36° to 86° F [2° to 30° C]).

• Monitor respirations closely until patient is fully recovered from neuromuscular blockade, as evidenced by tests of muscle strength (hand grip, head lift, and ability to cough).

• Because the drug has minimal vagolytic action, monitor for bradycardia during anesthesia.

• Know that a nerve stimulator and train-of-four monitoring are recommended to document antagonism of neuromuscular blockade and recovery of muscle strength. Before attempting pharmacologic reversal with neostigmine, some evidence of spontaneous recovery should be present.

• Be aware that experimental evidence suggests that acid-base and electrolyte balances may influence the actions of nondepolarizing neuromuscular blockers. Alkalosis may counteract the paralysis, and acidosis may enhance it.

☑ **PATIENT TEACHING**

• Explain the drug's purpose.

• Reassure the patient and family that he'll be monitored at all times.

## rocuronium bromide
Zemuron

*Pregnancy Risk Category: B*

**HOW SUPPLIED**
*Injection:* 10 mg/ml

## ACTION
Prevents acetylcholine from binding to receptors on the muscle end plate, thus blocking depolarization.

## ONSET, PEAK, DURATION
Onset occurs within 1 minute. Peak effects occur within 2 minutes in most patients. Duration is dose-dependent; 25% recovery of muscle twitch strength occurs within 22 to 67 minutes.

## INDICATIONS & DOSAGE
*Adjunct to general anesthesia to facilitate endotracheal intubation and to provide skeletal muscle relaxation during surgery or mechanical ventilation –*
Dosage depends on anesthetic used, individual needs, and response. Dosages are representative and must be adjusted.
**Adults and children:** initially, 0.6 mg/kg I.V. bolus. In most patients, tracheal intubation may be performed within 2 minutes; muscle paralysis should last about 22 minutes. A maintenance dosage of 0.1 mg/kg should provide an additional 12 minutes of muscle relaxation; 0.15 mg/kg will add 17 minutes; or 0.2 mg/kg will add 24 minutes to the duration of effect.

## ADVERSE REACTIONS
**CV:** tachycardia, abnormal ECG, arrhythmias (rare), transient hypotension and hypertension.
**GI:** nausea, vomiting.
**Respiratory:** asthma.
**Skin:** rash, edema, pruritus.
**Other:** hiccups.

## INTERACTIONS
*Aminoglycoside antibiotics (including amikacin, gentamicin, kanamycin, neomycin, streptomycin); polymyxin antibiotics (polymyxin B sulfate, colistin); anticonvulsants; clindamycin; tetracyclines; quinidine; general anesthetics (such as halothane, enflurane, isoflurane); opiate analgesics; succi-* *nylcholine:* potentiated neuromuscular blockade, leading to increased skeletal muscle relaxation and potentiated effect. Use cautiously during surgical and postoperative periods.

## CONTRAINDICATIONS
Contraindicated in patients with hypersensitivity to bromides.

## NURSING CONSIDERATIONS
● Use cautiously in patients with altered circulation time caused by CV disease, old age, and edematous states; hepatic disease; severe obesity; bronchogenic carcinoma; electrolyte disturbances; and neuromuscular disease.
● Administer sedatives or general anesthetics before neuromuscular blockers, as ordered. Neuromuscular blockers do not obtund consciousness or alter the pain threshold.
● Drug is not recommended for use during rapid sequence induction for cesarean section.
● Know that rocuronium should be used only by personnel skilled in airway management.
● Keep airway clear. Have emergency respiratory support equipment (endotracheal equipment, ventilator, oxygen, atropine, edrophonium, epinephrine, and neostigmine) available.
● **I.V. use:** Administer by rapid I.V. injection. Alternatively, give by continuous I.V. infusion. Infusion rates are highly individualized but have ranged from 0.004 to 0.16 mg/kg/minute. Compatible solutions include $D_5W$, 0.9% sodium chloride for injection, dextrose 5% in 0.9% sodium chloride for injection, sterile water for injection, and lactated Ringer's injection.
● Store reconstituted solution in refrigerator. Discard after 24 hours.
● Be alert that rocuronium provides conditions for intubation within 3 minutes. Effects last 25 to 40 minutes.
● Know that a nerve stimulator and train-of-four monitoring are recommended to confirm antagonism of

neuromuscular blockade and recovery of muscle strength. Before attempting pharmacologic reversal with neostigmine, some evidence of spontaneous recovery should be present.

• Keep in mind that prior administration of succinylcholine may enhance neuromuscular blocking effect and duration of action.

• Monitor patients with liver disease because they may require higher doses of the drug to achieve adequate muscle relaxation. However, such patients exhibit prolonged effects from the drug.

• Monitor respirations closely until patient is fully recovered from neuromuscular blockade, as evidenced by tests of muscle strength (hand grip, head lift, and ability to cough).

• Know that rocuronium is well tolerated in patients with renal failure.

• Give analgesics, as ordered, for pain.

## ☑ PATIENT TEACHING
• Explain all events and procedures to the patient because he can still hear.

• Answer the family's questions.

---

## succinylcholine chloride (suxamethonium chloride)
Anectine, Anectine Flo-Pack, Quelicin, Scoline‡, Sucostrin

*Pregnancy Risk Category: C*

### HOW SUPPLIED
*Injection:* 20 mg/ml, 50 mg/ml, 100 mg/ml; 100-mg vial, 500-mg vial, 1-g vial

### ACTION
Prolongs depolarization of the muscle end plate.

### ONSET, PEAK, DURATION
Onset occurs in 30 seconds to 1 minute after I.V. use; 2 to 3 minutes after I.M. use. Peak effects occur in 1 to 2 minutes after I.V. use. Effects persist for 4 to 10 minutes after I.V. use, 10 to 30 minutes after I.M. use.

### INDICATIONS & DOSAGE
*Adjunct to anesthesia to induce skeletal muscle relaxation; to facilitate intubation and assist with mechanical ventilation or orthopedic manipulations (drug of choice); to lessen muscle contractions in pharmacologically or electrically induced seizures –*
Dosage depends on anesthetic used, individual needs, and response. Dosages are representative only.
**Adults:** 25 to 75 mg I.V., then 2.5 mg/minute p.r.n., or 2.5 mg/kg I.M. up to maximum of 150 mg I.M. in deltoid muscle.
**Children:** 1 to 2 mg/kg I.M. or I.V. Maximum I.M. dosage is 150 mg. (Children may be less sensitive to succinylcholine than adults.)

### ADVERSE REACTIONS
**CV:** bradycardia, tachycardia, hypertension, hypotension, *arrhythmias,* flushing, *cardiac arrest.*
**EENT:** increased intraocular pressure.
**Respiratory:** *prolonged respiratory depression, apnea,* bronchostriction.
**Other:** *malignant hyperthermia,* muscle fasciculation, *postoperative muscle pain,* myoglobinemia, allergic or idiosyncratic hypersensitivity reactions *(anaphylaxis).*

### INTERACTIONS
*Aminoglycoside antibiotics (including amikacin, gentamicin, kanamycin, neomycin, streptomycin); polymyxin antibiotics (polymyxin B sulfate, colistin); cholinesterase inhibitors (such as neostigmine, pyridostigmine, edrophonium, physostigmine, or echothiophate); general anesthetics (such as halothane, enflurane, isoflurane):* potentiated neuromuscular blockade, leading to increased skeletal muscle relaxation and potentiated effect. Use cautiously during and after surgery.
*Cyclophosphamide, lithium, MAO inhibitors:* prolonged apnea. Use with caution.

---

*Digitalis glycosides:* may cause arrhythmias. Use together cautiously.

*Methotrimeprazine, opioid analgesics:* potentiated neuromuscular blockade, leading to increased skeletal muscle relaxation and possible respiratory paralysis. Use with extreme caution.

*Parenteral magnesium sulfate:* potentiated neuromuscular blockade, increased skeletal muscle relaxation, and possible respiratory paralysis. Use with caution, preferably with reduced doses.

## CONTRAINDICATIONS

Contraindicated in patients with hypersensitivity to the drug and in patients with abnormally low plasma pseudocholinesterase, angle-closure glaucoma, malignant hyperthermia, or penetrating eye injuries.

## NURSING CONSIDERATIONS

• Use cautiously in elderly or debilitated patients; in patients receiving quinidine or digitalis glycoside therapy; in patients with hepatic, renal, or pulmonary impairment; in those with respiratory depression, severe burns or trauma, electrolyte imbalances, hyperkalemia, paraplegia, spinal neuraxis injury, CVA, degenerative or dystrophic neuromuscular disease, myasthenia gravis, myasthenic syndrome of lung cancer or bronchogenic carcinoma, dehydration, thyroid disorders, collagen diseases, porphyria, fractures, muscle spasms, eye surgery, and pheochromocytoma. Also use large doses cautiously in patients undergoing cesarean section.

• Know that succinylcholine is the drug of choice for short procedures (less than 3 minutes) and for orthopedic manipulations; use caution in fractures or dislocations.

• Administer sedatives or general anesthetics before neuromuscular blockers, which do not obtund consciousness or alter the pain threshold.

• Be aware that succinylcholine

should be used only by personnel skilled in airway management.

• Keep airway clear. Have emergency respiratory support equipment (endotracheal equipment, ventilator, oxygen, atropine, and epinephrine) immediately available.

• **I.V. use:** Give test dose (10 mg I.M. or I.V.) after patient has been anesthetized. Normal response (no respiratory depression or transient depression for up to 5 minutes) indicates drug may be given. Do not give if patient develops respiratory paralysis sufficient to permit endotracheal intubation. (Recovery within 30 to 60 minutes.)

• When giving drug I.M., inject deeply, preferably high into deltoid muscle.

• Store injectable form in refrigerator. Store powder form at room temperature in tightly closed container. Use immediately after reconstitution. Do not mix with alkaline solutions (thiopental sodium, sodium bicarbonate, or barbiturates).

• Monitor baseline electrolyte determinations and vital signs (check respirations every 5 to 10 minutes during infusion).

• Monitor respirations closely until patient is fully recovered from neuromuscular blockade, as evidenced by tests of muscle strength (hand grip, head lift, and ability to cough).

• *Alert:* Don't use reversing agents. Unlike nondepolarizing agents, neostigmine or edrophonium may worsen neuromuscular blockade.

• Know that repeated or continuous infusions of succinylcholine are not advisable; they may cause reduced response or prolonged muscle relaxation and apnea.

• Give analgesics, as ordered, for pain.

## ☑ PATIENT TEACHING

• Explain all events and procedures to the patient because he can still hear.

• Reassure the patient that postoperative stiffness is normal and will soon subside.

# tubocurarine chloride
Tubarine†

*Pregnancy Risk Category: C*

## HOW SUPPLIED
*Injection:* 3 mg (20 units)/ml; 10 mg/ml‡

## ACTION
A nondepolarizing neuromuscular blocking agent that prevents acetylcholine from binding to receptors on the muscle end plate, thus blocking depolarization.

## ONSET, PEAK, DURATION
Onset occurs within 1 minute. Peak effects occur in 2 to 5 minutes. Effects persist for 20 to 40 minutes; 50% recovery of muscle twitch strength within 50 minutes, 90% recovery within 75 to 90 minutes.

## INDICATIONS & DOSAGE
*Adjunct to anesthesia to induce skeletal muscle relaxation; to facilitate intubation, orthopedic manipulations –*
Dosage depends on anesthetic used, individual needs, and response. Dosages listed are representative and must be adjusted.
**Adults:** 1 unit/kg or 0.15 mg/kg I.V. slowly over 60 to 90 seconds. Average dose is initially 40 to 60 units I.V. May give 20 to 30 units in 3 to 5 minutes. For longer procedures, give 20 units p.r.n.
**Children:** 1 unit/kg or 0.15 mg/kg.
*To assist with mechanical ventilation –*
**Adults and children:** initially, 0.0165 mg/kg I.V. (average 1 mg or 7 units); then adjust subsequent doses to patient response.
*To lessen muscle contractions in pharmacologically or electrically induced seizures –*
**Adults and children:** 1 unit/kg or

0.15 mg/kg over 60 to 90 seconds. Initial dose is 20 units (3 mg) less than calculated dose.
*Diagnosis of myasthenia gravis –*
**Adults:** 4 to 33 mcg/kg as a single I.V. dose.

## ADVERSE REACTIONS
**CV:** hypotension, arrhythmias, *cardiac arrest,* bradycardia.
**Respiratory:** *respiratory depression or apnea, bronchospasm.*
**Other:** profound and prolonged muscle relaxation, hypersensitivity reactions, idiosyncrasy, residual muscle weakness, increased salivation.

## INTERACTIONS
*Aminoglycoside antibiotics (including amikacin, gentamicin, kanamycin, neomycin, streptomycin); polymyxin antibiotics (polymyxin B sulfate, colistin); general anesthetics (such as halothane, enflurane, isoflurane):* potentiated neuromuscular blockade, leading to increased skeletal muscle relaxation and potentiated effect. Use cautiously during and after surgery.
*Amphotericin B, ethacrynic acid, furosemide, methotrimeprazine, opioid analgesics, propranolol, thiazide diuretics:* potentiated neuromuscular blockade, leading to increased skeletal muscle relaxation and possible respiratory paralysis. Use with extreme caution during surgical and postoperative periods.
*Quinidine:* prolonged neuromuscular blockade. Use together with caution. Monitor closely.

## CONTRAINDICATIONS
Contraindicated in patients with hypersensitivity to the drug and in patients for whom histamine release is a hazard (asthmatic patients).

## NURSING CONSIDERATIONS
● Use cautiously in elderly or debilitated patients and in those with hepatic or pulmonary impairment, hy-

pothermia, respiratory depression, myasthenia gravis, myasthenic syndrome of lung cancer or bronchogenic carcinoma, dehydration, thyroid disorders, collagen diseases, porphyria, electrolyte disturbances, fractures, and muscle spasms. Also use large doses cautiously in patients undergoing cesarean section.

● Keep airway clear. Have emergency respiratory support equipment (endotracheal equipment, ventilator, oxygen, atropine, edrophonium, epinephrine, and neostigmine) available.

● Know that only personnel skilled in airway management should administer tubocurarine.

● Allow succinylcholine effects to subside before giving tubocurarine.

● Administer sedatives or general anesthetics before neuromuscular blockers, which do not obtund consciousness or alter the pain threshold.

● Assess baseline electrolyte determinations (electrolyte imbalance can potentiate neuromuscular blocking effects).

● **I.V. use:** Give I.V. over 60 to 90 seconds.

● Do not mix with barbiturates (precipitate will form). Use only fresh solutions and discard if discolored.

● Check vital signs every 15 minutes. Notify the doctor at once of changes.

● Measure fluid intake and output; renal dysfunction prolongs duration of action because much of drug is unchanged before excretion.

● Know that a nerve stimulator and train-of-four monitoring are recommended to confirm antagonism of neuromuscular blockade and recovery of muscle strength. Before attempting pharmacologic reversal with neostigmine, some evidence of spontaneous recovery should be present.

● Monitor respirations closely until patient is fully recovered from neuromuscular blockade, as evidenced by tests of muscle strength (hand grip, head lift, and ability to cough).

● Give analgesics, as ordered, for pain.

☑ **PATIENT TEACHING**
● Explain all events and procedures to the patient because he still can hear.
● Answer the family's questions.

## vecuronium bromide
Norcuron

*Pregnancy Risk Category: C*

**HOW SUPPLIED**
*Injection:* 10-mg vial

**ACTION**
Prevents acetylcholine from binding to receptors on the muscle end plate, thus blocking depolarization.

**ONSET, PEAK, DURATION**
Onset occurs within 1 minute. Peak effects occur in 3 to 5 minutes. Effects persist for 25 to 30 minutes; 25% recovery of muscle twitch strength within 24 to 40 minutes, 95% recovery in 45 to 65 minutes.

**INDICATIONS & DOSAGE**
*Adjunct to general anesthesia to facilitate endotracheal intubation and to provide skeletal muscle relaxation during surgery or mechanical ventilation* –
Dosage depends on anesthetic used, individual needs, and response. Dosages are representative and must be adjusted.
**Adults and children over 9 years:** initially, 0.08 to 0.10 mg/kg I.V. bolus. Maintenance doses of 0.010 to 0.015 mg/kg within 25 to 40 minutes of initial dose should be administered during prolonged surgical procedures. Maintenance doses may be given q 12 to 15 minutes in patients receiving balanced anesthesia.
**Children under 9 years:** may require a slightly higher initial dose and also may require supplementation slightly more often than adults. Alternatively, drug may be given by continuous I.V. infu-

sion of 1 mcg/kg/minute initially, then 0.8 to 1.2 mcg/kg/minute.

## ADVERSE REACTIONS
**Respiratory:** *prolonged, dose-related respiratory insufficiency or apnea.* **Other:** skeletal muscle weakness.

## INTERACTIONS
*Aminoglycoside antibiotics (including amikacin, gentamicin, kanamycin, neomycin, streptomycin); polymyxin antibiotics (polymyxin B sulfate, colistin); clindamycin; bacitracin; tetracyclines; quinidine; general anesthetics (such as halothane, enflurane, isoflurane); other skeletal muscle relaxants:* potentiated neuromuscular blockade, leading to increased skeletal muscle relaxation and potentiated effect. Use cautiously during and after surgery. *Opioid analgesics:* potentiated neuromuscular blockade, leading to increased skeletal muscle relaxation and possible respiratory paralysis. Use with extreme caution, and reduce dose of vecuronium.

## CONTRAINDICATIONS
Contraindicated in patients with hypersensitivity to bromides.

## NURSING CONSIDERATIONS
● Use cautiously in elderly patients; in patients with altered circulation caused by CV disease and edematous states; and in those with hepatic disease, severe obesity, bronchogenic carcinoma, electrolyte disturbances, and neuromuscular disease.
● Keep airway clear. Have emergency respiratory support equipment (endotracheal equipment, ventilator, oxygen, atropine, edrophonium, epinephrine, and neostigmine) available.
● Know that the drug should be used only by personnel skilled in airway management.
● Administer sedatives or general anesthetics before neuromuscular blockers, which do not obtund consciousness or alter the pain threshold.
● **I.V. use:** Administer by rapid I.V. injection. Alternatively, 10 to 20 mg may be added to 100 ml of a compatible solution and given by I.V. infusion. Compatible solutions include $D_5W$, 0.9% sodium chloride for injection, dextrose 5% in 0.9% sodium chloride for injection, and lactated Ringer's injection.
● Do not mix with alkaline solutions.
● Store reconstituted solution in refrigerator. Discard after 24 hours.
● Know that a nerve stimulator and train-of-four monitoring are recommended to confirm antagonism of neuromuscular blockade and recovery of muscle strength. Before attempting pharmacologic reversal with neostigmine, some evidence of spontaneous recovery should be seen.
● Monitor respirations closely until patient is fully recovered from neuromuscular blockade as evidenced by tests of muscle strength (hand grip, head lift, and ability to cough).
● Keep in mind that prior administration of succinylcholine may enhance the neuromuscular blocking effect and duration of action.
● Know that vecuronium is well tolerated in patients with renal failure.
● Give analgesics, as ordered, for pain.

### ☑ PATIENT TEACHING
● Explain all events and procedures to the patient because he can still hear.
● Answer the family's questions.

# 43

## Antihistamines

astemizole
azatadine maleate
brompheniramine maleate
cetirizine hydrochloride
chlorpheniramine maleate
clemastine fumarate
cyproheptadine hydrochloride
dexchlorpheniramine maleate
diphenhydramine hydrochloride
loratadine
methdilazine hydrochloride
promethazine hydrochloride
promethazine theoclate
terfenadine
trimeprazine tartrate
tripelennamine citrate
tripelennamine hydrochloride
triprolidine hydrochloride

## COMBINATION PRODUCTS

ALLEREST MAXIMUM STRENGTH TABLETS◇: pseudoephedrine hydrochloride 30 mg and chlorpheniramine maleate 2 mg.

CHLOR-TRIMETON ALLERGY DECONGESTANT◇: chlorpheniramine maleate 4 mg and pseudoephedrine sulfate 60 mg.

CHLOR-TRIMETON DECONGESTANT REPETABS◇: chlorpheniramine maleate 8 mg and pseudoephedrine sulfate 120 mg.

CLARITIN-D: loratadine 5 mg and pseudoephedrine sulfate 120 mg.

CONDRIN-LA: phenylpropanolamine hydrochloride 75 mg and chlorpheniramine maleate 12 mg.

CONTAC CAPSULES◇: phenylpropanolamine 75 mg and chlorpheniramine maleate 8 mg.

CONTAC 12-HOUR CAPLETS◇: phenylpropanolamine 75 mg and chlorpheniramine maleate 8 mg.

CORICIDIN "D" TABLETS◇: chlorpheniramine maleate 2 mg, acetaminophen 325 mg, and phenylpropranolamine hydrochloride 12.5 mg.

DECONAMINE: pseudoephedrine hydrochloride 60 mg and chlorpheniramine maleate 4 mg.

DIMETAPP EXTENTABS: brompheniramine maleate 12 mg and phenylpropanolamine hydrochloride 75 mg.

DRIZE: phenylpropanolamine hydrochloride 75 mg and chlorpheniramine maleate 12 mg.

FEDAHIST: pseudoephedrine hydrochloride 60 mg and chlorpheniramine maleate 4 mg.

NALDECON: phenylephrine hydrochloride 10 mg, phenylpropanolamine hydrochloride 40 mg, phenyltoloxamine citrate 15 mg, and chlorpheniramine maleate 5 mg.

NOLAMINE: chlorpheniramine maleate 4 mg, phenindamine tartrate 24 mg, and phenylpropanolamine hydrochloride 50 mg.

NOVAFED A: pseudoephedrine hydrochloride 120 mg and chlorpheniramine maleate 8 mg.

NOVAHISTINE ELIXIR◇*: phenylephrine 5 mg, chlorpheniramine maleate 2 mg, and alcohol 5% per 5 ml.

ORNADE SPANSULES: phenylpropanolamine hydrochloride 75 mg and chlorpheniramine maleate 12 mg.

P-V-TUSSIN SYRUP*: chlorpheniramine maleate 2 mg/5 ml, phenindamine tartrate 5 mg/5 ml, phenylephrine hydrochloride 5 mg/5 ml, and pyrilamine maleate 6 mg/5 ml.

SELDANE-D: terfenadine 60 mg and pseudoephedrine hydrochloride 120 mg.

SUDAFED PLUS◇: pseudoephedrine hydrochloride 60 mg and chlorpheniramine maleate 4 mg.

TAVIST-D◇: clemastine fumarate 1.34 mg and phenylpropanolamine 75 mg.

TRIAMINIC-12: phenylpropanolamine

---

Reactions may be *common*, uncommon, *life-threatening*, or COMMON AND LIFE-THREATENING.

hydrochloride 75 mg and chlorpheniramine maleate 12 mg.

TRINALIN REPETABS: azatadine maleate 1 mg and pseudoephedrine sulfate 120 mg.

---

## astemizole
Hismanal

*Pregnancy Risk Category: C*

### HOW SUPPLIED
*Tablets:* 10 mg
*Oral suspension:* 2 mg/ml\*‡

### ACTION
Blocks effects of histamine at H₁ receptors. Astemizole is a nonsedating antihistamine; its chemical structure prevents entry into the CNS.

### ONSET, PEAK, DURATION
Onset is slow although exact time is unknown. Serum levels peak within 1 hour. Effects last up to 24 hours.

### INDICATIONS & DOSAGE
*Relief of symptoms associated with chronic idiopathic urticaria and seasonal allergic rhinitis –*
**Adults and children over 12 years:**
10 mg P.O. daily.

### ADVERSE REACTIONS
**CNS:** headache, nervousness, dizziness, drowsiness.
**CV:** *arrhythmias* (with high plasma levels).
**EENT:** dry mouth, pharyngitis, conjunctivitis.
**GI:** abdominal pain, increased appetite, nausea, diarrhea.
**Other:** arthralgia, weight gain, cholestatic jaundice.

### INTERACTIONS
*Fluvoxamine:* may alter astemizole's therapeutic effect. Monitor closely.
*Itraconazole, ketoconazole, macrolide antibiotics (such as erythromycin):*
risk of serious adverse cardiac reactions. Don't use together.

### CONTRAINDICATIONS
Contraindicated in patients with hypersensitivity to astemizole and in patients taking the antifungal agents itraconazole or ketoconazole or macrolide antibiotics, including erythromycin.

### NURSING CONSIDERATIONS
• Use cautiously in patients with hepatic or renal disease.
• Also use cautiously in patients with lower respiratory tract diseases (including asthma); drying effects can increase the risk of bronchial mucus plug formation.

### ☑ PATIENT TEACHING
• Ensure that patient knows to take astemizole only once a day. If symptoms persist or worsen, warn patient not to increase dosage without consulting doctor. High doses may increase risk of arrhythmias.
• Instruct patient to take drug on an empty stomach at least 2 hours after a meal and to avoid eating for at least 1 hour after dosing.
• Warn patient to stop drug 4 days before allergy skin tests to preserve accuracy of tests.

---

## azatadine maleate
Optimine, Zadine‡

*Pregnancy Risk Category: B*

### HOW SUPPLIED
*Tablets:* 1 mg
*Syrup:* 0.5 mg/5 ml‡

### ACTION
Competes with histamine for H₁-receptor sites on effector cells. Prevents, but does not reverse, histamine-mediated responses.

---

\*Liquid form contains alcohol.  \*\*May contain tartrazine.  †Canada only.  ‡Australia only.  ◇OTC.

## ONSET, PEAK, DURATION
Onset occurs within 15 to 60 minutes.
Plasma levels peak within 4 hours.
Effects persist for 12 hours.

## INDICATIONS & DOSAGE
*Rhinitis, allergy symptoms, chronic urticaria* —
**Adults and children 12 years and older:** 1 to 2 mg P.O. b.i.d. Maximum dosage is 4 mg daily.

## ADVERSE REACTIONS
**CNS:** *drowsiness, dizziness,* vertigo, disturbed coordination.
**CV:** hypotension, palpitations.
**GI:** anorexia, nausea, vomiting, *dry mouth and throat,* epigastric distress.
**GU:** urine retention.
**Hematologic:** *thrombocytopenia.*
**Respiratory:** thick bronchial secretions.
**Skin:** urticaria, rash.

## INTERACTIONS
*CNS depressants:* increased sedation.
Use together cautiously.
*MAO inhibitors:* increased anticholinergic effects. Don't use together.

## CONTRAINDICATIONS
Contraindicated in patients with acute asthmatic attacks and in breast-feeding patients.

## NURSING CONSIDERATIONS
• Use cautiously in elderly patients and in patients with increased intraocular pressure, hyperthyroidism, CV or renal disease, hypertension, bronchial asthma, urine retention, prostatic hyperplasia, bladder-neck obstruction, and stenosing peptic ulcerations.
• Monitor blood counts during long-term therapy, as ordered; watch for signs of blood dyscrasias.

## ☑ PATIENT TEACHING
• Instruct patient to reduce GI distress by taking drug with food or milk.
• Tell patient to stop drug 4 days before allergy skin tests to preserve accuracy of tests.
• Warn patient to avoid alcohol and activities that require alertness until drug's CNS effects are known.
• Inform patient that coffee or tea may reduce drowsiness. Sugarless gum, sugarless sour hard candy, or ice chips may relieve dry mouth.
• Tell patient to notify doctor if tolerance develops because a different antihistamine may need to be prescribed.

# brompheniramine maleate
Bromphen*◇, Chlorphed◇, Codimal-A, Conjec-B◇, Cophene-B, Dehist, Diamine T.D., Dimetane*◇, Dimetane Extentabs◇, Histaject Modified, Nasahist B, ND-Stat Revised, Oraminic II, Sinusol-B, Veltane

*Pregnancy Risk Category: C*

## HOW SUPPLIED
*Tablets:* 4 mg◇, 8 mg, 12 mg
*Tablets (extended-release):* 8 mg◇, 12 mg◇
*Elixir:* 2 mg/5 ml*◇
*Injection:* 10 mg/ml

## ACTION
Competes with histamine for $H_1$-receptor sites on effector cells. Prevents, but does not reverse, histamine-mediated responses.

## ONSET, PEAK, DURATION
Onset occurs in 15 to 60 minutes.
Peak levels occur within 2 to 5 hours.
Peak effects occur in 3 to 9 hours. Effects persist for 4 to 8 hours for regular release preparations, longer for extended-release preparations.

---

Reactions may be *common,* uncommon, *life-threatening,* or **COMMON AND LIFE-THREATENING.**

## INDICATIONS & DOSAGE

*Rhinitis, allergy symptoms –*

**Adults:** 4 to 8 mg P.O. t.i.d. or q.i.d.; or 8 to 12 mg extended-release P.O. b.i.d. or t.i.d.; or 5 to 20 mg q 6 to 12 hours I.M., I.V., or S.C. Maximum dosage is 40 mg daily.

**Children 6 years and over:** 2 to 4 mg P.O. t.i.d. or q.i.d.; or 8 to 12 mg extended-release P.O. q 12 hours; or 0.5 mg/kg I.M., I.V., or S.C. daily in divided doses t.i.d. or q.i.d.

**Children under 6 years:** 0.5 mg/kg P.O., I.M., I.V., or S.C. daily in divided doses t.i.d. or q.i.d.

*Note:* Children under 12 years should use only as directed by a doctor.

## ADVERSE REACTIONS

**CNS:** dizziness, tremors, irritability, insomnia, *drowsiness, stimulation.*
**CV:** hypotension, palpitations.
**GI:** anorexia, nausea, vomiting, *dry mouth and throat.*
**GU:** urine retention.
**Hematologic:** *thrombocytopenia, agranulocytosis.*
**Skin:** urticaria, rash.
**Other:** (after parenteral administration) local stinging, diaphoresis, syncope.

## INTERACTIONS

*CNS depressants:* increased sedation. Use together cautiously.
*MAO inhibitors:* increased anticholinergic effects. Don't use together.

## CONTRAINDICATIONS

Contraindicated in patients with hypersensitivity to any of the drug's ingredients; in those with acute asthma, severe hypertension or coronary artery disease, angle-closure glaucoma, urine retention, and peptic ulcer; and within 14 days of MAO inhibitor therapy.

## NURSING CONSIDERATIONS

● Use cautiously in elderly patients and in those with increased intraocular pressure, diabetes, ischemic heart disease, hyperthyroidism, hypertension, bronchial asthma, and prostatic hyperplasia.
● **I.V. use:** Injectable form containing 10 mg/ml can be given diluted or undiluted very slowly I.V.
● *Alert:* Do not give the 100 mg/ml injection I.V.
● Monitor blood count during long-term therapy, as ordered; observe for signs of blood dyscrasias.

## ☑ PATIENT TEACHING

● Instruct patient to reduce GI distress by taking drug with food or milk.
● Warn patient to avoid alcohol and activities that require alertness until drug's CNS effects are known.
● Tell patient that coffee or tea may reduce drowsiness. Causes less drowsiness than some other antihistamines.
● Inform patient that sugarless gum, sugarless sour hard candy, or ice chips may relieve dry mouth.
● Tell patient to notify doctor if tolerance develops because a different antihistamine may need to be prescribed.
● Instruct patient to stop drug 4 days before allergy skin tests to preserve accuracy of tests.

▼ *NEW DRUG*

## cetirizine hydrochloride
Zyrtec

*Pregnancy Risk Category: B*

## HOW SUPPLIED
*Tablets:* 5 mg, 10 mg

## ACTION
Selectively inhibits peripheral histamine-1 receptors.

---

## ONSET, PEAK, DURATION
Onset and duration are unknown. Peak plasma levels occur in 0.5 to 1.5 hours.

## INDICATIONS & DOSAGE
*Seasonal allergic rhinitis, perennial allergic rhinitis, chronic urticaria* –
**Adults and children 12 years and older:** 5 or 10 mg P.O. daily; 5 mg P.O. daily in those with renal or hepatic impairment.

## ADVERSE REACTIONS
**CNS:** *somnolence,* fatigue, dizziness.
**GI:** dry mouth.
**Other:** pharyngitis.

## INTERACTIONS
*Ethanol and other CNS depressants:* possible additive effect. Avoid concomitant use.
*Theophylline:* may cause decreased clearance of cetirizine. Monitor patient closely.

## CONTRAINDICATIONS
Contraindicated in patients with hypersensitivity to the drug or to hydroxyzine.

## NURSING CONSIDERATIONS
• Use cautiously in patients with renal impairment.
• Drug is not recommended for use in breast-feeding women.
• Safety of drug has not been established in children under age 12.

## ☑ PATIENT TEACHING
• Warn the patient not to drive or perform hazardous activities if he experiences somnolence, a common adverse reaction.
• Advise the patient not to use alcohol or other CNS depressants while taking the drug.

# chlorpheniramine maleate
Aller-Chlor*◊, Allergex‡, Chlo-Amine◊, Chlor-100◊, Chlorate◊, Chlor-Niramine◊, Chlor-Pro, Chlor-Pro 10, Chlorspan-12, Chlortab-4, Chlortab-8, Chlor-Trimeton*◊, Chlor-Trimeton 12 Hour Allergy◊, Chlor-Tripolon†◊, GenAllerate◊, Novopheniram‡◊, Pfeiffer's Allergy◊, Phenetron*, Piriton‡, Pyranistan◊, Telachlor, Teldrin◊, Trymegen◊

*Pregnancy Risk Category: B*

## HOW SUPPLIED
*Tablets:* 4 mg◊, 8 mg◊, 12 mg◊
*Tablets (chewable):* 2 mg◊
*Tablets (timed-release):* 8 mg◊, 12 mg◊
*Capsules (timed-release):* 6 mg◊, 8 mg◊, 12 mg◊
*Syrup:* 2 mg/5 ml*◊
*Injection:* 10 mg/ml, 100 mg/ml

## ACTION
Competes with histamine for $H_1$-receptor sites on effector cells. Prevents, but does not reverse, histamine-mediated responses.

## ONSET, PEAK, DURATION
Onset occurs in 15 to 60 minutes. Peak concentrations occur 2 to 6 hours after oral dose, immediately after I.V. injection, unknown after I.M. administration. Effects persist up to 24 hours.

## INDICATIONS & DOSAGE
*Rhinitis, allergy symptoms* –
**Adults:** 4 mg P.O. q 4 to 6 hours, not to exceed 24 mg/day; or 8 to 12 mg timed-release P.O. every 8 to 12 hours; or 5 to 40 mg I.M., I.V., or S.C. as a single dose.
**Children 6 to 12 years:** 2 mg P.O. q 4 to 6 hours, not to exceed 12 mg/day. Alternatively, may give 8 mg timed-release P.O. h.s.

---

Reactions may be *common,* uncommon, ***life-threatening,*** or **COMMON AND LIFE-THREATENING.**

**Children 2 to 6 years:** 1 mg P.O. q 4 to 6 hours, not to exceed 6 mg/day.

## ADVERSE REACTIONS
**CNS:** *stimulation,* sedation, *drowsiness,* excitability (in children).
**CV:** hypotension, palpitations.
**GI:** epigastric distress, *dry mouth.*
**GU:** urine retention.
**Respiratory:** thick bronchial secretions.
**Skin:** rash, urticaria.
**Other:** local stinging, burning sensation (after parenteral administration), pallor, weak pulse, transient hypotension.

## INTERACTIONS
*CNS depressants:* increased sedation. Use together cautiously.
*MAO inhibitors:* increased anticholinergic effects. Don't use together.

## CONTRAINDICATIONS
• Contraindicated in patients having acute asthmatic attacks.
• Antihistamines are not recommended for breast-feeding patients because small amounts of drug are excreted in breast milk.

## NURSING CONSIDERATIONS
• Use cautiously in elderly patients and in those with increased intraocular pressure, hyperthyroidism, CV or renal disease, hypertension, bronchial asthma, urine retention, prostatic hyperplasia, bladder-neck obstruction, and stenosing peptic ulcerations.
• **I.V. use:** Drug is available in 10 mg/ml ampules for I.V. use.
• **Alert:** Do not give the 100 mg/ml strength I.V. Chlorpheniramine is compatible with most I.V. solutions. Check with pharmacist before mixing with any I.V. solutions to verify specific compatibilities. Give injection over 1 minute.
• If symptoms occur during or after parenteral dose, discontinue drug. Notify the doctor.

☑ **PATIENT TEACHING**
• Warn patient to avoid alcohol and other CNS depressants and driving and other activities that require alertness until drug's CNS effects are known.
• Tell patient that coffee or tea may reduce drowsiness. Sugarless gum, sugarless sour hard candy, or ice chips may relieve dry mouth.
• Advise patient to stop drug 4 days before allergy skin tests to preserve accuracy of tests.
• Tell patient to notify doctor if tolerance develops because a different antihistamine may need to be prescribed.
• Tell parent that drug, including extended-release products, should not be used in children under 12 years unless directed by doctor.

# clemastine fumarate
Tavist, Tavist-1◇

*Pregnancy Risk Category: B*

## HOW SUPPLIED
*Tablets:* 1.34 mg◇, 2.68 mg
*Syrup:* 0.67 mg per 5 ml

## ACTION
Competes with histamine for $H_1$-receptor sites on effector cells. Prevents, but does not reverse, histamine-mediated responses.

## ONSET, PEAK, DURATION
Onset occurs in 15 to 60 minutes. Peak levels occur in 2 to 4 hours; peak effects occur in 5 to 7 hours. Effects persist for 12 hours.

## INDICATIONS & DOSAGE
*Rhinitis, allergy symptoms* −
**Adults and children 12 years and over:** 1.34 mg P.O. q 12 hours, or 2.68 mg P.O. once daily to t.i.d. as needed. Dosage should not exceed 8.04 mg/day.
**Children 6 to 12 years:** 0.67 to 1.34

mg P.O. b.i.d. Dosage should not exceed 4.02 mg/day.

## ADVERSE REACTIONS
**CNS:** *sedation, drowsiness, **seizures,*** nervousness, tremor, confusion, restlessness, vertigo, headache, *sleepiness, dizziness, incoordination,* fatigue.
**CV:** hypotension, palpitations, tachycardia.
**GI:** *epigastric distress,* anorexia, diarrhea, nausea, vomiting, constipation, *dry mouth.*
**GU:** urine retention, urinary frequency.
**Hematologic:** hemolytic anemia, ***thrombocytopenia, agranulocytosis.***
**Respiratory:** *thick bronchial secretions.*
**Skin:** rash, urticaria, photosensitivity, diaphoresis.
**Other:** *anaphylactic shock.*

## INTERACTIONS
*CNS depressants:* increased sedation. Use together cautiously.
*MAO inhibitors:* increased anticholinergic effects. Don't use together.

## CONTRAINDICATIONS
Contraindicated in patients with hypersensitivity to drug or other antihistamines of similar chemical structure, in those with acute asthma, and in neonates or premature infants and breast-feeding patients.

## NURSING CONSIDERATIONS
● Use cautiously in elderly patients and in those with angle-closure glaucoma, increased intraocular pressure, hyperthyroidism, CV disease, hypertension, bronchial asthma, prostatic hyperplasia, bladder-neck obstruction, pyloroduodenal obstruction, and stenosing peptic ulcerations.
● Know that children under 12 years should use only as directed by a doctor.
● Monitor blood counts during long-term therapy, as ordered; observe for signs of blood dyscrasias.

## ☑ PATIENT TEACHING
● Warn patient to avoid alcohol and driving or other activities that require alertness until drug's CNS effects are known.
● Tell patient that coffee or tea may reduce drowsiness. Sugarless gum, sugarless sour hard candy, or ice chips may relieve dry mouth.
● Advise patient to stop drug 4 days before allergy skin tests to preserve accuracy of tests.
● Tell patient to notify doctor if tolerance develops because a different antihistamine may need to be prescribed.

---

# cyproheptadine hydrochloride
Periactin

*Pregnancy Risk Category: B*

## HOW SUPPLIED
*Tablets:* 4 mg
*Syrup:* 2 mg/5 ml

## ACTION
Competes with histamine for $H_1$-receptor sites on effector cells. Prevents, but does not reverse, histamine-mediated responses.

## ONSET, PEAK, DURATION
Onset occurs in 15 to 60 minutes. Serum levels peak in 6 to 9 hours. Effects persist for 8 hours.

## INDICATIONS & DOSAGE
*Allergy symptoms, pruritus –*
**Adults:** 4 to 20 mg P.O. daily in divided doses. Maximum dosage is 0.5 mg/kg daily.
**Children 7 to 14 years:** 4 mg P.O. b.i.d. or t.i.d. Maximum dosage is 16 mg daily.
**Children 2 to 6 years:** 2 mg P.O.

---

b.i.d. or t.i.d. Maximum dosage is 12 mg daily.

## ADVERSE REACTIONS
**CNS:** *drowsiness,* dizziness, headache, fatigue, sedation, sleepiness, incoordination, confusion, restlessness, insomnia, nervousness, tremor, *seizures.*
**CV:** hypotension, palpitations, tachycardia.
**GI:** nausea, vomiting, epigastric distress, *dry mouth,* diarrhea, constipation.
**GU:** urine retention, urinary frequency.
**Hematologic:** hemolytic anemia, leukopenia, *agranulocytosis, thrombocytopenia.*
**Skin:** rash, urticaria, photosensitivity.
**Other:** weight gain, *anaphylactic shock.*

## INTERACTIONS
*CNS depressants:* increased sedation. Use together cautiously.
*MAO inhibitors:* increased anticholinergic effects. Don't use together.

## CONTRAINDICATIONS
Contraindicated in patients with hypersensitivity to drug or other drugs of similar chemical structure; in those with acute asthma, angle-closure glaucoma, stenosing peptic ulcer, symptomatic prostatic hyperplasia, bladder-neck obstruction, and pyloroduodenal obstruction; in concurrent therapy with MAO inhibitors; in neonates or premature infants; in elderly or debilitated patients, and in breastfeeding patients.

## NURSING CONSIDERATIONS
• Use cautiously in patients with increased intraocular pressure, hyperthyroidism, CV disease, hypertension, or bronchial asthma.
• Know that children under 14 years

should use only as directed by a doctor.

## ☑ PATIENT TEACHING
• Tell patient that GI distress can be reduced by taking drug with food or milk.
• Warn patient to avoid alcohol and driving or other activities that require alertness until drug's CNS effects are known.
• Tell patient that coffee or tea may reduce drowsiness. Sugarless gum, sugarless sour hard candy, or ice chips may relieve dry mouth.
• Advise patient to stop drug 4 days before allergy skin tests to preserve accuracy of tests.
• Instruct patient to notify doctor if tolerance develops because a different antihistamine may need to be prescribed.

---

## dexchlorpheniramine maleate
Dexchlor, Poladex T.D., Polaramine*, Polaramine Repetabs

*Pregnancy Risk Category: B*

## HOW SUPPLIED
*Tablets:* 2 mg
*Tablets (timed-release):* 4 mg, 6 mg
*Syrup:* 2 mg/5 ml*

## ACTION
Competes with histamine for $H_1$-receptor sites on effector cells. Prevents, but does not reverse, histamine-mediated responses.

## ONSET, PEAK, DURATION
Onset occurs in 15 to 60 minutes. Peak unknown. Effects persist for 4 to 8 hours.

## INDICATIONS & DOSAGE
*Rhinitis, allergy symptoms, contact dermatitis, pruritus –*
**Adults and children over 12 years:** 2 mg P.O. q 4 to 6 hours, not to exceed

---

*Liquid form contains alcohol.   **May contain tartrazine.   †Canada only.   ‡Australia only.   ◊OTC.   †

12 mg/day; or 4 to 6 mg timed-release
P.O. b.i.d. or t.i.d.
**Children 6 to 12 years:** 1 mg P.O. q 4
to 6 hours, not to exceed 6 mg/day; or
4 mg timed-release tablet P.O. h.s.
**Children 2 to 6 years:** 0.5 mg P.O.
q 4 to 6 hours, not to exceed 3 mg/
day.

## ADVERSE REACTIONS
**CNS:** *drowsiness,* dizziness, *stimulation.*
**GI:** nausea, *dry mouth.*
**GU:** polyuria, dysuria, urine retention.

## INTERACTIONS
*CNS depressants:* increased sedation.
Use together cautiously.
*MAO inhibitors:* increased anticholinergic effects. Don't use together.

## CONTRAINDICATIONS
• Contraindicated in patients with
acute asthmatic attacks.
• Antihistamines are not recommended for use in breast-feeding patients because small amounts of drug
are excreted in breast milk.

## NURSING CONSIDERATIONS
• Use cautiously in elderly patients
and in patients with increased intraocular pressure, hyperthyroidism, CV
or renal disease, hypertension, bronchial asthma, urine retention, prostatic hyperplasia, bladder-neck obstruction, and stenosing peptic ulcer.
• Know that children under 6 years
should use only as directed by a doctor. Timed-release tablets should not
be used for children younger than 6
years.

## ☑ PATIENT TEACHING
• Warn patient to avoid alcohol and
driving or other activities that require
alertness until drug's CNS effects are
known.
• Tell patient that coffee or tea may
reduce drowsiness. Sugarless gum,

sugarless sour hard candy, or ice chips
may relieve dry mouth.
• Advise patient to stop drug 4 days
before allergy skin tests to preserve
accuracy of tests.
• Tell patient to notify doctor if tolerance develops because a different antihistamine may need to be prescribed.

---

# diphenhydramine hydrochloride
Allerdryl†◇, AllerMax Caplets◇,
Aller-med◇, Banophen◇,
Banophen Caplets◇, Beldin◇,
Belix◇, Bena-D 10, Bena-D 50,
Benadryl◇, Benadryl 25◇,
Benadryl Kapseals◇, Benahist 10,
Benahist 50, Ben-Allergin-50,
Benoject-10, Benoject-50, Benylin
Cough◇, Bydramine Cough◇,
Compoz◇, Diphenacen-50,
Diphenadryl◇, Diphen Cough◇,
Diphenhist◇, Diphenhist Captabs◇,
Dormarex 2◇, Fynex◇, Genahist◇,
Gen-D-phen◇, Hydramine◇,
Hydramine Cough◇, Hydramyn◇,
Hydril◇, Hyrexin-50, Insomnal†◇,
Nervine Nighttime Sleep-Aid◇,
Nidryl◇, Noradryl◇, Nordryl◇
Nordryl Cough◇, Nytol Maximum
Strength◇, Nytol with DPH◇,
Phendry◇, Phendry Children's
Allergy Medicine◇, Sleep-Eze 3◇,
Sominex Formula 2◇, Tusstat◇,
Twilite Caplets◇, Uni-Bent Cough◇,
Wehdryl-10, Wehdryl-50

*Pregnancy Risk Category: B*

## HOW SUPPLIED
*Tablets:* 25 mg◇, 50 mg◇
*Capsules:* 25 mg◇, 50 mg◇
*Elixir:* 12.5 mg/5 ml (14% alcohol)\*◇
*Syrup:* 12.5 mg/5 ml◇
*Injection:* 10 mg/ml, 50 mg/ml

## ACTION
Competes with histamine for $H_1$-receptor sites on effector cells. Prevents, but does not reverse, hista-

---

mine-mediated responses, particularly histamine's effects on the smooth muscle of the bronchial tubes, GI tract, uterus, and blood vessels. Structurally related to local anesthetics, diphenhydramine provides local anesthesia by preventing initiation and transmission of nerve impulses. Also suppresses cough reflex by a direct effect in the medulla of the brain.

## ONSET, PEAK, DURATION
Onset occurs within 15 minutes of oral administration, immediately after I.V. administration, unknown after I.M. administration. Serum levels peak and drug effects occur 1 to 4 hours after administration. Effects persist for 6 to 8 hours.

## INDICATIONS & DOSAGE
*Rhinitis, allergy symptoms, motion sickness, Parkinson's disease –*
**Adults and children 12 years and over:** 25 to 50 mg P.O. t.i.d. or q.i.d.; or 10 to 50 mg deep I.M. or I.V. Maximum I.M. or I.V. dosage is 400 mg daily.
**Children under 12 years:** 5 mg/kg daily P.O., deep I.M., or I.V. in divided doses q.i.d. Maximum dosage is 300 mg daily.
*Sedation –*
**Adults:** 25 to 50 mg P.O., or deep I.M., p.r.n.
*Nighttime sleep aid –*
**Adults:** 50 mg P.O. h.s.
*Nonproductive cough –*
**Adults:** 25 mg P.O. q 4 to 6 hours (not to exceed 150 mg daily).
**Children 6 to 12 years:** 12.5 mg P.O. q 4 to 6 hours (not to exceed 75 mg daily).
**Children 2 to 6 years:** 6.25 mg P.O. q 4 to 6 hours (not to exceed 25 mg daily).

## ADVERSE REACTIONS
**CNS:** *drowsiness,* confusion, insomnia, headache, vertigo, *sedation, sleepiness, dizziness, incoordination,* fatigue, restlessness, tremor, nervousness, *seizures.*
**CV:** palpitations, hypotension, tachycardia.
**EENT:** diplopia, blurred vision, tinnitus.
**GI:** *nausea,* vomiting, diarrhea, *dry mouth,* constipation, *epigastric distress,* anorexia.
**GU:** dysuria, urine retention, urinary frequency.
**Hematologic:** hemolytic anemia, *thrombocytopenia, agranulocytosis.*
**Respiratory:** nasal congestion, *thickening of bronchial secretions.*
**Skin:** urticaria, photosensitivity, rash.
**Other:** *anaphylactic shock.*

## INTERACTIONS
*CNS depressants:* increased sedation. Use together cautiously.
*MAO inhibitors:* increased anticholinergic effects. Don't use together.

## CONTRAINDICATIONS
Contraindicated in patients with hypersensitivity to the drug, during acute asthmatic attacks, and in newborns or premature neonates and breast-feeding patients.

## NURSING CONSIDERATIONS
• Use with extreme caution in patients with angle-closure glaucoma, prostatic hyperplasia, pyloroduodenal and bladder-neck obstruction, asthma or COPD, increased intraocular pressure, hyperthyroidism, CV disease, hypertension, and stenosing peptic ulcer.
• Know that children under 12 years should use only as directed by a doctor.
• Alternate injection sites to prevent irritation. Administer I.M. injection deeply into large muscle.

**PATIENT TEACHING**
• Instruct patient to take 30 minutes before travel to prevent motion sickness.
• Tell patient to take drug with food or milk to reduce GI distress.
• Warn patient to avoid alcohol and driving or other hazardous activities that require alertness until drug's CNS effects are known.
• Tell patient that coffee or tea may reduce drowsiness. Sugarless gum, sugarless sour hard candy, or ice chips may relieve dry mouth.
• Advise patient to stop drug 4 days before allergy skin tests to preserve accuracy of tests.
• Tell patient to notify doctor if tolerance develops because a different antihistamine may need to be prescribed.
• Warn patient of possible photosensitivity. Advise use of a sunblock.

# loratadine
Claratyne‡, Claritin

*Pregnancy Risk Category: B*

**HOW SUPPLIED**
*Tablets:* 10 mg

**ACTION**
Blocks effects of histamine at $H_1$-receptor sites. Loratadine is a nonsedating antihistamine; its chemical structure prevents entry into the CNS.

**ONSET, PEAK, DURATION**
Onset occurs in 1 hour. Peak effects occur in 4 to 6 hours. Effects persist for at least 24 hours.

**INDICATIONS & DOSAGE**
*Symptomatic treatment of seasonal allergic rhinitis −*
**Adults and children 12 years and over:** 10 mg P.O. daily. Dosage for patients with hepatic failure is 10 mg P.O. every other day.

**ADVERSE REACTIONS**
**CNS:** headache, somnolence, fatigue, drowsiness.
**GI:** dry mouth.

**INTERACTIONS**
*Erythromycin:* increased loratadine plasma concentrations. Monitor patient closely.

**CONTRAINDICATIONS**
Contraindicated in patients with hypersensitivity to the drug.

**NURSING CONSIDERATIONS**
• Use cautiously in patients with liver impairment and in breast-feeding patients.
• Be aware that this drug can affect results of allergy skin tests.

☑ **PATIENT TEACHING**
• Instruct patient to take drug at least 2 hours after a meal and to avoid eating for at least 1 hour after taking drug.
• Ensure that patient knows to take drug only once daily. If symptoms persist or worsen, he should contact the doctor.
• Advise patient to stop taking drug 4 days before allergy skin tests to preserve accuracy of tests.

# methdilazine hydrochloride
Dilosyn †‡ Tacaryl*

*Pregnancy Risk Category: B*

**HOW SUPPLIED**
*Tablets:* 8 mg
*Tablets (chewable):* 3.6 mg methdilazine (equal to 4 mg methdilazine hydrochloride)
*Syrup:* 4 mg/5 ml*

**ACTION**
Competes with histamine for $H_1$-receptor sites on effector cells. Prevents, but does not reverse, hista-

---

mine-mediated responses. A phenothiazine derivative.

### ONSET, PEAK, DURATION
Onset occurs in 15 to 60 minutes.
Peak unknown. Effects persist for 6 to
12 hours.

### INDICATIONS & DOSAGE
*Allergic rhinitis, pruritus –*
**Adults:** 8 mg P.O. b.i.d. to q.i.d. or
7.2 mg chewable tablets P.O. b.i.d. to
q.i.d.
**Children over 3 years:** 4 mg P.O.
b.i.d. to q.i.d. or 3.6 mg chewable
tablets P.O. b.i.d. to q.i.d.

### ADVERSE REACTIONS
**CNS:** *drowsiness,* dizziness, head-
ache.
**GI:** nausea, *dry mouth and throat.*
**GU:** urine retention.
**Hepatic:** cholestatic jaundice.
**Skin:** rash.

### INTERACTIONS
*CNS depressants:* increased sedation.
Use together cautiously.
*Epinephrine:* methdilazine may block
or reverse the effects of epinephrine.
Use other pressor agents instead.
*MAO inhibitors:* increased anticholin-
ergic effects. Don't use together.
*Phenothiazines:* increased effects.
Don't use together.

### CONTRAINDICATIONS
Contraindicated in patients experiencing acute asthmatic attacks; in patients with hypersensitivity to the
drug; and in newborns or premature
neonates and breast-feeding patients.

### NURSING CONSIDERATIONS
• Use with extreme caution in patients with angle-closure glaucoma,
prostatic hyperplasia, pyloroduodenal
and bladder-neck obstructions, stenosing peptic ulcer, asthma or COPD,
increased intraocular pressure, hyper-

thyroidism, CV disease, and hypertension.
• Be aware that this drug can affect
results of allergy skin tests.

### ☑ PATIENT TEACHING
• Tell patient to reduce GI distress by
taking drug with food or milk.
• *Alert:* Available as chewable tablet
for children. Instruct child to chew
completely and swallow promptly;
may cause local anesthetic effect in
mouth, which increases the risk of
choking.
• Warn patient to avoid alcohol and
driving or other activities that require
alertness until drug's CNS effects are
known.
• Tell patient that coffee or tea may
reduce drowsiness. Sugarless gum,
sugarless sour hard candy, or ice chips
may relieve dry mouth.
• Advise patient to stop drug 4 days
before allergy skin tests to preserve
accuracy of tests.
• Tell patient to notify doctor if tolerance develops because a different antihistamine may need to be given.

---

## promethazine hydrochloride
Anergan 25, Anergan 50,
Histantil†, Pentazine, Phenameth,
Phenazine 25, Phenazine 50,
Phencen-50, Phenergan*,
Phenergan Fortis*, Phenergan
Plain*, Phenoject-50, PMS-
Promethazine†, Pro-50, Prometh-
25, Prometh-50, Promethegan,
Prorex-25, Prorex-50,
Prothazine†*, Prothazine Plain,
V-Gan-25, V-Gan-50

## promethazine theoclate
Avomine‡

*Pregnancy Risk Category: NR*

### HOW SUPPLIED
**promethazine hydrochloride**
*Tablets:* 12.5 mg, 25 mg, 50 mg

---

*Liquid form contains alcohol. **May contain tartrazine. †Canada only. ‡Australia only. ◇OTC.

*Syrup:* 5 mg/5 ml‡*, 6.25 mg/5 ml*,
10 mg/5 ml†*, 25 mg/5 ml*
*Injection:* 25 mg/ml, 50 mg/ml
*Suppositories:* 12.5 mg, 25 mg, 50 mg
**promethazine theoclate**
*Tablets:* 25 mg‡

## ACTION
Competes with histamine for $H_1$-receptor sites on effector cells. Prevents, but does not reverse, histamine-mediated responses. A phenothiazine derivative.

## ONSET, PEAK, DURATION
Onset occurs in 15 to 60 minutes after oral administration, 20 minutes after I.M. injection and P.R. administration, 3 to 5 minutes after I.V. administration. Peak unknown. Effects persist up to 12 hours.

## INDICATIONS & DOSAGE
*Motion sickness* –
**Adults:** 25 mg P.O. b.i.d.
**Children:** 12.5 to 25 mg P.O., I.M., or P.R. b.i.d.
*Nausea* –
**Adults:** 12.5 to 25 mg P.O., I.M., or P.R. q 4 to 6 hours, p.r.n.
**Children:** 12.5 to 25 mg I.M. or P.R. q 4 to 6 hours, p.r.n.
*Rhinitis, allergy symptoms* –
**Adults:** 12.5 mg P.O. q.i.d.; or 25 mg P.O. h.s.
**Children:** 6.25 to 12.5 mg P.O. t.i.d. or 25 mg P.O. or P.R. h.s.
*Sedation* –
**Adults:** 25 to 50 mg P.O. or I.M. h.s. or p.r.n.
**Children:** 12.5 to 25 mg P.O., I.M., or P.R. h.s.
*Routine preoperative or postoperative sedation or adjunct to analgesics* –
**Adults:** 25 to 50 mg I.M., I.V., or P.O.
**Children:** 12.5 to 25 mg I.M., I.V., or P.O.

## ADVERSE REACTIONS
**CNS:** *sedation,* confusion, sleepiness, dizziness, disorientation, extrapyramidal symptoms, *drowsiness.*
**CV:** hypotension, hypertension.
**EENT:** blurred vision.
**GI:** nausea, vomiting, *dry mouth.*
**GU:** urine retention.
**Hematologic:** leukopenia, *agranulocytosis, thrombocytopenia.*
**Other:** photosensitivity, rash.

## INTERACTIONS
*Anticholinergics, phenothiazines, tricyclic antidepressants:* increased effects. Don't give together.
*CNS depressants, ethanol:* increased sedation. Use together cautiously.
*Epinephrine:* promethazine may block or reverse the effects of epinephrine. Use other pressor agents instead.
*Levodopa:* promethazine may decrease levodopa's antiparkinsonian action. Avoid concomitant use.
*Lithium:* promethazine may reduce GI absorption or enhance renal elimination of lithium. Avoid concomitant use.
*MAO inhibitors:* increased extrapyramidal effects. Don't use together.

## CONTRAINDICATIONS
Contraindicated in patients with hypersensitivity to the drug; in those with intestinal obstruction, prostatic hyperplasia, bladder-neck obstruction, seizure disorders, coma, CNS depression, and stenosing peptic ulcerations; and in newborns and premature neonates, and breast-feeding patients; and in acutely ill or dehydrated children.

## NURSING CONSIDERATIONS
• Use cautiously in patients with pulmonary, hepatic, CV disease, or asthma.
• Know that pronounced sedative effect limits use in many ambulatory patients.
• Know that promethazine is used as

---

Reactions may be *common,* uncommon, *life-threatening,* or COMMON AND LIFE-THREATENING.

an adjunct to analgesics (usually to increase sedation) and that it has no analgesic activity.
- Reduce GI distress by giving drug with food or milk.
- **I.V. use:** Don't give in a concentration greater than 25 mg/ml or at a rate exceeding 25 mg/minute. Shield I.V. infusion from direct light.
- Inject deep I.M. into large muscle mass. Rotate injection sites.
- *Alert:* Don't administer via S.C. route.
- Be aware that drug may be safely mixed with meperidine in the same syringe.
- In patients scheduled for a myelogram, discontinue drug 48 hours before procedure and do not resume drug until 24 hours after procedure, as ordered, because of the risk of seizures.
- Know that drug may cause false-positive immunologic urine pregnancy test (Gravindex). Also may interfere with blood typing of ABO group.

☑ **PATIENT TEACHING**
- Tell patient to take oral form with food or milk.
- When treating motion sickness, tell patient to take first dose 30 to 60 minutes before travel. On succeeding days of travel, patient should take dose upon rising and with evening meal.
- Warn patient to avoid alcohol and driving or other activities that require alertness until drug's CNS effects are known.
- Tell patient that coffee or tea may reduce drowsiness. Sugarless gum, sugarless sour hard candy, or ice chips may relieve dry mouth.
- Warn patient about possible photosensitivity and precautions to avoid it.
- Advise patient to stop drug 4 days before allergy skin tests to preserve accuracy of tests.

# terfenadine
Seldane, Seldane Caplets†,
Teldane‡

*Pregnancy Risk Category: C*

**HOW SUPPLIED**
*Tablets:* 60 mg, 120 mg†
*Oral suspension†:* 6 mg/ml

**ACTION**
Competes with histamine for $H_1$-receptor sites on effector cells. Prevents, but does not reverse, histamine-mediated responses.

**ONSET, PEAK, DURATION**
Onset occurs in 1 to 2 hours. Serum levels peak in 2 hours. Time to peak effect occurs in 3 to 4 hours. Effects persist for over 12 hours.

**INDICATIONS & DOSAGE**
*Rhinitis, allergy symptoms* –
**Adults and children 12 years and over:** 60 mg P.O. b.i.d. or 120 mg once daily.

**ADVERSE REACTIONS**
**CNS:** fatigue, dizziness, *headache,* sedation, drowsiness, nervousness.
**CV:** *arrhythmias* (with high blood levels).
**GI:** abdominal distress, nausea, dry mouth, vomiting.
**Other:** cholestatic jaundice, rash, urticaria, cough, sore throat.

**INTERACTIONS**
*Cimetidine, ciprofloxacin, clarithromycin, itraconazole, ketoconazole, macrolide antibiotics (erythromycin, troleandomycin):* decreased hepatic metabolism of terfenadine, leading to increased serum levels and risk of serious arrhythmias. Avoid concomitant use.

**CONTRAINDICATIONS**
Contraindicated in patients with hypersensitivity to terfenadine; in those

---

taking the antifungal agents itraconazole or ketoconazole or macrolide antibiotics, including erythromycin; and in patients with significant hepatic impairment.

## NURSING CONSIDERATIONS
• Use cautiously in patients with cardiac disease.
• Be aware that terfenadine does not cause the degree of drowsiness and sedation associated with other antihistamines because it does not cross the blood-brain barrier; its anticholinergic and antiserotonin effects are mild.

## ☑ PATIENT TEACHING
• Instruct patient not to exceed prescribed dosage. If overdose occurs, monitor patient for arrhythmias.
• Instruct patient to keep well hydrated. Drug may cause a mild anticholinergic drying effect in patients with lower airway disease, such as asthma.

---

## trimeprazine tartrate
Panectyl†, Temaril*, Vallergan‡
*Pregnancy Risk Category: NR*

## HOW SUPPLIED
*Tablets:* 2.5 mg, 10 mg‡
*Spansule capsules (sustained-release):* 5 mg
*Syrup:* 2.5 mg/5 ml*, 7.5 mg/5 ml*‡, 30 mg/5 ml*‡

## ACTION
A phenothiazine derivative that competes with histamine for $H_1$-receptor sites on effector cells. Prevents, but does not reverse, histamine-mediated responses.

## ONSET, PEAK, DURATION
Onset occurs in 15 to 60 minutes. Peak unknown. Effects persist for 3 to 6 hours.

## INDICATIONS & DOSAGE
*Pruritus –*
**Adults:** 2.5 mg P.O. q.i.d.; or 5 mg sustained-release P.O. b.i.d.
**Children 3 years and over:** 2.5 mg P.O. h.s. or t.i.d., p.r.n.
**Children 6 months to 3 years:** 1.25 mg P.O. h.s. or t.i.d., p.r.n.

## ADVERSE REACTIONS
**CNS:** drowsiness, dizziness, confusion, headache, restlessness, tremor, irritability, insomnia, paradoxical excitation.
**CV:** hypotension, palpitations, tachycardia.
**GI:** anorexia, nausea, vomiting, *dry mouth and throat.*
**GU:** urinary frequency, urine retention.
**Hematologic:** *agranulocytosis,* leukopenia.
**Skin:** urticaria, rash, *photosensitivity.*

## INTERACTIONS
*Anticholinergics, MAO inhibitors, phenothiazines, tricyclic antidepressants:* increased anticholinergic effect. Don't use together.
*CNS depressants, ethanol:* increased sedation. Use together cautiously.
*Levodopa:* trimeprazine may block levodopa's antiparkinsonian effects. Don't use together.
*Lithium:* trimeprazine may decrease GI absorption and enhance renal excretion of lithium. Don't use together.

## CONTRAINDICATIONS
Contraindicated in patients with hypersensitivity to the drug or other phenothiazines; in those with acute asthma, coma, CNS depression, and bone marrow depression; in neonates or premature infants; and in acutely ill or dehydrated children; and in breast-feeding patients.

---

Reactions may be *common,* uncommon, *life-threatening,* or **COMMON AND LIFE-THREATENING.**

## NURSING CONSIDERATIONS
- Use with extreme caution in patients with angle-closure glaucoma, prostatic hyperplasia, stenosing peptic ulcer, pyloroduodenal or bladder-neck obstruction, and in patients receiving MAO inhibitors.
- Know that children under 12 years should use only as directed by a doctor.
- In patients scheduled for a myelogram, discontinue drug 48 hours before procedure, as ordered; do not resume drug until 24 hours after the procedure because of the risk of seizures.
- Monitor blood counts during long-term therapy, as ordered.

☑ **PATIENT TEACHING**
- Tell patient to take drug with food or milk to reduce GI distress.
- Warn patient to avoid alcohol and driving or other activities that require alertness until drug's CNS effects are known.
- Tell patient that coffee or tea may reduce drowsiness. Sugarless gum, sugarless sour hard candy, or ice chips may relieve dry mouth.
- Warn patient about risk of photosensitivity. Recommend use of a sunblock. If photosensitivity occurs, tell patient to discontinue drug and call the doctor.
- Advise patient to stop drug 4 days before allergy skin tests to preserve accuracy of tests.

---

# tripelennamine citrate
PBZ*

# tripelennamine hydrochloride
PBZ, PBZ-SR, Pelamine, Pyribenzamine

*Pregnancy Risk Category: NR*

## HOW SUPPLIED
**tripelennamine citrate**
*Elixir:* 37.5 mg/5 ml (equivalent to 25 mg/5 ml tripelennamine hydrochloride)*
**tripelennamine hydrochloride**
*Tablets:* 25 mg, 50 mg
*Tablets (extended-release):* 100 mg

## ACTION
Competes with histamine for $H_1$-receptor sites on effector cells. Prevents, but does not reverse, histamine-mediated responses.

## ONSET, PEAK, DURATION
Onset occurs in 15 to 60 minutes. Peak occurs in 2 to 3 hours. Effects persist for 4 to 6 hours.

## INDICATIONS & DOSAGE
*Rhinitis, allergy symptoms –*
**Adults:** 25 to 50 mg P.O. q 4 to 6 hours; or 100 mg extended-release P.O. b.i.d. or t.i.d. Maximum dosage is 600 mg daily.
**Children:** 5 mg/kg P.O. daily in four to six divided doses. Maximum dosage is 300 mg daily.

## ADVERSE REACTIONS
**CNS:** *drowsiness,* dizziness, confusion, restlessness, tremor, irritability, insomnia.
**CV:** palpitations.
**GI:** anorexia, diarrhea or constipation, *nausea, vomiting, dry mouth.*
**GU:** urinary frequency, urine retention.
**Skin:** urticaria, rash.
**Other:** thick bronchial secretions.

## INTERACTIONS
*CNS depressants:* increased sedation. Use together cautiously.
*MAO inhibitors:* increased anticholinergic effects. Don't use together.

## CONTRAINDICATIONS
Contraindicated in patients with hypersensitivity to the drug or any re-

---

*Liquid form contains alcohol.  **May contain tartrazine.  †Canada only.  ‡Australia only.  ◇OTC.

lated compounds; in those with angle-closure glaucoma, stenosing peptic ulcer, symptomatic prostatic hyperplasia, pyloroduodenal or bladder-neck obstruction, and lower respiratory tract symptoms, including asthma; and in premature infants, neonates, or breast-feeding patients.

## NURSING CONSIDERATIONS

• Use cautiously in elderly patients and in patients with increased intraocular pressure, hyperthyroidism, CV disease, hypertension, or history of bronchial asthma.
• Know that extended-release preparations should not be used in children.

## ☑ PATIENT TEACHING

• Tell patient to take drug with food or milk to reduce GI distress.
• Warn patient to avoid alcohol and driving or other activities that require alertness until drug's CNS effects are known.
• Tell patient that coffee or tea may reduce drowsiness. Sugarless gum or sour hard candy, or ice chips may relieve dry mouth.
• Advise patient to stop drug 4 days before allergy skin tests to preserve accuracy of tests.
• Tell patient to notify doctor if tolerance develops because a different antihistamine may need to be prescribed.

---

## triprolidine hydrochloride
Actidil◇, Alleract◇, Myidyl

*Pregnancy Risk Category: C*

## HOW SUPPLIED
*Tablets:* 2.5 mg◇
*Syrup\*:* 1.25 mg/5 ml◇

## ACTION
Competes with histamine for $H_1$-receptor sites on effector cells. Prevents, but does not reverse, histamine-mediated responses.

## ONSET, PEAK, DURATION
Onset occurs in 15 to 60 minutes. Peak levels occur in about 2 hours. Peak effects occur in 2 to 3 hours. Effects persist for 4 to 8 hours.

## INDICATIONS & DOSAGE
*Colds and allergy symptoms –*
**Adults and children 12 years and over:** 2.5 mg P.O. q 4 to 6 hours. Maximum dosage is 10 mg/day.
**Children 6 to 12 years:** 1.25 mg P.O. q 4 to 6 hours. Maximum dosage is 5 mg/day.
**Children 4 to 6 years:** 0.938 mg P.O. q 4 to 6 hours. Maximum dosage is 3.744 mg/day.
**Children 2 to 4 years:** 0.625 mg P.O. q 4 to 6 hours. Maximum dosage is 2.5 mg/day.
**Children 4 months to 2 years:** 0.313 mg P.O. q 4 to 6 hours. Maximum dosage is 1.252 mg/day.

## ADVERSE REACTIONS
**CNS:** *drowsiness, dizziness,* confusion, restlessness, insomnia, headache, *sedation, sleepiness, incoordination,* fatigue, anxiety, nervousness, tremor, **seizures, stimulation.**
**CV:** hypotension, palpitations, tachycardia.
**EENT:** *dry nose and throat.*
**GI:** anorexia, diarrhea or constipation, nausea, vomiting, *dry mouth,* epigastric distress.
**GU:** urinary frequency, urine retention.
**Hematologic:** hemolytic anemia, **thrombocytopenia, agranulocytosis.**
**Skin:** urticaria, rash, photosensitivity, diaphoresis.
**Other:** **anaphylactic shock,** chills, thickening of bronchial secretions.

## INTERACTIONS
*CNS depressants:* increased sedation. Use together cautiously.
*MAO inhibitors:* increased anticholinergic effects. Don't use together.

---

Reactions may be *common,* uncommon, *life-threatening,* or **COMMON AND LIFE-THREATENING.**

## CONTRAINDICATIONS

Contraindicated in patients with hypersensitivity to the drug, in those with acute asthma, and in neonates, premature infants, and breast-feeding patients.

## NURSING CONSIDERATIONS

● Use with extreme caution in patients with increased intraocular pressure, angle-closure glaucoma, hyperthyroidism, CV disease, hypertension, bronchial asthma, prostatic hyperplasia, bladder-neck obstruction, and stenosing peptic ulcerations.
● Know that children under 12 years should use only as directed by a doctor.

## ☑ PATIENT TEACHING

● Tell patient to take drug with food or milk to reduce GI distress.
● Warn patient to avoid alcohol and driving or other activities that require alertness until drug's CNS effects are known.
● Tell patient that coffee or tea may reduce drowsiness. Sugarless gum, sugarless sour hard candy, or ice chips may relieve dry mouth.
● Advise patient to stop drug 4 days before allergy skin tests to preserve accuracy of tests.

# 44

# Bronchodilators

albuterol
albuterol sulfate
aminophylline
atropine sulfate
(See Chapter 21, ANTIARRHYTHMICS.)
bitolterol mesylate
dyphylline
ephedrine sulfate
epinephrine
epinephrine bitartrate
epinephrine hydrochloride
ethylnorepinephrine
hydrochloride
ipratropium bromide
isoetharine hydrochloride
isoetharine mesylate
isoproterenol
isoproterenol hydrochloride
isoproterenol sulfate
metaproterenol sulfate
oxtriphylline
pirbuterol
salmeterol xinafoate
terbutaline sulfate
theophylline
theophylline sodium glycinate

## COMBINATION PRODUCTS
*Inhalants*
DUO-MEDIHALER: isoproterenol hydrochloride 0.16 mg and phenylephrine bitartrate 0.24 mg per dose.
*Oral bronchodilators*
BRONCHIAL CAPSULES: 150 mg theophylline and 90 mg guaifenesin.
DILOR-G TABLETS: 200 mg dyphylline and 200 mg guaifenesin.
DYFLEX-G TABLETS: 200 mg dyphylline and 200 mg guaifenesin.
DYLINE-GG TABLETS: 200 mg dyphylline and 200 mg guaifenesin.
GLYCERYL-T CAPSULES: 150 mg theophylline and 90 mg guaifenesin.
MARAX*: theophylline 130 mg, ephedrine sulfate 25 mg, and hydroxyzine hydrochloride 10 mg.

NEOTHYLLINE-GG TABLETS: 200 mg dyphylline and 200 mg guaifenesin.
QUIBRON CAPSULES: 150 mg theophylline and 90 mg guaifenesin.
SYNOPHYLATE-GG SYRUP*: 33.3 mg/5 ml guaifenesin and 100 mg/ml theophylline sodium glycinate.
THALFED◊: theophylline 120 mg, ephedrine hydrochloride 25 mg, and phenobarbital 8 mg.
*Decongestants*
ACTIFED◊: pseudoephedrine hydrochloride 60 mg and triprolidine hydrochloride 2.5 mg.
CONGESPIRIN◊: phenylephrine hydrochloride 1.25 mg and acetaminophen 81 mg.
DRISTAN◊: phenylephrine hydrochloride 5 mg, chlorpheniramine maleate 2 mg, and acetaminophen 325 mg.
NALDECON: phenylpropanolamine hydrochloride 40 mg, phenylephrine hydrochloride 10 mg, chlorpheniramine maleate 5 mg, and phenyltoloxamine citrate 15 mg.
ORNEX◊: phenylpropanolamine hydrochloride 18 mg and acetaminophen 325 mg.
SEMPREX-D: acrivastine 8 mg and pseudoephedrine hydrochloride 60 mg.

---

Reactions may be *common,* uncommon, *life-threatening,* or COMMON AND LIFE-THREATENING.

## albuterol (salbutamol)
Asmol‡, Proventil, Respolin‡,
Ventolin

## albuterol sulfate (salbutamol sulphate)
Proventil, Proventil Repetabs,
Respolin Autohaler Inhalation
Device‡, Respolin Inhaler‡,
Respolin Respirator Solution‡,
Ventolin, Ventolin Obstetric
Injection‡, Ventolin Rotacaps,
Volmax

*Pregnancy Risk Category: C*

### HOW SUPPLIED
**albuterol**
*Aerosol inhaler:* 90 mcg/metered
spray, 100 mcg/metered spray‡
**albuterol sulfate**
*Capsules for inhalation:* 200 mcg
*Tablets:* 2 mg, 4 mg
*Tablets (extended-release):* 4 mg, 8
mg
*Syrup:* 2 mg/5 ml
*Solution for inhalation:* 0.083%,
0.5%
*Injection:* 1 mg/ml‡

### ACTION
Relaxes bronchial and uterine smooth
muscle by acting on beta$_2$-adrenergic
receptors.

### ONSET, PEAK, DURATION
Onset occurs within 5 to 15 minutes
after inhalation, within 15 to 30 minutes after oral administration. Peak
effect occurs 1 to 1½ hours after inhalation, 2 to 3 hours after oral administration. Effects persist for 3 to 6
hours after inhalation, up to 6 hours
for syrup, up to 8 hours for tablets,
about 12 hours for extended-release
preparations.

### INDICATIONS & DOSAGE
*To prevent or treat bronchospasm in
patients with reversible obstructive
airway disease –*

**Adults and children 12 years and
older:** dosage and frequency vary
with dosage form.
*Aerosol inhalation –* 1 to 2 inhalations
q 4 to 6 hours. More frequent administration or a greater number of inhalations is not recommended.
*Solution for inhalation –* 2.5 mg t.i.d.
or q.i.d. by nebulizer. To prepare solution, use 0.5 ml of the 0.5% solution diluted with 2.5 ml of 0.9% sodium chloride. Alternatively, use 3 ml
of the 0.083% solution.
*Capsules for inhalation –* 200 mcg inhaled q 4 to 6 hours using a Rotahaler
inhalation device. Some patients may
need 400 mcg q 4 to 6 hours.
*Oral tablets –* 2 to 4 mg P.O. t.i.d. or
q.i.d. Maximum dosage is 8 mg
q.i.d.
*Extended-release tablets –* 4 to 8 mg
P.O. q 12 hours. Maximum dosage is
16 mg b.i.d.
**Children 6 to 13 years:** 2 mg (1 tsp)
P.O. t.i.d. or q.i.d.
**Children 2 to 5 years:** 0.1 mg/kg
P.O. t.i.d., not to exceed 2 mg (1 tsp)
t.i.d.
**Adults over 65 years:** 2 mg P.O.
t.i.d. or q.i.d.
*To prevent exercise-induced asthma –*
**Adults:** 2 inhalations 15 minutes be-
fore exercise.
*Prevention of premature labor‡ –*
**Adults:** initially, 10 mcg/minute by
continuous I.V. infusion (via an infu-
sion pump). Dosage should be in-
creased at 10-minute intervals until
desired response is achieved.

### ADVERSE REACTIONS
**CNS:** *tremor, nervousness,* dizziness,
insomnia, *headache, hyperactivity,*
weakness, CNS stimulation, malaise.
**CV:** *tachycardia, palpitations,* hypertension.
**EENT:** dry and irritated nose and
throat (with inhaled form), nasal congestion, epistaxis, hoarseness, bad
taste.

---

*Liquid form contains alcohol. **May contain tartrazine. †Canada only. ‡Australia only. ◇OTC.

**GI:** heartburn, *nausea, vomiting,* anorexia.
**Respiratory:** BRONCHOSPASM, cough, wheezing, dyspnea, bronchitis, increased sputum.
**Other:** muscle cramps, hypokalemia (with high doses), increased appetite, hypersensitivity reactions.

## INTERACTIONS
*CNS stimulants:* increased CNS stimulation. Avoid concomitant use.
*MAO inhibitors, tricyclic antidepressants:* increased adverse CV effects. Monitor patient closely.
*Propranolol and other beta blockers:* mutual antagonism. Monitor patient carefully.

## CONTRAINDICATIONS
Contraindicated in patients with hypersensitivity to the drug or any component of the formulation.

## NURSING CONSIDERATIONS
• Use cautiously in patients with CV disorders, including coronary insufficiency and hypertension; in patients with hyperthyroidism or diabetes mellitus; and in those who are unusually responsive to adrenergics.
• Use extended-release tablets cautiously in patients with preexisting GI narrowing.
• Know that pleasant-tasting syrup may be taken by children as young as 2 years. Contains no alcohol or sugar.
• Know that aerosol form may be prescribed for use 15 minutes before exercise to prevent exercise-induced bronchospasm.
• Know that patients may use tablets and aerosol concomitantly. Monitor closely for toxicity.
• **I.V. use:** Where available, I.V. form may be used to prepare infusion using sodium chloride for injection, dextrose for injection, or sodium chloride and dextrose for injection. Do not administer drug without dilution. Do not mix with any other medication. Dis-

card unused diluted solution after 24 hours.
• When used to prevent premature labor, monitor maternal heart rate closely. It should not exceed 140 beats/minute.
• After uterine contractions have ceased, drip rate of drug should be maintained for 1 hour, then gradually tapered at 50% increments in six hourly intervals. Do not continue infusions for more than 48 hours. If therapy needs to continue over 48 hours, doctor may prescribe 4 to 8 mg P.O. q.i.d.

## ☑ PATIENT TEACHING
• Warn patient about possibility of paradoxical bronchospasm. If this occurs, discontinue drug immediately.
• Teach patient to perform oral inhalation correctly. Give the following instructions for using metered-dose inhaler:
  – Clear nasal passages and throat.
  – Breathe out, expelling as much air from lungs as possible.
  – Place mouthpiece well into mouth as dose from inhaler is released, and inhale deeply.
  – Hold breath for several seconds, remove mouthpiece, and exhale slowly.
• If more than one inhalation is ordered, advise patient to wait at least 2 minutes before repeating procedure.
• Tell patient who is also using a steroid inhaler to use the bronchodilator first; then wait about 5 minutes before using the steroid. This allows bronchodilator to open air passages for maximum effectiveness.

---

Reactions may be *common,* uncommon, *life-threatening,* or COMMON AND LIFE-THREATENING.

# aminophylline (theophylline ethylenediamine)

Aminophyllin, Cardophyllin‡, Corophyllin†, Phyllocontin, Phyllocontin-350, Somophyllin, Somophyllin-DF, Truphylline

*Pregnancy Risk Category: C*

## HOW SUPPLIED

*Tablets:* 100 mg, 200 mg
*Tablets (extended-release):* 225 mg, 350 mg†
*Oral liquid:* 105 mg/5 ml
*Injection:* 250 mg/10 ml, 500 mg/20 ml, 100 mg/100 ml in 0.45% sodium chloride, 200 mg/100 ml in 0.45% sodium chloride
*Rectal suppositories:* 250 mg, 500 mg

## ACTION

Inhibits phosphodiesterase, the enzyme that degrades cAMP. Results in relaxation of smooth muscle of the bronchial airways and pulmonary blood vessels.

## ONSET, PEAK, DURATION

Onset occurs in 15 minutes after I.V. injection, 15 to 60 minutes after oral solution or tablets. Peak serum levels occur immediately after I.V. infusion; within 1 hour of oral solution; 2 hours after oral, uncoated tablets; 4 to 7 hours after extended-release capsules or tablets. Effects persist for variable lengths of time, depending on patient's age, concurrent illnesses, and smoking status.

## INDICATIONS & DOSAGE

*Symptomatic relief of bronchospasm –*
**Patients not currently receiving theophylline products who require rapid relief of symptoms:** loading dose is 6 mg/kg (equivalent to 4.7 mg/kg anhydrous theophylline) I.V. (less than or equal to 25 mg/minute); then maintenance infusion.
**Adults (nonsmokers):** 0.7 mg/kg/hour I.V. for 12 hours; then 0.5 mg/kg/hour.
**Otherwise healthy adult smokers:** 1 mg/kg/hour I.V. for 12 hours; then 0.8 mg/kg/hour.
**Older patients and adults with cor pulmonale:** 0.6 mg/kg/hour I.V. for 12 hours; then 0.3 mg/kg/hour.
**Adults with CHF or liver disease:** 0.5 mg/kg/hour I.V. for 12 hours; then 0.1 to 0.2 mg/kg/hour.
**Children 9 to 16 years:** 1 mg/kg/hour I.V. for 12 hours; then 0.8 mg/kg/hour.
**Children 6 months to 9 years:** 1.2 mg/kg/hour for 12 hours; then 1 mg/kg/hour.
**Patients currently receiving theophylline products:** aminophylline infusions of 0.63 mg/kg (0.5 mg/kg anhydrous theophylline) will increase plasma levels of theophylline by 1 mcg/ml. Some clinicians recommend a dose of 3.1 mg/kg (2.5 mg/kg anhydrous theophylline) if no obvious signs of theophylline toxicity are present.
*Chronic bronchial asthma –*
Dosage is highly individualized.
**Adults and children:** 16 mg/kg or 400 mg (whichever is less) P.O. daily in three or four divided doses q 6 to 8 hours if using rapidly absorbed dosage forms. Dosage may be increased, if tolerated, in increments of 25% q 2 to 3 days. Alternatively, 12 mg/kg or 400 mg (whichever is less) P.O. daily in two to three divided doses q 8 to 12 hours if using extended-release preparations. Dosage may be increased, if tolerated, by 2 to 3 mg/kg daily q 3 days.
Regardless of dosage form, dosage may be increased, if tolerated, up to the following maximum daily doses, without measurement of serum theophylline concentrations.
**Children up to 9 years:** 24 mg/kg daily.
**Children 9 to 12 years:** 20 mg/kg daily.

---

*Liquid form contains alcohol. **May contain tartrazine. †Canada only. ‡Australia only. ◇OTC.

**Children 12 to 16 years:** 18 mg/kg daily.

**Adults and children 16 years and older:** 13 mg/kg or 900 mg daily (whichever is less).

When the recommended maximum dosage is exceeded, dosage adjustment should be based on measurement of peak serum theophylline concentrations.

*Note:* Rectal dosage is the same as that recommended for oral dosage.

## ADVERSE REACTIONS
**CNS:** *nervousness, restlessness,* headache, *insomnia, seizures,* muscle twitching, irritability.
**CV:** *palpitations, sinus tachycardia,* extrasystoles, flushing, marked hypotension, arrhythmias.
**GI:** *nausea, vomiting,* diarrhea, epigastric pain, hematemesis.
**Respiratory:** tachypnea, *respiratory arrest.*
**Skin:** urticaria.
**Other:** irritation (with rectal suppositories), hyperglycemia, fever.

## INTERACTIONS
*Adenosine:* decreased antiarrhythmic effectiveness. Higher doses of adenosine may be necessary.
*Alkali-sensitive drugs:* reduced activity. Do not add to I.V. fluids containing aminophylline.
*Barbiturates, carbamazepine, nicotine, phenytoin, rifampin:* enhanced metabolism and decreased theophylline blood levels. Monitor for decreased aminophylline effect.
*Beta-adrenergic blockers:* antagonism. Propranolol and nadolol, especially, may cause bronchospasm in sensitive patients. Use together cautiously.
*Calcium channel blockers, cimetidine, disulfiran, influenza virus vaccine, interferon, macrolide antibiotics (such as erythromycin), oral contraceptives, quinolone antibiotics (such as ciprofloxacin):* decreased hepatic clearance of theophylline; elevated theophylline levels. Monitor for signs of toxicity.
*Ephedrine, other sympathomimetics:* theophylline may exhibit synergistic toxicity with these agents, predisposing patients to cardiac arrhythmias. Monitor patient closely.
*Lithium:* theophylline may increase excretion of lithium. Monitor patient closely.

## CONTRAINDICATIONS
Contraindicated in patients with hypersensitivity to xanthine compounds (caffeine, theobromine) and ethylenediamine and in patients with active peptic ulcer disease and seizure disorders (unless adequate anticonvulsant therapy is given). Rectal supppositories are also contraindicated in patients who have an irritation or infection of the rectum or lower colon.

## NURSING CONSIDERATIONS
• Use cautiously in neonates and infants under age 1, young children, and elderly patients; also use cautiously in patients with CHF or other cardiac or circulatory impairment, COPD, cor pulmonale, renal or hepatic disease, hyperthyroidism, diabetes mellitus, peptic ulcer, severe hypoxemia, and hypertension.
• Relieve GI symptoms by giving oral drug with full glass of water at meals, although food in stomach delays absorption. No evidence exists that antacids reduce adverse GI reactions. Know that enteric-coated tablets also may delay and impair absorption.
• **Alert:** Before giving loading dose, ensure that patient has not had recent theophylline therapy.
• **I.V. use:** I.V. drug administration can cause burning; dilute with compatible I.V. solution, and inject at a rate no faster than 25 mg/minute. Drug is compatible with most I.V. solutions except invert sugar, fructose, and fat emulsions.

---

Reactions may be *common*, uncommon, *life-threatening*, or **COMMON AND LIFE-THREATENING**.

- Suppositories are slowly and erratically absorbed. Administer rectal suppository if patients cannot take drug orally, as ordered. Schedule after evacuation, if possible; may be retained better if given before meal. Have patients remain recumbent 15 to 20 minutes after insertion.
- Monitor vital signs; measure and record fluid intake and output. Expected clinical effects include improved quality of pulse and respirations.
- Aminophylline is a soluble salt of theophylline. Know that dosage is adjusted by monitoring response, tolerance, pulmonary function, and serum theophylline levels. Monitor serum theophylline levels as ordered. Theophylline concentrations should range from 10 to 20 mcg/ml; toxicity has been reported with levels above 20 mcg/ml.
- Be aware that patients who experience urticaria may still tolerate other theophylline preparations. Urticaria may be caused by the ethylenediamine salt.

### ☑ PATIENT TEACHING
- Supply instructions for home care administration of form prescribed and dosage schedule. Some patients may require an around-the-clock dosage schedule.
- Warn elderly patient that dizziness, a common adverse reaction at start of therapy, may occur.
- Warn patient to check with the doctor or pharmacist before combining aminophylline with other drugs. OTC remedies may contain ephedrine in combination with theophylline salts; excessive CNS stimulation may result.
- Advise patient to avoid switching brand without first checking with the doctor.

# bitolterol mesylate
Tornalate

*Pregnancy Risk Category: C*

## HOW SUPPLIED
*Aerosol inhaler:* 370 mcg/metered spray

## ACTION
Relaxes bronchial smooth muscle by acting on beta$_2$-adrenergic receptors.

## ONSET, PEAK, DURATION
Onset occurs in 3 to 4 minutes. Peak effects occur within ½ to 1 hour. Effects persist for 5 to 8 hours, may be only 2½ to 5 hours in steroid-dependent patients.

## INDICATIONS & DOSAGE
*To prevent or treat bronchial asthma and bronchospasm–*
**Adults and children over 12 years:** to treat bronchospasm, two inhalations with an interval of at least 1 to 3 minutes, followed by a third inhalation, if needed. To prevent bronchospasm, the usual dosage is two inhalations q 8 hours. In either case, dosage should never exceed three inhalations q 6 hours or two inhalations q 4 hours.

## ADVERSE REACTIONS
**CNS:** *tremor,* nervousness, headache, dizziness, light-headedness.
**CV:** palpitations, chest discomfort, tachycardia.
**EENT:** throat irritation, cough.
**GI:** nausea, vomiting.
**Other:** dyspnea, hypersensitivity reactions.

## INTERACTIONS
*Adrenergic agents:* may cause serious CV effects. Use together cautiously. *Other sympathomimetic bronchodilators:* additive sympathomimetic effects. Avoid concurrent administration.

---

*Liquid form contains alcohol.  **May contain tartrazine.  †Canada only.  ‡Australia only.  ◇OTC.

## CONTRAINDICATIONS
Contraindicated in patients with hypersensitivity to the drug.

## NURSING CONSIDERATIONS
• Use cautiously in patients with ischemic heart disease or hypertension, hyperthyroidism, diabetes mellitus, arrhythmias, seizure disorders, and history of unusual responsiveness to beta-adrenergic agonists.
• Monitor blood pressure regularly.

## ☑ PATIENT TEACHING
• Advise patient not to exceed recommended dosages. Too frequent use may cause tachycardia.
• Remind patient that beneficial effects last for up to 8 hours, longer than most other similar bronchodilators.
• Teach patient to perform oral inhalation correctly. Give the following instructions for using a metered-dose inhaler:
  — Clear nasal passages and throat.
  — Breathe out, expelling as much air from lungs as possible.
  — Place mouthpiece well into mouth as dose from inhaler is released, and inhale deeply and slowly for about 10 seconds.
  — Hold breath for several seconds, remove mouthpiece, and exhale slowly.
• If more than one inhalation is ordered, tell patient to wait at least 2 minutes before repeating procedure.
• Tell patient who is also using a steroid inhaler to use bronchodilator first, then wait about 5 minutes before using steroid. This allows the bronchodilator to open air passages for maximum effectiveness.
• Tell patient that manufacturer recommends rinsing plastic mouthpiece daily with warm tap water, then drying it to ensure proper delivery of drug.

# dyphylline
Dilor*, Dilor-400, Dyflex, Lufyllin*, Lufyllin-400, Neothylline, Protophylline†

*Pregnancy Risk Category: C*

## HOW SUPPLIED
*Tablets:* 200 mg, 400 mg
*Elixir:* 100 mg/15 ml, 160 mg/15 ml*
*Injection:* 250 mg/ml

## ACTION
Unknown. Probably inhibits phosphodiesterase, the enzyme that degrades cAMP. Results in relaxation of smooth muscle of the bronchial airways and pulmonary blood vessels.

## ONSET, PEAK, DURATION
Onset occurs in 15 minutes to 1 hour. Peak levels occur within 1 hour. Effects persist for 4 to 6 hours.

## INDICATIONS & DOSAGE
*Relief of acute and chronic bronchial asthma and reversible bronchospasm associated with chronic bronchitis and emphysema –*
**Adults:** up to 15 mg/kg P.O. q 6 hours. I.M. route is rarely used, but patients may receive 250 to 500 mg I.M. injected slowly at 6-hour intervals.

## ADVERSE REACTIONS
**CNS:** *restlessness,* headache, *insomnia,* irritability, ***seizures,*** muscle twitching.
**CV:** *palpitations, sinus tachycardia,* extrasystoles, flushing, arrhythmias, marked hypotension.
**GI:** *nausea, vomiting,* epigastric pain, hematemesis.
**Respiratory:** tachypnea, ***respiratory arrest.***
**Other:** hyperglycemia, fever.

---

Reactions may be *common,* uncommon, *life-threatening,* or **COMMON AND LIFE-THREATENING.**

## INTERACTIONS
*Probenecid:* increased serum dyphylline levels. Monitor for adverse effects.

## CONTRAINDICATIONS
Contraindicated in patients with hypersensitivity to the drug or related xanthine compounds.

## NURSING CONSIDERATIONS
• Use cautiously in patients with severe cardiac disease, hypertension, hyperthyroidism, acute myocardial injury, or peptic ulcer.
• Know that dosage should be decreased in patients with renal insufficiency.
• Relieve gastric irritation by giving oral drug after meals; no evidence exists that antacids reduce this adverse reaction. May produce less gastric discomfort than theophylline.
• Do not administer I.V.
• Discard injectable dyphylline if precipitate is present. Protect from light.
• Monitor vital signs; measure and record fluid intake and output. Expected clinical effects include improved quality of pulse and respirations.
• Be aware that because dyphylline is a theophylline analog, unlike other derivatives (such as aminophylline); it is not converted to theophylline in the bloodstream. No routine plasma assays exist for determining effective blood levels.

## ☑ PATIENT TEACHING
• Supply instructions for home care and dosage schedule.
• Warn elderly patient that dizziness, a common adverse reaction at start of therapy, may occur.
• Warn patient to check with the doctor or pharmacist before taking any other drugs. OTC remedies may contain ephedrine in combination with theophylline salts; excessive CNS stimulation may result.

---

# ephedrine sulfate
Ephed II

*Pregnancy Risk Category: C*

## HOW SUPPLIED
*Tablets:* 30 mg‡
*Capsules:* 25 mg, 50 mg
*Injection:* 25 mg/ml, 50 mg/ml

## ACTION
Stimulates alpha- and beta-adrenergic receptors; a direct- and indirect-acting sympathomimetic.

## ONSET, PEAK, DURATION
Onset occurs within 5 minutes of I.V. use, 10 to 20 minutes of I.M. use, 15 to 60 minutes after oral use. Peak unknown. Effects persist for 30 minutes to 1 hour after I.M. or S.C. use, 3 to 5 hours after oral use.

## INDICATIONS & DOSAGE
*To correct hypotension –*
**Adults:** 25 to 50 mg I.M. or S.C., or 10 to 25 mg I.V. p.r.n. to maximum of 150 mg/24 hours.
**Children:** 3 mg/kg or 100 mg/m$^2$ S.C. or I.V. daily, in four to six divided doses.
*Bronchodilation or nasal decongestion –*
**Adults and children over 12 years:** 12.5 to 50 mg P.O. b.i.d., t.i.d., or q.i.d. Maximum dosage is 400 mg daily in six to eight divided doses.
**Children over 2 years:** 2 to 3 mg/kg P.O. daily in four to six divided doses.

## ADVERSE REACTIONS
**CNS:** *insomnia, nervousness,* dizziness, headache, muscle weakness, diaphoresis, euphoria, confusion, delirium.
**CV:** *palpitations,* tachycardia, hypertension, precordial pain.
**EENT:** dry nose and throat.

*Liquid form contains alcohol.   **May contain tartrazine.   †Canada only.   ‡Australia only.   ◊OTC.

**GI:** nausea, vomiting, anorexia.
**GU:** urine retention, painful urination due to visceral sphincter spasm.

## INTERACTIONS
*Acetazolamide:* increased serum ephedrine levels. Monitor for toxicity.
*Alpha-adrenergic blockers:* unopposed beta-adrenergic effects, resulting in hypotension. Avoid concomitant use.
*Antihypertensives:* decreased effects. Monitor blood pressure.
*Beta-adrenergic blockers:* unopposed alpha-adrenergic effects, resulting in hypertension. Monitor blood pressure.
*Digitalis glycosides, general anesthetics (halogenated hydrocarbons):* increased risk of ventricular arrhythmias. Monitor ECG closely.
*Ergot alkaloids:* enhanced vasoconstrictor activity. Monitor patient closely.
*Guanadrel, guanethidine:* enhanced pressor effects of ephedrine. Monitor patient closely.
*Levodopa:* enhanced risk of ventricular arrhythmias. Monitor ECG closely.
*MAO inhibitors, tricyclic antidepressants:* when given with sympathomimetics, may cause severe hypertension (hypertensive crisis). Monitor patient and blood pressure closely.
*Methyldopa, reserpine:* may inhibit effects of ephedrine. Use together cautiously.

## CONTRAINDICATIONS
Contraindicated in patients with hypersensitivity to ephedrine and other sympathomimetics; in those with porphyria, severe coronary artery disease, arrhythmias, angle-closure glaucoma, psychoneurosis, angina pectoris, substantial organic heart disease, and CV disease; and in those taking MAO inhibitors.

## NURSING CONSIDERATIONS
● Use with extreme caution in elderly men and in those with hypertension, hyperthyroidism, nervous or excitable states, diabetes, and prostatic hyperplasia.
● *Alert:* Know that hypoxia, hypercapnia, and acidosis, which may reduce effectiveness or increase the incidence of adverse reactions, must be identified and corrected before or during ephedrine administration.
● This drug is not a substitute for blood or fluid volume replenishment. Know that volume deficit must be corrected before administering vasopressors.
● **I.V. use:** Give 10 to 25 mg by I.V. injection slowly; repeat in 5 to 10 minutes if necessary. Compatible with most common I.V. solutions.
● To prevent insomnia, avoid giving within 2 hours of bedtime.
● Effectiveness decreases after 2 to 3 weeks, as tolerance develops. Doctor may need to increase dosage. Drug is not addictive.

## ☑ PATIENT TEACHING
● Tell patient taking oral form of drug at home to take last dose of day at least 2 hours before bedtime.
● Warn patient not to take OTC drugs that contain ephedrine without informing the doctor.

## epinephrine (adrenaline)
Adrenalin◇, Bronkaid Mist◇, Bronkaid Mistometer†, Primatene Mist◇

## epinephrine bitartrate
AsthmaHaler◇, Broniten Mist◇, Bronkaid Mist Suspension◇, Medihaler-Epi◇, Primatene Mist Suspension◇

## epinephrine hydrochloride
Adrenalin Chloride◇, Epi-Pen, Epi-Pen Jr., Sus-Phrine

*Pregnancy Risk Category: C*

### HOW SUPPLIED
*Aerosol inhaler:* 160 mcg◇, 200 mcg◇, 220 mcg◇, 250 mcg/metered spray◇
*Nebulizer inhaler:* 1% (1:100)†◇, 1.25%†◇, 2.25%†◇
*Injection:* 0.01 mg/ml (1:100,000), 0.1 mg/ml (1:10,000), 0.5 mg/ml (1:2,000), 1 mg/ml (1:1,000) parenteral; 5 mg/ml (1:200) parenteral suspension

### ACTION
Stimulates alpha- and beta-adrenergic receptors within the sympathetic nervous system.

### ONSET, PEAK, DURATION
Onset occurs immediately after I.V. injection, 3 to 5 minutes after inhalation, 6 to 15 minutes after S.C. injection, variable after I.M. use. Peak effects occur within 5 minutes of I.V. administration, within 30 minutes of S.C. injection. Effects persist for 1 to 3 hours after inhalation, less than 1 to about 4 hours after parenteral use.

### INDICATIONS & DOSAGE
*Bronchospasm, hypersensitivity reactions, anaphylaxis –*
**Adults:** 0.1 to 0.5 ml of 1:1,000 S.C. or I.M. Repeated q 10 to 15 minutes, p.r.n. Or 0.1 to 0.25 ml of 1:1,000 (1 to 2.5 ml of a commercially available 1:10,000 injection or of a 1:10,000 dilution prepared by diluting 1 ml of a commercially available 1:1,000 injection with 10 ml of water for injection or 0.9% sodium chloride for injection) I.V. slowly over 5 to 10 minutes.
**Children:** 0.01 ml (10 mcg) of 1:1,000/kg S.C.; repeated q 20 minutes to 4 hours p.r.n. Or, 0.005 ml/kg of 1:200 (Sus-Phrine) S.C.; repeated q 8 to 12 hours p.r.n.
*Hemostasis –*
**Adults:** 1:50,000 to 1:1,000, applied topically.
*Acute asthmatic attacks –*
**Adults and children 4 years and over:** 160 to 250 mcg (metered aerosol) which is equivalent to one inhalation, repeated once if necessary after at least 1 minute; subsequent doses should not be administered for at least 3 hours. Alternatively, 1% (1:100) solution of epinephrine or 2.25% solution of racepinephrine administered with a hand-bulb nebulizer as one to three deep inhalations, repeated q 3 hours as needed.
*To prolong local anesthetic effect –*
**Adults and children:** 0.1 to 0.2 mg (base) added to anesthetic spinal fluid mixture; 0.1 to 0.2 mg (base) in a 1:200,000 to 1:20,000 solution.
*To restore cardiac rhythm in cardiac arrest –*
**Adults:** 0.5 to 1 mg I.V. or into endotracheal tube. May be given intracardiac if no I.V. route or intratracheal route is available. Some clinicians advocate higher dose (up to 5 mg), especially in patients who don't respond to usual I.V dose. Following initial I.V. administration, may be infused I.V. at a rate of 1 to 4 mcg/minute.
**Children:** 10 mcg/kg I.V. or 5 to 10 mcg (0.05 to 0.1 ml of 1:10,000)/kg intracardiac.
*Note:* 1 mg equals 1 ml of 1:1,000 or 10 ml of 1:10,000.

### ADVERSE REACTIONS
**CNS:** *nervousness, tremor,* vertigo, *headache,* disorientation, agitation, *drowsiness,* fear, pallor, dizziness, weakness, ***cerebral hemorrhage,*** **CVA.** In patients with Parkinson's disease, the drug increases rigidity and tremor.
**CV:** *palpitations;* widened pulse pressure; ***hypertension; tachycardia; ventricular fibrillation; shock;*** anginal

pain; ECG changes, including a decreased T-wave amplitude.
**GI:** *nausea, vomiting.*
**Respiratory:** dyspnea.
**Skin:** urticaria, pain, hemorrhage at injection site.

## INTERACTIONS

*Alpha-adrenergic blockers:* hypotension due to unopposed beta-adrenergic effects. Avoid concomitant use.
*Antihistamines, thyroid hormones, tricyclic antidepressants:* when given with sympathomimetics, may cause severe adverse cardiac effects. Avoid giving together.
*Beta blockers, such as propranolol:* may cause vasoconstriction and reflex bradycardia. Monitor patient carefully.
*Digitalis glycosides, general anesthetics (halogenated hydrocarbons):* increased risk of ventricular arrhythmias. Monitor ECG closely.
*Doxapram, mazindol, methylphenidate:* enhanced CNS stimulation or pressor effects. Monitor patient closely.
*Ergot alkaloids:* enhanced vasoconstrictor activity. Monitor patient closely.
*Guanadrel, guanethidine:* enhanced pressor effects of epinephrine. Monitor patient closely.
*Levodopa:* enhanced risk of cardiac arrhythmias. Monitor ECG closely.
*MAO inhibitors:* increased risk of hypertensive crisis. Monitor blood pressure closely.

## CONTRAINDICATIONS

• Contraindicated in patients with angle-closure glaucoma, shock (other than anaphylactic shock), organic brain damage, cardiac dilation, arrhythmias, coronary insufficiency, or cerebral arteriosclerosis. Also contraindicated in patients during general anesthesia with halogenated hydrocarbons or cyclopropane and in patients in labor (may delay second stage).
• Some commercial products contain sulfites: contraindicated in patients with sulfite allergies except when epinephrine is being used for treatment of serious allergic reactions or other emergency situations.
• In conjunction with local anesthetics, epinephrine is contraindicated for use in fingers, toes, ears, nose, or genitalia.

## NURSING CONSIDERATIONS

• Use with extreme caution in patients with long-standing bronchial asthma and emphysema who have developed degenerative heart disease. Also use cautiously in elderly patients and in those with hyperthyroidism, CV disease, hypertension, psychoneurosis, and diabetes.
• Be aware that epinephrine is the drug of choice in emergency treatment of acute anaphylactic reactions.
• Discard epinephrine solutions after 24 hours or if solution is discolored or contains precipitate. Keep solution in light-resistant container, and don't remove before use.
• **I.V. use:** Don't mix with alkaline solutions. Use $D_5W$, 0.9% sodium chloride for injection, lactated Ringer's injection, or combinations of dextrose in sodium chloride. Mix just before use.
• When administering I.V., monitor blood pressure, heart rate, and ECG when therapy is initiated and frequently thereafter.
• **Alert:** Avoid I.M. administration of parenteral suspension into buttocks. Gas gangrene may occur because epinephrine reduces oxygen tension of the tissues, encouraging the growth of contaminating organisms.
• Massage site after I.M. injection to counteract possible vasoconstriction. Repeated local injection can cause necrosis resulting from vasoconstriction at injection site.

Reactions may be *common,* uncommon, **life-threatening,** or **COMMON AND LIFE-THREATENING.**

• Observe patients closely for adverse reactions. Notify doctor if adverse reactions develop; he may adjust dosage or discontinue drug.
• Know that if a sharp blood pressure rise occurs, rapid-acting vasodilators, such as nitrites or alpha-adrenergic blockers, can be given to counteract the marked pressor effect of large doses of epinephrine.
• Know that epinephrine is rapidly destroyed by oxidizing agents, such as iodine, chromates, nitrates, nitrites, oxygen, and salts of easily reducible metals (such as iron).

☑ **PATIENT TEACHING**
• Teach patient to perform oral inhalation correctly. Give the following instructions for using a metered-dose inhaler:
  — Clear nasal passages and throat.
  — Breathe out, expelling as much air from lungs as possible.
  — Place mouthpiece well into mouth as dose from inhaler is released, and inhale deeply.
  — Hold breath for several seconds, remove mouthpiece, and exhale slowly.
• If more than one inhalation is ordered, tell patient to wait at least 2 minutes before repeating procedure.
• Tell patient who is also using a steroid inhaler to use the bronchodilator first, then wait about 5 minutes before using steroid. This allows the bronchodilator to open air passages for maximum effectiveness.
• If patient has acute hypersensitivity reactions, such as to bee stings, it may be necessary to instruct him to self-inject epinephrine at home.

## ethylnorepinephrine hydrochloride
Bronkephrine

*Pregnancy Risk Category: C*

## HOW SUPPLIED
*Injection:* 2 mg/ml

## ACTION
Relaxes bronchial smooth muscle by acting on beta-adrenergic receptors.

## ONSET, PEAK, DURATION
Onset occurs in 6 to 12 minutes. Peak unknown. Effects persist for 1 to 2 hours.

## INDICATIONS & DOSAGE
*Bronchospasm caused by asthma –*
**Adults:** 0.5 to 1 ml (1 to 2 mg) S.C. or I.M.
**Children:** 0.1 to 0.5 ml (0.2 to 1 mg) S.C. or I.M.

## ADVERSE REACTIONS
**CNS:** *headache,* dizziness.
**CV:** changes in blood pressure, *increased pulse rate,* palpitations.
**GI:** nausea.

## INTERACTIONS
*Antihypertensives, nitrates:* decreased effects of these agents. Monitor blood pressure.
*Beta blockers:* mutual inhibition of clinical effects. Avoid concomitant use.
*CNS stimulants, xanthine derivatives:* enhanced CNS stimulation. Monitor patient closely.
*Digitalis glycosides, levodopa, halogenated inhalation anesthetics, cyclopropane:* increased risk of arrhythmias. Monitor closely.
*Rauwolfia alkaloids, sympathomimetics:* enhanced effects. Monitor patient closely.
*Thyroid hormones:* increased risk of coronary insufficiency. Use together cautiously.

## CONTRAINDICATIONS
Contraindicated in patients with hypersensitivity to the drug; in patients with tachyarrhythmias, tachycardia caused by digitalis toxicity, angle-clo-

sure glaucoma, or shock; and in those receiving general anesthesia with cyclopropane or halogenated inhalation anesthetics.

## NURSING CONSIDERATIONS
• Use cautiously in patients with CV disease or history of CVA.
• Know that drug is safer than epinephrine for use in hypertensive or severely ill patients in whom significant pressor effects are undesirable.
• Be aware that drug is valuable for use in children because of low incidence of adverse reactions; may be useful in diabetic asthmatic patients because of low glycogenolytic activity.
• Choose anatomic injection site carefully to avoid inadvertent intraneural or intravascular injection.

☑ **PATIENT TEACHING**
• Inform patient of need for drug and when and how it will be administered.
• Tell patient to report adverse reactions promptly.

---

# ipratropium bromide
Atrovent

*Pregnancy Risk Category: B*

## HOW SUPPLIED
*Inhaler:* each metered dose supplies 18 mcg
*Solution (for inhalation):* 0.02% (500 mg/vial)
*Solution (for nebulizer):* 0.025% (250 mcg/ml)‡
*Nasal spray:* each metered dose supplies 20 mcg†

## ACTION
Inhibits vagally mediated reflexes by antagonizing acetylcholine.

## ONSET, PEAK, DURATION
Onset occurs in 5 to 15 minutes. Peak effects occur in 1 to 2 hours. Effects

persist usually 3 to 4 hours; up to 6 hours in some patients.

## INDICATIONS & DOSAGE
*Bronchospasm associated with COPD –*
**Adults:** one to two inhalations q.i.d. Additional inhalations may be needed. However, total inhalations should not exceed 12 in 24 hours. Alternatively, use inhalation solution where available. Give 250 to 500 mcg dissolved in 0.9% sodium chloride and administer by nebulizer q 6 to 8 hours.
**Children 5 to 12 years:** give 125 to 250 mcg nebulizer solution dissolved in 0.9% sodium chloride and administer by nebulizer q 6 to 8 hours.
*Seasonal allergic rhinitis‡ –*
**Adults:** two sprays in each nostril b.i.d. Increase to t.i.d. or q.i.d. if needed. Maximum dosage is eight sprays in each nostril daily.

## ADVERSE REACTIONS
**CNS:** dizziness, headache, nervousness.
**CV:** palpitations.
**EENT:** cough, blurred vision, rhinitis, sinusitis.
**GI:** nausea, GI distress, dry mouth.
**Respiratory:** *upper respiratory tract infection, bronchitis,* cough, dyspnea, pharyngitis, bronchospasm, increased sputum.
**Skin:** rash.
**Other:** pain, back pain, chest pain, flulike symptoms.

## INTERACTIONS
*Anticholinergics:* increased anticholinergic effects. Avoid concomitant use.

## CONTRAINDICATIONS
Contraindicated in patients with hypersensitivity to the drug or to atropine or any of its derivatives and in those with a history of hypersensitivity to soyalecithin or related food

---

products, such as soybeans and peanuts.

## NURSING CONSIDERATIONS
• Use cautiously in patients with angle-closure glaucoma, prostatic hyperplasia, and bladder-neck obstruction.

☑ **PATIENT TEACHING**
• Warn patient that ipratropium bromide is not effective for treating acute episodes of bronchospasm where rapid response is required.
• Teach patient to perform oral inhalation correctly. Give the following instructions for using a metered-dose inhaler:
  – Clear nasal passages and throat.
  – Breathe out, expelling as much air from lungs as possible.
  – Place mouthpiece well into mouth as dose from inhaler is released, and inhale deeply.
  – Hold breath for several seconds, remove mouthpiece, and exhale slowly.
• Tell patient to avoid accidentally spraying into eyes. Temporary blurring of vision may result.
• If more than one inhalation is ordered, tell patient to wait at least 2 minutes before repeating procedure.
• Tell patient who is also using a steroid inhaler to use ipratropium first, then wait about 5 minutes before using the steroid. This allows the bronchodilator to open air passages for maximum effectiveness.
• Tell patient to take missed dose as soon as remembered unless it's almost time for the next dose. In that case, he should skip the missed dose and never double dose.

# isoetharine hydrochloride
Arm-a-Med Isoetharine, Bronkosol, Dey-Dose Isoetharine, Dey-Dose Isoetharine S/F, Dey-Lute Isoetharine S/F, Dispos-a-Med Isoetharine

# isoetharine mesylate
Bronkometer

*Pregnancy Risk Category: NR*

## HOW SUPPLIED
*Aerosol inhaler:* 340 mcg/metered spray
*Nebulizer inhaler:* 0.062%, 0.08%, 0.1%, 0.125%, 0.167%, 0.17%, 0.2%, 0.25%, 0.5%, 1% solution

## ACTION
Relaxes bronchial smooth muscle by acting on $beta_2$-adrenergic receptors.

## ONSET, PEAK, DURATION
Onset occurs in 1 to 6 minutes. Peak effects occur within 15 to 60 minutes. Effects persist 1 to 4 hours.

## INDICATIONS & DOSAGE
*Bronchial asthma and reversible bronchospasm that may occur with bronchitis and emphysema* –
**Adults:** *hydrochloride form* – administered by hand nebulizer, oxygen aerosolization, or IPPB; use chart below.

| Method | Dose | Dilutions |
| --- | --- | --- |
| Hand nebulizer | 3 to 7 inhalations | undiluted |
| Oxygen aerosolization | 0.5 ml | 1:3 with saline |
| IPPB | 0.5 ml | 1:3 with saline |

*mesylate form* – one or two inhalations. Occasionally, more may be required.

## ADVERSE REACTIONS
**CNS:** *tremor, headache,* dizziness, excitement, anxiety.

**CV:** *palpitations,* increased heart rate, alterations in blood pressure.
**GI:** nausea, vomiting.

### INTERACTIONS
*Cyclopropane, digitalis glycosides, halogenated inhalation anesthetics, levodopa:* increased risk of arrhythmias. Monitor closely.
*Epinephrine, other sympathomimetics:* may cause excessive tachycardia. Don't use together with isoetharine.
*Propranolol and other beta blockers:* blocked bronchodilating effect of isoetharine. Monitor patient carefully if used together.

### CONTRAINDICATIONS
Contraindicated in patients with hypersensitivity to the drug.

### NURSING CONSIDERATIONS
• Use cautiously in patients with hyperthyroidism, hypertension, or coronary disease and in those with hypersensitivity to sympathomimetics.
• Although isoetharine has minimal effects on the heart, know that it should be used cautiously in patients receiving general anesthetics that sensitize the myocardium to sympathomimetic drugs.
• **Alert:** Monitor for severe paradoxical bronchoconstriction after excessive use. If bronchoconstriction occurs, discontinue immediately and notify doctor.

### ☑ PATIENT TEACHING
• Teach patient to perform oral inhalation correctly. Give the following instructions for using a metered-dose inhaler:
  — Clear nasal passages and throat.
  — Breathe out, expelling as much air from lungs as possible.
  — Place mouthpiece well into mouth as dose from inhaler is released, and inhale deeply.
  — Hold breath for several seconds, remove mouthpiece, and exhale slowly.
• If more than one inhalation is ordered, tell patient to wait at least 2 minutes before repeating procedure.
• Tell patient who is also using a steroid inhaler to use the bronchodilator first, then wait about 5 minutes before using the steroid. This allows the bronchodilator to open air passages for maximum effectiveness.
• Because of oxidation of drug when diluted with water, pink sputum mimicking hemoptysis may occur after inhaling isoetharine solution. Tell patient not to be concerned.
• Warn patient that excessive use can lead to decreased effectiveness.

---

# isoproterenol (isoprenaline)
Aerolone, Dey-Dose Isoproterenol, Dispos-a-Med Isoproterenol, Isuprel, Vapo-Iso

## isoproterenol hydrochloride
Isuprel, Isuprel Glossets, Isuprel Mistometer, Norisodrine Aerotrol

## isoproterenol sulfate
Medihaler-Iso

*Pregnancy Risk Category: C*

---

### HOW SUPPLIED
**isoproterenol**
*Nebulizer inhaler:* 0.25%, 0.5%, 1%
**isoproterenol hydrochloride**
*Tablets (sublingual):* 10 mg, 15 mg
*Aerosol inhaler:* 120 mcg or 131 mcg/metered spray
*Injection:* 20 mcg/ml, 200 mcg/ml
**isoproterenol sulfate**
*Aerosol inhaler:* 80 mcg/metered spray

### ACTION
Relaxes bronchial smooth muscle by acting on beta$_2$-adrenergic receptors. As a cardiac stimulant, acts on beta$_1$-adrenergic receptors in the heart.

---

## ONSET, PEAK, DURATION
Onset occurs immediately after I.V. use, 2 to 5 minutes after inhalation, 15 to 30 minutes after S.L. use. Peak unknown. Effects persist for ½ to 2 hours after inhalation, less than 1 hour after I.V. use, 1 to 2 hours after S.L. use.

## INDICATIONS & DOSAGE
*Bronchial asthma and reversible bronchospasm –*
**Adults:** 10 to 15 mg hydrochloride S.L. t.i.d. or q.i.d. Daily S.L. dosage should not exceed 60 mg.
**Children:** 5 to 10 mg hydrochloride S.L. t.i.d. Daily S.L. dosage should not exceed 30 mg.
*Bronchospasm –*
**Adults and children:** acute dyspneic episodes: one inhalation of sulfate form initially. Repeated if needed after 2 to 5 minutes.

Maintenance dosage is one to two inhalations q.i.d. to six times daily. Repeated once more 10 minutes after second dose. No more than three doses should be administered for each attack.
*Bronchospasm in COPD –*
Administered via IPPB or for nebulization by compressed air or oxygen.
**Adults:** 2 ml of 0.125% or 2.5 ml of 0.1% solution (prepared by diluting 0.5 ml of 0.5% solution to 2 or 2.5 ml or by diluting 0.25 ml of 1% solution to 2 or 2.5 ml with water or 0.45% or 0.9% sodium chloride solution) up to five times daily.
**Children:** 2 ml of a 0.0625% solution or 2.5 ml of 0.05% solution (prepared by diluting 0.25 ml of 0.5% solution to 2 or 2.5 ml with water or 0.45%) or 0.9% sodium chloride solution) up to five times daily.
*Heart block and ventricular arrhythmias –*
**Adults:** (hydrochloride) initially, 0.02 to 0.06 mg I.V. Subsequent doses 0.01 to 0.2 mg I.V. or 5 mcg/minute I.V.; or 0.2 mg I.M. initially, then 0.02 to 1 mg, p.r.n.
**Children:** (hydrochloride) half of initial adult dose may be given.
*Shock –*
**Adults and children:** (hydrochloride) 0.5 to 5 mcg/minute by continuous I.V. infusion. Usual concentration is 1 mg (5 ml) in 500 ml $D_5W$. Rate adjusted according to heart rate, central venous pressure (CVP), blood pressure, and urine flow.

## ADVERSE REACTIONS
**CNS:** *headache, mild tremor,* weakness, dizziness, *nervousness,* insomnia, **Adams-Stokes seizures.**
**CV:** *palpitations, tachycardia, anginal pain, arrhythmias,* **cardiac arrest,** *rapid rise and fall in blood pressure.*
**GI:** *nausea, vomiting, heartburn.*
**Respiratory:** *bronchospasm,* bronchitis, sputum increase, pulmonary edema.
**Other:** diaphoresis, hyperglycemia; swelling of parotid glands with prolonged use.

## INTERACTIONS
*Epinephrine, other sympathomimetics:* increased risk of arrhythmias. Use together cautiously.
*Propranolol and other beta blockers:* blocked bronchodilating effect of isoproterenol. Monitor patient carefully if used together.

## CONTRAINDICATIONS
Contraindicated in patients with tachycardia caused by digitalis intoxication, in patients with preexisting arrhythmias (other than those that may respond to treatment with isoproterenol), and in those with angina pectoris.

## NURSING CONSIDERATIONS
• Use cautiously in elderly patients and in patients with renal or CV disease, coronary insufficiency, dia-

betes, hyperthyroidism, or history of sensitivity to sympathomimetic amines.

• Know that drug is not a substitute for blood or fluid volume deficit. Volume deficit should be corrected before administering vasopressors.

• Do not use injection or inhalation solution if it's discolored or contains precipitate.

• **I.V. use:** Give by direct injection or I.V. infusion. For infusion, drug may be diluted with most common I.V. solutions. However, do not use with sodium bicarbonate injection; drug decomposes rapidly in alkaline solutions.

• *Alert:* If heart rate exceeds 110 beats/minute with I.V. infusion, notify the doctor. Doses sufficient to increase the heart rate to more than 130 beats/minute may induce ventricular arrhythmias.

• When administering I.V. isoproterenol to treat shock, closely monitor blood pressure, CVP, ECG, arterial blood gas measurements, and urine output. Carefully adjust infusion rate according to these measurements, as ordered. Use a continuous infusion pump to regulate flow rate.

• If drug is administered via inhalation with oxygen, be sure oxygen concentration will not suppress respiratory drive.

• Follow same instructions for metered powder nebulizer, although deep inhalation is not necessary.

• Be aware that drug may aggravate ventilation-perfusion abnormalities; even while ease of breathing is improved, arterial oxygen tension may fall paradoxically.

• Be aware that isoproterenol may cause a slight rise in systolic blood pressure and a slight to marked drop in diastolic blood pressure.

• Monitor patient for adverse reactions.

☑ **PATIENT TEACHING**
• Teach patient to perform oral inhalation correctly. Give the following instructions for using a metered-dose inhaler:
  — Clear nasal passages and throat.
  — Breathe out, expelling as much air from lungs as possible.
  — Place mouthpiece well into mouth as dose from inhaler is released, and inhale deeply.
  — Hold breath for several seconds, remove mouthpiece, and exhale slowly.

• If more than one inhalation is ordered, tell patient to wait at least 2 minutes before repeating procedure.

• Tell patient who is also using a steroid inhaler to use the bronchodilator first, then wait about 5 minutes before using the steroid. This allows the bronchodilator to open air passages for maximum effectiveness.

• Warn patient using oral inhalant that drug may turn sputum and saliva pink.

• Teach patient to take S.L. tablet properly. Instruct patient to hold tablet under tongue and not to swallow saliva until tablet dissolves and is absorbed. Instruct him to rinse mouth with water between doses to help prevent oropharyngeal dryness.

• Caution patient that prolonged use of S.L. tablets can cause tooth decay.

• Tell patient not to use drug at bedtime if possible; it interrupts sleep patterns.

• Tell patient to discontinue drug immediately and notify doctor if drug causes precordial distress or anginal pain or if an increase in chest tightness or dyspnea occurs.

• Patient may develop a tolerance to this drug; warn against overuse.

---

Reactions may be *common,* uncommon, *life-threatening,* or COMMON AND LIFE-THREATENING.

# metaproterenol sulfate
Alupent, Arm-A-Med
Metaproterenol, Dey-Dose
Metaproterenol, Dey-Lute
Metaproterenol, Metaprel

*Pregnancy Risk Category: C*

## HOW SUPPLIED
*Tablets:* 10 mg, 20 mg
*Syrup:* 10 mg/5 ml
*Aerosol inhaler:* 0.65 mg/metered
spray
*Nebulizer inhaler:* 0.4%, 0.6%, 5%
solution

## ACTION
Relaxes bronchial smooth muscle by
acting on beta$_2$-adrenergic receptors.

## ONSET, PEAK, DURATION
Onset occurs in 1 minute with oral inhalation, in 5 to 30 minutes with aerosol nebulization, and in 15 minutes
with oral administration. Peak effects
occur within 1 hour. Effects persist
for 1½ hours after inhalation, 1 to 4
hours after oral use.

## INDICATIONS & DOSAGE
*Acute episodes of bronchial asthma –*
**Adults and children:** two to three inhalations. Do not repeat inhalations
more often than q 3 to 4 hours. Do not
exceed 12 inhalations daily.
*Bronchial asthma and reversible bron-
chospasm –*
**Adults:** 20 mg P.O. q 6 to 8 hours.
**Children over 9 years or over 27 kg:**
20 mg P.O. q 6 to 8 hours (0.4 mg to
0.9 mg/kg t.i.d.).
**Children 6 to 9 years or less than 27
kg:** 10 mg P.O. q 6 to 8 hours (0.4 mg
to 0.9 mg/kg t.i.d.).
  Alternatively, via IPPB or nebulizer:
**Adults and children 12 years and
over:** 0.2 to 0.3 ml of 5% solution diluted in approximately 2.5 ml of
0.45% or 0.9% sodium chloride or
2.5 ml of a commercially available

0.4% or 0.6% solution q 4 hours
p.r.n.
**Children 6 to 12 years:** 0.1 to 0.2 ml
of a 5% solution diluted in 0.9% sodium chloride to final volume of 3 ml
q 4 hours p.r.n.

## ADVERSE REACTIONS
**CNS:** *nervousness,* weakness, drowsiness, *tremor,* vertigo, headache.
**CV:** *tachycardia,* hypertension, palpitations; ***cardiac arrest*** (with excessive use).
**GI:** *vomiting, nausea,* heartburn, dry
mouth.
**Respiratory:** paradoxical bronchiolar
constriction with excessive use,
cough, dry and irritated throat.
**Skin:** rash, hypersensitivity reactions.

## INTERACTIONS
*Levodopa:* risk of arrhythmias. Avoid
concomitant use.
*Propranolol, other beta blockers:*
blocked bronchodilating effect of
metaproterenol. Monitor patient carefully if used together.

## CONTRAINDICATIONS
Contraindicated in patients with hypersensitivity to the drug or any of its
ingredients and in use during anesthesia with cyclopropane or halogenated
hydrocarbon general anesthetics and
in those with tachycardia and arrhythmias associated with tachycardia, peripheral or mesenteric vascular
thrombosis, profound hypoxia or hypercapnia.

## NURSING CONSIDERATIONS
● Use cautiously in patients with hypertension, hyperthyroidism, heart
disease, diabetes, or cirrhosis and in
those who are receiving digitalis glycosides.
● Be aware that patients may use tablets and aerosol concomitantly. Monitor closely for toxicity.
● Know that inhalant solution can be
administered by IPPB with drug di-

luted in 0.9% sodium chloride solution or with a hand nebulizer at full strength.

☑ **PATIENT TEACHING**
• Teach patient to perform oral inhalation correctly. Give the following instructions for using a metered-dose inhaler:
  — Clear nasal passages and throat.
  — Breathe out, expelling as much air from lungs as possible.
  — Place mouthpiece well into mouth as dose from inhaler is released, and inhale deeply.
  — Hold breath for several seconds, remove mouthpiece, and exhale slowly. Allow two minutes between inhalations.
• Store drug in light-resistant container.
• Tell patient that metaproterenol inhalations should precede steroid inhalations (when prescribed) by 10 to 15 minutes to maximize therapy.
• Tell patient who is also using a steroid inhaler to use the bronchodilator first, then wait about 5 minutes before using the steroid. This allows bronchodilator to open air passages for maximum effectiveness.
• If more than one inhalation is ordered, tell patient to wait at least 2 minutes before repeating procedure.
• Warn patient to discontinue immediately if paradoxical bronchospasm occurs and to notify doctor.
• Warn patient to notify doctor if no response is derived from dosage or to request dosage adjustment.

---

## oxtriphylline (choline salt of theophyllinate)
Choledyl*

*Pregnancy Risk Category: C*

**HOW SUPPLIED**
*Tablets:* 100 mg, 200 mg
*Tablets (extended-release):* 400 mg, 600 mg
*Tablets (delayed-release):* 200 mg
*Elixir*:* 100 mg/5 ml
*Syrup:* 50 mg/5 ml

**ACTION**
Inhibits phosphodiesterase, the enzyme that degrades cAMP. Results in relaxation of smooth muscle of the bronchial airways and pulmonary blood vessels. Oxtriphylline is equivalent to 64% anhydrous theophylline.

**ONSET, PEAK, DURATION**
Onset and duration unknown. Peak effects occur within 1 hour after oral solution, within 2 hours of oral tablets.

**INDICATIONS & DOSAGE**
*Acute bronchial asthma and reversible bronchospasm associated with chronic bronchitis and emphysema* —
**Adults (nonsmokers):** 4.7 mg/kg P.O. q 8 hours.
**Adults (smokers) and children 9 to 16 years:** 4.7 mg/kg q 6 hours.
**Children 1 to 9 years:** 6.2 mg/kg P.O. q 6 hours.
  If total daily maintenance dosage is established at approximately 800 to 1,200 mg, one sustained-action tablet q 12 hours may be substituted.

**ADVERSE REACTIONS**
**CNS:** *restlessness, dizziness,* headache, *insomnia,* irritability, *seizures,* muscle twitching.
**CV:** *palpitations, sinus tachycardia,* extrasystoles, flushing, marked hypotension, arrhythmias.
**GI:** *nausea, vomiting,* epigastric pain, diarrhea.
**Respiratory:** tachypnea, *respiratory arrest.*

**INTERACTIONS**
*Adenosine:* decreased antiarrhythmic effectiveness. Higher doses of adenosine may be necessary.
*Allopurinol (high-dose):* increased

---

Reactions may be *common,* uncommon, *life-threatening,* or **COMMON AND LIFE-THREATENING.**

serum theophylline levels. Monitor for toxicity.

*Barbiturates, carbamazepine, nicotine, phenytoin, rifampin:* enhanced metabolism and decreased theophylline blood levels. Monitor for decreased effect.

*Beta-adrenergic blockers:* antagonism. Propranolol and nadolol, especially, may cause bronchospasm in sensitive patients. Use together cautiously.

*Cimetidine, influenza virus vaccine, macrolide antibiotics (such as erythromycin), oral contraceptives, quinolone antibiotics (such as ciprofloxacin):* decreased hepatic clearance of theophylline; elevated theophylline levels. Monitor for signs of toxicity.

*Lithium:* increased renal excretion of lithium. Monitor for decreased effect.

## CONTRAINDICATIONS
Contraindicated in patients with hypersensitivity to xanthines (caffeine, theobromine) and in patients with preexisting arrhythmias, especially tachyarrhythmias.

## NURSING CONSIDERATIONS
• Use cautiously in young children, in elderly patients, and in those with peptic ulceration, COPD, cardiac failure, cor pulmonale, renal or hepatic impairment, glaucoma, severe hypoxemia, hypertension, compromised cardiac or circulatory function, angina, acute MI, sulfite sensitivity, hyperthyroidism, and diabetes mellitus.
• Do not combine with products containing ephedrine; excessive CNS stimulation (nervousness, tremor, akathisia) may result.
• Administer drug after meals and at bedtime.
• Know that oxtriphylline is a soluble salt of theophylline. Dosage is adjusted by monitoring response, tolerance, pulmonary function, and serum theophylline levels. Ensure that theophylline concentrations range from

10 to 20 mcg/ml; toxicity has been reported with levels above 20 mcg/ml.
• Monitor therapy carefully. Individuals metabolize theophyllines at different rates. Dosage adjustments are necessary in elderly patients; in those with CHF, cor pulmonale, and hepatic disease; and in smokers.
• Store at 15° to 30° C (59° to 86° F). Protect elixir from light and tablets from moisture.

## ☑ PATIENT TEACHING
• Tell patient to report GI distress, palpitations, irritability, restlessness, nervousness, or insomnia; may indicate excessive CNS stimulation.
• Tell patient that tablets should not be chewed, crushed, or dissolved. Instruct him when to take drug.

---

# pirbuterol
Maxair, Maxair Autohaler

*Pregnancy Risk Category: C*

## HOW SUPPLIED
*Inhaler:* 0.2 mg/metered dose

## ACTION
Relaxes bronchial smooth muscle by acting on beta$_2$-adrenergic receptors.

## ONSET, PEAK, DURATION
Onset occurs within 5 minutes. Peak effects occur in 30 to 60 minutes. Effects persist for 5 hours.

## INDICATIONS & DOSAGE
*Prevention and reversal of bronchospasm, asthma –*
**Adults and children 12 years and over:** one or two inhalations (0.2 to 0.4 mg) repeated q 4 to 6 hours. Not to exceed 12 inhalations daily.

## ADVERSE REACTIONS
**CNS:** tremor, nervousness, dizziness, insomnia, headache, vertigo.
**CV:** tachycardia, palpitations, chest tightness.

**EENT:** dry or irritated throat, dry mouth, cough.
**GI:** nausea, vomiting, diarrhea.

## INTERACTIONS
*MAO inhibitors, tricyclic antidepressants:* may potentiate action of beta-adrenergic agonist on vascular system. Use together cautiously.
*Propranolol, beta-adrenergic blockers:* decreased bronchodilating effects. Avoid concomitant use.

## CONTRAINDICATIONS
Contraindicated in patients with hypersensitivity to pirbuterol.

## NURSING CONSIDERATION
Use cautiously in patients with CV disorders, hyperthyroidism, diabetes, and seizure disorders or in those who are unusually responsive to sympathomimetic amines.

## ☑ PATIENT TEACHING
● Teach patient to perform oral inhalation correctly. Give the following instructions for using a metered-dose inhaler:
— Clear nasal passages and throat.
— Breathe out, expelling as much air from lungs as possible.
— Place mouthpiece well into mouth as dose from inhaler is released, and inhale deeply.
— Hold breath for several seconds, remove mouthpiece, and exhale slowly.
● If more than one inhalation is ordered, tell patient to wait at least 2 minutes before repeating procedure.
● Give the following instructions for using an autohaler:
— Remove mouthpiece cover by pulling down lip on back cover. Inspect mouthpiece for foreign objects. Locate "Up" arrows and air vents.
— Hold autohaler upright so arrows point up while raising lever until it snaps into place.

— Hold autohaler around the middle, and shake gently several times.
— Continue to hold upright and not block air vents at bottom. Exhale normally before use.
— Seal lips around mouthpiece. Inhale deeply through mouthpiece with steady, moderate force. A click will be heard and a soft puff will be felt when inhaling triggers the release of medication. Continue to take a full, deep breath.
— Take autohaler away from mouth when done inhaling. Hold breath for 10 seconds; then exhale slowly.
— Continue to hold autohaler upright while lowering lever. Lower lever after each puff. If additional puffs are ordered, wait one minute between each puff and repeat process.
● Tell patient who is also using a steroid inhaler to use the bronchodilator first, then wait about 5 minutes before using the steroid. This allows the bronchodilator to open air passages for maximum effectiveness.
● Tell patient who experiences increased bronchospasm after using drug to call the doctor.
● Advise patient to seek medical attention if a previously effective dosage does not control symptoms; this may signify worsening of the disease.

---

## salmeterol xinafoate
Serevent

*Pregnancy Risk Category: C*

### HOW SUPPLIED
*Inhalation aerosol:* 21 mcg/metered spray

### ACTION
Not clearly defined. Selectively activates beta$_2$-adrenergic receptors, which results in bronchodilation. Also

blocks the release of allergic mediators from mast cells lining the respiratory tract.

## ONSET, PEAK, DURATION
Onset occurs in 10 to 20 minutes. Peak effects occur after about 3 hours; plasma levels peak within 45 minutes, but drug acts locally in the lung and its action is not dependent on plasma levels. Effects persist about 12 hours.

## INDICATIONS & DOSAGE
*Long-term maintenance treatment of asthma; prevention of bronchospasm in patients with nocturnal asthma or reversible obstructive airway disease who require regular treatment with short-acting beta agonists –*
**Adults and children over 12 years:** two inhalations twice daily, one in the morning and one in the evening.

Not for use to treat acute symptoms.
*Prevention of exercise-induced bronchospasm –*
**Adults and children 12 years and over:** two inhalations at least 30 to 60 minutes before exercise.

## ADVERSE REACTIONS
**CNS:** *headache,* sinus headache, tremor, nervousness, giddiness.
**CV:** tachycardia, palpitations, ventricular arrhythmias.
**EENT:** *upper respiratory infection, nasopharyngitis,* nasal cavity or sinus disorder.
**GI:** nausea, vomiting, diarrhea, heartburn.
**Respiratory:** cough, lower respiratory infection, *bronchospasm.*
**Other:** hypersensitivity reactions (rash, urticaria), joint and back pain, myalgia.

## INTERACTIONS
*Beta-adrenergic agonists, theophylline, other methylxanthines:* possible adverse cardiac effects with excessive use. Monitor closely.
*MAO inhibitors:* risk of severe adverse CV effects. Avoid use within 14 days of MAO therapy.
*Tricyclic antidepressants:* risk of moderate to severe adverse CV effects. Use with extreme caution.

## CONTRAINDICATIONS
Contraindicated in patients with hypersensitivity to the drug or any component of the formulation.

## NURSING CONSIDERATION
Use cautiously in patients with coronary insufficiency, arrhythmias, hypertension, other CV disorders, thyrotoxicosis, or seizure disorders and in patients who are unusually responsive to sympathomimetics.

## ☑ PATIENT TEACHING
• Remind patient to take drug at approximately 12-hour intervals for optimum effect and to take the drug even when feeling better.
• If the patient is taking the drug to prevent exercise-induced bronchospasm, tell him he should take it 30 to 60 minutes before exercise.
• *Alert:* Tell patient that although this drug is a beta agonist, it should not be used to treat acute bronchospasm. He must be provided with a short-acting beta agonist (such as albuterol) to treat such exacerbations.
• Tell patient to contact the doctor if the short-acting agonist no longer provides sufficient relief or if more than four inhalations are needed per day. This may be a sign that the asthma symptoms are worsening. Tell him not to increase the dosage of salmeterol.
• If patient is taking an inhaled corticosteroid, he should continue to use it on a regular basis. Warn patient not to take any other medications without the doctor's consent.

---

*Liquid form contains alcohol.  **May contain tartrazine.  †Canada only.  ‡Australia only.  ◇OTC.

# terbutaline sulfate
Brethaire, Brethine, Bricanyl
*Pregnancy Risk Category: B*

## HOW SUPPLIED
*Tablets:* 2.5 mg, 5 mg
*Aerosol inhaler:* 200 mcg/metered spray
*Injection:* 1 mg/ml

## ACTION
Relaxes bronchial smooth muscle by acting on beta$_2$-adrenergic receptors. Also relaxes uterine muscle.

## ONSET, PEAK, DURATION
Onset occurs within 15 minutes of S.C. injection, 5 to 30 minutes after inhalation, 1 to 2 hours after oral use. Peak effects occur within 30 minutes to 1 hour of S.C. injection, 1 to 2 hours after inhalation, or 2 to 3 hours after oral use. Effects persist about 1½ to 4 hours after S.C. injection, 3 to 6 hours after inhalation, or 4 to 8 hours after oral use.

## INDICATIONS & DOSAGE
*Bronchospasm in patients with reversible obstructive airway disease –*
**Adults and children over 11 years:** dosage varies with dosage form.
*Aerosol inhaler –* two inhalations separated by 60-second interval, repeated q 4 to 6 hours.
*Injection –* 0.25 mg S.C. May be repeated in 15 to 30 minutes p.r.n. Dosage should not exceed 0.5 mg in 4 hours.
*Tablets in adults –* 2.5 to 5 mg P.O. q 6 hours t.i.d. during waking hours. Maximum dosage is 15 mg/day.
*Tablets in children 12 to 15 years –* 2.5 mg P.O. q 6 hours t.i.d. during waking hours. Maximum dosage is 7.5 mg/day.

## ADVERSE REACTIONS
**CNS:** *nervousness, tremor, drowsiness, dizziness, headache,* weakness.
**CV:** *palpitations,* tachycardia, arrhythmias, flushing.
**EENT:** dry and irritated nose and throat (with inhaled form).
**GI:** *vomiting, nausea,* heartburn.
**Respiratory:** *paradoxical bronchospasm with prolonged usage,* dyspnea.
**Other:** hypokalemia (with high doses), diaphoresis.

## INTERACTIONS
*CNS stimulants:* increased CNS stimulation. Avoid concomitant use.
*Cyclopropane, digitalis glycosides, halogenated inhalation anesthetics, levodopa:* increased risk of arrhythmias. Monitor closely, and avoid concomitant use with levodopa.
*MAO inhibitors:* when given with sympathomimetics, may cause severe hypertension (hypertensive crisis). Don't use together.
*Propranolol, other beta blockers:* blocked bronchodilating effects of terbutaline. Avoid concomitant use.

## CONTRAINDICATIONS
Contraindicated in patients with hypersensitivity to the drug or sympathomimetic amines.

## NURSING CONSIDERATIONS
• Use cautiously in patient with CV disorders, hyperthyroidism, diabetes, or seizure disorders.
• Give S.C. injections in lateral deltoid area.
• Protect injection from light. Do not use if discolored.
• Know that patients may use tablets and aerosol concomitantly. Monitor closely for toxicity.

## ☑ PATIENT TEACHING
• Ensure that patient and caregivers understand why drug is necessary.
• Teach patient to perform oral inhalation correctly. Give the following instructions for using a metered-dose inhaler:

---

Reactions may be *common,* uncommon, *life-threatening,* or **COMMON AND LIFE-THREATENING.**

- Clear nasal passages and throat.
- Breathe out, expelling as much air from lungs as possible.
- Place mouthpiece well into mouth as dose from inhaler is released, and inhale deeply.
- Hold breath for several seconds, remove mouthpiece, and exhale slowly.

• If more than one inhalation is ordered, tell patient to wait at least 2 minutes before repeating procedure.
• Tell patient who is also using a steroid inhaler to use bronchodilator first, then wait about 5 minutes before using steroid. This allows bronchodilator to open air passages for maximum effectiveness.
• Warn patient to discontinue the drug immediately and notify doctor if paradoxical bronchospasm occurs.
• Warn patient that tolerance may develop with prolonged use.

## theophylline

*Immediate-release liquids:*
Accurbron\*, Aquaphyllin, Asmalix\*, Bronkodyl\*, Elixicon, Elixomin\*, Elixophyllin\*, Lanophyllin\*, Lixolin, Slo-Phyllin, Theolair Liquid, Theon\*
*Immediate-release tablets and capsules:* Bronkodyl, Elixophyllin, Nuelin‡, Slo-Phyllin, Somophyllin-T
*Timed-release tablets:* Constant-T, Duraphyl, Quibron-T/SR, Respbid, Sustaire, Theo-Dur, Theolair-SR, Theo-Time, Uniphyl
*Timed-release capsules:* Aerolate, Elixophyllin SR, Nuelin-SR‡, Slo-bid Gyrocaps, Slo-Phyllin, Somophyllin-CRT, Theo-24, Theobid Duracaps, Theobid Jr. Duracaps, Theochron, Theo-Dur Sprinkle, Theospan-SR, Theovent Long-Acting

## theophylline sodium glycinate
Acet-Am†

*Pregnancy Risk Category: C*

## HOW SUPPLIED
**theophylline**
*Tablets:* 100 mg, 125 mg, 200 mg, 250 mg, 300 mg
*Tablets (chewable):* 100 mg
*Tablets (extended-release):* 100 mg, 200 mg, 250 mg, 300 mg, 400 mg, 450 mg, 500 mg
*Capsules:* 100 mg, 200 mg
*Capsules (extended-release):* 50 mg, 60 mg, 65 mg, 75 mg, 100 mg, 125 mg, 130 mg, 200 mg, 250 mg, 260 mg, 300 mg
*Elixir:* 27 mg/5 ml, 50 mg/5 ml\*
*Oral solution:* 27 mg/5 ml, 50 mg/5 ml
*Syrup:* 27 mg/5 ml, 50 mg/5 ml
*Dextrose 5% injection:* 200 mg in 50 ml or 100 ml; 400 mg in 100 ml, 250 ml, 500 ml, or 1,000 ml; 800 mg in 500 ml or 1,000 ml
**theophylline sodium glycinate**
*Elixir:* 110 mg/5 ml (equivalent to 55 mg anhydrous theophylline/5 ml)

## ACTION
Inhibits phosphodiesterase, the enzyme that degrades cAMP. Results in relaxation of smooth muscle of the bronchial airways and pulmonary blood vessels.

## ONSET, PEAK, DURATION
Onset occurs within 15 minutes of I.V. use, 15 minutes to 1 hour after oral use. Peak effects occur 15 to 30 minutes after I.V. use; 1 to 2 hours after oral use, except for enteric-coated tablets (peak in about 5 hours) and extended-release capsules and tablets (peak in 4 to 7 hours). Duration unknown.

---

## INDICATIONS & DOSAGE

*Oral theophylline for acute broncho-spasm in patients not currently receiving theophylline –*

**Adults:** (nonsmoker) 6 mg/kg P.O., followed by 2 to 3 mg/kg q 6 hours for 2 doses. Maintenance dosage is 3 mg/kg q 8 hours.

**Otherwise healthy adult smokers:** 6 mg/kg P.O., followed by 3 mg/kg q 6 hours for 3 doses. Maintenance dosage is 3 mg/kg q 6 hours.

**Older adults with cor pulmonale:** 6 mg/kg P.O., followed by 2 mg/kg q 6 hours for two doses. Maintenance dosage is 2 mg/kg q 8 hours.

**Adults with CHF or liver disease:** 6 mg/kg P.O., followed by 2 mg/kg q 8 hours for two doses. Maintenance dosage is 1 to 2 mg/kg q 12 hours.

**Children 9 to 16 years:** 6 mg/kg P.O., followed by 3 mg/kg q 6 hours for 3 doses. Maintenance dosage is 3 mg/kg q 6 hours.

**Children 6 months to 9 years:** 6 mg/kg P.O., followed by 4 mg/kg q 6 hours for 3 doses. Maintenance dosage is 4 mg/kg q 6 hours.

Extended-release preparations should not be used for the treatment of acute bronchospasm.

*Parenteral theophylline for patients not currently receiving theophylline –*

**Loading dose:** 4.7 mg/kg I.V. slowly; then maintenance infusion.

**Adults (nonsmokers):** 0.55 mg/kg/hour I.V. for 12 hours, then 0.39 mg/kg/hour.

**Otherwise healthy adult smokers:** 0.79 mg/kg/hour I.V. for 12 hours; then 0.63 mg/kg/hour.

**Older adults with cor pulmonale:** 0.47 mg/kg/hour I.V. for 12 hours; then 0.24 mg/kg/hour.

**Adults with CHF or liver disease:** 0.39 mg/kg/hour I.V. for 12 hours; then 0.08 to 0.16 mg/kg/hour.

**Children 9 to 16 years:** 0.79 mg/kg/hour I.V. for 12 hours; then 0.63 mg/kg/hour.

**Children 6 months to 9 years:** 0.95 mg/kg/hour I.V. for 12 hours; then 0.79 mg/kg/hour.

*Oral and parenteral theophylline for acute bronchospasm in patients currently receiving theophylline –*

**Adults and children:** each 0.5 mg/kg I.V. or P.O. (loading dose) will increase plasma levels by 1 mcg/ml. Ideally, dose is based on current theophylline level. In emergency situations, some clinicians recommend a 2.5 mg/kg P.O. dose of rapidly absorbed form if no obvious signs of theophylline toxicity are present.

*Chronic bronchospasm –*

**Adults and children:** 16 mg/kg or 400 mg P.O. daily (whichever is less) given in three or four divided doses at 6- to 8- hour intervals. Alternatively, 12 mg/kg or 400 mg P.O. daily (whichever is less) in an extended-release preparation given in two or three divided doses at 8- or 12-hour intervals. Dosage increased as tolerated at 2- to 3-day intervals to maximum dosage as follows:

**Adults and children 16 years and over:** 13 mg/kg or 900 mg P.O. daily (whichever is less).

**Children 12 to 16 years:** 18 mg/kg P.O. daily.

**Children 9 to 12 years:** 20 mg/kg P.O. daily.

**Children under 9 years:** 24 mg/kg P.O. daily.

## ADVERSE REACTIONS

**CNS:** *restlessness, dizziness,* headache, *insomnia,* irritability, *seizures,* muscle twitching.

**CV:** *palpitations, sinus tachycardia,* extrasystoles, flushing, marked hypotension, arrhythmias.

**GI:** *nausea, vomiting,* diarrhea, epigastric pain.

**Respiratory:** tachypnea, *respiratory arrest.*

---

Reactions may be *common*, uncommon, *life-threatening*, or **COMMON AND LIFE-THREATENING.**

## INTERACTIONS

*Adenosine:* decreased antiarrhythmic effectiveness. Higher doses of adenosine may be necessary.

*Barbiturates, carbamazepine, nicotine, phenytoin, rifampin:* enhanced metabolism and decreased theophylline blood levels. Monitor for decreased effect.

*Beta-adrenergic blockers:* antagonism. Propranolol and nadolol, especially, may cause bronchospasm in sensitive patients. Use together cautiously.

*Calcium channel blockers, cimetidine, disulfiram, influenza virus vaccine, interferon, macrolide antibiotics (such as erythromycin), oral contraceptives, quinolone antibiotics (such as ciprofloxacin), caffeine:* decreased hepatic clearance of theophylline; elevated theophylline levels. Monitor for signs of toxicity.

Patients taking Theo-24 should take it on an empty stomach because food accelerates the drug's absorption.

## CONTRAINDICATIONS

Contraindicated in patients with hypersensitivity to xanthine compounds (caffeine, theobromine) and in those with active peptic ulcer and seizure disorders.

## NURSING CONSIDERATIONS

• Use cautiously in young children, infants under 1 year, and neonates; in elderly patients; and in those with COPD, cardiac failure, cor pulmonale, renal or hepatic disease, peptic ulceration, hyperthyroidism, diabetes mellitus, glaucoma, severe hypoxemia, hypertension, compromised cardiac or circulatory function, angina, acute MI, or sulfite sensitivity.
• Be careful not to confuse extended-release dosage forms with regular-release dosage forms.
• **I.V. use:** Use commercially available infusion solution, or mix drug in D$_5$W. Use infusion pump for continuous infusion.
• Know that drug dosage may need to be increased in cigarette smokers and in habitual marijuana smokers because smoking causes the drug to be metabolized faster.
• Give drug around-the-clock, using extended-release product at bedtime, as ordered.
• Monitor vital signs; measure and record fluid intake and output. Expected clinical effects include improved quality of pulse and respirations.
• Know that individuals metabolize xanthines at different rates; dosage is determined by monitoring response, tolerance, pulmonary function, and serum theophylline levels. Serum theophylline concentrations should range from 10 to 20 mcg/ml; toxicity has been reported with levels above 20 mcg/ml.

## ☑ PATIENT TEACHING

• Supply instructions for home care and dosage schedule.
• Warn patient not to dissolve, crush, or chew extended-release products. Small children unable to swallow these can ingest (without chewing) the contents of bead-filled capsules sprinkled over soft food.
• Tell patient to relieve GI symptoms by taking oral drug with full glass of water after meals, although food in stomach delays absorption.
• Warn patient to take the drug regularly, as directed. Patients tend to want to take extra "breathing pills."
• Warn elderly patient that dizziness, a common adverse reaction at start of therapy, may occur.
• Warn patient to check with the doctor or pharmacist about *any* other drugs used. OTC remedies may contain ephedrine in combination with theophylline salts; excessive CNS stimulation may result.

---

*Liquid form contains alcohol.   **May contain tartrazine.   †Canada only.   ‡Australia only.   ◊OTC.

**benzonatate**
**codeine phosphate**
(See Chapter 28, NARCOTIC AND OPIOID
ANALGESICS.)
**codeine sulfate**
(See Chapter 28, NARCOTIC AND OPIOID
ANALGESICS.)
**dextromethorphan**
**hydrobromide**
**diphenhydramine hydrochloride**
(See Chapter 43, ANTIHISTAMINES.)
**guaifenesin**
**hydromorphone hydrochloride**
(See Chapter 28, NARCOTIC AND OPIOID
ANALGESICS.)

## COMBINATION PRODUCTS
Preparations are available in the following combinations:
● expectorants with decongestants or
antihistamines, or both
● antitussives with decongestants or
antihistamines, or both
● expectorants and antitussives
● expectorants and antitussives with
decongestants or antihistamines, or
both.

## benzonatate
Tessalon

*Pregnancy Risk Category: C*

## HOW SUPPLIED
*Capsules:* 100 mg

## ACTION
Suppresses the cough reflex by direct
action on the cough center in the medulla through an anesthetic action.

## ONSET, PEAK, DURATION
Onset occurs in 15 to 20 minutes.
Peak unknown. Effects persist for up
to 8 hours.

## INDICATIONS & DOSAGE
*Symptomatic relief of cough –*
**Adults and children over 10 years:**
100 mg P.O. t.i.d.; up to 600 mg daily
may be needed.

## ADVERSE REACTIONS
**CNS:** dizziness, headache, sedation.
**EENT:** nasal congestion, burning
sensation in eyes.
**GI:** nausea, constipation, GI upset.
**Skin:** hypersensitivity reactions
(rash).
**Other:** chills.

## INTERACTIONS
None significant.

## CONTRAINDICATIONS
Contraindicated in patients hypersensitive to the drug.

## NURSING CONSIDERATIONS
● Use cautiously in patients hypersensitive to paramino-benzoic acid anesthetics (procaine, tetracaine) because
cross sensitivity reactions may occur.
● Don't use benzonatate when cough
is a valuable diagnostic sign or is beneficial (as after thoracic surgery).
● Monitor cough type and frequency.
● Use with percussion and chest vibration.

## ☑ PATIENT TEACHING
● Warn patient not to chew capsules
or dissolve in mouth. Produces either
local anesthesia that may result in aspiration or CNS stimulation that may
cause restlessness, tremor, and seizures.
● Instruct patient to report adverse reactions.

---

# dextromethorphan hydrobromide

Balminil D.M.◇, Benylin DM◇, Broncho-Grippol-DM†, Children's Hold◇, DM Syrup◇, Hold◇, Koffex†, Mediquell◇, Neo-DM†, Ornex-DM 15◇, Ornex-DM 30◇, Pertussin Cough Suppressant◇, Pertussin CS◇, Pertussin ES◇, Robidex†, Robitussin Pediatric◇, Sedatuss†, St. Joseph Cough Suppressant for Children◇, Sucrets Cough Control Formula◇, Trocal◇, Vicks Formula 44 Pediatric Formula◇.
*More commonly available in combination products, such as:* Anti-Tuss DM Expectorant◇, Baytussin DM◇, Benylin Expectorant Cough Formula◇, Cheracol D Cough◇, Codistan No. 1◇, Efficol Cough Whip◇, Extra Action Cough◇, 2/G-DM Cough◇, Glycotuss dM◇, Guiamid D.M. Liquid◇, Guiatuss-DM◇, Halotussin-DM Expectorant◇, Kolephrin GG/DM◇, Mytussin DM◇, Naldecon Senior DX◇, Pertussin All-Night CS◇, Rhinosyn-DMX Expectorant◇, Robitussin-DM◇, Scot-Tussin DM Cough Chaser◇, Silexin Cough◇, Tolu-Sed DM◇, Tuss-DM◇, Unproco◇, Vicks Pediatric Formula 44E◇

*Pregnancy Risk Category: C*

## HOW SUPPLIED
*Liquid (extended-release):* 30 mg/5 ml◇
*Lozenges:* 5 mg◇, 7.5 mg◇
*Solution:* 3.5 mg/5 ml, 5 mg/5 ml*◇, 7.5 mg/5 ml*◇, 10 mg/5 ml*◇, 15 mg/5 ml*◇, 15 mg/15 ml*◇

## ACTION
An antitussive that suppresses the cough reflex by direct action on the cough center in the medulla.

## ONSET, PEAK, DURATION
Onset occurs within 30 minutes. Peak unknown. Effects persist 3 to 6 hours with conventional dosage forms; up to 12 hours with extended-release forms.

## INDICATIONS & DOSAGE
*Nonproductive cough –*
**Adults and children 12 years and over:** 10 to 20 mg P.O. q 4 hours, or 30 mg q 6 to 8 hours. Or, 60 mg extended-release liquid b.i.d. Maximum dosage is 120 mg daily.
**Children 6 to 12 years:** 5 to 10 mg P.O. q 4 hours, or 15 mg q 6 to 8 hours. Or, 30 mg extended-release liquid b.i.d. Maximum dosage is 60 mg daily.
**Children 2 to 6 years:** 2.5 to 5 mg P.O. q 4 hours, or 7.5 mg q 6 to 8 hours. Or, 15 mg extended-release liquid b.i.d. Maximum dosage is 30 mg daily.
  Dosages for children under 2 years must be individualized.

## ADVERSE REACTIONS
**CNS:** drowsiness, dizziness.
**GI:** nausea, vomiting, stomach pain.

## INTERACTIONS
*MAO inhibitors:* risk of hypotension, coma, hyperpyrexia, and death. Avoid concomitant use.

## CONTRAINDICATIONS
Contraindicated in patients currently taking MAO inhibitors or within 2 weeks of discontinuing MAO inhibitors.

## NURSING CONSIDERATIONS
• Use with caution in atopic children, sedated or debilitated patients, and in patients confined to the supine position. Also, use cautiously in patients with aspirin sensitivity.
• Don't use dextromethorphan when cough is a valuable diagnostic sign or is beneficial (as after thoracic surgery).

---

*Liquid form contains alcohol.   **May contain tartrazine.   †Canada only.   ‡Australia only.   ◇OTC.

• Know that dextromethorphan 15 to 30 mg is equivalent to 8 to 15 mg codeine as an antitussive.
• Be aware that drug produces no analgesia or addiction and little or no CNS depression.
• Use drug with chest percussion and vibration.
• Monitor cough type and frequency.

☑ **PATIENT TEACHING**
• Instruct patient to take exactly as prescribed.
• Tell patient to report adverse reactions.

---

## guaifenesin
### (glyceryl guaiacolate)

Anti-Tuss\*◇, Balminil Expectorant†, Baytussin◇, Breonesin◇, Cremacoat 2◇, Gee-Gee◇, GG-CEN\*◇, Glyate\*◇, Glycotuss◇, Glytuss◇, Guiatuss\*◇, Halotussin◇, Humibid L.A.◇, Hytuss◇, Hytuss-2X◇, Naldecon Senior EX◇, Neo-Spec†, Nortussin◇, Resyl†◇, Robafen◇, Robitussin\*◇, S-T Expectorant◇

*Pregnancy Risk Category: C*

### HOW SUPPLIED
*Tablets:* 100 mg◇, 200 mg◇
*Tablets (extended-release):* 600 mg
*Capsules:* 200 mg◇
*Capsules (extended-release):* 300 mg
*Solution:* 100 mg/5 ml\*◇, 200 mg/5 ml\*◇

### ACTION
Increases production of respiratory tract fluids to help liquefy and reduce the viscosity of tenacious secretions.

### ONSET, PEAK, DURATION
Unknown.

### INDICATIONS & DOSAGE
*Expectorant –*
**Adults and children 12 years and over:** 200 to 400 mg P.O. q 4 hours, or 600 to 1,200 mg extended-release capsules q 12 hours. Maximum dosage is 2,400 mg daily.
**Children 2 to 6 years:** 50 to 100 mg P.O. q 4 hours. Maximum dosage is 600 mg daily.
**Children 6 to 12 years:** 100 to 200 mg P.O. q 4 hours. Maximum dosage is 1,200 mg daily.

### ADVERSE REACTIONS
**CNS:** dizziness, headache.
**GI:** vomiting and nausea (with large doses).
**Skin:** rash.

### INTERACTIONS
None significant.

### CONTRAINDICATIONS
Contraindicated in patients hypersensitive to the drug.

### NURSING CONSIDERATIONS
• Be aware that drug is used to liquefy thick, tenacious sputum. Evidence that guaifenesin is effective as expectorant but no evidence to support role an antitussive.
• Know that drug may interfere with certain laboratory tests for 5-hydroxyindoleacetic acid and vanillylmandelic acid.
• Monitor cough type and frequency.

☑ **PATIENT TEACHING**
• *Alert:* Ensure that patient understands that persistent cough may indicate a serious condition and that he should contact a doctor if cough lasts longer than 1 week, recurs frequently, or is associated with high fever, rash, or severe headache.
• Advise patient to take each dose with a glass of water; increasing fluid intake may prove beneficial.
• Encourage deep-breathing exercises.

---

# 46

## Miscellaneous respiratory drugs

acetylcysteine
alpha₁ proteinase inhibitor
    (human)
beclomethasone dipropionate
beractant
colfosceril palmitate
cromolyn sodium
dexamethasone sodium
    phosphate inhalation
dornase alfa
epoprostenol sodium
flunisolide
nedocromil sodium
triamcinolone acetonide

**COMBINATION PRODUCTS**
None.

---

## acetylcysteine
Airbron†, Mucomyst,
Mucomyst-10, Mucosil-10,
Mucosil-20, Parvolex†‡

*Pregnancy Risk Category: NR*

**HOW SUPPLIED**
*Solution:* 10%, 20%
*Injection:* 200 mg/ml†‡

**ACTION**
A mucolytic that increases production
of respiratory tract fluids to help liquefy and reduce the viscosity of tenacious secretions. Also restores liver
stores of glutathione to treat acetaminophen toxicity.

**ONSET, PEAK, DURATION**
Unknown.

**INDICATIONS & DOSAGE**
*Pneumonia, bronchitis, tuberculosis,
cystic fibrosis, emphysema, atelectasis
(adjunct), complications of thoracic
surgery and CV surgery –*
**Adults and children:** 1 to 2 ml 10% or

20% solution by direct instillation into
trachea as often as every hour; or 3 to 5
ml of 20% solution or 6 to 10 ml of
10% solution by nebulization q 2 to 6
hours p.r.n. Alternatively, where available 300 mg/kg by I.V. infusion in divided doses.
*Acetaminophen toxicity –*
**Adults and children:** initially, 140
mg/kg P.O., followed by 70 mg/kg
P.O. q 4 hours for 17 doses. Or, where
available 300 mg/kg by I.V. infusion.

**ADVERSE REACTIONS**
**CV:** tachycardia, hypotension, hyper-
tension.
**EENT:** *rhinorrhea.*
**GI:** *stomatitis, nausea, vomiting.*
**Respiratory:** *bronchospasm* (espe-
cially in asthmatic patients).
**Other:** fever, clamminess, chest
tightness.

**INTERACTIONS**
*Activated charcoal:* limits acetylcysteine's effectiveness. Avoid concomitant
use in treating acetaminophen toxicity.

**CONTRAINDICATIONS**
Contraindicated in patients hypersensitive to the drug.

**NURSING CONSIDERATIONS**
• Use cautiously in elderly or debilitated patients with severe respiratory
insufficiency.
• Use plastic, glass, stainless steel, or
another nonreactive metal when administering by nebulization. Hand-
bulb nebulizers are not recommended
because output is too small and particle size too large.
• Physically or chemically incompatible with tetracyclines, erythromycin
lactobionate, amphotericin B, and ampicillin sodium. If administered by

---

*Liquid form contains alcohol. **May contain tartrazine. †Canada only. ‡Australia only. ◊OTC.

aerosol inhalation, these drugs should be nebulized separately. Iodized oil, trypsin, and hydrogen peroxide are physically incompatible with acetylcysteine; don't add to nebulizer.
• Monitor cough type and frequency.
• **I.V. use:** To prepare I.V. infusion, dilute calculated dose in $D_5W$. Dilute initial dose (150 mg/kg) in 200 ml of $D_5W$ and infuse over 15 minutes. Dilute second dose of 50 mg/kg in 500 ml of $D_5W$ and give over 4 hours. Dilute final dose of 100 mg/kg in 1,000 ml of $D_5W$ and infuse over 16 hours.
• After opening, store in refrigerator; use within 96 hours.
• **Alert:** Acetylcysteine is administered to treat acetaminophen overdose within 24 hours after ingestion. Start treatment immediately as prescribed; do not wait for results of acetaminophen blood levels.
• When used orally to treat acetaminophen overdose, dilute oral doses with cola, fruit juice, or water before administering. Dilute the 20% solution to a concentration of 5% (add 3 ml of diluent to each ml of acetylcysteine). If patient vomits within 1 hour of receiving loading or maintenance dose, repeat dose.

### ☑ PATIENT TEACHING
• Warn patient that drug may have a foul taste or smell that some patients find distressing.
• For maximum effect, instruct patient to clear his airway by coughing before aerosol administration.

---

## alpha₁ proteinase inhibitor (human)
Prolastin

*Pregnancy Risk Category: C*

### HOW SUPPLIED
*Injection:* 500 mg, 1,000 mg

### ACTION
Replaces alpha₁-proteinase in patients with alpha₁-antitrypsin deficiency.

### ONSET, PEAK, DURATION
Onset occurs within a few weeks. Serum levels peak immediately after I.V. infusion. Duration unknown.

### INDICATIONS & DOSAGE
*Chronic replacement therapy in patients with congenital alpha₁-antitrypsin deficiency and demonstrable panacinar emphysema* –
**Adults:** 60 mg/kg I.V. once weekly. May give at a rate of 0.08 ml/kg/minute or greater.

### ADVERSE REACTIONS
**CNS:** dizziness, light-headedness.
**Hematologic:** possible viral transmission, transient leukocytosis.
**Other:** delayed fever (transient).

### INTERACTIONS
*Cigarette smoke:* blocks drug's effects. Patients should not smoke.

### CONTRAINDICATIONS
Contraindicated in patients with selective immunoglobulin A (IgA) deficiency who have known antibodies against IgA.

### NURSING CONSIDERATIONS
• Use cautiously in patients at risk for circulatory overload.
• **I.V. use:** Store powder for injection in the refrigerator (36° to 46° F [2° to 8° C]). Reconstitute using the supplied diluent (sterile water for injection). After reconstitution, administer within 3 hours. Inject directly into vein; intermittent or continuous infusion is not recommended.
• Be aware that many commercial assays for alpha₁-proteinase inhibitor measure immunoreactivity of the protein and not inhibitor activity. Thus, monitoring serum level of the drug may not accurately reflect clinical response.

---

Reactions may be *common*, uncommon, *life-threatening*, or COMMON AND LIFE-THREATENING.

### ☑ PATIENT TEACHING
• Explain to patient that product has been treated to minimize the risk of transmission of hepatitis and AIDS. However, immunization against heptatitis B is recommended prior to drug therapy.
• Instruct patient to report adverse reactions promptly.
• Warn patient not to smoke throughout therapy.

---

## beclomethasone dipropionate
Aldecin Inhaler‡, Beclodisk†, Becloforte Inhaler‡, Beclovent, Beclovent Rotacaps†, Vanceril

*Pregnancy Risk Category: NR*

### HOW SUPPLIED
*Oral inhalation aerosol:* 42 mcg/metered spray, 50 mcg/metered spray‡

### ACTION
Unknown. Probably decreases inflammation, mainly by stabilizing leukocyte lysosomal membranes.

### ONSET, PEAK, DURATION
Onset occurs in 1 to 4 weeks. Peak and duration unknown.

### INDICATIONS & DOSAGE
*Steroid-dependent asthma –*
**Adults and children 12 years and over:** two to four inhalations t.i.d. or q.i.d. Maximum dosage is 20 inhalations daily.
**Children 6 to 12 years:** one to two inhalations t.i.d. or q.i.d. Maximum dosage is 10 inhalations daily.

### ADVERSE REACTIONS
**EENT:** hoarseness, fungal infection of throat, throat irritation.
**GI:** dry mouth, fungal infection of mouth.
**Skin:** hypersensitivity reactions (urticaria, rash).
**Other:** angioedema, bronchospasm, suppression of hypothalmic-pituitary-adrenal function, *adrenal insufficiency,* facial edema, wheezing.

### INTERACTIONS
None significant.

### CONTRAINDICATIONS
Contraindicated in patients hypersensitive to any component of the formulation (fluorocarbons, oleic acid) and in those with status asthmaticus.

### NURSING CONSIDERATIONS
• Use with extreme caution, if at all, in a patient with tuberculosis, fungal or bacterial infections, ocular herpes simplex or systemic viral infections.
• Not for use in patients with asthma controlled by bronchodilators or other noncorticosteroids alone or for those with nonasthmatic bronchial diseases.
• Use with caution in patients receiving systemic corticosteroid therapy.
• Be aware a spacer device may help ensure delivery of the proper dose.
• Check mucous membranes frequently for signs of fungal infection.
• Keep in mind that during times of stress (trauma, surgery, or infection) systemic corticosteroids may be needed to prevent adrenal insufficiency in previously steroid-dependent patients.
• Know that periodic measurement of growth and development may be necessary during high-dose or prolonged therapy in children.
• **Alert:** Taper oral glucocorticoid therapy slowly as ordered. Acute adrenal insufficiency and death have occurred in asthmatics who changed abruptly from oral corticosteroids to beclomethasone.

### ☑ PATIENT TEACHING
• Inform patient that beclomethasone doesn't provide relief for acute asthma attacks.
• Tell patient requiring a bronchodilator to use it several minutes before beclomethasone.

---

*Liquid form contains alcohol.   **May contain tartrazine.   †Canada only.   ‡Australia only.   ◇OTC.

- Instruct patient to carry a medical identification card indicating his need for supplemental systemic glucocorticoids during stress.
- Advise patient to allow 1 minute to elapse before taking subsequent puffs of medication and to hold his breath for a few seconds to enhance action of drug.
- Instruct patient to contact his doctor if response to therapy decreases or if symptoms don't improve within 3 weeks; dosage may need to be adjusted. Tell patient not to exceed recommended dosage on his own.
- Tell patient to keep inhaler clean and unobstructed. He should wash it with warm water and dry it thoroughly.
- Tell patient to prevent oral fungal infections by gargling or rinsing mouth with water after each use, but not to swallow the water.
- Tell patient to report symptoms associated with corticosteroid withdrawal, including fatigue, weakness, arthralgia, orthostatic hypotension, and dyspnea.
- Tell patient to store medication between 36° and 86° F (2° and 30° C). Advise patient to ensure delivery of the proper dose by gently warming canister to room temperature before using. Some patients carry the canister in a pocket to keep it warm.

## beractant (natural lung surfactant)
Survanta

### HOW SUPPLIED
*Suspension for intratracheal instillation:* 25 mg/ml

### ACTION
Lowers the surface tension on alveolar surfaces during respiration and stabilizes the alveoli against collapse. An extract of bovine lung containing neutral lipids, fatty acids, surfactant-associated proteins, and phospholipids, which mimics naturally occurring surfactant;

palmitic acid, tripalmitin, and colfosceril palmitate are added to standardize the solution's composition.

### ONSET, PEAK, DURATION
Onset occurs in ½ to 2 hours. Peak unknown. Effects persist for 2 to 3 days.

### INDICATIONS & DOSAGE
*Prevention of respiratory distress syndrome (RDS), also known as hyaline membrane disease, in premature neonates weighing 1,250 g or less at birth or having symptoms consistent with surfactant deficiency –*
**Neonates:** 4 ml/kg intratracheally; administer each dose in four quarter-doses, with a hand-held ventilator bag between quarter-doses at a rate of 60 breaths/minute and sufficient oxygen to prevent cyanosis. Give drug as soon as possible, preferably within 15 minutes of birth. Repeat in 6 hours if respiratory distress continues. Give no more than four doses in 48 hours.
*Rescue treatment of RDS in premature infants –*
**Neonates:** 4 ml/kg intratracheally; before administering, increase ventilator rate to 60 breaths/minute with an inspiratory time of 0.5 second and a fraction of inspired oxygen of 1. Administer each dose in four quarter-doses, using a hand-held resuscitation bag between quarter-doses at a rate of 60 breaths/minute and sufficient oxygen to prevent cyanosis. Give dose as soon as RDS is confirmed by X-ray, preferably within 8 hours of birth. Repeat in 6 hours if respiratory distress continues. Give no more than four doses in 48 hours.

### ADVERSE REACTIONS
**CV:** *transient bradycardia,* vasoconstriction, hypotension.
**Hematologic:** decreased oxygen saturation, hypocapnia, hypercapnia.
**Other:** endotracheal tube reflux or blockage, pallor, *apnea.*

Reactions may be *common,* uncommon, *life-threatening,* or COMMON AND LIFE-THREATENING.

**INTERACTIONS**
None significant.

**CONTRAINDICATIONS**
None known.

**NURSING CONSIDERATIONS**
• Beractant should be administered only by personnel experienced in the care of clinically unstable premature neonates. Such personnel should have knowledge of neonatal intubation and airway management.
• Accurate determination of weight is essential to proper measurement of dosage.
• Continuously monitor the neonate before, during, and after beractant administration. The endotracheal (ET) tube may be suctioned before giving the drug; allow the neonate to stabilize before proceeding with administration.
• Refrigerate at 36° to 46° F (2° to 8° C). Warm before administration by allowing drug to stand at room temperature for at least 20 minutes or by holding in hand for at least 8 minutes. Do not use artificial warming methods. Unopened vials that have been warmed to room temperature may be returned to the refrigerator within 8 hours; however, warm and return drug to the refrigerator only once. Vials are for single use only—discard unused drug.
• Beractant does not require sonication or reconstitution before use. Inspect contents before giving; ensure that the color is off-white to light brown and the contents are uniform. If settling occurs, swirl vial gently; do not shake. Some foaming is normal.
• Use a large-bore needle (20G or larger) to draw up drug; do not use a filter. Administer the drug using a #5 French end-hole catheter. Premeasure and shorten the catheter before use. Fill the catheter with beractant and discard any excess drug so that only the total dose to be given remains in the syringe. Insert catheter into the neonate's ET tube; make sure the catheter tip protrudes just beyond the end of the tube

above the neonate's carina. Do not instill drug into a mainstem bronchus.
• Homogeneous distribution of the drug is important. In clinical trials, each dose of the drug was given in four quarter-doses, with the patient positioned differently after each administration. Each quarter-dose was given over 2 to 3 seconds; the catheter was removed and the patient ventilated between quarter-doses. With the head and body inclined slightly downward, the first quarter-dose was given with the head turned to the right; the second quarter-dose, with the head turned to the left. Then the head and body were inclined slightly upward; the third quarter-dose was given with the head turned to the right; the fourth quarter-dose, with the head turned to the left.
• Immediately after administration, moist breath sounds and crackles can occur. *Do not* suction the neonate for 1 hour unless other signs of airway obstruction are evident.
• Continuous monitoring of ECG and transcutaneous oxygen saturation are essential; frequent arterial blood pressure monitoring and frequent arterial blood gas sampling are highly desirable.
• Transient bradycardia and oxygen desaturation are common after dosing.
• **Alert:** Know that beractant can rapidly affect oxygenation and lung compliance. Peak ventilator inspiratory pressures may need to be adjusted if chest expansion improves substantially after drug administration. Notify doctor and adjust immediately as directed because lung overdistention and fatal pulmonary air leakage may result.
• Know that audiovisual materials that describe dosage and administration procedures are available from the manufacturer.

☑ **PATIENT TEACHING**
• Inform parents of need for drug and explain drug action and administration.
• Encourage parents to ask questions

*Liquid form contains alcohol. **May contain tartrazine. †Canada only. ‡Australia only. ◇OTC.

and address any concerns raised by them.

## colfosceril palmitate
Exosurf Neonatal

### HOW SUPPLIED
*Suspension for intratracheal instillation:* 10 ml

### ACTION
Replaces a major component of naturally occurring lung surfactant (dipalmitoylphosphatidylcholine), which is deficient in premature neonates. The mixture also contains cetyl ethanol (which acts as a spreading agent between the air-fluid interface) and tyloxapol, a long chain ethanol polymer (which acts as a dispersant).

### ONSET, PEAK, DURATION
Unknown.

### INDICATIONS & DOSAGE
*Prevention of respiratory distress syndrome (RDS) in neonates weighing less than 1,350 g at risk for developing RDS; prophylactic treatment of neonates weighing more than 1,350 g with evidence of pulmonary insufficiency –*
**Neonates:** administer 5 ml/kg intratracheally as soon as possible after delivery. If neonate is maintained on a mechanical ventilator, repeat dosage 12 and 24 hours later.
*Rescue treatment of neonates with RDS –*
**Neonates:** administer 5 ml/kg intratracheally as soon as possible after diagnosis of RDS. If the neonate is still mechanically ventilated, administer a second dose of 5 ml/kg 12 hours later.

### ADVERSE REACTIONS
**CNS:** *seizures.*
**CV:** *intraventricular hemorrhage, patent ductus arteriosus, hypotension.*
**Hematologic:** *thrombocytopenia.*
**Respiratory:** PULMONARY HEMOR-RHAGE, APNEA, *pulmonary air leak, pneumonia.*
**Other:** *hyperbilirubinemia, sepsis,* meningitis, **death from sepsis.**

### INTERACTIONS
None significant.

### CONTRAINDICATIONS
None known.

### NURSING CONSIDERATIONS
• Colfosceril should be administered only by personnel experienced in the care of clinically unstable premature neonates. Such personnel should have knowledge of neonatal intubation and airway management.
• Accurate determination of weight is essential to proper measurement of dosage.
• Know that colfosceril can rapidly affect oxygenation and lung compliance. Peak ventilator inspiratory pressures may need to be adjusted if chest expansion improves substantially after drug administration. Notify doctor and adjust immediately as directed because lung overdistention and fatal pulmonary air leakage may result.
• Continuous monitoring of ECG and transcutaneous oxygen saturation are essential; frequent arterial blood pressure monitoring and arterial blood gas sampling are highly desirable. Continuously monitor the neonate before, during, and after drug administration.
• Reconstitute drug immediately before use with the supplied preservative-free sterile water for injection. Do not use solutions that contain antibacterial preservatives. After reconstitution, drug is stable for up to 12 hours at 36° to 86° F (2° to 30° C). Fill a 10-ml syringe with the supplied 8 ml of diluent, using an 18G or 19G needle. Then, pierce the top of the vial and allow the vacuum to draw in the sterile water. Do not use vials without a vacuum. Aspirate as much of the 8 ml as possible out of the vial while maintaining vacuum.

---

Reactions may be *common,* uncommon, *life-threatening,* or COMMON AND LIFE-THREATENING.

Quickly release the syringe plunger. Repeat this final step at least three or four times to ensure adequate mixing of the vial contents.

• When drawing up the dose, use liquid below the froth. Each 8-ml vial contains sufficient material to administer a 5 ml/kg dose to a neonate weighing up to 1,600 g.

• Note that the suspension should have a homogeneous, milky white appearance. Do not use vials that appear to contain large flakes. If the suspension appears to separate, the vial may be shaken gently or swirled to resuspend the material.

• Suction the neonate before administering drug. Do not suction for 2 hours after dosing unless it is necessary.

• Special endotracheal (ET) tube adapters are available with each kit of surfactant. Ensure that adapter used corresponds to the inside diameter of the neonate's ET tube. Insert the adapter into the tube with a twisting motion and connect it to the ventilator circuit. To administer the drug (in half-doses of 2.5 ml), remove the cap from side port of the adapter and attach syringe; do not interrupt mechanical ventilation. After dosing, remember to reattach cap.

• Instill each half-dose slowly over 1 to 2 minutes (30 to 50 mechanical breaths) in small bursts timed with inspiration. Administer first half-dose with the neonate in the midline position; then turn the neonate's head and torso 45 degrees to the right for 30 seconds to assist distribution of drug. Return the neonate to the midline position for the second half-dose, and again administer over 1 to 2 minutes. After the second half-dose, turn the neonate's head and torso 45 degrees to the left for 30 seconds.

• When administering, monitor the neonate's facial expressions, skin color, chest expansion, heart rate, and ET-tube patency and position. If the neonate becomes dusky or agitated,

heart rate slows, drug backs up in the ET tube, or oxygen saturation decreases by more than 15%, discontinue the drug and modify peak inspiratory pressure, ventilator rate, or fraction of inspired oxygen ($FIO_2$) as ordered. Note that rapid improvements in lung function may require rapid reductions in peak inspiratory pressure, ventilator rate, or $FIO_2$.

• *Alert:* Reduce ventilator rate immediately if the transcutaneous or arterial carbon dioxide measurements are less than 30 mm Hg. Failure to reduce the rate may result in hypocapnia, which can reduce blood flow to the brain.

• If the neonate becomes pink and the transcutaneous oxygen saturation exceeds 95%, reduce $FIO_2$ in a stepwise fashion until the saturation is 90% to 95%. Do so immediately because hyperoxia (an excess of systemic oxygen) may result.

• Monitor neonates for pulmonary hemorrhage.

☑ **PATIENT TEACHING**
• Inform parents of need for drug and explain drug action and administration.
• Encourage parents to ask questions and address any concerns raised by them.

## cromolyn sodium (sodium cromoglycate)
Crolom, Gastrocrom, Intal, Intal Aerosol Spray, Intal Nebulizer Solution, Nalcrom, Nasalcrom, Rynacrom†

*Pregnancy Risk Category: B*

**HOW SUPPLIED**
*Capsules (for oral solution):* 100 mg
*Aerosol:* 800 mcg/metered spray
*Nasal solution:* 5.2 mg/metered spray (40 mg/ml)
*Solution (for nebulization):* 20 mg/2 ml
*Ophthalmic solution:* 4%

---

*Liquid form contains alcohol.  **May contain tartrazine.  †Canada only.  ‡Australia only.  ◊OTC.

## ACTION
Inhibits the degranulation of sensitized mast cells that occurs after a patient's exposure to specific antigens. Also inhibits release of histamine and slow-reacting substance of anaphylaxis.

## ONSET, PEAK, DURATION
Unknown.

## INDICATIONS & DOSAGE
*Adjunct in severe perennial bronchial asthma –*
**Adults and children 5 years and over:** two metered sprays using inhaler q.i.d. at regular intervals. Alternatively, 20 mg via nebulization q.i.d. at regular intervals.
*Prevention and treatment of allergic rhinitis –*
**Adults and children over 5 years:** one spray in each nostril t.i.d. or q.i.d. Maximal administration is six times daily.
*Prevention of exercise-induced bronchospasm –*
**Adults and children 5 years or over:** two metered sprays inhaled no more than 1 hour before anticipated exercise.
*Conjunctivitis –*
**Adults and children 4 years and older:** 1 to 2 drops in each eye four to six times daily at regular intervals.
*Systemic mastocytosis –*
**Adults and children over 12 years:** 200 mg P.O. q.i.d. before meals and h.s.
**Children 2 to 12 years:** 100 mg P.O. q.i.d. 30 minutes before meals or h.s.

## ADVERSE REACTIONS
**CNS:** dizziness, headache.
**EENT:** *irritated throat and trachea,* nasal congestion, pharyngeal irritation, *sneezing,* nasal burning and irritation, epistaxis.
**GI:** nausea, esophagitis, abdominal pain.
**GU:** dysuria, urinary frequency.
**Respiratory:** *bronchospasm* (after inhalation of dry powder), *cough,* wheezing, *eosinophilic pneumonia.*

**Skin:** rash, urticaria.
**Other:** joint swelling and pain, lacrimation, swollen parotid gland, *angioedema,* bad taste in mouth.

## INTERACTIONS
None significant.

## CONTRAINDICATIONS
Contraindicated in patients experiencing acute asthma attacks and status asthmaticus and in patients with hypersensitivity to drug.

## NURSING CONSIDERATIONS
• Administer with caution in children. Use of cromolyn oral inhalation solution is *not* recommended in children under 2 years; cromolyn powder or aerosol for oral inhalation, not recommended in children under 5 years; cromolyn ophthalmic solution, not recommended in children under 4 years; and cromolyn nasal solution, not recommended in children under 6 years.
• Use inhalation form cautiously in patients with coronary artery disease or a history of arrhythmias.
• Know that drug (except for ophthalmic solution) should be used only when acute episode of asthma has been controlled, airway is cleared, and the patient can breathe independently.
• Be aware that oral cromolyn sodium should be used in full-term neonates and infants *only* for a severe, incapacitating disease, that is, when benefits clearly outweigh the risks.
• Dissolve powder in capsules for oral dose in hot water, and further dilute with cold water before ingestion. Do not mix with fruit juice, milk, or food.
• Discontinue drug if the patient develops eosinophilic pneumonia, indicated by eosinophilia and infiltrates on chest X-ray film.
• Watch for recurrence of asthmatic symptoms when dosage is decreased, especially when corticosteroids are also used.

---

Reactions may be *common,* uncommon, *life-threatening,* or COMMON AND LIFE-THREATENING.

## ☑ PATIENT TEACHING

• Instruct patient how to administer form of drug prescribed.
• Tell patient that esophagitis may be relieved by antacids or a glass of milk.
• Warn patient who is using the nasal solution that stinging or sneezing may occur upon administration.

---

# dexamethasone sodium phosphate inhalation

Decadron Phosphate Respihaler

*Pregnancy Risk Category: NR*

## HOW SUPPLIED

*Inhalation aerosol:* 100 mcg/metered spray

## ACTION

Unknown. Probably decreases inflammation, mainly by stabilizing leukocyte lysosomal membranes.

## ONSET, PEAK, DURATION

Onset occurs in 1 to 4 weeks. Peak and duration unknown.

## INDICATIONS & DOSAGE

*Steroid-dependent asthma –*
**Adults:** initially, three inhalations t.i.d. or q.i.d. Decreased as needed and tolerated; most patients respond to two inhalations b.i.d. Maximum dosage is 12 inhalations daily.
**Children:** two inhalations t.i.d. or q.i.d. Decreased as needed and tolerated; most patients respond to two inhalations b.i.d. Maximum dosage is eight inhalations daily.

## ADVERSE REACTIONS

**EENT:** hoarseness, fungal infection of throat, throat irritation.
**GI:** dry mouth, fungal infection of mouth.
**Other:** rash, wheezing, facial edema.

## INTERACTIONS

None significant.

## CONTRAINDICATIONS

Contraindicated in patients hypersensitive to any component of the formulation (fluorocarbons, ethanol) and in those with status asthmaticus, persistent positive sputum cultures for candida albicans, or systemic fungal infections.

## NURSING CONSIDERATIONS

• Not for use in patients with asthma controlled by bronchodilators or other noncorticosteroids alone or for those with nonasthmatic bronchial diseases.
• Use cautiously in patients with ocular herpes simplex, nonspecific ulcerative colitis, diverticulitis, fresh intestinal anastomoses, peptic ulcer, renal insufficiency, hypertension, osteoporosis, and myasthenia gravis.
• Know that a spacer device may help ensure delivery of the proper dose of medication.
• Check mucous membranes frequently for signs of fungal infection.
• Monitor patient for adverse effects. With prolonged use of high doses, systemic effects are likely because up to 50% of a dose is absorbed.
• Conduct periodic measurements of growth and development during high-dose or prolonged therapy in children.
• Know that during times of stress (trauma, surgery, or infection), systemic corticosteroids may be needed to prevent adrenal insufficiency in previously steroid-dependent patients.
• ***Alert:*** Taper oral glucocorticoid therapy slowly as ordered. Acute adrenal insufficiency and death have occurred in asthmatics who switched abruptly from oral corticosteroids to inhaled steroids. Be sure patients report symptoms associated with corticosteroid withdrawal, including fatigue, weakness, arthralgia, orthostatic hypotension, and dyspnea.

---

## ☑ PATIENT TEACHING

• Inform patient that dexamethasone doesn't provide relief for acute asthma attacks.

• Instruct patient to store medication between 36° and 86° F (2° and 30° C). Tell patient that this medication needs to be at room temperature when used. If the canister is cold, the proper dose may not be delivered.

• Advise patient to ensure delivery of the proper dose by gently warming the canister to room temperature before using. Some patients carry the canister in a pocket to keep it warm.

• Advise patient requiring bronchodilator to use it several minutes before dexamethasone.

• Tell patient to allow 1 minute to elapse before taking subsequent puffs of medication and to hold his breath for a few seconds to enhance action of drug.

• Instruct patient to contact the doctor if response to therapy decreases or if symptoms don't improve within 3 weeks of initiating therapy; the doctor may need to adjust the dosage. Tell patient not to exceed recommended dosage on his own.

• Advise patient to prevent oral fungal infection by gargling or rinsing mouth with water after each use, but not to swallow water.

• Teach patient to keep inhaler clean and unobstructed. He should wash it with warm water and dry it thoroughly.

• Instruct patient to carry a card indicating need for supplemental systemic glucocorticoids during stress.

## dornase alfa
Pulmozyme

*Pregnancy Risk Category: B*

### HOW SUPPLIED
*Inhalation solution:* 2.5-mg ampule (1 mg/ml)

### ACTION
Hydrolyzes DNA in sputum of cystic fibrosis patients, causing decreased viscosity and elasticity of pulmonary secretions.

### ONSET, PEAK, DURATION
Significant improvement in lung function occurs within 3 days to 1 week. Reduction in respiratory tract infections takes weeks to months. Peak increases in baseline measurement of amount of air exhaled in first second of expiration occur after about 9 days of therapy. Duration unknown.

### INDICATIONS & DOSAGE
*To improve pulmonary function and decrease the frequency of moderate to severe respiratory infections in patients with cystic fibrosis –*
**Adults and children 5 years and over:** one ampule (2.5 mg) inhaled once daily. Treatment usually takes 10 to 15 minutes. Use drug only with an approved nebulizer.

### ADVERSE REACTIONS
**EENT:** *pharyngitis, voice alteration,* laryngitis, conjunctivitis.
**Skin:** *rash,* urticaria.
**Other:** *chest pain.*

### INTERACTIONS
None significant.

### CONTRAINDICATIONS
Contraindicated in patients hypersensitive to the drug or Chinese hamster ovary cell-derived products.

### NURSING CONSIDERATIONS
• Know that drug is used in conjunction with other standard therapies for cystic fibrosis.

• Be aware that safety and efficacy in children under 5 years or with forced vital capacity of less than 40% of normal value have not been established.

• Administer only with the following nebulizers and compressors: the Hud-

son T Up-draft II disposable jet nebulizer and the Marquest Acorn II disposable jet nebulizer in conjunction with the Pulmo-Aide compressor or the PARI LC Jet⁺ reusable nebulizer in conjunction with the PARI PRO-NEB compressor.
• Discard cloudy or discolored solution.
• Do not mix with other drugs in the nebulizer. Doing so could lead to a physical or chemical reaction that may inactivate dornase alfa.
• Refrigerate drug in its protective foil pouch.

### ☑ PATIENT TEACHING
• Instruct patient how to administer drug at home.
• Remind the patient to breathe only through his mouth when using the nebulizer. If this is difficult, suggest use of a nose clip.
• Tell the patient that if he begins coughing during treatment to turn off the nebulizer without spilling the drug. To resume treatment, the patient should turn on the nebulizer and continue breathing through the mouthpiece until the nebulizer cup is empty or mist is no longer produced.

▼ NEW DRUG

## epoprostenol sodium
Flolan

*Pregnancy Risk Category: B*

### HOW SUPPLIED
*Injection:* 0.5 mg/17 ml, 1.5 mg/17 ml

### ACTION
Causes direct vasodilation of pulmonary and systemic arterial vascular beds and inhibits platelet aggregation.

### ONSET, PEAK, DURATION
Unknown.

### INDICATIONS & DOSAGE
*Long-term I.V. treatment of primary pulmonary hypertension in New York Heart Association (NYHA) Class III and Class IV patients –*
**Adults:** initially, 2 ng/kg/minute as I.V. infusion, increased in increments of 2 ng/kg/minute q 15 minutes or longer until dose-limiting pharmacologic effects are elicited. Maintenance dosing is begun with 4 ng/kg/minute less than the maximum tolerated rate determined during initial dosing. If the maximum rate is less than 5 ng/kg/minute, the maintenance infusion is started at one-half the maximum rate. Subsequent adjustments are made based on persistence, recurrence, or worsening of symptoms and occurrence of adverse events from excessive doses, but maintenance dose is usually increased in increments of 1 to 2 ng/kg/minute q 15 minutes or longer.

### ADVERSE REACTIONS
*After initial dosing –*
**CNS:** *headache, anxiety, nervousness, agitation,* dizziness, hypesthesia, paresthesia.
**CV:** *hypotension, chest pain,* bradycardia, tachycardia.
**GI:** *nausea, vomiting,* abdominal pain, dyspepsia.
**Respiratory:** dyspnea.
**Skin:** *flushing.*
**Other:** musculoskeletal pain, back pain, sweating.
*During maintenance dosing –*
**CNS:** *headache, anxiety, nervousness, dizziness, hypesthesia, hyperesthesia, paresthesia.*
**CV:** *tachycardia.*
**GI:** *nausea, vomiting, diarrhea.*
**Hematologic:** *thrombocytopenia.*
**Skin:** *flushing.*
**Other:** *jaw pain, flulike symptoms, chills, fever, sepsis, myalgia, nonspecific musculoskeletal pain.*

### INTERACTIONS
*Antihypertensive agents, diuretics, or other vasodilators:* additional reductions in blood pressure may occur. Monitor blood pressure closely.

---

*Liquid form contains alcohol.  **May contain tartrazine.  †Canada only.  ‡Australia only.  ◇OTC.

*Anticoagulants, antiplatelet agents:* may increase risk of bleeding. Monitor closely for bleeding.

## CONTRAINDICATIONS

Contraindicated in patients with hypersensitivity to drug or structurally related compounds. Chronic use is contraindicated in patients with CHF due to severe left ventricular systolic dysfunction and in patients who develop pulmonary edema during initial dosing.

## NURSING CONSIDERATIONS

• Use cautiously in elderly patients and in pregnant or breast-feeding women.
• Safety and efficacy in children have not been established.
• Drug should be used only by clinicians experienced in diagnosis and treatment of primary pulmonary hypertension. The appropriate dose must be determined in a setting with adequate personnel and equipment for physiologic monitoring and emergency care.
• **I.V. use:** Drug must be reconstituted only as directed, using sterile diluent for Flolan. Drug must not be reconstituted or mixed with any other parenteral medications or solutions before or during administration.
• Follow manufacturer guidelines for reconstituting drug. The prescribed concentration should be compatible with the infusion pump's minimum and maximum flow rates and reservoir capacity and with other criteria recommended by manufacturer. When used for maintenance infusion, drug should be prepared in a drug delivery reservoir appropriate for the infusion pump, with a total reservoir volume of at least 100 ml. Drug should be prepared using 2 vials of sterile diluent for use during 24 hours.
• Reconstituted solutions must be protected from light and refrigerated at 36° to 46° F (2° to 8° C) if not used immediately. Do not freeze reconstituted solutions. Discard frozen solution or solution that has been refrigerated for more than 48 hours.
• Maintenance dosing should be given by continuous I.V. infusion via a permanent indwelling central venous catheter using an ambulatory infusion pump. During establishment of dosing range, drug may be administered peripherally.
• To facilitate extended use at ambient temperatures above 77° F (25° C), a cold pouch with frozen gel packs can be used. The pouch must be able to maintain the drug at a temperature of 36° to 46° F for 12 hours. When such a pouch is used, the reconstituted solution should be used for no longer than 24 hours.
• After establishment of a maintenance infusion rate, observe the patient closely and monitor standing and supine blood pressure and heart rate for several hours to ensure tolerance.
• Avoid abrupt withdrawal of drug or sudden, large reductions in infusion rate. Ensure that a backup infusion pump and I.V. infusion set are available to avoid potential interruptions in drug delivery. A multilumen catheter should be considered if other I.V. therapies are routinely administered.
• Infusion rates should be adjusted only under a doctor's direction, except in life-threatening situations.
• Anticoagulant therapy should be administered during maintenance infusion, unless contraindicated. Monitor PT closely.
• To reduce risk of infection, aseptic technique must be used when reconstituting and administering the drug and when performing routine catheter care.

## ☑ PATIENT TEACHING

• Discuss the patient's long-term need for epoprostenol. Ensure that the patient or a family member can care for a permanent I.V. catheter and infusion pump.
• Show the patient and family how to reconstitute, administer, and store the

drug; how to use the infusion pump; and how to switch to a new pump in the event of pump failure. Stress the importance of maintaining continuous drug therapy.

• Urge the patient to report adverse reactions immediately; dosage adjustments may be necessary.

• Provide the patient with the telephone number of an organization that offers 24-hour support.

---

## flunisolide
AeroBid, AeroBid-M

*Pregnancy Risk Category: C*

### HOW SUPPLIED
*Oral inhalant:* 250 mcg/metered spray (at least 100 metered inhalations/container)

### ACTION
Unknown. Probably decreases inflammation, mainly by stabilizing leukocyte lysosomal membranes.

### ONSET, PEAK, DURATION
Onset occurs after 1 to 4 weeks of therapy. Peak and duration unknown.

### INDICATIONS & DOSAGE
*Steroid-dependent asthma –*
**Adults:** two inhalations (500 mcg) b.i.d. Maximum daily dose is four inhalations b.i.d.
**Children 6 to 15 years:** two inhalations (500 mcg) b.i.d. Higher dosages have not been studied.

### ADVERSE REACTIONS
**CNS:** dizziness, irritability, nervousness.
**CV:** palpitations.
**EENT:** throat irritation, hoarseness, nasopharyngeal fungal infections, *sore throat, nasal congestion.*
**GI:** *nausea, vomiting,* dry mouth, *diarrhea, upset stomach,* abdominal pain, decreased appetite.
**Other:** *upper respiratory tract infec-*tion, cold symptoms, flu, *edema, fe*ver, chest pain, rash, pruritus.

### INTERACTIONS
None significant.

### CONTRAINDICATIONS
Contraindicated in patients hypersensitive to the drug and in those with status asthmaticus or respiratory infections.

### NURSING CONSIDERATIONS
• Not recommended for use in patients with asthma controlled by bronchodilators or other noncorticosteroids alone or for those with nonasthmatic bronchial diseases.
• Know that a spacer device may help to ensure proper dosage administration.
• Store medication between 36° and 86° F (2° and 30° C).
• Withdraw drug slowly as ordered in patients who have received long-term oral corticosteroid therapy.
• Be aware that after withdrawal of systemic corticosteroids, patient may still need supplementation of systemic steroids if patient show signs and symptoms of adrenal insufficiency when exposed to trauma, surgery, or infections.

### ☑ PATIENT TEACHING
• Warn patient that flunisolide doesn't relieve emergency asthma attacks.
• Advise patient to ensure delivery of the proper dose by gently warming the canister to room temperature before using. Some patients carry the canister in a pocket to keep it warm.
• Tell patient who also is using a bronchodilator to use it several minutes before he uses flunisolide.
• Instruct patient to allow 1 minute to elapse before repeating inhalations and to hold his breath for a few seconds to enhance drug action.
• Teach patient to keep inhaler clean and unobstructed. He should wash it with warm water and dry it thoroughly after use.

---

*Liquid form contains alcohol.  **May contain tartrazine.  †Canada only.  ‡Australia only.  ◇OTC.

- Teach patient to check mucous membranes frequently for signs of fungal infection.
- The patient can prevent oral fungal infections by gargling or rinsing mouth with water after each inhaler use. Caution patient not to swallow the water.
- Advise parents of children receiving long-term therapy that the child should have periodic growth measurements and be checked for evidence of hypothalamic-pituitary-adrenal axis suppression.

# nedocromil sodium
Tilade

*Pregnancy Risk Category: B*

## HOW SUPPLIED
*Inhalation aerosol:* 1.75 mg/activation

## ACTION
Reduces inflammatory changes in the airway by blocking the release of inflammation mediators (such as leukotrienes, histamine, and prostaglandins) from mast cells, eosinophils, monocytes, neutrophils, macrophages, and other immune cells.

## ONSET, PEAK, DURATION
Onset occurs within days to 4 weeks. Time to peak concentration in an asthmatic patient occurs in 5 to 90 minutes. Effects persist for 6 to 12 hours.

## INDICATIONS & DOSAGE
*Maintenance in mild to moderate reversible obstructive airway disease –*
**Adults and children 12 years and over:** two inhalations q.i.d., preferably at regular intervals.

## ADVERSE REACTIONS
**CNS:** headache, dysphagia, fatigue.
**GI:** nausea, vomiting, dyspepsia, abdominal pain, dry mouth.
**Respiratory:** upper respiratory tract infection, rhinitis, cough, pharyngitis, increased sputum, bronchitis, dyspnea, bronchospasm.
**Other:** *unpleasant taste,* chest pain.

## INTERACTIONS
None significant.

## CONTRAINDICATIONS
Contraindicated in patients hypersensitive to the formulation or in patients experiencing an acute asthmatic attack or acute bronchospasm.

## NURSING CONSIDERATION
Know that drug should not be used during acute bronchospasm because drug action has a slow onset and is not therapeutic in aborting an acute attack.

## ☑ PATIENT TEACHING
- Warn the patient that nedocromil has no direct bronchodilating action and cannot replace bronchodilators during an acute asthmatic attack.
- Tell the patient that drug is an adjunct to the regular bronchodilator regimen and may reduce the need for corticosteroids or bronchodilators.
- Emphasize to the patient that regular use of the drug will help him feel better. Most patients report benefits after 1 week of use; some require longer treatment before any improvement.
- Teach the patient how to use the inhaler. Instruct him to shake canister immediately before use and to invert it just before actuation.
- Advise the patient to clean inhaler at least twice a week and to remove canister before rinsing inhaler in hot running water. He should let inhaler air-dry overnight.

# triamcinolone acetonide
Azmacort

*Pregnancy Risk Category: C*

## HOW SUPPLIED
*Inhalation aerosol:* 100 mcg/metered spray

---

Reactions may be *common,* uncommon, *life-threatening,* or **COMMON AND LIFE-THREATENING.**

## ACTION
Unknown. Probably decreases inflammation, mainly by stabilizing leukocyte lysosomal membranes.

## ONSET, PEAK, DURATION
Onset occurs in 1 to 4 weeks. Peak and duration unknown.

## INDICATIONS & DOSAGE
*Steroid-dependent asthma* –
**Adults:** two inhalations t.i.d. to q.i.d. Maximum dosage is 16 inhalations daily. In some patients, maintenance can be accomplished when total daily dosage is given b.i.d.
**Children 6 to 12 years:** one to two inhalations t.i.d. to q.i.d. Maximum dosage is 12 inhalations daily.

## ADVERSE REACTIONS
Most adverse reactions to corticosteroids are dose- or duration-dependent.
**EENT:** dry or irritated nose or throat, hoarseness.
**Respiratory:** cough, wheezing.
**Other:** *oral candidiasis,* dry or irritated tongue or mouth, facial edema.

## INTERACTIONS
None significant.

## CONTRAINDICATIONS
Contraindicated in patients hypersensitive to any component of the formulation and in those with status asthmaticus.

## NURSING CONSIDERATIONS
• It is not known if drug is excreted in breast milk. Because of the risk of severe adverse effects, breast-feeding is not recommended.
• Use with extreme caution, if at all, in patients with tuberculosis of the respiratory tract; untreated fungal, bacterial, or systemic viral infections; or ocular herpes simplex.
• Use cautiously in patients receiving systemic corticosteroids.
• Know that patients who have recently been switched from systemic administration of steroids to oral inhaled steroids may need to resume systemic steroid therapy during periods of stress or severe asthma attacks.
• Taper oral therapy slowly as ordered.
• Store medication between 36° and 86° F (2° and 30° C).

## ☑ PATIENT TEACHING
• Inform patient that inhaled corticosteroids don't provide relief for emergency asthma attacks.
• Advise patient to ensure delivery of the proper dose of medication by gently warming the canister to room temperature before using. Some patients carry the canister in a pocket to keep it warm.
• The patient requiring a bronchodilator should use it several minutes before triamcinolone. Tell patient to allow 1 minute to elapse before repeat inhalations and to hold breath for a few seconds to enhance drug action.
• Teach patient to check mucous membranes frequently for signs of fungal infection.
• Tell patient to prevent oral fungal infections by gargling or rinsing mouth with water after each use of the inhaler, but not to swallow the water.
• Tell patient to keep inhaler clean and unobstructed. He should wash it with warm water and dry it thoroughly after use.
• Instruct patient to contact the doctor if response to therapy decreases; the doctor may need to adjust the dosage. Tell patient not to exceed recommended dosage on his own.
• Instruct patient to carry a card indicating his need for supplemental systemic glucocorticoids during periods of stress.

# 47

# Antacids, adsorbents, and antiflatulents

**aluminum carbonate**
**aluminum hydroxide**
**aluminum phosphate**
**calcium carbonate**
**dihydroxyaluminum sodium carbonate**
**magaldrate**
**magnesium oxide**
**magnesium hydroxide**
   (See Chapter 50, LAXATIVES.)
**simethicone**
**sodium bicarbonate**
   (See Chapter 64, ACIDIFIER AND ALKALINIZERS.)

## COMBINATION PRODUCTS

ALKA-SELTZER WITH ASPIRIN,◊: sodium bicarbonate 1,916 mg, aspirin 325 mg, and citric acid 1,000 mg.
ALKA-SELTZER WITHOUT ASPIRIN◊: sodium bicarbonate 958 mg, citric acid 832 mg, and potassium bicarbonate 312 mg.
ALUDROX SUSPENSION◊: aluminum hydroxide 307 mg and magnesium hydroxide 103 mg.
CAMALOX TABLETS◊: aluminum hydroxide 225 mg, magnesium hydroxide 200 mg, and calcium carbonate 250 mg.
DI-GEL LIQUID◊: aluminum hydroxide 200 mg, magnesium hydroxide 200 mg, and simethicone 20 mg.
FLATULEX: simethicone 80 mg and activated charcoal 250 mg.
GAVISCON◊: aluminum hydroxide 31.7 mg and magnesium carbonate 137 mg.
GELUSIL◊: aluminum hydroxide 200 mg, magnesium hydroxide 200 mg, and simethicone 25 mg.
GELUSIL-II◊: aluminum hydroxide 400 mg, magnesium hydroxide 400 mg, and simethicone 30 mg.
MAALOX ◊: aluminum hydroxide 225

mg and magnesium hydroxide 200 mg.
MAALOX EXTRA STRENGTH TABLETS◊: aluminum hydroxide 400 mg and magnesium hydroxide 400 mg.
MAALOX PLUS TABLETS◊: aluminum hydroxide 200 mg, magnesium hydroxide 200 mg, and simethicone 25 mg.
MAALOX TC TABLETS◊: aluminum hydroxide 600 mg and magnesium hydroxide 300 mg.
MYLANTA TABLETS◊: aluminum hydroxide 200 mg, magnesium hydroxide 200 mg, and simethicone 20 mg.
MYLANTA-II TABLETS◊: aluminum hydroxide 400 mg, magnesium hydroxide 400 mg, and simethicone 40 mg.
RIOPAN PLUS CHEWABLE TABLETS◊: magaldrate 540 mg and simethicone 20 mg.
RIOPAN PLUS SUSPENSION◊: magaldrate 540 mg and simethicone 20 mg/5 ml.
TITRALAC PLUS SUSPENSION◊: calcium carbonate 500 mg and simethicone 20 mg.
TITRALAC TABLETS◊: calcium carbonate 420 mg and glycine 150 mg.
UNIVOL†: aluminum hydroxide and magnesium carbonate co-dried gel 300 mg and magnesium hydroxide 100 mg.
WINGEL◊: aluminum hydroxide 180 mg and magnesium hydroxide 160 mg.

## aluminum carbonate
Basaljel◊
*Pregnancy Risk Category: B*

## HOW SUPPLIED
*Tablets or capsules:* equivalent to aluminum hydroxide 500 mg◊

---

Reactions may be *common,* uncommon, *life-threatening,* or COMMON AND LIFE-THREATENING.

*Oral suspension:* equivalent to aluminum hydroxide 400 mg/5 ml◇

## ACTION
An antacid that reduces total acid load in the GI tract, elevates gastric pH to reduce pepsin activity, strengthens the gastric mucosal barrier, and increases esophageal sphincter tone.

## ONSET, PEAK, DURATION
Onset occurs in 20 minutes. Peak unknown. Effects persist for about 20 to 60 minutes in a fasting period and up to 3 hours if taken 1 hour after a meal.

## INDICATIONS & DOSAGE
*Antacid* –
**Adults:** 5 to 10 ml of suspension P.O. q 2 hours p.r.n.; or 1 to 2 tablets or capsules P.O. q 2 hours p.r.n. Maximum dosage is 24 capsules, tablets, or teaspoonfuls per 24 hours.
*To prevent formation of urinary phosphate stones (in conjunction with low-phosphate diet)* –
**Adults:** 15 to 30 ml of suspension in water or juice P.O. 1 hour after meals and h.s.; or 2 to 6 tablets or capsules 1 hour after meals and h.s.

## ADVERSE REACTIONS
**CNS:** encephalopathy.
**GI:** *constipation,* intestinal obstruction.
**Other:** hypophosphatemia, osteomalacia.

## INTERACTIONS
*Allopurinol, antibiotics (including quinolones and tetracyclines), corticosteroids, diflunisal, digoxin, ethambutol, histamine-2 antagonists, iron salts, isoniazid, penicillamine, phenothiazines, thyroid hormones, ticlopidine:* decreased pharmacologic effect because of possible impaired absorption. Separate administration times by 1 to 2 hours.
*Enteric-coated drugs:* may be released prematurely in stomach. Separate doses by at least 1 hour.

## CONTRAINDICATIONS
None known.

## NURSING CONSIDERATIONS
• Use cautiously in patients with chronic renal disease.
• When administering through nasogastric tube, make sure tube is placed correctly and is patent; after instilling, flush tube with water to ensure passage to stomach and to clear tube.
• Monitor long-term, high-dose use in patients on restricted sodium intake. Each tablet, capsule, or 5 ml of suspension contains about 3 mg of sodium.
• Record amount and consistency of stools. Manage constipation with laxatives or stool softeners as ordered. Alternate with magnesium-containing antacids (if the patient does not have renal disease).
• Monitor serum phosphate levels.
• Watch for symptoms of hypophosphatemia with prolonged use (anorexia, malaise, muscle weakness); can also lead to resorption of calcium and bone demineralization.
• Because drug contains aluminum, keep in mind that it is used in patients with renal failure to help control hyperphosphatemia by binding with phosphate in the GI tract.
• Know that Basaljel liquid contains no sugar.

## ☑ PATIENT TEACHING
• Warn patient not to take aluminum carbonate indiscriminately or to switch antacids without the doctor's advice.
• Instruct patient to shake suspension well and to take with small amount of water or fruit juice to facilitate passage.

---

*Liquid form contains alcohol. **May contain tartrazine. †Canada only. ‡Australia only. ◇OTC.

# aluminum hydroxide
AlternaGEL◇, Alu-Cap◇, Aluminum Hydroxide Gel Concentrated◇, Alu-Tab◇, Amphojel◇, Dialume◇, Nephrox◇

*Pregnancy Risk Category: C*

## HOW SUPPLIED
*Tablets:* 300 mg◇, 500 mg◇, 600 mg◇
*Capsules:* 475 mg◇, 500 mg◇
*Oral suspension:* 320 mg/5 ml◇, 450 mg/5ml◇, 600 mg/5 ml◇, 675 mg/5 ml◇

## ACTION
An antacid that reduces total acid load in the GI tract, elevates gastric pH to reduce pepsin activity, strengthens the gastric mucosal barrier, and increases esophageal sphincter tone.

## ONSET, PEAK, DURATION
Onset varies by dosage form; liquids are more rapid-acting than tablets or capsules. Peak unknown. Duration varies with gastric emptying time; 20 to 60 minutes in fasting patients, 3 hours when taken after meals.

## INDICATIONS & DOSAGE
*Antacid* –
**Adults:** 500 to 1500 mg P.O. (5 to 30 ml of most products) 1 hour after meals and h.s.; 300- or 600-mg tablet, chewed before swallowing, taken with milk or water five to six times daily after meals and h.s.

## ADVERSE REACTIONS
**CNS:** encephalopathy.
**GI:** *constipation,* intestinal obstruction.
**Other:** hypophosphatemia, osteomalacia.

## INTERACTIONS
*Allopurinol, antibiotics (including quinolones and tetracyclines), corticosteroids, diflunisal, digoxin, ethambutol, histamine-2 antagonists, iron salts, isoniazid, penicillamine, phenothiazines, thyroid hormones, ticlopidine:* decreased pharmacologic effect because of possible impaired absorption. Separate administration times.
*Enteric-coated drugs:* may be released prematurely in stomach. Separate doses by at least 1 hour.

## CONTRAINDICATIONS
None known.

## NURSING CONSIDERATIONS
• Use cautiously in patients with chronic renal disease.
• When administering through nasogastric tube, make sure tube is placed correctly and is patent; after instilling, flush tube with water to ensure passage to stomach and to clear tube.
• Monitor long-term, high-dose use in patient on restricted sodium intake. Each tablet, capsule, or 5 ml of suspension contains 2 to 3 mg of sodium.
• Record amount and consistency of stools. Manage constipation with laxatives or stool softeners as ordered; alternate with magnesium-containing antacids (if the patient does not have renal disease).
• Monitor serum phosphate levels.
• Watch for symptoms of hypophosphatemia with prolonged use (anorexia, malaise, and muscle weakness); can also lead to resorption of calcium and bone demineralization.
• Because drug contains aluminum, keep in mind that it is used in patients with renal failure to help control hyperphosphatemia by binding with phosphate in the GI tract.

## ☑ PATIENT TEACHING
• Instruct patient to shake suspension well and to follow with small amount of milk or water to facilitate passage.
• Advise patient not to take aluminum hydroxide indiscriminately or to switch antacids without the doctor's advice.

---

Reactions may be *common,* uncommon, ***life-threatening,*** or **COMMON AND LIFE-THREATENING.**

## aluminum phosphate
Phosphaljel◇

*Pregnancy Risk Category: NR*

**HOW SUPPLIED**
*Oral suspension:* 233 mg/5 ml◇

**ACTION**
Provides supplemental phosphate.

**ONSET, PEAK, DURATION**
Onset occurs in about 20 minutes. Peak unknown. Effects persist for 20 to 60 minutes in fasting patients, 3 hours when taken after meals.

**INDICATIONS & DOSAGE**
*To reduce fecal elimination of phosphorus –*
**Adults:** 15 to 30 ml undiluted P.O. q 2 hours between meals and h.s.

**ADVERSE REACTIONS**
**CNS:** encephalopathy.
**GI:** *constipation,* intestinal obstruction.
**Other:** hypophosphatemia, osteomalacia.

**INTERACTIONS**
*Ciprofloxacin and other quinolones, tetracyclines:* decreased antibiotic effect. Separate administration times.
*Enteric-coated drugs:* may be released prematurely in stomach. Separate doses by at least 1 hour.

**CONTRAINDICATIONS**
None known.

**NURSING CONSIDERATIONS**
• Use cautiously in patients with chronic renal disease.
• When administering through nasogastric tube, make sure tube is placed correctly and is patent; after instilling, flush tube with water to ensure passage to stomach and to clear tube.
• Record amount and consistency of stools. Manage constipation with laxatives or stool softeners as ordered; alternate with magnesium-containing antacids (if the patient does not have renal disease).
• Monitor patient closely, especially with long-term use. Also monitor long-term, high-dose use in patients on restricted sodium intake.
• *Alert:* Know that the drug can reverse hypophosphatemia induced by aluminum hydroxide.
• Be aware that Phosphaljel contains no sugar.

☑ **PATIENT TEACHING**
• Instruct patient to shake suspension well; it may be taken alone or with small amount of milk or water.
• Advise patient not to take aluminum phosphate indiscriminately or to switch antacids without the doctor's advice.

## calcium carbonate
Alka-Mints◇, Amitone◇, Calcilac◇, Calcimax‡, Calglycine◇, Cal-Sup‡, Chooz◇, Dicarbosil◇, Effercal-600‡, Equilet◇, Gencalc◇, Mallamint◇, Rolaids Calcium Rich◇, Titracid◇, Titralac◇,Titralac Extra Strength◇, Titralac Plus◇, Tums◇, Tums E-X◇, Tums Liquid Extra Strength◇

*Pregnancy Risk Category: NR*

**HOW SUPPLIED**
Calcium carbonate contains 40% calcium; 20 mEq calcium per gram.
*Tablets (chewable):* 350 mg◇, 420 mg◇, 500 mg◇, 750 mg, 850 mg, 1,000 mg, 1,250 mg‡
*Tablets:* 500 mg◇, 600 mg◇, 650 mg◇, 1,000 mg◇, 1,250 mg◇
*Chewing gum:* 500 mg/piece
*Oral suspension:* 1 g/5 ml◇, 250 mg/5 ml
*Lozenges:* 600 mg◇

---

*\*Liquid form contains alcohol. \*\*May contain tartrazine. †Canada only. ‡Australia only. ◇OTC.*

## ACTION
An antacid that reduces total acid load in the GI tract, elevates gastric pH to reduce pepsin activity, strengthens the gastric mucosal barrier, and increases esophageal sphincter tone.

## ONSET, PEAK, DURATION
Onset occurs within 20 minutes. Peak unknown. Effects persist for 20 to 60 minutes in fasting patients, 3 hours when taken after meals.

## INDICATIONS & DOSAGE
*Antacid, calcium supplement–*
**Adults:** 350 mg to 1.5 g P.O. or 2 pieces of chewing gum 1 hour after meals and h.s. p.r.n.

## ADVERSE REACTIONS
**CNS:** headache, irritability, weakness.
**GI:** rebound hyperacidity, *nausea.*

## INTERACTIONS
*Antibiotics (including quinolones and tetracyclines), hydantoins, iron salts, isoniazid, salicylates:* decreased pharmacologic effect because of possible impaired absorption. Separate administration times.
*Enteric-coated drugs:* may be released prematurely in stomach. Separate doses by at least 1 hour.
*Milk and other foods high in vitamin D:* possible milk-alkali syndrome (headache, confusion, distaste for food, nausea, vomiting, hypercalcemia, hypercalciuria, calcinosis, hypophosphatemia). Avoid concomitant use.

## CONTRAINDICATIONS
Contraindicated in patients with ventricular fibrillation or hypercalcemia.

## NURSING CONSIDERATIONS
• Use cautiously, if at all, in patients with sarcoidosis, renal or cardiac disease, and in patients receiving cardiac glycosides.

• Record amount and consistency of stools. Manage constipation with laxatives or stool softeners as ordered.
• Monitor serum calcium levels, especially in patients with mild renal impairment.
• Watch for symptoms of hypercalcemia (nausea, vomiting, headache, mental confusion, and anorexia).

## ☑ PATIENT TEACHING
• Advise patient not to take calcium carbonate indiscriminately or to switch antacids without the doctor's advice.
• Tell patient taking chewable tablets to chew thoroughly before swallowing and follow with a glass of water.
• Tell patient using suspension form to shake well and take with a small amount of water to facilitate passage.

# dihydroxyaluminum sodium carbonate
Rolaids◊

*Pregnancy Risk Category: NR*

## HOW SUPPLIED
*Tablets:* 334 mg◊

## ACTION
An antacid that reduces total acid load in the GI tract, elevates gastric pH to reduce pepsin activity, strengthens the gastric mucosal barrier, and increases esophageal sphincter tone.

## ONSET, PEAK, DURATION
Onset occurs in 20 minutes. Peak unknown. Effects persist for 20 to 60 minutes in fasting patients, 3 hours when taken after meals.

## INDICATIONS & DOSAGE
*Antacid–*
**Adults:** 1 to 2 tablets (334 to 668 mg) P.O., chewed well, p.r.n.

## ADVERSE REACTIONS
**CNS:** encephalopathy.
**GI:** *constipation,* intestinal obstruction.
**Other:** hypophosphatemia, osteomalacia.

## INTERACTIONS
*Allopurinol, antibiotics (including quinolones and tetracyclines), diflunisal, digoxin, iron, isoniazid, penicillamine, phenothiazines, quinidine:* decreased pharmacologic effect because of possible impaired absorption. Separate administration times.
*Enteric-coated drugs:* may be released prematurely in stomach. Separate doses by at least 1 hour.

## CONTRAINDICATIONS
None known.

## NURSING CONSIDERATIONS
• Use cautiously in patients with renal disease.
• Record amount and consistency of stools. Manage constipation with laxatives or stool softeners as ordered; alternate with magnesium-containing antacids (if the patient does not have renal disease).
• Monitor long-term, high-dose use in patients on restricted sodium intake. Has high sodium content (53 mg/tablet) and may increase sodium and water retention.

## ☑ PATIENT TEACHING
• Advise patient not to take dihydroxyaluminum sodium carbonate indiscriminately.
• Encourage patient to follow his prescribed diet, if applicable.

---

## magaldrate (aluminum-magnesium complex)
Antiflux†, Iosopan◇, Lowsium◇, Riopan◇

*Pregnancy Risk Category: NR*

## HOW SUPPLIED
*Tablets:* 480 mg◇
*Tablets (chewable):* 480 mg◇
*Oral suspension:* 540 mg/5 ml◇

## ACTION
An antacid that reduces total acid load in the GI tract, elevates gastric pH to reduce pepsin activity, strengthens the gastric mucosal barrier, and increases esophageal sphincter tone.

## ONSET, PEAK, DURATION
Onset occurs within 20 minutes. Peak unknown. Effects persist for 20 to 60 minutes in fasting patients, 3 hours when taken after meals.

## INDICATIONS & DOSAGE
*Antacid –*
**Adults:** 540 to 1,080 mg (5 to 10 ml) of suspension P.O. with water between meals and h.s.; or 480 to 960 mg tablets(1 to 2 tablets) P.O. with water between meals and h.s.; or 480 to 960 mg chewable tablets (1 to 2 tablets) P.O., chewed before swallowing, between meals and h.s.

## ADVERSE REACTIONS
**GI:** mild constipation or diarrhea.

## INTERACTIONS
*Allopurinol, antibiotics (including quinolones and tetracyclines), diflunisal, digoxin, iron salts, isoniazid, penicillamine, phenothiazines, quinidine, ticlopidine:* decreased pharmacologic effect because of possible impaired absorption. Separate administration times by 1 to 2 hours.
*Enteric-coated drugs:* may be released prematurely in stomach. Separate doses by at least 1 hour.

## CONTRAINDICATIONS
Contraindicated in patients with severe renal disease.

---

*Liquid form contains alcohol.  **May contain tartrazine.  †Canada only.  ‡Australia only.  ◇OTC.

## NURSING CONSIDERATIONS
• Use cautiously in patients with mild kidney impairment.
• When giving through nasogastric tube, make sure tube is placed properly and is patent. After instilling, flush tube with water to ensure passage to stomach and to clear tube.
• Record amount and consistency of stools.
• Monitor serum magnesium level in patients with mild kidney impairment. Symptomatic hypermagnesemia usually occurs only in severe renal failure.
• **Alert:** Keep in mind that drug is not typically used in patients with renal failure (although it contains aluminum) to help control hypophosphatemia because it contains magnesium, which may accumulate.
• Be aware that the drug has a very low sodium content and is good for patients on restricted sodium intake.

☑ **PATIENT TEACHING**
• Instruct patient to shake suspension well and to follow with water to facilitate passage.
• Tell patient taking chewable tablets to chew thoroughly and to follow with a glass of water.
• Advise patient not to take magaldrate indiscriminately or to switch antacids without the doctor's advice.

---

## magnesium oxide
Mag-Ox 400◊, Maox-420◊, Uro-Mag◊

*Pregnancy Risk Category: NR*

### HOW SUPPLIED
*Tablets:* 400 mg◊, 420 mg◊
*Capsules:* 140 mg◊

### ACTION
An antacid that reduces total acid load in the GI tract, elevates gastric pH to reduce pepsin activity, strengthens the gastric mucosal barrier, and increases esophageal sphincter tone.

### ONSET, PEAK, DURATION
Onset occurs within 20 minutes. Peak unknown. Effects persist for 20 to 60 minutes in fasting patients, 3 hours when taken after meals.

### INDICATIONS & DOSAGE
*Antacid –*
**Adults:** 140 mg P.O. with water or milk after meals and h.s.
*Laxative –*
**Adults:** 4 g P.O. with water or milk, usually h.s.
*Oral replacement therapy in mild hypomagnesemia –*
**Adults:** 400 to 840 mg P.O. daily. Monitor serum magnesium level.

### ADVERSE REACTIONS
**GI:** *diarrhea,* nausea, abdominal pain.
**Other:** hypermagnesemia.

### INTERACTIONS
*Allopurinol, antibiotics (including quinolones and tetracyclines), digoxin, iron salts, penicillamine, phenothiazines:* decreased pharmacologic effect because of possible impaired absorption. Separate administration times by 1 to 2 hours.
*Enteric-coated drugs:* may be released prematurely in stomach. Separate doses by at least 1 hour.

### CONTRAINDICATIONS
Contraindicated in patients with severe renal disease.

### NURSING CONSIDERATIONS
• Use cautiously in patients with mild renal impairment.
• When used as laxative, do not give other oral drugs 1 to 2 hours before or after treatment.
• Monitor serum magnesium levels. With prolonged use and some degree of renal impairment, watch for symp-

---

toms of hypermagnesemia (hypotension, nausea, vomiting, depressed reflexes, respiratory depression, and coma).
• If diarrhea occurs, be prepared to suggest alternative preparation.

☑ **PATIENT TEACHING**
• Advise patient not to take magnesium oxide indiscriminately or to switch antacids without the doctor's advice.

## simethicone
Extra Strength Gas-X◇, Gas-Relief◇, Gas-X◇, Maximum Strength Gas Relief◇, Maximum Strength Phazyme 125 Softgels◇, Mylanta Gas◇, Mylanta Gas Maximum Strength◇, Mylanta Gas Regular Strength◇, Mylicon◇, Ovol†, Ovol-40†, Ovol-80†, Phazyme◇, Phazyme 55†◇, Phazyme 95◇

*Pregnancy Risk Category: NR*

### HOW SUPPLIED
*Tablets:* 40 mg◇, 55 mg†◇, 60 mg◇, 80 mg◇, 95 mg◇, 125 mg◇
*Capsules:* 125 mg
*Drops:* 40 mg/0.6 ml◇

### ACTION
By its defoaming action, disperses or prevents formation of mucus-surrounded gas pockets in the GI tract.

### ONSET, PEAK, DURATION
Onset and peak is immediate. Duration unknown.

### INDICATIONS & DOSAGE
*Flatulence, functional gastric bloating–*
**Adults and children over 12 years:**
40 to 125 mg after each meal and h.s.

### ADVERSE REACTIONS
**GI:** expulsion of excessive liberated gas as belching, rectal flatus.

### INTERACTIONS
None significant.

### CONTRAINDICATIONS
Contraindicated in patients hypersensitive to the drug.

### NURSING CONSIDERATIONS
• Know that drug is not recommended for the treatment of infant colic because of limited information on its safety in infants and children.
• Be aware that medication does not prevent formation of gas.

☑ **PATIENT TEACHING**
• Tell patient to chew tablet before swallowing.
• Encourage patient to change positions frequently and ambulate to aid in passing flatus.

---

*Liquid form contains alcohol.   **May contain tartrazine.   †Canada only.   ‡Australia only.   ◇OTC.

# 48

# Digestive enzymes and gallstone solubilizers

chenodiol
monooctanoin
pancreatin
pancrelipase
ursodiol

## COMBINATION PRODUCTS
DONNAZYME TABLETS: pancreatin 300 mg, pepsin 150 mg, bile salts 150 mg, hyoscyamine sulfate 0.0518 mg, atropine sulfate 0.0097 mg, scopolamine hydrobromide 0.0033 mg, and phenobarbital 8.1 mg.
ENTOZYME TABLETS: pancreatin 300 mg, pepsin 250 mg, and bile salts 150 mg.
PANCREASE CAPSULES: lipase 4,000 units, protease 25,000 units, and amylase 20,000 units in enteric-coated microspheres.

---

## chenodiol
## (chenodeoxycholic acid)
Chenix

*Pregnancy Risk Category: X*

### HOW SUPPLIED
*Tablets:* 250 mg

### ACTION
Unknown. Probably suppresses hepatic synthesis of cholesterol and cholic acid, which contributes to biliary cholesterol desaturation and dissolution of gallstones.

### ONSET, PEAK, DURATION
Onset and duration unknown. Peak levels occur 50 minutes to 2 hours after a dose.

### INDICATIONS & DOSAGE
*Dissolution of radiolucent cholesterol stones (gallstones) when systemic disease or age precludes surgery –*

**Adults:** 250 mg P.O. b.i.d. for first 2 weeks, followed, as tolerated, by weekly increases of 250 mg/day, up to 13 to 16 mg/kg/day for up to 24 months.

### ADVERSE REACTIONS
**GI:** *diarrhea,* cramps, heartburn, constipation, nausea, vomiting, anorexia, epigastric distress.
**Hepatic:** reversible elevated hepatic enzymes, possible liver toxicity.

### INTERACTIONS
*Aluminum-containing antacids, cholestyramine, clofibrate, colestipol, estrogens, oral contraceptives:* decreased chenodiol effect.

### CONTRAINDICATIONS
Contraindicated in patients with known hepatocyte dysfunction, intrahepatic cholestasis, primary biliary cirrhosis, or sclerosing cholangitis, a gallbladder confirmed as nonvisualizing after two consecutive single doses of dye; radiopaque or radiolucent bile pigment stones; gallstone complications; or compelling reasons for gallbladder surgery, including unremitting acute cholecystitis, cholangitis, biliary obstruction, gallstone-induced pancreatitis, and biliary fistula; and during pregnancy.

### NURSING CONSIDERATIONS
• Know that treatment should be reserved for carefully selected patients.
• Monitor AST and ALT levels monthly for the first 3 months and every 3 months thereafter for duration of therapy, as ordered.
• Monitor the patient for diarrhea, which occurs in 30% to 40% of all patients. The doctor may reduce dosage until diarrhea subsides and may prescribe antidiarrheals. In some patients,

---

Reactions may be *common,* uncommon, *life-threatening*, or COMMON AND LIFE-THREATENING.

however, persistent diarrhea requires discontinuing chenodiol.
• Monitor oral cholecystogram or ultrasonogram every 6 to 9 months to observe for gallstone dissolution.
• Know that the drug is particularly effective in the dissolution of small, floatable gallstones.
• Keep in mind that the final dosage should not be less than 10 mg/kg/day; lower dosages are usually ineffective.

☑ **PATIENT TEACHING**
• Encourage compliance with the drug regimen and follow-up appointments.
• Tell patient to promptly report worsening symptoms (sudden right upper quadrant pain, nausea, vomiting).

---

# monooctanoin
Moctanin
*Pregnancy Risk Category: C*

## HOW SUPPLIED
*Infusion:* 120-ml bottles

## ACTION
Dissolves gallstones by rendering them more soluble.

## ONSET, PEAK, DURATION
Onset usually occurs within 72 hours. Peak and duration unknown.

## INDICATIONS & DOSAGE
*To solubilize cholesterol (radiolucent) gallstones that are retained in the biliary tract after cholecystectomy—*
**Adults:** administered as a continuous infusion for 2 to 10 days (for elimination or size reduction of stones) through a catheter inserted directly into the common bile duct via a T tube at a rate of 3 to 5 ml/hour and at a pressure of 10 cm $H_2O$.

## ADVERSE REACTIONS
**GI:** *pain, abdominal discomfort, nausea, vomiting, diarrhea,* anorexia, indigestion.

**Other:** fever.

## INTERACTIONS
None significant.

## CONTRAINDICATIONS
Contraindicated in patients with impaired hepatic function, biliary tract infection, or a history of recent duodenal ulceration or jejunitis; porto-systemic shunting; acute pancreatitis, or any active life-threatening problems that would be complicated by perfusion into the biliary tract.

## NURSING CONSIDERATIONS
• Be aware monooctanoin therapy should be initiated only by individuals experienced in infusion therapy.
• Because impaired liver function may lead to metabolic acidosis during monooctanoin administration, obtain routine liver function tests as ordered before perfusion therapy begins.
• *Alert:* Do not administer parenterally; for biliary tract infusion only.
• Dilute each vial with sterile water for injection. Dilution will reduce solution viscosity and enhance bathing of stone.
• Warm the solution to 60° to 80° F (16° to 27° C) before perfusion. Temperature should not fall below 65° F (18° C) during administration.
• Use a peristaltic infusion pump to regulate the infusion. Outpatients may use a battery-operated portable pump.
• Keep pump pressure at 10 cm $H_2O$ to minimize GI and biliary tract irritation. Pressure must be below 15 cm $H_2O$.
• Reduce GI symptoms by slowing the infusion rate or discontinuing infusion during meals, as ordered.

☑ **PATIENT TEACHING**
• Instruct outpatient on use of pump and drug administration.
• Inform patient of need for follow-up care and diagnostic studies.
• Tell patient to report adverse effects.

---

*Liquid form contains alcohol. **May contain tartrazine. †Canada only. ‡Australia only. ◊OTC.

# pancreatin

Bioglan Panazyme‡, Creon,
Dizymes Tablets◇, Donnazyme, 8X
Pancreatin 900 mg◇, Entozyme, 4X
Pancreatin 600 mg◇, Hi-Vegi-Lip
Tablets◇, Pancrezyme 4X Tablets◇

*Pregnancy Risk Category: C*

## HOW SUPPLIED
**Bioglan Panazyme‡**
*Tablets:* 468 mg pancreatin, 7,200 units lipase, 656 units protease, and 9,200 units amylase
**Creon**
*Capsules (enteric-coated microspheres):* 300 mg pancreatin, 8,000 units lipase, 13,000 units protease, and 30,000 units amylase
**Dizymes**
*Tablets (enteric-coated):* 250 mg pancreatin, 6,750 units lipase, 41,250 units protease, and 43,750 units amylase◇
**Donnazyme**
*Tablets:* 500 mg pancreatin, 1,000 units lipase, 12,500 units protease, and 12,500 units amylase
**8X Pancreatin 900 mg**
*Tablets (enteric-coated):* 7,200 mg pancreatin, 22,500 units lipase, 180,000 units protease, and 180,000 units amylase◇
**Entozyme**
*Tablets:* 500 mg pancreatin, 600 units lipase, 7,500 units protease, and 7,500 units amylase
**4X Pancreatin 600 mg**
*Tablets (enteric-coated):* 2,400 mg pancreatin, 12,000 units lipase, 60,000 units protease, and 60,000 units amylase◇
**Hi-Vegi-Lip**
*Tablets (enteric-coated):* 2,400 mg pancreatin, 4,800 units lipase, 60,000 units protease, and 60,000 units amylase◇
**Pancrezyme 4X**
*Tablets (enteric-coated):* 2,400 mg pancreatin, 12,000 units lipase, 60,000 units protease, and 60,000 units amylase◇

## ACTION
Replaces endogenous exocrine pancreatic enzymes and aids digestion of starches, fats, and proteins.

## ONSET, PEAK, DURATION
Onset and peak unknown. Effects persist for 1 to 2 hours.

## INDICATIONS & DOSAGE
*Exocrine pancreatic secretion insufficiency; digestive aid in diseases associated with deficiency of pancreatic enzymes, such as cystic fibrosis* —
**Adults and children:** dosage varies with condition being treated. Usual initial dosage is 8,000 to 24,000 units of lipase activity before or with each meal or snack. The total daily dose may also be given in divided doses at 1 to 2 hour intervals throughout the day.

## ADVERSE REACTIONS
**GI:** nausea, diarrhea (with high doses).
**Other:** allergic reactions, perianal irritation.

## INTERACTIONS
*Antacids:* may negate pancreatin's beneficial effect. Avoid concomitant use.
*Oral iron:* may decrease serum iron response. Monitor for decreased effectiveness.

## CONTRAINDICATIONS
Contraindicated in patients with hypersensitivity to the drug, or to pork protein or enzymes, acute pancreatitis, and acute exacerbations of chronic pancreatitis.

## NURSING CONSIDERATIONS
• Use with caution in pregnant or breast-feeding patients.
• Be aware that minimal USP standards dictate that each milligram of bovine or porcine pancreatin contain lipase 2 units, protease 25 units, and amylase 25 units.
• To avoid indigestion, monitor patient's dietary intake to ensure a proper balance of fat, protein, and starch in-

---

Reactions may be *common*, uncommon, ***life-threatening***, or **COMMON AND LIFE-THREATENING**.

take. Dosage varies according to degree of maldigestion and malabsorption, amount of fat in diet, and enzyme activity of individual preparations.
• Keep in mind that fewer bowel movements and improved stool consistency indicate effective therapy.
• Know that the drug is not effective in GI disorders unrelated to pancreatic enzyme deficiency.
• Know that enteric coating on some products may reduce available enzyme in upper portion of jejunum.

☑ **PATIENT TEACHING**
• Instruct patient to take before or with meals and snacks.
• Tell patient not to crush or chew enteric-coated forms. Capsules containing enteric-coated microspheres may be opened and sprinkled on a small quantity of cooled, soft food. Stress importance of swallowing immediately without chewing and following with glass of water or juice.
• Warn patient not to inhale powder form or powder from capsules; may irritate skin or mucous membranes.
• Tell patient to store in airtight containers at room temperature.
• Instruct patient not to change brands without consulting doctor.

---

## pancrelipase

Cotazym Capsules, Cotazym-S Capsules, Creon 10 Capsules, Creon 20 Capsules, Ilozyme Tablets, Ku-Zyme HP Capsules, Pancrease Capsules, Pancrease MT 4, Pancrease MT 10, Pancrease MT 16, Pancrease MT 20, Pancrelipase Capsules, Protilase Capsules, Ultrase MT 12, Ultrase MT 20, Ultrase MT 24, Viokase Powder, Viokase Tablets, Zymase Capsules

*Pregnancy Risk Category: C*

**HOW SUPPLIED**
**Cotazym**
*Capsules:* 8,000 units lipase, 30,000 units protease, 30,000 units amylase, and 25 mg calcium carbonate
**Cotazym-S**
*Capsules (enteric-coated spheres):* 5,000 units lipase, 20,000 units protease, and 20,000 units amylase
**Creon 10**
*Capsules (delayed-release):* 10,000 units lipase, 37,500 units protease, and 33,200 units amylase
**Creon 20**
*Capsules (delayed-release):* 20,000 units lipase, 75,000 units protease, and 66,400 units amylase
**Ilozyme**
*Tablets:* 11,000 units lipase, 30,000 units protease, and 30,000 units amylase
**Ku-Zyme HP**
*Capsules:* 8,000 units lipase, 30,000 units protease, and 30,000 units amylase
**Pancrease**
*Capsules (enteric-coated microspheres):* 4,000 units lipase, 25,000 units protease, and 20,000 units amylase
**Pancrease MT 4**
*Capsules (enteric-coated microtablets):* 4,500 units lipase, 12,000 units protease, and 12,000 units amylase
**Pancrease MT 10**
*Capsules (enteric-coated microtablets):* 10,000 units lipase, 30,000 units protease, and 30,000 units amylase
**Pancrease MT 16**
*Capsules (enteric-coated microtablets):* 16,000 units lipase, 48,000 units protease, and 48,000 units amylase
**Pancrease MT 20**
*Capsules (enteric-coated microtablets):* 20,000 units lipase, 44,000 units protease, and 56,000 units amylase
**Pancrelipase**
*Capsules (enteric-coated pellets):* 4,000 units lipase, 25,000 units protease, and 20,000 units amylase
**Protilase**
*Capsules (enteric-coated spheres):* 4,000 units lipase, 25,000 units protease, and 20,000 units amylase
**Ultrase MT 12**
*Capsules (delayed-release):* 12,000

---

*Liquid form contains alcohol. **May contain tartrazine. †Canada only. ‡Australia only. ◊OTC.

units lipase, 39,000 units protease, and 39,000 units amylase

**Ultrase MT 20**
*Capsules (delayed-release):* 20,000 units lipase, 65,000 units protease, and 65,000 units amylase

**Ultrase MT 24**
*Capsules (delayed-release):* 24,000 units lipase, 78,000 units protease, and 78,000 units amylase

**Viokase**
*Powder:* 16,800 units lipase, 70,000 units protease, and 70,000 units amylase per 0.7 g powder
*Tablets:* 8,000 units lipase, 30,000 units protease, and 30,000 units amylase

**Zymase**
*Capsules (enteric-coated spheres):* 12,000 units lipase, 24,000 units protease, and 24,000 units amylase

## ACTION
Replaces endogenous exocrine pancreatic enzymes and aids digestion of starches, fats, and proteins.

## ONSET, PEAK, DURATION
Variable.

## INDICATIONS & DOSAGE
*Exocrine pancreatic secretion insufficiency, cystic fibrosis in adults and children, steatorrhea and other disorders of fat metabolism secondary to insufficient pancreatic enzymes –*
**Adults and children 12 years and older:** dosage titrated to patient's response. Usual initial dosage 4,000 to 48,000 units of lipase with each meal.
**Children 7 to 12 years:** 4,000 to 12,000 units (more, if needed) of lipase activity with each meal or snack.
**Children 1 to 6 years:** 4,000 to 8,000 units of lipase with each meal and 4,000 units of lipase with each snack.
**Children 6 months to 1 year:** 2,000 units of lipase with each meal.
**Children under 6 months:** dosage not established.

## ADVERSE REACTIONS
**GI:** *nausea,* cramping, diarrhea (high doses).

## INTERACTIONS
*Antacids:* may destroy enteric coating and result in enhanced degradation of pancrelipase. Avoid concomitant use.
*Oral iron:* may decrease serum iron response. Monitor for decreased effectiveness.

## CONTRAINDICATIONS
Contraindicated in patients with severe hypersensitivity to pork, acute pancreatitis, or acute exacerbations of chronic pancreatic diseases.

## NURSING CONSIDERATIONS
● Know that drug should be used only after confirmed diagnosis of exocrine pancreatic insufficiency. It's not effective in GI disorders unrelated to enzyme deficiency.
● Know that lipase activity is greater than with other pancreatic enzymes.
● For infants, mix powder with applesauce and give with meals. Avoid contact with or inhalation of powder because it may be very irritating. Older children may take capsules with food.
● Monitor patient's stools. Adequate replacement decreases number of bowel movements and improves stool consistency.
● Know that minimal USP standards dictate that each milligram of pancrelipase contain 24 units lipase, 100 units protease, and 100 units amylase.
● Know that dosage varies with degree of maldigestion and malabsorption, amount of fat in diet, and enzyme activity of individual preparations.
● Know that enteric coating on some products may reduce available enzyme in upper portion of jejunum.

## ☑ PATIENT TEACHING
● Instruct patient to take before or with meals and snacks.
● Advise patient not to crush or chew

---

enteric-coated forms. Capsules containing enteric-coated microspheres may be opened and sprinkled on a small quantity of cooled, soft food. Stress importance of swallowing immediately without chewing and following with glass of water or juice.
• Warn patient not to inhale powder form or powder from capsules; it may irritate skin or mucous membranes.
• Tell patient to store in airtight containers at room temperature.
• Instruct patient not to change brands without consulting doctor.

## ursodiol
Actigall

*Pregnancy Risk Category: B*

### HOW SUPPLIED
*Capsules:* 300 mg

### ACTION
Unknown. A naturally occurring bile acid that probably suppresses hepatic synthesis and secretion of cholesterol as well as intestinal cholesterol absorption. After long-term use, ursodiol can solubilize cholesterol from gallstones.

### ONSET, PEAK, DURATION
Onset and duration unknown. Peak levels occur 1 to 3 hours after dose.

### INDICATIONS & DOSAGE
*Dissolution of gallstones less than 20 mm in diameter when surgery precluded –*
**Adults:** 8 to 10 mg/kg P.O. daily in two or three divided doses.

### ADVERSE REACTIONS
**CNS:** headache, fatigue, anxiety, depression, sleep disorders.
**EENT:** rhinitis.
**GI:** nausea, vomiting, dyspepsia, metallic taste, abdominal pain, biliary pain, cholecystitis, diarrhea, constipation, stomatitis, flatulence.
**Respiratory:** cough.

**Skin:** pruritus, rash, dry skin, urticaria, hair thinning, diaphoresis.
**Other:** arthralgia, myalgia, back pain.

### INTERACTIONS
*Aluminum-containing antacids, cholestyramine, colestipol:* bind ursodiol and prevent its absorption. Avoid concomitant use.
*Clofibrate, estrogens, oral contraceptives:* increased hepatic cholesterol secretion; may counteract the effects of ursodiol. Avoid concomitant use.

### CONTRAINDICATIONS
Contraindicated in patients hypersensitive to ursodiol or other bile acids and in those with chronic hepatic disease, unremitting acute cholecystitis, cholangitis, biliary obstruction, gallstone-induced pancreatitis, or biliary fistula.

### NURSING CONSIDERATIONS
• Know that drug won't dissolve calcified cholesterol stones, radiolucent bile pigment stones, or radiopaque stones.
• *Alert:* Monitor liver function test results, including AST and ALT, at the start of therapy and after 1 month, 3 months, and then every 6 months during therapy, as ordered. Abnormal tests may indicate a worsening of the disease. A theoretical risk exists that a hepatotoxic metabolite of ursodiol may form in some patients.
• Know that therapy usually is long-term, with ultrasound images of the gallbladder taken every 6 months. If partial stone dissolution does not occur within 12 months, eventual success is unlikely. Safety of use for longer than 24 months has not been established.

### ☑ PATIENT TEACHING
• Tell patient about alternative therapies, including "watchful waiting" (no intervention) and cholecystectomy because the relapse rate may be as high as 50% after 5 years.
• Tell patient to report adverse effects.

---

*Liquid form contains alcohol.  **May contain tartrazine.  †Canada only.  ‡Australia only.  ◇OTC.

# 49

## Antidiarrheals

**attapulgite**
**bismuth subsalicylate**
**calcium polycarbophil**
(See Chapter 50, LAXATIVES.)
**difenoxin hydrochloride and
   atropine sulfate**
**diphenoxylate hydrochloride and
   atropine sulfate**
**kaolin and pectin mixtures**
**loperamide**
**octreotide acetate**
**opium tincture**
**opium tincture, camphorated**

### COMBINATION PRODUCTS
K-C◊: 5.2 g kaolin, 260 mg pectin,
260 mg bismuth subsalicylate in 30-
ml suspension.
KAODENE NON-NARCOTIC◊: 3.9 g
kaolin and 194.4 mg pectin in 30-ml
bismuth subsalicylate liquid.

### attapulgite
Children's Kaopectate, Diar-Aid,
Diarrest, Diasorb, Diatrol,
Donnagel, Fowler's†, Kaopectate,
Kaopectate Advanced Formula,
Kaopectate Maximum Strength,
Kaopek, K-Pek, Parepectolin,
Rheaban

*Pregnancy Risk Category: NR*

### HOW SUPPLIED
*Tablets:* 300 mg, 600 mg†, 630 mg†,
750 mg
*Chewable tablets:* 300 mg, 600 mg
*Oral suspension:* 600 mg/15 ml, 750
mg/15 ml, 900 mg/15 ml†

### ACTION
A hydrated magnesium aluminum sil-
icate that is thought to adsorb large
numbers of bacteria and toxins and reduce water loss.

### ONSET, PEAK, DURATION
Unknown.

### INDICATIONS & DOSAGE
*Acute, nonspecific diarrhea –*
**Adults and adolescents:** 1.2 to 1.5 g
(up to 3 g if using Diasorb) P.O. after
each loose bowel movement, not to
exceed 9 g in 24 hours.
**Children 6 to 12 years:** 600 mg (suspension) or 750 mg (tablet) P.O. after
each loose bowel movement, not to
exceed 4.2 g (suspension) or 4.5 g
(tablet) in 24 hours.
**Children 3 to 6 years:** 300 mg P.O.
after each loose bowel movement, not
to exceed 2.1 g in 24 hours.

### ADVERSE REACTIONS
**GI:** constipation.

### INTERACTIONS
*Oral medications:* potential for impaired absorption of oral medications
when administered concurrently with
attapulgite. Administer attapulgite not
less than 2 hours before or 3 hours after these medications, and monitor for
decreased effectiveness.

### CONTRAINDICATIONS
Contraindicated in patients with dys-
entery or suspected bowel obstruction.

### NURSING CONSIDERATIONS
• Use cautiously in patients with dehydration. Promote adequate fluid intake to compensate for fluid loss from
diarrhea.
• Be aware that drug should not be
used if diarrhea is accompanied by fever or by blood or mucus in the stool.
If these signs occur during treatment,
withhold drug and notify doctor.

Reactions may be *common*, uncommon, *life-threatening*, or COMMON AND LIFE-THREATENING.

• Tell the patient to take the drug after each loose bowel movement until diarrhea is controlled.
• Instruct the patient to notify the doctor if diarrhea is not controlled within 48 hours or if fever develops.

---

## bismuth subsalicylate

Bismatrol◇, Bismatrol Extra Strength◇, Maximum Strength Pepto-Bismol Liquid◇, Pepto-Bismol◇, Pink Bismuth◇

*Pregnancy Risk Category: NR*

### HOW SUPPLIED
*Tablets (chewable):* 262 mg◇
*Caplets:* 262 mg
*Oral suspension:* 262 mg/15 ml◇, 130 mg/5 ml◇, 524 mg/15 ml◇

### ACTION
Unknown. Has a mild water-binding capacity; also may adsorb toxins and provide protective coating for mucosa.

### ONSET, PEAK, DURATION
Onset occurs within 1 hour. Peak and duration unknown.

### INDICATIONS & DOSAGE
*Mild, nonspecific diarrhea –*
**Adults:** 30 ml or 2 tablets P.O. q ½ to 1 hour, up to a maximum of eight doses and for no longer than 2 days.
**Children 3 to 6 years:** 5 ml or ⅓ tablet P.O.
**Children 6 to 9 years:** 10 ml or ⅔ tablet P.O.
**Children 9 to 12 years:** 15 ml or 1 tablet P.O.

### ADVERSE REACTIONS
**GI:** temporary darkening of tongue and stools.
**Other:** salicylism (with high doses).

### INTERACTIONS
*Aspirin, other salicylates:* risk of salicylate toxicity. Monitor closely.
*Oral anticoagulants, oral antidiabetic agents:* theoretical risk of increased effects of these agents after high doses of bismuth subsalicylate. Monitor the patient closely.
*Tetracycline:* decreased tetracycline absorption. Separate administration times by at least 2 hours.

### CONTRAINDICATIONS
Contraindicated in patients hypersensitive to salicylates.

### NURSING CONSIDERATIONS
• Use cautiously in patients already taking aspirin. Discontinue if tinnitus occurs.
• Avoid use before GI radiologic procedures because bismuth is radiopaque and may interfere with X-rays.

☑ PATIENT TEACHING
• Advise patient that bismuth subsalicylate contains a large amount of salicylate (each tablet has 102 mg salicylate; the regular-strength liquid has 130 mg/15 ml, and the extra-strength liquid has 230 mg/15 ml).
• Instruct patient to chew tablets well before swallowing or to shake liquid before measuring dose.
• Tell patient to call the doctor if diarrhea persists for more than 2 days or is accompanied by high fever.
• Tell patient to consult with the doctor before giving bismuth subsalicylate to children or teenagers during or after recovery from the flu or chicken pox.
• Inform patient that all forms of Pepto-Bismol are effective against traveler's diarrhea. Tablets and caplets may be more convenient to carry.

---

*Liquid form contains alcohol.   **May contain tartrazine.   †Canada only.   ‡Australia only.   ◇OTC.

# difenoxin hydrochloride and atropine sulfate
Lyspafen‡, Motofen
Controlled Substance Schedule IV

*Pregnancy Risk Category: C*

## HOW SUPPLIED
*Tablets:* 0.5 mg (with atropine sulphate 0.025 mg)‡, 1 mg (with atropine sulfate 0.025 mg)

## ACTION
Unknown. Probably exerts a direct effect on the intestinal wall to slow motility.

## ONSET, PEAK, DURATION
Onset occurs within 30 minutes. Peak levels occur within 40 to 60 minutes. Duration unknown.

## INDICATIONS & DOSAGE
*Adjunct in acute nonspecific diarrhea and acute exacerbations of chronic functional diarrhea –*
**Adults:** initially, 2 mg P.O., then 1 mg P.O. after each loose bowel movement or 1 mg q 3 to 4 hours p.r.n. Do not exceed total dosage of 8 mg daily. Not recommended for use longer than 2 days.

## ADVERSE REACTIONS
**CNS:** dizziness, light-headedness, drowsiness, headache, fatigue, nervousness, insomnia, confusion.
**EENT:** burning eyes, blurred vision.
**GI:** nausea, vomiting, dry mouth, epigastric distress, constipation.

## INTERACTIONS
*Barbiturates, CNS depressants, ethanol, narcotic agents, tranquilizers:* enhanced CNS depression. Closely monitor patient.
*MAO inhibitors:* possible hypertensive crisis. Avoid concomitant use.

## CONTRAINDICATIONS
Contraindicated in patients hypersensitive to difenoxin or atropine, in children under 2 years, in patients with diarrhea caused by pseudomembranous colitis associated with antibiotics, and in those with jaundice or diarrhea from organisms that may penetrate the intestinal mucosa (including toxigenic *Escherichia coli, Salmonella,* or *Shigella*).

## NURSING CONSIDERATIONS
• Use cautiously in patients with a history of drug abuse or in those currently receiving drugs with a high abuse potential. Difenoxin is the principal metabolite of diphenoxylate and is chemically related to meperidine.
• Know that atropine has been added to difenoxin to prevent abuse. The small dosage of atropine is unlikely to cause any significant clinical problems, but patients may experience dry mouth, tachycardia, urine retention, and flushing. Monitor for these effects.
• Monitor patients closely for fluid and electrolyte imbalance. Difenoxin-induced decreases in peristalsis may result in fluid retention in the colon with subsequent dehydration and possibly delayed difenoxin intoxication.
• *Alert:* For overdose, observe patient for at least 48 hours. Respiratory depression may occur up to 30 hours after ingestion. Use gastric lavage, establishment of a patent airway, and mechanically assisted ventilation to treat overdose and naloxone to reverse respiratory depression. Know that because difenoxin has a longer duration of action than naloxone, repeated injections of naloxone are necessary.

## ☑ PATIENT TEACHING
• Advise patient to avoid hazardous activities that require mental alertness, such as driving or operating heavy machinery, until CNS effects of the drug are known.

---

Reactions may be *common*, uncommon, ***life-threatening***, or **COMMON AND LIFE-THREATENING**.

- Advise patient to adhere to dosing schedule. Overdose with difenoxin may cause respiratory depression and coma. Encourage storing drug out of children's reach.

# diphenoxylate hydrochloride and atropine sulfate

Lofene, Logen, Lomenate, Lomotil*, Lonox

Controlled Substance Schedule V

*Pregnancy Risk Category: C*

## HOW SUPPLIED

*Tablets:* 2.5 mg (with atropine sulfate 0.025 mg)
*Liquid:* 2.5 mg/5 ml (with atropine sulfate 0.025 mg/5 ml)*

## ACTION

Unknown. Probably increases smooth muscle tone in the GI tract, inhibits motility and propulsion, and diminishes secretions.

## ONSET, PEAK, DURATION

Onset occurs in 45 to 60 minutes after ingestion. Plasma levels peak about 3 hours after ingestion. Effects persist for 3 to 4 hours.

## INDICATIONS & DOSAGE

*Acute, nonspecific diarrhea* –
**Adults:** initially, 5 mg P.O. q.i.d., then adjusted as needed.
**Children 2 to 12 years:** 0.3 to 0.4 mg/kg liquid form P.O. daily in four divided doses. For maintenance, initial dosage reduced, as needed, up to 75%.

## ADVERSE REACTIONS

**CNS:** *sedation, dizziness,* headache, drowsiness, lethargy, restlessness, depression, euphoria, malaise, confusion, numbness in extremities.
**CV:** tachycardia.
**EENT:** mydriasis.
**GI:** *dry mouth,* nausea, vomiting, abdominal discomfort or distention, *paralytic ileus,* anorexia, fluid retention in bowel or megacolon (may mask depletion of extracellular fluid and electrolytes, especially in young children treated for acute gastroenteritis), pancreatitis, swollen gums, possible physical dependence with long-term use.
**GU:** urine retention.
**Respiratory:** respiratory depression.
**Skin:** pruritus, rash, dry skin.
**Other:** *angioedema, anaphylaxis.*

## INTERACTIONS

*Barbiturates, CNS depressants, ethanol, narcotic agents, tranquilizers:* enhanced CNS depression. Closely monitor patient.
*MAO inhibitors:* possible hypertensive crisis. Avoid concomitant use.

## CONTRAINDICATIONS

Contraindicated in patients with hypersensitivity to diphenoxylate or atropine, acute diarrhea resulting from poison until toxic material is eliminated from GI tract, acute diarrhea caused by organisms that penetrate intestinal mucosa, or diarrhea resulting from antibiotic-induced pseudomembranous enterocolitis; also contraindicated in jaundiced patients and in children under 2 years.

## NURSING CONSIDERATIONS

- Use cautiously in children 2 years and over; in patients with hepatic disease, narcotic dependence, or acute ulcerative colitis; and in pregnant patients. Stop therapy immediately if abdominal distention or other signs of toxic megacolon develop and notify doctor.
- Monitor fluid and electrolyte balance. Correct fluid and electrolyte disturbances before starting drug. Dehydration, especially in young children, may increase risk of delayed toxicity.
- Keep in mind that a dose of 2.5 mg

---

*Liquid form contains alcohol.   **May contain tartrazine.   †Canada only.   ‡Australia only.   ◇OTC.

is as effective as 5 ml camphorated opium tincture.
• Know that the drug is not indicated for treating antibiotic-induced diarrhea.
• Be aware that drug is unlikely to be effective if no response occurs within 48 hours.
• Know that the risk of physical dependence increases with high dosage and long-term use. Atropine sulfate helps discourage abuse.

☑ **PATIENT TEACHING**
• Tell patient not to exceed recommended dosage.
• Warn patient not to use drug to treat acute diarrhea for longer than 2 days and to seek medical attention if diarrhea continues.
• Advise patient to avoid hazardous activities, such as driving, until CNS effects of the drug are known.

## kaolin and pectin mixtures
Kaolin with Pectin◇, Kao-Spen◇, Kapectolin◇

*Pregnancy Risk Category: NR*

### HOW SUPPLIED
*Oral suspension:* 5.2 mg kaolin and 260 mg pectin per 30 ml◇ (Kao-Spen◇); 90 g kaolin, 2 g pectin per 30 ml◇ (Kaolin with Pectin◇, Kapectolin◇)

### ACTION
Decreases fluid content of stools, although *total* water loss seems to remain the same.

### ONSET, PEAK, DURATION
Unknown.

### INDICATIONS & DOSAGE
*Mild, nonspecific diarrhea* –
**Adults and children 12 years and older:** 60 to 120 ml P.O. after each bowel movement.

**Children 3 to 6 years:** 15 to 30 ml P.O. after each bowel movement.
**Children 6 to 12 years:** 30 to 60 ml P.O. after each bowel movement.

### ADVERSE REACTIONS
**GI:** drug absorption of nutrients, other drugs, and enzymes; fecal impaction or ulceration in infants and elderly or debilitated patients after chronic use; constipation.

### INTERACTIONS
*Orally administered drugs:* adsorption may occur. Separate administration times by at least 2 to 3 hours.

### CONTRAINDICATIONS
None known.

### NURSING CONSIDERATION
Administer other oral drugs 2 to 3 hours before or after administration of a kaolin and pectin mixture.

☑ **PATIENT TEACHING**
• Warn patient not to use drug to replace specific therapy for underlying cause.
• Advise patient not to use drug for more than 2 days.

## loperamide
Imodium, Imodium A-D◇, Kaopectate II Caplets◇, Maalox Anti-Diarrheal Caplets◇, Pepto Diarrhea Control◇

*Pregnancy Risk Category: B*

### HOW SUPPLIED
*Caplets:* 2 mg◇
*Capsules:* 2 mg
*Oral liquid:* 1 mg/5 ml◇

### ACTION
Inhibits peristaltic activity, prolonging transit of intestinal contents.

## ONSET, PEAK, DURATION
Onset unknown. Peak plasma levels occur about 2½ hours after oral liquid, 4 to 5 hours after capsules. Effects persist for about 24 hours.

## INDICATIONS & DOSAGE
*Acute, nonspecific diarrhea –*
**Adults:** initially, 4 mg P.O., then 2 mg after each unformed stool. Maximum dosage is 16 mg daily.
**Children 2 to 6 years:** 5 ml P.O. t.i.d. on first day. If diarrhea persists, contact doctor.
**Children 6 to 8 years:** 10 ml (2 mg) P.O. b.i.d. on first day. If diarrhea persists, contact doctor.
**Children 8 to 12 years:** 10 ml (2 mg) t.i.d. P.O. on first day. (Subsequent doses of 5 ml (1 mg)/10 kg of body weight may be administered after each unformed stool.) Maximum dosage is 6 mg daily.
*Chronic diarrhea –*
**Adults:** initially, 4 mg P.O., then 2 mg after each unformed stool until diarrhea subsides. Dosage adjusted to individual response.

## ADVERSE REACTIONS
**CNS:** drowsiness, fatigue, dizziness.
**GI:** dry mouth; abdominal pain, distention, or discomfort; *constipation;* nausea; vomiting.
**Skin:** rash, hypersensitivity reactions.

## INTERACTIONS
None significant.

## CONTRAINDICATIONS
Contraindicated in patients with hypersensitivity and when constipation must be avoided. Also contraindicated in children under 2 years.

## NURSING CONSIDERATIONS
• Use cautiously in patients with hepatic disease.
• Be aware that the drug produces antidiarrheal action similar to diphenoxylate but without as many adverse CNS effects.
• ***Alert:*** Monitor children closely for CNS effects because they may be more sensitive to the CNS effects of the drug than adults.

## ☑ PATIENT TEACHING
• Advise patient not to exceed recommended dosage.
• In acute diarrhea, tell patient to discontinue drug and seek medical attention if no improvement occurs within 48 hours; in chronic diarrhea, he should notify doctor and discontinue drug if no improvement occurs after taking 16 mg daily for at least 10 days.
• Advise patient with acute colitis to stop drug immediately if abdominal distention or other symptoms develop and notify the doctor.

---

# octreotide acetate
Sandostatin

*Pregnancy Risk Category: B*

## HOW SUPPLIED
*Injection ampules:* 0.05 mg, 0.1 mg, 0.5 mg
*Injection-multidose vials:* 0.2 mg/ml, 1 mg/ml

## ACTION
Mimics the action of naturally occurring somatostatin.

## ONSET, PEAK, DURATION
Onset occurs within 30 minutes. Peak levels occur within ½ hour. Effects persist up to 12 hours.

## INDICATIONS & DOSAGE
*Flushing and diarrhea associated with carcinoid tumors –*
**Adults:** 0.1 to 0.6 mg daily S.C. in two to four divided doses for the first 2 weeks of therapy (usual daily dosage is 0.3 mg). Subsequent dosage based on individual response.

---

*Liquid form contains alcohol.  **May contain tartrazine.  †Canada only.  ‡Australia only.  ◊OTC.

*Watery diarrhea associated with vaso-active intestinal polypeptide secreting tumors (VIPomas)—*
**Adults:** 0.2 to 0.3 mg daily S.C. in two to four divided doses for the first 2 weeks of therapy. Subsequent dosage based on individual response; typically, don't exceed 0.45 mg daily.
*Acromegaly—*
**Adults:** initially, 50 mcg S.C. t.i.d., then adjusted according to somatomedin C levels q 2 weeks.

## ADVERSE REACTIONS
**CNS:** dizziness, light-headedness, fatigue, headache.
**CV:** sinus bradycardia, conduction abnormalities, arrhythmias.
**EENT:** blurred vision.
**GI:** *nausea, diarrhea, abdominal pain or discomfort, loose stools,* vomiting, fat malabsorption, gallbladder abnormalities, flatulence, constipation.
**GU:** pollakiuria, urinary tract infection.
**Skin:** flushing, edema, wheal, erythema or pain at injection site, alopecia.
**Other:** hyperglycemia, hypoglycemia, hypothyroidism, and pain, and/or burning at the S.C. injection site, cold symptoms, backache, joint pain, flulike symptoms.

## INTERACTIONS
*Cyclosporine:* may decrease plasma levels of cyclosporine. Monitor patient closely.

## CONTRAINDICATIONS
Contraindicated in patients hypersensitive to the drug or any of its components.

## NURSING CONSIDERATIONS
• Monitor baseline thyroid function tests as ordered.
• Monitor somatomedin C levels every 2 weeks as ordered. Know that

dosage adjustments are based on this level.
• Monitor laboratory tests periodically, such as thyroid function tests, urine 5-hydroxyindoleacetic acid, plasma serotonin, and plasma substance P (for carcinoid tumors), and plasma vasoactive intestinal peptide (for VIPomas).
• Monitor patients regularly for gallbladder disease. Octreotide therapy may be associated with development of cholelithiasis because of its effect on gallbladder motility or fat absorption.
• Monitor closely for symptoms of glucose imbalance. Be alert that insulin-dependent diabetic patients and patients receiving oral antidiabetic agents or oral diazoxide may require dosage adjustments during therapy.
• Keep in mind that octreotide therapy may alter fluid and electrolyte balance and may require adjustment of other drugs used to control symptoms of the disease, such as beta blockers.
• Be aware that half-life may be altered in patients in end-stage renal failure who are receiving dialysis.

☑ **PATIENT TEACHING**
• Instruct patient to report any signs of abdominal discomfort immediately.
• Stress importance of need for periodic laboratory testing during octreotide therapy.

# opium tincture*
Controlled Substance Schedule II

# opium tincture, camphorated* (paregoric)
Controlled Substance Schedule III
*Pregnancy Risk Category: NR*

---

## HOW SUPPLIED
**opium tincture**
*Oral solution:* equivalent to morphine 10 mg/ml*
**opium tincture, camphorated**
*Oral solution:* Each 5 ml contains morphine, 2 mg; anise oil, 0.2 ml; benzoic acid, 20 mg; camphor, 20 mg; glycerin, 0.2 ml; and ethanol to make 5 ml*

## ACTION
Increases smooth muscle tone in the GI tract, inhibits motility and propulsion, and diminishes secretions.

## ONSET, PEAK, DURATION
Unknown.

## INDICATIONS & DOSAGE
*Acute, nonspecific diarrhea –*
**Adults:** 0.6 ml opium tincture (range 0.3 to 1 ml) P.O. q.i.d. Maximum dosage is 6 ml daily. Or, 5 to 10 ml camphorated opium tincture once daily, b.i.d., t.i.d., or q.i.d. until diarrhea subsides.
**Children:** 0.25 to 0.5 ml/kg camphorated opium tincture P.O. once daily, b.i.d., t.i.d., or q.i.d. until diarrhea subsides.

## ADVERSE REACTIONS
**CNS:** dizziness, light-headedness.
**GI:** nausea, vomiting, physical dependence after long-term use.

## INTERACTIONS
None significant.

## CONTRAINDICATIONS
Contraindicated in patients with acute diarrhea caused by poisoning until toxic material is removed from GI tract or in those with diarrhea caused by organisms that penetrate intestinal mucosa.

## NURSING CONSIDERATIONS
• Use cautiously in patients with asthma, prostatic hyperplasia, hepatic disease, and history of opioid dependence.
• Mix with sufficient water to ensure passage to stomach.
• Know that a milky fluid forms when camphorated opium tincture is added to water.
• *Alert:* For overdose, use the narcotic antagonist naloxone, as ordered, to reverse respiratory depression.
• Keep in mind that opium content of opium tincture is 25 times greater than camphorated opium tincture. Camphorated opium tincture is more dilute, and teaspoonful doses are easier to measure than dropper quantities of opium tincture.
• Keep in mind that the drug is an effective and prompt-acting antidiarrheal, but unique because dosage can be adjusted precisely to patient's needs.
• Store in tightly capped, light-resistant container.

## ☑ PATIENT TEACHING
• Advise patient against using drug for more than 2 days; risk of physical dependence increases with long-term use.
• Instruct patient to measure dosage carefully to avoid overdose which can have serious consequences.

---

*Liquid form contains alcohol.  **May contain tartrazine.  †Canada only.  ‡Australia only.  ◇OTC.

# 50

# Laxatives

bisacodyl
calcium polycarbophil
cascara sagrada
cascara sagrada aromatic
 fluidextract
cascara sagrada fluidextract
castor oil
docusate calcium
docusate potassium
docusate sodium
glycerin
lactulose
magnesium citrate
magnesium hydroxide
magnesium sulfate
methylcellulose
mineral oil
phenolphthalein, white
phenolphthalein, yellow
polyethylene glycol and
 electrolyte solution
psyllium
senna
sodium phosphates

## COMBINATION PRODUCTS

AGORAL◇: mineral oil 28% and white phenolphthalein 1.3% in emulsion, with tragacanth, agar, egg albumin, acacia, and glycerin.
DIALOSE PLUS◇: docusate sodium 100 mg and casanthranol 30 mg.
DOXIDAN◇: docusate calcium 60 mg and phenolphthalein 65 mg.
D-S-S PLUS◇: docusate sodium 100 mg and casanthranol 30 mg.
HALEY'S M-O◇: mineral oil (25%) and magnesium hydroxide.
KONDREMUL WITH PHENOLPHTHA-LEIN◇: heavy mineral oil 55%, white phenolphthalein 150 mg/15 ml, and Irish moss as emulsifier.
MODANE PLUS◇: docusate sodium 100 mg and white phenolphthalein 65 mg.
PERI-COLACE CAPSULES◇: docusate sodium 100 mg and casanthranol 30 mg.
PERI-COLACE SYRUP◇: docusate sodium 60 mg and casanthranol 30 mg/15 ml.
SENOKOT-S◇: docusate sodium 50 mg and standardized senna concentrate 187 mg.
UNILAX SOFTGEL◇: docusate sodium 230 mg and yellow phenolphthalein 130 mg.

# bisacodyl

Bisac-Evac◇, Bisacolax†◇, Bisalax‡, Bisco-Lax**◇, Carter's Little Pills◇, Dacodyl◇, Deficol◇, Dulcagen◇, Dulcolax◇, Durolax‡, Fleet Bisacodyl◇, Fleet Bisacodyl Prep◇, Fleet Laxative◇, Laxit†◇, Theralax◇

*Pregnancy Risk Category: B*

## HOW SUPPLIED

*Tablets (enteric-coated):* 5 mg◇
*Enema:* 0.33 mg/dl◇, 10 mg/5 ml (microenema)‡
*Powder for rectal solution (bisacodyl tannex):* 1.5 mg bisacodyl and 2.5 g tannic acid
*Suppositories:* 5 mg◇, 10 mg◇

## ACTION

Unknown. A stimulant laxative that increases peristalsis probably by direct effect on the smooth muscle of the intestine. Thought to either irritate the musculature or stimulate the colonic intramural plexus. Also promotes fluid accumulation in the colon and small intestine.

## ONSET, PEAK, DURATION

Onset occurs 15 to 60 minutes after suppository, 6 to 12 hours after oral

---

Reactions may be *common*, uncommon, *life-threatening*, or COMMON AND LIFE-THREATENING.

administration. Peak and duration variable.

## INDICATIONS & DOSAGE

*Chronic constipation; preparation for delivery, surgery, or rectal or bowel examination –*

**Adults and children 12 years and over:** 10 to 15 mg P.O. in evening or before breakfast. Up to 30 mg P.O. as needed and ordered, or 10 mg P.R. for evacuation before examination or surgery.

**Children 6 to 12 years:** 5 mg P.O. or P.R. h.s. or before breakfast.

## ADVERSE REACTIONS

**CNS:** muscle weakness with excessive use, dizziness, faintness.
**GI:** *nausea, vomiting, abdominal cramps,* diarrhea (with high doses), *burning sensation in rectum* (with suppositories), laxative dependence with long-term or excessive use.
**Other:** alkalosis, hypokalemia, tetany, protein-losing enteropathy in excessive use, fluid and electrolyte imbalance.

## INTERACTIONS

*Milk or antacids:* gastric irritation or dyspepsia from premature dissolution of enteric coating. Do not administer together.

## CONTRAINDICATIONS

Contraindicated in patients with hypersensitivity, abdominal pain, nausea, vomiting, or other symptoms of appendicitis or acute surgical abdomen and in those with rectal bleeding, gastroenteritis, or intestinal obstruction.

## NURSING CONSIDERATIONS

• Time administration of drug so as not to interfere with scheduled activities or sleep. Soft, formed stools are usually produced 15 to 60 minutes after rectal administration.
• Before giving for constipation, de-

termine if the patient has adequate fluid intake, exercise, and diet.
• Know that tablets and suppositories are used together to clean the colon before and after surgery and before barium enema.
• Insert suppository as high as possible into the rectum, and try to position the suppository against the rectal wall. Avoid embedding within fecal material because this may delay the onset of action.
• Store tablets and suppositories at a temperature below 86° F (30° C).

## ☑ PATIENT TEACHING

• Advise the patient to swallow enteric-coated tablet whole to avoid GI irritation. Don't give within 1 hour of milk or antacid intake.
• Tell patient drug is for short-term treatment only (a stimulant laxative, this type is frequently abused). Discourage excessive use.
• Advise the patient to report adverse effects to the doctor.
• Teach the patient about dietary sources of bulk which include bran and other cereals, fresh fruit, and vegetables.

# calcium polycarbophil

Equalactin◇, Fiberall◇, FiberCon◇, FiberLax◇, FiberNorm◇, Mitrolan◇

*Pregnancy Risk Category: NR*

## HOW SUPPLIED

*Tablets:* 500 mg◇, 625 mg◇
*Tablets (chewable):* 500 mg◇, 1,250 mg◇

## ACTION

A bulk-forming laxative that absorbs water and expands to increase bulk and moisture content of stools. The increased bulk encourages peristalsis and bowel movement. As an antidiarrheal, absorbs free fecal water, thereby producing formed stools.

---

*Liquid form contains alcohol.   **May contain tartrazine.   †Canada only.   ‡Australia only.   ◇OTC.

**ONSET, PEAK, DURATION**
Onset occurs in 12 to 24 hours. Peak effects may not occur for up to 3 days. Duration variable.

**INDICATIONS & DOSAGE**
*Constipation –*
**Adults:** 1 g P.O. q.i.d. as required. Maximum dosage is 6 g in 24-hour period.
**Children 2 to 6 years:** use must be directed by doctor. 500 mg P.O. b.i.d. as required. Maximum dosage is 1.5 g in 24-hour period.
**Children 6 to 12 years:** 500 mg P.O. 1 to 3 times daily as required. Maximum dosage is 3 g in 24-hour period.
*Diarrhea associated with irritable bowel syndrome, as well as acute nonspecific diarrhea –*
**Adults:** 1 g P.O. q.i.d. as required. Maximum dosage is 6 g in 24-hour period.
**Children 2 to 6 years:** use must be directed by doctor. 500 mg P.O. b.i.d. as required. Maximum dosage is 1.5 g in 24-hour period.
**Children 6 to 12 years:** 500 mg P.O. t.i.d. as required. Maximum dosage is 3 g in 24-hour period.

**ADVERSE REACTIONS**
**GI:** abdominal fullness and increased flatus, intestinal obstruction.
**Other:** laxative dependence (with long-term or excessive use).

**INTERACTIONS**
*Tetracyclines:* impaired absorption of tetracyclines. Avoid using together.

**CONTRAINDICATIONS**
Contraindicated in patients with signs of GI obstruction.

**NURSING CONSIDERATIONS**
• Before giving for constipation, determine if the patient has adequate fluid intake, exercise, and diet.
• **Alert:** Be aware that rectal bleeding

or failure to respond to therapy may indicate need for surgery.

**☑ PATIENT TEACHING**
• Advise the patient to chew Equalactin or Mitrolan tablets thoroughly before swallowing and to drink a full glass of water with each dose. When used as an antidiarrheal, tell the patient not to drink a glass of water.
• Teach the patient about dietary sources of bulk, which include bran and other cereals, fresh fruit, and vegetables.
• For severe diarrhea, advise the patient to repeat dose every half hour, but not to exceed maximum daily dosage.

---

**cascara sagrada**

**cascara sagrada aromatic fluidextract***

**cascara sagrada fluidextract***

*Pregnancy Risk Category: C*

**HOW SUPPLIED**
*Tablets:* 325 mg
*Aromatic fluidextract:* 1 g/ml*
*Fluidextract:* 1 g/ml*

**ACTION**
Unknown. A stimulant laxative that increases peristalsis probably by direct effect on the smooth muscle of the intestine. Thought to either irritate the musculature or stimulate the colonic intramural plexus. Also promotes fluid accumulation in the colon and small intestine.

**ONSET, PEAK, DURATION**
Onset occurs in 6 to 10 hours. Peak and duration variable.

**INDICATIONS & DOSAGE**
*Acute constipation; preparation for bowel or rectal examination –*

---

**Adults and children 12 years and over:** one 325 mg tablet of cascara sagrada P.O. once daily h.s.; 200 to 400 mg of cascara sagrada extract P.O. once daily; 0.5 to 1.5 ml of cascara sagrada fluidextract P.O. once daily or 5 ml of aromatic cascara fluidextract P.O. once daily.

**Children under 2 years:** one-quarter adult dosage.

**Children 2 to 12 years:** one-half adult dosage.

### ADVERSE REACTIONS
**GI:** *nausea;* vomiting; diarrhea; loss of normal bowel function with excessive use; *abdominal cramps*, especially in severe constipation; malabsorption of nutrients; "cathartic colon" (syndrome resembling ulcerative colitis radiologically and pathologically) with chronic misuse; discoloration of rectal mucosa after long-term use.
**Other:** hypokalemia, protein enteropathy, electrolyte imbalance (with excessive use), laxative dependence (with long-term or excessive use).

### INTERACTIONS
None significant.

### CONTRAINDICATIONS
Contraindicated in patients with abdominal pain, nausea, vomiting, or other symptoms of appendicitis or acute surgical abdomen; acute surgical delirium; fecal impaction; and intestinal obstruction or perforation.

### NURSING CONSIDERATIONS
• Use cautiously when rectal bleeding is present.
• Before giving for constipation, determine if the patient has adequate fluid intake, exercise, and diet.
• Monitor serum electrolytes during prolonged use.
• Be aware that cascara sagrada aromatic fluidextract is less active and less bitter than the nonaromatic fluidextract.

• Know that liquid preparations are more reliable than solid dosage forms.

### ☑ PATIENT TEACHING
• Warn patient that drug may turn alkaline urine red-pink and acidic urine yellow-brown.
• Teach the patient about dietary sources of bulk, which include bran and other cereals, fresh fruit, and vegetables.

## castor oil
Alphamul◊, Emulsoil◊, Fleet Flavored Castor Oil◊, Kellogg's Castor Oil◊, Minims Castor Oil‡◊, Neoloid◊, Purge◊

*Pregnancy Risk Category: NR*

### HOW SUPPLIED
*Oral liquid:* 36.4% (Neoloid◊), 60% (Alphamul◊), 67% (Fleet◊), 95% (Emulsoil◊, Purge◊), 100% (Kellogg's◊, Minims◊)

### ACTION
Unknown. A stimulant laxative that increases peristalsis probably by direct effect on the smooth muscle of the intestine. Thought to either irritate the musculature or stimulate the colonic intramural plexus. Also promotes fluid accumulation in the colon and small intestine.

### ONSET, PEAK, DURATION
Onset occurs in 2 to 6 hours. Peak and duration variable.

### INDICATIONS & DOSAGE
*Preparation for rectal or bowel examination or for surgery –*
**Adults and children 12 years and older:** 15 to 60 ml P.O.
**Children under 2 years:** 2.5 to 7.5 ml P.O. Increased dose produces no greater effect.
**Children 2 to 12 years:** 5 to 15 ml P.O.
For all patients, administered as a

single dose about 16 hours before surgery or procedure.

**ADVERSE REACTIONS**
**GI:** *nausea;* vomiting; diarrhea; loss of normal bowel function with excessive use; *abdominal cramps,* especially in severe constipation; malabsorption of nutrients; "cathartic colon" (syndrome resembling ulcerative colitis radiologically and pathologically) with chronic misuse; laxative dependence with long-term or excessive use. May cause constipation after catharsis.
**Other:** hypokalemia, protein-losing enteropathy, other electrolyte imbalances (with excessive use).

**INTERACTIONS**
None significant.

**CONTRAINDICATIONS**
Contraindicated in patients with ulcerative bowel lesions; abdominal pain, nausea, vomiting, or other symptoms of appendicitis or acute surgical abdomen; and anal or rectal fissures, fecal impaction, or intestinal obstruction or perforation; and during menstruation or pregnancy.

**NURSING CONSIDERATIONS**
● Use cautiously in patients with rectal bleeding.
● Give castor oil with juice or carbonated beverage to mask oily taste. Have the patient stir mixture and drink it promptly. Ice held in the mouth before taking drug will help prevent tasting it.
● Shake emulsion well before measuring dose. Emulsion is better tolerated but is more expensive. Store below 40° F (4.4° C). Don't freeze.
● Give on empty stomach for best results.
● Time drug administration so that it doesn't interfere with scheduled activities or sleep.
● Know that increased intestinal mo-

tility lessens absorption of concomitantly administered oral drugs. Separate administration times.
● *Alert:* Be aware that failure to respond to drug may indicate acute condition requiring surgery.

☑ **PATIENT TEACHING**
● Tell the patient not to expect another bowel movement for 1 to 2 days after castor oil has emptied bowel.
● Warn patient about potential adverse reactions.

# docusate calcium (dioctyl calcium sulfosuccinate)
DC Softgels◇, Pro-Cal-Sof◇, Sulfalax Calcium◇, Surfak◇

# docusate potassium (dioctyl potassium sulfosuccinate)
Diocto-K◇, Kasof◇

# docusate sodium (dioctyl sodium sulfosuccinate)
Afko-Lube◇, Colace◇, Coloxyl‡, Coloxyl Enema Concentrate‡, Dialose◇, Diocto◇, Dioeze◇, Diosuccin◇, Dio-Sul◇, Disonate◇, Di-Sosul◇, Doss◇, Doxinate◇, D-S-S◇, Duosol◇, Genasoft◇, Laxinate 100◇, Modane Soft◇, Molatoc◇, Pro-Sof◇, Pro-Sof Liquid Concentrate◇, Pro-Sof Liquid Plus◇, Regulax SS◇, Regulex†◇, Regutol◇, Stulex◇, Therevac Plus◇, Therevac-SB◇

*Pregnancy Risk Category: C*

**HOW SUPPLIED**
**docusate calcium**
*Capsules:* 50 mg◇, 240 mg◇
**docusate potassium**
*Capsules:* 100 mg◇, 240 mg◇
**docusate sodium**
*Tablets:* 100 mg◇
*Capsules:* 50 mg◇, 60 mg◇, 100 mg◇, 240 mg◇, 250 mg◇

---

Reactions may be *common,* uncommon, *life-threatening,* or COMMON AND LIFE-THREATENING.

# Photoguide to tablets and capsules

One of the most critical responsibilities of any nurse is to ensure that the patient receives the right medication. This task becomes easier when the nurse can verify the appearance of drugs prescribed for the patient. The following photoguide provides full-color photographs of some of the most commonly prescribed tablets and capsules in the United States. Shown here in actual size, the tablets and capsules are organized alphabetically for quick reference.

**Accupril**
10 mg
20 mg

**acetaminophen and codeine**
300 mg/30 mg
300 mg/60 mg

**Adalat**
30 mg (extended-release)

**Altace**
2.5 mg
5 mg

**Ambien**
5 mg
10 mg

**amitriptyline hydrochloride**
25 mg
50 mg
75 mg
100 mg

**amoxicillin trihydrate**
250 mg
500 mg

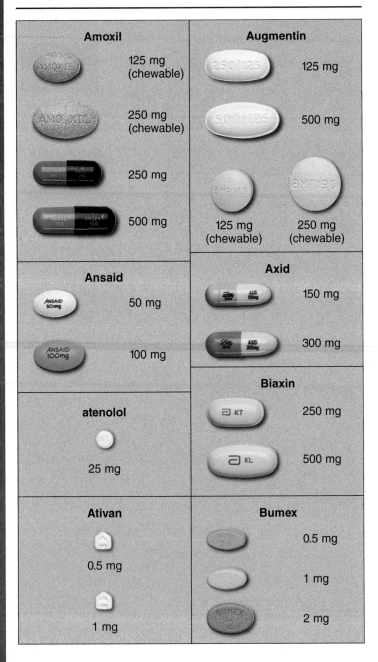

**Amoxil**

125 mg (chewable)

250 mg (chewable)

250 mg

500 mg

**Ansaid**

50 mg

100 mg

**atenolol**

25 mg

**Ativan**

0.5 mg

1 mg

**Augmentin**

125 mg

500 mg

125 mg (chewable)

250 mg (chewable)

**Axid**

150 mg

300 mg

**Biaxin**

250 mg

500 mg

**Bumex**

0.5 mg

1 mg

2 mg

**BuSpar**

5 mg     10 mg

**Calan**

40 mg     80 mg

120 mg

**Capoten**

12.5 mg     25 mg

**Carafate**

1 g

**Cardizem**

30 mg

60 mg

90 mg

**Cardizem CD**
(extended-release)

120 mg

180 mg

240 mg

**Cardizem SR**
(sustained-release)

60 mg

90 mg

120 mg

**Cardura**

1 mg     2 mg

4 mg

**Ceclor**

250 mg

500 mg

**Deltasone**

2.5 mg  5 mg

10 mg  20 mg

**Depakote**
(delayed-release)

125 mg  250 mg

500 mg

**Depakote Sprinkle**

125 mg

**DiaBeta**

1.25 mg  2.5 mg  5 mg

**dicyclomine hydrochloride**

10 mg

20 mg

**Diflucan**

100 mg  150 mg  200 mg

**Dilacor XR**

180 mg

240 mg

**Dilantin**

50 mg

**Dilantin Kapseals**

30 mg  100 mg

**doxepin hydrochloride**

75 mg

**Duricef**

500 mg

**Dyazide**

25 mg/37.5 mg

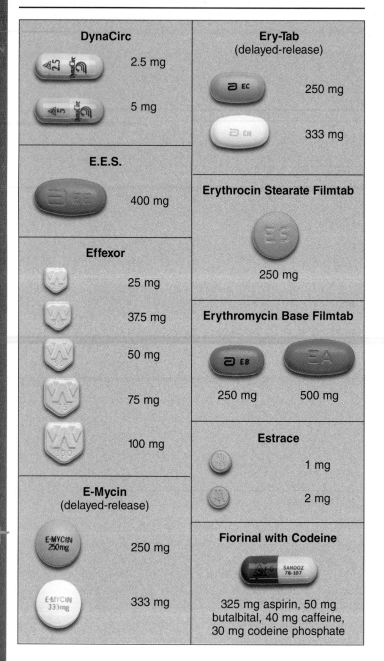

**DynaCirc**

2.5 mg

5 mg

**E.E.S.**

400 mg

**Effexor**

25 mg

37.5 mg

50 mg

75 mg

100 mg

**E-Mycin**
(delayed-release)

250 mg

333 mg

**Ery-Tab**
(delayed-release)

250 mg

333 mg

**Erythrocin Stearate Filmtab**

250 mg

**Erythromycin Base Filmtab**

250 mg          500 mg

**Estrace**

1 mg

2 mg

**Fiorinal with Codeine**

325 mg aspirin, 50 mg
butalbital, 40 mg caffeine,
30 mg codeine phosphate

**Floxin**

200 mg

300 mg

400 mg

**furosemide**

20 mg

**gemfibrozil**

600 mg

**glipizide**

10 mg

**Glucotrol**

5 mg          10 mg

**Glucotrol XL**

5 mg          10 mg

**Glynase**

3 mg          6 mg

**Halcion**

0.125 mg

0.25 mg

**Hismanal**

10 mg

**hydrocodone bitartrate and acetaminophen**

5 mg/ 500 mg

7.5 mg/ 500 mg

7.5 mg/ 750 mg

**Hytrin**

1 mg

2 mg

5 mg

10 mg

**Lodine**

200 mg

300 mg

400 mg

**Lopid**

600 mg

**Lorabid**

400 mg

**Lorcet 10/650**

10 mg/650 mg

**Lozol**

1.25 mg

2.5 mg

**Macrobid**

75 mg/25 mg

**methylphenidate hydrochloride**

5 mg

10 mg

20 mg

20 mg (extended-release)

**Mevacor**

10 mg    20 mg    40 mg

**Micro-K Extencaps**
(controlled-release)

10 mEq (750 mg)

**Micronase**
2.5 mg
5 mg

**Nitrostat**
0.3 mg
0.4 mg
0.6 mg

**Motrin**
400 mg
600 mg
800 mg

**Nolvadex**
10 mg

**nortriptyline hydrochloride**
10 mg
25 mg
50 mg

**Naprosyn**
250 mg
375 mg
500 mg

**Norvasc**
5 mg
10 mg

**naproxen**
375 mg
500 mg

**Ogen**
0.75 mg
(Ogen 0.625)
1.5 mg
(Ogen 1.25)

**Orasone**
1 mg

**Oruvail**
100 mg
150 mg
200 mg

**Pamelor**
10 mg
25 mg
50 mg
75 mg

**Paxil**
20 mg
30 mg

**PCE**
333 mg
500 mg

**Pepcid**
20 mg
40 mg

**Percocet**
5 mg/325 mg

**potassium chloride**
10 mEq (extended-release)

**Pravachol**
10 mg
20 mg
40 mg

| Seldane | | Sumycin | |
|---|---|---|---|
| | 60 mg | | 250 mg |

| Seldane-D | | Suprax | |
|---|---|---|---|
| | 60 mg/120 mg | | 400 mg |

| Sinemet | | Synthroid | |
|---|---|---|---|
| | 10 mg/100 mg | | 25 mcg |
| | 25 mg/250 mg | | 50 mcg |

| Sinemet CR | | | |
|---|---|---|---|
| | 25 mg/100 mg (extended-release) | | 75 mcg |
| | | | 88 mcg |

| Slo-bid Gyrocaps (extended-release) | | | |
|---|---|---|---|
| | | | 100 mcg |
| | 50 mg | | 112 mcg |
| | 75 mg | | 125 mcg |
| | 100 mg | | 150 mcg |
| | 200 mg | | 175 mcg |
| | 300 mg | | 200 mcg |
| | | | 300 mcg |

### Tagamet
200 mg

300 mg

### Tenormin
25 mg

50 mg

100 mg

### Theo-Dur
(timed-release)
100 mg

200 mg

300 mg

450 mg

### Toprol XL
50 mg

100 mg

150 mg

### Toradol
10 mg

### Trental
400 mg

### Trimox
250 mg

500 mg

| | |
|---|---|
| **Tylenol with Codeine No. 3** | 300 mg/30 mg |
| **Ultram** | 50 mg |
| **Valium** | 2 mg |
| | 5 mg |
| | 10 mg |
| **Vasotec** | 2.5 mg |
| | 5 mg |
| | 10 mg |
| | 20 mg |
| **Veetids** | 250 mg |
| | 500 mg |
| **verapamil hydrochloride** | 180 mg (sustained-release) |
| **Verelan** (sustained-release) | 120 mg |
| | 240 mg |
| **Vicodin** | 5 mg/500 mg |
| **Vicodin ES** | 7.5 mg/750 mg |

**Xanax**

0.25 mg

0.5 mg

1 mg

**Zantac**

150 mg

300 mg

**Zantac EFFERdose**

150 mg

**Zestril**

5 mg

10 mg

20 mg

40 mg

**Zithromax**

250 mg

**Zocor**

5 mg

10 mg

20 mg

**Zoloft**

50 mg

100 mg

**Zovirax**

200 mg

400 mg

800 mg

*Oral liquid:* 150 mg/15 ml◇
*Oral solution:* 50 mg/ml◇
*Syrup:* 50 mg/15 ml◇, 60 mg/15 ml◇
*Enema concentrate:* 18 g/100 ml
(must be diluted)‡

## ACTION
A stool softener that reduces surface tension of interfacing liquid contents of the bowel. This detergent activity promotes incorporation of additional liquid into stools, thus forming a softer mass.

## ONSET, PEAK, DURATION
Onset is variable; usually within 24 to 72 hours as is peak and duration.

## INDICATIONS & DOSAGE
*Stool softener –*
**Adults and children older than 12 years:** 50 to 500 mg P.O. daily until bowel movements are normal. Alternatively, give enema (where available). Dilute 1:24 with sterile water before administration, and give 100 to 150 ml (retention enema), 300 to 500 ml (evacuation enema), or 0.5 to 1.5 liters (flushing enema).
**Children under 3 years:** 10 to 40 mg docusate sodium P.O. daily.
**Children 3 to 6 years:** 20 to 60 mg docusate sodium P.O. daily.
**Children 6 to 12 years:** 40 to 120 mg docusate sodium P.O. daily.
   Higher dosages used for initial therapy. Dosage adjusted to individual response. Usual dosage in children and adults with minimal needs is 50 to 150 mg (calcium) P.O. daily.

## ADVERSE REACTIONS
**GI:** bitter taste, mild abdominal cramping, diarrhea, laxative dependence (with long-term or excessive use).

## INTERACTIONS
*Mineral oil:* may increase mineral oil absorption and cause toxicity and li-

poid pneumonia. Separate administration times.

## CONTRAINDICATIONS
Contraindicated in patients hypersensitive to the drug and in those with intestinal obstruction, undiagnosed abdominal pain, vomiting or other signs of appendicitis, fecal impaction, or acute surgical abdomen.

## NURSING CONSIDERATIONS
• Give liquid in milk, fruit juice, or infant formula to mask bitter taste.
• Before giving for constipation, determine if the patient has adequate fluid intake, exercise, and diet.
• Know that the drug is not for use in treating existing constipation but prevents constipation from developing.
• Be aware that the drug is laxative of choice for patients who should not strain during defecation, including patients recovering from MI or rectal surgery; for those with rectal or anal disease that makes passage of firm stools difficult; and for those with postpartum constipation.
• Store at 59° to 86° F (15° to 30° C), and protect liquid from light.

## ☑ PATIENT TEACHING
• Teach patient about dietary sources of bulk, which include bran and other cereals, fresh fruit, and vegetables.
• Instruct patient to use only occasionally and not for more than 1 week without the doctor's knowledge.
• Tell patient to discontinue if severe cramping occurs and to notify doctor.

## glycerin
Fleet Babylax◇, Sani-Supp◇
*Pregnancy Risk Category: NR*

## HOW SUPPLIED
*Enema (pediatric):* 4 ml/applicator◇
*Suppositories:* adult, children, and infant sizes◇

---

## ACTION
A hyperosmolar laxative that draws water from the tissues into the feces and thus stimulates evacuation.

## ONSET, PEAK, DURATION
Onset, peak and duration occur in 15 to 60 minutes.

## INDICATIONS & DOSAGE
*Constipation –*
**Adults and children 6 years and over:** 2 to 3 g as a rectal suppository or 5 to 15 ml as an enema.
**Children under 6 years:** 1 to 1.7 g as a rectal suppository; or 2 to 5 ml as an enema.

## ADVERSE REACTIONS
**GI:** *cramping pain,* rectal discomfort, hyperemia of rectal mucosa.

## INTERACTIONS
None significant.

## CONTRAINDICATIONS
Contraindicated in patients hypersensitive to the drug and in those with intestinal obstruction, undiagnosed abdominal pain, vomiting or other signs of appendicitis, fecal impaction, or acute surgical abdomen.

## NURSING CONSIDERATION
Know that drug is used mainly to re-establish proper toilet habits in laxative-dependent patients.

## ☑ PATIENT TEACHING
● Tell patient that the drug must be retained for at least 15 minutes; usually acts within 1 hour. Entire suppository need not melt to be effective.
● Warn patient about adverse GI reactions.

# lactulose
Cephulac, Cholac, Chronulac, Constilac, Duphalac, Enulose, Evalose, Generlac, Heptalac, Lactulax†, Portalac

*Pregnancy Risk Category: B*

## HOW SUPPLIED
*Syrup:* 10 g/15 ml

## ACTION
Produces an osmotic effect in the colon. Resulting distention promotes peristalsis. Also decreases blood ammonia, probably as a result of bacterial degradation, which decreases the pH of colon contents.

## ONSET, PEAK, DURATION
Onset occurs in 24 to 48 hours. Peak and duration variable.

## INDICATIONS & DOSAGE
*Constipation –*
**Adults:** 10 to 20 g (15 to 30 ml) P.O. daily, increased to 60 ml/day, if needed.
*To prevent and treat hepatic encephalopathy, including hepatic precoma and coma in patients with severe hepatic disease –*
**Adults:** initially, 20 to 30 g (30 to 45 ml) P.O. t.i.d. or q.i.d., until two or three soft stools are produced daily. Usual dosage is 60 to 100 g daily in divided doses. Alternatively, 200 g (300 ml) diluted with 700 ml of water or saline solution and administered as a retention enema q 4 to 6 hours p.r.n.

## ADVERSE REACTIONS
**GI:** *abdominal cramps, belching, diarrhea, gaseous distention, flatulence,* nausea, vomiting, diarrhea (with excessive dosage).

## INTERACTIONS
*Antacids, antibiotics, orally administered neomycin:* decreased effective-

---

Reactions may be *common,* uncommon, *life-threatening,* or COMMON AND LIFE-THREATENING.

ness of lactulose. Avoid concomitant use.

**CONTRAINDICATIONS**
Contraindicated in patients on a low-galactose diet.

**NURSING CONSIDERATIONS**
• Use cautiously in patients with diabetes mellitus.
• To minimize sweet taste, dilute with water or fruit juice or give with food.
• Prepare enema (not commercially available) by adding 200 g (300 ml) to 700 ml of water or 0.9% sodium chloride solution. The diluted solution is administered as a retention enema for 30 to 60 minutes. Use a rectal balloon catheter.
• If the enema is not retained for at least 30 minutes, be prepared to repeat dose.
• Monitor serum sodium level for possible hypernatremia, especially when giving in higher doses to treat hepatic encephalopathy.
• Be prepared to replace fluid loss.
• Store at room temperature, preferably below 86° F (30° C). Don't freeze.

☑ **PATIENT TEACHING**
• Instruct home care patient how to mix and then administer drug.
• Inform patient about adverse reactions and tell him to notify doctor if they become bothersome or if diarrhea occurs.
• Instruct patient not to take other laxatives while on lactulose therapy.

---

## magnesium citrate (citrate of magnesia)
Citroma◊, Citro-Mag†, Citro-Nesia◊

## magnesium hydroxide (milk of magnesia)
Milk of Magnesia◊, Phillips' Milk of Magnesia◊

# magnesium sulfate (epsom salts)◊
*Pregnancy Risk Category: NR*

**HOW SUPPLIED**
**magnesium citrate**
*Oral solution:* approximately 168 mEq magnesium/240 ml◊
**magnesium hydroxide**
*Oral suspension:* 7% to 8.5% (approximately 80 mEq magnesium/30 ml)◊
**magnesium sulfate**
*Granules:* approximately 40 mEq magnesium/5 g◊

**ACTION**
A saline laxative that produces an osmotic effect in the small intestine by drawing water into the intestinal lumen.

**ONSET, PEAK, DURATION**
Onset occurs in ½ to 3 hours. Peak and duration variable.

**INDICATIONS & DOSAGE**
*Constipation; to evacuate bowel before surgery –*
**Adults and children 12 years and older:** 11 to 25 g magnesium citrate P.O. daily as a single dose or divided; 2.4 to 4.8 g (30 to 60 ml) magnesium hydroxide P.O. daily as a single dose or divided; 10 to 30 g magnesium sulfate P.O. daily as a single dose or divided.
**Children 6 to 12 years:** 5.5 to 12.5 g magnesium citrate P.O. daily as a single dose or divided; 1.2 to 2.4 g (15 to 30 ml) magnesium hydroxide P.O. daily as a single dose or divided; 5 to 10 g magnesium sulfate P.O. daily as a single dose or divided.
**Children 2 to 6 years:** 2.7 to 6.25 g magnesium citrate P.O. daily as a single dose or divided; 0.4 to 1.2 g (5 to 15 ml) magnesium hydroxide P.O. daily as a single dose or divided; 2.5 to 5 g magnesium sulfate P.O. daily as a single dose or divided.

---

*Antacid –*
**Adults:** 5 to 15 ml milk of magnesia
P.O. t.i.d. or q.i.d.

## ADVERSE REACTIONS
**GI:** *abdominal cramping, nausea, diarrhea,* laxative dependence with long-term or excessive use.
**Other:** fluid and electrolyte disturbances with daily use.

## INTERACTIONS
*Orally administered drugs:* impaired absorption. Separate administration times.

## CONTRAINDICATIONS
Contraindicated in patients with abdominal pain, nausea, vomiting, or other symptoms of appendicitis or acute surgical abdomen and in those with myocardial damage, heart block, fecal impaction, rectal fissures, intestinal obstruction or perforation, renal disease, and patients about to deliver.

## NURSING CONSIDERATIONS
• Use cautiously in patients with rectal bleeding.
• Time drug administration so that it doesn't interfere with scheduled activities or sleep. Drug produces watery stools in 3 to 6 hours.
• Before giving for constipation, determine if the patient has adequate fluid intake, exercise, and diet.
• Chill magnesium citrate before use to make it more palatable.
• Shake suspension well; give with large amount of water when used as laxative. When administering through nasogastric tube, make sure tube is placed properly and is patent. After instilling, flush tube with water to ensure passage to stomach and maintain tube patency.
• *Alert:* Monitor serum electrolytes as ordered during prolonged use. Magnesium may accumulate in patients with renal insufficiency.

• Keep in mind that drug is for short-term therapy only.
• Know that magnesium sulfate is more potent than other saline laxatives.

☑ **PATIENT TEACHING**
• Instruct patient on drug administration.
• Teach patient about dietary sources of bulk, which include bran and other cereals, fresh fruit, and vegetables.
• Warn patient that frequent or prolonged use as a laxative may cause dependence.

## methylcellulose
Citrucel◊, Citrucel Orange
Flavor◊, Citrucel Sugar-Free
Orange Flavor◊, Cologel◊

*Pregnancy Risk Category: NR*

## HOW SUPPLIED
*Powder:* 2 g/tbs (heaping)◊
*Tablets:* 500 mg◊

## ACTION
A bulk-forming laxative that absorbs water and expands to increase bulk and moisture content of stools. The increased bulk encourages peristalsis and bowel movement.

## ONSET, PEAK, DURATION
Onset occurs in 12 to 24 hours. Peak effects may not occur for up to 3 days. Duration variable.

## INDICATIONS & DOSAGE
*Chronic constipation –*
**Adults:** 1 to 3 tbs (heaping) in 8 oz (240 ml) of cold water daily to t.i.d. Usual dose up to 6 g daily (3 tbs).
**Children 6 to 12 years:** 1 to 1½ level tbs in 4 oz (120 ml) of cold water daily to t.i.d. Usual dose up to 3 g daily (1½ tbs).

---

## ADVERSE REACTIONS
**GI:** *nausea,* vomiting, diarrhea (with excessive use); esophageal, gastric, small intestinal, or colonic strictures when drug is chewed or taken in dry form; *abdominal cramps,* especially in severe constipation; laxative dependence (with long-term or excessive use).

## INTERACTIONS
None significant.

## CONTRAINDICATIONS
Contraindicated in patients with abdominal pain, nausea, vomiting, or other symptoms of appendicitis or acute surgical abdomen and in those with intestinal obstruction or ulceration, disabling adhesions, or difficulty swallowing.

## NURSING CONSIDERATIONS
• Before giving for constipation, determine if the patient has adequate fluid intake, exercise, and diet.
• Be aware that the drug is especially useful in debilitated patients and in those with postpartum constipation, irritable bowel syndrome, diverticulitis, and colostomies. It's also used to treat laxative abuse and to empty colon before barium enema examinations.
• Know that the drug is not absorbed systemically and is nontoxic.

## ☑ PATIENT TEACHING
• Tell the patient to take drug with at least 8 oz of pleasant-tasting liquid to mask grittiness.
• Teach the patient about dietary sources of bulk, which include bran and other cereals, fresh fruit, and vegetables.

# mineral oil (liquid petrolatum)
Agoral Plain◇, Fleet Enema Mineral Oil◇, Kondremul◇, Kondremul Plain◇, Lansöyl†, Liqui-Doss◇, Milkinol◇, Neo-Cultol◇, Petrogalar Plain◇

*Pregnancy Risk Category: C*

## HOW SUPPLIED
*Emulsion:* 50%◇
*Oral liquid:* in pints, quarts, gallons◇
*Enema:* 120 ml◇, 133 ml◇

## ACTION
A lubricant laxative that increases water retention in stools by creating a barrier between colon wall and feces that prevents colonic reabsorption of fecal water.

## ONSET, PEAK, DURATION
Onset occurs in 6 to 8 hours. Peak and duration variable.

## INDICATIONS & DOSAGE
*Constipation; preparation for bowel studies or surgery –*
**Adults and children 12 years and older:** 5 to 45 ml P.O. h.s.; or 120 ml P.R. (as enema).
**Children 6 to 12 years:** 5 to 20 ml P.O. h.s.; or 30 to 60 ml P.R. (as enema).
**Children 2 to 6 years:** 30 to 60 ml P.R. (as enema).

## ADVERSE REACTIONS
**GI:** *nausea;* vomiting; diarrhea (with excessive use); *abdominal cramps,* especially in severe constipation; decreased absorption of nutrients and fat-soluble vitamins, resulting in deficiency; slowed healing after hemorrhoidectomy.
**Other:** laxative dependence (with long-term or excessive use), anal pruritus, anal irritation, hemorrhoids, perianal discomfort, *lipid pneumonia.*

## INTERACTIONS
*Docusate salts:* may increase mineral oil absorption and cause lipid pneumonia. Separate administration times.
*Fat-soluble vitamins (A, D, E, and K):* possible decreased absorption after prolonged administration. Monitor for vitamin deficiency.

## CONTRAINDICATIONS
Contraindicated in patients with abdominal pain, nausea, vomiting, or other symptoms of appendicitis or acute surgical abdomen and in those with fecal impaction or intestinal obstruction or perforation.

## NURSING CONSIDERATIONS
• Use cautiously in young children; in elderly or debilitated patients because of susceptibility to lipid pneumonia through aspiration, absorption, and transport from intestinal mucosa; and in patients with rectal bleeding.
• Before giving for constipation, determine if the patient has adequate fluid intake, exercise, and diet.
• Give drug on an empty stomach because it delays passage of food from stomach; drug is more active on an empty stomach.
• Give with fruit juice or carbonated drink to disguise taste.
• Keep in mind that drug may be used when the patient needs to ease the strain of evacuation.

## ☑ PATIENT TEACHING
• Advise the patient to take drug only at bedtime on an empty stomach and not to take it for more than 1 week. Tell him to take drug with fruit juice or carbonated drink to disguise taste.
• To avoid soiling clothing, advise the patient of possible rectal leakage from excessive dosages.
• Teach the patient about dietary sources of bulk, which include bran and other cereals, fresh fruit, and vegetables.

## phenolphthalein, white
Alophen◇, Medilax◇, Modane◇, Phenolax Wafers**◇, Prulet◇

## phenolphthalein, yellow
Espotabs◇, Evac-U-Gen◇, Evac-U-Lax◇, Ex-Lax◇, Ex-Lax Maximum Relief Formula◇, Ex-Lax Pills◇, Feen-A-Mint◇, Feen-A-Mint Gum◇, Lax-Pills◇

*Pregnancy Risk Category: NR*

## HOW SUPPLIED
**phenolphthalein, white**
*Tablets:* 60 mg◇, 65 mg◇, 130 mg◇
*Tablets (chewable):* 60 mg◇, 64.8 mg◇, 120 mg◇
**phenolphthalein, yellow**
*Tablets (chewable):* 80 mg◇, 90 mg◇, 97.2 mg◇
*Chewing gum:* 97.2 mg◇

## ACTION
Unknown. A stimulant laxative that increases peristalsis probably by direct effect on the smooth muscle of the intestine. Thought either to irritate the musculature or stimulate the colonic intramural plexus. Also promotes fluid accumulation in the colon and small intestine.

## ONSET, PEAK, DURATION
Onset occurs in 6 to 10 hours. Peak unknown. Effects persist for 3 to 4 days.

## INDICATIONS & DOSAGE
*Constipation –*
**Adults and children 12 years and over:** 30 to 270 mg P.O., preferably h.s.
**Children 6 to 12 years:** 30 to 60 mg P.O. h.s.
**Children 2 to 6 years:** 15 to 30 mg P.O. h.s.

## ADVERSE REACTIONS
**GI:** diarrhea; *colic (with large doses):* factitious nausea; vomiting; loss of

---

Reactions may be *common,* uncommon, *life-threatening,* or **COMMON AND LIFE-THREATENING.**

normal bowel function (with excessive use); *abdominal cramps,* especially in severe constipation; malabsorption of nutrients; "cathartic colon" (syndrome resembling ulcerative colitis radiologically and pathologically) with chronic misuse; reddish discoloration in alkaline feces or urine, laxative dependence (with long-term or excessive use).
**Skin:** dermatitis, pruritus, rash, increased pigmentation.
**Other:** hypersensitivity reactions.

## INTERACTIONS
None significant.

## CONTRAINDICATIONS
Contraindicated in patients with abdominal pain, nausea, vomiting, or other symptoms of appendicitis or acute surgical abdomen; in patients with fecal impaction or intestinal obstruction or perforation.

## NURSING CONSIDERATIONS
• Use cautiously in patients with rectal bleeding.
• Before giving for constipation, determine if the patient has adequate fluid intake, exercise, and diet.
• Time drug administration so that it doesn't interfere with scheduled activities or sleep.
• Be aware that yellow phenolphthalein has been reported to be two to three times as potent as white phenolphthalein, although this has not been proved in clinical studies.

## ☑ PATIENT TEACHING
• Tell parents that children may mistake for candy. Keep out of reach.
• Warn the patient to avoid excessive sun exposure, not to use drug with any other product containing phenolphthalein, and to discontinue use if dermatoses occur.
• Warn the patient that the drug may discolor alkaline urine red-pink and acidic urine yellow-brown.

• Teach the patient about dietary sources of bulk, which include bran and other cereals, fresh fruit, and vegetables.

## polyethylene glycol and electrolyte solution
Colovage, CoLyte, Co-Lav, Glycoprep‡, GoLYTELY, Go-Evac, Nulytely, OCL

*Pregnancy Risk Category: C*

## HOW SUPPLIED
*Powder for oral solution:* polyethylene glycol (PEG) 3350 (6 g), anhydrous sodium sulfate (568 mg), sodium chloride (146 mg), potassium chloride (74.5 mg) per 100 ml (Colovage); PEG 3350 (120 g), sodium sulfate (3.36 g), sodium chloride (2.92 g), potassium chloride (1.49 g) per 2 liters (CoLyte); PEG 3350 (60 g), sodium chloride (1.46 g), potassium chloride (0.745 g), sodium bicarbonate (1.68 g), sodium sulfate (5.68 g) per liter (Co-Lav); PEG 3350 (60 g), sodium chloride (1.46 g), potassium chloride (745 mg), sodium bicarbonate (1.68 g), sodium sulfate (5.68 g) per liter (Glycoprep‡); PEG 3350 (236 g), sodium sulfate (22.74 g), sodium bicarbonate (6.74g), sodium chloride (5.86 g), potassium chloride (2.97 g) per 4.8 liter (GoLYTELY); PEG 3350 (59 g), sodium sulfate (5.685 g), sodium bicarbonate (1.685 g), sodium chloride (1.465 g), potassium chloride (0.743 g) per liter (Go-Evac); PEG 3350 (420 g), sodium bicarbonate (5.72 g), sodium chloride (11.2 g), potassium chloride (1.48 g) per 4 liters (Nulytely); PEG 3350 (6 g), sodium sulfate decahydrate (1.29 g), sodium chloride (146 mg), potassium chloride (75 mg), polysorbate-80 (30 mg) per 100 ml (OCL)

## ACTION
PEG 3350, a nonabsorbable solution, acts as an osmotic agent. Sodium sul-

fate greatly reduces sodium absorption. The electrolyte concentration causes virtually no net absorption or secretion of ions.

### ONSET, PEAK, DURATION
Onset occurs within 1 hour. Peak and duration variable.

### INDICATIONS & DOSAGE
*Bowel preparation before GI examination –*
**Adults:** 240 ml P.O. q 10 minutes until 4 liters are consumed. Typically, administer 4 hours before examination, allowing 3 hours for drinking and 1 hour for bowel evacuation.

### ADVERSE REACTIONS
**GI:** *nausea, bloating, cramps, vomiting, abdominal fullness.*
**Skin:** urticaria, dermatitis, allergic reaction.
**Other:** anal irritation, rhinorrhea.

### INTERACTIONS
*Orally administered drugs:* decreased absorption if administered within 1 hour of starting therapy. Administer at least 2 to 3 hours before starting therapy.

### CONTRAINDICATIONS
Contraindicated in patients with GI obstruction or perforation, gastric retention, toxic colitis, or megacolon.

### NURSING CONSIDERATIONS
• Use tap water to reconstitute powder. Shake vigorously to ensure that all powder is dissolved. Refrigerate reconstituted solution but use within 48 hours.
• **Alert:** Do not add flavoring or additional ingredients to the solution or administer chilled solution. Hypothermia has been reported after ingestion of large amounts of chilled solution.
• Administer solution early in the morning if the patient is scheduled for a midmorning examination. Orally

administered solution induces diarrhea (onset 30 to 60 minutes) that rapidly cleans the bowel, usually within 4 hours.
• When used as preparation for barium enema, administer solution the evening before the examination to avoid interfering with barium coating of the colonic mucosa.
• If administered to semiconscious patients or to patients with impaired gag reflex, take care to prevent aspiration.
• Be aware that no major shifts in fluid or electrolyte balance have been reported.

### ☑ PATIENT TEACHING
• Tell the patient to fast for 3 to 4 hours before taking the solution and thereafter ingest only clear fluids until the examination is complete.
• Warn the patient about adverse reactions.

---

## psyllium
Cillium◇, Fiberall◇, Fibrepur†◇, Hydrocil Instant◇, Karacil†◇, Konsyl◇, Maalox Daily Fiber Therapy◇, Metamucil◇, Metamucil Instant Mix◇, Metamucil Sugar-Free◇, Modane Bulk◇, Mylanta Natural Fiber Supplement◇, Naturacil◇, Perdiem Plain◇, Prodiem Plain†◇, Pro-Lax◇, Reguloid Natural◇, Restore◇, Serutan◇, Siblin◇, Syllact◇, Versabran◇, V-Lax◇

*Pregnancy Risk Category: NR*

### HOW SUPPLIED
*Chewable pieces:* 1.7 g/piece◇
*Effervescent powder:* 3.4 g/packet◇, 3.7 g/packet◇
*Granules:* 2.5 g/tsp◇, 4.03 g/tsp◇
*Powder:* 3.3 g/tsp◇, 3.4 g/tsp◇, 3.5 g/tsp◇, 4.94 g/tsp◇
*Wafers:* 3.4 g/wafer◇

---

## ACTION

A bulk-forming laxative that absorbs water and expands to increase bulk and moisture content of the stool, thus encouraging peristalsis and bowel movement.

## ONSET, PEAK, DURATION

Onset occurs in 12 to 24 hours. Peak effects may not occur for 3 days. Duration variable.

## INDICATIONS & DOSAGE

*Constipation; bowel management—*
**Adults:** 1 to 2 tsp (rounded) P.O. in full glass of liquid once daily, b.i.d., or t.i.d., followed by second glass of liquid; or 1 packet dissolved in water once daily, b.i.d., or t.i.d.
**Children over 6 years:** 1 tsp (level) P.O. in half a glass of liquid h.s.

## ADVERSE REACTIONS

**GI:** nausea, vomiting, diarrhea (with excessive use); esophageal, gastric, small intestinal, and rectal obstruction when drug is taken in dry form; abdominal cramps, especially in severe constipation.

## INTERACTIONS

None significant.

## CONTRAINDICATIONS

Contraindicated in patients with hypersensitivity to drug, abdominal pain, nausea, vomiting, or other symptoms of appendicitis and in those with intestinal obstruction or ulceration, disabling adhesions, or difficulty swallowing.

## NURSING CONSIDERATIONS

● Before giving for constipation, determine if the patient has adequate fluid intake, exercise, and diet.
● Mix with at least 8 oz (240 ml) of cold, pleasant-tasting liquid, such as orange juice, to mask grittiness, and stir only a few seconds. Have the patient drink mixture immediately so it does not congeal. Follow with additional glass of liquid.
● For dosages in children under 6 years, consult the doctor.
● Know that drug may reduce appetite if taken before meals.
● Be aware that the drug is not absorbed systemically and is nontoxic. It is especially useful in debilitated patients and those with postpartum constipation, irritable bowel syndrome, and diverticular disease. It's also used to treat chronic laxative abuse and in combination with other laxatives to empty colon before barium enema examinations.

## ☑ PATIENT TEACHING

● Teach the patient how to properly mix medication. To enhance effect and prevent intestinal obstruction, tell him to take drug with plenty of water. Advise the patient that inhaling powder may cause allergic reactions.
● Tell the patient that laxative effect usually occurs in 12 to 24 hours but may be delayed 3 days.
● Advise the diabetic patient to check the label and use brand of psyllium that does not contain sugar.
● Teach the patient about dietary sources of bulk, which include bran and other cereals, fresh fruit, and vegetables.

---

## senna

Black-Draught◊, Fletcher's Castoria◊, Senexon◊, Senokot◊, Senolax◊, X-Prep Liquid*◊

*Pregnancy Risk Category: C*

## HOW SUPPLIED

*Tablets:* 187 mg◊, 217 mg◊, 600 mg◊
*Granules:* 326 mg/tsp◊, 1.65 g/½ tsp◊
*Suppositories:* 652 mg◊
*Syrup:* 218 mg/5 ml◊

---

*Liquid form contains alcohol.    **May contain tartrazine.    †Canada only.    ‡Australia only.    ◊OTC.

## ACTION

Unknown. A stimulant laxative that increases peristalsis probably by direct effect on the smooth muscle of the intestine. Thought to either irritate the musculature or stimulate the colonic intramural plexus. Also promotes fluid accumulation in the colon and small intestine.

## ONSET, PEAK, DURATION

Onset occurs in 6 to 10 hours. Peak and duration variable.

## INDICATIONS & DOSAGE

*Acute constipation; preparation for bowel or rectal examination* —
**Adults:** dosage range for Senokot is 1 to 8 tablets P.O.; ½ to 4 tsp of granules added to liquid P.O.; 1 to 2 suppositories P.R. h.s.; or 1 to 4 tsp syrup P.O. h.s. Dosage for Black-Draught is 2 tablets or ¼ to ½ tsp (level) of granules mixed with water.

X-Prep Liquid used solely as single dose for preradiographic bowel evacuation. Give 20 g powder dissolved in juice or 75 ml liquid P.O. between 2 p.m. and 4 p.m. on day before X-ray procedure. Use in divided doses, if needed, for elderly or debilitated patients.
**Children over 27 kg:** one-half adult dose of tablets, granules, or syrup (except Black-Draught tablets and granules — not recommended for children).
**Children 1 month to 1 year:** 1.25 to 2.5 ml Senokot syrup P.O. h.s.

## ADVERSE REACTIONS

**GI:** *nausea;* vomiting; diarrhea; loss of normal bowel function with excessive use; *abdominal cramps,* especially in severe constipation; malabsorption of nutrients; "cathartic colon" (syndrome resembling ulcerative colitis radiologically) with chronic misuse; possible constipation after catharsis; yellow or yellow-green cast to feces; diarrhea in breast-feeding infants of mothers receiving senna; darkened pigmentation of rectal mucosa with long-term use (usually reversible within 4 to 12 months after stopping drug); laxative dependence with excessive use.
**GU:** red-pink discoloration in alkaline urine; yellow-brown color to acidic urine.
**Other:** protein-losing enteropathy, electrolyte imbalance (such as hypokalemia).

## INTERACTIONS

None significant.

## CONTRAINDICATIONS

Contraindicated in patients with ulcerative bowel lesions; nausea, vomiting, abdominal pain, or other symptoms of appendicitis or acute surgical abdomen; fecal impaction; or intestinal obstruction or perforation.

## NURSING CONSIDERATIONS

● Before giving for constipation, determine if the patient has adequate fluid intake, exercise, and diet.
● Limit diet to clear liquids after X-Prep Liquid is taken.
● Avoid exposing product to excessive heat or light.
● Know that drug is used for short-term therapy.
● Know that senna is one of the most effective laxatives for counteracting constipation caused by narcotic analgesics.

## ☑ PATIENT TEACHING

● Teach the patient about dietary sources of bulk, including bran and other cereals, fresh fruit, and vegetables.
● Tell the patient to report persistent or severe reactions.

---

## sodium phosphates
Fleet Phospho-Soda◇
*Pregnancy Risk Category: NR*

---

Reactions may be *common,* uncommon, **life-threatening,** or COMMON AND LIFE-THREATENING.

## HOW SUPPLIED
*Liquid:* 2.4 g/5 ml sodium phosphate and 900 mg sodium biphosphate/5 ml◇
*Enema:* 160 mg/ml sodium phosphate and 60 mg/ml sodium biphosphate◇

## ACTION
A saline laxative that produces an osmotic effect in the small intestine by drawing water into the intestinal lumen.

## ONSET, PEAK, DURATION
Onset occurs in ½ to 3 hours after oral use, 5 to 10 minutes after enema. Peak and duration variable after oral dose, complete upon evacuation following enema.

## INDICATIONS & DOSAGE
*Constipation –*
**Adults:** 20 to 30 ml solution mixed with 120 ml cold water P.O.; or 60 to 135 ml P.R. (as enema).
**Children:** 5 to 15 ml solution mixed with 120 ml of cold water P.O.; or 67.5 ml P.R. (as enema).

## ADVERSE REACTIONS
**GI:** *abdominal cramping.*
**Other:** fluid and electrolyte disturbances (hypernatremia, hyperphosphatemia) with daily use; laxative dependence with long-term or excessive use.

## INTERACTIONS
None significant.

## CONTRAINDICATIONS
Contraindicated in patients with abdominal pain, nausea, vomiting, or other symptoms of appendicitis or acute surgical abdomen; intestinal obstruction or perforation; edema; CHF; megacolon; or impaired renal function and in patients on sodium-restricted diets.

## NURSING CONSIDERATIONS
● Use cautiously in patients with large hemorrhoids or anal excoriations.
● Before giving for constipation, determine if the patient has adequate fluid intake, exercise, and diet.
● *Alert:* Be aware that up to 10% of sodium content of drug may be absorbed.

## ☑ PATIENT TEACHING
● Teach patient about dietary sources of bulk, which include bran and other cereals, fresh fruit, and vegetables.
● Warn patient about adverse reactions and stress importance of using only for short-term therapy.

---

*Liquid form contains alcohol.   **May contain tartrazine.   †Canada only.   ‡Australia only.   ◇OTC.

# 51

# Antiemetics

benzquinamide hydrochloride
buclizine hydrochloride
chlorpromazine hydrochloride
(See Chapter 33, ANTIPSYCHOTICS.)
cyclizine hydrochloride
cyclizine lactate
dimenhydrinate
diphenidol hydrochloride
dronabinol
granisetron hydrochloride
meclizine hydrochloride
metoclopramide hydrochloride
ondansetron hydrochloride
perphenazine
(See Chapter 33, ANTIPSYCHOTICS.)
prochlorperazine
prochlorperazine edisylate
prochlorperazine maleate
promethazine hydrochloride
(See Chapter 43, ANTIHISTAMINES.)
scopolamine
(See Chapter 38, ANTICHOLINERGICS.)
thiethylperazine maleate
trimethobenzamide
hydrochloride

**COMBINATION PRODUCTS**
None.

---

## benzquinamide
## hydrochloride

*Pregnancy Risk Category: NR*

**HOW SUPPLIED**
*Injection:* 50 mg/vial

**ACTION**
Unknown. Thought to act on the chemoreceptor trigger zone to inhibit nausea and vomiting.

**ONSET, PEAK, DURATION**
Onset occurs within 15 minutes. Blood levels peak right after I.V. injection or within 30 minutes after I.M. injection. Effects last for 3 to 4 hours.

**INDICATIONS & DOSAGE**
*Nausea and vomiting associated with anesthesia and surgery –*
**Adults:** 50 mg I.M. (0.5 mg/kg to 1 mg/kg). Repeat in 1 hour, then q 3 to 4 hours, p.r.n.; or 25 mg (0.2 mg/kg to 0.4 mg/kg) I.V. as a single dose, given slowly (25 mg/minute).

**ADVERSE REACTIONS**
**CNS:** *drowsiness,* fatigue, insomnia, nervousness, restlessness, headache, excitation, tremor, twitching, dizziness.
**CV:** sudden rise in blood pressure and transient arrhythmias (premature atrial and ventricular contractions, atrial fibrillation) after I.V. administration; hypertension; hypotension.
**EENT:** salivation, blurred vision.
**GI:** anorexia, nausea, dry mouth.
**Skin:** urticaria, rash, diaphoresis, allergic reactions.
**Other:** muscle weakness, flushing, hiccups, diaphoresis, chills, fever.

**INTERACTIONS**
*CNS depressants, ethanol:* enhanced CNS effects. Avoid concomitant use.

**CONTRAINDICATIONS**
Contraindicated in patients with hypersensitivity to the drug as well as for I.V. use in patients with CV disease and within 15 minutes of administering preanesthetic or CV drugs.

**NURSING CONSIDERATIONS**
• Be aware that use during pregnancy is not recommended.
• **I.V. use:** Reconstitute with 2.2 ml of sterile water for injection or bacteriostatic water containing benzyl alcohol or propylparabens. Don't dilute further.

---

Reactions may be *common,* uncommon, *life-threatening,* or COMMON AND LIFE-THREATENING.

Inject directly and slowly (25 mg/minute).
• Do not reconstitute with 0.9% sodium chloride for injection.
• For I.M. use, give injections in large muscle mass. Use deltoid area only if well developed.
• Store dry powder and reconstituted solution in a light-resistant container. Reconstituted solution is stable for 14 days at room temperature.
• Monitor blood pressure frequently.
• Like other antiemetics, know that drug may mask symptoms of ototoxicity, brain tumor, or intestinal obstruction.

☑ **PATIENT TEACHING**
• Warn patient that drug usually causes drowsiness. Encourage patient to seek assistance when getting out of bed and during ambulation.
• Tell patient to report adverse effects.

## buclizine hydrochloride
Bucladin-S Softab**

*Pregnancy Risk Category: NR*

**HOW SUPPLIED**
*Tablets (chewable):* 50 mg

**ACTION**
Unknown. An antihistamine that may affect neural pathways originating in the labyrinth to inhibit nausea and vomiting.

**ONSET, PEAK, DURATION**
Onset and peak unknown. Effects persist for 4 to 6 hours.

**INDICATIONS & DOSAGE**
*Prevention of motion sickness –*
**Adults:** 50 mg P.O. at least ½ hour before beginning travel. If needed, repeat after 4 to 6 hours.
*Vertigo –*
**Adults:** 50 mg P.O., 1 to 3 times daily. Maintenance dosage is 50 mg b.i.d.

**ADVERSE REACTIONS**
**CNS:** *drowsiness,* headache, dizziness.
**GI:** dry mouth.

**INTERACTIONS**
*CNS depressants, ethanol:* additive CNS effects. Avoid concomitant use.

**CONTRAINDICATIONS**
Contraindicated in patients hypersensitive to the drug. Contains tartrazine, which may trigger allergic reactions in some, including those allergic to aspirin.

**NURSING CONSIDERATION**
Like other antiemetics, know that drug may mask symptoms of ototoxicity, intestinal obstruction, or brain tumor.

☑ **PATIENT TEACHING**
• Tell patient to place tablets in mouth and allow to dissolve without water, chew, or swallow them whole.
• Advise patient to avoid activities that require alertness until CNS effects of the drug are known.

## cyclizine hydrochloride
Marezine◇

## cyclizine lactate
Marezine, Marzine†

*Pregnancy Risk Category: B*

**HOW SUPPLIED**
**cyclizine hydrochloride**
*Tablets:* 50 mg◇
**cyclizine lactate**
*Injection:* 50 mg/ml

**ACTION**
Unknown. An antihistamine that may affect neural pathways originating in the labyrinth to inhibit nausea and vomiting.

**ONSET, PEAK, DURATION**
Onset may occur in ½ to 1 hour. Peak unknown. Effects last for 4 to 6 hours.

**INDICATIONS & DOSAGE**
*Prevention or treatment of motion sickness –*
**Adults and children 12 years and older:** 50 mg P.O. (hydrochloride) ½ hour before travel, then q 4 to 6 hours, p.r.n., to maximum of 200 mg daily; or 50 mg I.M. (lactate) q 4 to 6 hours, p.r.n.
**Children 6 to 12 years:** 25 mg (hydrochloride) P.O. q 4 to 6 hours, p.r.n., to a maximum of 75 mg daily.

**ADVERSE REACTIONS**
**CNS:** *drowsiness,* auditory and visual hallucinations, restlessness, excitation, nervousness.
**CV:** hypotension, palpitations, tachycardia.
**EENT:** blurred vision, diplopia, tinnitus, dry nose and throat.
**GI:** constipation, dry mouth, anorexia, nausea, vomiting, diarrhea, cholestatic jaundice.
**GU:** urine retention, urinary frequency.
**Skin:** urticaria, rash.

**INTERACTIONS**
*CNS depressants, ethanol:* additive CNS effects. Avoid concomitant use.

**CONTRAINDICATIONS**
Contraindicated in patients hypersensitive to the drug.

**NURSING CONSIDERATIONS**
• Use cautiously in patients with severe heart failure and after surgery.
• Like other antiemetics, know that drug may mask symptoms of ototoxicity, brain tumor, or intestinal obstruction.
• Store in cool place. When stored at room temperature, injection may turn slightly yellow; this change does not indicate loss of potency.

☑ **PATIENT TEACHING**
• Advise patient to avoid activities that require alertness until CNS effects of the drug are known.
• Instruct patient to report adverse reactions promptly.

---

**dimenhydrinate**
Andrumin‡, Apo-Dimenhydrinate†, Calm X◊, Children's Dramamine◊, Dimetabs, Dinate, Dommanate, Dramamine◊*, Dramamine Chewable◊**, Dramamine Liquid◊*, Dramanate, Dramilin, Dramocen, Dramoject, Dymenate, Gravol†, Gravol L/A†, Hydrate, Marmine◊, Nauseatol†, Nico-Vert◊, Novo-Dimenate†, PMS-Dimenhydrinate†, Tega-Vert◊, Travamine†, Travs‡, Triptone Caplets◊

*Pregnancy Risk Category: B*

**HOW SUPPLIED**
*Tablets:* 50 mg◊
*Tablets (chewable):* 50 mg◊
*Capsules:* 50 mg◊
*Elixir:* 15 mg/5 ml†
*Syrup:* 12.5 mg/4 ml*◊, 15.62 mg/5 ml
*Injection:* 50 mg/ml

**ACTION**
Unknown. An antihistamine that may affect neural pathways originating in the labyrinth to inhibit nausea and vomiting.

**ONSET, PEAK, DURATION**
Onset occurs right after I.V. administration, within 15 to 20 minutes of I.M. injection, within 20 to 30 minutes of oral administration. Peak unknown. Effects last for 3 to 6 hours.

**INDICATIONS & DOSAGE**
*Prevention and treatment of motion sickness –*
**Adults and children 12 years and over:** 50 to 100 mg P.O. q 4 to 6

---

hours; 50 mg I.M., p.r.n.; or 50 mg I.V. diluted in 10 ml sodium chloride for injection, injected over 2 minutes. Maximum dosage is 400 mg daily.
**Children 6 to 12 years:** 25 to 50 mg P.O. q 6 to 8 hours, not to exceed 150 mg in 24 hours.
**Children 2 to 6 years:** 12.5 to 25 mg P.O. q 6 to 8 hours, not to exceed 75 mg in 24 hours.

**ADVERSE REACTIONS**
**CNS:** *drowsiness,* headache, dizziness, confusion, nervousness, insomnia (especially in children), vertigo, tingling and weakness of hands, lassitude, excitation.
**CV:** palpitations, hypotension, tachycardia.
**EENT:** blurred vision, dry respiratory passages, diplopia, nasal congestion.
**GI:** dry mouth, nausea, vomiting, diarrhea, epigastric distress, constipation, anorexia.
**Respiratory:** wheezing, thickened bronchial secretions.
**Skin:** photosensitivity, urticaria, rash.
**Other:** *anaphylaxis,* tightness of chest.

**INTERACTIONS**
*CNS depressants, ethanol:* additive CNS depression. Avoid concomitant use.

**CONTRAINDICATIONS**
Contraindicated in patients hypersensitive to drug or its components.

**NURSING CONSIDERATIONS**
• Use cautiously in patients with seizures, acute angle-closure glaucoma, or enlarged prostate gland or in patients receiving ototoxic drugs.
• **I.V. use:** Before administration, dilute each ml of drug with 10 ml of sterile water for injection, $D_5W$, or 0.9% sodium chloride for injection.

Give by direct injection over not less than 2 minutes.
• Know that undiluted solution irritates veins and may cause sclerosis.
• Because incompatibilities are common, avoid mixing parenteral preparation with other drugs.
• *Alert:* Be aware that most I.V. products contain Benzyl Alcohol, which has been associated with a fatal "gasping syndrome" in premature infants and low birth weight infants.
• Like other antiemetics, know that drug may mask symptoms of ototoxicity, brain tumor, or intestinal obstruction.

☑ **PATIENT TEACHING**
• Advise patient to avoid activities that require alertness until CNS effects of the drug are known.
• Instruct patient to report adverse reactions promptly.

# diphenidol hydrochloride
Vontrol\*\*

*Pregnancy Risk Category: NR*

**HOW SUPPLIED**
*Tablets:* 25 mg

**ACTION**
Unknown. Probably diminishes labyrinthine function and vestibular stimulation and influences the chemoreceptor trigger zone to inhibit nausea and vomiting.

**ONSET, PEAK, DURATION**
Onset and duration unknown. Blood levels peak in 1½ to 3 hours.

**INDICATIONS & DOSAGE**
*Peripheral (labyrinthine) vertigo –*
**Adults:** 25 to 50 mg P.O. q 4 hours, p.r.n.
*Nausea and vomiting –*
**Adults:** 25 to 50 mg P.O. q 4 hours, p.r.n.
**Children over 23 kg:** 0.88 mg/kg

---

\*Liquid form contains alcohol.    \*\*May contain tartrazine.    †Canada only.    ‡Australia only.    ◊OTC.

P.O. q 4 hours, not to exceed 5.5 mg/kg/24 hours. Usual dose is 25 mg.

**ADVERSE REACTIONS**
**CNS:** *drowsiness,* dizziness, sleep disturbances, *confusion,* auditory and visual hallucinations, depression, malaise, headache, disorientation.
**CV:** transient hypotension.
**GI:** dry mouth, nausea, indigestion, heartburn.
**Skin:** urticaria.

**INTERACTIONS**
None significant.

**CONTRAINDICATIONS**
Contraindicated in patients with anuria and hypersensitivity to drug.

**NURSING CONSIDERATIONS**
• Use cautiously in patients with glaucoma, pyloric stenosis, pylorospasm, obstructive lesions of GI or GU tract, prostatic hyperplasia, or organic cardiospasm (achalasia).
• Closely supervise patients. Patients usually are hospitalized when receiving drug. Monitor fluid intake and output; report any changes.
• Like other antiemetics, be alert that drug may mask symptoms of ototoxicity, brain tumor, intestinal obstruction, or other conditions.
• **Alert:** Stop drug if auditory or visual hallucinations, disorientation, or confusion occur and notify doctor.

☑ **PATIENT TEACHING**
• Advise patient to ask for assistance when getting out of bed or during ambulation because of potential adverse CNS reactions.
• Instruct patient to report adverse reactions promptly.

# dronabinol (delta-g-tetrahydrocannabinol)
Marinol
Controlled Substance Schedule II

*Pregnancy Risk Category: C*

**HOW SUPPLIED**
*Capsules:* 2.5 mg, 5 mg, 10 mg

**ACTION**
Unknown. A derivative of marijuana.

**ONSET, PEAK, DURATION**
Onset unknown. Serum levels peak in 2 to 4 hours. Effects last 4 to 6 hours.

**INDICATIONS & DOSAGE**
*Nausea and vomiting associated with cancer chemotherapy –*
**Adults:** 5 mg/m² P.O. 1 to 3 hours before administration of chemotherapy. Then same dose q 2 to 4 hours after chemotherapy for a total of four to six doses per day. If needed, dosage increased in 2.5-mg/m² increments to a maximum of 15 mg/m² per dose.
*Anorexia and weight loss in patients with AIDS –*
**Adults:** 2.5 mg P.O. b.i.d. before lunch and dinner.

**ADVERSE REACTIONS**
**CNS:** *dizziness, drowsiness, euphoria, ataxia,* depersonalization, hallucinations, somnolence, headache, muddled thinking, asthenia, amnesia, confusion, *paranoia.*
**CV:** tachycardia, orthostatic hypotension, palpitations, vasodilation.
**GI:** *dry mouth, nausea, vomiting,* diarrhea.
**Other:** visual disturbances.

**INTERACTIONS**
*CNS depressants, ethanol, psychotomimetic substances, sedatives:* additive effects. Avoid concomitant use.

---

Reactions may be *common,* uncommon, *life-threatening,* or COMMON AND LIFE-THREATENING.

## CONTRAINDICATIONS
Contraindicated in patients hypersensitive to sesame oil or cannabinoids.

## NURSING CONSIDERATIONS
• Use cautiously in elderly, pregnant, or lactating patients and in those with heart disease, psychiatric illness, and history of drug abuse.
• Expect drug to be prescribed only for patients who have not responded satisfactorily to other antiemetics.
• Know that dronabinol is the principal active substance present in *Cannabis sativa* (marijuana). This substance can produce both physical and psychological dependence and has a high potential for abuse.
• Keep in mind that CNS effects are intensified at higher drug dosages.
• Be aware that drug's effects may persist for days after treatment ends.

## ☑ PATIENT TEACHING
• Tell the patient drug may induce unusual changes in mood or other adverse behavioral effects.
• Advise the patient against activities that require alertness until the CNS effects of the drug are known.
• Warn caregivers to supervise the patient during and immediately after treatment.

---

## granisetron hydrochloride
Kytril

*Pregnancy Risk Category: B*

## HOW SUPPLIED
*Injection:* 1 mg/ml
*Tablets:* 1 mg

## ACTION
A selective antagonist of a specific type of serotonin receptor ($5\text{-}HT_3$) located in the CNS in the chemoreceptor trigger zone and in the peripheral nervous system on nerve terminals of the vagus nerve. Drug's blocking action may occur at both sites.

## ONSET, PEAK, DURATION
Unknown.

## INDICATIONS & DOSAGE
*Prevention of nausea and vomiting associated with emetogenic cancer chemotherapy –*
**Adults and children 2 to 16 years:** 10 mcg/kg I.V. infused over 5 minutes. Begin infusion within 30 minutes before administration of chemotherapy. Alternatively, 1 mg P.O. up to 1 hour before chemotherapy and dosage repeated 12 hours later.

## ADVERSE REACTIONS
**CNS:** *headache, asthenia,* somnolence, dizziness, anxiety.
**CV:** hypertension.
**GI:** diarrhea, *constipation,* abdominal pain, *nausea,* vomiting, decreased appetite.
**Hematologic:** *leukopenia,* anemia, *thrombocytopenia.*
**Other:** fever, alopecia, elevated liver function tests.

## INTERACTIONS
None significant.

## CONTRAINDICATIONS
Contraindicated in patients hypersensitive to the drug.

## NURSING CONSIDERATIONS
• **I.V. use:** Dilute drug with 0.9% sodium chloride for injection or $D_5W$ to a volume of 20 to 50 ml. Infuse over 5 minutes, beginning within 30 minutes before initiating chemotherapy, and only on the days chemotherapy is given. Diluted solutions are stable for 24 hours at room temperature.
• Do not mix with other drugs; data regarding compatibility is limited.

## ☑ PATIENT TEACHING
• Stress to patient the importance of taking second dose of oral drug 12 hours later for maximum effectiveness.

---

*Liquid form contains alcohol. **May contain tartrazine. †Canada only. ‡Australia only. ◇OTC.

● Instruct patient to report adverse reactions immediately.

---

## meclizine hydrochloride (meclozine hydrochloride)
Ancolan‡, Antivert, Antivert/25◊, Antivert/50, Bonamine†, Bonine◊, Dizmiss◊, D-Vert 15, D-Vert 30, Meni-D, Ru-Vert M, Vergon◊

*Pregnancy Risk Category: B*

### HOW SUPPLIED
*Tablets:* 12.5 mg, 25 mg◊, 50 mg
*Tablets (chewable):* 25 mg◊
*Capsules:* 15 mg, 25 mg, 30 mg

### ACTION
Unknown. An antihistamine that may affect neural pathways originating in the labyrinth to inhibit nausea and vomiting.

### ONSET, PEAK, DURATION
Onset occurs in about 1 hour. Peak unknown. Effects persist 8 to 24 hours.

### INDICATIONS & DOSAGE
*Vertigo –*
**Adults:** 25 to 100 mg P.O. daily in divided doses. Dosage varies with patient response.
*Motion sickness –*
**Adults:** 25 to 50 mg P.O. 1 hour before travel, repeated daily for duration of journey.

### ADVERSE REACTIONS
**CNS:** *drowsiness,* restlessness, excitation, nervousness, auditory and visual hallucinations.
**CV:** hypotension, palpitations, tachycardia.
**EENT:** blurred vision, diplopia, tinnitus, dry nose and throat.
**GI:** dry mouth, constipation, anorexia, nausea, vomiting, diarrhea.
**GU:** urine retention, urinary frequency.
**Skin:** urticaria, rash.

### INTERACTIONS
*CNS depressants:* increased drowsiness. Use together cautiously.

### CONTRAINDICATIONS
Contraindicated in patients hypersensitive to the drug.

### NURSING CONSIDERATIONS
● Use cautiously in patients with asthma, glaucoma, or prostatic hyperplasia.
● Like other antiemetics, be alert that drug may mask symptoms of ototoxicity, brain tumor, or intestinal obstruction.

### ☑ PATIENT TEACHING
● Advise patient to avoid hazardous activities that require alertness until CNS effects of the drug are known.
● Instruct patient to report persistent or serious adverse reactions promptly.

---

## metoclopramide hydrochloride
Apo-Metoclop†, Clopra, Emex†, Maxeran†, Maxolon, Maxolon High Dose‡, Octamide, Octamide PFS, Pramin‡, Reclomide, Reglan

*Pregnancy Risk Category: B*

### HOW SUPPLIED
*Tablets:* 5 mg, 10 mg
*Syrup:* 5 mg/5 ml
*Injection:* 5 mg/ml

### ACTION
Stimulates motility of the upper GI tract by increasing lower esophageal sphincter tone and blocks dopamine receptors at the chemoreceptor trigger zone.

### ONSET, PEAK, DURATION
Onset occurs within 1 to 3 minutes of I.V. administration, 10 to 15 minutes after I.M. injection, 30 to 60 minutes after oral ingestion. Peak occurs in 1 to 2 hours after oral administration,

---

Reactions may be *common,* uncommon, *life-threatening,* or COMMON AND LIFE-THREATENING.

unknown for parenteral administration. Effects persist for 1 to 2 hours.

## INDICATIONS & DOSAGE

*Prevention or reduction of nausea and vomiting induced by cisplatin and other chemotherapeutic agents –*
**Adults:** 1 to 2 mg/kg I.V. 30 minutes before cancer chemotherapy, then repeated q 2 hours for two doses, then q 3 hours for three doses.
*Prevention or reduction of postoperative nausea and vomiting –*
**Adults:** 10 to 20 mg I.M. near the end of the surgical procedure, repeated q 4 to 6 hours p.r.n.
*To facilitate small-bowel intubation and to aid in radiologic examinations –*
**Adults and children over 14 years:** 10 mg (2 ml) I.V. as a single dose over 1 to 2 minutes.
**Children under 6 years:** 0.1 mg/kg I.V.
**Children 6 to 14 years:** 2.5 to 5 mg I.V. (0.5 to 1 ml).
*Delayed gastric emptying secondary to diabetic gastroparesis –*
**Adults:** 10 mg P.O. for mild symptoms, slow I.V. for severe symptoms 30 minutes before meals and h.s. for 2 to 8 weeks, depending on response.
*Gastroesophageal reflux disease –*
**Adults:** 10 to 15 mg P.O. q.i.d., p.r.n., 30 minutes before meals and h.s.

## ADVERSE REACTIONS

**CNS:** *restlessness, anxiety, drowsiness, fatigue, lassitude,* depression, akathisia, insomnia, confusion, *suicide ideation, seizures,* hallucinations, headache, dizziness, extrapyramidal symptoms, tardive dyskinesia, dystonic reactions.
**CV:** transient hypertension, hypotension.
**GI:** nausea, bowel disturbances, diarrhea.
**Hematologic:** neutropenia, *agranulocytosis.*
**Skin:** rash, urticaria.

**Other:** fever, prolactin secretion, loss of libido, urinary frequency, incontinence.

## INTERACTIONS

*Anticholinergics, opioid analgesics:* antagonized GI motility effects of metoclopramide. Use together cautiously.
*Butyrophenones, phenothiazines:* increased risk of extrapyramidal effects. Monitor closely.
*CNS depressants, ethanol:* additive CNS effects. Avoid concomitant use.

## CONTRAINDICATIONS

Contraindicated in patients in which stimulation of GI motility might be dangerous (for example, those with hemorrhage, obstruction, or perforation) and in those with hypersensitivity to drug, pheochromocytoma, or seizure disorders.

## NURSING CONSIDERATIONS

● Use cautiously in patients with history of depression, Parkinson's disease, and hypertension.
● **I.V. use:** Give lower doses (10 mg or less) by direct injection over 1 to 2 minutes. Dilute doses larger than 10 mg in 50 ml of a compatible diluent, and infuse over at least 15 minutes. Protection from light is unnecessary if the infusion mixture is administered within 24 hours.
● Know that the drug is compatible with $D_5W$, 0.9% sodium chloride for injection, and dextrose 5% in sodium chloride 0.45%.
● Closely monitor blood pressure in patients receiving I.V. form of the drug.
● *Alert:* Use diphenhydramine 25 mg I.V. as ordered to counteract the extrapyramidal adverse effects associated with high metoclopramide doses.
● Know that safety and effectiveness have not been established for therapy that continues longer than 12 weeks.

# ondansetron hydrochloride
Zofran

*Pregnancy Risk Category: B*

## HOW SUPPLIED
*Tablets:* 4 mg, 8 mg
*Injection:* 2 mg/ml, 4mg/ml
*Premixed injection:* 32 mg/50 ml

## ACTION
A selective antagonist of a specific type of serotonin receptor (5-HT$_3$) located in the CNS at the area postrema (chemoreceptor trigger zone) and in the peripheral nervous system on nerve terminals of the vagus nerve. Drug's blocking action may occur at both sites.

## ONSET, PEAK, DURATION
Unknown.

## INDICATIONS & DOSAGE
*Prevention of nausea and vomiting associated with emetogenic chemotherapy—*
**Adults and children 12 years and over:** 8 mg P.O. 30 minutes before start of chemotherapy. Follow with 8 mg P.O. 4 and 8 hours after first dose. Then follow with 8 mg q 8 hours for 1 to 2 days. Alternatively, administer a single dose of 32 mg by I.V. infusion over 15 minutes beginning 30 minutes before chemotherapy; or three divided doses of 0.15 mg/kg I.V. (first dose given 30 minutes before chemotherapy; subsequent doses given 4 and 8 hours after first dose). Infuse drug over 15 minutes.
**Children 4 to 12 years:** 4 mg P.O. 30 minutes before start of chemotherapy. Follow with 4 mg P.O. 4 and 8 hours after first dose. Then follow with 4 mg q 8 hours for 1 to 2 days. Alternatively, three doses of 0.15 mg/kg I.V. Give first dose 30 minutes before chemotherapy; administer subsequent doses 4 and 8 hours after first dose. Infuse drug over 15 minutes.
*Prevention of postoperative nausea and vomiting—*
**Adults:** 4 mg I.V. (undiluted) over 2 to 5 minutes. Alternatively, 16 mg P.O. 1 hour before induction of anesthesia.
*Prevention of nausea and vomiting associated with radiotherapy in patients receiving either total body irradiation, single high-dose fraction to the abdomen, or daily fractions to the abdomen—*
**Adults:** 8 mg P.O. t.i.d.

## ADVERSE REACTIONS
**CNS:** *headache, malaise, fatigue, dizziness, sedation.*
**GI:** *diarrhea, constipation,* abdominal pain, xerostomia.
**Hepatic:** transient elevations in AST and ALT levels.
**Skin:** rash.
**Other:** *musculoskeletal pain,* chills, urine retention, chest pain, injection-site reaction, fever, hypoxia, gynecologic disorders.

## INTERACTIONS
*Drugs that alter hepatic drug metabolizing enzymes, such as phenobarbital or cimetidine:* may alter pharmacokinetics of ondansetron. No dosage adjustment appears necessary.

## CONTRAINDICATIONS
Contraindicated in patients hypersensitive to the drug.

## NURSING CONSIDERATIONS
• Use cautiously in patients with liver failure.
• **I.V. use:** Dilute drug in 50 ml of D$_5$W injection or 0.9% sodium chlo-

ride for injection before administration.
- **Alert:** Administer as I.V. infusion over 15 minutes.
- Know that drug is also stable for up to 48 hours after dilution in 5% dextrose in 0.9% sodium chloride for injection, 5% dextrose in 0.45% sodium chloride for injection, and 3% sodium chloride for injection.

☑ **PATIENT TEACHING**
- Instruct patient to alert nurse immediately if difficulty breathing occurs after drug administration.
- Tell patient receiving drug I.V. to report discomfort at insertion site promptly.

---

## prochlorperazine
Compazine, PMS
Prochlorperazine†, Prorazin†,
Stemetil†

## prochlorperazine edisylate
Compa-Z, Compazine Syrup,
Cotranzine, Ultrazine-10

## prochlorperazine maleate
Anti-Naus‡, Compazine Spansule,
PMS Prochlorperazine†, Prorazin†,
Stemetil†

*Pregnancy Risk Category: NR*

### HOW SUPPLIED
**prochlorperazine**
*Tablets:* 5 mg, 10 mg
*Injection:* 5 mg/ml
*Suppositories:* 2.5 mg, 5 mg, 25 mg
**prochlorperazine edisylate**
*Syrup:* 5 mg/5 ml
*Injection:* 5mg/ml
**prochlorperazine maleate**
*Tablets:* 5 mg, 10 mg, 25 mg
*Capsules (sustained-release):* 10 mg,
15 mg, 30 mg

### ACTION
Acts on the chemoreceptor trigger zone to inhibit nausea and vomiting;
in larger doses, partially depresses the vomiting center.

### ONSET, PEAK, DURATION
Onset 30 to 40 minutes after oral use, 60 minutes after rectal use, 10 to 20 minutes after I.M. use. Peak unknown. Effects persist 3 to 4 hours after regular-release preparations, 10 to 12 hours after sustained-release preparations, 3 to 4 hours after rectal or I.M. use.

### INDICATIONS & DOSAGE
*Preoperative nausea control –*
**Adults:** 5 to 10 mg I.M. 1 to 2 hours before induction of anesthesia; repeat once in 30 minutes, if necessary. Or, 5 to 10 mg I.V. 15 to 30 minutes before induction of anesthesia; repeat once if necessary.
*Severe nausea and vomiting –*
**Adults:** 5 to 10 mg P.O., t.i.d. or q.i.d.; 15 mg sustained-release form P.O. on rising; 10 mg sustained-release form P.O. q 12 hours; 25 mg P.R., b.i.d.; or 5 to 10 mg I.M. repeated q 3 to 4 hours, p.r.n. Maximum I.M. dosage is 40 mg daily. Alternatively, 2.5 to 10 mg I.V. at a rate not to exceed 5 mg/minute.
**Children 9 to 13 kg:** 2.5 mg P.O. or P.R. once daily or b.i.d. Maximum dosage is 7.5 mg daily. Or give 0.132 mg/kg by deep I.M. injection. Control usually is obtained with one dose.
**Children 14 to 17 kg:** 2.5 mg P.O. or P.R., b.i.d. or t.i.d. Maximum dosage is 10 mg daily. Or give 0.132 mg/kg by deep I.M. injection. Control usually is obtained with one dose.
**Children 18 to 39 kg:** 2.5 mg P.O. or P.R., t.i.d.; or 5 mg P.O. or P.R., b.i.d. Maximum dosage is 15 mg daily. Or, give 0.132 mg/kg by deep I.M. injection. Control usually is obtained with one dose.
*To manage symptoms of psychotic disorders –*
**Adults:** 5 to 10 mg P.O., t.i.d. or q.i.d.

*Liquid form contains alcohol. **May contain tartrazine. †Canada only. ‡Australia only. ◊OTC.

**Children 2 to 12 years:** 2.5 mg P.O. or P.R., b.i.d. or t.i.d. Do not exceed 10 mg on day 1. Increase dosage gradually to recommended maximum (if necessary). In children 2 to 5 years, maximum daily dosage is 25 mg. In children 6 to 10 years, maximum daily dosage is 25 mg.

*To manage symptoms of severe psychoses –*

**Adults:** 10 to 20 mg I.M. repeated in 1 to 4 hours, if needed. Rarely, patients may receive 10 to 20 mg q 4 to 6 hours. Institute oral therapy after symptoms are controlled.

**Children 2 to 12 years:** 0.13 mg/kg I.M.

*Nonpsychotic anxiety –*

**Adults:** 5 to 10 mg by deep I.M. injection q 3 to 4 hours, not to exceed 40 mg daily; or 5 to 10 mg P.O., t.i.d. or q.i.d. Alternatively, give 15 mg extended-release capsule once daily or 10 mg extended-release capsule q 12 hours.

## ADVERSE REACTIONS

**CNS:** *extrapyramidal reactions,* sedation, pseudoparkinsonism, EEG changes, dizziness.
**CV:** *orthostatic hypotension,* tachycardia, ECG changes.
**EENT:** *ocular changes, blurred vision.*
**GI:** *dry mouth, constipation.*
**GU:** *urine retention,* dark urine, menstrual irregularities, inhibited ejaculation.
**Hematologic:** *transient leukopenia,* **agranulocytosis.**
**Hepatic:** *cholestatic jaundice.*
**Skin:** *mild photosensitivity,* allergic reactions, **exfoliative dermatitis.**
**Other:** hyperprolactinemia, gynecomastia, weight gain, increased appetite.

## INTERACTIONS

*Antacids:* inhibited absorption of oral phenothiazines. Separate antacid and phenothiazine doses by at least 2 hours.
*Anticholinergics, including antidepressants and antiparkinsonian agents:* increased anticholinergic activity and aggravated parkinsonian symptoms. Use together cautiously.
*Barbiturates:* may decrease phenothiazine effect. Monitor patient for decreased antiemetic effect.

## CONTRAINDICATIONS

Contraindicated in patients hypersensitive to phenothiazines and in those with CNS depression including coma; during pediatric surgery; when using spinal or epidural anesthetic, adrenergic blockers, or ethanol; and in children under 2 years.

## NURSING CONSIDERATIONS

• Use cautiously in patients with impaired CV function, glaucoma, seizure disorders; in those who have been exposed to extreme heat; and in children with acute illness.
• Dilute oral solution with tomato or fruit juice, milk, coffee, carbonated beverage, tea, water, or soup or mix with pudding.
• **I.V. use:** 15 to 30 minutes before induction, add 20 mg of prochlorperazine per liter of $D_5W$ and 0.9% sodium chloride solution. Infusion rate should not exceed 5 mg/minute. Maximum parenteral dosage is 40 mg daily. Infuse slowly, never as a bolus.
• For I.M. use, inject deeply into upper outer quadrant of gluteal region.
• Do not give S.C. or mix in syringe with another drug.
• To prevent contact dermatitis, avoid getting concentrate or injection solution on hands or clothing.
• Watch for orthostatic hypotension, especially when giving drug I.V.
• Monitor CBC and liver function studies during long-term therapy as ordered.
• *Alert:* Know that the drug is used only when vomiting can't be con-

---

Reactions may be *common,* uncommon, *life-threatening,* or **COMMON AND LIFE-THREATENING.**

trolled by other measures or when only a few doses are required. If more than four doses are needed in 24 hours, notify the doctor.
• Store in light-resistant container. Slight yellowing does not affect potency; discard extremely discolored solutions.

☑ **PATIENT TEACHING**
• Teach patient what to use to dilute oral solution.
• Advise patient to wear protective clothing when exposed to sunlight.
• Tell patient to call doctor if more than four doses are needed within 24 hours.

---

## thiethylperazine maleate
Norzine, Torecan**

*Pregnancy Risk Category: X*

### HOW SUPPLIED
*Tablets:* 10 mg
*Injection:* 5 mg/ml
*Suppositories:* 10 mg

### ACTION
Unknown. Probably acts on the chemoreceptor trigger zone to inhibit nausea and vomiting.

### ONSET, PEAK, DURATION
Onset occurs in 30 minutes. Peak unknown. Effects persist 4 hours.

### INDICATIONS & DOSAGE
*Nausea and vomiting–*
**Adults:** 10 mg P.O., I.M., or P.R. once daily, b.i.d. or t.i.d.

### ADVERSE REACTIONS
**CNS:** *extrapyramidal reactions* (high incidence), sedation (low incidence), pseudoparkinsonism, EEG changes, dizziness, confusion (especially in elderly patients).
**CV:** *orthostatic hypotension,* tachycardia, ECG changes.

**EENT:** *ocular changes, blurred vision.*
**GI:** *dry mouth, constipation.*
**GU:** *urine retention,* dark urine, menstrual irregularities, inhibited ejaculation, gynecomastia.
**Hematologic:** *transient leukopenia,* **agranulocytosis.**
**Hepatic:** *cholestatic jaundice.*
**Skin:** *mild photosensitivity,* allergic reactions.
**Other:** hyperprolactinemia, weight gain, increased appetite.

### INTERACTIONS
*Antacids:* inhibited absorption of oral phenothiazines. Separate antacid and phenothiazine doses by at least 2 hours.
*Anticholinergics, including antidepressants and antiparkinsonian agents:* increased anticholinergic activity and increased risk of parkinsonian-like symptoms. Use together cautiously.
*Barbiturates:* may decrease phenothiazine effect. Monitor patient for decreased antiemetic effect.

### CONTRAINDICATIONS
Contraindicated in patients hypersensitive to phenothiazines, in those with severe CNS depression or hepatic disease, in patients experiencing coma, and in pregnancy.

### NURSING CONSIDERATIONS
• Use cautiously in patients with aspirin hypersensitivity.
• *Alert:* Don't give I.V. May cause severe hypotension.
• For nausea and vomiting associated with anesthesia and surgery, give deep I.M. injection shortly before or when terminating anesthesia.
• If drug gets on skin, wash off at once to prevent contact dermatitis.
• Use only when vomiting can't be controlled by other measures or when only a few doses are required.
• Store suppositories in tightly covered

---

container and at temperatures below 77° F (25° C).

### ☑ PATIENT TEACHING
• Warn patient about hypotension and suggest that he stay in bed for 1 hour after receiving drug.
• Instruct patient to report decreased urine output, visual changes, and any CNS effects immediately.

## trimethobenzamide hydrochloride
Arrestin, Benzacot, Bio-Gan, Stemetic, Tebamide, Tegamide, T-Gen, Ticon, Tigan, Triban, Tribenzagan, Trimazide

*Pregnancy Risk Category: NR*

### HOW SUPPLIED
*Capsules:* 100 mg, 250 mg
*Injection:* 100 mg/ml
*Suppositories:* 100 mg, 200 mg

### ACTION
Unknown. Probably acts on the chemoreceptor trigger zone to inhibit nausea and vomiting.

### ONSET, PEAK, DURATION
Onset occurs 10 to 20 minutes after oral administration, 15 to 35 minutes after I.M. administration. Peak unknown. Effects persist for 2 to 3 hours after I.M. administration, 3 to 4 hours after oral administration.

### INDICATIONS & DOSAGE
*Nausea and vomiting—*
**Adults:** 250 mg P.O., t.i.d. or q.i.d.; or 200 mg I.M. or P.R., t.i.d. or q.i.d.
*Prevention of postoperative nausea and vomiting—*
**Adults:** 200 mg I.M. or P.R. as a single dose before or during surgery; if needed, repeat 3 hours after termination of anesthesia, p.r.n. Limit use to prolonged vomiting of known etiology.

**Children under 13 kg:** 100 mg P.R. t.i.d. or q.i.d.
**Children 13 to 40 kg:** 100 to 200 mg P.O. or P.R. t.i.d. or q.i.d.

### ADVERSE REACTIONS
**CNS:** *drowsiness,* dizziness (in large doses), headache, disorientation, depression, parkinsonion-like symptoms, *coma, seizures.*
**CV:** hypotension.
**GI:** diarrhea.
**Hepatic:** jaundice.
**Other:** hypersensitivity reactions (pain, stinging, burning, redness, swelling at I.M. injection site); blurred vision; muscle cramps.

### INTERACTIONS
*CNS depressants, ethanol:* additive CNS depression. Avoid concomitant use.

### CONTRAINDICATIONS
Contraindicated in patients with hypersensitivity to drug. Suppositories are contraindicated in patients hypersensitive to benzocaine hydrochloride or similar local anesthetic.

### NURSING CONSIDERATIONS
• Use cautiously in children.
• For I.M. administration, inject deeply into upper outer quadrant of gluteal region to reduce pain and local irritation.
• Like other antiemetics, drug may mask signs of overdose of toxic agents or symptoms of intestinal obstruction, brain tumor, or other conditions.
• Withhold drug if skin hypersensitivity reaction occurs.

### ☑ PATIENT TEACHING
• Instruct patient to refrigerate suppositories.
• Advise patient of the possibility of drowsiness and dizziness, and caution against driving or other activities requiring alertness until CNS effects of the drug are known.

# 52

# Antiulcer drugs

cimetidine
famotidine
lansoprazole
misoprostol
nizatidine
omeprazole
ranitidine hydrochloride
sucralfate

**COMBINATION PRODUCTS**
None.

## cimetidine
Tagamet, Tagamet HB◦

*Pregnancy Risk Category: B*

### HOW SUPPLIED
*Tablets:* 100 mg◦, 200 mg, 300 mg, 400 mg, 800 mg
*Oral liquid:* 300 mg/5 ml
*Effervescent tablets:* 800 mg‡
*Injection:* 100 mg/ml‡, 300 mg/2 ml; 300 mg in 50 ml 0.9% sodium chloride solution

### ACTION
Competitively inhibits the action of histamine-2 at receptor sites of the parietal cells, decreasing gastric acid secretion.

### ONSET, PEAK, DURATION
Onset unknown. Peak levels occur right after I.V. administration, unknown for I.M. administration, 45 to 90 minutes after oral dose. Effects last 4 to 5 hours after oral dose, unknown after parenteral administration. Therapeutic effects last 4 to 5 hours.

### INDICATIONS & DOSAGE
*Duodenal ulcer (short-term treatment and maintenance) –*
**Adults and children 16 years and over:** 800 mg P.O. h.s. Alternatively, 400 mg P.O. b.i.d. or 300 mg q.i.d. (with meals and h.s.). Treatment continued for 4 to 6 weeks unless endoscopy shows healing. For maintenance therapy, 400 mg h.s. For parenteral therapy, 300 mg diluted to 20 ml with 0.9% sodium chloride solution or other compatible I.V. solution by I.V. push over 1 to 2 minutes q 6 hours; or 300 mg diluted in 50 ml $D_5W$ or other compatible I.V. solution by I.V. infusion over 15 to 20 minutes q 6 hours; or 300 mg I.M. q 6 hours (no dilution necessary). Parenteral dosage increased by giving 300-mg doses more frequently to maximum daily dosage of 2,400 mg as needed. Alternatively, 900 mg/day (37.5 mg/hour) I.V. diluted in 100 to 1,000 ml of compatible solution by continuous I.V. infusion.
*Active benign gastric ulceration –*
**Adults:** 800 mg P.O. h.s., or 300 mg P.O. q.i.d. (with meals and h.s.) for up to 8 weeks.
*Pathologic hypersecretory conditions (such as Zollinger-Ellison syndrome, systemic mastocytosis, and multiple endocrine adenomas) –*
**Adults and children 16 years and over:** 300 mg P.O. q.i.d. with meals and h.s.; adjusted to individual needs. Maximum oral daily dosage is 2,400 mg.
  For parenteral therapy, 300 mg diluted to 20 ml with 0.9% sodium chloride solution or other compatible I.V. solution by I.V. push over 1 to 2 minutes q 6 hours; or 300 mg diluted in 50 ml dextrose 5% solution or other compatible I.V. solution by I.V. infusion over 15 to 20 minutes q 6 hours. Parenteral dosage increased by giving 300-mg doses more frequently to maximum daily dosage of 2,400 mg as needed.
*Gastroesophageal reflux disease –*

---

*Liquid form contains alcohol.   **May contain tartrazine.   †Canada only.   ‡Australia only.   ◦OTC.

**Adults:** 800 mg P.O. b.i.d. or 400 mg q.i.d. before meals and h.s. for up to 12 weeks.
*Prevention of upper GI bleeding in critically ill patients –*
**Adults:** 50 mg/hour by continuous I.V. infusion for up to 7 days; 25 mg/hour to patients with creatinine clearance below 30 ml/minute/1.73 m$^2$.
*Heartburn –*
**Adults:** 200 mg (Tagament HB only) P.O. with water as symptoms occur, or as directed, up to b.i.d. Maximum dosage 400 mg daily. Drug shouldn't be taken daily for longer than 2 weeks.

## ADVERSE REACTIONS

**CNS:** confusion, dizziness, headache, peripheral neuropathy, somnolence, hallucinations.
**GI:** *mild and transient diarrhea.*
**GU:** transient elevations in serum creatinine levels, impotence, mild gynecomastia if used longer than 1 month.
**Hematologic:** *agranulocytosis* (rare), *neutropenia, thrombocytopenia* (rare), *aplastic anemia* (rare).
**Hepatic:** jaundice (rare).
**Other:** hypersensitivity reactions, muscle pain, arthralgia.

## INTERACTIONS

*Antacids:* interference with cimetidine absorption. Separate administration by at least 1 hour if possible.
*Lidocaine, phenytoin, propranolol, some benzodiazepines, theophylline, warfarin:* inhibited hepatic microsomal enzyme metabolism of these drugs; monitor serum levels.

## CONTRAINDICATIONS

Contraindicated in patients hypersensitive to the drug.

## NURSING CONSIDERATIONS

● Use cautiously in elderly or debilitated patients because they may be more susceptible to cimetidine-induced confusion.
● Identify tablet strength when obtaining a drug history.
● **I.V. use:** Dilute I.V. solutions with 0.9% sodium chloride solution, D$_5$W and dextrose 10% in water (and combinations of these), lactated Ringer's solution, or 5% sodium bicarbonate injection. Do not dilute with sterile water for injection.
● **Alert:** Don't infuse I.V. too rapidly; bradycardia may occur. When giving I.V. in 100 ml of diluent solution, don't infuse so rapidly that circulatory overload results. Some authorities recommend infusing drug over at least 30 minutes, to minimize risk of adverse cardiac effects. Sometimes given as continuous I.V. infusion. Use infusion pump if given in a total volume of 250 ml over 24 hours or less.
● Schedule cimetidine dose at end of hemodialysis treatment. Hemodialysis reduces blood levels of cimetidine. Adjust dosage as ordered in patients with renal failure.
● Keep in mind that effectiveness for treatment of gastric ulcer is not as great as for duodenal ulcer.
● Know that up to 10 g overdose can occur without adverse reactions.

## ☑ PATIENT TEACHING

● Remind patient taking cimetidine once daily to take it at bedtime. If drug is being taken more than once a day, instruct him to take it with meals.
● Instruct patient taking Tagament HB not to exceed recommended dosage and not to take daily for longer than 14 days.
● Warn patient receiving drug I.M. that injection may be painful.
● Urge patient to avoid cigarette smoking because it may increase gastric acid secretion and worsen disease.

---

## famotidine
Pepcid, Pepcid AC◇, Pepcidine‡
*Pregnancy Risk Category: B*

---

## HOW SUPPLIED
*Tablets:* 10 mg, 20 mg, 40 mg
*Powder for oral suspension:* 40 mg/5 ml after reconstitution
*Injection:* 10 mg/ml
*Premixed injection:* 20 mg/50 ml in 0.9% sodium chloride

## ACTION
Competitively inhibits the action of histamine-2 at receptor sites of the parietal cells, decreasing gastric acid secretion.

## ONSET, PEAK, DURATION
Onset occurs within 1 hour after oral or I.V. dose. Peak levels occur within 20 minutes of I.V. injection, 1 to 3 hours after oral dose. Effects persist up to 12 hours.

## INDICATIONS & DOSAGE
*Duodenal ulcer (short-term treatment) –*
**Adults:** For acute therapy, 40 mg P.O. once daily h.s. or 20 mg P.O. b.i.d. For maintenance therapy, give 20 mg P.O. once daily h.s.
*Benign gastric ulcer (short-term treatment) –*
**Adults:** 40 mg P.O. daily h.s. for 8 weeks.
*Pathologic hypersecretory conditions (such as Zollinger-Ellison syndrome) –*
**Adults:** 20 mg P.O. q 6 hours up to 160 mg q 6 hours.
*Hospitalized patients with intractable ulcerations or hypersecretory conditions or patients who cannot take oral medication –*
**Adults:** 20 mg I.V. q 12 hours.
*Gastroesophageal reflux disease (GERD) –*
**Adults:** 20 mg P.O. b.i.d. for up to 6 weeks. For esophagitis caused by GERD, 20 to 40 mg b.i.d. for up to 12 weeks.
*Prevention or treatment of heartburn –*
**Adults:** 10 mg (Pepcid AC only) P.O. 1 hour before meals (prevention) or 10 mg (Pepcid AC only) P.O. with water when symptoms occur. Maximum dosage is 20 mg daily. Drug should not be taken daily for longer than 2 weeks.

## ADVERSE REACTIONS
**CNS:** *headache,* dizziness, vertigo, malaise, paresthesia.
**EENT:** tinnitus, taste disorder, orbital edema.
**GI:** diarrhea, constipation, anorexia, dry mouth.
**GU:** increased BUN and creatinine levels.
**Skin:** acne, dry skin, flushing.
**Other:** transient irritation at I.V. site, musculoskeletal pain, palpitations, fever.

## INTERACTIONS
None significant.

## CONTRAINDICATIONS
Contraindicated in patients hypersensitive to the drug.

## NURSING CONSIDERATIONS
● **I.V. use:** To prepare I.V. injection, dilute 2 ml (20 mg) famotidine with compatible I.V. solution to a total volume of either 5 or 10 ml, and inject over at least 2 minutes. Compatible solutions include sterile water for injection, 0.9% sodium chloride for injection, D₅W or dextrose 10% in water injection, 5% sodium bicarbonate injection, and lactated Ringer's injection.
● Alternatively, give famotidine by intermittent I.V. infusion. Dilute 20 mg (2 ml) famotidine in 100 ml of compatible solution, and infuse over 15 to 30 minutes. Solution is stable for 48 hours at room temperature after dilution.
● Store I.V. injection in refrigerator at 36° to 46° F (2° to 8° C).
● Store reconstituted suspension below 86° F (30° C). Discard after 30 days.

☑ **PATIENT TEACHING**
• Instruct the patient on proper use of over-the-counter product (Pepcid AC), if appropriate.
• Tell the patient to take prescription drug with a snack if desired.
• Remind patient that the prescription drug is most effective if taken at bedtime. Tell patients taking 20 mg b.i.d. to take at least one dose at bedtime.
• Advise the patient not to take prescription drug for longer than 8 weeks, unless the doctor specifically orders it, and to limit use of OTC product to no more than 2 weeks.
• With doctor's knowledge, allow the patient to take antacids concomitantly, especially at the beginning of therapy when pain is severe.
• Urge the patient to avoid cigarette smoking because it may increase gastric acid secretion and worsen disease.

---

# lansoprazole
Prevacid

*Pregnancy Risk Category: B*

## HOW SUPPLIED
*Capsules (delayed release):* 15 mg, 30 mg

## ACTION
Inhibits the activity of the proton pump and binds to hydrogen-potassium adenosine triphosphatase, located at the secretory surface of the gastric parietal cells, to block the formation of gastric acid.

## ONSET, PEAK, DURATION
Onset and duration unknown. Peak effects occur in 1.7 hours.

## INDICATIONS & DOSAGE
*Short-term treatment of active duodenal ulcer—*
**Adults:** 15 mg P.O. daily before eating for 4 weeks.
*Short-term treatment of erosive esophagitis—*
**Adults:** 30 mg P.O. before eating for

up to 8 weeks. If healing doesn't occur, 8 more weeks of therapy may be given.
*Long-term treatment of pathologic hypersecretory conditions, including Zollinger-Ellison syndrome—*
**Adults:** initially, 60 mg P.O. once daily. Dosage increased as needed. Daily dosages of more than 120 mg should be given in divided doses.

## ADVERSE REACTIONS
**CNS:** headache, agitation, amnesia, anxiety, apathy, confusion, depression, dizziness or syncope, hallucinations, hemiplegia, aggravated hostility, decreased libido, nervousness, paresthesia, thinking abnormality.
**CV:** chest pain, edema, angina, CVA, hypertension or hypotension, *MI,* palpitations, *shock,* vasodilation, cardiospasm.
**EENT:** amblyopia, deafness, eye pain, visual field deficits, otitis media, taste perversion, tinnitus.
**GI:** *diarrhea, nausea, abdominal pain,* halitosis, melena, anorexia, cholelithiasis, constipation, dry mouth, thirst, dyspepsia, dysphagia, eructation, esophageal stenosis, esophageal ulcer, esophagitis, fecal discoloration, flatulence, gastric nodules, fundic gland polyps, gastroenteritis, GI hemorrhage, hematemesis, increased appetite, increased salivation, rectal hemorrhage, stomatitis, tenesmus, ulcerative colitis.
**GU:** hematuria, impotence, renal calculi, albuminuria, abnormal menses, gynecomastia, breast tenderness.
**Hematologic:** anemia, hemolysis.
**Metabolic:** diabetes mellitus, goiter, hyperglycemia, hypoglycemia, gout, weight gain or loss.
**Musculoskeletal:** arthritis or arthralgia, musculoskeletal pain, myalgia.
**Respiratory:** asthma, bronchitis, increased cough, dyspnea, epistaxis, hemoptysis, hiccups, pneumonia, upper respiratory tract inflammation.
**Skin:** acne, alopecia, pruritus, rash, urticaria.

---

Reactions may be *common,* uncommon, *life-threatening,* or **COMMON AND LIFE-THREATENING.**

**Other:** asthenia, candidiasis, fever, flulike syndrome, infection, malaise.

## INTERACTIONS
*Ampicillin esters, digoxin, iron salts, ketoconazole:* lansoprazole may inhibit absorption. Monitor patient closely.
*Sucralfate:* delayed lansoprazole absorption. Give lansoprazole at least 30 minutes prior to sucralfate.
*Theophylline:* may cause mild increase in theophylline clearance. Use together cautiously. Dosage adjustment of theophylline may be needed when lansoprazole is started or stopped.

## CONTRAINDICATIONS
Contraindicated in patients hypersensitive to the drug.

## NURSING CONSIDERATIONS
• Know that no dosage adjustment is necessary in patients with renal insufficiency or in elderly patients. For patients with severe liver disease, dosage adjustment may be necessary.
• Be aware that lansoprazole should not to be used as maintenance therapy for treatment of patients with duodenal ulcer or erosive esophagitis.
• Because it is not known if lansoprazole is excreted in breast milk, be aware that a decision to discontinue breast-feeding or the drug should be made when drug is prescribed for breast-feeding women.

## ☑ PATIENT TEACHING
• Instruct patient to take the drug before eating.
• Tell patient who has trouble swallowing capsules to open and sprinkle contents over applesauce.

---

## misoprostol
Cytotec

*Pregnancy Risk Category: X*

## HOW SUPPLIED
*Tablets:* 100 mcg, 200 mcg

## ACTION
A synthetic prostaglandin $E_1$ analogue that replaces gastric prostaglandins depleted by NSAID therapy. Misoprostol also decreases basal and stimulated gastric acid secretion and may increase gastric mucus and bicarbonate production.

## ONSET, PEAK, DURATION
Onset occurs in 30 minutes. Plasma levels peak within 10 to 15 minutes. Effects persist about 3 hours.

## INDICATIONS & DOSAGE
*Prevention of NSAID-induced gastric ulcer in elderly or debilitated patients at high risk for complications from gastric ulcer and in patients with a history of NSAID-induced ulcer —*
**Adults:** 200 mcg P.O. q.i.d. with food; if not tolerated, may be decreased to 100 mcg P.O. q.i.d. Dosage should be given for duration of NSAID therapy.

## ADVERSE REACTIONS
**CNS:** headache.
**GI:** *diarrhea, abdominal pain,* nausea, flatulence, dyspepsia, vomiting, constipation.
**Other:** hypermenorrhea, dysmenorrhea, spotting, cramps, menstrual disorders.

## INTERACTIONS
*Antacids:* reduced plasma levels when administered concomitantly. Not considered significant.

## CONTRAINDICATIONS
Contraindicated in pregnant or lactating patients.

## NURSING CONSIDERATIONS
• Know that drug should not be routinely given to women of childbearing age unless they are at high risk for developing ulcers or complications from NSAID-induced ulcers.
• **Alert:** Take special precautions to prevent use of drug during pregnancy.

---

*Liquid form contains alcohol.   **May contain tartrazine.   †Canada only.   ‡Australia only.   ◇OTC.

Make sure the patient understands the dangers of misoprostol to a fetus and that she receives both oral and written warnings about these dangers. Also ensure that she can comply with effective contraception and that she has a negative serum pregnancy test within 2 weeks of initiating therapy.

### ☑ PATIENT TEACHING
• Instruct all patients not to share misoprostol. Remind them that when taken by a pregnant patient this drug may cause miscarriage, often with potentially life-threatening bleeding.
• Advise patient not to begin misoprostol therapy until the second or third day of the next normal menstrual period.

## nizatidine
Axid, Tazac‡

*Pregnancy Risk Category: C*

### HOW SUPPLIED
*Capsules:* 150 mg, 300 mg

### ACTION
Competitively inhibits the action of histamine-2 ($H_2$) at receptor sites of the parietal cells, decreasing gastric acid secretion.

### ONSET, PEAK, DURATION
Onset occurs within 30 minutes. Peak levels occur in ½ to 3 hours. Effects persist up to 12 hours.

### INDICATIONS & DOSAGE
*Active duodenal ulcer –*
**Adults:** 300 mg P.O. daily h.s. Alternatively, 150 mg P.O. b.i.d.
*Maintenance therapy for duodenal ulcer –*
**Adults:** 150 mg P.O. daily h.s.
*Benign gastric ulcer –*
**Adults:** 150 mg P.O. b.i.d. or 300 mg h.s. for 8 weeks.
*Gastroesophageal reflux disease –*
**Adults:** 150 mg P.O. b.i.d.
In patients with impaired renal func-

tion: If creatinine clearance is 20 to 50 ml/minute/1.73 m², 150 mg P.O. daily for treatment of active duodenal ulcer, or 150 mg every other day for maintenance therapy; if creatinine clearance is below 20 ml/minute/1.73 m², 150 mg P.O. every other day for treatment, or 150 mg every third day for maintenance.

### ADVERSE REACTIONS
**CNS:** *somnolence.*
**CV:** arrhythmias.
**Hematologic:** eosinophilia.
**Skin:** *diaphoresis,* rash, urticaria.
**Other:** hyperuricemia, fever, hepatocellular injury, elevated liver function tests.

### INTERACTIONS
*Aspirin:* possibly elevated serum salicylate levels (with high doses).
*Tomato-based mixed-vegetable juices:* may decrease potency of the drug when used concomitantly.

### CONTRAINDICATIONS
Contraindicated in patients hypersensitive to $H_2$-receptor antagonists.

### NURSING CONSIDERATIONS
• Use cautiously and in reduced dosages in patients with renal impairment.
• If necessary, open capsules and mix contents with apple juice. However, be aware that drug loses some potency when combined with tomato-based mixed-vegetable juices. Ask pharmacist about compatibility.
• Be aware that false-positive test results for urobilinogen may occur.

### ☑ PATIENT TEACHING
• Tell patient who has difficulty swallowing capsules that contents may be mixed with apple juice but not with tomato-based mixed vegetable juices.
• Urge patient to avoid cigarette smoking because it may increase gastric acid secretion and worsen disease.

---

Reactions may be *common,* uncommon, *life-threatening,* or **COMMON AND LIFE-THREATENING.**

## omeprazole
Losect‡, Prilosec

*Pregnancy Risk Category: C*

### HOW SUPPLIED
*Capsules (delayed-release):* 10 mg, 20 mg

### ACTION
Inhibits the activity of the acid (proton) pump, and binds to hydrogen-potassium adenosine triphosphatase, located at the secretory surface of the gastric parietal cells to block the formation of gastric acid.

### ONSET, PEAK, DURATION
Onset occurs within 1 hour. Peak effects occur within 2 hours. Effects persist 3 days or more; may take 4 days for gastric acid production to return to normal.

### INDICATIONS & DOSAGE
*Severe erosive esophagitis; poorly responsive gastroesophageal reflux disease (GERD) –*
**Adults:** 20 mg P.O. daily for 4 to 8 weeks. Patients with GERD should have failed initial therapy with a histamine-2 antagonist.
*Maintenance of healing erosive esophagitis –*
**Adults:** 20 mg P.O. daily.
*Pathologic hypersecretory conditions (such as Zollinger-Ellison syndrome) –*
**Adults:** initially, 60 mg P.O. daily; dosage titrated according to patient response. If daily dosage exceeds 80 mg, administer in divided doses. Dosages up to 120 mg t.i.d. have been given. Continue therapy as long as clinically indicated.
*Duodenal ulcer (short-term treatment) –*
**Adults:** 20 mg P.O. daily for 4 to 8 weeks.

### ADVERSE REACTIONS
**CNS:** headache, dizziness, asthenia.
**GI:** diarrhea, abdominal pain, nausea, vomiting, constipation, flatulence.
**Respiratory:** cough, upper respiratory infection.
**Skin:** rash.
**Other:** back pain.

### INTERACTIONS
*Ampicillin esters, iron derivatives, ketoconazole:* may exhibit poor bioavailability in patients taking omeprazole because optimal absorption of these drugs requires a low gastric pH. Avoid concomitant use.
*Diazepam, phenytoin, warfarin:* decreased hepatic clearance, possibly leading to increased serum levels. Monitor closely.

### CONTRAINDICATIONS
Contraindicated in patients hypersensitive to the drug or any component of the formulation.

### NURSING CONSIDERATIONS
• Know that dosage adjustments aren't needed for renal or hepatic impairment.
• Know that omeprazole increases its own bioavailability with repeated dosages. Drug is labile in gastric acid; less drug is lost to hydrolysis because the drug increases gastric pH.

### ☑ PATIENT TEACHING
• Tell the patient to swallow capsules whole and not to open or crush them.
• Caution patient not to perform hazardous activities if dizziness occurs.

## ranitidine hydrochloride
Apo-Ranitidine†, Zantac*, Zantac-C†, Zantac EFFERdose, Zantac 75◊

*Pregnancy Risk Category: B*

### HOW SUPPLIED
*Tablets:* 75 mg◊, 150 mg, 300 mg
*Dispersible tablets:* 150 mg‡

---

*Liquid form contains alcohol.   **May contain tartrazine.   †Canada only.   ‡Australia only.   ◊OTC.

*Effervescent tablets:* 150 mg
*Effervescent granules:* 150 mg
*Syrup:* 15 mg/ml*
*Injection:* 25 mg/ml
*Infusion:* 0.5 mg/ml in 100-ml containers

## ACTION

Competitively inhibits the action of histamine-2 at receptor sites of the parietal cells, decreasing gastric acid secretion.

## ONSET, PEAK, DURATION

Onset occurs within 1 hour. Peak effects occur in 1 to 3 hours. Effects persist up to 13 hours.

## INDICATIONS & DOSAGE

*Duodenal and gastric ulcer (short-term treatment); pathologic hypersecretory conditions, such as Zollinger-Ellison syndrome –*
**Adults:** 150 mg P.O. b.i.d. or 300 mg daily h.s. Alternatively, 50 mg I.V. or I.M. q 6 to 8 hours. Patients with Zollinger-Ellison syndrome may require dosages up to 6 g P.O. daily.
*Maintenance therapy for duodenal or gastric ulcer –*
**Adults:** 150 mg P.O. h.s.
*Gastroesophageal reflux disease –*
**Adults:** 150 mg P.O. b.i.d.
*Erosive esophagitis –*
**Adults:** 150 mg P.O. q.i.d. Maintenance therapy is 150 mg P.O. b.i.d.
*Treatment for heartburn –*
**Adults:** 75 mg (Zantac 75 only) P.O. as symptoms occur, not to exceed 150 mg daily.

## ADVERSE REACTIONS

**CNS:** vertigo, malaise.
**EENT:** blurred vision.
**Hematologic:** reversible leukopenia, pancytopenia.
**Hepatic:** elevated liver enzymes, jaundice.

**Other:** burning and itching at injection site, ***anaphylaxis,*** angioneurotic edema.

## INTERACTIONS

*Antacids:* may interfere with ranitidine absorption. Stagger doses if possible.
*Diazepam:* decreased absorption of diazepam. Monitor closely.
*Glipizide:* possible increased hypoglycemic effect. Adjust glipizide dosage as necessary.
*Procainamide:* possible decreased renal clearance of procainamide. Monitor patient closely for toxicity.
*Warfarin:* possible interference with warfarin clearance. Monitor closely.

## CONTRAINDICATIONS

Contraindicated in patients hypersensitive to the drug.

## NURSING CONSIDERATIONS

● Use cautiously in patients with hepatic dysfunction. Adjust dosage in patients with impaired renal function as ordered.
● Avoid using aluminum-based needles or other equipment when mixing or administering drug. Drug is incompatible with aluminum.
● **I.V. use:** When administering by I.V. push, dilute to a total volume of 20 ml, and inject over a period of 5 minutes. No dilution is necessary when administering I.M.
● To prepare I.V. injection, dilute 50 mg (2 ml) in 100 ml of compatible solution, and infuse over 15 to 20 minutes. Compatible solutions include 0.9% sodium chloride for injection, $D_5W$ or $D_{10}W$ injection, 5% sodium bicarbonate injection, or lactated Ringer's injection.
● When giving by intermittent I.V. infusion, dilute 50 mg ranitidine in 100 ml of $D_5W$, and infuse over 15 to 20 minutes. Or, give by continuous I.V. infusion: 150 mg in 250 ml of com-

patible solution. Administer at 6.25 mg/hour using an infusion pump.
• When administering premixed I.V. infusion, give by slow I.V. drip (over 15 to 20 minutes). Don't add other drugs to the solution. If used with a primary I.V. fluid system, discontinue the primary solution during the infusion.

☑ **PATIENT TEACHING**
• Instruct patient on proper use of OTC preparation, as indicated.
• Remind patient taking prescription drug once daily to take it at bedtime for best results.
• Instruct patient to take without regard to meals because absorption is not affected by food.
• Tell patient taking EFFERdose to dissolve drug in 6 to 8 ounces of water before taking it.
• Urge patient to avoid cigarette smoking because it may increase gastric acid secretion and worsen disease.

---

### sucralfate
Carafate, SCF‡, Sulcrate†
*Pregnancy Risk Category: B*

**HOW SUPPLIED**
*Tablets:* 1 g
*Suspension:* 1 g/10 ml

**ACTION**
Unknown. Probably adheres to and protects the ulcer's surface by forming a barrier.

**ONSET, PEAK, DURATION**
Onset and peak unknown. Effects persist for up to 6 hours.

**INDICATIONS & DOSAGE**
*Short-term (up to 8 weeks) treatment of duodenal ulcer –*
**Adults:** 1 g P.O. q.i.d. 1 hour before meals and h.s.
*Maintenance therapy for duodenal ulcer –*
**Adults:** 1 g P.O. b.i.d.

**ADVERSE REACTIONS**
**CNS:** dizziness, sleepiness, headache, vertigo.
**GI:** *constipation,* nausea, gastric discomfort, diarrhea, bezoar formation, vomiting, flatulence, dry mouth, indigestion.
**Skin:** rash, pruritus.
**Other:** back pain.

**INTERACTIONS**
*Antacids:* may decrease binding of drug to gastroduodenal mucosa, impairing effectiveness. Don't administer within 30 minutes of each other.
*Cimetidine, ciprofloxacin, digoxin, ketoconazole, norfloxacin, phenytoin, quinidine, ranitidine, tetracycline, theophylline:* decreased absorption. Separate administration times by at least 2 hours.

**CONTRAINDICATIONS**
None known.

**NURSING CONSIDERATIONS**
• Use with caution in patients with chronic renal failure.
• Know that drug is minimally absorbed and has a low incidence of adverse reactions.
• Monitor for severe, persistent constipation.
• Be aware that studies suggest that sucralfate is as effective as cimetidine in healing duodenal ulcer.
• Know that drug contains aluminum but isn't classified as an antacid.

☑ **PATIENT TEACHING**
• Tell patient to take sucralfate on an empty stomach (1 hour before each meal and at bedtime).
• Tell patient to continue prescribed regimen to ensure complete healing. Pain and ulcerative symptoms may subside within first few weeks of therapy.
• Urge patient to avoid cigarette smoking because it may increase gastric acid secretion and worsen disease.

---

betamethasone
betamethasone acetate and
  betamethasone sodium
  phosphate
betamethasone sodium
  phosphate
cortisone acetate
dexamethasone
dexamethasone acetate
dexamethasone sodium
  phosphate
fludrocortisone acetate
hydrocortisone
hydrocortisone acetate
hydrocortisone cypionate
hydrocortisone sodium
  phosphate
hydrocortisone sodium
  succinate
methylprednisolone
methylprednisolone acetate
methylprednisolone sodium
  succinate
prednisolone
prednisolone acetate
prednisolone sodium phosphate
prednisolone steaglate
prednisolone tebutate
prednisone
triamcinolone
triamcinolone acetonide
triamcinolone diacetate
triamcinolone hexacetonide

### COMBINATION PRODUCTS
DECADRON PHOSPHATE WITH XY-
LOCAINE: dexamethasone phosphate
4 mg and lidocaine hydrochloride 10
mg per ml.
PREDNISOLONE ACETATE AND
PREDNISOLONE SODIUM PHOS-
PHATE: prednisolone acetate 80 mg/
ml and prednisolone sodium phos-
phate 20 mg/ml

### betamethasone
Betnelan†, Betnesol†, Celestone*

### betamethasone acetate and betamethasone sodium phosphate
Celestone Chronodose‡,
Celestone Soluspan

### betamethasone sodium phosphate
Celestone Phosphate, Selestoject

*Pregnancy Risk Category: NR*

### HOW SUPPLIED
**betamethasone**
*Tablets:* 600 mcg
*Tablets (effervescent):* 500 mcg†
*Syrup:* 600 mcg/5 ml
**betamethasone acetate and beta-
methasone sodium phosphate**
*Injection (suspension):* betamethasone
acetate 3 mg and betamethasone sodium phosphate (equivalent to 3-mg
base) per ml
**betamethasone sodium phosphate**
*Injection:* 4 mg (equivalent to 3-mg
base)/ml in 5-ml vials

### ACTION
Not completely defined. Decreases
inflammation, mainly by stabilizing
leukocyte lysosomal membranes; suppresses the immune response; stimulates bone marrow; and influences
protein, fat, and carbohydrate metabolism.

### ONSET, PEAK, DURATION
Onset prompt. Peak unknown. Duration variable but thought to persist for
3.25 days after oral administration, 7
to 14 days after parenteral administration.

Reactions may be *common,* uncommon, *life-threatening,* or COMMON AND LIFE-THREATENING.

## INDICATIONS & DOSAGE

*Conditions with severe inflammation; conditions requiring immunosuppression —*

**Adults:** 0.6 to 7.2 mg P.O. daily; or 0.5 to 9 mg I.M., I.V., or into joint or soft tissue daily; or 1.5 to 12 mg of sodium phosphate-acetate suspension into joint or soft tissue q 1 to 2 weeks, p.r.n.

## ADVERSE REACTIONS

Most adverse reactions to corticosteroids are dose- or duration-dependent.

**CNS:** *euphoria, insomnia,* psychotic behavior, pseudotumor cerebri, vertigo, headache, paresthesia, *seizures.*
**CV:** *CHF,* hypertension, edema, arrhythmias, thrombophlebitis, ***thromboembolism.***
**EENT:** cataracts, glaucoma.
**Endocrine:** menstrual irregularities, cushingoid state (moonface, buffalo hump, central obesity).
**GI:** *peptic ulceration,* GI irritation, increased appetite, pancreatitis, nausea, vomiting.
**Skin:** delayed wound healing, acne, various skin eruptions.
**Other:** muscle weakness, osteoporosis, hirsutism, susceptibility to infections; hypokalemia, hyperglycemia, and carbohydrate intolerance; growth suppression in children; *acute adrenal insufficiency may follow increased stress (infection, surgery, or trauma) or abrupt withdrawal after long-term therapy.*
**After abrupt withdrawal:** rebound inflammation, fatigue, weakness, arthralgia, fever, dizziness, lethargy, depression, fainting, orthostatic hypotension, dyspnea, anorexia, hypoglycemia. *After prolonged use, sudden withdrawal may be fatal.*

## INTERACTIONS

*Aspirin, indomethacin, and other NSAIDs:* increased risk of GI distress and bleeding. Give together cautiously.
*Barbiturates, phenytoin, rifampin:* decreased corticosteroid effect. Corticosteroid dosage may need to be increased.
*Oral anticoagulants:* altered dosage requirements. Monitor PT closely.
*Potassium-depleting drugs, such as thiazide diuretics:* enhanced potassium-wasting effects of betamethasone. Monitor serum potassium levels.
*Skin-test antigens:* decreased response. Defer skin testing until therapy is completed.
*Toxoids and vaccines:* decreased antibody response and increased risk of neurologic complications. Avoid concomitant use.

## CONTRAINDICATIONS

Contraindicated in patients hypersensitive to the drug and in those with viral or bacterial infections (except in life-threatening situations) or systemic fungal infections.

## NURSING CONSIDERATIONS

• Use with extreme caution in a patient with recent MI or peptic ulcer (used only in life-threatening situations).
• Use cautiously in patients with renal disease, hypertension, osteoporosis, diabetes mellitus, hypothyroidism, cirrhosis, diverticulitis, nonspecific ulcerative colitis, recent intestinal anastomoses, thromboembolic disorders, seizures, myasthenia gravis, CHF, tuberculosis, ocular herpes simplex, emotional instability, and psychotic tendencies. Because some formulations contain sulfite preservatives, also use cautiously in patients with hypersensitivity to sulfites.
• ***Alert:*** Know that drug should not be used for alternate-day therapy.
• Obtain baseline weight before starting therapy, and weigh patients daily;

---

report any sudden weight gain to the doctor.
- For better results and less toxicity, give a once-daily dose in the morning.
- To reduce GI irritation, give with milk or food.
- To prevent muscle atrophy, give I.M. injection deeply. Rotate injection sites.
- **I.V. use:** Compatible with 0.9% sodium chloride, $D_5W$, lactated Ringer's injection, dextrose 5% in lactated Ringer's injection, and dextrose 5% in Ringer's injection.
- Be aware that drug should always be titrated to lowest effective dose.
- Monitor blood glucose and serum potassium levels regularly, as ordered. Diabetic patients may require adjustments in insulin dosage.
- Monitor for depression or mood changes, especially in patients receiving long-term therapy.
- A calorie- or sodium-restricted diet with protein supplementation may be necessary for patients receiving long-term therapy.
- Know that elderly patients may be more susceptible to osteoporosis.
- Adrenal suppression may last up to 1 year after drug is stopped.
- Gradually reduce drug dosage after long-term therapy, as ordered.
- Observe for signs of infection, especially after steroid withdrawal.

☑ **PATIENT TEACHING**
- Tell patient not to stop drug abruptly or without the doctor's consent.
- Tell patient to take drug with food or milk; tell patient using effervescent tablets to dissolve them in water immediately before ingestion.
- Teach patient about the drug's effects. Warn patient on long-term therapy about cushingoid symptoms and to report sudden weight gain or swelling to the doctor.
- Make sure patient reports symptoms associated with corticosteroid

withdrawal, including fatigue, weakness, arthralgia, orthostatic hypotension, and dyspnea.
- Make sure patient understands to contact the doctor if symptoms are worsening or the medication is no longer effective. Tell patient not to increase dosage without the doctor's consent.
- Advise elderly patient receiving long-term therapy to consider exercise or physical therapy. Also tell him to ask his doctor about vitamin D or calcium supplement.
- Advise patients receiving prolonged therapy to have periodic ophthalmic examinations.
- Tell patient to report slow healing.
- Instruct patient to carry a card indicating his need for supplemental glucocorticoids during stress.

## cortisone acetate
Cortate‡, Cortone Acetate

*Pregnancy Risk Category: NR*

### HOW SUPPLIED
*Tablets:* 5 mg, 10 mg, 25 mg
*Injection (suspension):* 25 mg/ml, 50 mg/ml

### ACTION
Not completely defined. Decreases inflammation, mainly by stabilizing leukocyte lysosomal membranes; suppresses the immune response; stimulates bone marrow; and influences protein, fat, and carbohydrate metabolism.

### ONSET, PEAK, DURATION
Highly variable.

### INDICATIONS & DOSAGE
*Adrenal insufficiency, allergy, inflammation* –
**Adults:** 25 to 300 mg P.O. or 20 to 300 mg I.M. daily or on alternate days. Dosages are highly individual-

---

Reactions may be *common,* uncommon, *life-threatening,* or **COMMON AND LIFE-THREATENING.**

ized, depending on severity of disease.

## ADVERSE REACTIONS
Most adverse reactions to corticosteroids are dose- or duration-dependent.

**CNS:** *euphoria, insomnia,* psychotic behavior, pseudotumor cerebri, vertigo, headache, paresthesia, *seizures.*
**CV:** *CHF,* hypertension, edema, arrhythmias, thrombophlebitis, *thromboembolism.*
**EENT:** cataracts, glaucoma.
**Endocrine:** menstrual irregularities, cushingoid state (moonface, buffalo hump, central obesity).
**GI:** *peptic ulceration,* GI irritation, increased appetite, pancreatitis, nausea, vomiting.
**Skin:** delayed wound healing, acne, various skin eruptions; atrophy at I.M. injection sites.
**Other:** muscle weakness, osteoporosis, hirsutism, susceptibility to infections; possible hypokalemia, hyperglycemia, and carbohydrate intolerance; growth suppression in children; *acute adrenal insufficiency may follow increased stress (infection, surgery, or trauma) or abrupt withdrawal after long-term therapy.*
**After abrupt withdrawal:** rebound inflammation, fatigue, weakness, arthralgia, fever, dizziness, lethargy, depression, fainting, orthostatic hypotension, dyspnea, anorexia, hypoglycemia. *After prolonged use, sudden withdrawal may be fatal.*

## INTERACTIONS
*Aspirin, indomethacin, and other NSAIDS:* increased risk of GI distress and bleeding. Give together cautiously.
*Barbiturates, phenytoin, rifampin:* decreased corticosteroid effect. Increase corticosteroid dosage, as ordered.
*Live attenuated virus vaccines, other toxoids and vaccines:* decreased antibody response and increased risk of neurologic complications. Avoid concomitant use.
*Oral anticoagulants:* altered dosage requirements. Monitor PT closely.
*Potassium-depleting drugs, such as thiazide diuretics:* enhanced potassium-wasting effects of cortisone. Monitor serum potassium levels.
*Skin-test antigens:* decreased response. Defer skin testing until therapy is completed.

## CONTRAINDICATIONS
Contraindicated in patients with hypersensitivity to drug or any of its ingredients or systemic fungal infections.

## NURSING CONSIDERATIONS
• Use with extreme caution in a patient with recent MI.
• Use cautiously in patients with GI ulcer, renal disease, hypertension, osteoporosis, diabetes mellitus, hypothyroidism, cirrhosis, diverticulitis, nonspecific ulcerative colitis, recent intestinal anastomoses, thromboembolic disorders, seizures, myasthenia gravis, CHF, tuberculosis, ocular herpes simplex, emotional instability, and psychotic tendencies.
• To reduce GI irritation, give with milk or food.
• For better results and less toxicity, give a once-daily dose in the morning.
• I.M. route causes slow onset of action. Should not be used in acute conditions where a rapid effect is required. May be used on a twice-daily schedule matching diurnal variation. Rotate injection sites to prevent muscle atrophy.
• Mixing or diluting parenteral suspension may alter absorption rate and decrease the drug's effectiveness.
• **Alert:** Know that drug is not for I.V. use.
• Know that drug should always be titrated to lowest effective dose.
• Monitor serum electrolyte and blood glucose levels as ordered.

---

*Liquid form contains alcohol.   **May contain tartrazine.   †Canada only.   ‡Australia only.   ◊OTC.

• Monitor patient for fluid and electrolyte imbalances. Patients may need low-sodium diet and potassium supplements.

• Know that elderly patients may be more susceptible to osteoporosis.

• Gradually reduce drug dosage after long-term therapy, as ordered.

• Observe for signs of infection, especially after steroid withdrawal.

☑ **PATIENT TEACHING**

• Tell patient not to discontinue drug abruptly or without the doctor's consent.

• Instruct patient to take drug with milk or food.

• Advise patient receiving long-term therapy to consider exercise or physical therapy. Also tell him to ask his doctor about vitamin D or calcium supplement.

• Tell patient to report slow healing.

• Warn patient on long-term therapy about cushingoid symptoms and to report sudden weight gain or swelling to the doctor.

• Instruct patient to carry a card indicating his need for supplemental glucocorticoids during stress.

---

## dexamethasone

Decadron*, Deronil†, Dexamethasone Intensol*, Dexasone†, Dexone 0.5, Dexone 0.75, Dexone 1.5, Dexone 4, Hexadrol*, Mymethasone*

## dexamethasone acetate

Dalalone D.P., Dalalone L.A., Decadron-LA, Decaject-L.A., Dexacen LA-8, Dexasone-LA, Dexone LA, Solurex-LA

## dexamethasone sodium phosphate

Ak-Dex, Dalalone, Decadrol, Decadron Phosphate, Decaject, Dexacen-4, Dexone, Hexadrol Phosphate, Solurex

*Pregnancy Risk Category: NR*

### HOW SUPPLIED
**dexamethasone**
*Tablets:* 0.25 mg, 0.5 mg, 0.75 mg, 1 mg, 1.5 mg, 2 mg, 4 mg, 6 mg
*Oral solution:* 0.5 mg/5 ml, 1 mg/ml
*Elixir:* 0.5 mg/5 ml*
**dexamethasone acetate**
*Injection:* 8 mg/ml, 16 mg/ml suspension
**dexamethasone sodium phosphate**
*Injection:* 4 mg/ml, 10 mg/ml, 20 mg/ml, 24 mg/ml

### ACTION
Not clearly defined. Decreases inflammation, mainly by stabilizing leukocyte lysosomal membranes; suppresses the immune response; stimulates bone marrow; and influences protein, fat, and carbohydrate metabolism.

### ONSET, PEAK, DURATION
Onset occurs within 1 hour after I.M. or I.V. administration; 1 to 2 hours after oral administration. Peak effects occur within 1 hour after I.M. or I.V. administration, within 1 to 2 hours after oral administration, or within 8 hours after use of the injectable suspension (acetate). Effects persist about 2½ days after oral use, 6 days after I.M. use (acetate), and up to 3 weeks after intralesional or intra-articular use (acetate or sodium phosphate).

### INDICATIONS & DOSAGE
*Cerebral edema –*
**Adults:** initially, 10 mg (phosphate) I.V.; then 4 to 6 mg I.M. q 6 hours until symptoms subside (usually 2 to 4 days); then tapered over 5 to 7 days.

---

Reactions may be *common,* uncommon, *life-threatening,* or COMMON AND LIFE-THREATENING.

*Inflammatory conditions, allergic reactions, neoplasias –*
**Adults:** 0.75 to 9 mg/day P.O. or 0.5 to 9 mg/day (phosphate) I.M.; or 4 to 16 mg (acetate) I.M. into joint or soft tissue q 1 to 3 weeks; or 0.8 to 1.6 mg (acetate) into lesions q 1 to 3 weeks.
*Shock –*
**Adults:** 1 to 6 mg/kg (phosphate) I.V. as a single dose; or 40 mg I.V. q 2 to 6 hours, p.r.n.
*Dexamethasone suppression test for Cushing's syndrome –*
**Adults:** after determining baseline 24-hour urine levels of 17-hydroxycorticosteroids, 0.5 mg P.O. q 6 hours for 48 hours; 24-hour urine collection made for determination of 17-hydroxycorticosteroid excretion again during second 24 hours of dexamethasone administration.

## ADVERSE REACTIONS
Most adverse reactions to corticosteroids are dose- or duration-dependent.
**CNS:** *euphoria, insomnia,* psychotic behavior, pseudotumor cerebri, vertigo, headache, paresthesia, *seizures.*
**CV:** *CHF,* hypertension, edema, arrhythmias, thrombophlebitis, *thromboembolism.*
**EENT:** cataracts, glaucoma.
**Endocrine:** menstrual irregularities, cushingoid state (moonface, buffalo hump, central obesity).
**GI:** *peptic ulceration,* GI irritation, increased appetite, pancreatitis, nausea, vomiting.
**Skin:** delayed wound healing, acne, various skin eruptions; atrophy at I.M. injection sites.
**Other:** muscle weakness, osteoporosis, hirsutism, susceptibility to infections; hypokalemia, hyperglycemia, and carbohydrate intolerance; growth suppression in children; *acute adrenal insufficiency may follow increased stress (infection, surgery, or trauma) or abrupt withdrawal after long-term therapy.*

**After abrupt withdrawal:** rebound inflammation, fatigue, weakness, arthralgia, fever, dizziness, lethargy, depression, fainting, orthostatic hypotension, dyspnea, anorexia, hypoglycemia. *After prolonged use, sudden withdrawal may be fatal.*

## INTERACTIONS
*Aspirin, indomethacin, and other NSAIDs:* increased risk of GI distress and bleeding. Give together cautiously.
*Barbiturates, phenytoin, rifampin:* decreased corticosteroid effect. Increase corticosteroid dosage, as ordered.
*Oral anticoagulants:* altered dosage requirements. Monitor PT closely.
*Potassium-depleting drugs, such as thiazide diuretics:* enhanced potassium-wasting effects of dexamethasone. Monitor serum potassium levels.
*Skin-test antigens:* decreased response. Defer skin testing until therapy is completed.
*Toxoids and vaccines:* decreased antibody response and increased risk of neurologic complications. Avoid concomitant use.

## CONTRAINDICATIONS
Contraindicated in patients hypersensitive to any component of the drug and in those with systemic fungal infections.

## NURSING CONSIDERATIONS
• Use with extreme caution in patient with recent MI.
• Use cautiously in patients with GI ulcer, renal disease, hypertension, osteoporosis, diabetes mellitus, hypothyroidism, cirrhosis, diverticulitis, nonspecific ulcerative colitis, recent intestinal anastomoses, thromboembolic disorders, seizures, myasthenia gravis, CHF, tuberculosis, ocular herpes simplex, emotional instability, and psychotic tendencies. Because some formulations contain sulfite pre-

---

*Liquid form contains alcohol. **May contain tartrazine. †Canada only. ‡Australia only. ◇OTC.

servatives, also use cautiously in patients sensitive to sulfites.

• For better results and less toxicity, give a once-daily dose in the morning.

• Give oral dose with food when possible.

• Give I.M. injection deeply into gluteal muscle. Rotate injection sites to prevent muscle atrophy. Avoid S.C. injection because atrophy and sterile abscesses may occur.

• **I.V. use:** When administering as direct injection, inject undiluted over at least 1 minute. When administering as an intermittent or continuous infusion, dilute solution according to the manufacturer's instructions and give over the prescribed duration. If used for continuous infusion, change solution every 24 hours.

• Always titrate to lowest effective dose as ordered.

• Monitor patients' weight, blood pressure, and serum electrolyte levels.

• Watch for depression or psychotic episodes, especially in high-dose therapy.

• Diabetic patients may need increased insulin; monitor blood glucose levels.

• Know that drug may mask or exacerbate infections, including latent amebiasis.

• Know that elderly patients may be more susceptible to osteoporosis.

• Inspect patient's skin for petechiae.

• Gradually reduce drug dosage after long-term therapy as ordered.

☑ **PATIENT TEACHING**
• Tell patient not to discontinue drug abruptly or without the doctor's consent.

• Instruct patient to take drug with food or milk.

• Teach patient the signs of early adrenal insufficiency: fatigue, muscular weakness, joint pain, fever, anorexia, nausea, dyspnea, dizziness, and fainting.

• Instruct patient to carry a card indicating his need for supplemental sys-

temic glucocorticoids during stress, especially when dosage is decreased.

• Warn patient on long-term therapy about cushingoid symptoms and to report sudden weight gain or swelling to the doctor.

• Warn patient about easy bruising.

• Advise patient receiving long-term therapy to consider exercise or physical therapy. Give vitamin D or calcium supplement as ordered.

• Advise patient receiving long-term therapy to have periodic ophthalmic examinations.

# fludrocortisone acetate
Florinef

*Pregnancy Risk Category: C*

**HOW SUPPLIED**
*Tablets:* 0.1 mg

**ACTION**
Increases sodium reabsorption and potassium and hydrogen secretion at the nephrons' distal convoluted tubules.

**ONSET, PEAK, DURATION**
Onset variable. Peak levels occur in 1.7 hours. Effects persist for 1 to 2 days.

**INDICATIONS & DOSAGE**
*Adrenal insufficiency (partial replacement), adrenogenital syndrome* –
**Adults:** 0.1 to 0.2 mg P.O. daily.

**ADVERSE REACTIONS**
**CV:** *sodium and water retention,* hypertension, cardiac hypertrophy, edema, CHF.
**Skin:** bruising, diaphoresis, urticaria, or allergic rash.
**Other:** hypokalemia.

**INTERACTIONS**
*Potassium-depleting drugs, such as thiazide diuretics:* enhanced potassium-wasting effects of fludrocorti-

---

Reactions may be *common,* uncommon, *life-threatening,* or COMMON AND LIFE-THREATENING.

sone. Monitor serum potassium levels.

## CONTRAINDICATIONS
Contraindicated in patients with hypersensitivity to drug or in patients with systemic fungal infections.

## NURSING CONSIDERATIONS
• Use cautiously in patients with hypothyroidism, cirrhosis, ocular herpes simplex, emotional instability, and psychotic tendencies, nonspecific ulcerative colitis, diverticulitis, fresh intestinal anastomoses, active or latent peptic ulcer, renal insufficiency, hypertension, osteoporosis, and myasthenia gravis.
• Be aware that drug is used with cortisone or hydrocortisone in adrenal insufficiency.
• *Alert:* Monitor patient's blood pressure and serum electrolyte levels. If hypertension occurs, notify doctor and expect dosage to be decreased by 50%.
• Weigh patients daily; report sudden weight gain to the doctor.
• Unless contraindicated, give low-sodium diet that's high in potassium and protein. Be aware that potassium supplements may be needed.

☑ **PATIENT TEACHING**
• Tell patients to report worsening symptoms, such as hypotension, weakness, cramping, and palpitations, to the doctor.
• Warn patient that mild peripheral edema is common.

---

## hydrocortisone
Cortef, Cortenema, Hydrocortone

## hydrocortisone acetate
Cortifoam, Hydrocortone Acetate

## hydrocortisone cypionate
Cortef

## hydrocortisone sodium phosphate
Hydrocortone Phosphate

## hydrocortisone sodium succinate
A-hydroCort, Solu-Cortef
*Pregnancy Risk Category: NR*

## HOW SUPPLIED
**hydrocortisone**
*Tablets:* 5 mg, 10 mg, 20 mg
*Enema:* 100 mg/60 ml
**hydrocortisone acetate**
*Injection:* 25 mg/ml\*, 50 mg/ml\* suspension
*Enema:* 10% aerosol foam (provides 90 mg/application)
*Suppositories:* 25 mg
**hydrocortisone cypionate**
*Oral suspension:* 10 mg/5 ml
**hydrocortisone sodium phosphate**
*Injection:* 50 mg/ml solution
**hydrocortisone sodium succinate**
*Injection:* 100-mg vial\*, 250-mg vial\*, 500-mg vial\*, 1,000-mg vial\*

## ACTION
Not clearly defined. Decreases inflammation, mainly by stabilizing leukocyte lysosomal membranes; suppresses the immune response; stimulates bone marrow; and influences protein, fat, and carbohydrate metabolism.

## ONSET, PEAK, DURATION
Highly variable.

## INDICATIONS & DOSAGE
*Severe inflammation, adrenal insufficiency –*
**Adults:** 5 to 30 mg P.O. b.i.d., t.i.d., or q.i.d. (as much as 80 mg q.i.d. may be given in acute situations); or initially, 100 to 250 mg succinate I.M. or I.V., and then 50 to 100 mg I.M., as indicated; or 15 to 240 mg phosphate I.M. or I.V. q 12 hours; or 5 to 75 mg acetate into joints or soft tissue. Dosage varies with size of

---

\*Liquid form contains alcohol.  \*\*May contain tartrazine.  †Canada only.  ‡Australia only.  ◇OTC.

joint. Local anesthetics often are injected with dose.

*Shock—*

**Adults:** initially, 50 mg/kg succinate I.V., repeated in 4 hours. Repeat dosage q 24 hours as needed. Alternatively, 100 to 500 mg to 2 g q 2 to 6 hours.

**Children:** 186 to 280 mcg/kg phosphate or succinate I.M. or I.V. t.i.d.

*Adjunct for ulcerative colitis and proctitis—*

**Adults:** 1 enema (100 mg) P.R. nightly for 21 days. Alternatively, 1 applicator (90-mg foam) P.R. daily or b.i.d. for 14 to 21 days.

## ADVERSE REACTIONS

Most adverse reactions to corticosteroids are dose- or duration-dependent.

**CNS:** *euphoria, insomnia,* psychotic behavior, pseudotumor cerebri, vertigo, headache, paresthesia, *seizures.*
**CV:** *CHF,* hypertension, edema, arrhythmias, thrombophlebitis, thromboembolism.
**EENT:** cataracts, glaucoma.
**Endocrine:** menstrual irregularities, cushingoid state (moonface, buffalo hump, central obesity).
**GI:** *peptic ulceration,* GI irritation, increased appetite, pancreatitis, nausea, vomiting.
**Skin:** delayed wound healing, acne, various skin eruptions, easy bruising.
**Other:** muscle weakness, osteoporosis, hirsutism, susceptibility to infections; possible hypokalemia, hyperglycemia, and carbohydrate intolerance; growth suppression in children; *acute adrenal insufficiency may occur with increased stress (infection, surgery, or trauma) or abrupt withdrawal after long-term therapy.*
**After abrupt withdrawal:** rebound inflammation, fatigue, weakness, arthralgia, fever, dizziness, lethargy, depression, fainting, orthostatic hypotension, dyspnea, anorexia, hypo-

glycemia. *After prolonged use, sudden withdrawal may be fatal.*

## INTERACTIONS

*Aspirin, indomethacin, and other NSAIDs:* increased risk of GI distress and bleeding. Give together cautiously.
*Barbiturates, phenytoin, rifampin:* decreased corticosteroid effect. Increase corticosteroid dosage, as ordered.
*Live attenuated virus vaccines, other toxoids and vaccines:* decreased antibody response and increased risk of neurologic complications. Avoid concomitant use.
*Oral anticoagulants:* altered dosage requirements. Monitor PT closely.
*Potassium-depleting drugs, such as thiazide diuretics:* enhanced potassium-wasting effects of hydrocortisone. Monitor serum potassium levels.
*Skin-test antigens:* decreased response. Defer skin testing until therapy is completed.

## CONTRAINDICATIONS

Contraindicated in patients allergic to any component of the formulation, in those with systemic fungal infections, and in premature infants (succinate).

## NURSING CONSIDERATIONS

● Use with extreme caution in patient with recent MI.
● Use cautiously in patients with GI ulcer, renal disease, hypertension, osteoporosis, diabetes mellitus, hypothyroidism, cirrhosis, diverticulitis, nonspecific ulcerative colitis, recent intestinal anastomoses, thromboembolic disorders, seizures, myasthenia gravis, CHF, tuberculosis, ocular herpes simplex, emotional instability, and psychotic tendencies.
● For better results and less toxicity, give a once-daily dose in the morning.
● Give oral dose with food when possible.
● **I.V. use:** Do not use the acetate or suspension form for I.V. use. When

---

Reactions may be *common,* uncommon, *life-threatening,* or **COMMON AND LIFE-THREATENING.**

administering as direct injection, inject directly into vein or an I.V. line containing a free-flowing compatible solution over 30 seconds to several minutes. When administering as an intermittent or continuous infusion, dilute solution according to manufacturer's instructions, and give over the prescribed duration. If used for continuous infusion, change solution every 24 hours.

• Hydrocortisone sodium phosphate may be added directly to $D_5W$ or 0.9% sodium chloride for I.V. administration.

• Reconstitute hydrocortisone sodium succinate with bacteriostatic water or bacteriostatic sodium chloride solution before adding to I.V. solutions. When giving by direct I.V. injection, inject over at least 30 seconds. For infusion, dilute with $D_5W$, 0.9% sodium chloride, or dextrose 5% in 0.9% sodium chloride to a concentration of 1 mg/ml or less.

• Give I.M. injection deeply into gluteal muscle. Rotate injection sites to prevent muscle atrophy. Avoid S.C. injection because atrophy and sterile abscesses may occur.

• *Alert:* Do not confuse Solu-Cortef with Solu-Medrol (methylprednisolone sodium succinate).

• Know that injectable forms are not used for alternate-day therapy.

• Enema may produce same systemic effects as other forms of hydrocortisone. If enema therapy must exceed 21 days, discontinue gradually by reducing administration to every other night for 2 or 3 weeks, as ordered.

• Be aware high-dose therapy is usually not continued beyond 48 hours.

• Always titrate to lowest effective dose as ordered.

• Monitor patients' weight, blood pressure, and serum electrolyte levels.

• Unless contraindicated, give low-sodium diet that's high in potassium and protein. Administer potassium supplements as ordered.

• Know that drug may mask or exacerbate infections, including latent amebiasis.

• Stress (fever, trauma, surgery, and emotional problems) may increase adrenal insufficiency. Increase dosage, as ordered.

• Watch for depression or psychotic episodes, especially during high-dose therapy.

• Inspect patients' skin for petechiae.

• Diabetic patients may need increased insulin; monitor blood glucose levels.

• Periodic measurement of growth and development may be necessary during high-dose or prolonged therapy in children.

• Know that elderly patients may be more susceptible to osteoporosis.

• Gradually reduce drug dosage after long-term therapy, as ordered.

☑ **PATIENT TEACHING**
• Tell patient not to discontinue the drug abruptly or without the doctor's consent.

• Instruct patient to take oral form of drug with milk or food.

• Warn patient on long-term therapy about cushingoid symptoms and to report sudden weight gain or swelling to the doctor.

• Teach patient the signs of early adrenal insufficiency: fatigue, muscular weakness, joint pain, fever, anorexia, nausea, dyspnea, dizziness, and fainting.

• Instruct patient to carry a card identifying his need for supplemental systemic glucocorticoids during stress.

• Warn patient about easy bruising.

• Advise patient receiving long-term therapy to consider exercise or physical therapy. Also tell him to ask his doctor about vitamin D or calcium supplement.

• Advise patient receiving long-term therapy to have periodic ophthalmic examinations.

---

*Liquid form contains alcohol.   **May contain tartrazine.   †Canada only.   ‡Australia only.   ◇OTC.

## methylprednisolone
Medrol**, Meprolone

## methylprednisolone acetate
depMedalone-40, depMedalone-80, Depoject-40, Depoject-80, Depo-Medrol, Depopred-40, Depopred-80, Depo-Predate 40, Depo-Predate 80, Duralone-40, Duralone-80, Medralone-40, Medralone-80, Medrol Enpak, Rep-pred 40, Rep-pred 80

## methylprednisolone sodium succinate
A-metha-Pred, Solu-Medrol

*Pregnancy Risk Category: NR*

**HOW SUPPLIED**
**methylprednisolone**
*Tablets:* 2 mg, 4 mg, 8 mg, 16 mg, 24 mg, 32 mg
**methylprednisolone acetate**
*Injection (suspension):* 20 mg/ml, 40 mg/ml, 80 mg/ml
*Enema:* 40 mg
**methylprednisolone sodium succinate**
*Injection:* 40-mg vial, 125-mg vial, 500-mg vial, 1,000-mg vial, 2,000-mg vial

**ACTION**
Not clearly defined. Decreases inflammation, mainly by stabilizing leukocyte lysosomal membranes; suppresses the immune response; stimulates bone marrow; and influences protein, fat, and carbohydrate metabolism.

**ONSET, PEAK, DURATION**
Onset occurs rapidly after I.V. or oral administration; slowly (6 to 48 hours) after I.M. injection of acetate suspension. Peak effects occur immediately after I.V. injection, within 1 to 2 hours after oral administration, 4 to 8 days after I.M. use, or 7 days after intralesional or intra-articular administration. Effects persist for 30 to 36 hours after oral administration, 1 to 4 weeks after I.M. use, or 1 to 5 weeks after intralesional or intra-articular administration.

**INDICATIONS & DOSAGE**
*Severe inflammation or immunosuppression –*
**Adults:** 2 to 60 mg P.O. daily in four divided doses; 40 to 80 mg acetate I.M. daily, or 10 to 250 mg succinate I.M. or I.V. q 4 hours; or 4 to 30 mg acetate into joint or soft tissue p.r.n.
**Children:** 0.5 mg/kg succinate I.V. daily in divided doses.
*Shock –*
**Adults:** 100 to 250 mg succinate I.V. at 2- to 6-hour intervals; or 30 mg/kg I.V. initially, repeated q 4 to 6 hours p.r.n. Continue therapy for 2 to 3 days or until the patient is stable.
*Proctitis –*
**Adults:** 40 mg P.R. (as retention enema) or by continuous I.V. drip three to seven times a week for at least 2 weeks.
**Children:** 500 mcg to 1 mg/kg or 15 to 30 mg/m² P.R. q 1 to 2 days for at least 2 weeks.

**ADVERSE REACTIONS**
Most adverse reactions to corticosteroids are dose- or duration-dependent.
**CNS:** *euphoria, insomnia,* psychotic behavior, pseudotumor cerebri, vertigo, headache, paresthesia, *seizures.*
**CV:** *CHF,* hypertension, edema, arrhythmias, thrombophlebitis, *thromboembolism, fatal arrest or circulatory collapse* (following rapid administration of large I.V. doses).
**EENT:** cataracts, glaucoma.
**Endocrine:** menstrual irregularities, cushingoid state (moonface, buffalo hump, central obesity).
**GI:** *peptic ulceration,* GI irritation, increased appetite, pancreatitis, nausea, vomiting.

Reactions may be *common,* uncommon, *life-threatening,* or **COMMON AND LIFE-THREATENING.**

**Skin:** delayed wound healing, acne, various skin eruptions.

**Other:** muscle weakness, osteoporosis, hirsutism, susceptibility to infections; hypokalemia, hyperglycemia, and carbohydrate intolerance; growth suppression in children; *acute adrenal insufficiency may occur with increased stress (infection, surgery, or trauma) or abrupt withdrawal after long-term therapy.*

**After abrupt withdrawal:** rebound inflammation, fatigue, weakness, arthralgia, fever, dizziness, lethargy, depression, fainting, orthostatic hypotension, dyspnea, anorexia, hypoglycemia. *After prolonged use, sudden withdrawal may be fatal.*

## INTERACTIONS

*Aspirin, indomethacin, and other NSAIDs:* increased risk of GI distress and bleeding. Give together cautiously.

*Barbiturates, phenytoin, rifampin:* decreased corticosteroid effect. Increase corticosteroid dosage, as ordered.

*Oral anticoagulants:* altered dosage requirements. Monitor PT closely.

*Potassium-depleting drugs, such as thiazide diuretics:* enhanced potassium-wasting effects of methylprednisolone. Monitor serum potassium levels.

*Skin-test antigens:* decreased response. Defer skin testing until therapy is completed.

*Toxoids and vaccines:* decreased antibody response and increased risk of neurologic complications. Avoid concomitant use.

## CONTRAINDICATIONS

Contraindicated in patients allergic to any component of the formulation, in those with systemic fungal infections and in premature infants (acetate and succinate).

## NURSING CONSIDERATIONS

● Use cautiously in patients with GI ulceration or renal disease, hypertension, osteoporosis, diabetes mellitus, hypothyroidism, cirrhosis, diverticulitis, nonspecific ulcerative colitis, recent intestinal anastomoses, thromboembolic disorders, seizures, myasthenia gravis, CHF, tuberculosis, ocular herpes simplex, emotional instability, and psychotic tendencies.

● Know that drug may be used for alternate-day therapy..

● For better results and less toxicity, give a once-daily dose in the morning.

● Give oral dose with food when possible. Know that critically ill patients may require concomitant antacid or histamine-2-receptor antagonist therapy.

● **I.V. use:** Use only methylprednisolone sodium succinate; never use acetate form for I.V. use. Reconstitute according to the manufacturer's directions using the supplied diluent, or use bacteriostatic water for injection with benzyl alcohol.

● When administering as direct injection, inject diluted drug into a vein or free-flowing compatible I.V. solution over at least 1 minute. For treatment of shock, give massive doses over at least 10 minutes to prevent arrhythmias and circulatory collapse. When administering as an intermittent or continuous infusion, dilute solution according to the manufacturer's instructions, and give over the prescribed duration. If used for continuous infusion, change solution every 24 hours.

● Compatible solutions include $D_5W$, 0.9% sodium chloride, and dextrose 5% in 0.9% sodium chloride.

● Do not confuse Solu-Medrol with Solu-Cortef (hydrocortisone sodium succinate).

● *Alert:* The manufacturers of Solu-Medrol state that the drug should not be given intrathecally because severe adverse reactions have been reported.

---

*Liquid form contains alcohol.   **May contain tartrazine.   †Canada only.   ‡Australia only.   ◇OTC.

• Give I.M. injection deeply into gluteal muscle. Avoid S.C. injection because atrophy and sterile abscesses may occur.

• Dermal atrophy may occur with large doses of acetate salt. Use multiple small injections rather than a single large dose and rotate injection sites.

• Don't use acetate salt when immediate onset of action is needed.

• Discard reconstituted solutions after 48 hours.

• Always titrate to lowest effective dose, as ordered.

• Monitor patients' weight, blood pressure, serum electrolyte levels, and sleep patterns. Euphoria may initially interfere with sleep, but patients generally adjust to the medication after 1 to 3 weeks.

• Know that drug may mask or exacerbate infections, including latent amebiasis.

• Watch for depression or psychotic episodes, especially in high-dose therapy.

• Diabetic patients may need increased insulin; monitor blood glucose levels.

• Watch for an enhanced response to drug in patients with hypothyroidism or cirrhosis.

• Unless contraindicated, give low-sodium diet that's high in potassium and protein. Administer potassium supplements as needed.

• Know that elderly patients may be more susceptible to osteoporosis.

• Gradually reduce drug dosage after long-term therapy, as ordered.

☑ **PATIENT TEACHING**
• Tell patient not to discontinue drug abruptly or without the doctor's consent.

• Instruct patient to take oral form of drug with milk or food.

• Teach patient the signs of early adrenal insufficiency: fatigue, muscular weakness, joint pain, fever, anorexia, nausea, dyspnea, dizziness, and fainting.

• Instruct patient to carry a card identifying his need for supplemental systemic glucocorticoids during stress.

• Warn patient on long-term therapy about cushingoid symptoms and to report sudden weight gain or swelling to the doctor.

• Advise patient receiving long-term therapy to consider exercise or physical therapy. Also tell patient to ask doctor about vitamin D or calcium supplement.

# prednisolone
Delta-Cortef, Deltasolone‡, Panafcortelone‡, Prelone, Solone‡

# prednisolone acetate
Articulose-50, Key-Pred 25, Key-Pred 50, Predaject-50, Predalone 50, Predate 50, Predcor-25, Predcor-50, Predicort-50

# prednisolone sodium phosphate
Hydeltrasol, Key-Pred-SP, Pediapred, Predate-S, Predicort RP, Predsol Retention Enema‡, Predsol Suppositories‡

# prednisolone steaglate
Sintisone‡

# prednisolone tebutate
Hydeltra-TBA, Nor-Pred TBA, Predalone TBA, Predate TBA, Predcor TBA

*Pregnancy Risk Category: NR*

**HOW SUPPLIED**
**prednisolone**
*Tablets:* 1 mg‡, 5 mg, 25 mg‡
*Syrup:* 15 mg/5 ml
**prednisolone acetate**
*Injection (suspension):* 25 mg/ml, 50 mg/ml, 100 mg/ml
**prednisolone sodium phosphate**
*Oral solution:* 5 mg/5 ml

---

Reactions may be *common,* uncommon, *life-threatening*, or **COMMON AND LIFE-THREATENING.**

*Injection:* 20 mg/ml
*Retention enema:* 20 mg/100 ml‡
*Suppositories:* 5 mg‡
**prednisolone steaglate**
*Tablets:* 6.65 mg (equal to 3.5 mg prednisolone)‡
**prednisolone tebutate**
*Injection (suspension):* 20 mg/ml

## ACTION
Not clearly defined. Decreases inflammation, mainly by stabilizing leukocyte lysosomal membranes; suppresses the immune response; stimulates bone marrow; and influences protein, fat, and carbohydrate metabolism.

## ONSET, PEAK, DURATION
Onset occurs rapidly after I.V., I.M., or oral administration; 1 to 2 days after intralesional or intra-articular use of tebutate suspension. Peak levels occur within 1 hour after I.M. or I.V. injection or within 1 to 2 hours after oral administration. Effects persist for 30 to 36 hours after oral use; up to 4 weeks after I.M. use, or 3 days to 4 weeks after intralesional or intra-articular use.

## INDICATIONS & DOSAGE
*Severe inflammation or immunosuppression –*
**Adults:** 2.5 to 15 mg P.O. b.i.d., t.i.d., or q.i.d.; 2 to 30 mg I.M. (acetate, phosphate) or I.V. (phosphate) q 12 hours; or 2 to 30 mg (phosphate) into joints, lesions, or soft tissue; or 4 to 40 mg (tebutate) into joints and lesions p.r.n.
*Proctitis‡ –*
**Adults:** 1 suppository b.i.d., preferably in the morning and h.s.
*Ulcerative colitis‡ –*
**Adults:** 1 retention enema h.s. nightly for 2 to 4 weeks. The contents of the enema should be retained overnight.

## ADVERSE REACTIONS
Most adverse reactions to corticosteroids are dose- or duration-dependent.
**CNS:** *euphoria, insomnia,* psychotic behavior, pseudotumor cerebri, vertigo, headache, paresthesia, *seizures.*
**CV:** *CHF,* hypertension, edema, arrhythmias, thrombophlebitis, ***thromboembolism.***
**EENT:** cataracts, glaucoma.
**Endocrine:** menstrual irregularities, cushingoid state (moonface, buffalo hump, central obesity).
**GI:** *peptic ulceration,* GI irritation, increased appetite, pancreatitis, nausea, vomiting.
**Skin:** delayed wound healing, acne, various skin eruptions.
**Other:** muscle weakness, osteoporosis, hirsutism, susceptibility to infections; hypokalemia, hyperglycemia, and carbohydrate intolerance; growth suppression in children; ***acute adrenal insufficiency may occur with increased stress (infection, surgery, or trauma) or abrupt withdrawal after long-term therapy.***
**After abrupt withdrawal:** rebound inflammation, fatigue, weakness, arthralgia, fever, dizziness, lethargy, depression, fainting, orthostatic hypotension, dyspnea, anorexia, hypoglycemia. *After prolonged use, sudden withdrawal may be fatal.*

## INTERACTIONS
*Aspirin, indomethacin, and other NSAIDs:* increased risk of GI distress and bleeding. Give together cautiously.
*Barbiturates, phenytoin, rifampin:* decreased corticosteroid effect. Increase corticosteroid dosage, as ordered.
*Oral anticoagulants:* altered dosage requirements. Monitor PT closely.
*Potassium-depleting drugs, such as thiazide diuretics:* enhanced potas-

---

sium-wasting effects of prednisolone. Monitor serum potassium levels.
*Skin-test antigens:* decreased response. Defer skin testing until therapy is completed.
*Toxoids and vaccines:* decreased antibody response and increased risk of neurologic complications. Avoid concomitant use.

## CONTRAINDICATIONS
Contraindicated in patients with hypersensitivity to drug or any of its ingredients and systemic fungal infections.

## NURSING CONSIDERATIONS
• Use with extreme caution in a patient with recent MI.
• Use cautiously in patients with GI ulcer, renal disease, hypertension, osteoporosis, diabetes mellitus, hypothyroidism, cirrhosis, diverticulitis, nonspecific ulcerative colitis, recent intestinal anastomoses, thromboembolic disorders, seizures, myasthenia gravis, CHF, tuberculosis, ocular herpes simplex, emotional instability, and psychotic tendencies.
• *Alert:* Don't confuse with prednisone.
• Always titrate to lowest effective dose, as ordered.
• Be aware that prednisolone salts (acetate, sodium phosphate, and tebutate) are used parenterally less often than other corticosteroids that have more potent anti-inflammatory action.
• Know that drug may be used for alternate-day therapy.
• Give oral dose with food when possible to reduce GI irritation.
• Give I.M. injection deeply into gluteal muscle. Rotate injection sites to prevent muscle atrophy. Avoid S.C. injection because atrophy and sterile abscesses may occur.
• **I.V. use:** Use only prednisolone sodium phosphate; never give acetate form I.V. When administering as di-

rect injection, inject undiluted over at least 1 minute. When administering as an intermittent or continuous infusion, dilute solution according to the manufacturer's instructions, and give over the prescribed duration. $D_5W$ or 0.9% sodium chloride are recommended as diluents for I.V. infusions.
• Monitor patients' weight, blood pressure, and serum electrolyte levels.
• Watch for depression or psychotic episodes, especially in high-dose therapy.
• Diabetic patients may need increased insulin; monitor blood glucose levels.
• Unless contraindicated, give low-sodium diet that's high in potassium and protein. Administer potassium supplements as needed.
• Know that drug may mask or exacerbate infections, including latent amebiasis.
• Know that elderly patients may be more susceptible to osteoporosis.
• Gradually reduce drug dosage after long-term therapy as ordered.

## ☑ PATIENT TEACHING
• Tell patient not to discontinue drug abruptly or without the doctor's consent.
• Instruct patient to take oral form of drug with food or milk.
• Teach patient the signs of early adrenal insufficiency: fatigue, muscular weakness, joint pain, fever, anorexia, nausea, dyspnea, dizziness, and fainting.
• Instruct patient to carry a card identifying his need for supplemental systemic glucocorticoids during stress.
• Warn patient on long-term therapy about cushingoid symptoms and to report sudden weight gain or swelling to the doctor.
• Tell patient to report slow healing.
• Advise patient receiving long-term therapy to consider exercise or physical therapy. Also tell patient to ask

---

doctor about vitamin D or calcium supplement.

## prednisone
Apo-Prednisone†, Deltasone, Liquid Pred*, Meticorten, Novo-prednisone†, Orasone, Panafcort‡, Panasol, Prednicen-M, Prednisone Intensol*, Sone‡, Sterapred, Winpred†

*Pregnancy Risk Category: NR*

### HOW SUPPLIED
*Tablets:* 1 mg, 2.5 mg, 5 mg, 10 mg, 20 mg, 25 mg, 50 mg
*Oral solution:* 5 mg/5 ml*, 5 mg/ml (concentrate)*
*Syrup:* 5 mg/5 ml*

### ACTION
Not clearly defined. Decreases inflammation, mainly by stabilizing leukocyte lysosomal membranes; suppresses the immune response; stimulates bone marrow; and influences protein, fat, and carbohydrate metabolism.

### ONSET, PEAK, DURATION
Variable.

### INDICATIONS & DOSAGE
*Severe inflammation or immunosuppression –*
**Adults:** 5 to 60 mg P.O. daily in divided doses. Maintenance dosage given once daily or every other day. Dosage must be individualized.
*Acute exacerbations of multiple sclerosis –*
**Adults:** 200 mg P.O. daily for 1 week; then 80 mg P.O. every other day for 1 month.

### ADVERSE REACTIONS
Most adverse reactions to corticosteroids are dose- or duration-dependent.
**CNS:** *euphoria, insomnia,* psychotic behavior, pseudotumor cerebri, vertigo, headache, paresthesia, *seizures.*
**CV:** *CHF,* hypertension, edema, arrhythmias, thrombophlebitis, ***thromboembolism.***
**EENT:** cataracts, glaucoma.
**Endocrine:** menstrual irregularities, cushingoid state (moonface, buffalo hump, central obesity).
**GI:** *peptic ulceration,* GI irritation, increased appetite, pancreatitis, nausea, vomiting.
**Skin:** delayed wound healing, acne, various skin eruptions.
**Other:** muscle weakness, osteoporosis, hirsutism, susceptibility to infections; hypokalemia, hyperglycemia, and carbohydrate intolerance; growth suppression in children; *acute adrenal insufficiency may occur with increased stress (infection, surgery, or trauma) or abrupt withdrawal after long-term therapy.*
**After abrupt withdrawal:** rebound inflammation, fatigue, weakness, arthralgia, fever, dizziness, lethargy, depression, fainting, orthostatic hypotension, dyspnea, anorexia, hypoglycemia. *After prolonged use, sudden withdrawal may be fatal.*

### INTERACTIONS
*Aspirin, indomethacin, and other NSAIDs:* increased risk of GI distress and bleeding. Give together cautiously.
*Barbiturates, phenytoin, rifampin:* decreased corticosteroid effect. Increase corticosteroid dosage, as ordered.
*Oral anticoagulants:* altered dosage requirements. Monitor PT closely.
*Potassium-depleting drugs, such as thiazide diuretics:* enhanced potassium-wasting effects of prednisone. Monitor serum potassium levels.
*Skin-test antigens:* decreased response. Defer skin testing until therapy is completed.
*Toxoids and vaccines:* decreased antibody response and increased risk of

---

*Liquid form contains alcohol.  **May contain tartrazine.  †Canada only.  ‡Australia only.  ◊OTC.

neurologic complications. Avoid concomitant use.

**CONTRAINDICATIONS**
Contraindicated in patients with hypersensitivity to drug or systemic fungal infections.

**NURSING CONSIDERATIONS**
• Use cautiously in patients with GI ulcer, renal disease, hypertension, osteoporosis, diabetes mellitus, hypothyroidism, cirrhosis, diverticulitis, nonspecific ulcerative colitis, recent intestinal anastomoses, thromboembolic disorders, seizures, myasthenia gravis, CHF, tuberculosis, ocular herpes simplex, emotional instability, and psychotic tendencies.
• *Alert:* Don't confuse with prednisolone.
• Know that drug may be used for alternate-day therapy.
• Always titrate to lowest effective dose as ordered.
• For better results and less toxicity, give a once-daily dose in the morning.
• Unless contraindicated, give oral dose with food when possible to reduce GI irritation.
• Monitor patients' blood pressure, sleep patterns, and serum potassium levels.
• Weigh patients daily; report sudden weight gain to the doctor.
• Watch for depression or psychotic episodes, especially in high-dose therapy.
• Diabetic patients may need increased insulin; monitor blood glucose levels.
• Know that elderly patients may be more susceptible to osteoporosis.
• Know that drug may mask or exacerbate infections, including latent amebiasis.
• Unless contraindicated, give lowsodium diet that's high in potassium and protein. Administer potassium supplements as needed.

• Gradually reduce drug dosage after long-term therapy, as ordered.

☑ **PATIENT TEACHING**
• Tell patient not to discontinue drug abruptly or without the doctor's consent.
• Instruct patient to take drug with food or milk.
• Teach patient signs of early adrenal insufficiency: fatigue, muscular weakness, joint pain, fever, anorexia, nausea, dyspnea, dizziness, and fainting.
• Instruct patient to carry a card identifying his need for supplemental systemic glucocorticoids during stress.
• Warn patient on long-term therapy about cushingoid symptoms and to report sudden weight gain or swelling to the doctor.
• Advise patient receiving long-term therapy to consider exercise or physical therapy. Also tell patient to ask doctor about vitamin D or calcium supplement.
• Tell patient to report slow healing.
• Advise patient receiving long-term therapy to have periodic ophthalmic examinations.

# triamcinolone
Aristocort, Atolone, Kenacort**

# triamcinolone acetonide
Cenocort A-40, Cinonide 40, Kenaject-40, Kenalog-10, Kenalog-40, Tac-3, Triam-A, Triamonide 40, Tri-Kort, Trilog

# triamcinolone diacetate
Amcort, Aristocort, Aristocort Forte, Aristocort Intralesional, Articulose-L.A., Cenocort Forte, Cinalone 40, Kenacort Diacetate, Triam-Forte, Triamolone 40, Trilone, Tristoject

# triamcinolone hexacetonide

Aristospan Intra-articular,
Aristospan Intralesional

*Pregnancy Risk Category: C*

## HOW SUPPLIED
**triamcinolone**
*Tablets:* 1 mg, 2 mg, 4 mg, 8 mg
**triamcinolone acetonide**
*Injection (suspension):* 3 mg/ml, 10 mg/ml, 40 mg/ml
**triamcinolone diacetate**
*Injection (suspension):* 25 mg/ml, 40 mg/ml
*Syrup:* 2 mg/5 ml, 4 mg/5 ml
**triamcinolone hexacetonide**
*Injection (suspension):* 5 mg/ml, 20 mg/ml

## ACTION
Not clearly defined. Decreases inflammation, mainly by stabilizing leukocyte lysosomal membranes; suppresses the immune response; stimulates bone marrow; and influences protein, fat, and carbohydrate metabolism.

## ONSET, PEAK, DURATION
Highly variable.

## INDICATIONS & DOSAGE
*Severe inflammation or immunosuppression –*
**Adults:** 4 to 48 mg P.O. daily in divided doses; 40 mg I.M. (diacetate, acetonide) weekly; 5 to 48 mg (diacetate) or 1 mg (acetonide) into lesions; 2 to 40 mg (diacetate) or 2.5 to 40 mg (acetonide) into joints or soft tissue; up to 0.5 mg (hexacetonide) per square inch of affected skin intralesionally; or 2 to 20 mg (hexacetonide) by intra-articular or intrasynovial use into soft tissue or into joint or lesion. A local anesthetic often is injected along with triamcinolone into the joint.

## ADVERSE REACTIONS
Most adverse reactions to corticosteroids are dose- or duration-dependent.
**CNS:** *euphoria, insomnia,* psychotic behavior, pseudotumor cerebri, vertigo, headache, paresthesia, *seizures.*
**CV:** *CHF,* hypertension, edema, arrhythmias, thrombophlebitis, ***thromboembolism.***
**EENT:** cataracts, glaucoma.
**Endocrine:** menstrual irregularities, cushingoid state (moonface, buffalo hump, central obesity).
**GI:** *peptic ulceration,* GI irritation, increased appetite, pancreatitis, nausea, vomiting.
**Skin:** delayed wound healing, acne, various skin eruptions.
**Other:** muscle weakness, osteoporosis, hirsutism, susceptibility to infections; hypokalemia, hyperglycemia, and carbohydrate intolerance; growth suppression in children; *acute adrenal insufficiency may occur with increased stress (infection, surgery, or trauma) or abrupt withdrawal after long-term therapy.*
**After abrupt withdrawal:** rebound inflammation, fatigue, weakness, arthralgia, fever, dizziness, lethargy, depression, fainting, orthostatic hypotension, dyspnea, anorexia, hypoglycemia. *After prolonged use, sudden withdrawal may be fatal.*

## INTERACTIONS
*Aspirin, indomethacin, and other NSAIDs:* increased risk of GI distress and bleeding. Give together cautiously.
*Barbiturates, phenytoin, rifampin:* decreased corticosteroid effect. Increase corticosteroid dosage, as ordered.
*Oral anticoagulants:* altered dosage requirements. Monitor PT closely.
*Potassium-depleting drugs, such as thiazide diuretics:* enhanced potassium-wasting effects of triamcinolone. Monitor serum potassium levels.
*Skin-test antigens:* decreased re-

---

*Liquid form contains alcohol.    **May contain tartrazine.    †Canada only.    ‡Australia only.    ◊OTC.

sponse. Defer skin testing until therapy is completed.
*Toxoids and vaccines:* decreased antibody response and increased risk of neurologic complications. Avoid concomitant use.

## CONTRAINDICATIONS

Contraindicated in patients hypersensitive to any component of the formulation or in those with systemic fungal infections.

## NURSING CONSIDERATIONS

• Use cautiously in patients with GI ulcer, renal disease, hypertension, osteoporosis, diabetes mellitus, hypothyroidism, cirrhosis, diverticulitis, nonspecific ulcerative colitis, recent intestinal anastomoses, thromboembolic disorders, seizures, myasthenia gravis, CHF, tuberculosis, ocular herpes simplex, emotional instability, and psychotic tendencies.
• Know that drug is not used for alternate-day therapy.
• Always titrate to lowest effective dose, as ordered.
• For better results and less toxicity, give a once-daily dose in the morning.
• Give oral dose with food when possible to reduce GI irritation.
• Parenteral form is *not* for I.V. use.
• Don't use diluents that contain preservatives; flocculation may occur.
• Give I.M. injection deeply into gluteal muscle. Rotate injection sites to prevent muscle atrophy.
• Monitor patients' weight, blood pressure, and serum electrolyte levels.
• Watch for depression or psychotic episodes, especially in high-dose therapy.
• Diabetic patients may need increased insulin; monitor blood glucose levels.
• Know that drug may mask or exacerbate infections, including latent amebiasis.
• Know that elderly patients may be more susceptible to osteoporosis.

• Unless contraindicated, give low-sodium diet that's high in potassium and protein. Administer potassium supplements as needed.
• Gradually reduce drug dosage after long-term therapy, as ordered.

## ☑ PATIENT TEACHING

• Tell patient not to discontinue drug abruptly or without the doctor's consent.
• Instruct patient to take drug with food or milk.
• Teach patient the signs of early adrenal insufficiency: fatigue, muscular weakness, joint pain, fever, anorexia, nausea, dyspnea, dizziness, and fainting.
• Instruct patient to carry a card identifying his need for supplemental systemic glucocorticoids during stress.
• Warn patient on long-term therapy about cushingoid symptoms and to report sudden weight gain and swelling to the doctor.
• Tell patient to report slow healing.
• Advise patient receiving long-term therapy to consider exercise or physical therapy. Also tell patient to ask doctor about vitamin D or calcium supplement.

---

Reactions may be *common,* uncommon, *life-threatening,* or COMMON AND LIFE-THREATENING.

# 54

## Androgens and anabolic steroids

danazol
fluoxymesterone
methyltestosterone
nandrolone decanoate
nandrolone phenpropionate
oxandrolone
oxymetholone
stanozolol
testosterone
testosterone cypionate
testosterone enanthate
testosterone propionate
testosterone transdermal system

### COMBINATION PRODUCTS

ANDROGYN L.A., DELADUMONE, VAL-
ERTEST NO. 1: testosterone enanthate
90 mg/ml and estradiol valerate 4 mg/
ml in sesame oil.
DEPANDROGEN, DEPO-TESTADIOL,
DEPOTESTOGEN, DUO-CYP, DURATES-
TRIN, TEST EST CYP (oil): testosterone
cypionate 50 mg and estradiol cypionate 2 mg.
ESTRATEST: esterified estrogens 1.25
mg and methyltestosterone 2.5 mg.
ESTRATEST H.S.: esterified estrogens
0.625 mg and methyltestosterone
1.25 mg.
HALODRIN: fluoxymesterone 1 mg
with ethinyl estradiol 0.02 mg.
PREMARIN WITH METHYLTESTOSTER-
ONE: conjugated estrogens 0.625 mg
and methyltestosterone 5 mg; or conjugated estrogens 1.25 mg and methyltestosterone 10 mg.

---

### danazol
Cyclomen†, Danocrine

*Pregnancy Risk Category: X*

### HOW SUPPLIED
*Capsules:* 50 mg, 100 mg, 200 mg

### ACTION
Not clearly defined. Gonadotropin inhibitor that suppresses the pituitary-
ovarian axis and inhibits estrogenic
effects.

### ONSET, PEAK, DURATION
Onset for pain relief in fibrocystic
breast disease occurs within 1 month.
Unknown for other indications. Peak
effects occur in 6 to 8 weeks when
treating endometriosis and in 2 to 3
months when treating fibrocystic
breast disease. Unknown for treatment of angioedema. Duration variable.

### INDICATIONS & DOSAGE
*Mild endometriosis –*
**Women:** initially, 100 to 200 mg P.O.
b.i.d. Subsequent dosage based on
patient response.
*Moderate to severe endometriosis –*
**Women:** 400 mg P.O. b.i.d. uninterrupted for 3 to 6 months; may be continued for 9 months.
*Fibrocystic breast disease –*
**Women:** 100 to 400 mg P.O. daily in
two divided doses uninterrupted for 2
to 6 months.
*Prevention of hereditary angio-
edema –*
**Adults:** 200 mg P.O. b.i.d to t.i.d.,
continued until favorable response is
achieved. Then dosage decreased by
50% at 1- to 3-month intervals.

### ADVERSE REACTIONS
**CNS:** dizziness, headache, sleep dis-
orders, fatigue, tremor, irritability,
excitation, lethargy, mental depres-
sion, chills, paresthesia.
**CV:** elevated blood pressure.
**EENT:** visual disturbances.
**GI:** gastric irritation, nausea, vomit-

---

*Liquid form contains alcohol.   **May contain tartrazine.   †Canada only.   ‡Australia only.   ◇OTC.

ing, diarrhea, constipation, change in appetite.

**GU:** hematuria, *hypoestrogenic effects (flushing, diaphoresis, vaginitis [including itching, dryness, and burning]; vaginal bleeding, nervousness, emotional lability, menstrual irregularities).*

**Hepatic:** reversible jaundice, elevated liver enzyme levels, hepatic dysfunction.

**Other:** muscle cramps or spasms; androgenic effects in women *(weight gain, hirsutism,* hoarseness, clitoral enlargement, *decreased breast size,* acne, edema, changes in libido, *oily skin or hair,* voice deepening).

### INTERACTIONS
*Carbamazepine:* may increase carbamazepine levels. Monitor carbamazepine levels closely.
*Warfarin:* May prolong PT in patients stabilized on warfarin. Monitor PT.

### CONTRAINDICATIONS
Contraindicated in patients with undiagnosed abnormal genital bleeding; porphyria; or impaired renal, cardiac, or hepatic function; during pregnancy; and in breast-feeding patients.

### NURSING CONSIDERATIONS
• Use cautiously in patients with seizure disorders or migraine headache.
• **Alert:** Avoid use in women of childbearing age until pregnancy is ruled out.
• Unless contraindicated, use with diet high in calories and protein.
• Monitor closely for signs of virilization. Some androgenic effects, such as deepening of voice, may not be reversible upon discontinuation of drug.
• Periodically evaluate hepatic function as ordered. Semen evaluation is routinely performed every 3 to 4 months, especially in adolescent boys.
• Know that periodic dosage decreases or gradual drug withdrawal is best.

• After withdrawal of treatment, ovulation and cyclic menstrual bleeding usually return in 2 to 3 months; fibrocystic disease symptoms return within 1 year for 50% of patients.

### ☑ PATIENT TEACHING
• Advise patient taking danazol for fibrocystic breast disease to examine breasts regularly and to call the doctor immediately if breast nodules enlarge during treatment.
• Make sure patient understands the importance of using an effective nonhormonal contraceptive during therapy.
• Instruct patient to report adverse reactions, especially signs of virilization, promptly.
• Advise washing after intercourse to decrease the risk of vaginitis. Instruct patient to wear only cotton underwear.

## fluoxymesterone
Android-F, Halotestin**
Controlled Substance Schedule III
*Pregnancy Risk Category: X*

### HOW SUPPLIED
*Tablets:* 2 mg, 5 mg, 10 mg

### ACTION
Stimulates target tissues to develop normally in androgen-deficient men.

### ONSET, PEAK, DURATION
Unknown.

### INDICATIONS & DOSAGE
*Hypogonadism caused by testicular deficiency* –
**Adults:** 5 to 20 mg P.O. daily.
*Delayed puberty* –
**Adolescent:** highly individualized; duration of therapy 4 to 6 months.
*Palliation of breast cancer in women* –
**Adults:** 10 to 40 mg P.O. daily in divided doses. All dosages are individu-

alized and reduced to minimum when effect is noted.

**ADVERSE REACTIONS**
**CNS:** headache, anxiety, depression, paresthesia, sleep apnea syndrome.
**CV:** edema.
**GI:** nausea.
**GU:** *hypoestrogenic effects in women (flushing; diaphoresis; vaginitis, including itching, dryness, and burning; vaginal bleeding; nervousness; emotional lability; menstrual irregularities); excessive hormonal effects in men (prepubertal – premature epiphyseal closure, acne,* priapism, *growth of body and facial hair,* phallic enlargement; postpubertal – testicular atrophy, oligospermia, decreased ejaculatory volume, impotence, gynecomastia, epididymitis).
**Hematologic:** polycythemia, elevated serum lipid levels, suppression of clotting factors.
**Hepatic:** reversible jaundice, peliosis hepatis, elevated liver enzyme levels, *liver cell tumors.*
**Other:** hypercalcemia; hypersensitivity skin manifestations; androgenic effects in women (acne, edema, *weight gain, hirsutism,* hoarseness, clitoral enlargement, deepening voice, *decreased breast size,* changes in libido, male-pattern baldness, *oily skin or hair).*

**INTERACTIONS**
*Hepatotoxic medications:* increased risk of hepatotoxicity. Monitor closely.
*Insulin, oral antidiabetic agents:* altered dosage requirements. Monitor blood glucose levels in diabetic patients.
*Oral anticoagulants:* altered dosage requirements. Monitor PT.

**CONTRAINDICATIONS**
Contraindicated in patients with hypersensitivity to drug, in males with breast cancer or prostate cancer, in those with cardiac, hepatic, or renal decompensation; during pregnancy; and in breast-feeding patients.

**NURSING CONSIDERATIONS**
• Use cautiously in prepubertal males, benign prostatic hyperplasia, and aspirin sensitivity.
• *Alert:* Avoid use in women of childbearing age until pregnancy is ruled out.
• Unless contraindicated, use with diet high in calories and protein. Give small, frequent feedings.
• Watch for symptoms of jaundice and periodically evaluate hepatic function, as ordered. Dosage adjustment may reverse condition. If liver function test results are abnormal, notify doctor because therapy should be stopped.
• Know that edema can be controlled with sodium restriction or diuretics. Monitor weight routinely.
• Monitor male patients for signs of excessive sexual stimulation or priapism.
• Be aware that semen evaluation is routinely performed every 3 to 4 months, especially in adolescent boys.
• *Alert:* Know that hypercalcemia symptoms may be difficult to distinguish from symptoms associated with condition being treated, unless anticipated and thought of as a symptom cluster. Hypercalcemia is particularly likely to occur in patients with metastatic breast cancer and may indicate bone metastases.
• Watch for symptoms of hypoglycemia in diabetic patients. Check blood glucose levels. Dosage of antidiabetic drug may need adjustment.
• When used in breast cancer, subjective effects may not occur for about 1 month; objective effects on clinical symptoms may take 3 months.

☑ **PATIENT TEACHING**
• If GI upset occurs, tell patient to take drug with food or meals.

• Make sure patient understands the importance of using an effective non-hormonal contraceptive during therapy.

• Advise washing after intercourse to decrease the risk of vaginitis. Instruct patient to wear only cotton underwear.

• Tell women to report menstrual irregularities and to discontinue therapy pending etiologic determination.

• Explain to patient taking drug for palliation of breast cancer that virilization usually occurs. Give emotional support. Tell patient to report androgenic effects immediately. Stopping drug will prevent further androgenic changes but will probably not reverse existing effects.

---

## methyltestosterone
Android, Metandren**, Metandren†, Oreton Methyl, Testomet‡, Testred, Virilon
Controlled Substance Schedule III

*Pregnancy Risk Category: X*

### HOW SUPPLIED
*Tablets:* 5 mg‡, 10 mg, 25 mg, 50 mg‡
*Tablets (buccal):* 10 mg, 25 mg†
*Capsules:* 10 mg

### ACTION
Stimulates target tissues to develop normally in androgen-deficient men.

### ONSET, PEAK, DURATION
Onset and duration unknown. Serum levels peak in 1 hour after buccal administration and 2 hours after oral administration.

### INDICATIONS & DOSAGE
*Postpartum breast engorgement in non-breast-feeding women* –
**Adults:** 80 mg P.O. daily, or 40 mg buccally daily for 3 to 5 days.
*Breast cancer in women 1 to 5 years postmenopausal* –

**Adults:** 50 to 200 mg P.O. daily; or 25 to 100 mg buccally daily.
*Male hypogonadism* –
**Adults:** 10 to 50 mg P.O. daily; or 5 to 25 mg buccally daily.
*Postpubertal cryptorchidism* –
**Adults:** 30 mg P.O. daily; or 15 mg buccally daily.

### ADVERSE REACTIONS
**CNS:** headache, anxiety, depression, paresthesia, sleep apnea syndrome.
**CV:** edema.
**EENT:** irritation of oral mucosa (with buccal administration).
**GI:** nausea.
**GU:** *hypoestrogenic effects in women (flushing; diaphoresis; vaginitis, including itching, dryness, and burning; vaginal bleeding; nervousness; emotional lability; menstrual irregularities); excessive hormonal effects in men (prepubertal – premature epiphyseal closure, acne, priapism, growth of body and facial hair, phallic enlargement; postpubertal – testicular atrophy, oligospermia, decreased ejaculatory volume, impotence, gynecomastia, epididymitis).*
**Hepatic:** reversible jaundice, cholestatic hepatitis, abnormal liver enzyme levels.
**Other:** hypercalcemia; polycythemia; hypersensitivity skin manifestations; suppression of clotting factors; muscle cramps or spasms; androgenic effects in women (acne, edema, *weight gain, hirsutism,* hoarseness, clitoral enlargement, *decreased breast size,* deepening voice, changes in libido, male-pattern baldness, *oily skin or hair*).

### INTERACTIONS
*Hepatotoxic medications:* increased risk of hepatotoxicity. Monitor closely.
*Insulin, oral antidiabetic agents:* altered dosage requirements. Monitor blood glucose levels in diabetic patients.

---

Reactions may be *common,* uncommon, *life-threatening,* or COMMON AND LIFE-THREATENING.

*Oral anticoagulants:* altered dosage requirements. Monitor PT.

### CONTRAINDICATIONS
Contraindicated in pregnant and breast-feeding patients or in males with breast cancer or prostate cancer.

### NURSING CONSIDERATIONS
• Use cautiously in elderly patients; patients with cardiac, renal, or hepatic disease; or healthy males with delayed puberty.
• Avoid use in women of childbearing age until pregnancy is ruled out.
• In children, X-rays of the wrist bones should be taken before therapy begins to establish the level of bone maturation. During treatment, bone maturation may proceed more rapidly than linear growth; ensure intermittent dosage and periodically review X-ray results to monitor bone maturation.
• Typically used only for intermittent therapy. Because of potential hepatotoxicity, watch closely for jaundice.
• Promptly report signs of virilization in women.
• Unless contraindicated, use with diet high in calories and protein. Give small, frequent feedings.
• Periodically check hemoglobin and hematocrit values, serum cholesterol and calcium levels, and cardiac and liver function test results, as ordered.
• Check weight regularly. Edema can be controlled with sodium restriction or diuretics.
• *Alert:* Therapeutic response in breast cancer is usually apparent within 3 months. Know therapy should be stopped if signs of disease progression appear.
• Report signs of hypercalcemia. In metastatic breast cancer, hypercalcemia may indicate progression of bone metastases.
• Know that semen evaluation is routinely performed every 3 to 4 months, especially in adolescent boys.

☑ **PATIENT TEACHING**
• Make sure patient understands the importance of using an effective non-hormonal contraceptive during therapy.
• Buccal tablets are twice as potent as oral tablets. Tell patient to avoid eating, drinking, chewing, or smoking while buccal tablet is in place and not to swallow tablet. Place in upper or lower buccal pouch between cheek and gum; tablet requires 30 to 60 minutes to dissolve. Instruct patient to change tablet absorption site with each dose to minimize risk of buccal irritation.
• Review signs and symptoms of virilization with female patient and instruct her to notify doctor immediately if any occur.
• Drug enhances hypoglycemia; teach patient the signs of hypoglycemia and method for checking blood glucose level. Instruct patient to report hypoglycemia immediately.
• Advise washing after intercourse to decrease the risk of vaginitis. Instruct patient to wear only cotton underwear.

## nandrolone decanoate
Anabolin LA, Androlone-D, Deca-Durabolin, Decolone, Hybolin Decanoate, Kabolin, Nandrobolic L.A., Neo-Durabolic

## nandrolone phenpropionate
Anabolin IM, Androlone, Durabolin, Hybolin Improved, Nandrobolic

Controlled Substance Schedule III

*Pregnancy Risk Category: X*

### HOW SUPPLIED
**nandrolone decanoate**
*Injection (in oil):* 50 mg/ml, 100 mg/ml, 200 mg/ml
**nandrolone phenpropionate**
*Injection (in oil):* 25 mg/ml, 50 mg/ml

---

*Liquid form contains alcohol.   **May contain tartrazine.   †Canada only.   ‡Australia only.   ◇OTC.

## ACTION
Anabolic steroid that promotes tissue-building processes, reverses catabolism, and stimulates erythropoiesis.

## ONSET, PEAK, DURATION
Onset and duration unknown. Serum levels peak in 1 to 2 days (phenpropionate) or 3 to 6 days (decanoate).

## INDICATIONS & DOSAGE
*Severe debility or disease states, refractory anemias—*
**Adults:** 50 to 100 mg decanoate I.M. at 1 to 4 week intervals for females; 50 to 200 mg decanoate I.M. at 1 to 4 week intervals for males. Therapy should be intermittent.
**Children 2 to 13 years:** 25 to 50 mg decanoate I.M. q 3 to 4 weeks.
*Control of metastatic breast cancer—*
**Adults:** 25 to 50 mg phenpropionate I.M. weekly.

## ADVERSE REACTIONS
**CNS:** excitation, insomnia, habituation, depression.
**CV:** edema.
**GI:** nausea, vomiting, diarrhea.
**GU:** bladder irritability, *hypoestrogenic effects in women (flushing; diaphoresis; vaginitis, including itching, dryness, and burning; vaginal bleeding; nervousness; emotional lability; menstrual irregularities); excessive hormonal effects in men (prepubertal—premature epiphyseal closure,* acne, priapism, *growth of body and facial hair,* phallic enlargement; postpubertal—testicular atrophy, oligospermia, decreased ejaculatory volume, impotence, gynecomastia, epididymitis).
**Hematologic:** elevated serum lipid levels, suppression of clotting factors.
**Hepatic:** reversible jaundice, peliosis hepatis, elevated liver enzyme levels, *liver cell tumors.*
**Skin:** pain and induration at injection site.
**Other:** androgenic effects in women (acne, edema, *weight gain, hirsutism,* hoarseness, clitoral enlargement, *decreased breast size,* changes in libido, male-pattern baldness, *oily skin or hair).*

## INTERACTIONS
*Hepatotoxic medications:* increased risk of hepatotoxicity. Monitor closely.
*Insulin, oral antidiabetic agents:* altered dosage requirements. Monitor blood glucose levels in diabetic patients.
*Oral anticoagulants:* altered dosage requirements. Monitor PT.

## CONTRAINDICATIONS
Contraindicated in patients with hypersensitivity to anabolic steroids; in males with breast cancer or prostate cancer; in those with nephrosis; in those experiencing the nephrotic phase of nephritis; in women with breast cancer and hypercalcemia; during pregnancy; or in breast-feeding patients.

## NURSING CONSIDERATIONS
● Use cautiously in patients with diabetes; cardiac, renal, or hepatic disease; epilepsy; or migraine or other conditions that may be aggravated by fluid retention.
● Avoid use in women of childbearing age until pregnancy is ruled out.
● In children, X-rays of the wrist bones should be taken before surgery to establish the level of bone maturation. During treatment, bone maturation may proceed more rapidly than linear growth; ensure intermittent dosage and periodically review X-ray results to monitor bone maturation.
● Inject I.M. drug deeply, preferably into upper outer quadrant of gluteal muscle in adults. Rotate injection sites to prevent muscle atrophy.
● Unless contraindicated, use with diet high in calories and protein. Give small, frequent feedings.

Reactions may be *common,* uncommon, *life-threatening,* or COMMON AND LIFE-THREATENING.

• Watch for signs of virilization, which may be irreversible despite prompt discontinuation of therapy.

• Closely observe boys under 7 years for precocious development of male sexual characteristics.

• Know that semen evaluation is routinely performed every 3 to 4 months, especially in adolescent boys.

• *Alert:* Periodically evaluate hepatic function, as ordered. Watch for jaundice; dosage adjustment may reverse condition. If liver function test results are abnormal, therapy should be stopped.

• Check weight regularly. Edema generally can be controlled with sodium restrictions or diuretics.

• Watch for symptoms of hypoglycemia in diabetic patients. Check blood glucose levels. Adjust dosage of antidiabetic agent, as ordered.

• Check quantitative urine and serum calcium levels. Hypercalcemia is most likely to occur in patients with breast cancer.

• When used to promote erythropoiesis in refractory anemias, make sure patients have adequate daily iron intake.

• Be aware that anabolic steroids may alter results of laboratory studies performed during therapy and for 2 to 3 weeks after therapy ends.

☑ **PATIENT TEACHING**

• Make sure patient understands the importance of using an effective nonhormonal contraceptive during therapy.

• Review signs and symptoms of virilization with female patient, and instruct her to notify doctor immediately if any occur.

• Advise washing after intercourse to decrease the risk of vaginitis. Instruct patients to wear only cotton underwear.

• Tell women to report menstrual irregularities and to discontinue therapy pending etiologic determination.

## oxandrolone
Lonavar‡, Oxandrin
Controlled Substance Schedule III

*Pregnancy Risk Category: X*

**HOW SUPPLIED**
*Tablets:* 2.5 mg

**ACTION**
Anabolic steroid that promotes tissue-building processes, reverses catabolism, and stimulates erythropoiesis.

**ONSET, PEAK, DURATION**
Unknown.

**INDICATIONS & DOSAGE**
*To combat catabolic effects of corticosteroid therapy, osteoporosis, prolonged immobilization, and debilitated states —*
**Adults:** 2.5 mg P.O. b.i.d., t.i.d., or q.i.d., up to 20 mg daily.
**Children:** 0.25 mg/kg P.O. daily

**ADVERSE REACTIONS**
**CNS:** excitation, insomnia, habituation, depression.
**CV:** edema.
**GI:** nausea, vomiting, constipation, diarrhea.
**GU:** bladder irritability, *hypoestrogenic effects in women (flushing; diaphoresis; vaginitis, including itching, dryness, and burning; vaginal bleeding; nervousness; emotional lability; menstrual irregularities); excessive hormonal effects in men (prepubertal — premature epiphyseal closure, acne,* priapism, *growth of body and facial hair,* phallic enlargement; postpubertal — testicular atrophy, oligospermia, decreased ejaculatory volume, impotence, gynecomastia, epididymitis).
**Hematologic:** elevated serum lipid levels, suppression of clotting factors.
**Hepatic:** reversible jaundice, peliosis hepatis, elevated liver enzyme levels, *liver cell tumors.*

**Other:** androgenic effects in women (acne, edema, *weight gain, hirsutism,* hoarseness, clitoral enlargement, *decreased breast size,* changes in libido, male-pattern baldness, *oily skin or hair*).

## INTERACTIONS
*Hepatotoxic medications:* increased risk of hepatotoxicity. Monitor closely.
*Insulin, oral antidiabetic agents:* altered dosage requirements. Monitor blood glucose levels in diabetic patients.
*Oral anticoagulants:* altered dosage requirements. Monitor PT.

## CONTRAINDICATIONS
Contraindicated in patients with hypersensitivity to anabolic steroids, in males with breast cancer or prostate cancer; in those with nephrosis or nephrotic phase of nephritis; in women with breast cancer and hypercalcemia; during pregnancy; and in breast-feeding patients.

## NURSING CONSIDERATIONS
● Use cautiously in patients with diabetes; cardiac, renal, or hepatic disease, epilepsy; or migraine or other conditions that may be aggravated by fluid retention.
● Avoid use in women of childbearing age until pregnancy is ruled out.
● In children, X-rays of the wrist bones should be taken before therapy begins to establish the level of bone maturation. During treatment, bone maturation may proceed more rapidly than linear growth; ensure intermittent dosage and review X-ray results periodically to monitor bone maturation.
● Unless contraindicated, use with diet high in calories and protein. Give small, frequent feedings.
● When used to promote erythropoiesis, make sure patients have adequate daily iron intake.

● Watch for signs of virilization, which may be irreversible despite prompt discontinuation of therapy. Doctor must decide if benefits outweigh adverse effects.
● Closely observe boys under 7 years for precocious development of male sexual characteristics.
● Know that semen evaluation is routinely performed every 3 to 4 months, especially in adolescent boys.
● Monitor weight routinely. Edema generally can be controlled with sodium restriction or diuretics.
● Periodically monitor hepatic function. Watch for jaundice. Dosage adjustment may reverse condition. Periodically check liver function test results.
● Watch for symptoms of hypoglycemia in diabetic patients. Check blood glucose levels. Adjust dosage of antidiabetic agent as necessary.
● Know that anabolic steroids may alter results of laboratory studies performed during therapy and for 2 to 3 weeks after therapy ends.
● **Alert:** Be aware that hypercalcemia symptoms may be difficult to distinguish from symptoms of condition being treated, unless anticipated and thought of as a cluster. Hypercalcemia is most likely to occur in patients with metastatic breast cancer and may indicate bone metastases.

## ☑ PATIENT TEACHING
● If GI upset occurs, tell patient to take drug with food or meals.
● Make sure patient understands the importance of using an effective nonhormonal contraceptive during therapy.
● Review signs and symptoms of virilization with female patient, and instruct her to notify doctor immediately if any occur.
● Advise washing after intercourse to decrease the risk of vaginitis. Instruct patient to wear only cotton underwear.

---

Reactions may be *common,* uncommon, *life-threatening,* or COMMON AND LIFE-THREATENING.

• Tell women to report menstrual irregularities and to discontinue therapy pending etiologic determination.

---

## oxymetholone
Anadrol-50, Anapolon 50†‡
Controlled Substance Schedule III

*Pregnancy Risk Category: X*

### HOW SUPPLIED
*Tablets:* 50 mg

### ACTION
Anabolic steroid that promotes tissue-building processes, reverses catabolism, and stimulates erythropoiesis.

### ONSET, PEAK, DURATION
Unknown.

### INDICATIONS & DOSAGE
*Aplastic anemia –*
**Adults and children:** 1 to 5 mg/kg P.O. daily. Dosage is highly individualized; and response is not immediate. A trial of 3 to 6 months is required.

### ADVERSE REACTIONS
**CNS:** excitation, insomnia, habituation, depression.
**CV:** edema.
**GI:** nausea, vomiting, constipation, diarrhea.
**GU:** bladder irritability, hypoestrogenic effects in women (flushing; diaphoresis; vaginitis, including itching, dryness, and burning; vaginal bleeding; nervousness; emotional lability; menstrual irregularities); excessive hormonal effects in men (prepubertal — premature epiphyseal closure, *acne,* priapism, *growth of body and facial hair,* phallic enlargement; postpubertal — testicular atrophy, oligospermia, decreased ejaculatory volume, impotence, gynecomastia, epididymitis).
**Hematologic:** elevated serum lipid levels, suppression of clotting factors.
**Hepatic:** reversible jaundice, peliosis hepatis, elevated liver enzyme levels, *liver cell tumors.*
**Other:** androgenic effects in women (acne, edema, *weight gain, hirsutism,* hoarseness, clitoral enlargement, *decreased breast size,* changes in libido, male-pattern baldness, *oily skin or hair).*

### INTERACTIONS
*Hepatotoxic medications:* increased risk of hepatotoxicity. Monitor closely.
*Insulin, oral antidiabetic agents:* altered dosage requirements. Monitor blood glucose levels in diabetic patients.
*Oral anticoagulants:* altered dosage requirements. Monitor PT.

### CONTRAINDICATIONS
Contraindicated in patients with hypersensitivity to anabolic steroids; in males with breast cancer or prostate cancer; in nephrosis or nephrotic phase of nephritis; in women with breast cancer and hypercalcemia; during pregnancy; and in breast-feeding patients.

### NURSING CONSIDERATIONS
• Use cautiously in patients with diabetes; cardiac, renal or hepatic disease; epilepsy; or migraine or other conditions that may be aggravated by fluid retention.
• Avoid use in women of childbearing age until pregnancy is ruled out.
• In children, X-rays of the wrist bones should be taken before therapy to establish the level of bone maturation. During treatment, bone maturation may proceed more rapidly than linear growth; ensure intermittent dosage and review X-ray results periodically to monitor bone maturation. Epiphyseal development may continue 6 months after therapy ends.
• Unless contraindicated, use with diet high in calories and protein. Give small, frequent feedings.

---

*Liquid form contains alcohol. **May contain tartrazine. †Canada only. ‡Australia only. ◊OTC.

• When used to promote erythropoiesis, make sure patients have adequate daily iron intake.

• Watch for signs of virilization, which may be irreversible despite prompt discontinuation of therapy. Doctor must decide if benefits outweigh adverse effects.

• Closely observe boys under 7 years for precocious development of male sexual characteristics.

• Know that semen evaluation is routinely performed every 3 to 4 months, especially in adolescent boys.

• Periodically evaluate hepatic function. Watch for symptoms of jaundice; dosage adjustment may reverse condition. If liver function test results are abnormal, therapy should be stopped.

• Monitor weight routinely. Edema generally can be controlled with sodium restriction or diuretics.

• Watch for symptoms of hypoglycemia in diabetic patients. Check blood glucose levels. Adjust dosage of antidiabetic agent as necessary.

• Know that anabolic steroids may alter results of laboratory studies performed during therapy and for 2 to 3 weeks after therapy ends.

• *Alert:* Know that hypercalcemia symptoms may be difficult to distinguish from symptoms of condition being treated, unless anticipated and thought of as a cluster. Hypercalcemia is most likely to occur in patients with metastatic breast cancer and may indicate bone metastases.

☑ **PATIENT TEACHING**
• If GI upset occurs, tell patient to take with food or meals.

• Make sure patient understands the importance of using an effective nonhormonal contraceptive during therapy.

• Review signs and symptoms of virilization with female patient and instruct her to notify doctor immediately if any occur.

• Advise washing after intercourse to decrease the risk of vaginitis. Instruct patients to wear only cotton underwear.

• Tell women to report menstrual irregularities and to discontinue therapy pending etiologic determination.

## stanozolol
Winstrol
Controlled Substance Schedule III

*Pregnancy Risk Category: X*

**HOW SUPPLIED**
*Tablets:* 2 mg

**ACTION**
Anabolic steroid that promotes tissue-building processes, reverses catabolism, and stimulates erythropoiesis.

**ONSET, PEAK, DURATION**
Unknown.

**INDICATIONS & DOSAGE**
*Prevention of hereditary angioedema—*
**Adults:** initially, 2 mg P.O. t.i.d. to 4 mg q.i.d for 5 days. Dosage gradually reduced at 1- to 3-month intervals to a dosage of 2 mg P.O. daily.
**Children under 6 years:** 1 mg P.O. daily.
**Children 6 to 12 years:** up to 2 mg P.O. daily.
*Note:* Stanozolol is used in children only during an acute attack.

**ADVERSE REACTIONS**
**CNS:** excitation, insomnia, habituation, depression.
**CV:** edema.
**GI:** nausea, vomiting, constipation, diarrhea.
**GU:** bladder irritability, hypoestrogenic effects in women (flushing; diaphoresis; vaginitis, including itching, dryness, and burning; vaginal bleeding; nervousness; emotional lability; menstrual irregularities); excessive hormonal effects in men (prepubertal—premature epiphyseal closure,

---

Reactions may be *common,* uncommon, *life-threatening,* or **COMMON AND LIFE-THREATENING.**

*acne,* priapism, *growth of body and facial hair,* phallic enlargement; post-pubertal—testicular atrophy, oligospermia, decreased ejaculatory volume, impotence, gynecomastia, epididymitis).

**Hematologic:** elevated serum lipid levels, suppression of clotting factors.
**Hepatic:** reversible jaundice, peliosis hepatis, elevated liver enzyme levels, *liver cell tumors.*
**Other:** androgenic effects in women (acne, edema, *weight gain, hirsutism,* hoarseness, clitoral enlargement, *decreased breast size,* changes in libido, male-pattern baldness, *oily skin or hair*).

## INTERACTIONS
*Hepatotoxic medications:* increased risk of hepatotoxicity. Monitor closely.
*Insulin, oral antidiabetic agents:* altered dosage requirements. Monitor blood glucose levels in diabetic patients.
*Oral anticoagulants:* altered dosage requirements. Monitor PT.

## CONTRAINDICATIONS
Contraindicated in patients with hypersensitivity to anabolic steroids; in males with breast cancer or prostate cancer; in nephrosis or nephrotic phase of nephritis; in women with breast cancer and with hypercalcemia; during pregnancy; and in breast-feeding patients.

## NURSING CONSIDERATIONS
• Use cautiously in patients with diabetes; cardiac, renal, or hepatic disease; epilepsy; or migraine or other conditions that may be aggravated by fluid retention.
• Avoid use in women of childbearing age until pregnancy is ruled out.
• In children, X-rays of the wrist bones should be taken before therapy begins to establish the level of bone maturation. During treatment, bone

maturation may proceed more rapidly than linear growth; ensure intermittent dosage and review X-ray results periodically to monitor bone maturation.
• Know that a lower dosage in young women (2 mg b.i.d.) is recommended to avoid virilization. Watch for signs of virilization, which may be irreversible despite prompt discontinuation of therapy. Doctor must decide if benefits of therapy outweigh adverse effects.
• To minimize GI distress, administer before or with meals.
• Unless contraindicated, use with diet high in calories and protein. Give small, frequent feedings.
• Closely observe boys under 7 years for precocious development of male sexual characteristics.
• Know that semen evaluation is routinely performed every 3 to 4 months, especially in adolescent boys.
• Monitor weight routinely. Edema is generally controllable with sodium restriction or diuretics.
• **Alert:** Periodically evaluate hepatic function. Watch for symptoms of jaundice; dosage adjustment may reverse condition. Check liver function test results regularly; if they are abnormal, therapy should be discontinued.
• Monitor serum cholesterol levels.
• Watch for symptoms of hypoglycemia in diabetic patients. Check blood glucose levels. Adjust dosage of antidiabetic agent, as ordered.
• Know that anabolic steroids may alter results of laboratory studies performed during therapy and for 2 to 3 weeks after therapy ends.

## ☑ PATIENT TEACHING
• Make sure patient understands the importance of using an effective non-hormonal contraceptive during therapy.
• Instruct patient to take drug before or with meals.
• Review signs and symptoms of virili-

---

zation with female patient, and instruct her to notify doctor immediately if any occur.

• Advise washing after intercourse to decrease the risk of vaginitis. Instruct patients to wear only cotton underwear.

• Tell women to report menstrual irregularities and to discontinue therapy pending etiologic determination.

---

## testosterone
Andro 100, Andronaq-50, Histerone-50, Histerone-100, Testamone 100, Testaqua, Testoject-50

## testosterone cypionate
Andro-Cyp 100, Andro-Cyp 200, Andronaq-LA, Andronate 100, Andronate 200, depAndro 100, depAndro 200, Depotest, Depo-Testosterone, Duratest-100, Duratest-200, T-Cypionate, Testa-C, Testoject-LA, Testred Cypionate 200, Virilon IM

## testosterone enanthate
Andro-L.A. 200, Andropository 100, Andryl 200, Delatest, Delatestryl, Durathate-200, Everone, Malogex†, Testone L.A. 200, Testrin-P.A.

## testosterone propionate
Malogen†, Testex

Controlled Substance Schedule III
*Pregnancy Risk Category: X*

### HOW SUPPLIED
**testosterone**
*Injection (aqueous suspension):* 25 mg/ml, 50 mg/ml, 100 mg/ml
**testosterone cypionate**
*Injection (in oil):* 50 mg/ml, 100 mg/ml, 200 mg/ml
**testosterone enanthate**
*Injection (in oil):* 100 mg/ml, 200 mg/ml

**testosterone propionate**
*Injection (in oil):* 25 mg/ml, 50 mg/ml, 100 mg/ml

### ACTION
Stimulates target tissues to develop normally in androgen-deficient men. Testosterone may have some antiestrogen properties, making it useful to treat certain estrogen-dependent breast cancers. Its action in postpartum breast engorgement is not known because testosterone does not suppress lactation.

### ONSET, PEAK, DURATION
Unknown.

### INDICATIONS & DOSAGE
*Male hypogonadism –*
**Adults:** 10 to 25 mg I.M. two to three times weekly, or 50 to 400 mg (cypionate, enanthate) I.M. q 2 to 4 weeks, or 10 to 25 mg (propionate) I.M. two to four times weekly.
*Delayed puberty in males –*
**Adolescent:** 12.5 to 25 mg (propionate) I.M. two or three times weekly for up to 6 months.
*Metastatic breast cancer in women 1 to 5 years post menopausal –*
**Adults:** 100 mg I.M. three times weekly; 50 to 100 mg (propionate) I.M. three times weekly; or 200 to 400 mg (cypionate, enanthate) I.M. q 2 to 4 weeks.
*Postpartum breast pain and engorgement –*
**Adults:** 25 to 50 mg I.M. of testosterone or testosterone propionate daily for 3 to 4 days.

### ADVERSE REACTIONS
**CNS:** headache, anxiety, depression, paresthesia, sleep apnea syndrome.
**CV:** edema.
**GI:** nausea.
**GU:** hypoestrogenic effects in women (flushing; diaphoresis; vaginitis, including itching, drying, and burning; vaginal bleeding; menstrual irregular-

---

Reactions may be *common,* uncommon, *life-threatening,* or COMMON AND LIFE-THREATENING.

ities); excessive hormonal effects in men (prepubertal — premature epiphyseal closure, *acne*, priapism, *growth of body and facial hair,* phallic enlargement; postpubertal — testicular atrophy, oligospermia, decreased ejaculatory volume, impotence, gynecomastia, epididymitis).

**Hepatic:** reversible jaundice, cholestatic hepatitis, abnormal liver enzyme levels.

**Skin:** pain and induration at injection site, local edema.

**Other:** hypercalcemia; polycythemia; hypersensitivity skin manifestations; suppression of clotting factors; androgenic effects in women (*acne, edema, oily skin, weight gain, hirsutism, hoarseness,* clitoral enlargement, deepening voice, decreased or increased libido).

## INTERACTIONS

*Hepatotoxic medications:* increased risk of hepatotoxicity. Monitor closely.

*Insulin, oral antidiabetic agents:* altered dosage requirements. Monitor blood glucose levels in diabetic patients.

*Oral anticoagulants:* altered dosage requirements. Monitor PT.

## CONTRAINDICATIONS

Contraindicated in male patients with breast or prostate cancer; in patients with hypercalcemia; in those with cardiac, hepatic, or renal decompensation; during pregnancy, and in breast-feeding patients.

## NURSING CONSIDERATIONS

• Use cautiously in elderly patients.
• Avoid use in women of childbearing age until pregnancy is ruled out.
• Administer daily dosage requirement in divided doses for best results.
• Store I.M. preparations at room temperature. If crystals appear, warm and shake the bottle to disperse them.
• Inject deep into upper outer quad-

rant of gluteal muscle. Rotate injection sites to prevent muscle atrophy. Report soreness at site because of the possibility of postinfection furunculosis.
• Unless contraindicated, use with diet high in calories and protein. Give small, frequent feedings.
• Monitor periodic liver function test results, as ordered.
• In patients with metastatic breast cancer, hypercalcemia usually indicates progression of bone metastases. Report signs of hypercalcemia.
• Report signs of virilization in women; doctor will need to reevaluate treatment.
• Monitor weight routinely. Edema generally can be controlled with sodium restriction or diuretics.
• Monitor prepubertal boys by X-ray for rate of bone maturation.
• **Alert:** Therapeutic response in breast cancer is usually apparent within 3 months. Know that therapy should be stopped if signs of disease progression appear.
• Know that androgens may alter results of laboratory studies during therapy and for 2 to 3 weeks after therapy ends.

## ☑ PATIENT TEACHING

• Make sure patient understands the importance of using an effective nonhormonal contraceptive during therapy.
• Review signs and symptoms of virilization with female patient and instruct her to notify doctor immediately if any occur.
• Advise washing after intercourse to decrease the risk of vaginitis. Instruct patients to wear only cotton underwear.
• Instruct men to report priapism, reduced ejaculatory volume, and gynecomastia. Notify doctor if these occur as drug needs to be stopped.
• Enhances hypoglycemia; teach pa-

---

tient to recognize signs of hypoglycemia and immediately report them.

# testosterone transdermal system

Androderm, Testoderm
Controlled Substance Schedule III

*Pregnancy Risk Category: X*

## HOW SUPPLIED
*Transdermal system:* 4 mg/day, 6 mg/day

## ACTION
Releases testosterone, which stimulates target tissues to develop normally in androgen-deficient men.

## ONSET, PEAK, DURATION
Onset unknown. Serum levels peak within 2 to 4 hours after application. Steady-state levels are reached after 3 to 4 weeks of therapy. Testosterone levels decline toward baseline within 2 hours after removal.

## INDICATIONS & DOSAGE
*Primary or hypogonadotropic hypogonadism in men 18 years and older* —
**Adults:** one 6-mg/day patch applied to the scrotal area daily. If scrotal area is too small for the 6-mg/day patch, therapy started with the smaller sized 4-mg/day patch. Patch worn for 22 to 24 hours daily.

## ADVERSE REACTIONS
**CNS:** *CVA.*
**GU:** *gynecomastia,* prostatitis, urinary tract infection, breast tenderness.
**Skin:** acne.
**Other:** *pruritus,* discomfort, irritation.

## INTERACTIONS
*Antidiabetic agents:* altered antidiabetic agent dosage requirements. Monitor blood glucose levels.
*Oral anticoagulants:* altered anticoagulant dosage requirements. Monitor PT.
*Oxyphenbutazone:* may elevate serum levels of oxyphenbutazone. Monitor patients for adverse reactions.

## CONTRAINDICATIONS
Contraindicated in patients hypersensitive to the drug, in women, and men with known or suspected breast or prostate cancer.

## NURSING CONSIDERATIONS
• Use cautiously in elderly men because they may be at greater risk for developing prostatic hyperplasia or prostate cancer. Also use cautiously in patients with preexisting renal, hepatic, or cardiac disease.
• Because chronic use of systemic androgens is associated with polycythemia, monitor hematocrit and hemoglobin values periodically in patients on long-term therapy, as ordered.
• Periodically assess liver function tests, serum lipid profiles, and prostatic acid phosphatase and prostate-specific antigen levels as ordered.

## ☑ PATIENT TEACHING
• Teach patient how to apply the transdermal system. Warn patient that adequate serum levels will not be attained if the patch is not applied to genital skin.
• Tell patient that topical testosterone preparations used by men have caused virilization in female partners. These women should report acne or changes in body hair distribution.
• Advise patient to report persistent erections, nausea, vomiting, changes in skin color, or ankle edema to the doctor.

---

Reactions may be *common*, uncommon, *life-threatening*, or COMMON AND LIFE-THREATENING.

# 55

# Estrogens and progestins

chlorotrianisene
dienestrol
diethylstilbestrol
diethylstilbestrol diphosphate
esterified estrogens
estradiol
estradiol cypionate
estradiol valerate
estrogens, conjugated
estrone
estropipate
ethinyl estradiol
ethinyl estradiol and
desogestrel
ethinyl estradiol and
ethynodiol diacetate
ethinyl estradiol and
levonorgestrel
ethinyl estradiol and
norethindrone
ethinyl estradiol and
norethindrone acetate
ethinyl estradiol and
norgestimate
ethinyl estradiol and
norgestrel
ethinyl estradiol, norethindrone
acetate, and ferrous fumarate
mestranol and norethindrone
mestranol and norethynodrel
hydroxyprogesterone caproate
levonorgestrel
medroxyprogesterone acetate
norethindrone
norethindrone acetate
norgestrel
progesterone
quinestrol

## COMBINATION PRODUCTS
MENRIUM 5-2: chlordiazepoxide 5
mg and esterified estrogens 0.2 mg.
MENRIUM 5-4: chlordiazepoxide 5
mg and esterified estrogens 0.4 mg.
MENRIUM 10-4: chlordiazepoxide
10 mg and esterified estrogens 0.4 mg.

PMB-200: conjugated estrogens 0.45
mg and meprobamate 200 mg.
PMB-400: conjugated estrogens 0.45
mg and meprobamate 400 mg.

---

## chlorotrianisene
TACE**

*Pregnancy Risk Category: X*

**HOW SUPPLIED**
*Capsules:* 12 mg, 25 mg

**ACTION**
Increases the synthesis of DNA,
RNA, and protein in responsive tissues and reduces release of follicle-
stimulating hormone and luteinizing
hormone from the pituitary gland.

**ONSET, PEAK, DURATION**
Onset and peak unknown. Effects persist for about 24 hours.

**INDICATIONS & DOSAGE**
*Prostate cancer–*
**Adults:** 12 to 25 mg P.O. daily.
*Female hypogonadism–*
**Adults:** 12 to 25 mg P.O. for 21 days,
followed by one dose of progesterone
100 mg I.M. or 5 days of oral proges-
togen concurrently with last 5 days of
chlorotrianisene (for example, medroxyprogesterone 5 to 10 mg).
*Vasomotor symptoms associated with
menopausal symptoms, atrophic vaginitis, kraurosis vulvae–*
**Adults:** 12 to 25 mg P.O. daily for 30
days or cyclic (3 weeks on, 1 week off).

**ADVERSE REACTIONS**
**CNS:** headache, dizziness, chorea,
migraine, depression, *seizures.*
**CV:** thrombophlebitis; *thromboembolism;* hypertension; edema; *increased*

---

*risk of CVA, pulmonary embolism, MI.*

**EENT:** worsening of myopia or astigmatism, intolerance of contact lenses.
**GI:** *nausea,* vomiting, abdominal cramps, bloating, colitis, acute pancreatitis, anorexia, increased appetite, excessive thirst, weight changes.
**GU:** in women — breakthrough bleeding, altered menstrual flow, dysmenorrhea, *increased risk of endometrial cancer, possibility of increased risk of breast cancer,* amenorrhea, cervical erosion or abnormal secretions, enlargement of uterine fibromas, vaginal candidiasis; in men — *gynecomastia, testicular atrophy, impotence.*
**Hepatic:** cholestatic jaundice, *hepatic adenoma.*
**Skin:** melasma, urticaria, hirsutism or hair loss, erythema nodosum, dermatitis.
**Other:** breast changes (tenderness, enlargement, secretion), hypercalcemia, gallbladder disease.

## INTERACTIONS

*Carbamazepine, phenobarbital, rifampin:* decreased effectiveness of estrogen therapy. Monitor closely.
*Corticosteroids:* possible enhanced effects. Monitor closely.
*Cyclosporine:* increased risk of toxicity. Use together with caution and frequently monitor cyclosporine levels.
*Dantrolene, other hepatotoxic medications:* increased risk of hepatotoxicity. Monitor closely.
*Oral anticoagulants:* dosage adjustments may be necessary. Monitor PT.
*Tamoxifen:* estrogens may interfere with effectiveness of tamoxifen. Avoid concomitant use.

## CONTRAINDICATIONS

Contraindicated in patients with thrombophlebitis or thromboembolic disorders; in those with breast, reproductive organ, or genital cancer; in those with undiagnosed abnormal genital bleeding; and during pregnancy.

## NURSING CONSIDERATIONS

● Use cautiously in patients with cerebrovascular or coronary artery disease; asthma; bone disease; migraine; seizures; cardiac, hepatic, or renal dysfunction; hypercalcemia from metastatic breast disease; and family history (mother, grandmother, sister) of breast or genital tract cancer, or who have breast nodules, fibrocystic disease, or abnormal mammographic findings.
● Ensure that patients have a thorough physical examination before initiating estrogen therapy. Periodically monitor blood pressure, hepatic function, and serum lipid levels.
● Monitor weight regularly and recommend sodium restriction, as needed. May cause fluid retention and edema.
● Notify the pathologist about any patients receiving estrogen therapy when specimens are obtained and sent to pathology for evaluation.
● Because of the risk of thromboembolism, know that therapy should be stopped at least 1 month before procedures associated with prolonged immobilization or thromboembolism, such as knee or hip surgery.

## ☑ PATIENT TEACHING

● Tell patient that patient package insert that describes estrogen's adverse effects is available; however, also give patient verbal explanation.
● *Alert:* Warn patient to immediately report suspected pregnancy; abdominal pain; pain, numbness, or stiffness in legs or buttocks; pressure or pain in chest; shortness of breath; severe headaches; visual disturbances, such as blind spots, flashing lights, or blurriness; vaginal bleeding or discharge; breast lumps; swelling of hands or feet; yellow skin and sclera; dark urine; and light-colored stools.
● Explain to patient on cyclic therapy for postmenopausal symptoms that, although withdrawal bleeding may oc-

cur during week off drug, fertility is not restored. Pregnancy cannot occur because patient does not ovulate.
• Teach women how to perform routine breast self-examination.
• Tell diabetic patient to report elevated blood glucose test results so that antidiabetic medication dosage can be adjusted.
• Emphasize the importance of regular physical examinations. Studies suggest that postmenopausal women who use estrogen replacement for more than 5 years to treat menopausal symptoms may be at increased risk for endometrial cancer. This risk is reduced by using cyclic rather than continuous therapy and the lowest possible dosages of estrogen. Adding progestins to the regimen decreases the incidence of endometrial hyperplasia; however, it isn't known if progestins affect the incidence of endometrial cancer. Most studies show no increased risk of breast cancer.

---

## dienestrol (dienoestrol)
DV, Ortho Dienestrol

*Pregnancy Risk Category: X*

**HOW SUPPLIED**
*Vaginal cream:* 0.01%

**ACTION**
Unknown.

**ONSET, PEAK, DURATION**
Unknown.

**INDICATIONS & DOSAGE**
*Atrophic vaginitis and kraurosis vulvae (short-term)—*
**Postmenopausal women:** 1 to 2 intravaginal applications of vaginal cream daily for 1 to 2 weeks (as directed); then half that dose for the same period. Doctor may prescribe a maintenance dosage of 1 applicatorful one to three times a week.

**ADVERSE REACTIONS**
**GU:** vaginal discharge, increased intravaginal discomfort, uterine bleeding (with excessive use), burning sensation.
**Other:** systemic effects (breast tenderness, peripheral edema).

**INTERACTIONS**
*Carbamazepine, phenobarbital, rifampin:* decreased effectiveness of estrogen therapy. Monitor closely.
*Corticosteroids:* possible enhanced effects. Monitor closely.
*Cyclosporine:* increased risk of toxicity. Use together with caution and frequently monitor cyclosporine levels.
*Dantrolene, other hepatotoxic medications:* increased risk of hepatotoxicity. Monitor closely.
*Oral anticoagulants:* dosage adjustments may be necessary. Monitor PT.
*Tamoxifen:* estrogens may interfere with effectiveness of tamoxifen. Avoid concomitant use.

**CONTRAINDICATIONS**
Contraindicated in patients with active thrombophlebitis or thromboembolic disorders associated with estrogen therapy or past history of such events; in those with breast, reproductive organ, or genital cancer; or in those with undiagnosed abnormal genital bleeding; and during pregnancy.

**NURSING CONSIDERATIONS**
• Use cautiously in patients with cerebral vascular or coronary artery disease, diabetes, hypertension, epilepsy, migraine; strong family history of breast cancer or who have breast nodules, fibrocystic disease, or abnormal mammograms; cardiac or renal dysfunction; history of depression; liver dysfunction; metabolic bone diseases; and young patients in whom bone growth is not complete.
• Ensure that patients have a thorough physical examination before initiating estrogen therapy. Patients receiving

---

*Liquid form contains alcohol.    **May contain tartrazine.    †Canada only.    ‡Australia only.    ◊OTC.

long-term therapy should have examinations yearly. Periodically monitor body weight, blood pressure, hepatic function, and serum lipid levels as ordered.
• Monitor closely. Systemic reactions may occur with normal intravaginal use.

☑ **PATIENT TEACHING**
• Tell patient that patient package insert that describes estrogen's adverse effects is available; however, also give patient verbal explanation.
• Instruct patient to apply drug at bedtime to increase effectiveness.
• Teach patient how to insert suppositories or cream, and tell her to wash vaginal area with soap and water before application.
• Instruct patient to remain recumbent for 30 minutes after administration to prevent loss of drug.
• Tell patient not to wear a tampon while receiving vaginal therapy. She may need to wear a sanitary pad to protect clothing.
• Instruct patient to report systemic reactions (breast pain or tenderness, swelling of the hands or feet) or vaginal discharge or bleeding.
• Teach women how to perform routine breast self-examination.
• Warn patient not to exceed the prescribed dosage.
• Inform patient withdrawal bleeding may occur if estrogen is suddenly stopped.

## diethylstilbestrol (stilboestrol)
DES

## diethylstilbestrol diphosphate
DES, Honvol†, Stilphostrol

*Pregnancy Risk Category: X*

## HOW SUPPLIED
**diethylstilbestrol**
*Tablets:* 1 mg, 5 mg
**diethylstilbestrol diphosphate**
*Tablets:* 50 mg, 83 mg†
*Injection:* 50 mg/ml†

## ACTION
Increases the synthesis of DNA, RNA, and protein in responsive tissues. Also reduces release of follicle-stimulating hormone and luteinizing hormone from the pituitary gland.

## ONSET, PEAK, DURATION
Unknown.

## INDICATIONS & DOSAGE
*Prostate cancer—*
**Men:** initially, 1 to 3 mg P.O. daily; may be reduced to 1 mg daily, or 50 mg P.O. diphosphate t.i.d. Then increased up to 200 mg or more as needed t.i.d. or 0.5 g I.V., followed by 1 g daily for 5 or more days as needed. Maintenance dosage 0.25 to 0.5 g I.V. once or twice weekly.
*Metastatic, advanced breast cancer—*
**Men and postmenopausal women:** 15 mg P.O. daily.

## ADVERSE REACTIONS
**CNS:** headache, dizziness, chorea, depression, *seizures.*
**CV:** thrombophlebitis; *thromboembolism;* hypertension; edema; *increased risk of CVA, pulmonary embolism, MI.*
**EENT:** worsening of myopia or astigmatism, intolerance of contact lenses.
**GI:** *nausea,* vomiting, abdominal cramps, bloating, anorexia, increased appetite, excessive thirst, weight changes, pancreatitis.
**GU:** in women—breakthrough bleeding, altered menstrual flow, dysmenorrhea, amenorrhea, cervical erosion, *increased risk of endometrial cancer, possibility of increased risk of breast cancer,* altered cervical secretions, enlargement of uterine fibromas, vag-

---

Reactions may be *common,* uncommon, *life-threatening,* or COMMON AND LIFE-THREATENING.

inal candidiasis, loss of libido; in men—gynecomastia, testicular atrophy, impotence.

**Hepatic:** cholestatic jaundice, *hepatic adenoma*.

**Skin:** melasma, urticaria, hirsutism or hair loss, erythema nodosum, dermatitis.

**Other:** breast tenderness or enlargement, hypercalcemia, gallbladder disease.

## INTERACTIONS

*Carbamazepine, phenobarbital, rifampin:* decreased effectiveness of estrogen therapy. Monitor closely.

*Corticosteroids:* possible enhanced effects. Monitor closely.

*Cyclosporine:* increased risk of toxicity. Use together with caution and frequently monitor cyclosporine levels.

*Dantrolene, other hepatotoxic medications:* increased risk of hepatotoxicity. Monitor closely.

*Oral anticoagulants:* dosage adjustments may be necessary. Monitor PT.

*Tamoxifen:* estrogens may interfere with effectiveness of tamoxifen. Avoid concomitant use.

## CONTRAINDICATIONS

Contraindicated in men with known or suspected breast cancer except in selected patients being treated for metastatic disease, in patients with active thrombophlebitis or thromboembolic disorders, estrogen-dependent neoplasia, undiagnosed abnormal genital bleeding, during pregnancy, and history of thrombophlebitis, thrombosis, or thromboembolic disorders associated with estrogen use.

## NURSING CONSIDERATIONS

• Use cautiously in patients with hypertension, mental depression, bone disease, migraine, seizures, diabetes mellitus, cardiac, hepatic, or renal dysfunction, and cerebrovascular or coronary artery disease.

• Ensure that patients have a thorough physical examination before initiating estrogen therapy. Patients receiving long-term therapy should have examinations yearly. Periodically monitor body weight, blood pressure, hepatic function, and serum lipid levels.

• *Alert:* Know that high incidence of gross nonmalignant genital changes may occur in offspring of women taking drug during pregnancy. Female offspring have a higher than normal risk of developing cervical and vaginal adenocarcinoma. Male offspring may have a higher than normal risk of developing testicular tumors, epididymal cysts, and impaired fertility.

• If patients experience GI upset, give drug with or immediately after meals.

• **I.V. use:** Mix ordered dose in 250 to 500 ml of $D_5W$ or 0.9% sodium chloride. Infuse at 1 to 2 ml/minute for the first 15 minutes; if no adverse reactions occur, increase infusion rate to administer entire dose within 1 hour.

• Notify the pathologist about any patients receiving estrogen therapy when specimens are obtained and sent to pathology for evaluation.

• Know that increased number of CV deaths reported in men taking diethylstilbestrol tablet (5 mg daily) for prostate cancer for a long time. This effect is not associated with 1-mg daily dose.

• Because of the risk of thromboembolism, know that therapy should be discontinued at least 1 month before procedures associated with prolonged immobilization or thromboembolism, such as knee or hip surgery.

## ☑ PATIENT TEACHING

• Tell patient that patient package insert that describes estrogen's adverse effects is available; however, also give patient verbal explanation.

• Tell patient not to crush, break, or chew enteric-coated tablets. Instruct

---

*Liquid form contains alcohol.   **May contain tartrazine.   †Canada only.   ‡Australia only.   ◇OTC.

patient to take with food if stomach upset occurs.

• **Alert:** Warn patient to immediately report abdominal pain; pain, numbness, or stiffness in legs or buttocks; pressure or pain in chest; shortness of breath; severe headache; visual disturbances, such as blind spots, flashing lights, or blurriness; vaginal bleeding or discharge; breast lumps; sudden weight gain; swelling of hands or feet; yellow sclera or skin; dark urine; and light-colored stools.

• Teach women how to perform routine breast self-examination.

• Tell diabetic patient to report elevated blood glucose test results so that antidiabetic medication dosage can be adjusted.

---

## esterified estrogens
Estratab, Menest, Neo-Estrone†

*Pregnancy Risk Category: X*

### HOW SUPPLIED
*Tablets:* 0.3 mg, 0.625 mg, 1.25 mg, 2.5 mg
*Tablets (film-coated):* 0.3 mg, 0.625 mg, 1.25 mg, 2.5 mg

### ACTION
Increases the synthesis of DNA, RNA, and protein in responsive tissues. Also reduces release of follicle-stimulating hormone and luteinizing hormone from the pituitary gland.

### ONSET, PEAK, DURATION
Unknown.

### INDICATIONS & DOSAGE
*Inoperable prostate cancer* –
**Men:** 1.25 to 2.5 mg P.O. t.i.d.
*Breast cancer* –
**Men and postmenopausal women:** 10 mg P.O. t.i.d. for 3 or more months.
*Female hypogonadism* –
**Women:** 2.5 mg P.O. daily to t.i.d. in cycles of 20 days, 10 days off.

*Castration, primary ovarian failure* –
**Women:** 2.5 mg P.O. daily to t.i.d. in cycles of 3 weeks on, 1 week off.
*Vasomotor menopausal symptoms* –
**Women:** average dosage is 1.25 mg P.O. daily in cycles of 3 weeks on, 1 week off.
*Atrophic vaginitis and atrophic urethritis* –
**Women:** 0.3 to 1.25 mg or more P.O. daily in cycles of 3 weeks on, 1 week off.

### ADVERSE REACTIONS
**CNS:** headache, dizziness, chorea, depression, *seizures*.
**CV:** thrombophlebitis; *thromboembolism;* hypertension; edema; *increased risk of CVA, pulmonary embolism, MI.*
**EENT:** worsening of myopia or astigmatism, intolerance of contact lenses.
**GI:** *nausea,* vomiting, abdominal cramps, bloating, anorexia, increased appetite, weight changes, pancreatitis.
**GU:** in women – breakthrough bleeding, altered menstrual flow, dysmenorrhea, amenorrhea, *increased risk of endometrial cancer, possibility of increased risk of breast cancer,* cervical erosion, altered cervical secretions, enlargement of uterine fibromas, vaginal candidiasis; in men – gynecomastia, testicular atrophy, impotence.
**Hepatic:** cholestatic jaundice, *hepatic adenoma.*
**Skin:** melasma, rash, hirsutism or hair loss, erythema nodosum, dermatitis.
**Other:** breast changes (tenderness, enlargement, secretion), gallbladder disease, hypercalcemia.

### INTERACTIONS
*Carbamazepine, phenobarbital, rifampin:* decreased effectiveness of estrogen therapy. Monitor closely.
*Corticosteroids:* possible enhanced effects. Monitor closely.
*Cyclosporine:* increased risk of toxic-

---

Reactions may be *common,* uncommon, *life-threatening,* or COMMON AND LIFE-THREATENING.

ity. Use together with caution and frequently monitor cyclosporine levels.
*Dantrolene, other hepatotoxic medications:* increased risk of hepatotoxicity. Monitor closely.
*Oral anticoagulants:* dosage adjustments may be necessary. Monitor PT.
*Tamoxifen:* estrogens may interfere with effectiveness of tamoxifen. Avoid concomitant use.

## CONTRAINDICATIONS
Contraindicated in patients with breast cancer (except metastatic disease), estrogen-dependent neoplasia, active thrombophlebitis or thromboembolic disorders, undiagnosed abnormal genital bleeding, hypersensitivity to drug, history of thromboembolic disease, or during pregnancy.

## NURSING CONSIDERATIONS
• Use cautiously in patients with history of hypertension, mental depression, cardiac or renal dysfunction, liver impairment, or bone diseases, migraine, seizures, or diabetes mellitus.
• Ensure that patients have a thorough physical examination before initiating estrogen therapy. Patients receiving long-term therapy should have repeat examinations yearly. Periodically monitor body weight, blood pressure, serum lipid levels, and hepatic function as ordered.
• Notify the pathologist about any patients receiving estrogen therapy when specimens are obtained and sent to pathology for evaluation.
• Because of the risk of thromboembolism, know that therapy should be discontinued at least one month before procedures associated with prolonged immobilization or thromboembolism, such as knee or hip surgery.

## ☑ PATIENT TEACHING
• Tell patient that patient package insert that describes estrogen's adverse effects is available; however, also give patient verbal explanation.

• Emphasize the importance of regular physical examinations. Studies suggest that postmenopausal women who use estrogen replacement for more than 5 years to treat menopausal symptoms may be at increased risk for endometrial cancer. This risk is reduced by using cyclic rather than continuous therapy and the lowest possible dosages of estrogen. Adding progestins to the regimen decreases the incidence of endometrial hyperplasia; however, it isn't known if progestins affect the incidence of endometrial cancer. Most studies show no increased risk of breast cancer.
• *Alert:* Warn patient to immediately report abdominal pain; pain, numbness, or stiffness in legs or buttocks; pressure or pain in chest; shortness of breath; severe headaches; visual disturbances, such as blind spots, flashing lights, or blurriness; vaginal bleeding or discharge; breast lumps; swelling of hands or feet; yellow skin or sclera; dark urine; and light-colored stools.
• Tell diabetic patient to report elevated blood glucose test results so that antidiabetic medication dosage can be adjusted.
• Explain to patient on cyclic therapy for postmenopausal symptoms that, although she may experience withdrawal bleeding during week off drug, fertility is not restored. Pregnancy cannot occur because patient does not ovulate.
• Teach women how to perform routine breast self-examination.

## estradiol (oestradiol)
Climara, Estrace**, Estrace
Vaginal Cream, Estraderm

## estradiol cypionate
depGynogen, Depo-Estradiol,
Dura-Estrin, E-Cypionate, Estro-
Cyp, Estrofem, Estroject-L.A.

---

*Liquid form contains alcohol.   **May contain tartrazine.   †Canada only.   ‡Australia only.   ◇OTC.

## estradiol valerate (oestradiol valerate)
Delestrogen, Dioval, Duragen-10, Duragen-20, Duragen-40, Estradiol L.A., Estra-L 20, Estra-L 40, Estraval, Estraval P.A., Feminate, Femogex, Gynogen L.A., L.A.E., Menaval, Primogyn Depot‡, Ru-Est-Span 20, Ru-Est-Span 40, Valergen-10, Valergen-20, Valergen-40

*Pregnancy Risk Category: X*

## HOW SUPPLIED
**estradiol**
*Tablets (micronized):* 0.5 mg, 1 mg, 2 mg
*Transdermal:* 4 mg/10 cm² (delivers 0.05 mg/24 hours); 8 mg/20 cm² (delivers 0.1 mg/24 hours)
*Vaginal cream (in nonliquefying base):* 0.1 mg/g
**estradiol cypionate**
*Injection (in oil):* 1 mg/ml, 5 mg/ml
**estradiol valerate**
*Injection (in oil):* 10 mg/ml, 20 mg/ml, 40 mg/ml

## ACTION
Increases the synthesis of DNA, RNA, and protein in responsive tissues. Also reduces release of follicle-stimulating hormone and luteinizing hormone from the pituitary gland.

## ONSET, PEAK, DURATION
Unknown.

## INDICATIONS & DOSAGE
*Vasomotor menopausal symptoms, female hypogonadism, female castration, primary ovarian failure –*
**Adults:** 1 to 2 mg P.O. (estradiol) daily in cycles of 21 days on and 7 days off, or cycles of 5 days on and 2 days off; or 1 transdermal system delivering 0.05 mg/24 hours, applied twice weekly in cycles of 3 weeks on and 1 week off. Alternatively, 1 to 5 mg (cypionate) I.M. q 3 to 4 weeks or 10 to 20 mg (valerate) I.M. q 4 weeks p.r.n.
*Atrophic vaginitis, kraurosis vulvae –*
**Adults:** 2 to 4 g intravaginal applications of cream daily for 1 to 2 weeks. When vaginal mucosa is restored, maintenance dosage is 1 g one to three times weekly in a cyclic regimen. Alternatively, 10 to 20 mg (valerate) I.M. q 4 weeks p.r.n.
*Palliative treatment of advanced, inoperable breast cancer –*
**Men and postmenopausal women:** 10 mg P.O. (estradiol) t.i.d. for 3 months.
*Palliative treatment of advanced inoperable prostate cancer –*
**Men:** 30 mg (valerate) I.M. q 1 to 2 weeks, or 1 to 2 mg P.O. (estradiol) t.i.d.

## ADVERSE REACTIONS
**CNS:** headache, dizziness, chorea, depression, *seizures.*
**CV:** thrombophlebitis, *thromboembolism,* hypertension, edema.
**EENT:** worsening of myopia or astigmatism, intolerance of contact lenses.
**GI:** *nausea,* vomiting, abdominal cramps, bloating, increased appetite, weight changes, pancreatitis.
**GU:** in women – breakthrough bleeding, altered menstrual flow, dysmenorrhea, amenorrhea, *increased risk of endometrial cancer, possibility of increased risk of breast cancer,* cervical erosion, altered cervical secretions, enlargement of uterine fibromas, vaginal candidiasis; in men – gynecomastia, testicular atrophy, impotence.
**Hepatic:** cholestatic jaundice, *hepatic adenoma.*
**Skin:** melasma, urticaria, erythema nodosum, dermatitis, hirsutism or hair loss.
**Other:** breast changes (tenderness, enlargement, secretion), gallbladder disease, hypercalcemia.

---

Reactions may be *common*, uncommon, *life-threatening*, or **COMMON AND LIFE-THREATENING**.

## INTERACTIONS

*Carbamazepine, phenobarbital, rifampin:* decreased effectiveness of estrogen therapy. Monitor closely.
*Corticosteroids:* possible enhanced effects. Monitor closely.
*Cyclosporine:* increased risk of toxicity. Use together with caution and frequently monitor cyclosporine levels.
*Dantrolene, other hepatotoxic medications:* increased risk of hepatotoxicity. Monitor closely.
*Oral anticoagulants:* dosage adjustments may be necessary. Monitor PT.
*Tamoxifen:* estrogens may interfere with effectiveness of tamoxifen. Avoid concomitant use.

## CONTRAINDICATIONS

Contraindicated in patients with thrombophlebitis or thromboembolic disorders, estrogen-dependent neoplasia, breast or reproductive organ cancer (except for palliative treatment), or undiagnosed abnormal genital bleeding and during pregnancy. Also contraindicated in patients with history of thrombophlebitis or thromboembolic disorders associated with previous estrogen use (except for palliative treatment of breast and prostate cancer).

## NURSING CONSIDERATIONS

● Use cautiously in patients with cerebrovascular or coronary artery disease; asthma; bone diseases; migraine; seizures; cardiac, hepatic or renal dysfunction; or in women with a strong family history of breast cancer or who have breast nodules, fibrocystic disease, or abnormal mammographic findings.
● Ensure that patients have a thorough physical examination before initiating estrogen therapy. Patients receiving long-term therapy should have repeat examinations yearly. Periodically monitor serum lipid levels, blood pressure, body weight, and hepatic function as ordered.

● Ask patients about allergies, especially to foods or plants. Estradiol is available as an aqueous solution or as a solution in peanut oil; estradiol cypionate, as a solution in cottonseed oil or vegetable oil; estradiol valerate, as a solution in castor oil, sesame oil, or vegetable oil.
● To administer as an I.M. injection, make sure drug is well dispersed in solution by rolling vial between palms. Inject deep I.M. into large muscle. Rotate injection sites to prevent muscle atrophy. Never give drug I.V..
● Apply the transdermal patch to clean, dry, hairless, intact skin on abdomen or buttocks. Do not apply it to breasts, waistline, or other areas where clothing can loosen the patch. When applying, ensure good contact with the skin, especially around the edges, and hold in place with the palm for about 10 seconds. Rotate application sites.
● Know that in women who are currently taking oral estrogen, treatment with the Estraderm transdermal patch can begin 1 week after withdrawal of oral therapy or sooner if menopausal symptoms appear before the end of the week.
● Because of the risk of thromboembolism, know that therapy should be discontinued at least 1 month before procedures associated with prolonged immobilization or thromboembolism, such as knee or hip surgery.
● Notify the pathologist about any patients receiving estrogen therapy when specimens are obtained and sent to pathology for evaluation.

### ☑ PATIENT TEACHING

● Tell patient that patient package insert that describes estrogen's adverse effects is available; however, also give patient verbal explanation.
● Emphasize the importance of regular physical examinations. Studies suggest that postmenopausal women

---

*Liquid form contains alcohol.  **May contain tartrazine.  †Canada only.  ‡Australia only.  ◇OTC.

who use estrogen replacement for more than 5 years to treat menopausal symptoms may be at increased risk for endometrial cancer. This risk is reduced by using cyclic rather than continuous therapy and the lowest possible dosages of estrogen. Adding progestins to the regimen decreases the incidence of endometrial hyperplasia; however, it isn't known if progestins affect the incidence of endometrial cancer. Most studies show no increased risk of breast cancer.

• Teach patient how to use vaginal cream. Patient should wash vaginal area with soap and water before applying. Tell her to take drug at bedtime or to lie flat for 30 minutes after instillation to minimize drug loss.

• *Alert:* Warn patient to immediately report abdominal pain; pain, numbness, or stiffness in legs or buttocks; pressure or pain in chest; shortness of breath; severe headaches; visual disturbances, such as blind spots, flashing lights, or blurriness; vaginal bleeding or discharge; breast lumps; swelling of hands or feet; yellow skin or sclera; dark urine; and light-colored stools.

• Explain to patient on cyclic therapy for postmenopausal symptoms that, although withdrawal bleeding may occur during week off drug, fertility is not restored. Pregnancy cannot occur because patient does not ovulate.

• Tell diabetic patient to report elevated blood glucose test results so that antidiabetic medication dosage can be adjusted.

• Teach women how to perform routine breast self-examination.

# estrogens, conjugated (estrogenic substances, conjugated; oestrogens, conjugated)

C.E.S.†, Premarin, Premarin Intravenous

*Pregnancy Risk Category: X*

## HOW SUPPLIED
*Tablets:* 0.3 mg, 0.625 mg, 0.9 mg, 1.25 mg, 2.5 mg
*Injection:* 25 mg/5 ml
*Vaginal cream:* 0.625 mg/g

## ACTION
Increases the synthesis of DNA, RNA, and protein in responsive tissues. Also reduces release of follicle-stimulating hormone and luteinizing hormone from the pituitary gland.

## ONSET, PEAK, DURATION
Unknown.

## INDICATIONS & DOSAGE
*Abnormal uterine bleeding (hormonal imbalance) –*
**Women:** 25 mg I.V. or I.M., repeated in 6 to 12 hours as needed.
*Palliative treatment of breast cancer (at least 5 years after menopause) –*
**Men and postmenopausal women:** 10 mg P.O. t.i.d. for 3 months or more.
*Female castration, primary ovarian failure –*
**Women:** 1.25 mg P.O. daily in cycles of 3 weeks on and 1 week off.
*Osteoporosis –*
**Postmenopausal women:** 0.625 mg P.O. daily in cyclic regimen (3 weeks on, 1 week off)
*Hypogonadism –*
**Women:** 2.5 mg P.O. b.i.d. or t.i.d. for 20 consecutive days each month.
*Vasomotor menopausal symptoms –*
**Women:** 0.3 to 1.25 mg P.O. daily in cycles of 3 weeks on and 1 week off.
*Atrophic vaginitis, kraurosis vulvae –*
**Women:** 0.5 to 2 g intravaginally

---

Reactions may be *common*, uncommon, *life-threatening*, or COMMON AND LIFE-THREATENING.

once daily on a cyclical basis (3 weeks on and 1 week off).
*Palliative treatment of inoperable prostate cancer—*
**Men:** 1.25 to 2.5 mg P.O. t.i.d.

## ADVERSE REACTIONS
**CNS:** headache, dizziness, chorea, depression, *seizures.*
**CV:** thrombophlebitis; *thromboembolism;* hypertension; edema; *increased risk of CVA, pulmonary embolism, MI.*
**EENT:** worsening of myopia or astigmatism, intolerance of contact lenses.
**GI:** *nausea,* vomiting, abdominal cramps, bloating, anorexia, increased appetite, weight changes, pancreatitis.
**GU:** in women—breakthrough bleeding, altered menstrual flow, dysmenorrhea, amenorrhea, *increased risk of endometrial cancer, possibility of increased risk of breast cancer,* cervical erosion, altered cervical secretions, enlargement of uterine fibromas, vaginal candidiasis; in men—gynecomastia, testicular atrophy, impotence.
**Hepatic:** cholestatic jaundice, *hepatic adenoma.*
**Skin:** melasma, urticaria, flushing (with rapid I.V. administration), hirsutism or hair loss, erythema nodosum, dermatitis.
**Other:** breast changes (tenderness, enlargement, secretion), hypercalcemia, gallbladder disease.

## INTERACTIONS
*Carbamazepine, phenobarbital, rifampin:* decreased effectiveness of estrogen therapy. Monitor closely.
*Corticosteroids:* possible enhanced effects. Monitor closely.
*Cyclosporine:* increased risk of toxicity. Use together with caution and frequently monitor cyclosporine levels.
*Dantrolene, other hepatotoxic medications:* increased risk of hepatotoxicity. Monitor closely.

*Oral anticoagulants:* dosage adjustments may be necessary. Monitor PT.
*Tamoxifen:* estrogens may interfere with effectiveness of tamoxifen. Avoid concomitant use.

## CONTRAINDICATIONS
Contraindicated in patients with thrombophlebitis or thromboembolic disorders, estrogen-dependent neoplasia, breast or reproductive organ cancer (except for palliative treatment), or undiagnosed abnormal genital bleeding and during pregnancy.

## NURSING CONSIDERATIONS
• Use cautiously in patients with cerebrovascular or coronary artery disease; asthma; bone disease; migraine; seizures; cardiac, hepatic, or renal dysfunction; or in women with family history (mother, grandmother, sister) of breast or genital tract cancer or who have breast nodules, fibrocystic disease, or abnormal mammographic findings.
• Ensure that patients have a thorough physical examination before initiating estrogen therapy. Patients receiving long-term therapy should have examinations yearly. Periodically monitor serum lipid levels, blood pressure, body weight, and hepatic function, as ordered.
• Know that I.M. or I.V. use preferred for rapid treatment of dysfunctional uterine bleeding or reduction of surgical bleeding.
• Refrigerate before reconstituting. Agitate gently after adding diluent.
• **I.V. use:** When giving by direct I.V. injection, administer slowly to avoid flushing reaction. For infusion, mix with $D_5W$, 0.9% sodium chloride for injection, or invert sugar solutions. Avoid mixing with solutions of acidic pH to prevent incompatibility.
• When administering by I.M. injection, inject deeply into large muscle. Rotate injection sites to prevent muscle atrophy.

• Notify the pathologist about any patients receiving estrogen therapy when specimens are obtained and sent to pathology for evaluation.
• Because of the risk of thromboembolism, know that therapy should be discontinued at least 1 month before procedures associated with prolonged immobilization or thromboembolism, such as knee or hip surgery.

## ☑ PATIENT TEACHING
• Tell patient that patient package insert that describes estrogen's adverse effects is available; however, also give patient verbal explanation.
• Emphasize the importance of regular physical examinations. Studies suggest that postmenopausal women who use estrogen replacement for more than 5 years to treat menopausal symptoms may be at increased risk for endometrial cancer. This risk is reduced by using cyclic rather than continuous therapy and the lowest possible dosages of estrogen. Adding progestins to the regimen decreases the incidence of endometrial hyperplasia; however, it isn't known if progestins affect the incidence of endometrial cancer. Most studies show no increased risk of breast cancer.
• Teach patient how to use vaginal cream. Patient should wash the vaginal area with soap and water before applying. Tell her to use drug at bedtime or to lie flat for 30 minutes after instillation to minimize drug loss.
• Explain to patient on cyclic therapy for postmenopausal symptoms that, although withdrawal bleeding may occur during week off drug, fertility is not restored. Pregnancy cannot occur because she does not ovulate.
• *Alert:* Warn patient to immediately report abdominal pain; pain, numbness, or stiffness in legs or buttocks; pressure or pain in chest; shortness of breath; severe headaches; visual disturbances, such as blind spots, flashing lights, or blurriness; vaginal

bleeding or discharge; breast lumps; swelling of hands or feet; yellow skin or sclera; dark urine; and light-colored stools.
• Tell diabetic patient to report elevated blood glucose test results so that antidiabetic medication dosage can be adjusted.
• Teach women how to perform routine breast self-examination.

## estrone (oestrone)
Estroject-2, Estrone A, Estrone 5, Femogen Forte†, Gynogen, Kestrin Aqueous, Kestrone 5, Theelin Aqueous, Unigen, Wehgen-V

*Pregnancy Risk Category: X*

## HOW SUPPLIED
*Injection (aqueous suspension):* 2 mg/ml, 5 mg/ml

## ACTION
Increases the synthesis of DNA, RNA, and protein in responsive tissues. Also reduces release of follicle-stimulating hormone and luteinizing hormone from the pituitary.

## ONSET, PEAK, DURATION
Unknown.

## INDICATIONS & DOSAGE
*Atrophic vaginitis, kraurosis vulvae, and vasomotor menopausal symptoms* –
**Women:** 0.1 to 0.5 mg I.M. two or three times weekly.
*Female hypogonadism, castration, and primary ovarian failure* –
**Women:** 0.1 to 1 mg I.M. weekly as a single dose or in divided doses.
*Palliative treatment of inoperable prostate cancer* –
**Men:** 2 to 4 mg I.M. two to three times weekly.

## ADVERSE REACTIONS

**CNS:** headache, dizziness, chorea, depression, *seizures.*

**CV:** *increased risk of CVA, pulmonary embolism, MI;* thrombophlebitis; *thromboembolism;* hypertension; edema.

**EENT:** worsening of myopia or astigmatism, intolerance of contact lenses.

**GI:** *nausea,* vomiting, abdominal cramps, bloating, anorexia, increased appetite, weight changes, pancreatitis.

**GU:** in women — breakthrough bleeding, altered menstrual flow, dysmenorrhea, amenorrhea, cervical erosion, altered cervical secretions, *increased risk of endometrial cancer, possibility of increased risk of breast cancer,* enlargement of uterine fibromas, vaginal candidiasis; in men — gynecomastia, testicular atrophy, impotence.

**Hepatic:** cholestatic jaundice, *hepatic adenoma.*

**Skin:** melasma, urticaria, hirsutism or hair loss, erythema nodosum, dermatitis.

**Other:** breast changes (tenderness, enlargement, secretion), hypercalcemia, gallbladder disease.

## INTERACTIONS

*Carbamazepine, phenobarbital, rifampin:* decreased effectiveness of estrogen therapy. Monitor closely.

*Corticosteroids:* possible enhanced effects. Monitor closely.

*Cyclosporine:* increased risk of toxicity. Use together with caution and frequently monitor cyclosporine levels.

*Dantrolene, other hepatotoxic medications:* increased risk of hepatotoxicity. Monitor closely.

*Oral anticoagulants:* dosage adjustments may be necessary. Monitor PT.

*Tamoxifen:* estrogens may interfere with effectiveness of tamoxifen. Avoid concomitant use.

## CONTRAINDICATIONS

Contraindicated in patients with thrombophlebitis or thromboembolic disorders, estrogen-dependent neoplasia, breast or reproductive organ cancer (except for palliative treatment), or undiagnosed abnormal genital bleeding and during pregnancy.

## NURSING CONSIDERATIONS

● Use cautiously in patients with cerebrovascular or coronary artery disease; asthma; bone diseases; mental depression; migraine; seizures; cardiac, hepatic, or renal dysfunction; or in women with family history (mother, grandmother, sister) of breast or genital tract cancer or who have breast nodules, fibrocystic disease, or abnormal mammographic findings.

● Ensure that patients have a thorough physical examination before initiating estrogen therapy. Patients receiving long-term therapy should have examinations yearly. Periodically monitor serum lipid levels, blood pressure, body weight, and hepatic function, as ordered.

● Administer estrone I.M. Rotate injection sites to prevent muscle atrophy.

● Notify the pathologist about any patients receiving estrogen therapy when specimens are obtained and sent to pathology for evaluation.

● Because of the risk of thromboembolism, know that therapy should be discontinued at least 1 month before procedures associated with prolonged immobilization or thromboembolism, such as knee or hip surgery.

## ☑ PATIENT TEACHING

● Inform patient that patient package insert that describes estrogen's adverse effects is available; however, also give patient verbal explanation.

● Emphasize the importance of regular physical examinations. Studies suggest that postmenopausal women who use estrogen replacement for more than 5 years to treat menopausal symptoms may be at increased risk for endometrial cancer. This risk is reduced by using cyclic rather than continuous therapy and the lowest possible dosages of estrogen. Adding progestins to the regimen decreases the incidence of endometrial hyperplasia; however, it isn't known if progestins affect the incidence of endometrial cancer. Most studies show no increased risk of breast cancer.

• Explain to patient on cyclic therapy for postmenopausal symptoms that, although withdrawal bleeding may occur during week off drug, fertility is not restored. Pregnancy cannot occur because patient does not ovulate.

• *Alert:* Warn patient to immediately report abdominal pain; pain, numbness, or stiffness in legs or buttocks; pressure or pain in chest; shortness of breath; severe headaches; visual disturbances, such as blind spots, flashing lights, or blurriness; vaginal bleeding or discharge; breast lumps; swelling of hands or feet; yellow skin and sclera; dark urine; and light-colored stools.

• Tell diabetic patient to report elevated blood glucose test results so that antidiabetic medication dosage can be adjusted.

• Teach women how to perform routine breast self-examination.

## estropipate (piperazine estrone sulfate)
Ogen, OrthoEST

*Pregnancy Risk Category: X*

### HOW SUPPLIED
*Tablets:* 0.75 mg, 1.5 mg, 3 mg, 6 mg
*Vaginal cream:* 1.5 mg/g

### ACTION
Increases the synthesis of DNA, RNA, and proteins in responsive tissues. Also reduces release of follicle-stimulating hormone and luteinizing hormone from the pituitary gland.

### ONSET, PEAK, DURATION
Unknown.

### INDICATIONS & DOSAGE
*Vulval and vaginal atrophy –*
**Women:** 0.625 to 5 mg P.O. daily 3 weeks on, 1 week off, or 2 to 4 g of vaginal cream daily. Typically, dosage given on a cyclical, short-term basis.
*Primary ovarian failure, female castration, female hypogonadism –*
**Women:** administered on a cyclical basis – 1.25 to 7.5 mg P.O. daily for the first 3 weeks, followed by a rest period of 8 to 10 days. If bleeding does not occur by the end of the rest period, cycle repeated.
*Vasomotor menopausal symptoms –*
**Women:** 0.625 mg to 5 mg P.O. daily in cyclic method of 3 weeks on, 1 week off.
*Prevention of osteoporosis –*
**Women:** 0.625 mg P.O. daily for 25 days of a 31-day cycle.

### ADVERSE REACTIONS
**CNS:** depression, headache, dizziness, migraine, *seizures.*
**CV:** edema; thrombophlebitis; *increased risk of CVA, pulmonary embolism, MI; thromboembolism.*
**GI:** nausea, vomiting, abdominal cramps, bloating, weight changes.
**GU:** increased size of uterine fibromas, *increased risk of endometrial cancer, possibility of increased risk of breast cancer,* vaginal candidiasis, cystitis-like syndrome, dysmenorrhea, amenorrhea, breakthrough bleeding, condition resembling premenstrual syndrome.
**Hepatic:** cholestatic jaundice, *hepatic adenoma.*
**Skin:** hemorrhagic eruption, erythema nodosum, *erythema multiforme,* hirsutism, melasma, hair loss.
**Other:** breast engorgement or enlargement, hypercalcemia, gallbladder disease, aggravation of porphyria, libido changes.

---

Reactions may be *common,* uncommon, *life-threatening,* or **COMMON AND LIFE-THREATENING.**

## INTERACTIONS

*Carbamazepine, phenobarbital, rifampin:* decreased effectiveness of estrogen therapy. Monitor closely.

*Corticosteroids:* possible enhanced effects. Monitor closely.

*Cyclosporine:* increased risk of toxicity. Use together with caution and frequently monitor cyclosporine levels.

*Dantrolene, other hepatotoxic medications:* increased risk of hepatotoxicity. Monitor closely.

*Oral anticoagulants:* dosage adjustments may be necessary. Monitor PT.

*Tamoxifen:* estrogens may interfere with effectiveness of tamoxifen. Avoid concomitant use.

## CONTRAINDICATIONS

Contraindicated in patients with active thrombophlebitis or thromboembolic disorders; in those with estrogen-dependent neoplasia, breast, reproductive organ, or genital cancer; in those with undiagnosed genital bleeding; and during pregnancy.

## NURSING CONSIDERATIONS

● Use cautiously in patients with cerebrovascular or coronary artery disease; asthma; mental depression; bone disease; migraine; seizures; cardiac, hepatic, or renal dysfunction; and in women with a family history (mother, grandmother, sister) of breast or genital tract cancer or who have breast nodules, fibrocystic disease, or abnormal mammographic findings.

● Ensure that patients have a thorough physical examination before initiating estrogen therapy. Patients receiving long-term therapy should have examinations yearly. Periodically monitor serum lipid levels, blood pressure, body weight, and hepatic function as ordered.

● Know that when used to treat hypogonadism, the duration of therapy necessary to produce withdrawal bleeding depends on the patient's endometrial response to the drug. If satisfactory withdrawal bleeding does not occur, an oral progestin is added to the regimen, as ordered. Explain to the patient that, despite the return of withdrawal bleeding, pregnancy cannot occur because she does not ovulate.

● Be aware of the following estropipate/estrone equivalents:

| | | |
|---|---|---|
| 0.75 mg estropipate | = | 0.625 mg estrone |
| 1.5 mg estropipate | = | 1.25 mg estrone |
| 3 mg estropipate | = | 2.5 mg estrone |
| 6 mg estropipate | = | 5 mg estrone |

● Because of the risk of thromboembolism, know that therapy should be discontinued at least 1 month before procedures associated with prolonged immobilization or thromboembolism, such as knee or hip surgery.

## ☑ PATIENT TEACHING

● Tell patient that patient package insert that describes estrogen's adverse effects is available; however, also give patient verbal explanation.

● Stress the importance of regular physical examinations. Studies suggest that postmenopausal women who use estrogen replacement for more than 5 years to treat menopausal symptoms may be at increased risk for endometrial cancer. This risk is reduced by using cyclic rather than continuous therapy and the lowest possible dosages of estrogen. Adding progestins to the regimen decreases the incidence of endometrial hyperplasia; however, it isn't known if progestins affect the incidence of endometrial cancer. Most studies show no increased risk of breast cancer.

● *Alert:* Warn patient to immediately report abdominal pain; pain, stiffness, or numbness in the legs or buttocks; pressure or pain in the chest; shortness of breath; severe headaches; visual disturbances, such as blind spots or flashing lights; vaginal bleeding or discharge; breast lumps; swelling of the hands or feet; yellow skin or sclera; dark urine; and light-colored stools.

---

*Liquid form contains alcohol.  **May contain tartrazine.  †Canada only.  ‡Australia only.  ◊OTC.

• Teach women how to perform routine breast self-examination.

---

# ethinyl estradiol (ethinyloestradiol)

Estinyl**, Feminone

*Pregnancy Risk Category: X*

## HOW SUPPLIED
*Tablets:* 0.02 mg, 0.05 mg, 0.5 mg

## ACTION
Increases the synthesis of DNA, RNA, and protein in responsive tissues. Also reduces release of follicle-stimulating hormone and luteinizing hormone from the pituitary gland.

## ONSET, PEAK, DURATION
Unknown.

## INDICATIONS & DOSAGE
*Palliative treatment of metastatic breast cancer (at least 5 years after menopause)* –
**Women:** 1 mg P.O. t.i.d. for at least 3 months.
*Female hypogonadism* –
**Women:** 0.05 mg P.O. once daily to t.i.d. 2 weeks a month, followed by 2 weeks of progesterone therapy; continued for three to six monthly dosing cycles, followed by 2 months off.
*Vasomotor menopausal symptoms* –
**Women:** 0.02 to 0.05 mg P.O. daily for cycles of 3 weeks on and 1 week off.
*Palliative treatment of metastatic inoperable prostate cancer* –
**Men:** 0.15 to 2 mg P.O. daily.

## ADVERSE REACTIONS
**CNS:** headache, dizziness, chorea, depression, *seizures*.
**CV:** thrombophlebitis; *thromboembolism;* hypertension; edema, *increased risk of CVA, pulmonary embolism, MI.*
**EENT:** worsening of myopia or astigmatism, intolerance to contact lenses.

**GI:** *nausea,* vomiting, abdominal cramps, bloating, anorexia, increased appetite, weight changes.
**GU:** in women – breakthrough bleeding, altered menstrual flow, dysmenorrhea, amenorrhea, cervical erosion, *increased risk of endometrial cancer, possibility of increased risk of breast cancer,* altered cervical secretions, enlargement of uterine fibromas, vaginal candidiasis; in men – gynecomastia, testicular atrophy, impotence.
**Hepatic:** cholestatic jaundice, *hepatic adenoma.*
**Skin:** melasma, urticaria, acne, seborrhea, oily skin, hirsutism or hair loss, erythema nodosum, dermatitis.
**Other:** breast changes (tenderness, enlargement, secretion), hypercalcemia, gallbladder disease.

## INTERACTIONS
*Carbamazepine, phenobarbital, rifampin:* decreased effectiveness of estrogen therapy. Monitor closely.
*Corticosteroids:* possible enhanced effects. Monitor closely.
*Cyclosporine:* increased risk of toxicity. Use together with caution and frequently monitor cyclosporine levels.
*Dantrolene, other hepatotoxic medications:* increased risk of hepatotoxicity. Monitor closely.
*Oral anticoagulants:* dosage adjustments may be necessary. Monitor PT.
*Tamoxifen:* estrogens may interfere with effectiveness of tamoxifen. Avoid concomitant use.

## CONTRAINDICATIONS
Contraindicated in patients with thrombophlebitis or thromboembolic disorders, estrogen-dependent neoplasia, breast or reproductive organ cancer (except for palliative treatment), or undiagnosed abnormal genital bleeding and during pregnancy.

## NURSING CONSIDERATIONS
• Use cautiously in patients with cerebrovascular or coronary artery disease;

---

Reactions may be *common,* uncommon, *life-threatening,* or **COMMON AND LIFE-THREATENING.**

asthma; mental depression; bone disease; cardiac, hepatic, or renal dysfunction; or in women with a family history (mother, grandmother, sister) of breast or genital tract cancer, or who have breast nodules, fibrocystic disease, or abnormal mammographic findings.

• Ensure that patients have a thorough physical examination before initiating estrogen therapy. Patients receiving long-term therapy should have examinations yearly. Periodically monitor serum lipid levels, blood pressure, body weight, and hepatic function as ordered.

• Because of the risk of thromboembolism, know that therapy should be discontinued at least 1 month before procedures associated with prolonged immobilization or thromboembolism, such as knee or hip surgery.

• Notify the pathologist about any patients receiving estrogen therapy when specimens are obtained and sent to pathology for evaluation.

☑ **PATIENT TEACHING**

• Tell patient that patient package insert that describes estrogen's adverse effects is available; however, also give patient verbal explanation.

• Emphasize the importance of regular physical examinations. Studies suggest that postmenopausal women who use estrogen replacement for more than 5 years to treat menopausal symptoms may be at increased risk for endometrial cancer. This risk is reduced by using cyclic rather than continuous therapy and the lowest possible dosages of estrogen. Adding progestins to the regimen decreases the incidence of endometrial hyperplasia; however, it isn't known if progestins affect the incidence of endometrial cancer. Most studies show no increased risk of breast cancer.

• Explain to patient on cyclic therapy for postmenopausal symptoms that, although withdrawal bleeding may occur during week off drug, fertility is not restored. Pregnancy cannot occur because patient does not ovulate.

• **Alert:** Warn patient to immediately report abdominal pain; pain, numbness, or stiffness in legs or buttocks; pressure or pain in chest; shortness of breath; severe headaches; visual disturbances, such as blind spots, flashing lights, or blurriness; vaginal bleeding or discharge; breast lumps; swelling of hands or feet; yellow skin or sclera; dark urine; or light-colored stools.

• Tell diabetic patient to report elevated blood glucose test results so that antidiabetic medication dosage can be adjusted.

• Teach women how to perform routine breast self-examination.

---

## ethinyl estradiol and desogestrel
monophasic: Desogen, Ortho-Cept

## ethinyl estradiol and ethynodiol diacetate
monophasic: Demulen 1/35, Demulen 1/50

## ethinyl estradiol and levonorgestrel
monophasic: Levlen, Nordette
triphasic: Tri-Levlen, Triphasil

## ethinyl estradiol and norethindrone
monophasic: Brevicon, Genora 0.5/35, Genora 1/35, ModiCon, N.E.E. 1/35, Nelova 0.5/35 E, Nelova1/35 E, Norcept-E 1/35, Norethin 1/35 E, Norinyl 1 + 35, Ortho-Novum 1/35, Ovcon-35, Ovcon-50
biphasic: Jenset-28, Nelova 10/11, Ortho-Novum 10/11
triphasic: Ortho-Novum 7/7/7, Tri-Norinyl

---

*Liquid form contains alcohol. **May contain tartrazine. †Canada only. ‡Australia only. ◊OTC.

## ethinyl estradiol and norethindrone acetate

monophasic: Loestrin 21 1/20, Loestrin 21 1.5/30, Norlestrin 21 1/50, Norlestrin 21 2.5/50

## ethinyl estradiol and norgestimate

monophasic: Ortho Cyclen
triphasic: Ortho Tri-Cyclen

## ethinyl estradiol and norgestrel

monophasic: Lo/Ovral, Ovral

## ethinyl estradiol, norethindrone acetate, and ferrous fumarate

monophasic: Loestrin Fe 1/20, Loestrin Fe 1.5/30, Norlestrin Fe 1/50, Norlestrin Fe 2.5/50

## mestranol and norethindrone

monophasic: Genora 1/50, Nelova 1/50 M, Norethin 1/50 M, Norinyl 1 + 50, Ortho-Novum 1/50

## mestranol and norethynodrel

monophasic: Enovid 5 mg, Enovid 10 mg

*Pregnancy Risk Category: X*

---

**HOW SUPPLIED**
*Monophasic oral contraceptives*
**ethinyl estradiol and desogestrel**
*Tablets:* ethinyl estradiol 30 mcg and desogestrel 0.15 mg (Desogen, Ortho-Cept)
**ethinyl estradiol and ethynodiol diacetate**
*Tablets:* ethinyl estradiol 35 mcg and ethynodiol diacetate 1 mg (Demulen 1/35); ethinyl estradiol 50 mcg and ethynodiol diacetate 1 mg (Demulen 1/50)
**ethinyl estradiol and levonorgestrel**
*Tablets:* ethinyl estradiol 30 mcg and levonorgestrel 0.15 mg (Levlen, Nordette)

**ethinyl estradiol and norethindrone**
*Tablets:* ethinyl estradiol 35 mcg and norethindrone 0.4 mg (Ovcon-35); ethinyl estradiol 35 mcg and norethindrone 0.5 mg (Brevicon, Genora 0.5/35, ModiCon, Nelova 0.5/35 E); ethinyl estradiol 35 mcg and norethindrone 1 mg (Genora 1/35, N.E.E. 1/35, Nelova 1/35 E, Norcept-E 1/35, Norethin 1/35 E, Norinyl 1 + 35, Ortho-Novum 1/35); ethinyl estradiol 50 mcg and norethindrone 1 mg (Ovcon-50)
**ethinyl estradiol and norethindrone acetate**
*Tablets:* ethinyl estradiol 20 mcg and norethindrone acetate 1 mg (Loestrin 21 1/20); ethinyl estradiol 30 mcg and norethindrone acetate 1.5 mg (Loestrin 21 1.5/30); ethinyl estradiol 50 mcg and norethindrone acetate 1 mg (Norlestrin 21 1/50); ethinyl estradiol 50 mcg and norethindrone acetate 2.5 mg (Norlestrin 21 2.5/50)
**ethinyl estradiol and norgestimate**
*Tablets:* ethinyl estradiol 35 mcg and norgestimate 0.25 mg (Ortho Cyclen)
**ethinyl estradiol and norgestrel**
*Tablets:* ethinyl estradiol 30 mcg and norgestrel 0.3 mg (Lo/Ovral); ethinyl estradiol 50 mcg and norgestrel 0.5 mg (Ovral)
**ethinyl estradiol, norethindrone acetate, and ferrous fumarate**
*Tablets:* ethinyl estradiol 20 mcg, norethindrone acetate 1 mg, and ferrous fumarate 75 mg (Loestrin Fe 1/20); ethinyl estradiol 30 mcg, norethindrone acetate 1.5 mg, and ferrous fumarate 75 mg (Loestrin Fe 1.5/30); ethinyl estradiol 50 mcg, norethindrone acetate 1 mg, and ferrous fumarate 75 mg (Norlestrin Fe 1/50); ethinyl estradiol 50 mcg, norethindrone acetate 2.5 mg, and ferrous fumarate 75 mg (Norlestrin Fe 2.5/50)
**mestranol and norethindrone**
*Tablets:* mestranol 50 mcg and norethindrone 1 mg (Genora 1/50, Nelova 1/50 M, Norethin 1/50 M, Norinyl 1 + 50, Ortho-Novum 1/50)

---

**mestranol and norethynodrel**
*Tablets:* mestranol 75 mg and norethynodrel 5 mg (Enovid 5 mg); mestranol 150 mg and norethynodrel 9.85
mg (Enovid 10 mg).
**Biphasic oral contraceptives**
**ethinyl estradiol and norethindrone**
*Tablets:* ethinyl estradiol 35 mcg and
norethindrone 0.5 mg during phase 1
[10 days]; ethinyl estradiol 35 mcg
and norethindrone 1 mg during phase
2 [11 days] (Jenset-28, Nelova 10/11,
Ortho-Novum 10/11)
**Triphasic oral contraceptives**
**ethinyl estradiol and levonorgestrel**
*Tablets:* (Tri-Levlen, Triphasil) ethinyl estradiol 35 mcg and levonorgestrel 0.05 mg during phase 1 [6 days];
ethinyl estradiol 35 mcg and levonorgestrel 0.075 mg during phase 2 [5
days]; ethinyl estradiol 35 mcg and levonorgestrel 0.125 mg during phase 3
[10 days]
**ethinyl estradiol and norethindrone**
*Tablets:* (Tri-Norinyl) ethinyl estradiol
35 mcg and norethindrone 0.5 mg
during phase 1 [7 days]; ethinyl estradiol 35 mcg and norethindrone 1 mg
during phase 2 [9 days]; ethinyl estradiol 35 mcg and norethindrone 0.5 mg
during phase 3 [5 days]; (Ortho-
Novum 7/7/7) ethinyl estradiol 35
mcg and norethindrone 0.5 mg during
phase 1 [7 days]; ethinyl estradiol 35
mcg and norethindrone 0.75 mg during phase 2 [7 days]; ethinyl estradiol
35 mcg and norethindrone 1 mg during phase 3 [7 days]
**ethinyl estradiol and norgestimate**
*Tablets:* (Ortho Tri-Cyclen) ethinyl
estradiol 35 mcg and norgestimate
0.18 mg during phase 1 [7 days]; ethinyl estradiol 35 mcg and norgestimate
0.215 mg during phase 2 [7 days];
ethinyl estradiol 35 mcg and norgestimate 0.25 mg during phase 3 [7 days]

**ACTION**
Oral contraceptives inhibit ovulation
through a negative feedback mechanism directed at the hypothalamus.

They also may prevent transport of
the ovum through the fallopian tubes.
  Estrogen suppresses secretion of
follicle-stimulating hormone, blocking follicular development and ovulation.
  Progestin suppresses secretion of
luteinizing hormone so ovulation cannot occur even if the follicle develops.
Progestin thickens cervical mucus,
which interferes with sperm migration, and also causes endometrial
changes that prevent implantation of
the fertilized ovum.

**ONSET, PEAK, DURATION**
Onset and duration unknown. Plasma
levels of ethinyl estradiol peak within
1 to 2 hours; of norethindrone, within
½ to 4 hours.

**INDICATIONS & DOSAGE**
*Contraception –*
**Adults:** *Monophasic oral contraceptives* – 1 tablet P.O. daily, beginning
on day 5 of menstrual cycle (first day
of menstrual flow is day 1). With 20-
and 21-tablet packages, new dosing
cycle begins 7 days after last tablet
taken. With 28-tablet packages, dosage is 1 tablet daily without interruption; extra tablets are placebos or contain iron.
*Biphasic oral contraceptives –*
1 color tablet P.O. daily for 10 days;
then next color tablet for 11 days.
*Triphasic oral contraceptives –*
1 tablet P.O. daily in the sequence
specified by the brand.
*Endometriosis –*
**Adults:** 1 tablet Enovid 5 mg or 10
mg P.O. daily for 2 weeks starting on
day 5 of menstrual cycle. Continued
without interruption for 6 to 9
months, increasing dosage by 5 to 10
mg q 2 weeks, up to 20 mg daily; up
to 40 mg daily as needed and ordered
if breakthrough bleeding occurs.

---

*Liquid form contains alcohol.  **May contain tartrazine.  †Canada only.  ‡Australia only.  ◇OTC.

## ADVERSE REACTIONS

**CNS:** *headache, dizziness,* depression, lethargy, migraine.
**CV:** *thromboembolism,* hypertension, edema, *pulmonary embolism, CVA.*
**EENT:** worsening of myopia or astigmatism, intolerance of contact lenses, exophthalmos, diplopia.
**GI:** *nausea,* vomiting, abdominal cramps, bloating, anorexia, changes in appetite, weight gain, *bowel ischemia,* pancreatitis.
**GU:** *breakthrough bleeding,* granulomatous colitis, dysmenorrhea, amenorrhea, cervical erosion or abnormal secretions, enlargement of uterine fibromas, vaginal candidiasis.
**Hepatic:** gallbladder disease, cholestatic jaundice, *liver tumors.*
**Skin:** rash, acne, *erythema multiforme.*
**Other:** breast changes *(tenderness, enlargement, secretion);* hypercalcemia.

## INTERACTIONS

*Carbamazepine, phenobarbital, phenytoin, rifampin:* decreased effectiveness of estrogen therapy. Monitor closely.
*Corticosteroids:* possible enhanced effects. Monitor closely.
*Griseofulvin, penicillins, tetracyclines:* may decrease effectiveness of oral contraceptives. Avoid concomitant use, if possible.
*Oral anticoagulants:* dosage adjustments may be necessary. Monitor PT.
*Tamoxifen:* estrogens may interfere with effectiveness of tamoxifen. Avoid concomitant use.

## CONTRAINDICATIONS

Contraindicated in patients with thromboembolic disorders, cerebrovascular or coronary artery disease, diplopia or any ocular lesion arising from ophthalmic vascular disease, classical migraine, MI, known or suspected breast cancer, known or suspected estrogen-dependent neoplasia, benign or malignant liver tumors, active liver disease or history of cholestatic jaundice with pregnancy or prior use of oral contraceptives, and undiagnosed abnormal vaginal bleeding; in known or suspected pregnancy; and in breast-feeding patients.

## NURSING CONSIDERATIONS

● Use cautiously in patients with cardiac, renal, or hepatic insufficiency; hyperlipidemia; hypertension; migraine; seizure disorders; or asthma.
● Be aware that triphasic oral contraceptives may cause fewer adverse reactions, such as breakthrough bleeding and spotting.
● Know that the Centers for Disease Control and Prevention reports that the use of oral contraceptives *may decrease* the incidence of ovarian and endometrial cancers. Also, oral contraceptives do not appear to increase a woman's risk of breast cancer. However, the FDA reports that oral contraceptives may be linked to an increased risk of cervical cancer.
● Periodically monitor serum lipid levels, blood pressure, body weight, and hepatic function as ordered.
● Know that many laboratory tests are affected by oral contraceptives.
● Estrogens and progestins may alter glucose tolerance, thus changing dosage requirements for antidiabetic drugs. Monitor blood glucose levels.
● Discontinue if patients develop granulomatous colitis while on oral contraceptives and notify doctor.
● Know that drug should be discontinued at least 1 week before surgery to decrease risk of thromboembolism. Tell patient to use an alternative method of birth control.

☑ **PATIENT TEACHING**
● Tell patient to take tablets at same time each day; nighttime dosing may reduce nausea and headaches.
● Advise patient to use an additional

method of birth control, such as condoms or a diaphragm with spermicide, for the first week of administration in the initial cycle.

• Tell patient missed doses in midcycle greatly increase likelihood of pregnancy.

• If one tablet is missed, tell patient to take it as soon as she remembers or to take two tablets the next day and continue regular schedule. If patient misses 2 consecutive days, instruct her to take two tablets daily for 2 days and then resume normal schedule. Also advise her to use an additional method of birth control for 7 days after two missed doses. If three or more doses are missed, tell patient to discard remaining tablets in monthly package and to substitute another contraceptive method. If next menstrual period doesn't begin on schedule, warn patient to rule out pregnancy before starting new dosing cycle. If menstrual period begins, have patient start new dosing cycle 7 days after last tablet was taken.

• Warn patient that headache, nausea, dizziness, breast tenderness, spotting, and breakthrough bleeding are common at first. These effects should diminish after three to six dosing cycles (months).

• Instruct patient to weigh herself at least twice a week and to report any sudden weight gain or edema to the doctor.

• Warn patient to avoid exposure to ultraviolet light or prolonged exposure to sunlight.

• *Alert:* Warn patient to immediately report abdominal pain; numbness, stiffness, or pain in legs or buttocks; pressure or pain in chest; shortness of breath; severe headache; visual disturbances, such as blind spots, blurriness, or flashing lights; undiagnosed vaginal bleeding or discharge; two consecutive, missed menstrual periods; lumps in the breast; swelling of hands or feet; or severe pain in the abdomen (tumor rupture in the liver).

• Advise patient of increased risks associated with simultaneous use of cigarettes and oral contraceptives.

• If one menstrual period is missed and tablets have been taken on schedule, tell patient to continue taking them. If two consecutive menstrual periods are missed, tell patient to stop drug and have pregnancy test. Progestins may cause birth defects if taken early in pregnancy.

• Advise patient not to take same drug for longer than 12 months without consulting the doctor. Stress importance of Papanicolaou tests and annual gynecologic examinations.

• Advise patient to check with the doctor about how soon pregnancy may be attempted after hormonal therapy is stopped. Many doctors recommend that women not become pregnant within 2 months after stopping drug.

• Warn patient of possible delay in achieving pregnancy when drug is discontinued.

• Tell patient many doctors advise women on long-term therapy (5 years or longer) to stop drug and use other birth control methods. Periodically reassess patient while off hormone therapy.

• Teach patient how to perform routine breast self-examination.

# hydroxyprogesterone caproate

Delta-Lutin, Duralutin, Gesterol L.A. 250, Hy/Gestrone, Hylutin, Hyprogest 250, Pro-Depo, Prodrox 250, Pro-Span

*Pregnancy Risk Category: X*

## HOW SUPPLIED
*Injection:* 125 mg/ml, 250 mg/ml

---

## ACTION

Suppresses ovulation, possibly by inhibiting pituitary gonadotropin secretion, and forms thick cervical mucus.

## ONSET, PEAK, DURATION

Onset and peak unknown. Effects persist for 9 to 17 days.

## INDICATIONS & DOSAGE

*Amenorrhea, uterine bleeding –*
**Adults:** 375 mg I.M. q 4 weeks. Stop after four cycles.
*Palliative treatment of advanced inoperable endometrial cancer –*
**Adults:** 1 to 7 g I.M. weekly.

## ADVERSE REACTIONS

**CNS:** depression.
**CV:** thrombophlebitis, *thromboembolism, CVA, pulmonary embolism,* edema.
**EENT:** exophthalmos, diplopia.
**GU:** breakthrough bleeding, dysmenorrhea, amenorrhea, cervical erosion, abnormal secretions.
**Hepatic:** cholestatic jaundice.
**Skin:** rash, acne, pruritus, melasma, irritation and pain at injection site.
**Other:** breast tenderness, enlargement, or secretion; changes in weight.

## INTERACTIONS

None significant.

## CONTRAINDICATIONS

Contraindicated in patients with hypersensitivity to drug, thromboembolic disorders, cerebral apoplexy, breast or genital organ cancer, undiagnosed abnormal vaginal bleeding, severe hepatic disease, or missed abortion and during pregnancy.

## NURSING CONSIDERATIONS

• Use cautiously in patients with diabetes mellitus, seizures, migraine, cardiac or renal disease, asthma, mental depression, or impaired liver function.
• Know that drug should not be used

to induce withdrawal bleeding or as a test for pregnancy; drug may cause birth defects and masculinization of female fetus.
• Give oil solutions (sesame oil and castor oil) via deep I.M. injection in gluteal muscle. Rotate injection sites to prevent muscle atrophy.

## ☑ PATIENT TEACHING

• FDA regulations require that, before receiving first dose, patient reads package insert explaining possible adverse effects of progestin. Also give patient verbal explanation.
• *Alert:* Tell patient to report any unusual symptoms immediately and to stop drug and call the doctor if visual disturbances or migraine occur.
• Warn patient that edema and weight gain are likely. Tell her to monitor weight routinely, and recommend sodium-restricted diet as needed.
• Instruct patient to report breast pain or tenderness, vaginal discharge or bleeding, and swelling of the hands or feet.
• Teach patient how to perform routine breast self-examination.
• Instruct patient that normal menstrual cycles may not resume for 2 to 3 months after drug is stopped.

## levonorgestrel
Norplant System

*Pregnancy Risk Category: X*

## HOW SUPPLIED

*Implants:* 36 mg per capsule; each kit contains six capsules

## ACTION

Slowly releases the synthetic progestin levonorgestrel into the bloodstream. How progestins provide contraception is not fully understood, but they alter the mucus covering the cervix, prevent implantation of the egg, and, in some patients, prevent ovulation.

## ONSET, PEAK, DURATION
Onset and peak levels occur within 24 hours. Effects persist about 5 years.

## INDICATIONS & DOSAGE
*Prevention of pregnancy –*
**Women:** six capsules implanted subdermally in the midportion of the upper arm, about 8 cm above the elbow crease, during the first 7 days of the onset of menses. Capsules are placed in fanlike position, 15 degrees apart (total of 75 degrees). Contraceptive efficacy lasts for 5 years.

## ADVERSE REACTIONS
**CNS:** headache, nervousness, dizziness.
**GI:** nausea, *abdominal discomfort,* appetite change.
**GU:** *amenorrhea, many days of bleeding or prolonged bleeding, spotting, irregular onset of bleeding, frequent onset of bleeding, scanty bleeding, cervicitis, vaginitis, leukorrhea.*
**Skin:** dermatitis, acne, hirsutism, hypertrichosis, alopecia, infection at implant site, transient pain or itching at implant site.
**Other:** adnexal enlargement, mastalgia, weight gain, *musculoskeletal pain, removal difficulty, breast discharge.*

## INTERACTIONS
*Carbamazepine, phenytoin, rifampin:* may reduce the contraceptive efficacy of levonorgestrel implants. Monitor closely.

## CONTRAINDICATIONS
Contraindicated in patients with active thrombophlebitis or thromboembolic disorders, undiagnosed abnormal genital bleeding, acute liver disease, malignant or benign liver tumors, known or suspected breast cancer, and in known or suspected pregnancy.

## NURSING CONSIDERATIONS
• Use cautiously in patients with a history of depression, in diabetic and prediabetic patients, and in patients with hyperlipidemia.
• Know that most patients develop variations in menstrual bleeding patterns, including irregular bleeding, prolonged bleeding, spotting, and amenorrhea. In most patients, these irregularities diminish over time.
• Be aware that irregular bleeding may mask symptoms of cervical or endometrial cancer.
• Closely monitor patients with conditions that may be aggravated by fluid retention because steroid hormones may cause fluid retention.
• Be aware laboratory tests for sex hormone-binding globulin and thyroxine ($T_4$) concentrations may show decreased values; for triiodothyronine ($T_3$) uptake, increased values.
• Know implants do not contain estrogen. Levonorgestrel is a totally synthetic progestin.
• Expect implants to be removed if patients develop active thrombophlebitis or thromboembolic disease or will be immobilized for a significant length of time because of illness or some other factor.
• If jaundice develops, expect implants to be removed because steroid hormone metabolism is impaired in patients with liver failure.
• Although retinal thrombosis after use of oral contraceptives has been reported, no similar incidents have been documented after use of the implant system. However, patients with sudden unexplained vision problems, including users of contact lenses who develop vision changes or changes in lens tolerance, should be immediately evaluated by an ophthalmologist.

## ☑ PATIENT TEACHING
• *Alert:* Tell patient to report to the doctor immediately if one of the implanted capsules falls out (before the

---

skin heals over the implant). Contraceptive efficacy may be impaired.
• Warn patient that missed menstrual periods are not an accurate indicator of early pregnancy because drug may induce amenorrhea. Advise patient that 6 weeks or more of amenorrhea (after a pattern of regular menstrual periods) could indicate pregnancy. If pregnancy is confirmed, the implants must be removed.
• Encourage regular (at least annual) physical examinations.

# medroxyprogesterone acetate

Amen, Curretab, Cycrin, Depo-Provera, Provera

*Pregnancy Risk Category: X*

## HOW SUPPLIED
*Tablets:* 2.5 mg, 5 mg, 10 mg
*Injection (suspension):* 100 mg/ml, 150 mg/ml, 400 mg/ml

## ACTION
Suppresses ovulation, possibly by inhibiting pituitary gonadotropin secretion, thus preventing follicular maturation and causing endometrial thinning.

## ONSET, PEAK, DURATION
Unknown.

## INDICATIONS & DOSAGE
*Abnormal uterine bleeding caused by hormonal imbalance –*
**Adults:** 5 to 10 mg P.O. daily for 5 to 10 days beginning on sixteenth day of menstrual cycle. If the patient also has received estrogen – 10 mg P.O. daily for 10 days beginning on sixteenth day of cycle.
*Secondary amenorrhea –*
**Adults:** 5 to 10 mg P.O. daily for 5 to 10 days.
*Endometrial or renal cancer –*
**Adults:** 400 to 1,000 mg I.M. weekly.

*Contraception in women –*
**Adults:** 150 mg I.M. once q 3 months.

## ADVERSE REACTIONS
**CNS:** depression.
**CV:** thrombophlebitis, *pulmonary embolism,* edema, *thromboembolism, CVA.*
**EENT:** exophthalmos, diplopia.
**GU:** breakthrough bleeding, dysmenorrhea, amenorrhea, cervical erosion, abnormal secretions.
**Hepatic:** cholestatic jaundice.
**Skin:** rash, pain, induration, sterile abscesses, acne, pruritus, melasma, alopecia, hirsutism.
**Other:** breast tenderness, enlargement, or secretion; changes in weight.

## INTERACTIONS
*Aminoglutethimide, rifampin:* decreased progestin effects. Monitor for diminished therapeutic response. Patient should use a nonhormonal contraceptive during therapy with these drugs.

## CONTRAINDICATIONS
Contraindicated in patients with hypersensitivity to drug, active thromboembolic disorders, or past history of thromboembolic disorders or of cerebral vascular disease or apoplexy, breast cancer, undiagnosed abnormal vaginal bleeding, missed abortion, or hepatic dysfunction and during pregnancy. Tablets are also contraindicated in patients with liver dysfunction or known or suspected malignant disease of the genital organs.

## NURSING CONSIDERATIONS
• Use cautiously in patients with diabetes mellitus, seizures, migraine, cardiac or renal disease, asthma, and mental depression.
• Know that the drug should not be used as test for pregnancy; drug may cause birth defects and masculinization of female fetus.

---

Reactions may be *common,* uncommon, *life-threatening,* or COMMON AND LIFE-THREATENING.

• I.M. injection may be painful. Monitor sites for evidence of sterile abscess. Rotate injection sites to prevent muscle atrophy.

☑ **PATIENT TEACHING**
• FDA regulations require that, before receiving first dose, patient reads package insert explaining possible adverse effects of progestins. Also, give patient verbal explanation.
• *Alert:* Tell patient to report any unusual symptoms immediately and to stop drug and call the doctor if visual disturbances or migraine occurs.
• Teach patient how to perform routine monthly breast self-examination.

---

## norethindrone
Micronor, Norlutin, Nor-Q.D.

## norethindrone acetate
Aygestin, Aygestin Cycle Pack, Norlutate

*Pregnancy Risk Category: X*

## HOW SUPPLIED
**norethindrone**
*Tablets:* 0.35 mg, 5 mg
**norethindrone acetate**
*Tablets:* 5 mg

## ACTION
Suppresses ovulation, possibly by inhibiting pituitary gonadotropin secretion, and forms thick cervical mucus.

## ONSET, PEAK, DURATION
Unknown.

## INDICATIONS & DOSAGE
*Amenorrhea, abnormal uterine bleeding –*
**Adults:** 5 to 20 mg norethindrone or 2.5 to 10 mg norethindrone acetate P.O. daily on days 5 to 25 of menstrual cycle.
*Endometriosis –*
**Adults:** 10 mg norethindrone P.O. daily for 14 days; then increased by 5

mg daily q 2 weeks up to 30 mg daily. Or 5 mg norethindrone acetate P.O. daily for 14 days; then increased by 2.5 mg daily q 2 weeks, up to 15 mg daily.
*Contraception in women –*
**Adults:** initially, 0.35 mg norethindrone P.O. on the first day of menstruation; then 0.35 mg daily.

## ADVERSE REACTIONS
**CNS:** depression.
**CV:** thrombophlebitis, *pulmonary embolism,* edema, *thromboembolism, CVA.*
**EENT:** exophthalmos, diplopia.
**GU:** breakthrough bleeding, dysmenorrhea, amenorrhea, cervical erosion, abnormal secretions.
**Hepatic:** cholestatic jaundice.
**Skin:** melasma, rash, acne, pruritus.
**Other:** breast tenderness, enlargement, or secretion; changes in weight.

## INTERACTIONS
*Barbiturates, carbamazepine, rifampin:* decreased progestin effects. Monitor for diminished therapeutic response.

## CONTRAINDICATIONS
Contraindicated in patients with thromboembolic disorders, cerebral apoplexy, or history of these conditions; hypersensitivity to drug; breast cancer, undiagnosed abnormal vaginal bleeding, severe hepatic disease, or missed abortion and during pregnancy.

## NURSING CONSIDERATIONS
• Use cautiously in patients with diabetes mellitus, seizures, migraine, cardiac or renal disease, asthma, and mental depression.
• Norethindrone acetate is twice as potent as norethindrone. Know that norethindrone acetate should not be used for contraception.
• Know that use as test for pregnancy is not appropriate; drug may cause

---

*Liquid form contains alcohol.  **May contain tartrazine.  †Canada only.  ‡Australia only.  ◇OTC.

birth defects and masculinization of female fetus.
- Know that preliminary estrogen treatment is usually needed in menstrual disorders.
- Watch patients carefully for signs of edema.

☑ **PATIENT TEACHING**
- FDA regulations require that, before receiving first dose, patient reads package insert explaining possible adverse effects of progestin. Also give patient verbal explanation.
- *Alert:* Tell patient to report any unusual symptoms immediately and to stop drug and call the doctor if visual disturbances or migraine occurs.
- Teach patient how to perform routine monthly breast self-examination.

---

## norgestrel
Ovrette\*\*

*Pregnancy Risk Category: X*

### HOW SUPPLIED
*Tablets:* 0.075 mg

### ACTION
Unknown. Probably suppresses ovulation, possibly by inhibiting pituitary gonadotropin secretion, and forms thick cervical mucus.

### ONSET, PEAK, DURATION
Unknown.

### INDICATIONS & DOSAGE
*Contraception in women –*
**Adults:** 0.075 mg P.O. daily.

### ADVERSE REACTIONS
**CNS:** cerebral thrombosis or hemorrhage, migraine, depression.
**CV:** thrombophlebitis, *pulmonary embolism,* edema, *thromboembolism, CVA.*
**EENT:** exophthalmos, diplopia.
**GU:** *breakthrough bleeding, change in menstrual flow,* dysmenorrhea,

spotting, amenorrhea, cervical erosion.
**Hepatic:** cholestatic jaundice.
**Skin:** melasma, rash, acne, pruritus.
**Other:** breast tenderness, enlargement, or secretion; changes in weight.

### INTERACTIONS
*Barbiturates, carbamazepine, rifampin:* decreased progestin effects. Monitor for diminished therapeutic response.

### CONTRAINDICATIONS
Contraindicated in patients with thromboembolic disorders, cerebral apoplexy, or history of these conditions; hypersensitivity to drug; breast cancer, undiagnosed abnormal vaginal bleeding, severe hepatic disease, and missed abortion, and during pregnancy.

### NURSING CONSIDERATIONS
- Use cautiously in patients with diabetes mellitus, seizures, migraine, cardiac or renal disease, asthma, and mental depression.
- Be aware that norgestrel is a progestin-only oral contraceptive known as the "minipill."

☑ **PATIENT TEACHING**
- FDA regulations require that, before receiving first dose, patient reads package insert explaining possible adverse effects of progestins. Also provide verbal explanation.
- Tell patient to take pill every day, at the same time, even if menstruating.
- Risk of pregnancy increases with each tablet missed. Tell patient who misses one tablet to take it as soon as she remembers and then to take the next tablet at the regular time. Advise patient who misses two tablets to take one as soon as she remembers and then to take the next regular dose at the usual time and also to use a nonhormonal method of contraception in addition to norgestrel until 14 tablets

---

have been taken. Instruct patient who misses three or more tablets to discontinue drug and use a nonhormonal method of contraception until after menses. If menstrual period does not occur within 45 days, pregnancy testing is necessary.
• Advise patient using oral contraceptives of the increased risk of serious adverse CV reactions associated with heavy cigarette smoking (15 or more cigarettes per day). These risks are quite marked in women over age 35.
• Instruct patient to immediately report excessive bleeding or bleeding between menstrual cycles, breast pain or tenderness, vaginal discharge, or swelling of the hands or feet.
• *Alert:* Tell patient to report any unusual symptoms immediately and to stop drug and call the doctor if visual disturbances, migraine, or numbness or tingling in limbs occurs.
• Teach patient how to perform routine breast self-examination.

## progesterone
Gesterol 50, Progestilin†

*Pregnancy Risk Category: X*

### HOW SUPPLIED
*Injection (in oil):* 50 mg/ml

### ACTION
Suppresses ovulation, possibly by inhibiting pituitary gonadotropin secretion, and forms thick cervical mucus.

### ONSET, PEAK, DURATION
Unknown.

### INDICATIONS & DOSAGE
*Amenorrhea –*
**Adults:** 5 to 10 mg I.M. daily for 6 to 8 days, usually beginning 8 to 10 days before the anticipated start of menstruation.
*Dysfunctional uterine bleeding –*
**Adults:** 5 to 10 mg I.M. daily for six doses.

### ADVERSE REACTIONS
**CNS:** depression.
**CV:** thrombophlebitis, *thromboembolism, CVA, pulmonary embolism,* edema.
**GU:** breakthrough bleeding, dysmenorrhea, amenorrhea, cervical erosion, abnormal secretions.
**Hepatic:** cholestatic jaundice.
**Skin:** melasma, rash, acne, pruritus, pain at injection site.
**Other:** breast tenderness, enlargement, or secretion.

### INTERACTIONS
*Barbiturates, carbamazepine, rifampin:* decreased progestin effects. Monitor for diminished therapeutic response.

### CONTRAINDICATIONS
Contraindicated in patients with thromboembolic disorders, cerebral apoplexy, or history of these conditions; hypersensitivity to drug; breast cancer, undiagnosed abnormal vaginal bleeding, severe hepatic disease, and missed abortion.

### NURSING CONSIDERATIONS
• Use cautiously in patients with diabetes mellitus, seizures, migraine, cardiac or renal disease, asthma, and mental depression.
• Know preliminary estrogen treatment is usually needed in menstrual disorders.
• Give oil solutions (peanut oil or sesame oil) via deep I.M. injection. Check sites frequently for irritation. Rotate injection sites.

### ☑ PATIENT TEACHING
• FDA regulations require that, before receiving first dose, patient reads package insert explaining possible adverse effects of progestins. Also give patient verbal explanation.
• *Alert:* Tell patient to report any unusual symptoms immediately and to

stop drug and call the doctor if visual disturbances or migraine occurs.
• Teach patient how to perform routine breast self-examination.

---

# quinestrol
Estrovis

*Pregnancy Risk Category: X*

## HOW SUPPLIED
*Tablets:* 100 mcg

## ACTION
Increases the synthesis of DNA, RNA, and protein in responsive tissues. Also reduces release of follicle-stimulating hormone and luteinizing hormone from the pituitary gland.

## ONSET, PEAK, DURATION
Unknown.

## INDICATIONS & DOSAGE
*Moderate to severe vasomotor symptoms associated with menopause, atrophic vaginitis, kraurosis vulvae, female hypogonadism, female castration, primary ovarian failure* —
**Adults:** 100 mcg P.O. once daily for 7 days, followed by 100 mcg weekly as maintenance dosage, beginning 2 weeks after start of treatment. Dosage increased to 200 mcg weekly if necessary.

## ADVERSE REACTIONS
**CNS:** headache, dizziness, chorea, migraine, depression, *seizures.*
**CV:** thrombophlebitis; *thromboembolism;* hypertension; edema; *increased risk of CVA, pulmonary embolism, MI.*
**EENT:** worsening of myopia or astigmatism, intolerance of contact lenses.
**GI:** *nausea,* vomiting, abdominal cramps, bloating, anorexia, increased appetite, excessive thirst.
**GU:** breakthrough bleeding, altered menstrual flow, dysmenorrhea, amenorrhea, cervical erosion or abnormal secretions, *increased risk of endometrial cancer, possibility of increased risk of breast cancer,* enlargement of uterine fibromas, vaginal candidiasis.
**Hepatic:** cholestatic jaundice, *hepatic adenoma.*
**Skin:** melasma, urticaria, hirsutism or hair loss, erythema nodosum, dermatitis.
**Other:** breast changes (tenderness, enlargement, secretion), hypercalcemia, gallbladder disease, weight changes.

## INTERACTIONS
*Carbamazepine, phenobarbital, rifampin:* decreased effectiveness of estrogen therapy. Monitor closely.
*Corticosteroids:* possible enhanced effects. Monitor closely.
*Cyclosporine:* increased risk of toxicity. Use together with caution and frequently monitor cyclosporine levels.
*Dantrolene, other hepatotoxic medications:* increased risk of hepatotoxicity. Monitor closely.
*Oral anticoagulants:* dosage adjustments may be necessary. Monitor PT.
*Tamoxifen:* estrogens may interfere with effectiveness of tamoxifen. Avoid concomitant use.

## CONTRAINDICATIONS
Contraindicated in patients with thrombophlebitis or thromboembolic disorders, breast or reproductive organ cancer, or undiagnosed abnormal genital bleeding and during pregnancy.

## NURSING CONSIDERATIONS
• Use cautiously in patients with asthma; cerebrovascular or coronary artery disease, mental depression; migraine; seizures; bone diseases associated with hypercalcemia; cardiac, hepatic, or renal dysfunction; or in women with family history (mother, grandmother, sister) of breast or genital tract cancer, or who have breast

---

Reactions may be *common,* uncommon, *life-threatening,* or COMMON AND LIFE-THREATENING.

nodules, fibrocystic disease, or abnormal mammographic findings.

• Ensure that patients have a thorough physical examination before initiating estrogen therapy. Patients receiving long-term therapy should have examinations yearly. Periodically monitor body weight, blood pressure, hepatic function, and serum lipid levels, as ordered.

• Be aware that quinestrol is similar in effectiveness to conjugated estrogens in treating postmenopausal symptoms. Its biggest advantage is that it can be taken once a week.

• Notify the pathologist about any patients receiving estrogen therapy when specimens are obtained and sent to pathology for evaluation.

• Know that attempts to discontinue medication should be made at 3- to 6-month intervals.

### ☑ PATIENT TEACHING

• Tell patient that patient package insert that describes estrogen's adverse effects is available; however, also give patient verbal explanation.

• Stress the importance of regular physical examinations. Studies suggest that postmenopausal women who use estrogen replacement for more than 5 years to treat menopausal symptoms may be at increased risk for endometrial cancer. This risk is reduced by using cyclic rather than continuous therapy and the lowest possible dosages of estrogen. Adding progestins to the regimen decreases the incidence of endometrial hyperplasia; however, it isn't known if progestins affect the incidence of endometrial cancer. Most studies show no increased risk of breast cancer.

• Explain to patient on replacement therapy for postmenopausal symptoms that, although menstrual-like bleeding or spotting may occur, fertility is not restored. Pregnancy cannot occur because patient does not ovulate.

• **Alert:** Warn patient to immediately report abdominal pain; pain, numbness, or stiffness in legs or buttocks; pressure or pain in chest; shortness of breath; severe headaches; visual disturbances, such as blind spots, flashing lights, or blurriness; vaginal bleeding or discharge; breast lumps; swelling of hands or feet; yellow skin or sclera; dark urine; or light-colored stools.

• Tell diabetic patient to report elevated blood glucose test results so that antidiabetic medication dosage can be adjusted.

• Teach patient how to perform routine breast self-examination.

# 56

## Gonadotropins

**gonadorelin acetate**
**histrelin acetate**
**menotropins**
**nafarelin acetate**

**COMBINATION PRODUCTS**
None.

---

### gonadorelin acetate
Lutrepulse

*Pregnancy Risk Category: B*

**HOW SUPPLIED**
*Injection:* 0.8 mg/10 ml, 3.2 mg/10 ml vials; supplied as kit with I.V. supplies and ambulatory infusion pump

**ACTION**
Mimics action of gonadotropin-releasing hormone, resulting in the synthesis and release of luteinizing hormone (LH) from anterior pituitary gland. LH then acts upon reproductive organs to regulate hormone synthesis.

**ONSET, PEAK, DURATION**
Unknown.

**INDICATIONS & DOSAGE**
*Induction of ovulation in women with primary hypothalamic amenorrhea—*
**Adults:** 5 mcg I.V. q 90 minutes for 21 days. If no response follows three treatment intervals, increase dosage as ordered.

**ADVERSE REACTIONS**
**Skin:** hematoma, local infection, inflammation, mild phlebitis.
**Other:** multiple pregnancy, ovarian hyperstimulation.

**INTERACTIONS**
*Other ovulation stimulators:* Additive effects. Avoid concomitant use.

**CONTRAINDICATIONS**
Contraindicated in patients hypersensitive to the drug, in women with conditions that could be complicated by pregnancy (such as prolactinoma), in those who are anovulatory from any cause other than a hypothalamic disorder, and in those with ovarian cysts.

**NURSING CONSIDERATIONS**
• **I.V. use:** To mimic the naturally occurring hormone, administer gonadorelin in a pulsatile fashion with the available ambulatory infusion pump. Set the pulse period at 1 minute (infuse drug over 1 minute) and the pulse interval at 90 minutes.
• To give 2.5 mcg/pulse, reconstitute the 0.8-mg vial with 8 ml of supplied diluent, and set the pump to deliver 25 microliters/pulse. To administer 5 mcg/pulse, use the same dosage strength and dilution, but set the pump to deliver 50 microliters/pulse.
• Some patients may need higher I.V. doses. To give 10 mcg/pulse, reconstitute the 3.2-mg vial with 8 ml of supplied diluent, and set pump to deliver 25 microliters/pulse. To give 20 mcg/pulse, use same dosage strength and dilution, but set pump to deliver 50 microliters/pulse.
• Inspect the I.V. site at each visit.
• Know that patients usually need pelvic ultrasound on days 7 and 14 after a baseline scan. Some doctors prefer shorter intervals between scans.

**☑ PATIENT TEACHING**
• Ensure that patient understands that multiple pregnancy is possible (incidence is about 12%). Monitoring of dosage and ovarian ultrasonography to monitor drug response are needed.
• Instruct patient about proper aseptic technique and care of the I.V. site.

---

Reactions may be *common,* uncommon, *life-threatening,* or COMMON AND LIFE-THREATENING.

Cannula and I.V. site should be changed every 48 hours. Written instructions are available for patient.

• Anaphylaxis has been reported with similar drugs. Teach patient symptoms of hypersensitivity reactions (hives, wheezing, difficulty breathing), and encourage her to report these at once.

• Tell patient to report signs of infection, hematoma, inflammation, or phlebitis at injection site. She also should report severe abdominal pain, bloating, swelling of the hands or feet, nausea, vomiting, diarrhea, substantial weight gain, or shortness of breath.

• Encourage patient to adhere to the close monitoring schedule required by the therapy. Regular pelvic examinations, midluteal-phase serum progesterone determinations, and multiple ovarian ultrasound scans are necessary.

---

## histrelin acetate
Supprelin

*Pregnancy Risk Category: X*

### HOW SUPPLIED
*Injection:* 120 mcg/0.6 ml, 300 mcg/0.6 ml, 600 mcg/0.6 ml

### ACTION
An agonist that mimics the effects of gonadotropin-releasing hormone (GnRH; also called luteinizing hormone-releasing hormone, or LHRH) but is more potent. Chronic administration desensitizes responsiveness of the pituitary gonadotropin, decreasing sex hormone production by the testes or ovaries.

### ONSET, PEAK, DURATION
Unknown.

### INDICATIONS & DOSAGE
*Centrally mediated (idiopathic or neurogenic) precocious puberty –*
**Children (girls 2 to 8 years; boys 2 to 9½ years):** 10 mcg/kg S.C. daily.

### ADVERSE REACTIONS
**CNS:** *mood changes, nervousness, dizziness, depression, headache, libido changes, insomnia, anxiety,* paresthesia, cognitive changes, syncope, somnolence, lethargy, impaired consciousness, tremor, hyperkinesia, *seizures,* hot flashes, conduct disorder, fatigue.
**CV:** *vasodilation,* edema, palpitations, pallor, tachycardia, hypertension.
**EENT:** epistaxis, ear congestion, abnormal pupillary function, otalgia, visual disturbances, hearing loss, polyopia, photophobia, rhinorrhea, sinusitis, nasal infections,.
**GI:** *abdominal pain, nausea, vomiting, diarrhea, flatulence, decreased appetite, dyspepsia,* cramps, constipation, thirst, gastritis, GI distress.
**GU:** *menstrual changes, vaginal dryness, leukorrhea, hypermenorrhea, vaginal bleeding, vaginitis, dysmenorrhea,* polyuria, incontinence, dysuria, hematuria, nocturia, tenderness of female genitalia, glycosuria.
**Hematologic:** hyperlipidemia, anemia.
**Respiratory:** *upper respiratory infection, respiratory congestion, cough,* asthma, breathing disorder, bronchitis, hyperventilation.
**Skin:** *redness, swelling, acne, rash, diaphoresis,* urticaria, pruritus, alopecia.
**Other:** *fever, arthralgia, muscle stiffness, muscle cramps, breast pain or edema,* breast discharge, decreased breast size, *weight gain, body pains,* chills, malaise, purpura, acute hypersensitivity reactions *(anaphylaxis, angioedema).*

### INTERACTIONS
None significant.

### CONTRAINDICATIONS
Contraindicated in patients hypersensitive to any component of drug and in pregnant or breast-feeding patients. Safety and efficacy haven't been established in children under 2 years.

---

## NURSING CONSIDERATIONS

• Be aware drug is indicated only for patients who will comply with the daily schedule. Noncompliance or inadequate dosing may result in inadequate control of the pubertal process, which can result in recurrence of symptoms, including onset of menses, breast development, or testicular growth; long-term consequences may involve decreased adult height.

• A complete physical and endocrinologic evaluation should be performed before initiating drug therapy; several indices should be reexamined at 3 months, then every 6 to 12 months thereafter. Such evaluations should include determinations of height and weight, hand and wrist X-rays for bone-age determination, sex steroid (estradiol or testosterone) levels, and GnRH stimulation test. Monitor these tests periodically to determine effectiveness of therapy.

• Further tests to rule out other causes of precocious puberty include beta human chorionic gonadotropin levels (to detect chorionic gonadotropin-secreting tumor); pelvic/adrenal/testicular ultrasound (to detect steroid-secreting tumor); and computed tomography scan of the head (to detect any previously undiagnosed intracranial tumor). Workup also sets baseline of gonad size for serial monitoring.

• Refrigerate drug (36° to 46° F [2° to 8° C]) and protect from light in its original container. Use vials only once because drug does not contain preservatives. Allow drug to reach room temperature before giving.

• Give S.C. and rotate injection sites to minimize local reactions.

• Know that decreases in follicle-stimulating hormone, leutinizing hormone, and sex steroid levels occur within 3 months.

• Patients should be reevaluated if prepubertal levels of sex steroids or GnRH test responses are not achieved within 3 months of therapy.

### ☑ PATIENT TEACHING

• Before therapy, make sure patient and caregivers understand the importance of adhering to the daily schedules. Tell parents to give drug at the same time each day to aid compliance and ensure adequate dosing.

• Drug is dispensed as a 30-day kit that contains a patient information leaflet. Ensure that caregivers read and understand the leaflet.

• Inform patient that because drug is a peptide, it's destroyed in the GI tract and so must be given parenterally.

• Explain to patient the importance of rotating injection sites daily. Sites should include upper arms, thighs, and abdomen.

• Warn patient of the potential risks of therapy and potential adverse effects. During the first month of treatment, girls commonly experience a slight menstrual flow, which probably is related to decreasing estrogen levels brought on by treatment. As estrogen levels drop, menses begins because estrogens support the endometrium.

• Advise patient to seek medical attention at once if any signs of hypersensitivity reactions occur—sudden development of skin rash, difficulty in breathing or swallowing, or rapid heartbeat. Notify the doctor if severe or persistent swelling, redness, or irritation appears at the injection site.

---

# menotropins
Pergonal

*Pregnancy Risk Category: X*

## HOW SUPPLIED
*Injection:* 75 international units of luteinizing hormone (LH) and 75 units of follicle-stimulating hormone (FSH) activity per ampule; 150 units of LH and 150 units of FSH activity per ampule

---

## ACTION
When given to women who have not had primary ovarian failure, mimics FSH in inducing follicular growth and LH in aiding follicular maturation; induces spermatogenesis in men.

## ONSET, PEAK, DURATION
Onset for follicular growth and maturation, 9 to 12 days. Peak and duration unknown.

## INDICATIONS & DOSAGE
*Anovulation –*
**Women:** 75 units each of FSH and LH I.M. daily for 7 to 12 days, followed by 5,000 to 10,000 units of human chorionic gonadotropin (HCG) I.M. 1 day after last dose of menotropins. Repeated for one to three menstrual cycles until ovulation occurs.
*Infertility with ovulation –*
**Women:** 75 units each of FSH and LH I.M. daily for 7 to 12 days, then 5,000 to 10,000 units HCG I.M. 1 day after last dose of menotropins. Repeated for two menstrual cycles, then increased to 150 units each of FSH and LH daily for 7 to 12 days, followed by 5,000 to 10,000 units HCG I.M. 1 day after last dose of menotropins. Repeated for two menstrual cycles.
*Infertility in men –*
**Men:** prior treatment with HCG of 5,000 units three times a week for 4 to 6 months; then 75 units each of FSH and LH I.M. three times weekly (given with 2,000 units of HCG twice weekly) for at least 4 months. If increased spermatogenesis does not occur, dosage increased to 150 units each of FSH and LH three times weekly (dosage of HCG remains unchanged).

## ADVERSE REACTIONS
**CNS:** headache, malaise, dizziness.
**CV:** *stroke,* tachycardia.
**GI:** nausea, vomiting, diarrhea, abdominal cramps, bloating.
**GU:** *ovarian enlargement with pain and abdominal distention,* multiple births, ovarian hyperstimulation syndrome (sudden ovarian enlargement, ascites with or without pain, or pleural effusion), ovarian cysts.
**Respiratory:** *atelectasis, acute respiratory distress syndrome, pulmonary embolism, pulmonary infarction, arterial occlusion,* dyspnea, tachypnea.
**Other:** fever, *gynecomastia, hypersensitivity and anaphylactic reactions,* chills, musculoskeletal aches, joint pains, rash, ectopic pregnancy.

## INTERACTIONS
None significant.

## CONTRAINDICATIONS
Contraindicated in patients hypersensitive to the drug; in women with primary ovarian failure, uncontrolled thyroid or adrenal dysfunction, pituitary tumor, abnormal uterine bleeding, uterine fibromas, or ovarian cysts or enlargement; in pregnant patients; and in men with normal pituitary function, primary testicular failure, or infertility disorders other than hypogonadotropic hypogonadism.

## NURSING CONSIDERATIONS
• Close monitoring is critical to ensure adequate ovarian stimulation without hyperstimulation.
• Reconstitute with 1 to 2 ml of sterile 0.9% sodium chloride for injection. Use immediately.
• Rotate injection sites.

## ☑ PATIENT TEACHING
• Tell patient about possibility of multiple births.
• In infertility, encourage daily intercourse from day before HCG is given until ovulation occurs.
• Tell patient that pregnancy usually occurs 4 to 6 weeks after therapy.
• Instruct patient to immediately report severe abdominal pain, bloating, swelling of the hands or feet, nausea, vomiting, diarrhea, substantial weight gain, or shortness of breath.

---

*Liquid form contains alcohol.   **May contain tartrazine.   †Canada only.   ‡Australia only.   ◇OTC.

# nafarelin acetate
Synarel

*Pregnancy Risk Category: X*

## HOW SUPPLIED
*Nasal solution:* 200 mcg/spray in metered-dose spray bottle (2 mg/ml)

## ACTION
A gonadotropin-releasing hormone (GnRH) analogue that acts on the pituitary to decrease release of follicle-stimulating hormone and luteinizing hormone, thus decreasing ovarian stimulation, lowering circulating estrogens, and improving symptoms associated with endometriosis.

## ONSET, PEAK, DURATION
Decreased levels of sex hormones occur after 4 weeks. Serum levels peak 10 to 40 minutes after dose. Effects persist for up to 3 to 6 months.

## INDICATIONS & DOSAGE
*Management of endometriosis –*
**Women 18 years and older:** 1 spray in one nostril b.i.d. Treatment begun on day 2, 3, or 4 of menstrual cycle. Maximum duration of therapy is 6 months.
*Central precocious puberty –*
**Children:** 2 sprays in each nostril in the morning and evening. Total daily dosage is 8 sprays (1,600 mcg).

## ADVERSE REACTIONS
**CNS:** *headaches, emotional lability, insomnia,* depression.
**CV:** *edema.*
**EENT:** *nasal irritation.*
**Skin:** *acne,* seborrhea, hirsutism.
**Other:** *hot flashes, decreased libido, myalgia, reduced breast size,* weight gain or loss, increased libido, decreased bone density, *vaginal dryness.*

## INTERACTIONS
None significant.

## CONTRAINDICATIONS
Contraindicated in patients hypersensitive to GnRH analogs or any components of the formulation (benzalkonium chloride, sorbitol, purified water, glacial acetic acid, hydrochloric acid, or sodium hydroxide), in those with undiagnosed vaginal bleeding, in breast-feeding patients, and during pregnancy.

## NURSING CONSIDERATIONS
● Be aware that studies have confirmed a small loss in bone density after 6 months of therapy, probably caused by drug-induced hypoestrogenic state. Patients with major risk factors for osteoporosis (chronic alcohol or tobacco use, strong family history of osteoporosis, or use of drugs that may reduce bone mass) should not receive additional courses of therapy and should strongly weigh the risks and benefits before an initial trial of the drug.

## ☑ PATIENT TEACHING
● Teach patient that menstruation will stop with regular use of drug and to call the doctor if menstruation persists or breakthrough bleeding occurs.
● Advise patient to use a nonhormonal form of contraception (such as barrier contraception). Although drug will usually inhibit ovulation, it's not a reliable contraceptive, particularly if patient misses a few doses. Tell patient to stop the drug and call the doctor if she thinks she is pregnant.
● Instruct patient to immediately report severe abdominal pain, bloating, swelling of the hands or feet, nausea, vomiting, diarrhea, substantial weight gain, or shortness of breath.
● Tell patient who develops a cold or rhinitis during therapy to call the doctor. If a topical nasal decongestant is needed, the manufacturer suggests that it be used at least 30 minutes after nafarelin treatment to reduce possible interference with nafarelin absorption.

---

Reactions may be *common,* uncommon, *life-threatening,* or **COMMON AND LIFE-THREATENING.**

**57**

# Antidiabetic drugs and glucagon

acarbose
acetohexamide
chlorpropamide
glipizide
glucagon
glyburide
insulins
metformin hydrochloride
tolazamide
tolbutamide

## COMBINATION PRODUCTS
HUMULIN 50/50◇: isophane insulin suspension (human) 50% and insulin injection (human) 50%, 100 units/ml.
HUMULIN 70/30◇, MIXTARD HUMAN‡, NOVOLIN 70/30◇): isophane insulin suspension (human) 70% and insulin injection (human) 30%, 100 units/ml.

▼ NEW DRUG

## acarbose
Precose
*Pregnancy Risk Category: B*

### HOW SUPPLIED
*Tablets:* 50 mg, 100 mg

### ACTION
An alpha-glucosidase inhibitor that delays digestion of carbohydrates, resulting in a smaller rise in blood glucose concentration.

### ONSET, PEAK, DURATION
Onset and duration are unknown. Plasma level peaks in 1 hour.

### INDICATIONS & DOSAGE
*Adjunct to diet to lower blood glucose in patients with non-insulin-dependent diabetes mellitus whose hyperglycemia cannot be managed by diet alone or by diet and a sulfonylurea –*

**Adults:** 25 mg P.O. t.i.d. at start of each main meal. Subsequent dosage adjustment made q 4 to 8 weeks, based on 1-hour postprandial glucose level and tolerance. Maintenance dosage is 50 mg to 100 mg P.O. t.i.d., depending on patient's weight.

### ADVERSE REACTIONS
**GI:** *abdominal pain, diarrhea, flatulence.*
**Other:** elevated serum transaminase level.

### INTERACTIONS
*Calcium channel blockers, corticosteroids, estrogens, isoniazid, nicotinic acid, oral contraceptives, phenothiazines, phenytoin, sympathomimetics, thiazides and other diuretics, thyroid products:* may cause hyperglycemia during concomitant use or hypoglycemia when withdrawn. Monitor blood glucose level.
*Intestinal adsorbents (such as activated charcoal) and digestive enzyme preparations containing carbohydrate-splitting enzymes (such as amylase and pancreatin):* may reduce the effect of acarbose. Do not administer concomitantly.

### CONTRAINDICATIONS
Contraindicated in patients with hypersensitivity to the drug, diabetic ketoacidosis, cirrhosis, inflammatory bowel disease, colonic ulceration, partial intestinal obstruction, predisposition to intestinal obstruction, chronic intestinal disease associated with marked disorder of digestion or absorption, and any condition that may deteriorate because of increased intestinal gas formation.

---

*Liquid form contains alcohol. **May contain tartrazine. †Canada only. ‡Australia only. ◇OTC.

## NURSING CONSIDERATIONS

• Drug is not recommended for use in patients with serum creatinine levels greater than 2.0 mg/dl and in pregnant or breast-feeding women.
• Use cautiously in patients with mild to moderate renal impairment and in those receiving a sulfonylurea or insulin. Acarbose may increase hypoglycemic potential of the sulfonylurea. Monitor a patient receiving both drugs closely. If hypoglycemia occurs, treat patient with oral glucose (dextrose). Severe hypoglycemia may require I.V. glucose infusion or glucagon administration. Dosage adjustments may be needed to prevent further hypoglycemia, so report hypoglycemia and treatment required to the doctor. Insulin therapy may be needed in times of increased stress (infection, fever, surgery, or trauma). Monitor the patient closely for hyperglycemia.
• Safety and efficacy of drug have not been established in children.
• Monitor the patient's 1-hour postprandial plasma glucose level to determine therapeutic effectiveness of acarbose and to identify appropriate dose. Report hyperglycemia to the doctor. Thereafter, glycosylated hemoglobin should be measured every 3 months.
• Monitor serum transaminase level every 3 months in the first year of therapy and periodically thereafter in patients receiving doses in excess of 50 mg t.i.d. Report abnormalities; dosage adjustment or drug withdrawal may be needed.

☑ **PATIENT TEACHING**
• Have patient take the drug daily with first bite of each of three main meals.
• Explain to patient that therapy relieves symptoms but doesn't cure the disease.
• Stress importance of adhering to specific diet, weight reduction, exercise, and hygiene programs. Show the patient how to monitor blood glucose level and how to recognize and treat hyperglycemia.
• Teach patient taking a sulfonylurea how to recognize hypoglycemia. Advise him to treat symptoms with a form of dextrose rather than with a product containing table sugar.
• Urge patient to carry medical identification at all times.

---

## acetohexamide
Dimelor†, Dymelor

*Pregnancy Risk Category: NR*

### HOW SUPPLIED
*Tablets:* 250 mg, 500 mg

### ACTION
Unknown. A sulfonylurea that probably stimulates insulin release from the pancreatic beta cells and reduces glucose output by the liver. An extrapancreatic effect increases peripheral sensitivity to insulin.

### ONSET, PEAK, DURATION
Onset within 1 hour. Plasma levels of acetohexamide peak within 2 hours; plasma levels of insulin, within 1 to 2 hours. Effects last 12 to 24 hours.

### INDICATIONS & DOSAGE
*Adjunct to diet to lower blood glucose level in patients with type II diabetes (non-insulin-dependent)* –
**Adults:** initially, 250 mg P.O. daily before breakfast; dosage increased q 5 to 7 days (by 250 to 500 mg), as needed, to maximum of 1.5 g daily in divided doses b.i.d. or t.i.d. before meals.
*To replace insulin therapy in patients with type II diabetes* –
**Adults:** if insulin dosage is less than 20 units daily, insulin is stopped and oral therapy started with 250 mg P.O. daily before breakfast, increased as above, if needed. If insulin dosage is 20 to 40 units daily, oral therapy is

---

started with 250 mg P.O. daily before breakfast, while insulin dosage is reduced by 25% to 30% daily or every other day, depending on response to oral therapy.

## ADVERSE REACTIONS

**CNS:** paresthesia, fatigue, dizziness, vertigo, malaise, headache.
**EENT:** tinnitus.
**GI:** nausea, heartburn, epigastric distress.
**Hematologic:** leukopenia, *thrombocytopenia, aplastic anemia, agranulocytosis,* hemolytic anemia.
**Skin:** rash, pruritus, erythema, urticaria.
**Other:** *hypersensitivity reactions, hypoglycemia.*

## INTERACTIONS

*Anabolic steroids, chloramphenicol, clofibrate, guanethidine, MAO inhibitors, phenylbutazone, salicylates, sulfonamides:* increased hypoglycemic activity. Monitor blood glucose level.
*Beta blockers, clonidine:* prolonged hypoglycemic effect and masked symptoms of hypoglycemia. Use together cautiously.
*Corticosteroids, glucagon, rifampin, thiazide diuretics:* decreased hypoglycemic response. Monitor blood glucose level.
*Ethanol:* possible disulfiram-like reaction. Avoid concomitant use.
*Hydantoins:* increased blood levels of hydantoins. Monitor blood levels.
*Oral anticoagulants:* increased hypoglycemic activity or enhanced anticoagulant effect. Monitor blood glucose level and PT.

## CONTRAINDICATIONS

Contraindicated for treating patients with type I diabetes (insulin-dependent) or diabetes that can be adequately controlled by diet. Also contraindicated in patients with type II diabetes complicated by ketosis, acidosis, diabetic coma; hyperglycemia associated with primary renal disease; pregnancy or lactation; major surgery; severe infections; severe trauma; or hypersensitivity to sulfonylureas.

## NURSING CONSIDERATIONS

• Use cautiously in patients with a history of porphyria, impaired hepatic or renal function, or in debilitated, malnourished, or elderly patients.
• During periods of increased stress, such as infection, fever, surgery, or trauma, patients may require insulin therapy. Monitor patients closely for hyperglycemia in these situations.
• Know that patients transferring from another oral agent usually need no transition period.
• Be aware that patients transferring from insulin therapy to an oral antidiabetic agent require blood glucose monitoring at least three times a day before meals. Patients may require hospitalization during transition.

## ☑ PATIENT TEACHING

• Instruct patient about nature of disease, importance of following therapeutic regimen, adhering to specific diet, weight reduction, exercise, and personal hygiene programs and about avoiding infection. Explain how and when to perform self-monitoring of blood glucose level, and teach recognition of and intervention for hypoglycemia and hyperglycemia.
• Make sure patient understands that therapy only relieves symptoms.
• Tell patient not to change drug dosage without the doctor's consent and to report abnormal blood or urine glucose test results.
• Teach patient to carry candy or other simple sugars to treat mild hypoglycemic episodes. Severe episodes may require hospital treatment.
• Advise patient not to take any other medication, including OTC drugs, without checking with the doctor.
• Advise patient to avoid moderate to

---

*Liquid form contains alcohol. **May contain tartrazine. †Canada only. ‡Australia only. ◇OTC.

large intake of alcohol because of possible disulfiram-like reaction.
• Advise patient to carry medical identification at all times.

---

## chlorpropamide
Apo-Chlorpropamide†, Diabinese, Glucamide, Novo-Propamide†

*Pregnancy Risk Category: C*

### HOW SUPPLIED
*Tablets:* 100 mg, 250 mg

### ACTION
Unknown. A sulfonylurea that probably stimulates insulin release from the pancreatic beta cells and reduces glucose output by the liver. An extrapancreatic effect increases peripheral sensitivity to insulin. Also exerts an antidiuretic effect in patients with diabetes insipidus.

### ONSET, PEAK, DURATION
Onset occurs within 1 hour. Peak levels occur in 2 to 4 hours; peak hypoglycemic effect, within 3 to 6 hours. Effects persist for up to 60 hours.

### INDICATIONS & DOSAGE
*Adjunct to diet to lower blood glucose level in patients with type II diabetes (non-insulin-dependent)* –
**Adults:** 250 mg P.O. daily with breakfast or in divided doses if GI disturbances occur. Initial dosage increased after 5 to 7 days because of extended duration of action; then increased q 3 to 5 days by 50 to 125 mg, if needed, to a maximum of 750 mg daily. On the other hand, some patients with mild diabetes respond well to dosages of 100 mg or less daily.
**Adults over 65 years:** initially, 100 to 125 mg P.O. daily.
*To change from insulin to oral therapy* –
**Adults:** if insulin dosage is less than 40 units daily, insulin is stopped and oral therapy started as above. If insulin dosage is 40 units or more daily,

oral therapy started as above with insulin reduced 50%. Insulin dosage reduced further according to response.

### ADVERSE REACTIONS
**CNS:** paresthesia, fatigue, dizziness, vertigo, malaise, headache.
**EENT:** tinnitis.
**GI:** nausea, heartburn, epigastric distress.
**GU:** tea-colored urine.
**Hematologic:** leukopenia, *thrombocytopenia, aplastic anemia, agranulocytosis,* hemolytic anemia.
**Skin:** rash, pruritus, erythema, urticaria.
**Other:** *hypersensitivity reactions, prolonged hypoglycemia, dilutional hyponatremia.*

### INTERACTIONS
*Anabolic steroids, chloramphenicol, clofibrate, guanethidine, MAO inhibitors, phenylbutazone, salicylates, sulfonamides:* increased hypoglycemic activity. Monitor blood glucose level.
*Beta blockers, clonidine:* prolonged hypoglycemic effect and masked symptoms of hypoglycemia. Use together cautiously.
*Corticosteroids, glucagon, rifampin, thiazide diuretics:* decreased hypoglycemic response. Monitor blood glucose level.
*Ethanol:* possible disulfiram-like reaction. Avoid concomitant use.
*Hydantoins:* increased blood levels of hydantoins. Monitor blood levels.
*Oral anticoagulants:* increased hypoglycemic activity or enhanced anticoagulant effect. Monitor blood glucose level and PT.

### CONTRAINDICATIONS
Contraindicated for treating type I diabetes (insulin-dependent) or diabetes that can be adequately controlled by diet. Also contraindicated in patients with type II diabetes complicated by ketosis, acidosis, diabetic coma, major surgery, severe infec-

---

Reactions may be *common,* uncommon, *life-threatening,* or **COMMON AND LIFE-THREATENING.**

tions, severe trauma, during pregnancy or breast-feeding; and in patients with hypersensitivity to the drug.

## NURSING CONSIDERATIONS
• Use cautiously in patients with porphyria, impaired hepatic or renal function or in debilitated, malnourished or elderly patients.
• Know that elderly patients may be more sensitive to adverse effects.
• Know that drug may accumulate in patients with renal insufficiency. Watch for and report signs of impending renal insufficiency, such as dysuria, anuria, and hematuria.
• *Alert:* Know adverse effects of chlorpropamide, especially hypoglycemia, may be more frequent or severe than with some other sulfonylureas because of its long duration of action. If hypoglycemia occurs, monitor patients closely for a minimum of 3 to 5 days.
• Monitor serum alkaline phosphatase levels routinely, as ordered. Progressive increases may indicate the need to discontinue drug.
• Patients transferring from another oral antidiabetic agent usually need no transition period.
• Patients may require hospitalization during transition from insulin therapy to an oral antidiabetic agent. Monitor patients' blood glucose levels at least three times a day before meals.

## ☑ PATIENT TEACHING
• Instruct patient about nature of the disease, importance of following therapeutic regimen, adhering to specific diet, weight reduction, exercise, and personal hygiene programs, and about avoiding infection. Explain how and when to perform self-monitoring of blood glucose level, and teach recognition of and intervention for hypoglycemia and hyperglycemia.
• Make sure patient understands that therapy only relieves symptoms.

• Tell patient not to change drug dosage without the doctor's consent and to report abnormal blood or urine glucose test results.
• Teach patient to carry candy or other simple sugars to treat mild hypoglycemic episodes. Severe episodes may require hospital treatment.
• Advise patient not to take any other drugs, including OTC drugs, without checking with the doctor.
• Advise patient to avoid intake of alcohol. Chlorpropamide-alcohol flush is characterized by facial flushing, light-headedness, headache, and occasional breathlessness. Even very small amounts of alcohol can produce this reaction.
• Advise patient to carry medical identification at all times.

---

# glipizide
Glucotrol, Glucotrol XL, Minidiab‡
*Pregnancy Risk Category: C*

## HOW SUPPLIED
*Tablets:* 5 mg, 10 mg
*Tablets (extended-release):* 5 mg, 10 mg

## ACTION
Unknown. A sulfonylurea that probably stimulates insulin release from the pancreatic beta cells and reduces glucose output by the liver. An extrapancreatic effect increases peripheral sensitivity to insulin.

## ONSET, PEAK, DURATION
Onset occurs within 15 to 30 minutes. Serum drug levels peak 1 to 3 hours after oral dose; peak insulin levels occur in ½ to 2 hours. Effects persist for 10 to 16 hours.

## INDICATIONS & DOSAGE
*Adjunct to diet to lower blood glucose level in patients with type II diabetes (non-insulin-dependent)* –
**Adults:** initially, 5 mg P.O. daily before breakfast. Elderly patients or

those with liver disease may be started on 2.5 mg. Usual maintenance dosage is 10 to 15 mg. Maximum recommended daily dosage is 40 mg.
*To replace insulin therapy –*
**Adults:** if insulin dosage is more than 20 units daily, the patient is started at usual dosage in addition to 50% of the insulin. If insulin dosage is less than 20 units, insulin may be discontinued.

### ADVERSE REACTIONS
**CNS:** dizziness, drowsiness, headache.
**GI:** nausea, constipation, diarrhea.
**Hematologic:** leukopenia, hemolytic anemia, *agranulocytosis, thrombocytopenia, aplastic anemia.*
**Hepatic:** cholestatic jaundice.
**Skin:** rash, pruritus.
**Other:** *hypoglycemia.*

### INTERACTIONS
*Anabolic steroids, chloramphenicol, clofibrate, guanethidine, MAO inhibitors, phenylbutazone, probenecid, salicylates, sulfonamides:* increased hypoglycemic activity. Monitor blood glucose level.
*Beta blockers, clonidine:* prolonged hypoglycemic effect and masked symptoms of hypoglycemia. Use together cautiously.
*Corticosteroids, glucagon, rifampin, thiazide diuretics:* decreased hypoglycemic response. Monitor blood glucose level.
*Ethanol:* possible disulfiram-like reaction. Avoid concomitant use.
*Hydantoins:* increased blood levels of hydantoins. Monitor blood levels.
*Oral anticoagulants:* increased hypoglycemic activity or enhanced anticoagulant effect. Monitor blood glucose levels and PT.

### CONTRAINDICATIONS
Contraindicated in patients with hypersensitivity to drug, diabetic ketoacidosis with or without coma, and during pregnancy or breast-feeding.

### NURSING CONSIDERATIONS
• Use cautiously in patients with renal and hepatic disease and in debilitated, malnourished, or elderly patients.
• Know that elderly patients may be more sensitive to adverse effects.
• Give about 30 minutes before meals.
• Know that some patients taking glipizide may attain effective control on a once-daily regimen; others show a better response with divided dosing.
• Be aware that glipizide is a second-generation sulfonylurea. The frequency of adverse reactions appears to be lower than with first-generation drugs, such as chlorpropamide.
• During periods of increased stress, such as infection, fever, surgery, or trauma, patients may require insulin therapy. Monitor patients closely for hyperglycemia in these situations.
• Patients transferring from insulin therapy to an oral antidiabetic agent require blood glucose monitoring at least three times daily before meals. Patients may require hospitalization during transition.

### ☑ PATIENT TEACHING
• Instruct patient about nature of disease, importance of following therapeutic regimen, adhering to specific diet, weight reduction, exercise, personal hygiene programs, and about avoiding infection. Explain how and when to perform self-monitoring of blood glucose level, and teach recognition of hypoglycemia and hyperglycemia.
• Tell patient not to change drug dosage without the doctor's consent and to report abnormal blood or urine glucose test results.
• Tell patient not to take any other medication, including OTC drugs, without checking with the doctor.
• Advise patient to carry medical identification at all times.

---

Reactions may be *common,* uncommon, *life-threatening,* or **COMMON AND LIFE-THREATENING.**

# glucagon

*Pregnancy Risk Category: B*

## HOW SUPPLIED

*Powder for injection:* 1 mg (1 unit)-vial, 10 mg (10 units)-vial

## ACTION

Raises blood glucose level by promoting catalytic depolymerization of hepatic glycogen to glucose.

## ONSET, PEAK, DURATION

Onset almost immediate after parenteral administration. Peak hyperglycemic effect occurs within 30 minutes. Hyperglycemic effects persist 1 to 2 hours. Onset, peak and duration variable when used to relax GI smooth muscle but occur more quickly and last for shorter duration.

## INDICATIONS & DOSAGE

*Hypoglycemia –*
**Adults and children weighing more than 20 kg:** 1 mg S.C., I.M., or I.V.
**Children weighing 20 kg or less:** 0.5 mg S.C., I.M., or I.V.
*Note:* May repeat in 15 minutes, if necessary. I.V. glucose must be given if patient fails to respond. When patient responds, supplemental carbohydrate needs to be given immediately.
*Diagnostic aid for radiologic examination –*
**Adults:** 0.25 to 2 mg I.V. or I.M. before radiologic procedure.

## ADVERSE REACTIONS

**CV:** hypotension.
**GI:** nausea, vomiting.
**Respiratory:** respiratory distress.
**Other:** hypersensitivity reactions (***bronchospasm,*** rash, dizziness, light-headedness).

## INTERACTIONS

*Phenytoin:* inhibited glucagon-induced insulin release. Use cautiously.

## CONTRAINDICATIONS

Contraindicated in patients with hypersensitivity to drug or with pheochromocytoma.

## NURSING CONSIDERATIONS

• Use cautiously in those with history of insulinoma or pheochromocytoma.
• **I.V. use:** Reconstitute 1-unit vial with 1 ml of diluent; reconstitute 10-unit vial with 10 ml of diluent. Use only the diluent supplied by the manufacturer when preparing doses of 2 mg or less. For larger doses, dilute with sterile water for injection.
• For I.V. drip infusion, use dextrose solution, which is compatible with glucagon (drug forms a precipitate in chloride solutions). Inject directly into vein or into I.V. tubing of a free-flowing compatible solution over 2 to 5 minutes. Interrupt primary infusion during glucagon injection if using the same I.V. line.
• *Alert:* Arouse patients from coma as quickly as possible and give additional carbohydrates orally to prevent secondary hypoglycemic reactions.
• Unstable hypoglycemic diabetic patients may not respond to glucagon; give dextrose I.V. instead as ordered.

## ☑ PATIENT TEACHING

• Instruct patient and caregivers in proper glucagon administration and recognition of hypoglycemia.
• Explain importance of calling the doctor at once in emergencies.

# glyburide (glibenclamide)

DiaBeta**, Euglucon†, Glynase PresTab, Micronase

*Pregnancy Risk Category: B*

## HOW SUPPLIED

*Tablets:* 1.25 mg, 2.5 mg, 5 mg
*Tablets (micronized):* 1.5 mg, 3 mg, 5 mg

## ACTION

Unknown. A sulfonylurea that probably stimulates insulin release from the pancreatic beta cells and reduces glucose output by the liver. An extrapancreatic effect increases peripheral sensitivity to insulin and causes a mild diuretic effect.

## ONSET, PEAK, DURATION

Onset occurs in 1 hour for micronized form, 2 to 4 hours for nonmicronized form. Peak levels of glyburide occur in 2 to 4 hours; maximum increases in insulin levels are seen in 1 to 2 hours. Effects persist for 24 hours.

## INDICATIONS & DOSAGE

*Adjunct to diet to lower blood glucose level in patients with type II diabetes (non-insulin-dependent)* –
**Adults:** initially, 2.5 to 5 mg regular tablets P.O. once daily with breakfast. Patients who are more sensitive to antidiabetic agents should be started at 1.25 mg daily. Usual maintenance dosage is 1.25 to 20 mg daily as a single dose or in divided doses.

Alternatively, micronized formulation may be used. Initial dosage is 1.5 to 3 mg daily. Patients who are more sensitive to antidiabetic agents should be started at 0.75 mg daily.
*To replace insulin therapy* –
**Adults:** if insulin dosage is more than 40 units daily, patient is started on 5 mg regular tablets or 3 mg micronized formulation P.O. once daily in addition to 50% of the insulin dosage.

## ADVERSE REACTIONS

**EENT:** changes in accommodation or blurred vision.
**GI:** nausea, epigastric fullness, heartburn.
**Hematologic:** leukopenia, hemolytic anemia, *agranulocytosis, thrombocytopenia, aplastic anemia.*
**Hepatic:** cholestatic jaundice, hepatitis, abnormal liver function.

**Skin:** rash, pruritus, other allergic reactions.
**Other:** *hypoglycemia,* arthralgia, myalgia, angioedema.

## INTERACTIONS

*Anabolic steroids, chloramphenicol, clofibrate, guanethidine, MAO inhibitors, phenylbutazone, salicylates, sulfonamides:* increased hypoglycemic activity. Monitor blood glucose level.
*Beta blockers, clonidine:* prolonged hypoglycemic effect and masked symptoms of hypoglycemia. Use together cautiously.
*Corticosteroids, glucagon, rifampin, thiazide diuretics:* decreased hypoglycemic response. Monitor blood glucose level.
*Ethanol:* possible disulfiram-like reaction. Avoid concomitant use.
*Hydantoins:* increased blood levels of hydantoins. Monitor blood levels.
*Oral anticoagulants:* increased hypoglycemic activity or enhanced anticoagulant effect. Monitor blood glucose level and PT.

## CONTRAINDICATIONS

Contraindicated in patients with hypersensitivity to the drug or diabetic ketoacidosis with or without coma, and during pregnancy or breast-feeding.

## NURSING CONSIDERATIONS

● Use cautiously in patients with hepatic or renal impairment, or in debilitated, malnourished, or elderly patients.
● Know that elderly patients may be more sensitive to adverse effects.
● *Alert:* Know that micronized glyburide (Glynase PresTab) contains drug in a smaller particle size and is not bioequivalent to regular glyburide tablets. Patients who have been taking Micronase or DiaBeta need to be retitrated.
● Know that although most patients may take glyburide once daily, those taking more than 10 mg daily may

---

Reactions may be *common,* uncommon, *life-threatening,* or COMMON AND LIFE-THREATENING.

achieve better results with twice-daily dosage.

• Know that glyburide is a second-generation sulfonylurea. The frequency of adverse effects appears to be lower than with first-generation drugs, such as chlorpropamide.

• During periods of increased stress, such as infection, fever, surgery, or trauma, patients may require insulin therapy. Monitor patients closely for hyperglycemia in these situations.

• Patients transferring from insulin to an oral antidiabetic agent require blood glucose monitoring at least three times a day before meals. Patients may require hospitalization during transition.

☑ **PATIENT TEACHING**
• Instruct patient about nature of disease, importance of following therapeutic regimen, adhering to specific diet, weight reduction, exercise, and personal hygiene programs, and about avoiding infection. Explain how and when to perform self-monitoring of blood glucose levels, and teach recognition of and intervention for hypoglycemia and hyperglycemia.

• Tell patient not to change drug dosage without the doctor's consent and to report abnormal blood or urine glucose test results.

• Teach patient to carry candy or other simple sugars to treat mild hypoglycemic episodes. Severe episodes may require hospital treatment.

• Advise patient not to take any other medication, including OTC drugs, without first checking with the doctor.

• Advise patient to carry medical identification at all times.

## insulins

### insulin injection (regular insulin, crystalline zinc insulin)

Actrapid HM‡, Actrapid HM Penfill‡, Actrapid MC‡, Actrapid MC Penfill‡, Humulin R◇, Hypurin Neutral‡, Insulin 2‡, Novolin R◇, Novolin R PenFill◇, Pork Regular Iletin II◇, Regular (Concentrated) Iletin II, Regular Iletin I◇, Regular Purified Pork Insulin◇, Velosulin Human‡, Velosulin Insuject‡

### insulin zinc suspension, prompt (semilente)

Semilente MC‡

### isophane insulin suspension (neutral protamine Hagedorn insulin, NPH)

Humulin N◇, Humulin NPH‡, Hypurin Isophane‡, Insulatard‡, Insulatard Human†, Isotard MC‡, Novolin N◇, Novolin N PenFill◇, NPH Insulin◇, NPH Purified Pork◇, Pork NPH Iletin II◇, Protaphane HM‡, Protaphane HM Penfill‡, Protaphane MC‡

### isophane insulin suspension with insulin injection

Actraphane HM‡, Actraphane HM Penfill‡, Actraphane MC‡, Humulin 50/50◇, Humulin 70/30◇, Novolin 70/30, Novolin 70/30 PenFill◇

### insulin zinc suspension (lente)

Humulin L◇, Lente Iletin II◇, Lente Insulin◇, Lente MC‡, Lente Purified Pork Insulin◇, Monotard HM‡, Monotard MC‡, Novolin L◇

---

*Liquid form contains alcohol.  **May contain tartrazine.  †Canada only.  ‡Australia only.  ◇OTC.

## protamine zinc suspension (PZI)

Protamine Zinc Insulin MC‡

## insulin zinc suspension, extended (ultralente)

Humulin U◇, Ultralente Insulin◇, Ultratard HM‡, Ultratard MC‡

*Pregnancy Risk Category: NR*

## HOW SUPPLIED
**insulin injection**
*Injection (human):* 100 units/ml (Actrapid HM‡, Humulin R◇, Novolin R◇, Velosulin Human‡); 100 units/ml in 1.5-ml cartridge system◇ (Actrapid HM Penfill‡, Novolin R PenFill◇)
*Injection (from pork):* 100 units/ml◇
*Injection (purified beef):* 100 units/ml (Hypurin Neutral‡, Insulin 2‡)
*Injection (purified pork):* 100 units/ml (Actrapid MC‡, Pork Regular Iletin II◇, Regular Purified Pork Insulin◇); 100 units/ml in 1.5-ml cartridge system‡ (Actrapid MC Penfill‡); 100 units/ml in 2-ml cartridge system‡; 500 units/ml (Regular [Concentrated] Iletin II)
**insulin zinc suspension, prompt**
*Injection (purified pork):* 100 units/ml◇ (Semilente MC‡)
**isophane insulin suspension**
*Injection (from beef):* 100 units/ml◇ (NPH Insulin◇)
*Injection (human, recombinant):* 100 units/ml (Humulin N◇, Humulin NPH‡, Insulatard Human†, Novolin N◇, Protaphane HM‡); 100 units/ml in 1.5-ml cartridge system (Protaphane HM PenFill‡, Novolin N PenFill◇)
*Injection (purified beef):* 100 units/ml (Hypurin Isophane‡, Isotard MC‡)
*Injection (purified pork):* 100 units/ml (Insulatard‡, NPH Purified Pork◇, Pork NPH Iletin II, Protaphane MC‡)
**isophane insulin suspension 50% with insulin injection 50%**
*Injection (human):* 100 units/ml (Humulin 50/50◇)

**isophane insulin suspension 70% with insulin injection 30%**
*Injection (human):* 100 units/ml (Actraphane HM‡, Humulin 70/30‡, Novolin 70/30◇); 100 units/ml in 1.5-ml cartridge system (Actraphane HM Penfill‡, Novolin 70/30 PenFill◇)
*Injection (purified pork):* 100 units/ml (Actraphane MC‡)
**insulin zinc suspension**
*Injection (from beef):* 100 units/ml (Lente Insulin◇, Lente MC‡)
*Injection (purified beef):* 100 units/ml (Lente MC‡)
*Injection (purified pork):* 100 units/ml (Lente Iletin II, Monotard MC‡, Lente Purified Pork Insulin◇)
*Injection (human):* 100 units/ml◇ (Humulin L◇, Monotard HM‡, Novolin I◇)
**protamine zinc suspension**
*Injection (purified pork):* 100 units/ml Protamine Zinc Insulin MC‡
**insulin zinc suspension, extended**
*Injection (from beef):* 100 units/ml◇ (Ultralente Insulin◇)
*Injection (human):* 100 units/ml (Ultratard HM‡, Humulin U◇)
*Injection (purified pork):* 100 units/ml‡ (Ultratard MC‡)

## ACTION
Increases glucose transport across muscle and fat cell membranes to reduce blood glucose level. Promotes conversion of glucose to its storage form, glycogen; triggers amino acid uptake and conversion to protein in muscle cells and inhibits protein degradation; stimulates triglyceride formation and inhibits release of free fatty acids from adipose tissue; and stimulates lipoprotein lipase activity, which converts circulating lipoproteins to fatty acids.

## ONSET, PEAK, DURATION
Highly variable. Onset occurs within ½ to 1½ hours with S.C. rapid-acting insulin, 1 to 2½ hours with S.C. intermediate-acting insulins, and 4 to 8

---

Reactions may be *common,* uncommon, *life-threatening,* or **COMMON AND LIFE-THREATENING.**

hours with S.C. long-acting insulins. Serum levels peak in 2 to 3 hours with S.C. rapid-acting regular insulins, 4 to 10 hours with S.C. rapid-acting semilente insulin, 4 to 15 hours with S.C. intermediate-acting insulins, and 10 to 30 hours with S.C. long-acting insulins. Effects persist for 5 to 7 hours with S.C. rapid-acting regular insulin, 12 to 16 hours with S.C. rapid-acting semilente insulin, 18 to 24 hours with S.C. intermediate-acting insulins, and 36 hours for S.C. long-acting insulins.

## INDICATIONS & DOSAGE
*Diabetic ketoacidosis (use regular insulin only)* –
**Adults:** 0.33 units/kg as an I.V. bolus, followed by 0.1 units/kg/hour by continuous infusion. Continue infusion until blood glucose level drops to 250 mg/dl; then S.C. insulin is begun with dosage and dosage interval adjusted according to patient's blood glucose concentration.

Alternatively, 50 to 100 units I.V. and 50 to 100 units S.C. stat; then additional doses q 2 to 6 hours based on blood glucose levels.

To prepare infusion, add 100 units of regular insulin and 1 g of albumin to 100 ml of 0.9% sodium chloride solution. Insulin concentration will be 1 unit/ml. (The albumin will adhere to plastic, preventing insulin from adhering to plastic.)
**Children:** 0.1 unit/kg as an I.V. bolus, then 0.1 unit/kg hourly by continuous infusion until blood glucose level drops to 250 mg/dl; then S.C. insulin started. Alternatively, 1 to 2 units/kg in two divided doses, one I.V. and the other S.C., followed by 0.5 to 1 unit/kg I.V. q 1 to 2 hours based on blood glucose levels.
*Type I diabetes (insulin-dependent), adjunct to type II diabetes (noninsulin-dependent) inadequately controlled by diet and oral antidiabetic agents* –
**Adults and children:** therapeutic regimen is prescribed by the doctor and adjusted according to patient's blood glucose concentrations.

## ADVERSE REACTIONS
**Skin:** urticaria, pruritus, swelling, redness, stinging, warmth at injection site.
**Other:** *lipoatrophy, lipohypertrophy,* hypersensitivity reactions (**anaphylaxis,** rash), **hypoglycemia,** hyperglycemia (rebound, or Somogyi, effect).

## INTERACTIONS
*Anabolic steroids, beta blockers, clofibrate, ethanol, fenfluramine, guanethidine, MAO inhibitors, salicylates, tetracycline:* prolonged hypoglycemic effect. Monitor blood glucose level carefully.
*Corticosteroids, dextrothyroxine, epinephrine, smoking, thiazide diuretics, thyroid hormone:* diminished insulin response. Monitor for hyperglycemia.
*Diazoxide, phenytoin (high doses):* may inhibit endogenous insulin secretion and cause hypoglycemia in diabetic patients. Carefully adjust insulin dosage when using with these drugs.
*Oral contraceptives:* may decrease glucose tolerance in diabetic patients. Monitor blood glucose levels and adjust insulin dosage carefully.

## CONTRAINDICATIONS
None known.

## NURSING CONSIDERATIONS
• Know that insulin is the drug of choice to treat diabetes during pregnancy. Insulin requirements increase in pregnant diabetic patients and then decline immediately postpartum. Monitor patient closely.
• Dosage is always expressed in USP units. Remember to use only the syringes calibrated for the particular concentration of insulin administered. U-500 insulin must be administered with a U-100 syringe because no syringes are made for this strength.

*Liquid form contains alcohol. **May contain tartrazine. †Canada only. ‡Australia only. ◇OTC.

• Be aware some patients may develop insulin resistance and require large insulin doses to control symptoms of diabetes. U-500 insulin is available as Regular (Concentrated) Iletin II for such patients. Although every pharmacy may not stock it, it is available. Nurses should give the hospital pharmacy sufficient notice before requesting refill of in-house prescription. Never store U-500 insulin in same area with other insulin preparations because of danger of severe overdose if given accidentally to other patients.

• To mix insulin suspension, swirl vial gently or rotate between palms or between palm and thigh. Don't shake vigorously: this causes bubbling and air in syringe.

• Know that lente, semilente, and ultralente insulins may be mixed in any proportion. Regular insulin may be mixed with NPH or lente insulins in any proportion. When mixing regular insulin with intermediate or long acting insulin, always draw up regular insulin into syringe first.

• Note that switching from separate injections to a prepared mixture may alter patient response. Whenever NPH or lente is mixed with regular insulin in the same syringe, give it immediately to avoid loss of potency.

• Don't use insulin that changes color or becomes clumped or granular in appearance.

• Check expiration date on vial before using contents.

• Know that usual administration route is S.C. For proper S.C. administration, remember to pinch a fold of skin with the fingers at least 3″ (7.6 cm) apart, and insert the needle at a 45- to 90-degree angle.

• Press but do not rub site after injection. Rotate injection sites and chart to avoid overuse of one area. Know that diabetic patients may achieve better control if injection site is rotated within same anatomic region.

• *Alert:* Know that regular insulin is used in patients with circulatory collapse, diabetic ketoacidosis, or hyperkalemia. Do not use regular insulin (Concentrated), 500 units/ml, I.V. Do not use intermediate or long-acting insulins for coma or other emergency requiring rapid drug action. Also know that ketosis-prone type I severely ill, and newly diagnosed diabetic patients with very high blood glucose levels may require hospitalization and I.V. treatment with regular fast-acting insulin.

• **I.V. use:** Only administer regular insulin I.V. Inject directly, at ordered rate, into vein through an intermittent infusion device or into a port close to I.V. access site. Intermittent infusion is not recommended. If given by continuous infusion, infuse drug diluted in 0.9% sodium chloride at the prescribed rate.

• Store insulin in cool area. Refrigeration is desirable but not essential, except with regular insulin concentrated.

## ☑ PATIENT TEACHING

• Make sure patient knows that therapy only relieves symptoms.

• Instruct patient about nature of disease, importance of following the therapeutic regimen, adhering to specific diet, weight reduction, exercise, and personal hygiene program, and about avoiding infection. Emphasize the importance of the timing of injections and eating and that meals must not be omitted.

• Stress to patient that accuracy of measurement is important, especially with concentrated regular insulin. Aids, such as magnifying sleeve or dose magnifier, may improve accuracy. Instruct patient and caregivers how to measure and administer insulin.

• Advise patient not to alter the order of mixing insulins or change the model or brand of insulin, syringe, or needle.

• Teach that self-monitoring of blood glucose levels and urine ketone tests

---

Reactions may be *common,* uncommon, *life-threatening,* or **COMMON AND LIFE-THREATENING.**

are essential guides to dosage and success of therapy. It's important to recognize hypoglycemic symptoms because insulin-induced hypoglycemia is hazardous and may cause brain damage if prolonged; most adverse effects are self-limiting and temporary.

• Instruct patient on proper use of equipment for performing self-monitoring of blood glucose levels.

• Advise patient not to smoke within 30 minutes after insulin injection. Cigarette smoking decreases the amount of absorption of insulin administered subcutaneously.

• Tell patient that marijuana use may increase insulin requirements.

• Advise patient to wear a medical identification bracelet at all times, to carry ample insulin and syringes on trips, to have carbohydrates (lump of sugar or candy) on hand for emergencies, and to note time zone changes for dosage schedule when traveling.

---

## metformin hydrochloride
Glucophage

*Pregnancy Risk Category: B*

### HOW SUPPLIED
*Tablets:* 500 mg, 850 mg

### ACTION
Decreases hepatic glucose production and intestinal absorption of glucose and improves insulin sensitivity (increases peripheral glucose uptake and utilization).

### ONSET, PEAK, DURATION
Not clearly defined, although food does delay onset and peak of the drug.

### INDICATIONS & DOSAGE
*Adjunct to diet to lower blood glucose level in patients with type II diabetes (non-insulin-dependent)* –
**Adults:** initially, 500 mg P.O. b.i.d. given with morning and evening meals, or 850 mg P.O. once daily given with morning meal. When 500-mg dose form used, dosage increased 500 mg weekly to maximum dosage of 2,500 mg P.O. daily in divided doses as needed. When 850-mg dose form used, dosage increased 850 mg every other week to a maximum dosage of 2,550 mg P.O. daily in divided doses as needed.

### ADVERSE REACTIONS
**GI:** diarrhea, nausea, vomiting, abdominal bloating, flatulence, anorexia.
**Hematologic:** megaloblastic anemia.
**Other:** *lactic acidosis,* unpleasant or metallic taste.

### INTERACTIONS
*Calcium channel blockers, corticosteroids, estrogens, isoniazid, nicotinic acid, oral contraceptives, phenothiazines, phenytoin, sympathomimetics, thiazide and other diuretics, thyroid agents:* may produce hyperglycemia. Monitor patient's glycemic control. Metformin dosage may need to be increased.
*Cationic drugs, such as amiloride, cimetidine, digoxin, morphine, procainamide, quinidine, quinine, ranitidine, triamterene, trimethoprim, vancomycin:* have the potential to compete for common renal tubular transport systems, which may increase metformin plasma levels. Monitor patient's blood glucose level.
*Nifedipine:* increased metformin plasma levels. Monitor patient closely. Metformin dosage may need to be decreased.

### CONTRAINDICATIONS
Contraindicated in patients with hypersensitivity to the drug, renal disease, or metabolic acidosis. Metformin should be temporarily withheld in patients undergoing radiologic studies involving parenteral administration of iodinated contrast materials because use of such products may result in acute renal dys-

---

*Liquid form contains alcohol.   **May contain tartrazine.   †Canada only.   ‡Australia only.   ◊OTC.

function. The drug should also be promptly discontinued if the patient enters a hypoxic state. Metformin generally should be avoided in patients with hepatic disease.

## NURSING CONSIDERATIONS

● Use caution when giving drug to elderly, debilitated, or malnourished patients and to those with adrenal or pituitary insufficiency because of increased risk of hypoglycemia.
● Know that before therapy begins, the patient's renal function should be assessed and then assessed at least annually thereafter. If renal impairment is detected, expect the doctor to switch the patient to a different antidiabetic agent.
● Administer with meals; once-daily dosage should be given with breakfast and twice-daily dosage with breakfast and dinner.
● Know that when transferring patients from standard oral hypoglycemic agents (except chlorpropamide) to metformin, no transition period generally is necessary. When switching patients from chlorpropamide to metformin, care should be exercised during the first 2 weeks of metformin therapy because the prolonged retention of chlorpropamide increases the risk of hypoglycemia during this time.
● Monitor patient's blood glucose levels regularly to evaluate effectiveness of therapy. Notify doctor if blood glucose levels become elevated despite therapy.
● Be aware that if the patient has not responded to 4 weeks of therapy using the maximum dosage, the doctor may add an oral sulfonylurea while continuing metformin at the maximum dosage. If the patient still does not respond after several months of concomitant therapy at maximum dosages, the doctor may discontinue both agents and institute insulin therapy.
● Monitor patient closely during times of increased stress, such as infection,

fever, surgery, or trauma. Insulin therapy may be needed in these situations.
● Be aware that the incidence of metformin-induced lactic acidosis is very low. Reported cases have occurred primarily in diabetic patients with significant renal insufficiency; with multiple, concomitant medical or surgical problems; and with multiple, concomitant drug regimens. The risk increases with the degree of renal impairment and the patient's age.
● *Alert:* Know that metformin should be discontinued immediately and the doctor notified if the patient develops any condition associated with hypoxemia or dehydration because of the risk of lactic acidosis associated with these conditions.
● Expect metformin therapy to be temporarily suspended for any surgical procedure (except minor procedures not associated with restricted intake of food and fluids) and should not be restarted until the patient's oral intake has resumed and renal function has been evaluated as normal.
● Monitor the patient's hematologic status for evidence of megaloblastic anemia. Patients with inadequate vitamin $B_{12}$ or calcium intake or absorption appear to be predisposed to developing subnormal vitamin $B_{12}$ levels. These patients should have routine serum vitamin $B_{12}$ level determinations every 2 to 3 years.

## ☑ PATIENT TEACHING

● *Alert:* Instruct patient about nature of diabetes, importance of following therapeutic regimen, adhering to specific diet, weight reduction, exercise, personal hygiene programs, and avoiding infection. Explain how and when to perform self-monitoring of blood glucose level, and teach signs of hypoglycemia and hyperglycemia.
● Instruct patient to discontinue drug and notify the doctor immediately if unexplained hyperventilation, myalgia, malaise, unusual somnolence, or

---

Reactions may be *common*, uncommon, *life-threatening*, or COMMON AND LIFE-THREATENING.

other nonspecific symptoms of early lactic acidosis occur.
- Warn patient not to consume excessive alcohol while taking metformin.
- Tell patient not to change drug dosage without the doctor's consent. Encourage patient to report abnormal blood glucose results.
- Advise patient not to take any other medication, including OTC drugs, without checking with the doctor.
- Instruct patient to carry medical identification at all times.

---

## tolazamide
Tolamide, Tolinase
*Pregnancy Risk Category: C*

### HOW SUPPLIED
*Tablets:* 100 mg, 250 mg, 500 mg

### ACTION
Unknown. A sulfonylurea that probably stimulates insulin release from the pancreatic beta cells and reduces glucose output by the liver. An extrapancreatic effect increases peripheral sensitivity to insulin.

### ONSET, PEAK, DURATION
Onset occurs in 4 to 6 hours. Peak hypoglycemic effect within 4 to 6 hours. Effects persist for 12 to 24 hours.

### INDICATIONS & DOSAGE
*Adjunct to diet to lower blood glucose levels in patients with type II diabetes (non-insulin-dependent)* –
**Adults:** initially, 100 mg P.O. daily with breakfast if fasting blood sugar (FBS) is under 200 mg/dl, or 250 mg P.O. if FBS is over 200 mg/dl. Dosage adjusted at weekly intervals by 100 to 250 mg as needed. Maximum daily dosage is 500 mg b.i.d. before meals.
**Adults over 65 years:** 100 mg P.O. once daily.
*To change from insulin to oral therapy* –
**Adults:** if insulin dosage is under 20 units daily, insulin is stopped and oral

therapy started at 100 mg P.O. daily with breakfast. If insulin dosage is 20 to 40 units daily, insulin is stopped and oral therapy started at 250 mg P.O. daily with breakfast. If insulin dosage is over 40 units daily, insulin is decreased by 50% and oral therapy started at 250 mg P.O. daily with breakfast. Dosage may be adjusted by 100 to 250 mg.

### ADVERSE REACTIONS
**CNS:** paresthesia, fatigue, dizziness, vertigo, malaise, headache.
**GI:** nausea, vomiting, epigastric distress.
**Hematologic:** leukopenia, hemolytic anemia, ***thrombocytopenia, aplastic anemia, agranulocytosis.***
**Skin:** rash, urticaria, pruritus, erythema.
**Other:** *hypersensitivity reactions, hypoglycemia.*

### INTERACTIONS
*Anabolic steroids, chloramphenicol, clofibrate, guanethidine, MAO inhibitors, phenylbutazone, salicylates, sulfonamides:* increased hypoglycemic activity. Monitor blood glucose level.
*Beta blockers, clonidine:* prolonged hypoglycemic effect and masked symptoms of hypoglycemia. Use together cautiously.
*Corticosteroids, glucagon, rifampin, thiazide diuretics:* decreased hypoglycemic response. Monitor blood glucose level.
*Ethanol:* possible disulfiram-like reaction. Avoid concomitant use of moderate to large amounts of ethanol.
*Hydantoins:* increased blood levels of hydantoins. Monitor blood levels.
*Oral anticoagulants:* increased hypoglycemic activity or enhanced anticoagulant effect. Monitor blood glucose levels and PT.

### CONTRAINDICATIONS
Contraindicated for treating type I diabetes (insulin-dependent) or diabetes that can be adequately con-

---

\*Liquid form contains alcohol. \*\*May contain tartrazine. †Canada only. ‡Australia only. ◊OTC.

trolled by diet. Also contraindicated in patients with type II diabetes complicated by ketosis, acidosis, coma, or other acute complications such as major surgery, severe infection, or severe trauma; in patients with uremia or hypersensitivity to drug; and during pregnancy or breast-feeding.

## NURSING CONSIDERATIONS
• Use cautiously in elderly, debilitated, or malnourished patients or patients with impaired hepatic or renal function or porphyria.
• Know that elderly patients may be more sensitive to adverse effects.
• Be aware that patients transferring from another oral antidiabetic agent usually need no transition period.
• Patients transferring from insulin therapy to an oral antidiabetic agent require blood glucose level testing at least three times a day before meals. Hospitalization may be required during the transition.

## ☑ PATIENT TEACHING
• Make sure patient knows that therapy relieves symptoms but doesn't cure disease.
• Instruct patient about nature of disease, importance of following therapeutic regimen, adhering to specific diet, weight reduction, exercise, and personal hygiene programs, and about avoiding infection. Explain how and when to perform self-monitoring of blood glucose levels, and teach recognition of and intervention for hypoglycemia and hyperglycemia.
• Tell patient not to change drug dosage without the doctor's consent and to report abnormal blood or urine glucose test results.
• Teach patient to carry candy or other simple sugars to treat mild hypoglycemic episodes. Severe episodes may require hospital treatment.
• Advise patient not to take any other medication, including OTC drugs, without checking with the doctor.

• Advise patient to avoid moderate to large intake of alcohol because of possible disulfiram-like reaction.
• Advise patient to carry medical identification at all times.

---

## tolbutamide
Apo-Tolbutamide, Mobenol†, Novo-Butamide†, Oramide, Orinase

*Pregnancy Risk Category: C*

### HOW SUPPLIED
*Tablets:* 250 mg, 500 mg

### ACTION
Unknown. A sulfonylurea that probably stimulates insulin release from the pancreatic beta cells and reduces glucose output by the liver. An extrapancreatic effect increases peripheral sensitivity to insulin.

### ONSET, PEAK, DURATION
Onset occurs within 1 hour. Plasma levels peak in 3 to 5 hours; peak hypoglycemic effects within 5 to 8 hours. Effects persist for 6 to 12 hours.

### INDICATIONS & DOSAGE
*Adjunct to diet to lower blood glucose levels in patients with type II diabetes (non-insulin-dependent)* –
**Adults:** initially, 1 to 2 g P.O. daily as a single dose or in divided doses b.i.d. to t.i.d. Dosage adjusted, if necessary, to maximum of 3 g daily; however, the manufacturer states that little benefit occurs with doses greater than 2 g daily.
*To change from insulin to oral therapy* –
**Adults:** if insulin dosage is under 20 units daily, insulin is stopped and oral therapy started at 1 to 2 g P.O. daily. If insulin dosage is 20 to 40 units daily, insulin is reduced by 30% to 50% and oral therapy started as above. If insulin dosage is over 40 units daily, insulin is reduced by 20% and oral therapy started as above.

---

Reactions may be *common*, uncommon, *life-threatening*, or **COMMON AND LIFE-THREATENING**.

Further reductions are based on patient's response to oral therapy.

## ADVERSE REACTIONS
**CNS:** paresthesia, fatigue, dizziness, vertigo, malaise, headache.
**GI:** nausea, heartburn, epigastric distress.
**Hematologic:** leukopenia, hemolytic anemia, *thrombocytopenia, aplastic anemia, agranulocytosis.*
**Skin:** rash, pruritus, erythema, urticaria.
**Other:** *hypersensitivity reactions, hypoglycemia, dilutional hyponatremia.*

## INTERACTIONS
*Anabolic steroids, chloramphenicol, clofibrate, guanethidine, MAO inhibitors, phenylbutazone, salicylates, sulfonamides:* increased hypoglycemic activity. Monitor blood glucose level.
*Beta blockers, clonidine:* prolonged hypoglycemic effect and masked symptoms of hypoglycemia. Use together cautiously.
*Corticosteroids, glucagon, rifampin, thiazide diuretics:* decreased hypoglycemic response. Monitor blood glucose level.
*Ethanol:* possible disulfiram-like reaction. Avoid concomitant use of moderate to large amount of ethanol.
*Hydantoins:* increased blood levels of hydantoins. Monitor blood levels closely.
*Oral anticoagulants:* increased hypoglycemic activity or enhanced anticoagulant effect. Monitor blood glucose levels and PT.

## CONTRAINDICATIONS
Contraindicated for treating type I diabetes (insulin-dependent) or diabetes that can be adequately controlled by diet. Also contraindicated in patients with type II diabetes complicated by fever, ketosis, acidosis, coma, or other acute complications such as major surgery, severe infection, or severe trauma; in patients with hypersensitivity to drug or severe renal insufficiency; and during pregnancy or breast-feeding.

## NURSING CONSIDERATIONS
● Use cautiously in elderly, debilitated, or malnourished patients or patients with impaired hepatic or renal function or porphyria.
● Know that elderly patients may be more sensitive to adverse effects.
● Know that patients transferring from another oral antidiabetic agent usually need no transition period.
● Be aware that patients transferring from insulin therapy to an oral antidiabetic agent require blood glucose level testing at least three times a day before meals. Hospitalization may be required during the transition.

☑ **PATIENT TEACHING**
● Instruct patient about nature of disease, importance of following therapeutic regimen, adhering to specific diet, weight reduction, exercise, and personal hygiene program, and about avoiding infection. Explain how and when to perform self-monitoring of blood glucose levels, and teach recognition of and intervention for hypoglycemia and hyperglycemia.
● Tell him that therapy relieves symptoms but doesn't cure disease.
● Tell patient not to change dosage without doctor's consent and to report abnormal glucose test results.
● Teach patient to carry candy or other simple sugars to treat mild hypoglycemic episodes.
● Advise patient not to take any other medication, including OTC drugs, without checking with the doctor.
● Advise patient to avoid moderate to large intake of alcohol because of possible disulfiram-like reaction.
● Advise patient to carry medical identification at all times.

*Liquid form contains alcohol.   **May contain tartrazine.   †Canada only.   ‡Australia only.   ◊OTC.

# 58

## Thyroid hormones

**levothyroxine sodium**
**liothyronine sodium**
**liotrix**
**thyroid**
**thyrotropin**

**COMBINATION PRODUCTS**
None.

---

## levothyroxine sodium
## (T₄ or L-thyroxine sodium)
Eltroxin†, Levo-T, Levothroid,
Levoxine, Levoxyl, Oroxine‡,
Synthroid**

*Pregnancy Risk Category: A*

---

### HOW SUPPLIED
*Tablets:* 0.025 mg, 0.05 mg, 0.075
mg, 0.088 mg, 0.1 mg, 0.112 mg,
0.125 mg, 0.137 mg, 0.15 mg, 0.175
mg, 0.2 mg, 0.3 mg.
*Injection:* 200 mcg-vial, 500 mcg-vial

### ACTION
Not completely defined. Stimulates metabolism of all body tissues by accelerating rate of cellular oxidation.

### ONSET, PEAK, DURATION
Onset in 24 hours. Time to peak therapeutic effect is 3 to 4 weeks. Effects
persist for 1 to 3 weeks.

### INDICATIONS & DOSAGE
*Cretinism—*
**Children under 1 year:** initially,
0.025 to 0.05 mg P.O. daily, increased by 0.05 mg P.O. q 4 to 6
weeks as needed.
*Myxedema coma—*
**Adults:** 200 to 500 mcg I.V.; then 100
to 300 mcg given on second day, followed by parenteral maintenance dosage of 50 to 200 mcg I.V. daily. Pa-

tient should be switched to oral maintenance as soon as possible.
*Thyroid hormone replacement—*
**Adults:** initially, 0.025 to 0.05 mg
P.O. daily, increased by 0.025 mg
P.O. q 2 to 4 weeks until desired response occurs. Maintenance dosage is
0.1 to 0.4 mg P.O. daily. May administer I.V. or I.M. when P.O. ingestion
is precluded for long periods. However, dosage adjustment is necessary.
**Adults over 65 years:** 0.0125 mg to
0.025 mg P.O. daily. Increased by
0.025 mg at 3- to 8-week intervals depending on response.
**Children:** initially, 0.025 to 0.05 mg
in children younger than 1 year or 3 to
5 mcg/kg in children 1 year and older
P.O. daily, gradually increased by
0.025 to 0.05 mg q 2 to 4 weeks until
desired response occurs.

### ADVERSE REACTIONS
**CNS:** *nervousness, insomnia, tremor,*
headache.
**CV:** *tachycardia, palpitations, **ar-**
**rhythmias,** angina pectoris, **cardiac ar-**
**rest.***
**GI:** diarrhea, vomiting.
**Other:** weight loss, diaphoresis, heat
intolerance, fever, menstrual irregularities, allergic skin reactions.

### INTERACTIONS
*Cholestyramine, colestipol:* impaired
levothyroxine absorption. Separate
doses by 4 to 5 hours.
*Insulin, oral antidiabetic agents:* altered serum glucose levels. Monitor
blood glucose levels. Dosage adjustments may be necessary.
*I.V. phenytoin:* free thyroid released.
Monitor for tachycardia.
*Oral anticoagulants:* altered PT.
Monitor PT. Dosage adjustments may
be necessary.

---

Reactions may be *common,* uncommon, ***life-threatening,*** or **COMMON AND LIFE-THREATENING.**

*Sympathomimetics, such as epinephrine:* increased risk of coronary insufficiency. Monitor closely.

## CONTRAINDICATIONS

Contraindicated in patients with hypersensitivity to drug, acute MI uncomplicated by hypothyroidism, untreated thyrotoxicosis, or uncorrected adrenal insufficiency.

## NURSING CONSIDERATIONS

• Use with extreme caution in elderly patients and those with angina pectoris, hypertension, other CV disorders, renal insufficiency, or ischemia.
• Use cautiously in those with diabetes mellitus or insipidus or myxedema.
• Rapid replacement in patients with arteriosclerosis may precipitate angina, coronary occlusion, or CVA. Use cautiously in these patients. Also, in patients with coronary artery disease who must receive thyroid hormone, observe carefully for possible coronary insufficiency.
• Know that thyroid hormone replacement requirements are about 25% lower in patients over age 60 than in young adults.
• Also know that patients with adult hypothyroidism are unusually sensitive to thyroid hormone. Patient should be started at lowest dosage and titrated to higher dosages according to patients' symptoms and laboratory data until euthyroid state is reached.
• **I.V. use:** Prepare I.V. dose immediately before injection. Do not mix with other solutions. Inject into vein over 1 to 2 minutes.
• When changing from levothyroxine to liothyronine ($T_3$), levothyroxine should be stopped and liothyronine begun. Dosage should be increased in small increments after residual effects of levothyroxine have disappeared. When changing from liothyronine to levothyroxine, levothyroxine is started several days before withdrawing liothyronine to avoid relapse.

• Monitor blood pressure and heart rate closely. High initial I.V dosage is usually well tolerated by patients in myxedema coma. Normal serum levels of $T_4$ should occur within 24 hours, followed by a threefold increase in serum $T_3$ in 3 days.
• Know that thyroid hormones alter thyroid function test results.
• Know that patients taking levothyroxine who need to have radioactive iodine uptake studies performed must discontinue drug 4 weeks before test.

## ☑ PATIENT TEACHING

• Make sure patient understands the importance of compliance. Tell patient to take thyroid hormones at the same time each day, preferably before breakfast, to maintain constant hormone levels. Suggest morning dosage to prevent insomnia.
• Warn patient (especially elderly patient) to tell the doctor at once if chest pain, palpitations, sweating, nervousness, shortness of breath, or other signs of overdose or aggravated CV disease occur.
• Advise patient who has achieved stable response not to change brands.
• Tell patient to report unusual bleeding and bruising.

## liothyronine sodium ($T_3$)

Cyronine, Cytomel, Tertroxin‡, Triostat

*Pregnancy Risk Category: A*

### HOW SUPPLIED

*Tablets:* 5 mcg, 25 mcg, 50 mcg
*Injection:* 10 mcg/ml

### ACTION

Not clearly defined. Enhances oxygen consumption by most tissues of the body, increases the basal metabolic rate and the metabolism of carbohydrates, lipids, and proteins.

## ONSET, PEAK, DURATION
Onset unknown. Peak occurs in 2 to 3 days. Effects persist about 3 days.

## INDICATIONS & DOSAGE
*Congenital hypothyroidism* –
**Children:** 5 mcg P.O. daily with a 5-mcg increase q 3 to 4 days until desired response achieved.
*Myxedema* –
**Adults:** initially, 5 mcg P.O. daily, increased by 5 to 10 mcg q 1 or 2 weeks until daily dosage reaches 25 mcg. Then, increased by 12.5 to 25 mcg daily q 1 to 2 weeks. Maintenance dosage is 50 to 100 mcg daily.
*Myxedema coma, premyxedema coma* –
**Adults:** initially, 10 to 20 mcg I.V. for patients with known or suspected CV disease; 25 to 50 mcg I.V. for patients not known to have CV disease. Subsequent dosage adjustments made as indicated by patient's condition and response. Patient should be switched to oral therapy as soon as possible.
*Nontoxic goiter* –
**Adults:** initially, 5 mcg P.O. daily; may increase by 5 to 10 mcg daily q 1 to 2 weeks, until daily dosage reaches 25 mcg. Then, increase by 12.5 to 25 mcg daily q 1 to 2 weeks. Usual maintenance dosage is 75 mcg daily.
*Thyroid hormone replacement* –
**Adults:** initially, 25 mcg P.O. daily, increased by 12.5 to 25 mcg q 1 to 2 weeks until satisfactory response occurs. Usual maintenance dosage is 25 to 75 mcg daily.
*$T_3$ suppression test to differentiate hyperthyroidism from euthyroidism* –
**Adults:** 75 to 100 mcg P.O. daily for 7 days.

## ADVERSE REACTIONS
**CNS:** *nervousness, insomnia, tremor,* headache.
**CV:** *tachycardia, **arrhythmias,*** angina pectoris, ***cardiac decompensation and collapse.***
**GI:** diarrhea, vomiting.

**Other:** weight loss, heat intolerance, diaphoresis, accelerated bone maturation in infants and children, menstrual irregularities, skin reactions.

## INTERACTIONS
*Cholestyramine, colestipol:* impaired liothyronine absorption. Separate doses by 4 to 5 hours.
*Insulin, oral antidiabetic agents:* initial thyroid replacement therapy may cause increases in insulin or oral hypoglycemic requirements. Monitor blood glucose levels. Dosage adjustments may be necessary.
*Oral anticoagulants:* altered PT. Monitor PT. Dosage adjustments may be necessary.
*Sympathomimetics, such as epinephrine:* increased risk of coronary insufficiency. Monitor closely.

## CONTRAINDICATIONS
Contraindicated in patients with hypersensitivity to drug, acute MI uncomplicated by hypothyroidism, untreated thyrotoxicosis, or uncorrected adrenal insufficiency.

## NURSING CONSIDERATIONS
● Use with extreme caution in elderly patients and those with angina pectoris, hypertension, other CV disorders, renal insufficiency, or ischemia.
● Use cautiously in patients with diabetes mellitus or insipidus or myxedema.
● Rapid replacement in patients with arteriosclerosis may precipitate angina, coronary occlusion, or CVA. Use cautiously in these patients. In patients with coronary artery disease who must receive thyroid hormones, observe carefully for possible coronary insufficiency.
● *Alert:* Know that levothyroxine is usually the preferred agent for thyroid hormone replacement therapy. Liothyronine may be used when a rapid onset or a rapidly reversible agent is desirable or in patients with impaired

peripheral conversion of levothyroxine to liothyronine.

• Be aware that regulation of liothyronine dosage is difficult.

• Know that thyroid hormone replacement requirements are about 25% lower in patients over age 60 than in young adults.

• **I.V. use:** Repeat dosages should be administered longer than 4 hours apart but less than 12 hours apart. Do not administer injection I.M. or S.C.

• Monitor pulse and blood pressure.

• Know that thyroid hormones alter thyroid function tests. Monitor PT; patients taking these hormones usually require decreased anticoagulant dosage.

• When changing from levothyroxine to liothyronine, levothyroxine should be stopped and liothyronine begun at a low dosage. Dosage should be increased in small increments after residual effects of levothyroxine have disappeared. When changing from liothyronine to levothyroxine, levothyroxine is started several days before withdrawing liothyronine to avoid relapse.

• Know that patients taking liothyronine who need radioactive iodine uptake studies done must discontinue drug 7 to 10 days before test.

☑ **PATIENT TEACHING**

• Make sure patient understands the importance of compliance. Tell patient to take thyroid hormones at the same time each day, preferably before breakfast, to maintain constant hormone levels. Suggest morning dosage to prevent insomnia.

• Advise patient who has achieved a stable response not to change brands.

• Warn patient (especially elderly patient) to tell the doctor at once if chest pain, palpitations, sweating, nervousness, or other signs of overdose or aggravated CV disease occur.

• Tell patient to report unusual bleeding and bruising.

# liotrix
Euthroid**, Thyrolar

*Pregnancy Risk Category: A*

## HOW SUPPLIED
*Tablets:* levothyroxine sodium ($T_4$) 30 mcg and liothyronine sodium ($T_3$) 7.5 mcg (Euthroid-½); levothyroxine sodium 60 mcg and liothyronine sodium 15 mcg (Euthroid-1); levothyroxine sodium 120 mcg and liothyronine sodium 30 mcg (Euthroid-2); levothyroxine sodium 180 mcg and liothyronine sodium 45 mcg (Euthroid-3); levothyroxine sodium 12.5 mcg and liothyronine sodium 3.1 mcg (Thyrolar-¼); levothyroxine sodium 25 mcg and liothyronine sodium 6.25 mcg (Thyrolar-½); levothyroxine sodium 50 mcg and liothyronine sodium 12.5 mcg (Thyrolar-1); levothyroxine sodium 100 mcg and liothyronine sodium 25 mcg (Thyrolar-2); levothyroxine sodium 150 mcg and liothyronine sodium 37.5 mcg (Thyrolar-3)

## ACTION
Not clearly defined. Stimulates metabolism of all body tissues by accelerating the rate of cellular oxidation and provides both $T_3$ and $T_4$ to the tissues.

## ONSET, PEAK, DURATION
Unknown.

## INDICATIONS & DOSAGE
*Hypothyroidism –*
Dosages are expressed in thyroid equivalents and must be individualized to approximate the deficit in the patient's thyroid secretion.

**Adults and children:** initially, 12.5 mcg of levothyroxine and 3.1 mcg of liothyronine P.O. daily, or 25 mcg of levothyroxine and 6.25 mcg of liothyronine daily, or 30 mcg of levothyroxine and 7.5 mcg of liothyronine daily. Dosage is increased in increments of the initial dose at 2-week intervals to achieve desired response.

## ADVERSE REACTIONS

**CNS:** *nervousness, insomnia, tremor,* headache.
**CV:** *tachycardia,* **arrhythmias,** angina pectoris, **cardiac decompensation and collapse.**
**GI:** *diarrhea, vomiting.*
**Other:** weight loss, heat intolerance, diaphoresis, accelerated rate of bone maturation in infants and children, menstrual irregularities, allergic skin reactions.

## INTERACTIONS

*Cholestyramine, colestipol:* impaired liotrix absorption. Separate doses by 4 to 5 hours.
*Insulin, oral antidiabetic agents:* altered serum glucose levels. Monitor blood glucose levels. Dosage adjustments may be necessary.
*I.V. phenytoin:* free thyroid released. Monitor for tachycardia.
*Oral anticoagulants:* altered PT. Monitor PT. Dosage adjustments may be necessary.
*Sympathomimetics, such as epinephrine:* increased risk of coronary insufficiency. Monitor closely.

## CONTRAINDICATIONS

Contraindicated in patients with hypersensitivity to drug, acute MI uncomplicated by hypothyroidism, untreated thyrotoxicosis, or uncorrected adrenal insufficiency.

## NURSING CONSIDERATIONS

• Use with extreme caution in elderly patients and those with angina pectoris, hypertension, other CV disorders, renal insufficiency, or ischemia.
• Use cautiously in patients with myxedema or diabetes mellitus or insipidus.
• Rapid replacement in arteriosclerosis may precipitate angina, coronary occlusion, or CVA. Use cautiously in these patients.

• In patients with coronary artery disease who must receive thyroid hormones, observe carefully for possible coronary insufficiency. Also observe carefully during surgery because arrhythmias can be precipitated.
• Know that thyroid hormone replacement requirements are about 25% lower in patients over age 60 than in young adults.
• Monitor pulse and blood pressure.
• Know that thyroid hormones alter thyroid function test results.

### ☑ PATIENT TEACHING

• Make sure patient understands the importance of compliance. Tell patient to take thyroid hormones at the same time each day, preferably before breakfast, to maintain constant hormone levels. Suggest morning dosage to prevent insomnia.
• Warn patient (especially elderly patient) to tell the doctor at once if chest pain, palpitations, sweating, nervousness, or other signs of overdose or aggravated CV disease occur.
• The two commercially prepared liotrix drugs contain different amounts of each ingredient; tell patient not to change from one brand to the other.
• Tell patient to report unusual bleeding and bruising.

---

## thyroid

Armour Thyroid, S-P-T, Thyrar, Thyroid Strong, Thyroid USP Enseals, Thyro-Teric, Westhroid

*Pregnancy Risk Category: A*

### HOW SUPPLIED

*Tablets:* 15 mg, 30 mg, 60 mg, 65 mg, 90 mg, 120 mg, 130 mg, 180 mg, 240 mg, 300 mg
*Tablets (bovine origin):* 30 mg, 60 mg, 120 mg
*Tablets (pork origin):* 15 mg, 30 mg, 60 mg, 120 mg, 200 mg, 250 mg, 300 mg

---

Reactions may be *common,* uncommon, **life-threatening,** or **COMMON AND LIFE-THREATENING.**

*Tablets (enteric-coated):* 60 mg, 120 mg

*Strong tablets (50% stronger than thyroid USP, and containing 0.3% iodine):* 32.5 mg, 65 mg, 130 mg, 200 mg

*Capsules (porcine origin):* 60 mg, 120 mg, 180 mg, 300 mg

## ACTION
Not clearly defined. Stimulates metabolism of all body tissues by accelerating the rate of cellular oxidation.

## ONSET, PEAK, DURATION
Unknown.

## INDICATIONS & DOSAGE
*Mild hypothyroidism—*
**Adults:** initially, 60 mg P.O. daily, increased by 60 mg q 30 days until desired response occurs. Usual maintenance dosage is 60 to 180 mg daily as a single dose.
*Severe hypothyroidism—*
**Adults:** initially, 15 mg P.O. daily, increased by 30 mg daily after 2 weeks, and 2 weeks later increased to 60 mg daily. After 2 months, dosage increased to 120 mg daily, as needed, for 2 months. Then increased to 180 mg daily as needed.
*Congenital or severe hypothyroidism in children—*
**Children:** same as adults with severe hypothyroidism.

## ADVERSE REACTIONS
**CNS:** *nervousness, insomnia,* tremor, headache.
**CV:** *tachycardia,* **arrhythmias,** angina pectoris, **cardiac decompensation and collapse.**
**GI:** diarrhea, vomiting.
**Other:** weight loss, heat intolerance, diaphoresis, accelerated rate of bone maturation in infants and children, menstrual irregularities, allergic skin reactions.

## INTERACTIONS
*Cholestyramine:* impaired thyroid absorption. Separate doses by 4 to 5 hours.
*Insulin, oral antidiabetic agents:* altered serum glucose levels. Monitor blood glucose levels. Dosage adjustments may be necessary.
*Oral anticoagulants:* altered PT. Monitor PT. Dosage adjustments may be necessary.
*Sympathomimetics, such as epinephrine:* increased risk of coronary insufficiency. Monitor closely.

## CONTRAINDICATIONS
Contraindicated in patients with hypersensitivity to drug, acute MI uncomplicated by hypothyroidism, untreated thyrotoxicosis, or uncorrected adrenal insufficiency.

## NURSING CONSIDERATIONS
• Use with extreme caution in elderly patients and those with angina pectoris, hypertension, other CV disorders, renal insufficiency, or ischemia.
• Use cautiously in patients with myxedema or diabetes mellitus or insipidus.
• In patients with coronary artery disease who must receive thyroid hormones, observe carefully for possible coronary insufficiency.
• Know that thyroid hormone replacement requirements are about 25% lower in patients over age 60 than in young adults.
• Monitor pulse and blood pressure.
• **Alert:** Know that in children, sleeping pulse rate and basal morning temperature are guides to treatment.
• Know that thyroid hormones alter thyroid function test results.

## ☑ PATIENT TEACHING
• Tell patient to take thyroid hormones at the same time each day, preferably before breakfast, to maintain constant hormone levels. Suggest morning dosage to prevent insomnia.

---

*Liquid form contains alcohol.   **May contain tartrazine.   †Canada only.   ‡Australia only.   ◇OTC.

• Advise patient who has achieved stable response not to change brands.
• Warn patient (especially elderly patient) to tell the doctor at once if chest pain, palpitations, sweating, nervousness, or other signs of overdose or aggravated CV disease occur.
• Tell patient to report unusual bleeding and bruising.

# thyrotropin (thyroid-stimulating hormone, or TSH)
Thytropar

*Pregnancy Risk Category: C*

## HOW SUPPLIED
*Powder for injection:* 10 IU-vial

## ACTION
Stimulates uptake of radioactive iodine ($^{131}$I) in patients with thyroid cancer and promotes thyroid hormone production by the anterior pituitary gland.

## ONSET, PEAK, DURATION
Onset occurs in minutes. Hypertrophy and hyperplasia of the thyroid gland occur within 24 hours. Effects rapidly reverse after withdrawal.

## INDICATIONS & DOSAGE
*Diagnosis of thyroid cancer remnant with $^{131}$I after surgery –*
**Adults:** 10 IU I.M. or S.C. for 3 to 7 days.
*Differential diagnosis of primary and secondary hypothyroidism –*
**Adults:** 10 IU I.M. or S.C. for 1 to 3 days.
*In protein-bound iodine or $^{131}$I uptake determinations for differential diagnosis of subclinical hypothyroidism or low thyroid reserve –*
**Adults:** 10 IU I.M. or S.C.
*Therapy for thyroid cancer (local or metastatic) with $^{131}$I –*
**Adults:** 10 IU I.M. or S.C. for 3 to 8 days.

*To determine thyroid status of patient receiving thyroid hormone –*
**Adults:** 10 units I.M. or S.C. for 1 to 3 days.

## ADVERSE REACTIONS
**CNS:** headache.
**CV:** *tachycardia,* hypotension.
**GI:** nausea, vomiting.
**Other:** thyroid hyperplasia (with large doses), hypersensitivity reactions (postinjection flare, urticaria, *anaphylaxis*).

## INTERACTIONS
*Insulin, oral antidiabetic agents:* altered serum glucose levels. Monitor blood glucose levels. Dosage adjustments may be necessary.
*Oral anticoagulants:* altered PT. Monitor PT. Dosage adjustments may be necessary.
*Sympathomimetics such as epinephrine:* increased risk of coronary insufficiency. Monitor closely.

## CONTRAINDICATIONS
Contraindicated in patients with hypersensitivity to the drug, coronary thrombosis, or untreated Addison's disease.

## NURSING CONSIDERATIONS
• Use cautiously in patients with angina pectoris, CHF, hypopituitarism, and adrenocortical suppression.
• Know that 3-day dosage schedule may be used in long-standing pituitary myxedema or with prolonged use of thyroid medication.

## ☑ PATIENT TEACHING
• Explain to patient how drug is used as diagnostic agent, if indicated.
• Instruct patient to report adverse reactions promptly.

---

Reactions may be *common,* uncommon, *life-threatening,* or COMMON AND LIFE-THREATENING.

methimazole
potassium iodide
potassium iodide, saturated
    solution
strong iodine solution
propylthiouracil
radioactive iodine (sodium
    iodide) $^{131}$I

## COMBINATION PRODUCTS
None.

## methimazole
Tapazole

*Pregnancy Risk Category: D*

### HOW SUPPLIED
*Tablets:* 5 mg, 10 mg

### ACTION
Inhibits oxidation of iodine in thyroid gland, blocking iodine's ability to combine with tyrosine to form thyroxine. Also may prevent coupling of monoiodotyrosine and diiodotyrosine to form thyroxine and triiodothyronine.

### ONSET, PEAK, DURATION
Onset occurs within 5 days. Plasma levels peak in ½ to 1 hour. Duration unknown.

### INDICATIONS & DOSAGE
*Hyperthyroidism* –
**Adults:** if mild, 15 mg P.O. daily; if moderately severe, 30 to 45 mg daily ; if severe, 60 mg daily. Daily dose divided into three doses at 8-hour intervals. Maintenance dosage is 5 to 15 mg daily.
**Children:** 0.4 mg/kg P.O. daily in divided doses q 8 hours. Maintenance dosage is 0.2 mg/kg daily in divided doses q 8 hours.

### ADVERSE REACTIONS
**CNS:** headache, drowsiness, vertigo, paresthesia, neuritis, neuropathies, CNS stimulation, depression.
**EENT:** loss of taste.
**GI:** diarrhea, nausea, vomiting (may be dose-related), salivary gland enlargement, epigastric distress.
**GU:** nephritis.
**Hematologic:** *agranulocytosis,* leukopenia, *thrombocytopenia, aplastic anemia.*
**Hepatic:** jaundice, hepatic dysfunction, hepatitis.
**Skin:** rash, urticaria, discoloration, pruritus, erythema nodosum, exfoliative dermatitis, lupuslike syndrome.
**Other:** arthralgia, myalgia, fever, lymphadenopathy, hypothyroidism (mental depression; cold intolerance; hard, nonpitting edema; hypoprothrombinemia and bleeding).

### INTERACTIONS
None significant.

### CONTRAINDICATIONS
Contraindicated in patients with hypersensitivity to drug and in breast-feeding patients.

### NURSING CONSIDERATIONS
● Use with extreme caution during pregnancy. Pregnant women may require less drug as pregnancy progresses. Monitor thyroid function studies closely. Thyroid may be added to regimen. Drug may be stopped during last few weeks of pregnancy.
● Monitor CBC periodically as ordered to detect impending leukopenia, thrombocytopenia, and agranulocytosis. Also monitor hepatic function.
● ***Alert:*** Dosages over 30 mg/day increase the risk of agranulocytosis.
● Watch for signs of hypothyroidism

(mental depression; cold intolerance; hard, nonpitting edema); notify doctor because dosage may need to be adjusted as necessary.

• Discontinue drug and notify doctor if severe rash or enlarged cervical lymph nodes develop.

### ☑ PATIENT TEACHING

• Tell patient to take drug with meals to reduce adverse GI reactions.
• Warn patient to report fever, sore throat, mouth sores, skin eruptions, anorexia, pruritus, right upper quadrant pain, yellow skin or sclera.
• Tell him to ask the doctor about using iodized salt and eating shellfish.
• Warn patient against OTC cough medicines; many contain iodine.
• Instruct patient to store drug in light-resistant container.

---

## potassium iodide
Iostat, Pima, Thyro-Block

## potassium iodide, saturated solution (SSKI)

## strong iodine solution (Lugol's solution)
*Pregnancy Risk Category: D*

### HOW SUPPLIED
**potassium iodide**
*Tablets:* 130 mg
*Tablets (enteric-coated):* 300 mg
*Oral solution:* 500 mg/15 ml
*Syrup:* 325 mg/5 ml
**potassium iodide, saturated solution**
*Oral solution:* 1 g/ml
**strong iodine solution**
*Oral solution:* iodine 50 mg/ml and potassium iodide 100 mg/ml

### ACTION
Inhibits thyroid hormone formation, limits iodide transport into the thyroid gland, and blocks thyroid hormone release.

### ONSET, PEAK, DURATION
Onset occurs within 24 hours. Peak occurs in 10 to 15 days. Duration unknown.

### INDICATIONS & DOSAGE
*Preparation for thyroidectomy –*
**Adults and children:** strong iodine solution (USP), 0.1 to 0.3 ml P.O. t.i.d., or potassium iodide, saturated solution (SSKI), 1 to 5 drops in water P.O. t.i.d. after meals for 10 to 14 days before surgery.
*Thyrotoxic crisis –*
**Adults and children:** 500 mg P.O. q 4 hours (about 10 drops of SSKI).
*Radiation protectant for thyroid gland –*
**Adults and children 1 year and over:** 130 mg P.O. daily for 10 days after radiation exposure.
**Children up to 1 year:** 65 mg P.O. daily for 10 days after exposure.

### ADVERSE REACTIONS
**EENT:** inflammation of salivary glands, periorbital edema.
**GI:** diarrhea, burning mouth and throat, sore teeth and gums, *metallic taste.*
**Skin:** acneiform rash.
**Other:** fever; *hypersensitivity reactions.*

### INTERACTIONS
*ACE inhibitors, potassium-sparing diuretics:* risk of hyperkalemia. Avoid concomitant use.
*Antithyroid medications:* potassium iodide may potentiate hypothyroid or goitrogenic effects. Monitor closely.
*Lithium carbonate:* hypothyroidism may occur. Use with caution.

### CONTRAINDICATIONS
Contraindicated in patients with tuberculosis, acute bronchitis, iodide hypersensitivity, or hyperkalemia. Some formulations contain sulfites, which may precipitate allergic reactions in hypersensitive individuals.

---

Reactions may be *common,* uncommon, *life-threatening,* or **COMMON AND LIFE-THREATENING.**

## NURSING CONSIDERATIONS

• Use cautiously in patients with hypocomplementemic vasculitis, goiter, or autoimmune thyroid disease.
• Know that drug is usually given with other antithyroid drugs.
• Know that doctor may avoid prescribing enteric-coated tablets, which have been associated with small-bowel lesions and can lead to serious complications, including perforation, hemorrhage, or obstruction.
• Dilute oral solutions in water, milk, or fruit juice, and give after meals to prevent gastric irritation, to hydrate the patient, and to mask salty taste.
• Give iodides through straw to avoid tooth discoloration.
• *Alert:* Know that earliest signs of delayed hypersensitivity reactions caused by iodides are irritation and swollen eyelids.
• Store in light-resistant container.

☑ **PATIENT TEACHING**
• Instruct patient how to mask salty taste of oral solution. Tell him to take all forms of the drug after meals.
• Warn patient that sudden withdrawal may precipitate thyroid crisis.
• Tell him to ask the doctor about using iodized salt and eating shellfish.

---

## propylthiouracil (PTU)
Propyl-Thyracil†

*Pregnancy Risk Category: D*

### HOW SUPPLIED
*Tablets:* 50 mg, 100 mg†

### ACTION
Inhibits oxidation of iodine in thyroid gland, blocking iodine's ability to combine with tyrosine to form thyroxine, and may prevent coupling of monoiodotyrosine and diiodotyrosine to form thyroxine and triiodothyronine.

### ONSET, PEAK, DURATION
Onset and duration unknown. Plasma levels peak 1 to 1½ hours after oral administration.

### INDICATIONS & DOSAGE
*Hyperthyroidism –*
**Adults:** 100 to 150 mg P.O. t.i.d.; up to 1,200 mg daily have been used in severe cases. Maintenance dosage is 100 to 150 mg once daily in divided doses t.i.d.
**Children over 10 years:** 150 to 300 mg P.O. daily in divided doses t.i.d. Maintenance dosage determined by patient response.
**Children 6 to 10 years:** 50 to 150 mg P.O. daily in divided doses t.i.d. Maintenance dosage determined by patient's response.
*Preparation for thyroidectomy –*
**Adults:** 200 mg q 4 to 6 hours on first day; once full control of symptoms is achieved, dosage is gradually reduced to usual maintenance levels.
*Thyrotoxic crisis –*
**Adults and children:** 200 mg P.O. q 4 to 6 hours on first day; once full control of symptoms is achieved, dosage is gradually reduced to usual maintenance levels.

### ADVERSE REACTIONS
**CNS:** headache, drowsiness, vertigo, paresthesia, neuritis, neuropathies, CNS stimulation, depression.
**CV:** vasculitis.
**EENT:** visual disturbances.
**GI:** diarrhea, *nausea, vomiting* (may be dose-related), epigastric distress, salivary gland enlargement, loss of taste.
**GU:** nephritis.
**Hematologic:** *agranulocytosis,* leukopenia, *thrombocytopenia, aplastic anemia.*
**Hepatic:** jaundice, *hepatotoxicity.*
**Skin:** rash, urticaria, skin discoloration, pruritus, erythema nodosum, exfoliative dermatitis, lupuslike syndrome.

---

**Other:** arthralgia, myalgia, fever, lymphadenopathy; dose-related hypothyroidism (mental depression; hypoprothrombinemia and bleeding; cold intolerance; hard, nonpitting edema).

### INTERACTIONS
*Anticoagulants:* anticoagulant effects may be increased. Monitor PT.

### CONTRAINDICATIONS
Contraindicated in patients with hypersensitivity to drug and in breast-feeding patients.

### NURSING CONSIDERATIONS
● Use cautiously in pregnant patients. Pregnant women may require less drug as pregnancy progresses. Monitor thyroid function studies closely. Thyroid may be added to regimen. Drug may be stopped during last few weeks of pregnancy.
● Give drug with meals to reduce adverse GI reactions.
● Watch for signs of hypothyroidism (mental depression; cold intolerance; hard, nonpitting edema); adjust dosage as ordered.
● Monitor CBC periodically to detect impending leukopenia, thrombocytopenia, and agranulocytosis.
● *Alert:* Discontinue drug and notify doctor if severe rash or enlarged cervical lymph nodes develop.
● Store drug in light-resistant container.

### ☑ PATIENT TEACHING
● Instruct patient to take drug with meals.
● Warn patient to report fever, sore throat, mouth sores, and skin eruptions.
● Tell him to ask the doctor about using iodized salt and eating shellfish.
● Warn patient against OTC cough medicines; many contain iodine.

## radioactive iodine (sodium iodide) $^{131}$I
Iodotope Therapeutic, Sodium Iodide $^{131}$I Therapeutic

*Pregnancy Risk Category: X*

### HOW SUPPLIED
All radioactivity concentrations are determined at the time of calibration.
**Iodotope Therapeutic**
*Capsules:* radioactivity range is 1 to 50 millicuries (mCi)/capsule at time of calibration
*Oral solution:* radioactivity concentration is 7.05 mCi/ml at time of calibration; in vials containing approximately 7, 14, 28, 70, or 106 mCi at time of calibration
**Sodium Iodide $^{131}$I Therapeutic**
*Capsules:* radioactivity range is 0.8 to 100 mCi/capsule at the time of calibration
*Oral solution:* radioactivity range is 3.5 to 150 mCi/vial at the time of calibration

### ACTION
Limits thyroid hormone secretion by destroying thyroid tissue. The affinity of thyroid tissue for radioactive iodine facilitates uptake of drug by cancerous thyroid tissue that has metastasized to other sites in the body.

### ONSET, PEAK, DURATION
Onset occurs in 2 to 4 weeks. Peak effect occurs in 2 to 4 months. Duration unknown.

### INDICATIONS & DOSAGE
*Hyperthyroidism –*
**Adults:** usual dosage is 4 to 10 mCi P.O. Dosage is based on estimated weight of thyroid gland and thyroid uptake. Treatment repeated after 6 weeks, based on serum thyroxine level.
*Thyroid cancer –*
**Adults:** 50 to 150 mCi P.O. Dosage is based on estimated malignant thyroid tissue and metastatic tissue as deter-

---

Reactions may be *common,* uncommon, *life-threatening,* or COMMON AND LIFE-THREATENING.

mined by total body scan. Treatment repeated according to clinical status.

## ADVERSE REACTIONS
**CV:** chest pain, tachycardia.
**EENT:** *fullness in neck,* pain on swallowing, sore throat, cough.
**Hematologic:** anemia; blood dyscrasia; leukopenia; ***thrombocytopenia;*** possible increased risk of **leukemia** later (after sufficient [131]I dose for thyroid ablation following cancer surgery).
**Skin:** rash, pruritus, urticaria.
**Other:** hypothyroidism; radiation-induced thyroiditis; radiation sickness (nausea, vomiting); ***death;*** temporary thinning of hair; allergic type reactions; possible increased risk of birth defects in offspring after sufficient [131]I dose for thyroid ablation after cancer surgery.

## INTERACTIONS
*Lithium carbonate:* hypothyroidism may occur. Use with caution.

The following drugs can interfere with the action of [131]I and should be withheld the specified time before administering the [131]I dose:
*Adrenocorticoids:* 1 week.
*Benzodiazepines:* 1 month.
*Cholecystographic agents:* 6 to 9 months.
*Contrast media containing iodine:* 1 to 2 months.
*Iodine-containing products, including vitamins, expectorants, antitussives, and topical agents:* 2 weeks.
*Salicylates:* 1 to 2 weeks.

## CONTRAINDICATIONS
Contraindicated in pregnant patients except to treat thyroid cancer and in breast-feeding patients.

## NURSING CONSIDERATIONS
• Know that all antithyroid medications and thyroid preparations need to be stopped 1 week before [131]I dose. If medications are not stopped, patients may receive thyroid-stimulating hormone for 3 days before [131]I dose. When treating women of childbearing age, give dose during menstruation or within 7 days after menstruation.
• Know that after therapy for hyperthyroidism, patients should not resume antithyroid drugs, but should continue propranolol or other drugs used to treat symptoms of hyperthyroidism until onset of full [131]I effect occurs (usually 6 weeks).
• Monitor thyroid function via serum thyroxine levels, as ordered.
• Institute full radiation precautions. Have patient use disposal methods when coughing and expectorating. After dose for hyperthyroidism, patient's urine and saliva are slightly radioactive for 24 hours; vomitus is highly radioactive for 6 to 8 hours.
• After dose for thyroid cancer, patient's urine, saliva, and perspiration are radioactive for 3 days. Isolate patient and observe these precautions: Do not allow pregnant personnel to care for patient; use disposable eating utensils and linens; instruct patient to save urine in lead container for 24 to 48 hours so that amount of radioactive material can be determined. Limit contact with patient to 30 minutes per shift per person the first day, and increase time, as necessary, to 1 hour second day and longer on third day.

## ☑ PATIENT TEACHING
• Tell patient to fast overnight before administration and to drink as much fluid as possible for 48 hours after administration.
• Instruct patient on radiation precautions to use after drug administration.
• Warn patient who is discharged less than 7 days after [131]I dose for thyroid cancer to avoid close contact with small children and not to sleep in the same room with spouse for 7 days after treatment.

---

corticotropin
repository corticotropin
cosyntropin
desmopressin acetate
leuprolide acetate
(See Chapter 72, ANTINEOPLASTICS THAT
ALTER HORMONE BALANCE.)
lypressin
sermorelin acetate
somatrem
somatropin
vasopressin

**COMBINATION PRODUCTS**
None.

---

## corticotropin (adrenocorticotropic hormone, ACTH)
ACTH, Acthar

### repository corticotropin
Acthar Gel (H.P.)†, ACTH Gel,
H.P. Acthar Gel

*Pregnancy Risk Category: C*

### HOW SUPPLIED
*Aqueous injection:* 25 unit-vial, 40
units/vial
*Repository injection:* 40 units/ml, 80
units/ml

### ACTION
By replacing the body's own tropic
hormone, stimulates the adrenal cortex to secrete its entire spectrum of
hormones.

### ONSET, PEAK, DURATION
Variable.

### INDICATIONS & DOSAGE
*Diagnostic test of adrenocortical func-
tion –*
**Adults:** up to 80 units repository form

I.M. or S.C. in divided doses or as a
single dose; or 10 to 25 units aqueous
form in 500 ml of D₅W I.V. over 8
hours, between blood samplings.

Individual dosages generally vary
with adrenal glands' sensitivity to
stimulation as well as with specific
disease. Infants and younger children
require larger doses per kilogram than
do older children and adults.
*For therapeutic use –*
**Adults:** 40 units aqueous form S.C.
or I.M. in four divided doses; or 40 to
80 units q 24 to 72 hours (repository
form).

### ADVERSE REACTIONS
**CNS:** *seizures, dizziness,* vertigo, increased intracranial pressure with
papilledema, pseudotumor cerebri.
**CV:** hypertension, CHF, necrotizing
angiitis, *shock.*
**EENT:** cataracts, glaucoma.
**GI:** peptic ulceration with perforation
and hemorrhage, pancreatitis, abdominal distention, ulcerative esophagitis,
nausea, vomiting.
**Skin:** impaired wound healing, thin
fragile skin, petechiae, ecchymoses,
facial erythema, diaphoresis, acne,
hyperpigmentation, allergic reactions,
hirsutism.
**Other:** muscle weakness, steroid myopathy, loss of muscle mass, osteoporosis, vertebral compression fractures, pneumonia, abscess and septic
infection, cushingoid symptoms, suppression of growth in children, activation of latent diabetes mellitus, progressive increase in antibodies, loss of
corticotropin stimulatory effect, hypersensitivity reactions (rash, *bronchospasm*), *sodium and fluid retention,* calcium and potassium loss, hypokalemic alkalosis, negative nitrogen balance, menstrual irregularities.

---

Reactions may be *common,* uncommon, *life-threatening,* or **COMMON AND LIFE-THREATENING.**

## INTERACTIONS

*Anticonvulsants, barbiturates, rifampin:* increased metabolism of corticotropin and decreased effectiveness. Monitor for lack of effect.

*Antidiabetic agents:* may increase requirments of antidiabetic agents due to intrinsic hyperglycemic activity of corticotropin. Monitor blood glucose levels closely.

*Estrogens:* may potentiate the effects of cortisol. Dosage adjustments may be necessary.

*NSAIDs, salicylates:* increased risk of GI bleeding. Avoid concomitant use.

*Oral anticoagulants:* altered PT. Monitor PT. Dosage adjustments may be necessary.

*Potassium-wasting diuretics, amphotericin B:* increased risk of hypokalemia. Monitor serum potassium levels.

## CONTRAINDICATIONS

Contraindicated in patients with peptic ulcer, scleroderma, osteoporosis, systemic fungal infections, ocular herpes simplex, peptic ulceration, CHF, hypertension, sensitivity to pork and pork products, adrenocortical hyperfunction or primary insufficiency, or Cushing's syndrome. Also contraindicated in those who have had recent surgery.

## NURSING CONSIDERATIONS

• Use cautiously in pregnant patients and in women of childbearing age. Also use cautiously in patients being immunized and in those patients with latent tuberculosis or tuberculin reactivity, hypothyroidism, cirrhosis, acute gouty arthritis, psychotic tendencies, renal insufficiency, diverticulitis, nonspecific ulcerative colitis, thromboembolic disorders, seizures, uncontrolled hypertension, or myasthenia gravis.

• Know that corticotropin treatment should be preceded by verification of adrenal responsiveness and test for hypersensitivity and allergic reactions.

• Be aware that corticotropin should be adjunctive, not sole, therapy. Oral agents are preferred for long-term therapy.

• **I.V. use:** Use only the aqueous form for I.V. administration. Dilute in 500 ml of $D_5W$ and infuse over 8 hours.

• If administering gel, warm it to room temperature, draw into large needle, and give slowly as deep I.M. injection with 21G or 22G needle.

• Refrigerate reconstituted solution and use within 24 hours.

• Know that corticotropin may mask signs of chronic disease and decrease host resistance and ability to localize infection.

• Note and record weight changes, fluid exchange, and resting blood pressures until minimal effective dosage is achieved.

• Watch neonates of corticotropin-treated mothers for signs of hypoadrenalism.

• Unusual stress may require additional use of rapidly acting corticosteroids. When possible, gradually reduce corticotropin dosage to smallest effective dose as ordered to minimize induced adrenocortical insufficiency. Know that therapy can be reinstituted if stressful situation (trauma, surgery, severe illness) occurs shortly after stopping drug.

## ☑ PATIENT TEACHING

• Warn patient that injection is painful.

• Stress importance of informing all members of health care team about therapeutic use of drug because unusual stress may require additional use of rapidly acting corticosteroids.

• Instruct patient how to handle troublesome adverse reactions, such as limiting sodium intake to reduce severity of edema and increasing protein intake to combat nitrogen loss.

---

*Liquid form contains alcohol.  **May contain tartrazine.  †Canada only.  ‡Australia only.  ◇OTC.

• Advise patient about need for close follow up care.

# cosyntropin
Cortrosyn

*Pregnancy Risk Category: C*

## HOW SUPPLIED
*Injection:* 0.25 mg-vial

## ACTION
By replacing the body's own tropic hormone, stimulates the adrenal cortex to secrete its entire spectrum of hormones.

## ONSET, PEAK, DURATION
Onset occurs within 5 minutes of I.V. use. Peak cortisol levels occur within 1 hour of I.M. or I.V. use. Duration unknown.

## INDICATIONS & DOSAGE
*Diagnostic test of adrenocortical function –*
**Adults and children 2 years and over:** 0.25 to 1 mg I.M. or I.V. (unless label prohibits I.V. administration) between blood samplings.
**Children under 2 years:** 0.125 mg I.M. or I.V.

## ADVERSE REACTIONS
**CNS:** *seizures,* dizziness, vertigo, increased intracranial pressure with papilledema, pseudotumor cerebri.
**EENT:** cataracts, glaucoma.
**GI:** peptic ulceration, pancreatitis, abdominal distension, ulcerative esophagitis, nausea, vomiting.
**Skin:** pruritus; impaired wound healing; thin, fragile skin; petechiae; ecchymoses; facial erythema; diaphoresis; acne; hyperpigmentation; hirsutism.
**Other:** flushing, hypersensitivity reactions, muscle weakness, steroid myopathy, loss of muscle mass, osteoporosis, vertebral compression, fractures, cushingoid symptoms, menstrual irregularities.

## INTERACTIONS
*Cortisone, hydrocortisone:* may interfere with test results of cortisol levels if administered on test day.
*Spironolactone:* may interfere with fluorometric analysis of cortisol levels. Avoid concomitant use.

## CONTRAINDICATIONS
Contraindicated in patients with hypersensitivity to drug.

## NURSING CONSIDERATIONS
• Use cautiously in patients hypersensitive to natural corticotropin.
• **I.V. use:** Reconstitute with 1 ml of supplied diluent. For direct injection, administer over at least 2 minutes. May be further diluted with D₅W or 0.9% sodium chloride and infused over 6 hours. Solution is stable for 12 hours at room temperature.
• Know that drug is synthetic duplication of the biologically active part of the corticotropin molecule. It is less likely to produce sensitivity than natural corticotropin derived from animal sources.
• Monitor patients for allergic reactions, rashes, dyspnea, wheezing, or evidence of anaphylaxis.

## ☑ PATIENT TEACHING
• Explain test procedure to patient.
• Tell patient to report adverse reactions immediately.

# desmopressin acetate
DDAVP, Minirin‡, Stimate

*Pregnancy Risk Category: B*

## HOW SUPPLIED
*Nasal solution:* 0.1 mg/ml
*Injection:* 4 mcg/ml

---

## ACTION

Increases the permeability of the renal tubular epithelium to adenosine monophosphate and water; the epithelium promotes reabsorption of water and produces a concentrated urine (ADH effect). Desmopressin also increases factor VIII activity by releasing endogenous factor VIII from plasma storage sites.

## ONSET, PEAK, DURATION

Onset occurs within 1 hour for antidiuretic action, within 15 to 30 minutes for antihemorrhagic action. Peak antidiuretic effects occur within 1 to 5 hours, peak antihemorrhagic action in 1½ to 2 hours. Antidiuretic effects persist for 8 to 12 hours, antihemorrhagic effects for 4 to 12 hours.

## INDICATIONS & DOSAGE

*Nonnephrogenic diabetes insipidus, temporary polyuria and polydipsia associated with pituitary trauma –*
**Adults:** 0.1 to 0.4 ml intranasally daily in one to three doses. Morning and evening doses adjusted separately for adequate diurnal rhythm of water turnover. Alternatively, injectable form administered in dosage of 0.5 to 1 ml I.V. or S.C. daily, usually in two divided doses.
**Children 3 months to 12 years:** 0.05 to 0.3 ml intranasally daily in one or two doses.
*Hemophilia A and von Willebrand's disease –*
**Adults and children:** 0.3 mcg/kg diluted in 0.9% sodium chloride and infused I.V. over 15 to 30 minutes. Dose repeated if necessary as indicated by laboratory response and the patient's clinical condition.
*Primary nocturnal enuresis –*
**Children 6 years and over:** initially, 20 mcg intranasally h.s. Dosage adjusted according to response. Maximum recommended dosage is 40 mcg daily.

## ADVERSE REACTIONS

**CNS:** headache.
**CV:** slight rise in blood pressure at high dosage.
**EENT:** rhinitis, epistaxis, sore throat, cough.
**GI:** nausea, abdominal cramps.
**GU:** vulval pain.
**Other:** flushing, local erythema, swelling or burning after injection.

## INTERACTIONS

*Clofibrate:* enhanced and prolonged effects of desmopressin. Monitor carefully.
*Demeclocycline, epinephrine, ethanol, heparin, lithium:* increased risk of adverse effects. Monitor closely.

## CONTRAINDICATIONS

Contraindicated in patients hypersensitive to the drug, and in patients with Type IIB von Willebrand's disease.

## NURSING CONSIDERATIONS

• Use cautiously in patients with coronary artery insufficiency or hypertensive CV disease or in patients with conditions associated with fluid and electrolyte imbalances, such as cystic fibrosis, because these patients are prone to hyponatremia.
• Know that desmopressin injection should not be used to treat hemophilia A with factor VIII levels of 0% to 5% or severe cases of von Willebrand's disease.
• Intranasal use can cause changes in the nasal mucosa resulting in erratic, unreliable absorption. Report a worsening condition to the doctor, who may prescribe injectable DDAVP.
• Adjust fluid intake to reduce risk of water intoxication and sodium depletion, especially in children or elderly patients.
• *Alert:* Overdose may cause oxytocic or vasopressor activity. Withhold drug and notify doctor. Use furosemide if

fluid retention is excessive, as ordered.

### ☑ PATIENT TEACHING
• Instruct patient to clear nasal passages before administering drug.
• Some patients may have difficulty measuring and inhaling drug into nostrils. Teach patient and caregivers correct method of administration.
• Nasal congestion, allergic rhinitis, or upper respiratory infections may impair drug absorption. Advise patient to report such conditions to the doctor; they may require a dosage adjustment.
• Teach patient using S.C. desmopressin to rotate injection sites to prevent tissue damage.
• Warn patient to drink only enough water to satisfy thirst.
• Inform patient that, when treating hemophilia A and von Willebrand's disease, taking desmopressin may avoid the hazards of using blood products.
• Advise patient to wear medical identification indicating his use of this drug.

---

## lypressin
Diapid

*Pregnancy Risk Category: B*

### HOW SUPPLIED
*Nasal spray:* 0.185 mg/ml

### ACTION
Increases the permeability of the renal tubular epithelium to adenosine monophosphate and water; the epithelium promotes reabsorption of water and produces a concentrated urine (ADH effect).

### ONSET, PEAK, DURATION
Onset occurs within 1 hour. Serum levels peak in 30 to 120 minutes. Effects persist for 3 to 4 hours.

### INDICATIONS & DOSAGE
*Nonnephrogenic diabetes insipidus* –
**Adults and children:** one or two sprays (approximately 2 USP posterior pituitary pressor units/spray) in either or both nostrils q.i.d. and an additional dose h.s., if needed, to prevent nocturia. If usual dosage is inadequate, frequency should be increased rather than number of sprays.

### ADVERSE REACTIONS
**CNS:** headache.
**EENT:** nasal congestion or ulceration, irritation or pruritus of nasal passages, periorbital edema with itching, rhinorrhea, conjunctivitis.
**GI:** heartburn caused by drip of excessive spray into pharynx, abdominal cramps, frequent bowel movements.
**GU:** possible transient fluid retention from overdose.
**Other:** hypersensitivity reaction.

### INTERACTIONS
None significant.

### CONTRAINDICATIONS
Contraindicated in patients hypersensitive to the drug.

### NURSING CONSIDERATIONS
• Use cautiously in patients with coronary artery disease, hypertension, allergic rhinitis, or upper airway infection.
• Test patients sensitive to ADH for sensitivity to lypressin as ordered.
• Know that drug is particularly useful when diabetes insipidus is unresponsive to other therapy or when ADH of animal origin causes adverse reactions.
• To administer a uniform, well-diffused spray, hold bottle upright with patient in vertical position holding head upright.
• Know that nasal congestion, allergic rhinitis, or upper respiratory infections may diminish drug absorp-

---

tion and require larger dose or adjunctive therapy.

## ☑ PATIENT TEACHING
• Ensure that patient understands drug is for topical application to the nasal mucosa and should not be inhaled.
• Instruct patient to clear nasal passage before administering drug.
• Warn patient that inadvertent inhalation of spray may cause tightness in chest, coughing, and transient dyspnea.
• Instruct patient to wear medical identification indicating his condition.

---

## sermorelin acetate
Geref

*Pregnancy Risk Category: C*

### HOW SUPPLIED
*Powder for injection:* 50 mcg-ampule

### ACTION
A synthetic polypeptide that mimics the aminoterminal segment of the naturally occurring human growth hormone (GH).

### ONSET, PEAK, DURATION
Onset and duration unknown. Peak levels of GH occur in about 30 minutes after injection in children; 35 minutes after injection in adults.

### INDICATIONS & DOSAGE
*Diagnostic aid to determine the pituitary gland's ability to secrete GH –*
**Adults and children:** 1 mcg/kg as a single I.V. injection.

### ADVERSE REACTIONS
**CNS:** headache.
**EENT:** unusual taste in mouth.
**GI:** nausea, vomiting.
**Skin:** pain, redness, or swelling at injection site.
**Other:** transient warmth or flushing

of face, antibody formation, paleness, tightness in chest.

### INTERACTIONS
*Anticholinergics, antithyroid medications (such as propylthiouracil):* decreased response to sermorelin. Avoid concomitant use.
*Clonidine, insulin-induced hypoglycemia, levodopa:* may elevate somatotropin levels.
*Corticosteroids, cyclooxygenase inhibitors (for example, acetaminophen, aspirin, or NSAIDs), insulin:* altered pituitary gland secretion of somatotropin. Don't perform the test in patients receiving these drugs.

### CONTRAINDICATIONS
Contraindicated in patients with hypersensitivity to the drug or any components of the formulation.

### NURSING CONSIDERATIONS
• Know that GH therapy should be discontinued 1 week before the test.
• Know that response to drug may be blunted in hypothyroid patients.
• Be aware although hypersensitivity reactions have been reported with administration of other polypeptide hormones, none have been reported with sermorelin. About 25% of patients develop antibody formation with prolonged use; however, no symptomatic allergic reactions have been reported.
• Be aware that baseline GH levels generally are low ( less than 4 ng/ml). Provocative tests, such as sermorelin, are useful in determining that the pituitary somatotroph can respond. However, a normal response doesn't rule out GH deficiency if the deficit is caused by hypothalamic dysfunction. This test is most easily interpreted if patients have had a subnormal response to conventional provocative testing (such as clonidine, levodopa, or arginine) and a normal response to sermorelin, thus suggesting that the cause of GH deficiency is hypotha-

---

*Liquid form contains alcohol.   **May contain tartrazine.   †Canada only.   ‡Australia only.   ◇OTC.

lamic dysfunction. Abnormal results from both conventional tests and sermorelin can't pinpoint the location of the dysfunction.

• Draw venous blood samples for GH determinations 15 minutes before and immediately before injection. Administer bolus injection (1 mcg/kg I.V.) and follow with 3 ml of 0.9% sodium chloride injection flush. Venous samples for GH determinations should be drawn at 15-minute intervals after injection (15 minutes, 30 minutes, 45 minutes, and 60 minutes).

• **I.V. use:** Reconstitute each ampule with a minimum of 0.5 ml of the supplied diluent. One ampule contains 50 mcg of drug, which is sufficient to test a 110-lb (50-kg) patient. Larger patients require the use of multiple ampules.

### ☑ PATIENT TEACHING

• Make sure patient understands that the test must be performed in the morning after an overnight fast. He shouldn't take anything by mouth after midnight.

• Instruct patient to report adverse reactions immediately.

---

## somatrem
Protropin

*Pregnancy Risk Category: C*

### HOW SUPPLIED
*Injectable lyophilized powder:* 5-mg (about 15-IU) vial, 10-mg (about 30-IU) vial

### ACTION
Purified growth hormone (GH) of recombinant DNA origin that stimulates linear, skeletal muscle, and organ growth.

### ONSET, PEAK, DURATION
Onset. Peak levels occur in about 7.5 hours. Effects persist for 12 to 48 hours.

### INDICATIONS & DOSAGE
*Long-term treatment of children who have growth failure because of lack of adequate endogenous GH secretion* –
**Children (prepuberty):** highly individualized; up to 0.1 mg/kg I.M. or S.C. three times weekly.

### ADVERSE REACTIONS
**Other:** hypothyroidism, hyperglycemia, *antibodies to GH.*

### INTERACTIONS
*Glucocorticoids:* may inhibit growth-promoting action of somatrem. Adjust glucocorticoid dosage as necessary.

### CONTRAINDICATIONS
Contraindicated in patients with epiphyseal closure, active neoplasia, or hypersensitivity to benzyl alcohol.

### NURSING CONSIDERATIONS
• Use cautiously in patients with hypothyroidism and in those whose GH deficiency is caused by an intracranial lesion.

• Be sure to check this product's expiration date.

• To prepare the solution, inject the supplied bacteriostatic water for injection into the vial containing the drug. Then swirl the vial with a gentle rotary motion until the contents are completely dissolved. *Don't shake* the vial.

• After reconstitution, vial solution should be clear. Don't inject solution if it is cloudy or contains any particles.

• If drug is administered to neonates, reconstitute immediately before use with sterile water for injection (without bacteriostat). Use the vial once; then discard.

• Store reconstituted vial in refrigerator; use within 7 days.

• *Alert:* Know that toxicity in neonates has occurred from exposure to benzyl alcohol used in the drug as a preservative.

---

Reactions may be *common,* uncommon, *life-threatening,* or COMMON AND LIFE-THREATENING.

- Know that regular checkups, including monitoring of height and of blood and radiologic studies, are necessary.
- Observe patients for signs of glucose intolerance and hyperglycemia.
- Monitor periodic thyroid function tests for hypothyroidism as ordered, which may require treatment with a thyroid hormone.

☑ **PATIENT TEACHING**
- Reassure patient and caregivers that somatrem is *pure* and *safe*. Drug replaces pituitary-derived human GH, which was removed from the market in 1985 because of its association with a rare but fatal viral infection (Jakob-Creutzfeldt disease).
- Review the signs and symptoms of hypothyroidism and hyperglycemia. Instruct patient and parents to report any such signs or symptoms promptly.

---

## somatropin
Humatrope, Nutropin

*Pregnancy Risk Category: C*

### HOW SUPPLIED
*Injection:* 2-mg (about 6-IU [Humatrope]) vial†, 5-mg (about 15-IU [Humatrope]) vial, 10-mg (about 30-IU [Nutropin]) vial

### ACTION
Purified growth hormone (GH) of recombinant DNA origin that stimulates skeletal, linear, muscle, and organ growth.

### ONSET, PEAK, DURATION
Onset and duration unknown. Plasma levels peak in about 7.5 hours.

### INDICATIONS & DOSAGE
*Long-term treatment of growth failure in children with inadequate secretion of endogenous GH –*
**Children:** up to 0.06 mg/kg body weight S.C. or I.M. three times weekly using Humatrope or 0.30 mg/kg body weight S.C. weekly in daily divided doses using Nutropin.
*Growth failure in children associated with chronic renal insufficiency up to the time of renal transplantation (Nutropin only) –*
**Children:** 0.35 mg/kg body weight S.C. weekly in daily divided doses.

### ADVERSE REACTIONS
**CNS:** headache, weakness.
**CV:** mild, transient edema.
**Hematologic:** *leukemia.*
**Metabolic:** mild hyperglycemia, hypothyroidism.
**Other:** injection site pain, localized muscle pain, antibodies to GH.

### INTERACTIONS
None significant.

### CONTRAINDICATIONS
Contraindicated in patients with closed epiphyses or an active underlying intracranial lesion. Humatrope should not be reconstituted with the supplied diluent for patients with a known sensitivity to either *m*-cresol or glycerin.

### NURSING CONSIDERATIONS
- Use cautiously in children with hypothyroidism and in those whose GH deficiency is caused by an intracranial lesion. Be aware that these children should be examined frequently for progression or recurrence of the underlying disease.
- To prepare the solution, inject the supplied diluent into the vial containing the drug by aiming the stream of the liquid against the glass wall of the vial. Then swirl the vial with a gentle rotary motion until the contents are completely dissolved. *Don't shake* the vial.
- After reconstitution, vial solution should be clear. Don't inject solution if it is cloudy or contains particles.
- Know that patients on dialysis re-

---

*Liquid form contains alcohol.   **May contain tartrazine.   †Canada only.   ‡Australia only.   ◇OTC.

quire changes in drug administration schedule as follows:

—Hemodialysis: administer prior to bedtime or 3 to 4 hours after dialysis.

—Chronic Cycling Peritoneal dialysis: administer in the morning after competion of dialysis.

—Chronic Ambulatory Peritoneal Dialysis: administer in the evening at the time of the overnight exchange.

• Store reconstituted vial in refrigerator; use within 14 days.

• If sensitivity to the diluent should occur, the vials may be reconstituted with sterile water for injection. When drug is reconstituted in this manner, use only 1 reconstituted dose per vial, refrigerate the solution if it is not used immediately after reconstitution, use the reconstituted dose within 24 hours, and discard the unused portion.

• Monitor child's height regularly. Know that regular checkups, including monitoring of blood and radiologic studies, also are necessary.

• Monitor patient's blood glucose levels regularly because GH may induce a state of insulin resistance.

• Know that excessive glucocorticoid therapy will inhibit the growth-promoting effect of somatropin. Patients with a coexisting corticotropin deficiency should have their glucocorticoid replacement dosage carefully adjusted to avoid an inhibitory effect on growth.

• Monitor periodic thyroid function tests, as ordered, for hypothyroidism, which may require treatment with a thyroid hormone.

☑ **PATIENT TEACHING**

• Inform parents that child with endocrine disorders (including GH deficiency) may develop slipped capital epiphyses more frequently. Tell them that if they notice their child is limping, they should notify the doctor.

• Stress importance of close follow-up care.

## vasopressin (ADH)
Pitressin

*Pregnancy Risk Category: C*

### HOW SUPPLIED
*Injection:* 0.5-ml and 1-ml ampules, 20 units/ml

### ACTION
Increases the permeability of the renal tubular epithelium to adenosine monophosphate and water; the epithelium promotes reabsorption of water and produces a concentrated urine (ADH effect).

### ONSET, PEAK, DURATION
Onset and peak unknown. Effects persist for 2 to 8 hours.

### INDICATIONS & DOSAGE
*Nonnephrogenic, nonpsychogenic diabetes insipidus—*
**Adults:** 5 to 10 units I.M. or S.C. b.i.d. to q.i.d., p.r.n.; or intranasally (aqueous solution used as spray or applied to cotton balls) in individualized dosages, based on response.
**Children:** 2.5 to 10 units I.M. or S.C. b.i.d. to q.i.d., p.r.n.; or intranasally (aqueous solution used as spray or applied to cotton balls) in individualized doses.
*Postoperative abdominal distention—*
**Adults:** initially, 5 units (aqueous) I.M.; then q 3 to 4 hours, increased to 10 units, if needed. Dosage reduced proportionally for children.
*To expel gas before abdominal X-ray—*
**Adults:** 5 to 15 units S.C. at 2 hours; then again at 30 minutes before X-ray.

### ADVERSE REACTIONS
**CNS:** tremor, headache, vertigo.
**CV:** angina in patients with vascular disease; vasoconstriction, *arrhythmias, cardiac arrest,* myocardial ischemia, circumoral pallor, decreased cardiac output.

---

Reactions may be *common,* uncommon, *life-threatening,* or COMMON AND LIFE-THREATENING.

**GI:** abdominal cramps, nausea, vomiting, flatulence.

**Other:** water intoxication (drowsiness, listlessness, headache, confusion, weight gain, *seizures, coma),* hypersensitivity reactions (urticaria, angioedema, *bronchoconstriction, anaphylaxis*), diaphoresis, cutaneous gangrene.

## INTERACTIONS

*Carbamazepine, chlorpropamide, clofibrate, fludrocortisone, tricyclic antidepressants:* increased antidiuretic response. Use together cautiously.

*Demeclocycline, ethanol, heparin, lithium, norepinephrine:* reduced antidiuretic activity. Use together cautiously.

## CONTRAINDICATIONS

Contraindicated in patients with chronic nephritis accompanied by nitrogen retention.

## NURSING CONSIDERATIONS

● Use cautiously in children, elderly patients, pregnant patients, preoperative and postoperative polyuric patients, and in those with seizure disorders, migraine headache, asthma, CV disease, heart failure, renal disease, goiter with cardiac complications, arteriosclerosis, or fluid overload.

● Know that synthetic desmopressin is sometimes preferred because of its longer duration of action and less frequent adverse reactions. Desmopressin also is commercially available as a nasal solution.

● May be used for transient polyuria resulting from ADH deficiency related to neurosurgery or head injury.

● *Alert:* Never inject during first stage of labor; may cause ruptured uterus.

● Know that minimum effective dosage should be used to reduce adverse reactions.

● Give with 1 to 2 glasses of water to reduce adverse reactions and to improve therapeutic response.

● Monitor specific gravity of urine and fluid intake and output to aid evaluation of drug effectiveness.

● To prevent possible seizures, coma, and death, observe patients closely for early signs of water intoxication.

● Monitor blood pressure of patients taking vasopressin twice daily. Watch for excessively elevated blood pressure or lack of response to drug, which may be indicated by hypotension. Also monitor daily weight.

● A rectal tube will facilitate gas expulsion after vasopressin injection.

## ☑ PATIENT TEACHING

● Instruct patient to rotate injection sites to prevent tissue damage.

● Tell patient to report adverse reactions promptly.

# Parathyroid-like drugs

**calcifediol**
**calcitonin (human)**
**calcitonin (salmon)**
**calcitriol**
**dihydrotachysterol**
**etidronate disodium**

## COMBINATION PRODUCTS
None.

---

## calcifediol
Calderol

*Pregnancy Risk Category: C*

### HOW SUPPLIED
*Capsules:* 20 mcg, 50 mcg

### ACTION
A vitamin D analogue that stimulates calcium absorption from the GI tract and promotes secretion of calcium from bone to blood.

### ONSET, PEAK, DURATION
Onset unknown. Peak levels occur in 4 hours. Effects persist for 15 to 20 days.

### INDICATIONS & DOSAGE
*Metabolic bone disease and hypocalcemia associated with chronic renal failure –*
**Adults:** initially, 300 to 350 mcg P.O. weekly. Dosage increased at 4-week intervals if necessary.

### ADVERSE REACTIONS
Vitamin D intoxication associated with hypercalcemia
**CNS:** headache, somnolence, weakness, irritability, psychosis (rare).
**CV:** hypertension, arrhythmias.
**EENT:** conjunctivitis, photosensitivity reactions, rhinorrhea.
**GI:** constipation, nausea, vomiting, polydipsia, pancreatitis, metallic taste, dry mouth, anorexia, diarrhea.
**GU:** polyuria, nocturia.
**Skin:** pruritus.
**Other:** bone and muscle pain, weight loss, hyperthermia, nephrocalcinosis, decreased libido.

### INTERACTIONS
*Cholestyramine, colestipol:* decreased absorption of orally administered vitamin D analogues. Avoid concomitant use.
*Corticosteroids:* counteract vitamin D analogue effects. Don't use together.
*Digitalis glycosides:* increased risk of arrhythmias. Avoid concomitant use.
*Magnesium-containing antacids:* possible hypermagnesemia, especially in patients with chronic renal failure. Avoid concomitant use.
*Other vitamin D analogues:* increased toxicity. Avoid concomitant use.

### CONTRAINDICATIONS
Contraindicated in patients with hypercalcemia or vitamin D toxicity.

### NURSING CONSIDERATIONS
● Monitor serum calcium level as ordered; serum calcium level multiplied by serum phosphate level should not exceed 70. During titration, serum calcium level should be determined at least weekly.
● If hypercalcemia occurs, discontinue calcifediol and notify doctor. Drug may be resumed after serum calcium level returns to normal.

### ☑ PATIENT TEACHING
● Teach the patient to report signs and symptoms of hypercalcemia.
● Instruct the patient about importance of getting an adequate daily intake of calcium. Inform the patient

---

Reactions may be *common,* uncommon, *life-threatening,* or **COMMON AND LIFE-THREATENING.**

about foods high in calcium and how much should be consumed daily to meet RDA.

## calcitonin (human)
Cibacalcin

## calcitonin (salmon)
Calcimar, Miacalcin, Miacalcin Nasal Spray

*Pregnancy Risk Category: C*

### HOW SUPPLIED
**calcitonin human**
*Injection:* 0.5 mg/vial
**calcitonin salmon**
*Injection:* 100 IU/ml, 1-ml ampules; 200 IU/ml, 2-ml ampules
*Nasal spray:* 200 I.U./activation in 2-ml bottle

### ACTION
Decreases osteoclastic activity by inhibiting osteocytic osteolysis and decreases mineral release and matrix or collagen breakdown in bone.

### ONSET, PEAK, DURATION
Onset immediate after I.V. injection, within 15 minutes after I.M. or S.C. injection. Plasma levels peak immediately after I.V. injection, within 4 hours after I.M. or S.C. injection. Effects persist for 30 minutes to 12 hours after I.V. administration, 8 to 24 hours after I.M. or S.C. injection.

### INDICATIONS & DOSAGE
*Paget's disease of bone (osteitis deformans) –*
**Adults:** initially, 100 IU of calcitonin (salmon) daily S.C. or I.M.; maintenance dosage is 50 to 100 IU daily or every other day. Alternatively, calcitonin (human) 0.5 mg S.C. daily. If the patient improves sufficiently, dosage reduced to 0.25 mg. daily 2 or 3 times per week. Some patients may need as much as 1 mg daily.
*Hypercalcemia –*

**Adults:** 4 IU/kg of calcitonin (salmon) q 12 hours I.M. If response inadequate after 1 or 2 days dose increased to 8 IU/kg I.M. q 12 hours. If response remains unsatisfactory after 2 more days, dosage increased to maximum of 8 IU/kg I.M. q 6 hours.
*Postmenopausal osteoporosis –*
**Adults:** 100 IU of calcitonin (salmon) daily I.M. or S.C. Alternatively, 200 IU (1 activation) of calcitonin (salmon) daily intranasally.

### ADVERSE REACTIONS
**CNS:** headache, weakness, dizziness, paresthesia.
**EENT:** eye pain, nasal congestion.
**GI:** transient *nausea,* unusual taste, diarrhea, anorexia, *vomiting,* epigastric discomfort, abdominal pain.
**GU:** *increased urinary frequency,* nocturia.
**Skin:** *facial flushing,* rashes, pruritus of ear lobes, *inflammation at injection site.*
**Other:** hypersensitivity reactions *(anaphylaxis),* edema of feet, chills, chest pressure, shortness of breath, tender palms and soles.

### INTERACTIONS
None significant.

### CONTRAINDICATIONS
Contraindicated in patients hypersensitive to salmon calcitonin. Human calcitonin has no contraindications.

### NURSING CONSIDERATIONS
• Be aware that skin test is usually done before therapy.
• Systemic allergic reactions possible since hormone is protein. Keep epinephrine handy.
• Know that calcitonin (human) is especially indicated in patients who have developed resistance to calcitonin (salmon). Calcitonin (human) is associated with risk of diminishing efficacy caused by antibody formation or hypersensitivity reactions.

---

*Liquid form contains alcohol.  **May contain tartrazine.  †Canada only.  ‡Australia only.  ◇OTC.

• Administer at bedtime when possible to minimize nausea and vomiting.
• I.M. route is preferred if the volume of the dose to be administered exceeds 2 ml.
• Use freshly reconstituted solution within 2 hours.
• Observe the patient for signs of hypocalcemic tetany during therapy (muscle twitching, tetanic spasms, and seizures when hypocalcemia is severe).
• Monitor serum calcium level closely. Watch for signs of hypercalcemia relapse: bone pain, renal calculi, polyuria, anorexia, nausea, vomiting, thirst, constipation, lethargy, bradycardia, muscle hypotonicity, pathologic fracture, psychosis, and coma.
• Know that periodic examinations of urine sediment are advisable.
• Monitor periodic serum alkaline phosphatase and 24-hour urine hydroxyproline levels to evaluate drug effect as ordered.
• In patients with good initial clinical response to calcitonin who suffer relapse, expect to evaluate for antibody response to the hormone protein.
• If symptoms have been relieved after 6 months, know that treatment may be discontinued until symptoms or radiologic signs recur.
• Store calcitonin (human) at room temperature (77° F [25° C]); refrigerate calcitonin (salmon) at 36° to 46° F (2° to 8° C).
• When administered for postmenopausal osteoporosis, remind the patient to take adequate calcium and vitamin D supplements.

☑ **PATIENT TEACHING**
• Instruct the home care patient or family member on how to administer drug. Tell them to administer drug at bedtime if only one dose is required daily. If nasal spray is prescribed, tell patient to alternate nostrils daily.
• Facial flushing and warmth occur in 20% to 30% of all patients within minutes of injection and usually last about 1 hour. Reassure the patient that this is a transient effect.
• Tell the patient to report signs and symptoms of hypercalcemia promptly. Inform them that if calcitonin loses its hypocalcemic activity, further medication or increased dosages will be of no value.

---

## calcitriol (1,25-dihydroxy-cholecalciferol)
Calcijex, Rocaltrol
*Pregnancy Risk Category: C*

### HOW SUPPLIED
*Capsules:* 0.25 mcg, 0.5 mcg
*Injection:* 1 mcg/ml, 2 mcg/ml

### ACTION
A vitamin D analogue that stimulates calcium absorption from the GI tract and promotes secretion of calcium from bone to blood.

### ONSET, PEAK, DURATION
Onset occurs within 2 to 6 hours. Plasma levels peak in 3 to 6 hours. Effects persist for 3 to 5 days.

### INDICATIONS & DOSAGE
*Hypocalcemia in patients undergoing chronic dialysis –*
**Adults:** initially, 0.25 mcg P.O. daily. Dosage may be increased by 0.25 mcg daily at 4- to 8-week intervals. Maintenance dosage is 0.25 mcg every other day, up to 1.25 mcg daily.
*Hypoparathyroidism and pseudohypoparathyroidism –*
**Adults and children 6 years and over:** initially, 0.25 mcg P.O. daily. Dosage may be increased at 2- to 4-week intervals. Maintenance dosage is 0.25 to 2 mcg daily.

---

Reactions may be *common,* uncommon, *life-threatening,* or **COMMON AND LIFE-THREATENING.**

*Hypoparathyroidism –*
**Children 1 to 6 years:** 0.25 to 0.75 mcg P.O. daily.
*Hypercalcemia –*
**Adults:** 0.5 mcg or 0.01 mcg/kg I.V. rapidly three times a week. Dosage may be increased at 2- to 4-week intervals as needed. Maintenance dosage is 0.5 to 3 mcg or 0.01 to 0.05 mcg/kg I.V. rapidly three times a week.

### ADVERSE REACTIONS
Vitamin D intoxication associated with hypercalcemia
**CNS:** headache, somnolence, weakness, irritability, psychosis (rare).
**CV:** hypertension, arrhythmias.
**EENT:** conjunctivitis, photophobia, rhinorrhea.
**GI:** nausea, vomiting, constipation, polydipsia, pancreatitis, metallic taste, dry mouth, anorexia.
**GU:** polyuria, nocturia.
**Skin:** pruritus.
**Other:** bone and muscle pain, weight loss, hyperthermia, nephrocalcinosis, decreased libido.

### INTERACTIONS
*Cholestyramine, colestipol, excessive use of mineral oil:* decreased absorption of orally administered vitamin D analogues. Avoid concomitant use.
*Corticosteroids:* counteract vitamin D analogue effects. Don't use together.
*Digitalis glycosides:* increased risk of arrhythmias. Avoid concomitant use.
*Magnesium-containing antacids:* may induce hypermagnesemia, especially in patients with chronic renal failure. Avoid concomitant use.

### CONTRAINDICATIONS
Contraindicated in patients with hypercalcemia or vitamin D toxicity. Withhold all preparations containing vitamin D.

### NURSING CONSIDERATIONS
• Monitor serum calcium level; serum calcium level multiplied by the serum phosphate level should not exceed 70. During titration, determine serum calcium level twice weekly. Discontinue if hypercalcemia occurs and notify doctor, but resume after serum calcium level returns to normal. The patient should receive adequate daily intake (1,000 mg) of calcium.
• Protect from heat and light.

### ☑ PATIENT TEACHING
• Tell the patient to immediately report early symptoms of vitamin D intoxication: weakness, nausea, vomiting, dry mouth, constipation, muscle or bone pain, or metallic taste.
• Instruct the patient to adhere to diet and calcium supplementation and to avoid unapproved OTC drugs and magnesium-containing antacids.
• *Alert:* Tell the patient that this drug must not be taken by anyone for whom it was not prescribed because of its potentially serious toxic effects. It is the most potent form of vitamin D available.

## dihydrotachysterol
AT-10‡, DHT Intensol*, Hytakerol
*Pregnancy Risk Category: C*

### HOW SUPPLIED
*Tablets:* 0.125 mg, 0.2 mg, 0.4 mg
*Capsules:* 0.125 mg
*Oral solution:* 0.2 mg/5 ml, 0.2 mg/ml* (DHT Intensol*), 0.25 mg/ml (in sesame oil)
*Note:* 1 mg of dihydrotachysterol is equal to 120,000 units ergocalciferol (vitamin $D_2$).

### ACTION
A vitamin D analogue that stimulates calcium absorption from the GI tract and promotes secretion of calcium from bone to blood.

---

*Liquid form contains alcohol.  **May contain tartrazine.  †Canada only.  ‡Australia only.  ◇OTC.

## ONSET, PEAK, DURATION
Onset occurs in several hours. Peak effects occur in 1 to 2 weeks. Effects persist up to 9 weeks.

## INDICATIONS & DOSAGE
*Hypocalcemia associated with hypoparathyroidism and pseudohypoparathyroidism —*
**Adults:** initially, 0.75 to 2.5 mg P.O. daily for several days. Maintenance dosage is 0.2 to 1.5 mg daily.
**Children:** initially, 1 to 5 mg P.O. for several days. Maintenance dosage is 0.5 to 1.5 mg daily.
*Prophylaxis of hypocalcemic tetany following thyroid surgery —*
**Adults:** 0.25 mg P.O. daily (with calcium supplements).

## ADVERSE REACTIONS
Vitamin D intoxication associated with hypercalcemia
**CNS:** headache, somnolence, irritability, psychosis (rare).
**CV:** hypertension, arrhythmias.
**EENT:** conjunctivitis, photophobia, rhinorrhea.
**GI:** nausea, vomiting, constipation, polydipsia, pancreatitis, metallic taste, dry mouth, anorexia, diarrhea.
**GU:** polyuria, nocturia.
**Other:** weakness, bone and muscle pain, thirst, weight loss, hyperthermia, decreased libido, nephrocalcinosis.

## INTERACTIONS
*Cholestyramine, colestipol, excessive use of mineral oil:* decreased absorption of orally administered vitamin D analogues. Avoid concomitant use.
*Corticosteroids:* counteract vitamin D analogue effects. Don't use together.
*Digitalis glycosides:* increased risk of arrhythmias. Avoid concomitant use.
*Magnesium-containing antacids:* possible hypermagnesemia, especially in patients with chronic renal failure. Avoid concomitant use.

*Other vitamin D analogues:* increased toxicity. Avoid concomitant use.

## CONTRAINDICATIONS
Contraindicated in patients with hypercalcemia or vitamin D toxicity.

## NURSING CONSIDERATIONS
• Monitor serum calcium level as ordered; the serum calcium level multiplied by serum phosphate level should not exceed 70. During titration, determine serum calcium level twice weekly. Discontinue if hypercalcemia occurs and notify doctor. Know that drug can be resumed after serum calcium level returns to normal. Adequate daily intake of calcium is 1,000 mg.
• Monitor urine calcium level.
• Store in tightly closed, light-resistant container. Don't refrigerate.

### ☑ PATIENT TEACHING
• Tell the patient to report any early signs of hypercalcemia: thirst, headache, vertigo, tinnitus, or anorexia promptly.
• Instruct the patient to adhere to diet and calcium supplementation and to avoid unapproved OTC drugs and magnesium-containing antacids.

---

# etidronate disodium
Didronel

*Pregnancy Risk Category: C*

## HOW SUPPLIED
*Tablets:* 200 mg, 400 mg
*Injection:* 50 mg/ml

## ACTION
Decreases osteoclastic activity by inhibiting osteocytic osteolysis and decreases mineral release and matrix or collagen breakdown in bone.

## ONSET, PEAK, DURATION
Highly variable.

---

Reactions may be *common,* uncommon, *life-threatening,* or COMMON AND LIFE-THREATENING.

## INDICATIONS & DOSAGE

*Symptomatic Paget's disease of bone (osteitis deformans)* –
**Adults:** 5 to 10 mg/kg P.O. daily (not to exceed 6 months of therapy) or 11 to 20 mg/kg P.O. daily (not to exceed 3 months of therapy) in single dose 2 hours before a meal with water or juice.
*Heterotopic ossification in spinal cord injuries* –
**Adults:** 20 mg/kg P.O. daily for 2 weeks, then 10 mg/kg daily for 10 weeks. Total treatment period is 12 weeks.
*Heterotopic ossification after total hip replacement* –
**Adults:** 20 mg/kg P.O. daily for 1 month before total hip replacement and for 3 months afterward.
*Malignancy-associated hypercalcemia* –
**Adults:** 7.5 mg/kg I.V. daily for 3 consecutive days. Maintenance dosage is 20 mg/kg P.O. daily for 30 days. May be used for a maximum of 90 days.

## ADVERSE REACTIONS

**GI:** occur most frequently at dosage of 20 mg/kg daily – diarrhea, increased frequency of bowel movements, nausea, constipation, stomatitis.
**Other:** increased or recurrent bone pain, pain at previously asymptomatic sites, increased risk of fracture, *elevated serum phosphate level,* fever, fluid overload, dyspnea, *seizures,* abnormal hepatic function, hypersensitivity reactions.

## INTERACTIONS
None significant.

## CONTRAINDICATIONS
Contraindicated in patients with known hypersensitivity to drug or in patients with clinically overt osteomalacia.

## NURSING CONSIDERATIONS
• Use cautiously in patients with impaired renal function.
• Know that some patients may receive I.V. etidronate for up to 7 days. However, the risk of hypokalemia increases after 3 days of treatment.
• Monitor renal function before and during therapy as ordered.
• Don't give drug with food, milk, or antacids; may reduce absorption.
• **I.V. use:** Dilute daily dose in at least 250 ml of 0.9% sodium chloride solution or $D_5W$, and infuse over at least 2 hours.
• To monitor drug effect, review serum alkaline phosphatase and urinary hydroxyproline excretion; both will decrease if therapy is effective.
• Be aware that elevated serum phosphate level may occur, especially in patients receiving higher doses. However, the phosphate level usually returns to normal 2 to 4 weeks after drug is discontinued.

## ☑ PATIENT TEACHING
• Stress importance of a diet high in calcium and vitamin D.
• Tell the patient not to eat for 2 hours after daily dose.
• Tell the patient that improvement may not occur for up to 3 months and may continue for months after drug is stopped.

---

\*Liquid form contains alcohol.   \*\*May contain tartrazine.   †Canada only.   ‡Australia only.   ◇OTC.

acetazolamide
acetazolamide sodium
amiloride hydrochloride
bendroflumethiazide
bumetanide
chlorothiazide
chlorothiazide sodium
chlorthalidone
dichlorphenamide
ethacrynate sodium
ethacrynic acid
furosemide
hydrochlorothiazide
indapamide
mannitol
methazolamide
methyclothiazide
metolazone
polythiazide
quinethazone
spironolactone
torsemide
triamterene
trichlormethiazide
urea

## COMBINATION PRODUCTS

ALDACTAZIDE 25/25: spironolactone 25 mg and hydrochlorothiazide 25 mg.
ALDACTAZIDE 50/50: spironolactone 50 mg and hydrochlorothiazide 50 mg.
DYAZIDE: triamterene 37.5 mg and hydrochlorothiazide 25 mg.
MAXZIDE: triamterene 75 mg and hydrochlorothiazide 50 mg.
MAXZIDE-25MG: triamterene 37.5 mg and hydrochlorothiazide 25 mg.
MODURETIC: amiloride hydrochloride 5 mg and hydrochlorothiazide 50 mg.
SPIROZIDE: spironolactone 25 mg and hydrochlorothiazide 25 mg.
ZIAC 2.5: bisoprolol fumarate 2.5 mg and hydrochlorothiazide 6.25 mg.

ZIAC 5: bisoprolol fumarate 5 mg and hydrochlorothiazide 6.25 mg.
ZIAC 10: bisoprolol fumarate 10 mg and hydrochlorothiazide 6.25 mg.

---

## acetazolamide
Acetazolam†, AK-Zol, Apo-Acetazolamide†, Dazamide, Diamox, Diamox Sequels

## acetazolamide sodium
Diamox Parenteral, Diamox Sodium†

*Pregnancy Risk Category: C*

### HOW SUPPLIED
**acetazolamide**
*Tablets:* 125 mg, 250 mg
*Capsules (extended-release):* 500 mg
**acetazolamide sodium**
*Injection:* 500 mg-vial

### ACTION
Blocks the action of carbonic anhydrase, promoting renal excretion of sodium, potassium, bicarbonate, and water, and decreases secretion of aqueous humor in the eye, thereby lowering intraocular pressure. As an anticonvulsant, may inhibit carbonic anhydrase in the CNS and decrease abnormal paroxysmal or excessive neuronal discharge. In acute mountain sickness, carbonic anhydrase inhibitors produce a respiratory and metabolic acidosis that may stimulate ventilation, increase cerebral blood flow, promote the release of oxygen from hemoglobin, and increase ventilation.

### ONSET, PEAK, DURATION
Onset occurs 1 to 1½ hours after tablets, 2 hours after capsules, 2 minutes after I.V. injection. Peak effects occur

---

Reactions may be *common*, uncommon, **life-threatening**, or COMMON AND LIFE-THREATENING.

2 to 4 hours after tablets, 8 to 12 hours after capsules, 15 minutes after I.V. injection. Effects persist for 8 to 12 hours after tablets, 18 to 24 hours after capsules, 4 to 5 hours after I.V. injection.

## INDICATIONS & DOSAGE
*Secondary glaucoma and preoperative treatment of acute angle-closure glaucoma* –
**Adults:** 250 mg P.O. q 4 hours; or 250 mg P.O. b.i.d. for short-term therapy. To rapidly lower intraocular pressure, initially, 500 mg I.V., then 125 to 250 mg I.V. q 4 hours.
*Edema in CHF* –
**Adults:** 250 to 375 mg P.O., or I.V. daily in the morning.
*Chronic open-angle glaucoma* –
**Adults:** 250 mg to 1 g P.O. daily in divided doses q.i.d., or 500 mg (extended-release) P.O. b.i.d.
*Prevention or amelioration of acute mountain sickness* –
**Adults:** 500 mg to 1 g P.O. daily in divided doses q 8 to 12 hours, or 500 mg (extended-release) P.O. b.i.d. Treatment started 24 to 48 hours before ascent, and continued for 48 hours while at high altitude.
*Adjunctive treatment of myoclonic, refractory generalized tonic-clonic, absence, or mixed seizures* –
**Adults and children:** 8 to 30 mg/kg P.O. daily in divided doses. For adults, the optimum dosage range is 375 mg to 1 g daily. Usually given with other anticonvulsants.

## ADVERSE REACTIONS
**CNS:** drowsiness, paresthesia, confusion.
**EENT:** transient myopia, hearing dysfunction, tinnitus.
**GI:** nausea, vomiting, anorexia, altered taste, diarrhea.
**GU:** polyuria, hematuria.
**Hematologic:** *aplastic anemia,* hemolytic anemia, leukopenia.
**Skin:** rash.

**Other:** *pain at injection site,* sterile abscesses, hyperchloremic acidosis, hypokalemia, asymptomatic hyperuricemia.

## INTERACTIONS
*Amphetamines, anticholinergics, mecamylamine, quinidine:* decreased renal clearance of these agents, increasing toxicity. Monitor closely.
*Cyclosporine:* increased cyclosporine levels which may cause nephrotoxicity and neurotoxicity. Monitor closely.
*Lithium:* increased excretion of lithium resulting in decreased effectiveness. Monitor closely.
*Methenamine:* reduced effectiveness of acetazolamide. Avoid concomitant use.
*Primidone:* serum and urine concentrations of primidone may be decreased. Monitor patient closely.
*Salicylates:* possible accumulation and toxicity of acetazolamide, including CNS depression and metabolic acidosis. Monitor closely.

## CONTRAINDICATIONS
Contraindicated in patients with hypersensitivity to the drug; in longterm therapy for chronic noncongestive angle-closure glaucoma; and in those with hyponatremia or hypokalemia, renal or hepatic disease or dysfunction, adrenal gland failure, and hyperchloremic acidosis.

## NURSING CONSIDERATIONS
• Use cautiously in patients with respiratory acidosis, emphysema, or chronic pulmonary disease, and in patients receiving other diuretics.
• Reconstitute 500-mg vial with at least 5 ml of sterile water for injection. Use within 24 hours of reconstitution.
• **I.V. use:** Inject 100 to 500 mg/minute into a large vein using a 21G or 23G needle. Intermittent or continuous infusion is not recommended.
• If the patient is unable to swallow

---

*Liquid form contains alcohol. **May contain tartrazine. †Canada only. ‡Australia only. ◊OTC.

oral forms, check with the pharmacist. He may make a suspension using crushed acetazolamide tablets in a highly flavored syrup, such as cherry, raspberry, or chocolate. Although concentrations up to 500 mg/5 ml are feasible, concentrations of 250 mg/5 ml are more palatable. Refrigeration improves palatability but doesn't improve stability. Suspensions are stable for 1 week.

• Monitor fluid intake and output and electrolytes, especially serum potassium, bicarbonate, and chloride. When used in diuretic therapy, consult the doctor and dietitian about providing a high-potassium diet.

• Monitor elderly patients closely because they are especially susceptible to excessive diuresis.

• Weigh the patient daily. Rapid or excessive fluid loss causes weight loss and hypotension.

• Keep in mind that the diuretic effect decreases when acidosis occurs but can be reestablished by withdrawing drug, as ordered, for several days and then restarting, or by using intermittent administration schedules.

• Because bicarbonate ion excretion makes the patient's urine alkaline, be aware that the drug may cause false-positive urine protein tests.

☑ **PATIENT TEACHING**
• Tell patient to take oral form with food if GI upset occurs.
• Caution patient not to perform hazardous activities if adverse CNS reactions occur.

---

# amiloride hydrochloride
Kaluril‡, Midamor

*Pregnancy Risk Category: B*

## HOW SUPPLIED
*Tablets:* 5 mg

## ACTION
A potassium-sparing diuretic that inhibits sodium reabsorption and potassium excretion in the distal tubules.

## ONSET, PEAK, DURATION
Onset occurs within 2 hours. Peak effects occur in 6 to 10 hours. Effects persist for 24 hours.

## INDICATIONS & DOSAGE
*Hypertension; edema associated with CHF, usually in patients also taking thiazide or other potassium-wasting diuretics –*
**Adults:** usual dosage is 5 mg P.O. daily. Increased to 10 mg daily, if necessary. Maximum dosage is 20 mg daily.

## ADVERSE REACTIONS
**CNS:** *headache,* weakness, dizziness, encephalopathy.
**CV:** orthostatic hypotension.
**GI:** *nausea, anorexia, diarrhea, vomiting,* abdominal pain, constipation, appetite changes.
**GU:** impotence.
**Hematologic:** *aplastic anemia,* neutropenia.
**Other:** hyperkalemia, fatigue, muscle cramps, dyspnea.

## INTERACTIONS
*ACE inhibitors, potassium-containing salt substitutes, potassium-sparing diuretics, potassium supplements:* possible hyperkalemia. Avoid concomitant use.
*Lithium:* decreased lithium clearance, increasing risk of lithium toxicity. Monitor lithium level.
*NSAIDs:* decreased diuretic effectiveness. Avoid concomitant use.

## CONTRAINDICATIONS
Contraindicated in patients with elevated serum potassium level (greater than 5.5 mEq/L). Don't administer to patients receiving other potassium-sparing diuretics, such as spironolac-

---

Reactions may be *common,* uncommon, *life-threatening,* or **COMMON AND LIFE-THREATENING.**

tone and triamterene. Also contraindicated in patients with anuria, acute or chronic renal insufficiency, diabetic nephropathy, and hypersensitivity to the drug.

## NURSING CONSIDERATIONS
• Use with extreme caution, if at all, in patients with diabetes mellitus.
• Use cautiously in patients with severe, existing hepatic insufficiency and in elderly or debilitated patients.
• To prevent nausea, administer amiloride with meals.
• If amiloride is not taken concurrently with a potassium-wasting drug, monitor potassium level because of increased risk of hyperkalemia. Alert doctor immediately if potassium level exceeds 6.5 mEq/L, and expect drug to be discontinued.

## ☑ PATIENT TEACHING
• Advise the patient to avoid sudden posture changes and to rise slowly to avoid orthostatic hypotension.
• Caution the patient not to perform hazardous activities if adverse CNS reactions occur.
• To prevent serious hyperkalemia, warn the patient to avoid excessive ingestion of potassium-rich foods, potassium-containing salt substitutes, and potassium supplements.

---

## bendroflumethiazide (bendrofluazide)
Aprinox‡, Aprinox-M‡, Benzide‡, Naturetin

*Pregnancy Risk Category: C*

## HOW SUPPLIED
*Tablets:* 5 mg, 10 mg

## ACTION
A thiazide diuretic that increases sodium and water excretion by inhibiting sodium and chloride reabsorption in the nephron's distal segment.

## ONSET, PEAK, DURATION
Onset occurs in 1 to 2 hours. Peak effects occur in 4 hours. Effects persist for 6 to 12 hours.

## INDICATIONS & DOSAGE
*Edema, hypertension –*
**Adults:** initially, 5 to 20 mg P.O. daily or divided b.i.d. Maintenance dosage is 2.5 to 15 mg P.O. daily.
**Children:** initially, 0.1 to 0.4 mg/kg (3 to 12 mg/m²) P.O. daily or divided b.i.d. Maintenance dosage is 0.05 to 0.1 mg/kg (1.5 to 3 mg/m²) P.O. daily or divided b.i.d.

## ADVERSE REACTIONS
**CNS:** dizziness, vertigo, headache, paresthesia, weakness, restlessness, blurred vision.
**CV:** volume depletion and dehydration, orthostatic hypotension.
**GI:** anorexia, nausea, diarrhea, pancreatitis, vomiting, constipation.
**GU:** allergic glomerulonephritis, glycosuria, anuria.
**Hematologic:** *aplastic anemia, agranulocytosis,* leukopenia, *thrombocytopenia,* hemolytic anemia.
**Hepatic:** jaundice.
**Skin:** dermatitis, photosensitivity, rash, ecchymoses; purpura, pruritus.
**Other:** impotence; hypokalemia; asymptomatic hyperuricemia; hyperglycemia and impairment of glucose tolerance; fluid and electrolyte imbalances, including dilutional hyponatremia and hypochloremia, metabolic alkalosis (in diabetics), hypercalcemia; gout; muscle cramps; *anaphylaxis;* pneumonitis and vasculitis.

## INTERACTIONS
*Cholestyramine, colestipol:* decreased intestinal absorption of thiazides. Separate doses.
*Diazoxide:* increased antihypertensive, hyperglycemic, and hyperuricemic effects. Use together cautiously.
*Digitalis glycosides:* increased risk of

---

*Liquid form contains alcohol.   **May contain tartrazine.   †Canada only.   ‡Australia only.   ◇OTC.

digitalis toxicity from bendroflume-thiazide-induced hypokalemia. Monitor potassium and digitalis levels.
*Ethanol, barbiturates, opiates:* increased orthostatic hypotensive effect. Monitor closely.
*Lithium:* decreased lithium clearance, increasing risk of lithium toxicity. Monitor lithium level.
*NSAIDs:* increased risk of NSAID-induced renal failure. Monitor closely.

## CONTRAINDICATIONS
Contraindicated in patients with anuria or hypersensitivity to other thiazides or other sulfonamide-derived drugs.

## NURSING CONSIDERATIONS
• Use cautiously in patients with severe renal disease and impaired hepatic function.
• To prevent nocturia, give in the morning.
• Monitor fluid intake and output, weight, serum electrolyte levels, serum creatinine, and BUN regularly. Drug is not as effective if serum creatinine and BUN are more than twice normal.
• Watch for signs of hypokalemia, such as muscle weakness and cramps. Know that drug may be used with potassium-sparing diuretic to prevent potassium loss.
• Consult the doctor and dietitian to provide high-potassium diet. Foods rich in potassium include citrus fruits, bananas, tomatoes, dates, and apricots.
• Monitor blood glucose levels, and check insulin requirements in diabetic patients.
• Monitor blood uric acid levels, especially in patients with a history of gout.
• Monitor elderly patients, who are especially susceptible to excessive diuresis.
• As ordered, discontinue thiazides and thiazide-like diuretics before parathyroid function tests are performed.

• In hypertension, be aware that therapeutic response may be delayed several days.
• Be aware that drug may produce false-negative results in phentolamine, phenolsulfonphthalein, and tyramine tests.

## ☑ PATIENT TEACHING
• Instruct the patient to take drug in morning to prevent nocturia.
• Advise the patient to avoid sudden posture changes and to rise slowly to avoid orthostatic hypotension.
• Advise the patient to use a sunblock to prevent photosensitivity reactions.

---

# bumetanide
Bumex, Burinex‡

*Pregnancy Risk Category: C*

## HOW SUPPLIED
*Tablets:* 0.5 mg, 1 mg, 2 mg
*Injection:* 0.25 mg/ml

## ACTION
A potent loop diuretic that inhibits sodium and chloride reabsorption at the ascending portion of the loop of Henle.

## ONSET, PEAK, DURATION
Onset occurs within minutes after I.V. administration, 40 minutes after I.M. injection, 30 to 60 minutes after oral use. Peak effects occur 15 to 30 minutes after I.V. administration, 1 to 2 hours after oral use. Effects persist for 4 to 6 hours after oral use, 3½ to 4 hours after I.V. administration.

## INDICATIONS & DOSAGE
*Edema in CHF, or hepatic or renal disease—*
**Adults:** 0.5 to 2 mg P.O. once daily. If diuretic response is not adequate, a second or third dose may be given at 4- to 5-hour intervals. Maximum dosage is 10 mg/day. May be administered parenterally if P.O. not feasible.

---

Usual initial dose is 0.5 to 1 mg given I.V. or I.M. If response is not adequate, a second or third dose may be given at 2- to 3-hour intervals. Maximum dosage is 10 mg/day.

## ADVERSE REACTIONS
**CNS:** dizziness, headache, vertigo.
**CV:** volume depletion and dehydration, orthostatic hypotension, ECG changes, chest pain.
**EENT:** transient deafness, tinnitus.
**GI:** nausea, vomiting, upset stomach, dry mouth, diarrhea, pain.
**GU:** *renal failure,* premature ejaculation, difficulty maintaining erection, oliguria.
**Hematologic:** azotemia, *thrombocytopenia.*
**Skin:** rash, pruritus, diaphoresis.
**Other:** hypokalemia; hypochloremic alkalosis; asymptomatic hyperuricemia; weakness; arthritic pain; fluid and electrolyte imbalances, including dilutional hyponatremia, hypocalcemia, hyperglycemia and glucose intolerance impairment; muscle pain and tenderness.

## INTERACTIONS
*Aminoglycoside antibiotics:* potentiated ototoxicity. Use together cautiously.
*Antihypertensives:* increased risk of hypotension. Use together cautiously.
*Digitalis glycosides:* increased risk of digitalis toxicity from bumetanide-induced hypokalemia. Monitor potassium and digitalis levels.
*Indomethacin, NSAIDs, probenecid:* inhibited diuretic response. Use together cautiously.
*Lithium:* decreased lithium clearance, increasing risk of lithium toxicity. Monitor lithium level.
*Metolazone:* profound diuresis and potential electrolyte loss. Monitor the patient for fluid and electrolyte disorders.
*Other potassium-wasting drugs:* increased risk of hypokalemia. Use together cautiously.

## CONTRAINDICATIONS
Contraindicated in patients with hypersensitivity to the drug or to sulfonamides (possible cross-sensitivity), in those with anuria or hepatic coma, and in patients in states of severe electrolyte depletion.

## NURSING CONSIDERATIONS
• Use cautiously in patients with hepatic cirrhosis and ascites and in those with depressed renal function.
• **I.V. use:** Give I.V. doses directly, using a 21G or 23G needle over 1 to 2 minutes. For intermittent infusion, give diluted drug through an intermittent infusion device or piggyback into an I.V. line containing a free-flowing, compatible solution. Infuse at ordered rate. Continuous infusion not recommended.
• To prevent nocturia, give in the morning. If second dose is necessary, give in early afternoon.
• Be aware that the safest and most effective dosage schedule for control of edema is intermittent dosage given on alternate days, or for 3 to 4 days with 1 or 2 days of rest periods.
• Monitor fluid intake and output, weight, and serum electrolyte, BUN, and carbon dioxide levels frequently.
• Watch for signs of hypokalemia, such as muscle weakness and cramps.
• Consult the doctor and dietitian about providing a high-potassium diet. Foods rich in potassium include citrus fruits, tomatoes, bananas, dates, and apricots.
• Monitor blood glucose levels in diabetic patients.
• Monitor blood uric acid levels, especially in patients with a history of gout.
• Monitor blood pressure and pulse rate during rapid diuresis. Bumetanide can lead to profound water and electrolyte depletion.
• If oliguria or azotemia develops or increases, know that the doctor may stop drug.

---

*Liquid form contains alcohol. **May contain tartrazine. †Canada only. ‡Australia only. ◇OTC.

• Keep in mind that bumetanide can be safely used in patients allergic to furosemide; 1 mg of bumetanide equals 40 mg of furosemide.

☑ **PATIENT TEACHING**
• Tell patient to take drug in morning to prevent nocturia and if second dose is prescribed to take it in early afternoon. Also instruct patient to take drug with food or milk if adverse GI reactions occur.
• Advise patient to stand up slowly to prevent dizziness, and to limit alcohol intake and strenuous exercise in hot weather to avoid exacerbating orthostatic hypotension.

---

# chlorothiazide
Azide‡, Chlotride‡, Diuret‡, Diurigen, Diuril

# chlorothiazide sodium
Sodium Diuril

*Pregnancy Risk Category: C*

## HOW SUPPLIED
**chlorothiazide**
*Tablets:* 250 mg, 500 mg
*Oral suspension:* 250 mg/5 ml
**chlorothiazide sodium**
*Injection:* 500-mg vial

## ACTION
A thiazide diuretic that increases sodium and water excretion by inhibiting sodium reabsorption in the nephron's cortical diluting site.

## ONSET, PEAK, DURATION
Onset occurs 2 hours after an oral dose, 15 minutes after I.V. use. Peak effects occur in about 4 hours after an oral dose, 30 minutes after I.V. use. Effects persist for 6 to 12 hours.

## INDICATIONS & DOSAGE
*Edema, hypertension –*
**Adults:** 500 mg to 2 g P.O. or I.V. daily or in divided doses.

*Diuresis, hypertension –*
**Children 2 to 12 years:** 1 g P.O. daily or in divided doses.
**Children 6 months to 2 years:** 10 to 20 mg/kg P.O. daily or in two divided doses.
**Children under 6 months:** up to 30 mg/kg P.O. daily in two divided doses.

## ADVERSE REACTIONS
**CNS:** dizziness, vertigo, headache, paresthesia, weakness, restlessness.
**CV:** volume depletion and dehydration, orthostatic hypotension, vasculitis.
**GI:** anorexia, nausea, pancreatitis, vomiting, epigastric distress, abdominal pain, diarrhea, constipation.
**GU:** impotence, *renal failure,* interstitial nephritis, hematuria.
**Hematologic:** *aplastic anemia, agranulocytosis,* leukopenia, *thrombocytopenia,* hemolytic anemia.
**Hepatic:** jaundice.
**Skin:** dermatitis, photosensitivity, rash, urticaria, alopecia.
**Other:** impotence, hypersensitivity reactions; hypokalemia; asymptomatic hyperuricemia; hyperglycemia and impairment of glucose tolerance; fluid and electrolyte imbalances, including dilutional hyponatremia and hypochloremia, metabolic alkalosis, hypercalcemia; gout; *anaphylaxis,* pneumonitis.

## INTERACTIONS
*Antidiabetic agents:* decreased effectiveness; dosage adjustments may be necessary. Monitor blood glucose levels.
*Cholestyramine, colestipol:* decreased intestinal absorption of thiazides. Separate doses.
*Diazoxide:* increased antihypertensive, hyperglycemic, and hyperuricemic effects. Use together cautiously.
*Digitalis glycosides:* increased risk of digitalis toxicity from chlorothiazide-

---

Reactions may be *common*, uncommon, *life-threatening*, or **COMMON AND LIFE-THREATENING.**

induced hypokalemia. Monitor potassium and digitalis levels.
*Ethanol, barbiturates, opiates:* increased orthostatic hypotensive effect. Monitor closely.
*Lithium:* decreased lithium clearance, increasing risk of lithium toxicity. Monitor lithium level.
*NSAIDs:* increased risk of NSAID-induced renal failure. Monitor the patient for renal failure.

## CONTRAINDICATIONS
Contraindicated in patients with anuria or hypersensitivity to other thiazides or other sulfonamide-derived drugs.

## NURSING CONSIDERATIONS
• Use cautiously in patients with severe renal disease and impaired hepatic function.
• To prevent nocturia, give in the morning. If second dose is necessary give in early afternoon.
• Administer oral form with food to enhance absorption.
• **I.V. use:** Reconstitute 500 mg with 18 ml of sterile water for injection. Inject reconstituted drug directly into vein, through an I.V. line containing a free-flowing, compatible solution, or through an intermittent infusion device. Store reconstituted solutions at room temperature up to 24 hours. Compatible with I.V. dextrose or sodium chloride solutions.
• Never inject I.M. or S.C.
• Avoid I.V. infiltration; can be very painful.
• Avoid simultaneous administration with whole blood and its derivatives.
• Monitor fluid intake and output, weight, blood pressure, and serum electrolyte levels.
• Watch for signs of hypokalemia, such as muscle weakness and cramps. Drug may be used with potassium-sparing diuretic to prevent potassium loss.
• Consult the doctor and dietitian

about providing a high-potassium diet. Foods rich in potassium include citrus fruits, tomatoes, bananas, dates, and apricots.
• Monitor blood glucose levels, and check insulin requirements in diabetic patients.
• Monitor serum creatinine and BUN regularly. Drug not as effective if these levels are more than twice normal.
• Monitor blood uric acid level, especially in patients with a history of gout.
• Monitor serum calcium and watch for progressive renal impairment.
• Monitor elderly patients, who are especially susceptible to excessive diuresis.
• As ordered, discontinue thiazides and thiazide-like diuretics before parathyroid function tests.
• In patients with hypertension, be aware that therapeutic response may be delayed several days.

## ☑ PATIENT TEACHING
• Instruct the patient to take drug with food and in morning to prevent nocturia. If second dose is necessary tell the patient to take it in early afternoon.
• Advise the patient to avoid sudden posture changes and to rise slowly to avoid orthostatic hypotension.
• Advise the patient to use a sunblock to prevent photosensitivity reactions.

# chlorthalidone
Apo-Chlorthalidone†, Hygroton, Novo-Thalidone†, Thalitone, Uridon†

*Pregnancy Risk Category: B*

## HOW SUPPLIED
*Tablets:* 15 mg, 25 mg, 50 mg, 100 mg

## ACTION
Although not a thiazide, chlorthalidone acts similarly, increasing sodium

---

and water excretion by inhibiting sodium and chloride reabsorption in the nephron's distal segment.

## ONSET, PEAK, DURATION
Onset occurs in 2 to 3 hours. Peak effects occur in 2 to 6 hours. Effects persist for 2 to 3 days.

## INDICATIONS & DOSAGE
*Edema, hypertension –*
**Adults:** initially, 25 to 100 mg P.O. daily, or up to 200 mg P.O. on alternate days.
**Children:** 2 mg/kg or 60 mg/m² P.O. three times weekly.

## ADVERSE REACTIONS
**CNS:** dizziness, vertigo, headache, paresthesia, weakness, restlessness.
**CV:** volume depletion and dehydration, vasculitis.
**GI:** anorexia, nausea, pancreatitis, vomiting, abdominal pain, diarrhea, constipation.
**GU:** impotence.
**Hematologic:** *aplastic anemia, agranulocytosis,* leukopenia, thrombocytopenia.
**Hepatic:** jaundice.
**Skin:** dermatitis, photosensitivity, rash, purpura, urticaria.
**Other:** hypersensitivity reactions; hypokalemia; asymptomatic hyperuricemia; hyperglycemia and impairment of glucose tolerance; fluid and electrolyte imbalances, including dilutional hyponatremia and hypochloremia, metabolic alkalosis, hypercalcemia; gout.

## INTERACTIONS
*Antidiabetic agents:* decreased effectiveness; dosage adjustments may be necessary. Monitor blood glucose levels.
*Cholestyramine, colestipol:* decreased intestinal absorption of thiazides. Separate doses.
*Diazoxide:* increased antihypertensive, hyperglycemic, and hyperuricemic effects. Use together cautiously.
*Digitalis glycosides:* increased risk of digitalis toxicity from chlorthalidone-induced hypokalemia. Monitor potassium and digitalis levels.
*Ethanol, barbiturates, opiates:* increased orthostatic hypotensive effect. Monitor closely.
*Lithium:* decreased lithium clearance, increasing risk of lithium toxicity. Monitor lithium level.
*NSAIDs:* increased risk of NSAID-induced renal failure. Monitor closely.

## CONTRAINDICATIONS
Contraindicated in patients with anuria or hypersensitivity to thiazides or other sulfonamide-derived drugs.

## NURSING CONSIDERATIONS
• Use cautiously in patients with severe renal disease and impaired hepatic function.
• To prevent nocturia, give in the morning.
• Monitor fluid intake and output, weight, blood pressure, and serum electrolyte levels.
• Watch for signs of hypokalemia, such as muscle weakness, and cramps. Know that drug may be used with potassium-sparing diuretic to prevent potassium loss.
• Consult the doctor and dietitian about a high-potassium diet. Foods rich in potassium include citrus fruits, tomatoes, bananas, and dates.
• Monitor serum creatinine and BUN levels regularly. Drug is not as effective if these levels are more than twice normal.
• Monitor blood uric acid levels, especially in patients with a history of gout.
• Monitor blood glucose levels, and check insulin requirements in diabetic patients.
• Monitor elderly patients, who are especially susceptible to excessive diuresis.

---

Reactions may be *common,* uncommon, *life-threatening,* or **COMMON AND LIFE-THREATENING.**

• As ordered, discontinue thiazides and thiazide-like diuretics before parathyroid function tests.
• In patients with hypertension, be aware that therapeutic response may be delayed several days.
• *Alert:* Do not confuse Uridon tablets (available in Canada only) with the urinary anti-infective Uridon Modified (available in the United States).

☑ **PATIENT TEACHING**
• Instruct the patient to take in morning to prevent nocturia.
• Advise the patient to avoid sudden posture changes and to rise slowly to avoid orthostatic hypotension.
• Advise the patient to use a sunblock to prevent photosensitivity reactions.

## dichlorphenamide
Daranide

*Pregnancy Risk Category: C*

**HOW SUPPLIED**
*Tablets:* 50 mg

**ACTION**
Not clearly understood. A carbonic anhydrase inhibitor that appears to decrease secretion of aqueous humor, lowering intraocular pressure.

**ONSET, PEAK, DURATION**
Onset occurs in ½ to 1 hour. Peak effects occur in 2 to 4 hours. Effects persist for 6 to 12 hours.

**INDICATIONS & DOSAGE**
*Adjunct in glaucoma –*
**Adults:** initially, 100 to 200 mg P.O., followed by 100 mg q 12 hours until desired response obtained. Maintenance dosage is 25 to 50 mg P.O. daily, b.i.d., or t.i.d., given concomitantly with miotics.

**ADVERSE REACTIONS**
**CNS:** drowsiness, ataxia, tremor, tinnitus, headache, weakness, nervousness, depression, confusion.
**GI:** nausea, vomiting, anorexia, constipation.
**GU:** renal calculi, urinary frequency.
**Hematologic:** leukopenia, *thrombocytopenia, agranulocytosis.*
**Skin:** rash.
**Other:** hyperchloremic acidosis, hypokalemia, asymptomatic hyperuricemia.

**INTERACTIONS**
*Amphetamines, anticholinergics, mecamylamine, quinidine:* decreased renal clearance of these agents, increasing toxicity. Avoid concomitant use.
*Methenamine:* reduced effectiveness of dichlorphenamide. Avoid concomitant use.
*Salicylates:* possible accumulation and toxicity of dichlorphenamide. Monitor closely.

**CONTRAINDICATIONS**
Contraindicated in patients with hypersensitivity to the drug and in those with hepatic insufficiency, renal failure, adrenocortical insufficiency, hyperchloremic acidosis, depressed sodium or potassium level, and severe pulmonary obstruction with inability to increase alveolar ventilation.

**NURSING CONSIDERATIONS**
• Use cautiously in patients with respiratory acidosis.
• Monitor electrolyte levels, especially serum potassium, in initial treatment; know that potassium supplements may be necessary.
• In patients with respiratory acidosis, monitor blood pH and arterial blood gases.
• Be aware that drug may cause false-positive results in urine protein tests.
• Evaluate patients for eye pain to determine if drug is effective.

---

*Liquid form contains alcohol. **May contain tartrazine. †Canada only. ‡Australia only. ◊OTC.

## ☑ PATIENT TEACHING
● Tell patient to take drug with food if GI upset occurs.
● Caution patient not to perform hazardous activities if adverse CNS reactions occur.

## ethacrynate sodium
Sodium Edecrin

## ethacrynic acid
Edecril‡, Edecrin

*Pregnancy Risk Category: B*

## HOW SUPPLIED
**ethacrynic acid**
*Tablets:* 25 mg, 50 mg
**ethacrynate sodium**
*Injection:* 50 mg (with 62.5 mg of mannitol and 0.1 mg of thimerosal)

## ACTION
A potent loop diuretic that inhibits sodium and chloride reabsorption at the proximal and distal tubules and the ascending loop of Henle.

## ONSET, PEAK, DURATION
Onset occurs in 5 minutes after I.V. use, 30 minutes after oral use. Peak effects occur 15 to 30 minutes after I.V. use, 2 hours after oral use. Effects persist for 2 hours after I.V use, 6 to 8 hours after oral use.

## INDICATIONS & DOSAGE
*Acute pulmonary edema –*
**Adults:** 50 mg or 0.5 to 1 mg/kg I.V. Usually only one dose is necessary; occasionally, a second dose may be required.
*Edema –*
**Adults:** 50 to 200 mg P.O. daily. Refractory cases may require up to 200 mg b.i.d.
**Children:** initial dose is 25 mg P.O., increased cautiously in 25-mg increments daily until desired effect is achieved.

## ADVERSE REACTIONS
**CNS:** confusion, fatigue, vertigo, headache.
**CV:** volume depletion and dehydration, orthostatic hypotension.
**EENT:** transient deafness with too-rapid I.V. injection, blurred vision, tinnitus, hearing loss.
**GI:** diarrhea, anorexia, nausea, vomiting, GI bleeding, pancreatitis.
**GU:** oliguria, hematuria, nocturia, polyuria, frequent urination.
**Hematologic:** *agranulocytosis,* neutropenia, *thrombocytopenia,* azotemia.
**Other:** hypokalemia; hypochloremic alkalosis; asymptomatic hyperuricemia; fever; chills; malaise; fluid and electrolyte imbalances, including dilutional hyponatremia, hypocalcemia, hypomagnesemia; hyperglycemia and impaired glucose tolerance.

## INTERACTIONS
*Aminoglycoside antibiotics:* potentiated ototoxic adverse reactions of both drugs. Use together cautiously.
*Antihypertensives:* increased risk of hypotension. Use together cautiously.
*Cisplatin:* increased risk of ototoxicity. Avoid concomitant use.
*Digitalis glycosides:* increased risk of digitalis toxicity from ethacrynate-induced hypokalemia. Monitor potassium and digitalis levels.
*Lithium:* decreased lithium clearance, increasing risk of lithium toxicity. Monitor lithium level.
*Metolazone:* profound diuresis and enhanced electrolyte loss. Use together cautiously.
*NSAIDs:* decreased diuretic effectiveness. Use together cautiously.
*Warfarin:* potentiated anticoagulant effect. Use together cautiously.

## CONTRAINDICATIONS
Contraindicated in patients with hypersensitivity to the drug, in those with anuria, and in infants.

---

Reactions may be *common,* uncommon, *life-threatening,* or COMMON AND LIFE-THREATENING.

## NURSING CONSIDERATIONS
• Use cautiously in patients with electrolyte abnormalities or hepatic impairment.
• To prevent nocturia, give oral doses in the morning.
• **I.V. use:** Reconstitute vacuum vial with 50 ml of $D_5W$ or 0.9% sodium chloride solution. Give slowly through tubing of running infusion over several minutes. Discard unused solution after 24 hours. Don't use cloudy or opalescent solutions.
• If more than one I.V. dose is necessary, use a new injection site to avoid thrombophlebitis.
• Don't mix with whole blood or its derivatives.
• Don't give S.C. or I.M. because of local pain and irritation.
• Monitor fluid intake and output, weight, blood pressure, and serum electrolyte levels.
• Watch for signs of hypokalemia, such as muscle weakness and cramps.
• Consult the doctor and dietitian about providing a high-potassium diet. Foods rich in potassium include citrus fruits, tomatoes, bananas, dates, and apricots. Know that potassium chloride and sodium supplements may be needed.
• Monitor elderly patients, who are especially susceptible to excessive diuresis.
• Monitor blood uric acid levels, especially in patients with a history of gout.
• *Alert:* Be aware that severe diarrhea will necessitate discontinuing drug. Know that patient should not receive drug again after diarrhea has resolved.

## ☑ PATIENT TEACHING
• Instruct patient to take oral form of drug in morning to prevent nocturia and if second dose is required to take it in early afternoon. Also tell patient to take drug with food or milk if adverse GI reactions occur.

• Advise patient to avoid sudden posture changes and to rise slowly to avoid orthostatic hypotension.
• Caution patient not to perform hazardous activities if drowsiness occurs.
• Advise diabetic patient to closely monitor blood glucose levels.

---

# furosemide (frusemide†‡)
Apo-Furosemide†, Furoside†, Lasix*, Lasix Special†, Myrosemide*, Novosemide†, Urex‡, Urex-M‡, Uritol†

*Pregnancy Risk Category: C*

## HOW SUPPLIED
*Tablets:* 20 mg, 40 mg, 80 mg, 500 mg†‡
*Oral solution:* 8 mg/ml, 10 mg/ml, 40 mg/5 ml
*Injection:* 10 mg/ml

## ACTION
A potent loop diuretic that inhibits sodium and chloride reabsorption at the proximal and distal tubules and the ascending loop of Henle.

## ONSET, PEAK, DURATION
Onset occurs about 5 minutes after I.V. administration, about 20 to 60 minutes after oral administration. Peak effects occur within 30 minutes of I.V. administration, within 1 to 2 hours of oral administration. Effects persist about 2 hours after I.V. administration, 6 to 8 hours after oral administration.

## INDICATIONS & DOSAGE
*Acute pulmonary edema –*
**Adults:** 40 mg I.V. injected slowly over 1 to 2 minutes; then 80 mg I.V. in 1 to 1½ hours if needed.
*Edema –*
**Adults:** 20 to 80 mg P.O. daily in the morning, second dose in 6 to 8 hours; carefully titrated up to 600 mg daily if needed. Or, 20 to 40 mg I.M. or I.V., increased by 20 mg q 2 hours until de-

---

*Liquid form contains alcohol.   **May contain tartrazine.   †Canada only.   ‡Australia only.   ◇OTC.

sired response is achieved. Give I.V. dose slowly over 1 to 2 minutes.

**Infants and children:** 2 mg/kg P.O. daily, increased by 1 to 2 mg/kg in 6 to 8 hours if needed; carefully titrated up to 6 mg/kg daily if needed.

*Hypertension—*

**Adults:** 40 mg P.O. b.i.d. Dosage adjusted according to response.

## ADVERSE REACTIONS

**CNS:** vertigo, headache, dizziness, paresthesia, restlessness.

**CV:** volume depletion and dehydration, orthostatic hypotension.

**EENT:** transient deafness with too rapid I.V. injection, blurred vision.

**GI:** abdominal discomfort and pain, diarrhea, anorexia, nausea, vomiting, constipation, pancreatitis.

**GU:** nocturia, polyuria, frequent urination, oliguria.

**Hematologic:** *agranulocytosis,* leukopenia, *thrombocytopenia,* azotemia, anemia, *aplastic anemia.*

**Skin:** dermatitis, purpura.

**Other:** hypokalemia; hypochloremic alkalosis; asymptomatic hyperuricemia; fever; muscle spasm; weakness; fluid and electrolyte imbalances, including dilutional hyponatremia, hypocalcemia, hypomagnesemia; hyperglycemia and impaired glucose tolerance; transient pain at injection site with I.M. administration; thrombophlebitis with I.V. administration.

## INTERACTIONS

*Aminoglycoside antibiotics, cisplatin:* potentiated ototoxicity. Use together cautiously.

*Antidiabetic agents:* decreased hypoglycemic effects. Monitor blood glucose levels.

*Antihypertensives:* increased risk of hypotension. Use together cautiously.

*Corticosteroids, corticotropin, amphotericin B, metolazone:* increased risk of hypokalemia. Monitor potassium levels closely.

*Digitalis glycosides, neuromuscular blockers:* increased toxicity of these agents from furosemide-induced hypokalemia. Monitor potassium levels.

*Ethacrynic acid:* may increase risk of ototoxicty. Do not use concomitantly.

*Lithium:* decreased lithium excretion, resulting in lithium toxicity. Monitor lithium level.

*NSAIDs:* inhibited diuretic response. Use together cautiously.

## CONTRAINDICATIONS

Contraindicated in patients with anuria or in patients with a history of hypersensitivity to the drug.

## NURSING CONSIDERATIONS

● Use cautiously in patients with hepatic cirrhosis. Know that furosemide should be used during pregnancy only if potential benefits clearly outweigh possible risks to fetus.

● To prevent nocturia, give P.O. and I.M. preparations in the morning. Give second doses in early afternoon.

● **I.V. use:** Given by direct injection over 1 to 2 minutes. Alternatively, dilute with $D_5W$, 0.9% sodium chloride solution, or lactated Ringer's solution, and infuse no faster than 4 mg/minute to avoid ototoxicity. Use prepared infusion solution within 24 hours.

● *Alert:* Monitor weight, blood pressure, and pulse rate routinely with chronic use and during rapid diuresis. Furosemide can lead to profound water and electrolyte depletion.

● Be aware that if oliguria or azotemia develops or increases, it may require stopping drug.

● Monitor fluid intake and output and serum electrolyte, BUN, and carbon dioxide levels frequently.

● Watch for signs of hypokalemia, such as muscle weakness and cramps.

● Consult the doctor and dietitian about a high-potassium diet. Foods rich in potassium include citrus fruits, tomatoes, bananas, and dates.

● Monitor blood glucose levels in diabetic patients.

Reactions may be *common,* uncommon, *life-threatening,* or COMMON AND LIFE-THREATENING.

- Monitor blood uric acid, especially in patients with a history of gout.
- Monitor elderly patients, who are especially susceptible to excessive diuresis, with potential for circulatory collapse and thromboembolic complications.
- Store tablets in light-resistant container to prevent discoloration (doesn't affect potency). Don't use discolored (yellow) injectable preparation. Refrigerate oral furosemide solution to ensure drug stability.

☑ **PATIENT TEACHING**
- Advise patient to take the drug with food to prevent GI upset. Also tell patient to take drug in morning to prevent nocturia; if second dose is required, tell patient to take the second dose in early afternoon.
- Advise patient to stand slowly to prevent dizziness and to limit alcohol intake and strenuous exercise in hot weather to avoid exacerbating orthostatic hypotension.
- Advise patient to immediately report ringing in ears, severe abdominal pain, or sore throat and fever; may indicate furosemide toxicity.
- Discourage patient taking furosemide at home from storing different types of medication in the same container, increasing the risk of drug errors. The most popular strengths of furosemide and digoxin are white tablets approximately equal in size.
- Tell patient to check with the doctor or pharmacist before taking any OTC medications.

## hydrochlorothiazide
Apo-Hydro†, Aquazide-H, Diaqua, Dichlotride‡, Diuchlor H†, Esidrix, Ezide, Hydro-D, HydroDIURIL, Hydro-Par, Mictrin, Neo-Codema†, Novo-Hydrazide†, Oretic, Urozide†
*Pregnancy Risk Category: D*

**HOW SUPPLIED**
*Tablets:* 25 mg, 50 mg, 100 mg
*Oral solution:* 10 mg/ml, 50 mg/5 ml, 100 mg/ml

**ACTION**
A thiazide diuretic that increases sodium and water excretion by inhibiting sodium and chloride reabsorption in the nephron's distal segment.

**ONSET, PEAK, DURATION**
Onset occurs in 2 hours. Peak effects occur within 4 to 6 hours. Effects persist for 6 to 12 hours.

**INDICATIONS & DOSAGE**
*Edema –*
**Adults:** 25 to 100 mg P.O. daily or intermittently.
**Children 2 to 12 years:** 37.5 to 100 mg P.O. daily in two divided doses.
**Children 6 months to 2 years:** 12.5 to 37.5 mg P.O. daily in two divided doses.
**Infants under 6 months:** up to 3.3 mg/kg P.O. daily in two divided doses. Total daily dosage may range from 12.5 to 37.5 mg.
*Hypertension –*
**Adults:** 25 to 50 mg P.O. daily as a single dose or divided b.i.d. Daily dosage increased or decreased according to blood pressure.

Doses greater than 50 mg/day are not required when combined with other antihypertensives.

**ADVERSE REACTIONS**
**CNS:** dizziness, vertigo, headache, paresthesia, weakness, restlessness.
**CV:** volume depletion and dehydration, orthostatic hypotension, allergic myocarditis, vasculitis.
**GI:** anorexia, nausea, pancreatitis, epigastric distress, vomiting, abdominal pain, diarrhea, constipation.
**GU:** polyuria, frequent urination, *renal failure,* interstitial nephritis.
**Hematologic:** *aplastic anemia,*

---

*Liquid form contains alcohol. **May contain tartrazine. †Canada only. ‡Australia only. ◇OTC.

*agranulocytosis,* leukopenia, ***thrombocytopenia,*** hemolytic anemia.
**Hepatic:** jaundice.
**Respiratory:** respiratory distress, pneumonitis.
**Skin:** dermatitis, photosensitivity, rash, purpura, alopecia.
**Other:** hypersensitivity reactions; hypokalemia; asymptomatic hyperuricemia; hyperglycemia and impaired glucose tolerance; fluid and electrolyte imbalances, including dilutional hyponatremia and hypochloremia, metabolic alkalosis, hypercalcemia; gout; muscle cramps; ***anaphylactic reactions.***

## INTERACTIONS
*Antidiabetic agents:* decreased effectiveness of hypoglycemic agents; dosage adjustments may be necessary. Monitor blood glucose levels.
*Antihypertensives:* additive antihypertensive effect. Use together cautiously.
*Cholestyramine, colestipol:* decreased intestinal absorption of thiazides. Separate doses.
*Diazoxide:* increased antihypertensive, hyperglycemic, and hyperuricemic effects. Use together cautiously.
*Digitalis glycosides:* increased risk of digitalis toxicity from hydrochlorothiazide-induced hypokalemia. Monitor potassium and digitalis levels.
*Ethanol, barbiturates, opiates:* increased orthostatic hypotensive effect. Monitor closely.
*Lithium:* decreased lithium excretion, increasing risk of lithium toxicity. Monitor lithium level.
*NSAIDs:* increased risk of NSAID-induced renal failure. Monitor closely.

## CONTRAINDICATIONS
Contraindicated in patients with anuria or hypersensitivity to other thiazides or other sulfonamide derivatives.

## NURSING CONSIDERATIONS
● Use cautiously in patients with severe renal disease, impaired hepatic function, and progressive hepatic disease.
● To prevent nocturia, give in the morning.
● Monitor fluid intake and output, weight, blood pressure, and serum electrolyte levels.
● Watch for signs of hypokalemia, such as muscle weakness and cramps. Drug may be used with potassium-sparing diuretic to prevent potassium loss.
● Consult the doctor and dietitian about a high-potassium diet. Foods rich in potassium include citrus fruits, tomatoes, bananas, and dates.
● Monitor serum creatinine and BUN levels regularly. Drug is not as effective if these levels are more than twice normal.
● Monitor blood uric acid levels, especially in patients with a history of gout.
● Monitor blood glucose levels, especially in diabetic patients.
● Monitor elderly patients, who are especially susceptible to excessive diuresis.
● As ordered, discontinue thiazides and thiazide-like diuretics before parathyroid function tests.
● In patients with hypertension, know that therapeutic response may be delayed several days.

## ☑ PATIENT TEACHING
● Advise the patient to take the drug with food to minimize GI upset. Also tell him to take drug in morning to avoid nocturia; if second dose is needed, have him take it in early afternoon.
● Advise the patient to avoid sudden posture changes and to rise slowly to avoid orthostatic hypotension.
● Advise the patient to use a sunblock to prevent photosensitivity reactions.
● Tell the patient to check with the

---

Reactions may be *common,* uncommon, *life-threatening,* or **COMMON AND LIFE-THREATENING.**

doctor or pharmacist before taking any OTC medications.

## indapamide
Lozide†, Lozol, Natrilix‡

*Pregnancy Risk Category: B*

### HOW SUPPLIED
*Tablets:* 1.25 mg, 2.5 mg

### ACTION
Unknown. A thiazide-like diuretic that probably inhibits sodium reabsorption in the nephron's distal segment. Also has a direct vasodilating effect that may be a result of calcium channel-blocking action.

### ONSET, PEAK, DURATION
Onset occurs in 1 to 2 hours. Peak effects occur within 2 hours. Effects persist for up to 36 hours.

### INDICATIONS & DOSAGE
*Edema –*
**Adults:** initially, 2.5 mg P.O. daily in the morning. Increased to 5 mg daily after 1 week, if needed.
*Hypertension –*
**Adults:** initially, 1.25 mg P.O. daily in a.m. Increased to 2.5 mg daily after 4 weeks, if needed. Increased to 5 mg daily after 4 more weeks, if needed.

### ADVERSE REACTIONS
**CNS:** headache, nervousness, dizziness, light-headedness, weakness, vertigo, restlessness, drowsiness, fatigue, anxiety, depression, numbness of extremities, irritability, agitation.
**CV:** volume depletion and dehydration, orthostatic hypotension, palpitations, premature ventricular contractions, irregular heartbeat, vasculitis.
**GI:** anorexia, nausea, epigastric distress, vomiting, abdominal pain, diarrhea, constipation.
**GU:** nocturia, polyuria, frequent urination, impotence.

**Skin:** rash, pruritus, urticaria, flushing.
**Other:** muscle cramps and spasms; asymptomatic hyperuricemia; fluid and electrolyte imbalances, including dilutional hyponatremia and hypochloremia, metabolic alkalosis, hypokalemia; gout; rhinorrhea; weight loss.

### INTERACTIONS
*Diazoxide:* increased antihypertensive, hyperglycemic, and hyperuricemic effects. Use together cautiously.
*Digitalis glycosides:* increased risk of digitalis toxicity from indapamide-induced hypokalemia. Monitor potassium and digitalis levels.
*Lithium:* decreased lithium clearance which may increase lithium toxicity. Should not be administered concomitantly.
*NSAIDs:* increased risk of NSAID-induced renal failure. Monitor the patient for signs of renal failure.

### CONTRAINDICATIONS
Contraindicated in patients with anuria or hypersensitivity to other sulfonamide-derived drugs.

### NURSING CONSIDERATIONS
• Use cautiously in patients with severe renal disease, impaired hepatic function, and progressive hepatic disease.
• To prevent nocturia, give in the morning.
• Monitor fluid intake and output, weight, blood pressure, and serum electrolyte levels.
• Watch for signs of hypokalemia, such as muscle weakness and cramps. Know that drug may be used with potassium-sparing diuretic to prevent potassium loss.
• Consult the doctor and dietitian about a high-potassium diet. Foods rich in potassium include citrus fruits, tomatoes, bananas, and dates.
• Monitor serum creatinine and BUN

---

*Liquid form contains alcohol.   **May contain tartrazine.   †Canada only.   ‡Australia only.   ◇OTC.

levels regularly. Drug is not as effective if these levels are more than twice normal.
- Monitor blood uric acid levels, especially in patients with a history of gout.
- Monitor blood glucose levels, especially in diabetic patients.
- Monitor elderly patients, who are especially susceptible to excessive diuresis.
- As ordered, discontinue thiazides and thiazide-like diuretics before parathyroid function tests.
- In patients with hypertension, be aware that therapeutic response may be delayed several days.

☑ **PATIENT TEACHING**
- Instruct the patient to take drug in morning to prevent nocturia and with food if GI upset occurs.
- Advise the patient to avoid sudden posture changes and to rise slowly to avoid orthostatic hypotension.

## mannitol
Osmitrol

*Pregnancy Risk Category: C*

### HOW SUPPLIED
*Injection:* 5%, 10%, 15%, 20%, 25%

### ACTION
An osmotic diuretic that increases the osmotic pressure of glomerular filtrate, inhibiting tubular reabsorption of water and electrolytes, and that elevates blood plasma osmolality, resulting in enhanced water flow into extracellular fluid.

### ONSET, PEAK, DURATION
Onset occurs in 30 to 60 minutes. Peak effects occur within 1 hour. Effects persist for 6 to 8 hours.

### INDICATIONS & DOSAGE
*Test dose for marked oliguria or suspected inadequate renal function –*
**Adults and children over 12 years:**
200 mg/kg or 12.5 g as a 15% or 20% I.V. solution over 3 to 5 minutes. Response is adequate if 30 to 50 ml urine/hour is excreted over 2 to 3 hours; if response is inadequate, a second test dose is given. If still no response after the second dose, mannitol should not be continued.
*Oliguria –*
**Adults and children over 12 years:**
100 g I.V. as a 15% to 20% solution over 1½ to several hours.
*Prevention of oliguria or acute renal failure –*
**Adults and children over 12 years:**
50 to 100 g I.V. of a concentrated solution, followed by a 5% to 10% solution. Exact concentration determined by fluid requirements.
*Edema; ascites caused by renal, hepatic, or cardiac failure –*
**Adults and children over 12 years:**
100 g I.V. as a 10% to 20% solution over 2 to 6 hours.
*Reduction of intraocular or intracranial pressure –*
**Adults and children over 12 years:**
1.5 to 2 g/kg as a 15% to 25% I.V. solution over 30 to 60 minutes.
*Diuresis in drug intoxication –*
**Adults and children over 12 years:**
5% to 10% solution continuously up to 200 g I.V., while maintaining 100 to 500 ml urine output/hour and a positive fluid balance.
*Irrigating solution during transurethral resection of the prostate gland –*
**Adults:** 2.5% to 5% solution as needed.

### ADVERSE REACTIONS
**CNS:** *seizures,* dizziness, headache.
**CV:** edema, thrombophlebitis, hypotension, hypertension, CHF, tachycardia, angina-like chest pain.
**EENT:** blurred vision, rhinitis, dry mouth.
**GI:** thirst, nausea, vomiting, *diarrhea.*
**GU:** urine retention.
**Other:** fluid and electrolyte imbal-

---

Reactions may be *common,* uncommon, *life-threatening,* or **COMMON AND LIFE-THREATENING.**

ance, dehydration, local pain, fever, chills, urticaria.

### INTERACTIONS
*Lithium:* increased urinary excretion of lithium. Monitor closely.

### CONTRAINDICATIONS
Contraindicated in patients with hypersensitivity to the drug and in those with anuria, severe pulmonary congestion, frank pulmonary edema, severe CHF, severe dehydration, metabolic edema, progressive renal disease or dysfunction, or active intracranial bleeding except during craniotomy.

### NURSING CONSIDERATIONS
• To redissolve crystallized solution (occurs at low temperatures or in concentrations greater than 15%), warm bottle in hot water bath and shake vigorously. Cool to body temperature before giving. Do not use solution with undissolved crystals.
• **I.V. use:** Administer as intermittent or continuous infusion at prescribed rate, using an in-line filter and an infusion pump. Direct injection is not recommended. Check I.V. line patency at infusion site before and during administration.
• Avoid infiltration; if it occurs, observe for inflammation, edema, and necrosis.
• For maximum intraocular pressure reduction before surgery, give 1 to 1½ hours preoperatively, as ordered.
• Monitor vital signs, including central venous pressure, and fluid intake and output hourly. Report increasing oliguria. Check weight, renal function, fluid balance, and serum and urine sodium and potassium levels daily.
• Insert urethral catheter in comatose or incontinent patients because therapy is based on strict evaluation of fluid intake and output. In patients with urethral catheters, use an hourly urometer collection bag to facilitate accurate evaluation of output.
• Be aware that drug can be used to measure glomerular filtration rate.
• To relieve thirst, give frequent mouth care or fluids as permitted.
• When used as an irrigating solution for prostate surgery, keep in mind that concentrations of 3.5% or greater are needed to avoid hemolysis.

### ☑ PATIENT TEACHING
• Tell patient that he may feel thirsty or experience mouth dryness, and emphasize importance of drinking only the amount of fluids ordered.
• Instruct patient to report adverse reactions promptly and to alert nurse if discomfort occurs at I.V. site.

---

## methazolamide
Neptazane
*Pregnancy Risk Category: C*

### HOW SUPPLIED
*Tablets:* 25 mg, 50 mg

### ACTION
A carbonic anhydrase inhibitor that decreases secretion of aqueous humor, lowering intraocular pressure.

### ONSET, PEAK, DURATION
Onset occurs in 2 to 4 hours. Peak effects occur in 6 to 8 hours. Effects persist for 10 to 18 hours.

### INDICATIONS & DOSAGE
*Glaucoma (chronic open-angle or secondary, or preoperatively in obstructive or acute angle-closure)* —
**Adults:** 50 to 100 mg P.O. b.i.d. or t.i.d.

### ADVERSE REACTIONS
**CNS:** drowsiness, paresthesia, fatigue, malaise, confusion.
**EENT:** transient myopia, hearing dysfunction, tinnitus.

---

**GI:** nausea, vomiting, anorexia, taste alteration, diarrhea.
**GU:** crystalluria, renal calculi.
**Skin:** urticaria.
**Other:** metabolic acidosis, electrolyte imbalance.

## INTERACTIONS
*Amphetamines, anticholinergics, mecamylamine, quinidine:* decreased renal clearance of these agents, increasing the risk of toxicity. Avoid concomitant use.
*Methenamine compounds:* reduced methenamine effectiveness. Avoid concomitant use.
*Salicylates:* accumulation and toxicity of methazolamide may occur. Monitor closely.

## CONTRAINDICATIONS
Contraindicated for long-term use in acute angle-closure glaucoma and in patients with depressed serum sodium or potassium levels, renal or hepatic disease or dysfunction, adrenal gland dysfunction, or hyperchloremic acidosis.

## NURSING CONSIDERATIONS
• Use cautiously in patients with emphysema and pulmonary obstruction.
• Monitor fluid intake and output, weight, and serum electrolyte levels.
• Monitor elderly patients, who are especially susceptible to excessive diuresis.
• Know that this drug may cause false-positive urine protein tests by alkalinizing urine.
• Evaluate the patient for eye pain to ensure drug is effective in decreasing intraocular pressure.

## ☑ PATIENT TEACHING
• Caution the patient to comply with prescribed dosage to lessen risk of metabolic acidosis. Effects may decrease in acidosis.
• Warn the patient not to perform

hazardous activities if adverse CNS reactions occur.

---

# methyclothiazide
Aquatensen, Duretic†, Enduron, Enduron M‡
*Pregnancy Risk Category: B*

## HOW SUPPLIED
*Tablets:* 2.5 mg, 5 mg

## ACTION
A thiazide diuretic that increases sodium and water excretion by inhibiting sodium and chloride reabsorption in the nephron's distal segment.

## ONSET, PEAK, DURATION
Onset occurs in 2 hours. Peak effects occur in 6 hours. Effects persist for 24 or more hours.

## INDICATIONS & DOSAGE
*Edema –*
**Adults:** 2.5 to 10 mg P.O daily.
*Hypertension –*
**Adults:** 2.5 to 5 mg P.O daily.

## ADVERSE REACTIONS
**CNS:** dizziness, vertigo, headache, paresthesia, weakness, restlessness.
**CV:** volume depletion and dehydration, orthostatic hypotension, vasculitis.
**GI:** anorexia, nausea, pancreatitis, epigastric distress, vomiting, diarrhea, constipation.
**GU:** polyuria, frequent urination, impotence.
**Hematologic:** *aplastic anemia, agranulocytosis,* leukopenia, *thrombocytopenia,* hemolytic anemia.
**Hepatic:** jaundice.
**Respiratory:** respiratory distress, pneumonitis.
**Skin:** dermatitis, photosensitivity, rash, purpura, *anaphylaxis,* urticaria.
**Other:** asymptomatic hyperuricemia; gout; hyperglycemia and glucose tol-

---

Reactions may be *common,* uncommon, *life-threatening,* or **COMMON AND LIFE-THREATENING.**

erance impairment; fluid and electrolyte imbalances, including hypokalemia, dilutional hyponatremia and hypochloremia, metabolic alkalosis, hypercalcemia; fever; muscle cramps; inappropriate ADH secretion.

## INTERACTIONS
*Cholestyramine, colestipol:* decreased intestinal absorption of thiazides. Separate doses.
*Diazoxide:* increased antihypertensive, hyperglycemic, and hyperuricemic effects. Use together cautiously.
*Digitalis glycosides:* increased risk of digitalis toxicity from methyclothiazide-induced hypokalemia. Monitor potassium and digitalis levels.
*Ethanol, barbiturates, opiates:* increased orthostatic hypotensive effect. Monitor closely.
*Ganglionic or peripheral adrenergic blockers:* may potentiate effect of methyclothiazide. Monitor closely.
*Lithium:* decreased lithium clearance, increasing risk of lithium toxicity. Monitor lithium levels.
*NSAIDs:* increased risk of NSAID-induced renal failure. Monitor closely.

## CONTRAINDICATIONS
Contraindicated in patients with anuria or hypersensitivity to thiazides or other sulfonamide-derived drugs.

## NURSING CONSIDERATIONS
• Use cautiously in patients with renal disease or dysfunction, impaired hepatic function, and progressive hepatic disease.
• To prevent nocturia, give in the morning.
• Monitor fluid intake and output, weight, blood pressure, and serum electrolyte levels.
• Watch for signs of hypokalemia, such as muscle weakness and cramps. Know that drug may also be used with potassium-sparing diuretic to prevent potassium loss.

• Consult the doctor and dietitian about providing a high-potassium diet. Foods rich in potassium include citrus fruits, tomatoes, bananas, dates, and apricots.
• Monitor blood glucose levels, especially in diabetic patients.
• Monitor serum creatinine and BUN levels regularly. Drug is not as effective if these levels are more than twice normal.
• Monitor blood uric acid levels, especially in patients with a history of gout.
• As ordered, discontinue thiazides and thiazide-like diuretics before parathyroid function tests are performed.
• Monitor elderly patients, who are especially susceptible to excessive diuresis.
• In patients with hypertension, know that the therapeutic response may be delayed several days.

## ☑ PATIENT TEACHING
• Instruct the patient to take drug in morning to prevent nocturia.
• Advise the patient to avoid sudden posture changes and to rise slowly to avoid orthostatic hypotension.
• Advise the patient to use a sunblock to prevent photosensitivity reactions.

---

# metolazone
Diulo, Mykrox, Zaroxolyn**
*Pregnancy Risk Category: B*

## HOW SUPPLIED
*Tablets (extended-release):* 2.5 mg, 5 mg, 10 mg
*Tablets (prompt-release):* 0.5 mg

## ACTION
Increases sodium and water excretion by inhibiting sodium reabsorption in the cortical diluting site of the ascending loop of Henle.

---

*Liquid form contains alcohol.   **May contain tartrazine.   †Canada only.   ‡Australia only.   ◊OTC.

## ONSET, PEAK, DURATION

Onset occurs in 1 hour. Peak effects occur in about 2 to 4 hours after prompt-release tablets, 8 hours after extended-release tablets. Effects persist for 12 to 24 hours.

## INDICATIONS & DOSAGE

*Edema in CHF or renal disease* –
**Adults:** 5 to 20 mg (extended-release) P.O. daily.
*Hypertension* –
**Adults:** 2.5 to 5 mg (extended-release) P.O. daily. Maintenance dosage based on patient's blood pressure. Or 0.5 mg (prompt-release) P.O. once daily in a.m., increased to 1 mg P.O. daily as needed. If response is inadequate, another antihypertensive is added.

## ADVERSE REACTIONS

**CNS:** *dizziness,* headache, fatigue, vertigo, paresthesia, weakness, restlessness, drowsiness, anxiety, depression, nervousness, blurred vision.
**CV:** volume depletion and dehydration, orthostatic hypotension, palpitations, vasculitis.
**GI:** anorexia, nausea, pancreatitis, epigastric distress, vomiting, abdominal pain, diarrhea, constipation, dry mouth.
**GU:** nocturia, polyuria, frequent urination, impotence.
**Hematologic:** *aplastic anemia, agranulocytosis,* leukopenia.
**Hepatic:** jaundice, hepatitis.
**Skin:** dermatitis, photosensitivity, rash, purpura, pruritus, urticaria.
**Other:** hyperglycemia and glucose tolerance impairment; fluid and electrolyte imbalances, including hypokalemia, dilutional hyponatremia and hypochloremia, metabolic alkalosis, hypercalcemia; muscle cramps.

## INTERACTIONS

*Anticoagulants:* may affect hypoprothrombinemic response. Monitor PT.
*Antidiabetic agents:* may alter blood glucose level requiring dosage adjustment of antidiabetic agents. Monitor blood glucose levels.
*Cholestyramine, colestipol:* decreased intestinal absorption of thiazides. Separate doses.
*Diazoxide:* increased antihypertensive, hyperglycemic, and hyperuricemic effects. Use together cautiously.
*Digitalis glycosides:* increased risk of digitalis toxicity from metolazone-induced hypokalemia. Monitor potassium and digitalis levels.
*Ethanol, barbiturates, opiates:* increased orthostatic hypotensive effect. Monitor closely.
*Lithium:* decreased lithium clearance, increasing risk of lithium toxicity. Monitor lithium level.
*NSAIDs:* increased risk of NSAID-induced renal failure. Monitor the patient for signs of renal failure.
*Other antihypertensives:* may have additive effects. Use together cautiously.

## CONTRAINDICATIONS

Contraindicated in patients with anuria, hepatic coma or precoma, or hypersensitivity to thiazides or other sulfonamide-derived drugs.

## NURSING CONSIDERATIONS

● Use cautiously in patients with impaired renal or hepatic function.
● To prevent nocturia, give in the morning.
● Keep in mind that Mykrox (prompt-release) tablets are more rapidly and completely absorbed than other brands, mimicking an oral solution. Do not interchange Mykrox with Diulo (extended-release) or Zaroxolyn (extended-release) tablets.
● Monitor fluid intake and output, weight, blood pressure, and serum electrolyte levels.
● Watch for signs of hypokalemia, such as muscle weakness and cramps. Know that drug may be used with po-

tassium-sparing diuretic to prevent potassium loss.

- Consult the doctor and dietitian about providing a high-potassium diet. Foods rich in potassium include citrus fruits, tomatoes, bananas, dates, and apricots.
- Monitor blood glucose levels, especially in diabetic patients.
- Monitor blood uric acid levels, especially in patients with a history of gout.
- Monitor elderly patients, who are especially susceptible to excessive diuresis.
- In patients with hypertension, know that the therapeutic response may be delayed several days.
- Keep in mind that unlike thiazide diuretics, metolazone is effective in patients with decreased renal function.
- Be aware that drug is used as an adjunct in furosemide-resistant edema.
- As ordered, discontinue thiazides and thiazide-like diuretics before parathyroid function tests.

✓ **PATIENT TEACHING**
- Tell the patient to take drug in morning to prevent nocturia.
- Advise the patient to avoid sudden posture changes and to rise slowly to avoid orthostatic hypotension.
- Advise the patient to use a sunblock to prevent photosensitivity reactions.

---

## polythiazide
Renese

*Pregnancy Risk Category: C*

**HOW SUPPLIED**
*Tablets:* 1 mg, 2 mg, 4 mg

**ACTION**
A thiazide diuretic that increases sodium and water excretion by inhibiting sodium and chloride reabsorption in the nephron's distal segment.

**ONSET, PEAK, DURATION**
Onset occurs in 2 hours. Peak effects occur in about 6 hours. Effects persist for 24 to 48 hours.

**INDICATIONS & DOSAGE**
*Hypertension –*
**Adults:** 2 to 4 mg P.O. daily.
*Edema in heart or renal failure –*
**Adults:** 1 to 4 mg P.O. daily.

**ADVERSE REACTIONS**
**CNS:** dizziness, vertigo, headache, paresthesia, weakness, restlessness.
**CV:** volume depletion and dehydration, orthostatic hypotension, vasculitis.
**GI:** anorexia, nausea, pancreatitis, gastric irritation, vomiting, abdominal pain, diarrhea, constipation.
**GU:** polyuria, frequent urination, impotence.
**Hematologic:** *aplastic anemia, agranulocytosis,* leukopenia, *thrombocytopenia.*
**Hepatic:** jaundice.
**Skin:** photosensitivity, rash, purpura, urticaria.
**Other:** hypokalemia; asymptomatic hyperuricemia; hyperglycemia and glucose tolerance impairment; fluid and electrolyte imbalances, including dilutional hyponatremia and hypochloremia, metabolic alkalosis, hypercalcemia; gout.

**INTERACTIONS**
*Cholestyramine, colestipol:* decreased intestinal absorption of thiazides. Separate doses.
*Diazoxide:* increased antihypertensive, hyperglycemic, and hyperuricemic effects. Use together cautiously.
*Digitalis glycosides:* increased risk of digitalis toxicity from polythiazide-induced hypokalemia. Monitor potassium and digitalis levels.
*Ethanol, barbiturates, opiates:* increased orthostatic hypotensive effect. Monitor closely.
*Lithium:* decreased lithium clearance,

increasing risk of toxicity. Monitor lithium levels.

*NSAIDs:* increased risk of NSAID-induced renal failure. Monitor the patient for signs of renal failure.

**CONTRAINDICATIONS**
Contraindicated in patients with anuria or hypersensitivity to thiazides or other sulfonamide-derived drugs.

**NURSING CONSIDERATIONS**
• Use cautiously in patients with severe renal disease and impaired hepatic function.
• To prevent nocturia, give in the morning.
• Monitor fluid intake and output, weight, blood pressure, and serum electrolytes.
• Watch for signs of hypokalemia, such as muscle weakness and cramps. Know that drug may be used with potassium-sparing diuretic to prevent potassium loss.
• Consult the doctor and dietitian about providing a high-potassium diet. Foods rich in potassium include citrus fruits, tomatoes, bananas, dates, and apricots.
• Monitor blood uric acid levels, especially in patients with a history of gout.
• Check insulin requirements in diabetic patients.
• Monitor elderly patients, who are especially susceptible to excessive diuresis.
• As ordered, discontinue thiazides and thiazide-like diuretics before parathyroid function tests.
• In patients with hypertension, know that the therapeutic response may be delayed several days.

☑ **PATIENT TEACHING**
• Instruct the patient to take in morning to prevent nocturia.
• Advise the patient to avoid sudden posture changes and to rise slowly to avoid orthostatic hypotension.
• Advise the patient to use a sunblock to prevent photosensitivity reactions.

# quinethazone
Aquamox‡, Hydromox

*Pregnancy Risk Category: NR*

**HOW SUPPLIED**
*Tablets:* 50 mg

**ACTION**
Although not a thiazide diuretic, quinethazone acts similarly, increasing sodium and water excretion by inhibiting sodium reabsorption in the nephron's cortical diluting site.

**ONSET, PEAK, DURATION**
Onset occurs in 2 hours. Peak effects occur in 6 hours. Effects persist for 18 to 24 hours.

**INDICATIONS & DOSAGE**
*Management of edema or hypertension* —
**Adults:** 50 to 100 mg P.O. daily or 50 mg P.O. b.i.d. Occasionally, up to 150 to 200 mg P.O. daily may be needed.

**ADVERSE REACTIONS**
**CNS:** dizziness, vertigo, headache, paresthesia, weakness, restlessness.
**CV:** volume depletion and dehydration, orthostatic hypotension, vasculitis.
**GI:** anorexia, nausea, pancreatitis, epigastric distress, vomiting, abdominal pain, diarrhea, constipation.
**GU:** polyuria, frequent urination, impotence.
**Hematologic:** *aplastic anemia, agranulocytosis,* leukopenia, *thrombocytopenia.*
**Hepatic:** jaundice.
**Skin:** dermatitis, photosensitivity, rash, purpura, urticaria.
**Other:** hypokalemia; hyperglycemia and glucose tolerance impairment; fluid and electrolyte imbalances, in-

---

Reactions may be *common,* uncommon, *life-threatening,* or COMMON AND LIFE-THREATENING.

cluding dilutional hyponatremia and hypochloremia, metabolic alkalosis, hypercalcemia.

### INTERACTIONS
*Cholestyramine, colestipol:* decreased intestinal absorption of thiazides. Separate doses.
*Diazoxide:* increased antihypertensive, hyperglycemic, and hyperuricemic effects. Use together cautiously.
*Digitalis glycosides:* increased risk of digitalis toxicity from quinethazone-induced hypokalemia. Monitor potassium and digitalis levels.
*Ethanol, barbiturates, opiates:* increased orthostatic hypotensive effect. Monitor closely.
*Lithium:* decreased lithium clearance, increasing risk of lithium toxicity. Monitor lithium level.
*NSAIDs:* increased risk of NSAID-induced renal failure. Monitor the patient for signs of renal failure.

### CONTRAINDICATIONS
Contraindicated in patients with anuria or hypersensitivity to quinethazones, thiazides, or other sulfonamide-derived drugs.

### NURSING CONSIDERATIONS
• Use cautiously in patients with severe renal disease and impaired hepatic function.
• To prevent nocturia, give in the morning.
• Monitor fluid intake and output, weight, blood pressure, and serum electrolytes.
• Watch for signs of hypokalemia, such as muscle weakness and cramps. Know that drug may be used with potassium-sparing diuretic to prevent potassium loss.
• Consult the doctor and dietitian about providing a high-potassium diet. Foods rich in potassium include citrus fruits, tomatoes, bananas, dates, and apricots.

• Monitor serum creatinine, BUN, and blood glucose levels regularly.
• Monitor blood uric acid levels, especially in patients with a history of gout.
• Monitor elderly patients, who are especially susceptible to excessive diuresis.
• As ordered, discontinue thiazides and thiazide-like diuretics before parathyroid function tests.
• In patients with hypertension, know that the therapeutic response may be delayed several days.

### ☑ PATIENT TEACHING
• Tell the patient to take drug in morning to prevent nocturia; if second dose is needed daily, tell the patient to take it in early afternoon.
• Advise the patient to avoid sudden posture changes and to rise slowly to avoid orthostatic hypotension.
• Advise the patient to use a sunblock to prevent photosensitivity reactions.

---

## spironolactone
Aldactone, Novospiroton†, Spirotone‡

*Pregnancy Risk Category: NR*

### HOW SUPPLIED
*Tablets:* 25 mg, 50 mg, 100 mg

### ACTION
A potassium-sparing diuretic that antagonizes aldosterone in the distal tubules, increasing sodium and water excretion.

### ONSET, PEAK, DURATION
Onset occurs in 1 to 2 days. Peak effects occur within 2 to 3 days. Effects persist for 2 to 3 days.

### INDICATIONS & DOSAGE
*Edema –*
**Adults:** 25 to 200 mg P.O. daily or in divided doses.

**Children:** 3.3 mg/kg P.O. daily or in divided doses.
*Hypertension—*
**Adults:** 50 to 100 mg P.O. daily or in divided doses.
*Diuretic-induced hypokalemia—*
**Adults:** 25 to 100 mg P.O. daily when oral potassium supplements are contraindicated.
*Detection of primary hyperaldosteronism—*
**Adults:** 400 mg P.O. daily for 4 days (short test) or 3 to 4 weeks (long test). If hypokalemia and hypertension are corrected, a presumptive diagnosis of primary hyperaldosteronism is made.
*Management of primary hyperaldosteronism—*
**Adults:** 100 to 400 mg P.O. daily.

## ADVERSE REACTIONS
**CNS:** headache, drowsiness, lethargy, confusion, ataxia.
**GI:** diarrhea, gastric bleeding, ulceration, cramping, gastritis, vomiting.
**Skin:** urticaria, maculopapular eruptions.
**Other:** *hyperkalemia,* dehydration, hyponatremia, transient elevation in BUN, metabolic acidosis, inability to maintain erection, hirsutism, gynecomastia, breast soreness and menstrual disturbances in women, drug fever, *agranulocytosis.*

## INTERACTIONS
*ACE inhibitors, indomethacin, potassium-containing salt substitutes, potassium-rich foods, potassium supplements:* increased risk of hyperkalemia. Don't use together, especially in patients with renal impairment.
*Aspirin:* possible blocked diuretic effect of spironolactone. Watch for diminished spironolactone response.
*Digoxin:* may alter digoxin clearance, increasing risk of digoxin toxicity. Monitor digoxin levels.

## CONTRAINDICATIONS
Contraindicated in patients with anuria, acute or progressive renal insufficiency, or hyperkalemia.

## NURSING CONSIDERATIONS
• Use cautiously in patients with fluid or electrolyte imbalances, impaired renal function, and hepatic disease.
• To enhance absorption, give drug with meals.
• Protect drug from light.
• Monitor serum electrolytes, fluid intake and output, weight, and blood pressure.
• Monitor elderly patients, who are more susceptible to excessive diuresis.
• Inform the laboratory that patient is taking spironolactone because it may interfere with some laboratory tests that measure digoxin levels.
• Be aware that drug is less potent than thiazide and loop diuretics; useful as an adjunct to other diuretic therapy. Diuretic effect delayed 2 to 3 days when used alone.
• Keep in mind that maximum antihypertensive response may be delayed for up to 2 weeks.
• Watch for mild acidosis, which may occur during therapy, because of danger in patients with hepatic cirrhosis.
• Know that breast cancer has been reported in some patients taking spironolactone.

## ☑ PATIENT TEACHING
• Instruct the patient to take drug in morning to prevent nocturia; if second dose is needed, tell the patient to take it in early afternoon. Also tell the patient to take it with food.
• *Alert:* Warn the patient to avoid excessive ingestion of potassium-rich foods, potassium-containing salt substitutes, and potassium supplements to prevent serious hyperkalemia.
• Caution the patient not to perform hazardous activities if adverse CNS reactions occur.

---

Reactions may be *common,* uncommon, *life-threatening,* or **COMMON AND LIFE-THREATENING.**

# torsemide
Demadex

*Pregnancy Risk Category: B*

## HOW SUPPLIED
*Injection:* 10 mg/ml
*Tablets:* 5 mg, 10 mg, 20 mg, 100 mg

## ACTION
A loop diuretic that enhances excretion of sodium, chloride, and water by acting on the ascending portion of the loop of Henle.

## ONSET, PEAK, DURATION
Onset occurs within 10 minutes of I.V. use, 1 hour after oral use. Peak effects occur within 1 hour of I.V. use, 1 to 2 hours after oral use. Effects persist for 6 to 8 hours.

## INDICATIONS & DOSAGE
*Diuresis in patients with CHF* –
**Adults:** initially, 10 to 20 mg P.O. or I.V. once daily. If response is inadequate, the dose is doubled until a response is obtained. Maximum dosage is 200 mg daily.
*Diuresis in patients with chronic renal failure* –
**Adults:** initially, 20 mg P.O. or I.V. once daily. If response is inadequate, the dose is doubled until a response is obtained. Maximum dosage is 200 mg daily.
*Diuresis in patients with hepatic cirrhosis* –
**Adults:** initially, 5 to 10 mg P.O. or I.V. once daily with an aldosterone antagonist or a potassium-sparing diuretic. If response is inadequate, the dose is doubled until a response is obtained. Maximum dosage is 40 mg daily.
*Hypertension* –
**Adults:** initially, 5 mg P.O. daily. Increased to 10 mg if needed and tolerated. If response is still inadequate, within 4 to 6 weeks another antihypertensive should be added.

## ADVERSE REACTIONS
**CNS:** dizziness, headache, nervousness, insomnia, syncope.
**CV:** ECG abnormalities, chest pain, edema.
**EENT:** rhinitis, cough, sore throat.
**GI:** diarrhea, constipation, nausea, dyspepsia.
**GU:** *excessive urination.*
**Other:** asthenia, arthralgia, myalgia.

## INTERACTIONS
*Cholestyramine:* decreased absorption of torsemide. Separate administration times by at least 3 hours.
*Digoxin:* decreased torsemide clearance. No dosage adjustments are necessary.
*Indomethacin:* decreased diuretic effectiveness in sodium-restricted patients. Avoid concomitant use.
*Lithium, ototoxic drugs such as aminoglycosides or ethacrynic acid:* possible increased toxicity of these agents. Avoid concomitant use.
*NSAIDs:* may potentiate nephrotoxicity of NSAIDs. Use together cautiously.
*Probenecid:* decreased diuretic effectiveness. Avoid concomitant use.
*Salicylates:* decreased excretion, possibly leading to salicylate toxicity. Avoid concomitant use.
*Spironolactone:* decreased renal clearance of spironolactone. No dosage adjustments are necessary.

## CONTRAINDICATIONS
Contraindicated in patients with anuria or hypersensitivity to the drug or other sulfonylurea derivatives.

## NURSING CONSIDERATIONS
● Use cautiously in patients with hepatic disease and associated cirrhosis and ascites; sudden changes in fluid and electrolyte balance may precipitate hepatic coma in these patients.
● To prevent nocturia, give in the morning.

---

*Liquid form contains alcohol.   **May contain tartrazine.   †Canada only.   ‡Australia only.   ◇OTC.

- Inspect ampules for precipitate or discoloration before use.
- **I.V. use:** May be given by direct injection over at least 2 minutes. Rapid injection may cause ototoxicity. Don't give more than 200 mg at a time.
- Monitor fluid intake and output, serum electrolyte levels, blood pressure, weight, and pulse rate during rapid diuresis and routinely with chronic use. Drug can cause profound diuresis and water and electrolyte depletion.
- Watch for signs of hypokalemia, such as muscle weakness and cramps.
- Consult the doctor and dietitian about providing a high-potassium diet. Foods rich in potassium include citrus fruits, tomatoes, bananas, dates, and apricots.
- Monitor elderly patients, who are especially susceptible to excessive diuresis with potential for circulatory collapse and thromboembolic complications.

☑ **PATIENT TEACHING**
- Tell the patient to take drug in morning to prevent nocturia.
- To prevent orthostatic hypotehnsion, advise the patient to change positions slowly to prevent dizziness, and to limit alcohol intake and strenuous exercise in hot weather to prevent orthostatic hypotension.
- Advise the patient to immediately report ringing in ears. May indicate toxicity.
- Tell the patient to check with the doctor or pharmacist before taking any OTC medications.

---

## triamterene
Dyrenium, Dytac‡

*Pregnancy Risk Category: B*

### HOW SUPPLIED
*Tablets†:* 50 mg, 100 mg
*Capsules:* 50 mg, 100 mg

### ACTION
A potassium-sparing diuretic that inhibits sodium reabsorption and potassium and hydrogen excretion by direct action on the distal tubules.

### ONSET, PEAK, DURATION
Onset occurs in 2 to 4 hours. Peak effects occur in several days. Effects persist for 7 to 9 hours.

### INDICATIONS & DOSAGE
*Edema—*
**Adults:** initially, 100 mg P.O. b.i.d. after meals. Total dosage should not exceed 300 mg daily.

### ADVERSE REACTIONS
**CNS:** dizziness, weakness, fatigue, headache.
**CV:** hypotension.
**GI:** dry mouth, nausea, vomiting, diarrhea.
**Hematologic:** megaloblastic anemia related to low folic acid levels, ***thrombocytopenia.***
**Skin:** photosensitivity, rash.
**Other:** *anaphylaxis, hyperkalemia,* muscle cramps, transient elevation in BUNs or creatinine levels, acidosis, interstitial nephritis, hypokalemia, azotemia, jaundice, increased liver enzyme abnormalities.

### INTERACTIONS
*ACE inhibitors, potassium-containing salt substitutes, potassium-rich foods, potassium supplements:* increased risk of hyperkalemia. Don't use together.
*Amantadine:* increased risk of amantadine toxicity. Don't use together.
*Lithium:* decreased lithium clearance, increasing risk of lithium toxicity. Monitor lithium level.
*NSAIDs:* may enhance risk of nephrotoxicity. Avoid concomitant use.
*Quinidine:* may interfere with some laboratory tests that measure quinidine levels. Inform laboratory that patient is taking triamterene.

---

## CONTRAINDICATIONS
Contraindicated in patients with hypersensitivity to the drug and in those with anuria, severe or progressive renal disease or dysfunction, severe hepatic disease, or hyperkalemia.

## NURSING CONSIDERATIONS
• Use cautiously in patients with impaired hepatic function or diabetes mellitus and in elderly or debilitated patients.
• To minimize nausea, give medication after meals.
• Monitor blood pressure, BUN, and serum electrolyte levels.
• Watch for blood dyscrasia.
• To minimize excessive rebound potassium excretion, withdraw drug gradually, as ordered.
• Know that drug is less potent than thiazides and loop diuretics and is useful as an adjunct to other diuretic therapy. Usually used with potassium-wasting diuretics. Full effect is delayed 2 to 3 days when used alone.

## ☑ PATIENT TEACHING
• Tell the patient to take drug after meals to minimize nausea.
• *Alert:* Warn the patient to avoid excessive ingestion of potassium-rich foods, potassium-containing salt substitutes, and potassium supplements to prevent serious hyperkalemia.
• Teach the patient to avoid direct sunlight, wear protective clothing, and use a sunblock to prevent photosensitivity reactions.

---

# trichlormethiazide
Diurese, Metahydrin**, Naqua, Trichlorex**

*Pregnancy Risk Category: C*

## HOW SUPPLIED
*Tablets:* 2 mg, 4 mg

## ACTION
A thiazide diuretic that increases sodium and water excretion by inhibiting sodium and chloride reabsorption in the nephron's distal segment.

## ONSET, PEAK, DURATION
Onset occurs in 2 hours. Peak effects occur in about 6 hours. Effects persist for 24 hours or longer.

## INDICATIONS & DOSAGE
*Edema* –
**Adults:** 1 to 4 mg P.O. daily or b.i.d.
*Hypertension* –
**Adults:** 2 to 4 mg P.O. daily.

## ADVERSE REACTIONS
**CNS:** dizziness, vertigo, headache, paresthesia, weakness, restlessness.
**CV:** volume depletion and dehydration, orthostatic hypotension, palpitations, vasculitis.
**GI:** anorexia, nausea, pancreatitis, epigastric distress, vomiting, abdominal pain, diarrhea, constipation.
**GU:** polyuria, frequent urination, impotence.
**Hematologic:** *aplastic anemia, agranulocytosis,* leukopenia, *thrombocytopenia.*
**Hepatic:** jaundice.
**Skin:** dermatitis, photosensitivity, rash, purpura, urticaria.
**Other:** hypokalemia; asymptomatic hyperuricemia; hyperglycemia and glucose tolerance impairment; fluid and electrolyte imbalances, including dilutional hyponatremia and hypochloremia, metabolic alkalosis, hypercalcemia; gout; muscle cramps.

## INTERACTIONS
*Cholestyramine, colestipol:* decreased intestinal absorption of thiazides. Separate doses.
*Diazoxide:* increased antihypertensive, hyperglycemic, and hyperuricemic effects. Use together cautiously.
*Digitalis glycosides:* increased risk of

---

digitalis toxicity from trichlormethiazide-induced hypokalemia. Monitor potassium and digitalis levels.
*Ethanol, barbiturates, opiates:* increased orthostatic hypotensive effect. Monitor closely.
*Lithium:* decreased lithium clearance, increasing risk of lithium toxicity. Monitor lithium level.
*NSAIDs:* increased risk of NSAID-induced renal failure. Monitor the patient for signs of renal failure.

## CONTRAINDICATIONS
Contraindicated in patients with anuria or hypersensitivity to thiazides or other sulfonamide-derived drugs.

## NURSING CONSIDERATIONS
• Use cautiously in patients with severe renal disease and impaired hepatic function.
• To prevent nocturia, give in the morning.
• Monitor fluid intake and output, weight, blood pressure, and serum electrolyte levels.
• Watch for signs of hypokalemia, such as muscle weakness and cramps. Know that drug may be used with potassium-sparing diuretic to prevent hypokalemia.
• Consult the doctor and dietitian about providing a high-potassium diet. Foods rich in potassium include citrus fruits, tomatoes, bananas, dates, and apricots.
• Monitor serum creatinine, BUN, and blood glucose levels regularly. Drug is not as effective if these levels are more than twice normal.
• Monitor blood uric acid levels, especially in patients with a history of gout.
• As ordered, discontinue thiazides and thiazide-like diuretics before parathyroid function tests.
• Monitor elderly patients, who are especially susceptible to excessive diuresis.
• In patients with hypertension, know

that the therapeutic response may be delayed several days.

## ☑ PATIENT TEACHING
• Tell the patient to take drug in morning to prevent nocturia.
• Advise the patient to avoid sudden posture changes and to rise slowly to avoid orthostatic hypotension.
• Advise the patient to use a sunblock to prevent photosensitivity reactions.

# urea (carbamide)
Ureaphil

*Pregnancy Risk Category: C*

## HOW SUPPLIED
*Injection:* 40 g/150 ml

## ACTION
An osmotic diuretic that increases the osmotic pressure of glomerular filtrate, inhibiting tubular reabsorption of water and electrolytes. Also elevates blood plasma osmolality, resulting in enhanced water flow into extracellular fluid.

## ONSET, PEAK, DURATION
Onset occurs in 30 to 45 minutes. Peak effects occur in 1 to 2 hours. Diuresis and decreased CSF pressure last for 3 to 10 hours; decreased intraocular pressure lasts 5 to 6 hours.

## INDICATIONS & DOSAGE
*Elevated intracranial or intraocular pressure –*
**Adults:** 1 to 1.5 g/kg as a 30% solution by slow I.V. infusion over 1 to 2½ hours. Rate should not exceed 4 ml/minute. Maximum dosage is 120 g daily.
**Children:** 0.5 to 1.5 g/kg by slow I.V. infusion (rate not to exceed 4 ml/minute) or 35 g/m$^2$ in 24 hours. Children under 2 years may receive as little as 0.1 g/kg by slow I.V. infusion.

---

Reactions may be *common*, uncommon, *life-threatening*, or COMMON AND LIFE-THREATENING.

## ADVERSE REACTIONS
**CNS:** *headache,* syncope, disorientation.
**GI:** *nausea, vomiting.*
**Other:** irritation or necrotic sloughing with extravasation.

## INTERACTIONS
*Lithium:* increased lithium clearance and decreased lithium effectiveness. Monitor lithium level.

## CONTRAINDICATIONS
Contraindicated in patients with severely impaired renal function, marked dehydration, frank hepatic failure, active intracranial bleeding, and sickle-cell disease with CNS involvement.

## NURSING CONSIDERATIONS
• Use cautiously in patients with cardiac disease or hepatic or renal impairment and during pregnancy and breast-feeding.
• **I.V. use:** Avoid rapid I.V. infusion; may cause hemolysis or increased capillary bleeding. Maximum infusion rate is 4 ml/minute.
• *Alert:* Avoid extravasation; may cause reactions ranging from mild irritation to necrosis.
• To prepare 135 ml of 30% solution, mix contents of 40-g vial of urea with 105 ml of $D_5W$ or dextrose 10% in water or 10% invert sugar in water. Each ml of 30% solution provides 300 mg urea.
• Don't give through the same infusion set as blood or blood derivatives.
• Use freshly reconstituted urea only for I.V. infusion; solution becomes ammonia upon standing. Use within minutes of reconstitution and discard within 24 hours.
• Don't infuse into leg veins; may cause phlebitis or thrombosis, especially in elderly patients.
• Assess breath sounds for crackles, indicating pulmonary edema.
• Watch for signs of hyponatremia (nausea, vomiting, tachycardia) or hypokalemia (muscle weakness, lethargy); may indicate electrolyte depletion before serum levels are reduced.
• Maintain adequate hydration; monitor blood pressure, fluid intake and output, and serum electrolyte levels.
• In patients with renal disease, monitor BUN level.
• To ensure bladder emptying in comatose patients, use an indwelling urinary catheter, and use an hourly urometer collection bag for accurate evaluation of diuresis.
• If satisfactory diuresis does not occur in 6 to 12 hours, be aware that urea should be discontinued and renal function reevaluated.

## ☑ PATIENT TEACHING
• Instruct patient to report adverse reactions promptly.
• Tell patient to alert nurse if discomfort occurs at I.V. insertion site.

---

# 63

## Electrolytes and replacement solutions

calcium acetate
calcium carbonate
calcium chloride
calcium citrate
calcium glubionate
calcium gluceptate
calcium gluconate
calcium lactate
calcium phosphate, dibasic
calcium phosphate, tribasic
dextran, low molecular weight
dextran, high molecular weight
hetastarch
magnesium chloride
magnesium sulfate
potassium acetate
potassium bicarbonate
potassium chloride
potassium gluconate
Ringer's injection
Ringer's injection, lactated
sodium chloride

### COMBINATION PRODUCTS

KLORVESS*: 20 mEq each potassium and chloride (from potassium chloride, potassium bicarbonate, and l-lysine monohydrochloride).
K-LYTE-CL: 25 mEq potassium, 25 mEq chloride (from potassium chloride, potassium bicarbonate, and lysine hydrochloride).
NEUTRA-PHOS: phosphorus 250 mg, sodium 164 mg, potassium 278 mg (from dibasic and monobasic sodium and potassium phosphate).
TWIN-K: 15 ml supplies 20 mEq of potassium ions as a combination of potassium gluconate and potassium citrate.

### calcium acetate
Phos-Ex◇, Phos-Lo

### calcium carbonate
Apo-Cal†◇, BioCal◇, Calcarb 600◇, Cal-Carb-HD◇, Calci-Chew◇, Calciday 667◇, Calcilac◇, Calci-Mix◇, Calcite 500†◇, Calcium 500†◇, Calcium 600◇, Calglycine◇, Cal-Guard Softgels, Cal-Plus◇, Calsan†◇, Caltrate 300†◇, Caltrate 600†◇, Caltrate Chewable†◇, Chooz◇, Dicarbosil◇, Gencalc 600◇, Mallamint◇, Mega-Cal†◇, Nephro-Calci◇, Nu-Cal†◇, Os-Cal†◇, Os-Cal 500◇, Os-Cal Chewable†◇, Oysco◇, Oysco 500 Chewable◇, Oyst-Cal 500◇, Oyst-Cal 500 Chewable◇, Oystercal 500◇, Oyster Shell Calcium-500◇, Rolaids Calcium Rich◇, Super Calcium 1200◇, Titralac◇, Tums◇, Tums E-X◇

### calcium chloride◇
Calciject†

### calcium citrate◇
Citrical◇, Citrical Liquitabs†◇

### calcium glubionate◇
Calcium-Sandoz†, Neo-Calglucon

### calcium gluceptate◇

### calcium gluconate
Kalcinate

### calcium lactate◇

### calcium phosphate, dibasic◇

### calcium phosphate, tribasic
Posture◇

*Pregnancy Risk Category: C*

---

Reactions may be *common*, uncommon, *life-threatening*, or **COMMON AND LIFE-THREATENING.**

## HOW SUPPLIED
**calcium acetate**
*Contains 253 mg or 12.7 mEq of elemental calcium/g*
*Tablets:* 250 mg◇, 500 mg◇, 667 mg, 668 mg◇, 1,000 mg◇
*Injection:* 0.5 mEq Ca$^{++}$ per ml
**calcium carbonate**
*Contains 400 mg or 20 mEq of elemental calcium/g*
*Tablets:* 650 mg◇, 667 mg◇, 750 mg◇, 1.25 g◇, 1.5 g◇
*Tablets (chewable):* 350 mg◇, 420 mg◇, 500 mg◇, 625 mg◇†, 750 mg◇, 850 mg◇, 1.25 g◇
*Capsules:* 600 mg◇, 1.25 g◇
*Oral suspension:* 1.25 g/5 ml◇
*Powder packets:* 6.5 g (2,400 mg calcium) per packet◇
**calcium chloride**
*Contains 270 mg or 13.5 mEq of elemental calcium/g*
*Injection:* 10% solution in 10-ml ampules, vials, and syringes
**calcium citrate**
*Contains 211 mg or 10.6 mEq of elemental calcium/g*
*Tablets:* 950 mg◇
*Effervescent tablets:* 2376 mg◇
**calcium glubionate**
*Contains 64 mg or 3.2 mEq elemental calcium/g*
*Syrup:* 1.8 g/5 ml
**calcium glucceptate**
*Contains 82 mg or 4.1 mEq elemental calcium/g*
*Injection:* 1.1 g/5 ml in 5-ml ampules or 10-ml vials
**calcium gluconate**
*Contains 90 mg or 4.5 mEq of elemental calcium/g*
*Tablets:* 500 mg◇, 650 mg◇, 975 mg◇, 1 g◇
*Injection:* 10% solution in 10-ml ampules and vials, 10-ml or 50-ml vials
*Pharmacy bulk vials:* 100 ml, 200 ml
**calcium lactate**
*Contains 130 mg or 6.5 mEq of elemental calcium/g*
*Tablets:* 325 mg, 650 mg

**calcium phosphate, dibasic**
*Contains 230 mg or 11.5 mEq of elemental calcium/g*
*Tablets:* 500 mg◇
**calcium phosphate, tribasic**
*Contains 400 mg or 20 mEq of elemental calcium/g*
*Tablets:* 300 mg◇, 600 mg◇

## ACTION
Replaces and maintains calcium.

## ONSET, PEAK, DURATION
Onset and peak effects occur immediately after I.V. injection, return to normal within ½ to 2 hours.

## INDICATIONS & DOSAGE
*Hypocalcemic emergency–*
**Adults:** 7 to 14 mEq calcium I.V. May be given as a 10% calcium gluconate solution, 2% to 10% calcium chloride solution, or a 22% calcium glucceptate solution.
**Children:** 1 to 7 mEq calcium I.V.
**Infants:** up to 1 mEq calcium I.V.
*Hypocalcemic tetany–*
**Adults:** 4.5 to 16 mEq calcium I.V. Repeated until tetany is controlled.
**Children:** 0.5 to 0.7 mEq/kg calcium I.V. three to four times a day until tetany is controlled.
**Neonates:** 2.4 mEq/kg I.V. daily in divided doses.
*Adjunctive treatment of cardiac arrest–*
**Adults:** 0.027 to 0.054 mEq/kg calcium chloride I.V., 4.5 to 6.3 mEq calcium glucceptate I.V., or 2.3 to 3.7 mEq calcium gluconate I.V.
**Children:** 0.27 mEq/kg calcium chloride I.V. Repeated in 10 minutes if necessary; determine serum calcium levels before administering further doses.
*Adjunctive treatment of magnesium intoxication–*
**Adults:** initially, 7 mEq I.V. Subsequent doses must be based upon the patient's response.

*During exchange transfusions –*
**Adults:** 1.35 mEq concurrently with each 100 ml citrated blood.
**Neonates:** 0.45 mEq after each 100 ml citrated blood.
*Hyperphosphatemia –*
**Adults:** 1,334 to 2,000 mg P.O. calcium acetate t.i.d. with meals. Most dialysis patients will require three to four tablets with each meal.
*Dietary supplement –*
**Adults:** 500 mg to 2 g P.O. daily.

## ADVERSE REACTIONS
**CNS:** with I.V. use – tingling sensations, sense of oppression or heat waves; with rapid I.V. injection – syncope.
**CV:** mild fall in blood pressure; with rapid I.V. injection – vasodilation, bradycardia, *arrhythmias, cardiac arrest.*
**GI:** with oral use – irritation, hemorrhage, *constipation;* with I.V. use – chalky taste; with oral calcium chloride – hemorrhage, nausea, vomiting, thirst, abdominal pain.
**GU:** hypercalcemia, polyuria, renal calculi.
**Skin:** with I.M. use – local reactions including burning, necrosis, tissue sloughing, cellulitis, soft tissue calcification.
**Other:** with S.C. injection – pain and irritation; with I.V. use – *vein irritation.*

## INTERACTIONS
*Atenolol, tetracyclines, fluoroquinolones:* decreased bioavailability of these agents and calcium when oral preparations are taken together. Separate administration times.
*Calcium channel blockers:* decreased calcium effectiveness. Avoid concomitant use.
*Digitalis glycosides:* increased digitalis toxicity; give calcium cautiously (if at all) to digitalized patients.
*Sodium polystyrene sulfonate:* risk of metabolic acidosis in patients with renal disease. Avoid concomitant use.

*Thiazide diuretics:* risk of hypercalcemia. Avoid concomitant use.
*Foods containing oxalic acid (found in rhubarb and spinach), phytic acid (bran and whole cereals), and phosphorus (milk and dairy products):* may interfere with calcium absorption.

## CONTRAINDICATIONS
Contraindicated in patients with ventricular fibrillation, hypercalcemia, hypophosphatemia, or renal calculi.

## NURSING CONSIDERATIONS
• Use all calcium products with extreme caution in patients with sarcoidosis and renal or cardiac disease, and in digitalized patients. Use calcium chloride cautiously in patients with cor pulmonale, respiratory acidosis, and respiratory failure.
• Warm solutions to body temperature before administration.
• **I.V. use (direct injection):** Administer slowly through a small needle into a large vein or through an I.V. line containing a free-flowing, compatible solution at a rate not exceeding 1 ml/minute (1.5 mEq/minute) for calcium chloride, 1.5 to 5 ml/minute for calcium gluconate, and 2 ml/minute for calcium gluceptate. Do not use scalp veins in children.
• **I.V. use (intermittent infusion):** Infuse diluted solution through an I.V. line containing a compatible solution. Maximum rate of 200 mg/minute suggested for calcium gluceptate and calcium gluconate.
• Give calcium chloride I.V. only. When adding to parenteral solutions that contain other additives (especially phosphorus or phosphate), watch for precipitate. Use an in-line filter.
• Give calcium gluconate I.V. only.
• Monitor ECG when giving calcium I.V. Stop if the patient complains of discomfort and notify doctor. Following I.V. injection, the patient should remain recumbent for 15 minutes.
• Give I.M. injection in the gluteal

region in adults; lateral thigh in infants. Use I.M. route only in emergencies when no I.V. route available.
• Ensure that the doctor specifies the form of calcium he wants given; crash carts usually contain both calcium gluconate and calcium chloride.
• Monitor blood calcium levels frequently. Hypercalcemia may result after large doses in chronic renal failure. Report abnormalities.
• *Alert:* Be aware that severe necrosis and tissue sloughing can occur after extravasation. Calcium gluconate is less irritating to veins and tissues than calcium chloride.

### ✓ PATIENT TEACHING
• Tell patient to take oral calcium 1 to 1½ hours after meals if GI upset occurs.
• Warn patient to avoid oxalic acid (found in rhubarb and spinach), phytic acid (in bran and whole cereals), and phosphorus (in dairy products) in the meal preceding calcium consumption; these substances may interfere with calcium absorption.

---

## dextran, low molecular weight (dextran 40)
Dextran 40, Gentran 40, 10% LMD, Rheomacrodex

*Pregnancy Risk Category: C*

### HOW SUPPLIED
*Injection:* 10% dextran 40 in $D_5W$ or 0.9% sodium chloride solution

### ACTION
Expands plasma volume via colloidal osmotic effect, drawing fluid from interstitial to intravascular space, providing fluid replacement.

### ONSET, PEAK, DURATION
Onset and peak effects occur immediately after an I.V. infusion. Effects persist up to 3 hours.

### INDICATIONS & DOSAGE
*Plasma volume expansion –*
**Adults:** dosage by I.V. infusion depends on amount of fluid loss. First 10 ml/kg of dextran infused rapidly with central venous pressure monitoring, the remaining dose slowly. Total dosage not to exceed 20 ml/kg body weight daily. If therapy continues longer than 24 hours, do not exceed 10 ml/kg daily – continued for no longer than 5 days.
*Prophylaxis of venous thrombosis –*
**Adults:** 10 ml/kg (500 to 1,000 ml) I.V. on the day of the procedure; 500 ml on days 2 and 3.
*Hemodiluent in extracorporeal circulation –*
**Adults:** 10 to 20 ml/kg added to the perfusion circuit, not to exceed total dosage of 20 ml/kg.

### ADVERSE REACTIONS
**GI:** nausea, vomiting.
**GU:** tubular stasis and blocking, increased urine viscosity.
**Hematologic:** *decreased hemoglobin and hematocrit levels;* increased bleeding time (with higher doses).
**Hepatic:** increased AST and ALT levels.
**Skin:** hypersensitivity reactions, urticaria.
**Other:** *anaphylaxis,* thrombophlebitis.

### INTERACTIONS
None significant.

### CONTRAINDICATIONS
Contraindicated in patients with hypersensitivity to the drug and in those with marked hemostatic defects, marked cardiac decompensation, and renal disease with severe oliguria or anuria.

### NURSING CONSIDERATIONS
• Use cautiously in patients with active hemorrhage, thrombocytopenia, or diabetes mellitus.
• Assess hydration before starting therapy; otherwise, use urine or serum osmolarity because urine spe-

---

cific gravity is affected by urine dextran concentration.

● **I.V. use:** Observe the patient closely during early phase of infusion when most anaphylactic reactions occur.

● Watch for circulatory overload and a rise in central venous pressure. Provides plasma expansion slightly greater than volume infused.

● Monitor urine flow rate during administration. If oliguria or anuria occurs or is not relieved, stop dextran and give loop diuretic as ordered.

● Check hemoglobin and hematocrit levels; if values fall below 30% by volume, notify the doctor.

● As ordered, use D₅W solution instead of 0.9% sodium chloride solution for patients with heart failure.

● Be aware the doctor may order dextran 1 to protect against dextran-induced anaphylaxis. Administer 20 ml of dextran 1 (containing 150 mg/ml) I.V. over 60 seconds, 1 to 2 minutes before the I.V. infusion of dextran.

● Be aware that drug may interfere with analyses of blood grouping, crossmatching, bilirubin, blood glucose, and protein.

● Store at constant 77° F (25° C). May precipitate in storage but can be heated to dissolve if necessary.

☑ **PATIENT TEACHING**
● Explain use and administration of dextran to patient and family.
● Tell patient to report adverse effects.

---

## dextran, high molecular weight (dextran 70, dextran 75)

Dextran 75, Gentran 70, Gentran 75, Macrodex

*Pregnancy Risk Category: C*

### HOW SUPPLIED
*Injection:* 6% dextran 70 in 0.9% sodium chloride solution or dextrose 5%; 6% dextran 75 in 0.9% sodium chloride solution or dextrose 5%

### ACTION
Expands plasma volume via colloidal osmotic effect, drawing fluid from interstitial to intravascular space, providing fluid replacement.

### ONSET, PEAK, DURATION
Onset and peak effects occur right after infusion. Duration unknown.

### INDICATIONS & DOSAGE
*Plasma expander –*
**Adults:** 30 g (500 ml of 6% solution) I.V. In emergencies, may be given at 1.2 to 2.4 g (20 to 40 ml) per minute. In normovolemic or nearly normovolemic patients, rate of infusion should not exceed 240 mg (4 ml)/minute.

Total dosage during first 24 hours not to exceed 1.2 g/kg; actual dosage depends on amount of fluid loss and resultant hemoconcentration and must be determined for each patient.

### ADVERSE REACTIONS
**GI:** nausea, vomiting.
**GU:** increased specific gravity and viscosity of urine, tubular stasis and blocking. oliguria, anuria.
**Hematologic:** *decreased hemoglobin and hematocrit levels;* with doses of 15 ml/kg body weight, prolonged bleeding time and significant suppression of platelet function.
**Hepatic:** increased AST and ALT levels.
**Skin:** hypersensitivity reactions, urticaria.
**Other:** fever, arthralgia, nasal congestion, *anaphylaxis, thrombophlebitis.*

### INTERACTIONS
None significant.

### CONTRAINDICATIONS
Contraindicated in patients with hypersensitivity to dextran and in those with marked hemostatic defects, marked cardiac decompensation,

---

Reactions may be *common,* uncommon, *life-threatening,* or **COMMON AND LIFE-THREATENING.**

renal disease with severe oliguria or anuria, hypervolemic conditions, and severe bleeding disorders.

## NURSING CONSIDERATIONS
• Use cautiously in patients with active hemorrhage, thrombocytopenia, impaired renal clearance, chronic liver disease, and abdominal conditions or in patients undergoing bowel surgery.
• Assess hydration before starting therapy; otherwise, use urine or serum osmolarity because urine specific gravity is affected by the urine dextran concentration.
• Have blood samples drawn *before* starting infusion.
• *Alert:* I.V. use: Observe patient closely during early phase of infusion when most anaphylactic reactions occur.
• As ordered, use $D_5W$ solution instead of 0.9% sodium chloride solution for patients with heart failure.
• Monitor urine flow rate during administration. If oliguria or anuria occurs or is not relieved by infusion, stop dextran and give loop diuretic.
• Watch for circulatory overload. Provides plasma expansion slightly greater than volume infused.
• Monitor hemoglobin and hematocrit levels; if values fall below 30% by volume, notify the doctor.
• Be aware that the doctor may order dextran 1 to protect against dextran-induced anaphylaxis. Give 20 ml of dextran 1 (containing 150 mg/ml) I.V. over 60 seconds, 1 to 2 minutes before I.V. infusion of dextran 70.
• Be aware that the drug may interfere with analyses of blood grouping, crossmatching, bilirubin, blood glucose, and protein.
• Know that the drug may precipitate in storage but can be heated to dissolve if necessary.

☑ **PATIENT TEACHING**
• Explain use and administration of dextran to patient and family.
• Tell patient to report adverse effects.

---

# hetastarch
Hespan

*Pregnancy Risk Category: C*

## HOW SUPPLIED
*Injection:* 500 ml (6 g/100 ml in 0.9% sodium chloride solution)

## ACTION
Expands plasma volume and provides fluid replacement.

## ONSET, PEAK, DURATION
Onset and peak effects occur immediately after I.V. infusion. Duration unknown.

## INDICATIONS & DOSAGE
*Plasma expander –*
**Adults:** 500 to 1,000 ml I.V., depending on amount of blood lost and resultant hemoconcentration. Total dosage usually not to exceed 1,500 ml/day. Up to 20 ml/kg hourly may be used in hemorrhagic shock.

## ADVERSE REACTIONS
**CNS:** headache.
**CV:** peripheral edema of lower extremities.
**EENT:** periorbital edema.
**GI:** nausea, vomiting.
**Respiratory:** wheezing.
**Skin:** urticaria.
**Other:** wheezing, mild fever, chills, muscle pain.

## INTERACTIONS
None significant.

## CONTRAINDICATIONS
Contraindicated in patients with severe bleeding disorders, severe CHF, or renal failure with oliguria and anuria.

---

## NURSING CONSIDERATIONS
• Know that hetastarch is *not* a substitute for blood or plasma.
• To avoid circulatory overload, monitor patients with impaired renal function carefully.
• When used in continuous-flow centrifugation, know that leukapheresis ratio is usually one part hetastarch to eight parts venous whole blood.
• Discontinue if allergic or sensitivity reactions occur and notify doctor. If necessary, administer an antihistamine as ordered.
• Discard partially used bottles.

### ☑ PATIENT TEACHING
• Explain use and administration of drug to patient and family.
• Tell patient to report adverse reactions promptly.

---

# magnesium chloride
Slow-Mag◇

# magnesium sulfate
*Pregnancy Risk Category: NR*

## HOW SUPPLIED
**magnesium chloride**
*Tablets (delayed-release):* 64 mg
**magnesium sulfate**
*Injectable solutions:* 10%, 12.5%, 25%, 50% in 2-ml, 5-ml, 10-ml, 20-ml, and 30-ml ampules, vials, and prefilled syringes

## ACTION
Replaces and maintains magnesium levels; as an anticonvulsant, reduces muscle contractions by interfering with release of acetylcholine at myoneural junction.

## ONSET, PEAK, DURATION
Onset is immediate after I.V. administration; about 1 hour after I.M. administration; and unknown after oral administration. Serum levels peak within 4 hours of oral dose; unknown after I.V. and I.M. administration. Effects persist for about 30 minutes after I.V. administration; 3 to 4 hours after I.M. administration; and 4 to 6 hours after oral administration.

## INDICATIONS & DOSAGE
*Mild hypomagnesemia –*
**Adults:** 1 g I.M. q 6 hours for four doses, depending on serum magnesium level. Alternatively, 3 g P.O. q 6 hours for four doses.
*Severe hypomagnesemia (serum magnesium 0.8 mEq/L or less, with symptoms) –*
**Adults:** 5 g I.V. in 1 liter of solution over 3 hours.
   Subsequent doses depend on serum magnesium levels.
*Magnesium supplementation –*
**Adults:** 64 mg (one tablet) P.O. t.i.d.
*Magnesium supplementation in total parenteral nutrition (TPN) –*
**Adults:** 4 to 24 mEq I.V. daily added to TPN solution.
**Infants:** 2 to 10 mEq I.V. daily added to TPN solution.
   Each 2 ml of 50% solution contains 1 g, or 8.12 mEq, magnesium sulfate.
*Acute treatment of preeclampsia and eclampsia –*
**Adults:** loading dose: 2 to 4 g (4 to 8 ml of 50% solution), given by slow I.V. bolus (over 5 minutes). Maintenance dosage is 1 to 2 g hourly by constant infusion. Prepare by adding 8 ml of 50% solution to 250 ml D₅W.
*Hypomagnesemic seizures –*
**Adults:** 1 to 2 g of 10% solution I.V. over 15 minutes, then 1 g I.M. q 4 to 6 hours, based on the patient's response and magnesium blood level.
*Seizures secondary to hypomagnesemia in acute nephritis –*
**Children:** 0.2 ml/kg of 50% solution I.M. q 4 to 6 hours p.r.n., or 100 mg/kg of 1% to 3% solution I.V. very slowly. Titrate dosage based on magnesium blood level and seizure response.
*Paroxysmal atrial tachycardia unresponsive to other treatments –*

---

**Adults:** 3 to 4 g I.V. of 10% solution over 30 seconds, with close monitoring of ECG.

## ADVERSE REACTIONS
**CNS:** toxicity — *weak or absent deep tendon reflexes,* flaccid paralysis, hypothermia, drowsiness, stupor.
**CV:** slow, weak pulse; arrhythmias (caused by hypocalcemia); *hypotension; circulatory collapse* (with toxicity).
**Respiratory:** *respiratory paralysis*
**Skin:** flushing, diaphoresis.
**Other:** hypocalcemia.

## INTERACTIONS
*Digitalis glycosides:* possible serious cardiac conduction changes. Administer with extreme caution.
*Neuromuscular blockers:* possible increased neuromuscular blockage. Use cautiously.
*Nitrofurantoin, tetracyclines, penicillamine:* decreased bioavailability with oral magnesium supplements. Separate administration by 2 to 3 hours.

## CONTRAINDICATIONS
Contraindicated in patients with myocardial damage or heart block and in actively progressing labor.

## NURSING CONSIDERATIONS
● Use parenteral magnesium with extreme caution in patients with impaired renal function.
● **I.V. use:** Inject I.V. bolus dose slowly, using infusion pump for continuous infusion, if available, to avoid respiratory or cardiac arrest. Maximum infusion rate is 150 mg/minute. Rapid drip causes feeling of heat.
● *Alert:* When giving I.V. for severe hypomagnesemia, watch for respiratory depression and signs of heart block. Respirations should be over 16 breaths/minute before dose is given.
● Know that magnesium sulfate may form a precipitate when mixed with solutions containing ethanol, arsenates, barium, calcium, clindamycin, heavy metals, hydrocortisone sodium succinate, phosphates, polymyxin B sulfate, procaine, salicylates, or tartrates. Drug is also incompatible with alkalis, including carbonates and bicarbonates.
● Be aware that undiluted 50% solutions may be given by deep I.M. injection to adults. Dilute solutions to 20% or less for use in children.
● Keep I.V. calcium available to reverse magnesium intoxication.
● Test knee-jerk and patellar reflexes before each additional dose. If absent, notify doctor and give no more magnesium until reflexes return; otherwise, the patient may develop temporary respiratory failure and need cardiopulmonary resuscitation or I.V. administration of calcium.
● Check magnesium level after repeated doses.
● Monitor fluid intake and output. Output should be 100 ml or more during 4-hour period before dose.
● After giving to toxemic patients within 24 hours before delivery, watch neonate for signs of magnesium toxicity, including neuromuscular and respiratory depression.

☑ **PATIENT TEACHING**
● Explain use and administration of drug to patient and family.
● Tell patient to report adverse effects.

---

## potassium acetate
*Pregnancy Risk Category: C*

## HOW SUPPLIED
*Injection:* 2 mEq/ml in 20-ml, 30-ml vials; 4 mEq/ml in 50-ml vials.

## ACTION
Replaces and maintains potassium level.

## ONSET, PEAK, DURATION
Onset and peak levels occur right after I.V. infusion. Duration unknown.

## INDICATIONS & DOSAGE
*Treatment of hypokalemia –*
**Adults:** no more than 20 mEq hourly in concentration of 40 mEq/liter or less. Total 24-hour dosage should not exceed 150 mEq (3 mEq/kg in children). Potassium replacement should be done with ECG monitoring and frequent serum potassium determinations. I.V. route should be used only for life-threatening hypokalemia or when oral replacement not feasible.
*Prevention of hypokalemia –*
**Adults:** dosage is individualized to the patient's needs, not to exceed 150 mEq/day. Administered as an additive to I.V. infusions. Usual dose is 20 mEq/liter infused at a rate not to exceed 20 mEq/hour.
**Children:** individualized dosage not to exceed 3 mEq/kg/day. Administered as an additive to I.V. infusions.

## ADVERSE REACTIONS
*Signs of hyperkalemia –*
**CNS:** paresthesia of the extremities, listlessness, mental confusion, weakness or heaviness of legs, flaccid paralysis.
**CV:** hypotension, *arrhythmias,* heart block, ECG changes, *cardiac arrest.*
**GI:** nausea, vomiting, abdominal pain, diarrhea.
**Respiratory:** *respiratory paralysis.*
**Other:** pain and redness at infusion site, fever, hyperkalemia.

## INTERACTIONS
*ACE inhibitors, potassium-sparing diuretics:* increased risk of hyperkalemia. Use with extreme caution.

## CONTRAINDICATIONS
Contraindicated in patients with severe renal impairment with oliguria, anuria, or azotemia; in those with untreated Addison's disease; and in those with acute dehydration, heat cramps, hyperkalemia, hyperkalemic form of familial periodic paralysis, and conditions associated with extensive tissue breakdown.

## NURSING CONSIDERATIONS
● Use cautiously in patients with cardiac disease and in those with renal impairment.
● **I.V. use:** Give by I.V. infusion only, never I.V. push or I.M. Watch for pain and redness at infusion site. Large-bore needle reduces local irritation.
● **Alert:** Give slowly as diluted solution; potentially fatal hyperkalemia may result from too-rapid infusion.
● During therapy, monitor ECG, renal function, fluid intake and output, and serum potassium, serum creatinine, and BUN levels. Never give potassium postoperatively until urine flow is established.

## ☑ PATIENT TEACHING
● Explain use and administration to patient and family.
● Tell patient to report adverse effects.

---

# potassium bicarbonate
K⁺Care ET, K-Electrolyte Effervescent Tablets, K-Gen ET, K-Ide, Klor-Con/EF, K-Lyte

*Pregnancy Risk Category: NR*

## HOW SUPPLIED
*Effervescent tablets:* 6.5 mEq, 25 mEq

## ACTION
Replaces and maintains potassium.

## ONSET, PEAK, DURATION
Onset and duration unknown. Peak levels occur within 4 hours.

## INDICATIONS & DOSAGE
*Hypokalemia –*
**Adults:** 25 to 50 mEq dissolved in one-half to a full glass of water (120 to 240 ml) once daily to q.i.d.

---

Reactions may be *common,* uncommon, *life-threatening,* or COMMON AND LIFE-THREATENING.

## ADVERSE REACTIONS
**CNS:** paresthesia of the extremities, listlessness, mental confusion, weakness or heaviness of legs, flaccid paralysis.
**CV:** *arrhythmias,* ECG changes, hypotension.
**GI:** *nausea, vomiting, abdominal pain,* diarrhea.

## INTERACTIONS
*ACE inhibitors, potassium-sparing diuretics:* risk of hyperkalemia. Use with extreme caution.

## CONTRAINDICATIONS
Contraindicated in patients with severe renal impairment with oliguria, anuria, or azotemia; in those with untreated Addison's disease; and in patients with acute dehydration, heat cramps, hyperkalemia, hyperkalemic form of familial periodic paralysis, and other conditions associated with extensive tissue breakdown.

## NURSING CONSIDERATIONS
• Use cautiously in patients with cardiac disease and in those with renal impairment.
• Dissolve potassium bicarbonate tablets completely in 6 to 8 oz (180 to 240 ml) of cold water to minimize GI irritation.
• Ask the patient's flavor preference. Available in lime and orange flavors.
• Don't administer potassium supplements postoperatively until urine flow has been established.
• Never switch potassium products without a doctor's order. Potassium chloride cannot be given instead of potassium bicarbonate.
• Monitor BUN, serum potassium, and creatinine levels; and fluid intake and output.

## ☑ PATIENT TEACHING
• Tell patient to take drug with meals and sip slowly over 5 to 10 minutes.
• Tell patient to report adverse effects.

# potassium chloride
Cena-K, K⁺10, Kaochlor 10%*, Kaochlor S-F 10%*, Kaon-Cl, Kaon-Cl 20%*, Kato Powder, Kay Ciel*, K⁺Care, K-Dur, K-Lease, K-Lor, Klor-10%*, Klor-Con, Klorvess, Klotrix, K-Lyte/Cl, K-Norm, K-Tab, Micro-K Extencaps, Rum-K, Slow-K, Ten-K

*Pregnancy Risk Category: C*

## HOW SUPPLIED
*Tablets (controlled-release):* 6.7 mEq (500 mg), 8 mEq (600 mg), 10 mEq (750 mg), 20 mEq (1,500 mg)
*Tablets (film-coated):* 2.5 mEq (200 mg), 8 mEq (600 mg), 10 mEq (750 mg)
*Capsules (controlled-release):* 8 mEq (600 mg), 10 mEq (750 mg)
*Oral liquid:* 5% (10 mEq/15 ml), 7.5% (15 mEq/15 ml), 10% (20 mEq/15 ml), 15% (30 mEq/15 ml), 20% (40 mEq/15 ml)
*Powder for oral use:* 15-mEq packet, 20-mEq packet, 25-mEq packet, 25-mEq dose
*Injection:* 20-mEq, 40-mEq ampules; additive syringes containing 30-mEq or 40-mEq; 10-mEq, 20-mEq, 30-mEq, 40-mEq, 60-mEq, 100-mEq, 200-mEq, 400-mEq, or 1,000-mEq vials

## ACTION
Replaces and maintains potassium level.

## ONSET, PEAK, DURATION
Onset and serum levels peak immediately after I.V. infusion. Duration unknown.

## INDICATIONS & DOSAGE
*Hypokalemia –*
**Adults:** 40 to 100 mEq P.O. daily in three or four divided doses for treatment; 20 mEq for prevention. Further dosage based on serum potassium level.
**Children:** 3 mEq/kg daily. Total daily dosage not to exceed 40 mEq/m².

---

*Liquid form contains alcohol.   **May contain tartrazine.   †Canada only.   ‡Australia only.   ◊OTC.

Use I.V. route only when oral replacement is not feasible or when hypokalemia is life-threatening. If serum potassium is less than 2 mEq/ml, maximum infusion rate is 40 mEq/hour; maximum infusion concentration is 80 mEq/L; and maximum 24-hour dose is 400 mEq. If serum potassium level is greater than 2 mEq/ml, maximum infusion rate is 10 mEq/hour; maximum infusion concentration is 40 mEq/L; and maximum 24-hour dose is 200 mEq. For routine supplementation, the usual dose is 20 mEq hourly in concentration of 40 mEq/L or less.

## ADVERSE REACTIONS
*Signs of hyperkalemia –*
**CNS:** paresthesia of the extremities, listlessness, mental confusion, weakness or heaviness of limbs, flaccid paralysis.
**CV:** *arrhythmias, heart block, possible cardiac arrest,* ECG changes, hypotension.
**GI:** *nausea, vomiting, abdominal pain,* diarrhea.
**Respiratory:** *respiratory paralysis.*
**Other:** *postinfusion phlebitis,* hyperkalemia.

## INTERACTIONS
*ACE inhibitors, potassium-sparing diuretics:* risk of hyperkalemia. Use with extreme caution.

## CONTRAINDICATIONS
Contraindicated in patients with severe renal impairment with oliguria, anuria, or azotemia; in those with untreated Addison's disease; and in patients with acute dehydration, heat cramps, hyperkalemia, hyperkalemic form of familial periodic paralysis, and other conditions associated with extensive tissue breakdown.

## NURSING CONSIDERATIONS
● Use cautiously in patients with cardiac disease and in those with renal impairment.
● *Alert:* **I.V. use:** Give by infusion only, never I.V. push or I.M. Give slowly as dilute solution; potentially fatal hyperkalemia may result from too-rapid infusion.
● Give oral potassium supplements with extreme caution because different forms deliver varying amounts of potassium. Never switch products without a doctor's order.
● Make sure powders are completely dissolved before administering.
● Know that enteric-coated tablets are not recommended because of increased potential for GI bleeding and small-bowel ulcerations.
● Know that tablets in wax matrix sometimes lodge in esophagus and cause ulceration in cardiac patients who have esophageal compression from enlarged left atrium. Use liquid form in such patients and in those with esophageal stasis or obstruction.
● Know that drug is often used orally with potassium-wasting diuretics to maintain potassium levels.
● Be aware that sugar-free liquid is available (Kaochlor S-F 10%); use if tablet or capsule passage is likely to be delayed, such as in GI obstruction. Have patients sip slowly to minimize GI irritation.
● Don't crush sustained-release potassium products.
● Monitor ECG and serum electrolyte levels during therapy.
● Monitor renal function. Potassium should not be given during immediate postoperative period until urine flow is established.

## ☑ PATIENT TEACHING
● Instruct patient how to prepare (powders) and administer drug form prescribed. Tell patient to take with or after meals with full glass of water or fruit juice to lessen GI distress.

---

Reactions may be *common,* uncommon, *life-threatening,* or **COMMON AND LIFE-THREATENING.**

- Teach patient the signs and symptoms of hyperkalemia, and tell patient to notify doctor if they occur.
- Tell patient to alert nurse if discomfort occurs at I.V. insertion site.
- Warn patient not to use salt substitutes concurrently, except with the doctor's permission.

## potassium gluconate
Glu-K, Kaon Liquid*, Kaon Tablets, Kaylixir*, K-G Elixir*, Potassium-Rougier†

*Pregnancy Risk Category: C*

### HOW SUPPLIED
*Tablets:* 500 mg (2 mEq K⁺), 1,170 mg (5 mEq K⁺)
*Elixir:* 4.68 g (20 mEq K⁺)/15 ml*

### ACTION
Replaces and maintains intracellular and extracellular potassium.

### ONSET, PEAK, DURATION
Onset and duration unknown. Peak levels occur within 4 hours of oral dose.

### INDICATIONS & DOSAGE
*Hypokalemia –*
**Adults:** 40 to 100 mEq P.O. daily in three or four divided doses for treatment; 20 mEq daily for prevention. Further dosage adjustments are based on serum potassium determinations.

### ADVERSE REACTIONS
**CNS:** paresthesia of the extremities, listlessness, mental confusion, weakness or heaviness of legs, flaccid paralysis.
**CV:** *arrhythmias,* ECG changes.
**GI:** *nausea, vomiting, abdominal pain,* diarrhea.

### INTERACTIONS
*ACE inhibitors, potassium-sparing diuretics:* risk of hyperkalemia. Use with extreme caution.

### CONTRAINDICATIONS
Contraindicated in patients with severe renal impairment with oliguria, anuria, or azotemia; in those with untreated Addison's disease; and in patients with acute dehydration, heat cramps, hyperkalemia, hyperkalemic form of familial periodic paralysis, and other conditions associated with extensive tissue breakdown.

### NURSING CONSIDERATIONS
- Give oral potassium supplements with extreme caution because different forms deliver varying amounts of potassium. Never switch products without a doctor's order.
- Use cautiously in patients with cardiac disease and in those with renal impairment.
- Don't administer potassium supplements postoperatively until urine flow has been established.
- Monitor ECG, serum potassium and creatinine levels, BUN, and fluid intake and output.

### ☑ PATIENT TEACHING
- Advise the patient to sip liquid potassium slowly to minimize GI irritation. Also tell patient to take drug with or after meals with a full glass of water or fruit juice.
- Warn the patient not to use salt substitutes concurrently, except with the doctor's permission.

## Ringer's injection
*Pregnancy Risk Category: NR*

### HOW SUPPLIED
*Injection:* 250 ml, 500 ml, 1,000 ml

### ACTION
Replaces fluids and electrolytes.

### ONSET, PEAK, DURATION
Onset and serum levels peak immediately after I.V. infusion. Duration unknown.

## INDICATIONS & DOSAGE
*Fluid and electrolyte replacement—*
**Adults and children:** dosage highly individualized, but usually 1.5 to 3 liters (2% to 6% body weight), infused I.V. over 18 to 24 hours.

## ADVERSE REACTIONS
**CV:** fluid overload.

## INTERACTIONS
None significant.

## CONTRAINDICATIONS
Contraindicated in patients with renal failure, except as emergency volume expander.

## NURSING CONSIDERATIONS
• Use cautiously in patients with CHF, circulatory insufficiency, renal dysfunction, hypoproteinemia, and pulmonary edema.
• Know that Ringer's injection contains sodium, 147 mEq/liter; potassium, 4 mEq/liter; calcium, 4.5 mEq/liter; and chloride, 155.5 mEq/liter.
• Be aware that electrolyte content is insufficient for treating severe electrolyte deficiencies, but it does provide electrolytes in levels approximately equal to those of the blood.

☑ **PATIENT TEACHING**
• Explain use and administration of drug to patient and family.
• Tell patient to report any unusual signs or symptoms promptly.

---

## Ringer's injection, lactated (Hartmann's solution, Ringer's lactate solution)

*Pregnancy Risk Category: NR*

### HOW SUPPLIED
*Injection:* 150 ml, 250 ml, 500 ml, 1,000 ml

### ACTION
Replaces fluids and electrolytes.

## ONSET, PEAK, DURATION
Onset and serum levels peak immediately after I.V. infusion. Duration unknown.

## INDICATIONS & DOSAGE
*Fluid and electrolyte replacement—*
**Adults and children:** dosage highly individualized, but usually 1.5 to 3 liters (2% to 6% body weight) infused I.V. over 18 to 24 hours.

## ADVERSE REACTIONS
**CV:** fluid overload.

## INTERACTIONS
None significant.

## CONTRAINDICATIONS
Contraindicated in patients with renal failure, except as emergency volume expander.

## NURSING CONSIDERATIONS
• Use cautiously in patients with CHF, circulatory insufficiency, renal dysfunction, hypoproteinemia, and pulmonary edema.
• Know that lactated Ringer's injection contains sodium, 130 mEq/L; potassium, 4 mEq/L; calcium, 3 mEq/L; chloride, 109.7 mEq/L; and lactate, 28 mEq/L.
• Be aware that lactated Ringer's injection more closely approximates the electrolyte concentration in blood plasma.

☑ **PATIENT TEACHING**
• Explain use and administration of drug to patient and family.
• Tell patient to report any unusual signs or symptoms promptly.

---

## sodium chloride
*Pregnancy Risk Category: NR*

### HOW SUPPLIED
*Tablets:* 650 mg
*Tablets (slow-release):* 600 mg
*Injection:* 0.45% sodium chloride solu-

---

tion 25 ml, 50 ml, 150 ml, 250 ml, 500 ml, 1,000 ml; 0.9% sodium chloride solution 2 ml, 3 ml, 5 ml, 10 ml, 20 ml, 25 ml, 30 ml, 50 ml, 100 ml, 150 ml, 250 ml, 500 ml, 1,000 ml; 3% sodium chloride solution 500 ml; 5% sodium chloride solution 500 ml; 14.6% sodium chloride solution 20 ml, 40 ml, 200 ml; 23.4% sodium chloride solution 30 ml, 50 ml, and 200 ml.

### ACTION
Replaces and maintains sodium and chloride levels.

### ONSET, PEAK, DURATION
Onset and serum levels peak immediately after I.V. infusion. Duration unknown.

### INDICATIONS & DOSAGE
*Fluid and electrolyte replacement in hyponatremia caused by electrolyte loss or in severe salt depletion –*
**Adults:** dosage is highly individualized. 3% or 5% solution used only with frequent electrolyte determination and given only slow I.V. With 0.45% solution: 3% to 8% of body weight, according to deficiencies, over 18 to 24 hours; with 0.9% solution: 2% to 6% of body weight, according to deficiencies, over 18 to 24 hours.
*Management of heat cramp caused by excessive perspiration –*
**Adults:** 1 g P.O. with every glass of water.

### ADVERSE REACTIONS
**CV:** aggravation of CHF; edema if given too rapidly or in excess.
**Respiratory:** *pulmonary edema* if given too rapidly or in excess.
**Other:** hypernatremia and aggravation of existing metabolic acidosis with excessive infusion; serious electrolyte disturbances, loss of potassium; local tenderness, abscess, tissue necrosis at injection site; thrombophlebitis.

### INTERACTIONS
None significant.

### CONTRAINDICATIONS
Contraindicated in patients with conditions in which sodium and chloride administration is detrimental. Sodium chloride 3% and 5% injections are contraindicated in patients with increased, normal, or only slightly decreased serum electrolyte concentrations.

### NURSING CONSIDERATIONS
• Use cautiously in patients with CHF, circulatory insufficiency, renal dysfunction, and hypoproteinemia and in elderly or postoperative patients.
• *Alert:* **I.V. use:** Infuse 3% and 5% solutions slowly and cautiously to avoid pulmonary edema. Use only for critical situations, and observe the patient continually.
• Don't confuse concentrates (14.6%, 23.4%) available to add to parenteral nutrient solutions with 0.9% sodium chloride injection, and never give without diluting. Read labels carefully.
• Monitor serum electrolyte levels.

### ☑ PATIENT TEACHING
• Explain use and administration of drug to patient and family.
• Tell patient to report adverse reactions promptly.

---

# 64

# Acidifier and alkalinizers

**ammonium chloride**
**sodium bicarbonate**
**sodium lactate**
**tromethamine**

## COMBINATION PRODUCTS
None.

---

## ammonium chloride◇
*Pregnancy Risk Category: C*

### HOW SUPPLIED
*Tablets:* 500 mg◇
*Tablets (enteric-coated):* 500 mg◇
*Injection:* 2.14% (0.4 mEq/ml),
26.75% (5 mEq/ml)

### ACTION
Increases free hydrogen ion concentration, resulting in acidosis, and acts as an expectorant by causing reflex stimulation of bronchial mucous glands.

### ONSET, PEAK, DURATION
Onset and serum levels peak immediately after I.V. infusion. Duration unknown.

### INDICATIONS & DOSAGE
*Metabolic alkalosis; chloride replacement –*
**Adults and children:** I.V. dose (in mEq) is equal to the serum chloride deficit (in mEq/L) multiplied by the extracellular fluid volume (estimated as 20% of the body weight in kilograms). One-half the calculated volume should be given, then the patient reassessed.
*Acidifier –*
**Adults:** 4 to 12 g P.O. daily in divided doses q 4 to 6 hours.
**Children:** 75 mg/kg P.O. daily in four divided doses.

### ADVERSE REACTIONS
Adverse reactions usually result from ammonia toxicity or too-rapid I.V. administration.
**CNS:** *coma,* twitching, *tonic convulsions.*
**CV:** bradycardia, cardiac arrhythmias.
**Skin:** rash, pallor, diaphoresis.
**Respiratory:** irregular respirations with periods of apnea.
**Other:** *metabolic acidosis,* pain at injection site.

### INTERACTIONS
*Spironolactone:* increased systemic acidosis. Use together cautiously.

### CONTRAINDICATIONS
Contraindicated in patients with primary respiratory acidosis and high total carbon dioxide ($CO_2$) and buffer base and in those with severe hepatic or renal dysfunction (as self-medication).

### NURSING CONSIDERATIONS
• Use cautiously in patients with pulmonary insufficiency or cardiac edema and in infants.
• Determine $CO_2$ combining power and serum electrolytes before and during therapy to prevent acidosis. Each gram of ammonium chloride will reduce the $CO_2$ combining power by 1.1 volume percent.
• **I.V. use:** Dilute concentrated form (26.75%) before administration. Add 100 to 200 mEq (20 to 40 ml of the 26.75% solution) to 500 or 1,000 ml of 0.9% sodium chloride for injection. Administer via infusion pump, not exceeding 5 ml/minute in adults.
• Lessen pain of I.V. injection by decreasing infusion rate.
• To decrease GI adverse reactions,

---

Reactions may be *common,* uncommon, *life-threatening,* or **COMMON AND LIFE-THREATENING.**

give oral form after meals. Enteric-coated tablets may also minimize GI symptoms but are absorbed erratically.
• Do not administer drug with milk or other alkaline solutions; they are incompatible.
• Monitor urine pH and output. Diuresis is normal for first 2 days.
• Monitor rate and depth of respirations frequently.

☑ **PATIENT TEACHING**
• Instruct patient to take oral form after meals. Tell him not to ingest milk or milk-based products at the meal preceding drug administration.
• Tell patient to report adverse reactions promptly.

---

### sodium bicarbonate◊
Arm and Hammer Pure Baking Soda, Bell/ans, Citrocarbonate, Soda Mint

*Pregnancy Risk Category: NR*

#### HOW SUPPLIED
*Tablets◊:* 325 mg, 520 mg, 650 mg
*Injection:* 4% (2.4 mEq/5 ml), 4.2% (5 mEq/10 ml), 5% (297.5 mEq/500 ml), 7.5% (8.92 mEq/10 ml and 44.6 mEq/50 ml), 8.4% (10 mEq/10 ml and 50 mEq/50 ml)

#### ACTION
Restores body's buffering capacity of the body and neutralizes excess acid.

#### ONSET, PEAK, DURATION
Onset and peak serum levels occur immediately after I.V. infusion. Duration unknown after I.V. infusion. Onset, peak, and duration unknown after oral administration.

#### INDICATIONS & DOSAGE
*Cardiac arrest –*
**Adults and children:** 1 mEq/kg I.V. of 7.5% or 8.4% solution, followed by 0.5 mEq/kg I.V. every 10 minutes, depending on arterial blood gases

(ABGs). Further dosages based on results of ABG analysis. If ABG results are unavailable, use 0.5 mEq/kg I.V. every 10 minutes until spontaneous circulation returns.
**Infants up to 2 years:** not to exceed 8 mEq/kg I.V. daily of 4.2% solution.
*Metabolic acidosis –*
**Adults and children:** dosage depends on blood $CO_2$ content, pH, and the patient's clinical condition. Generally, 2 to 5 mEq/kg I.V. infused over 4- to 8-hour period.
*Systemic or urinary alkalinization –*
**Adults:** initially, 4 g P.O., followed by 1 to 2 g q 4 hours.
**Children:** 84 to 840 mg/kg P.O. daily.
*Antacid –*
**Adults:** 300 mg to 2 g P.O. up to q.i.d. taken with glass of water.

#### ADVERSE REACTIONS
**GI:** gastric distention, belching, flatulence.
**Other:** with overdose – *metabolic alkalosis,* hypernatremia, hyperosmolarity; local pain and irritation at injection site.

#### INTERACTIONS
*Anorexients, flecainide, mecamylamine, quinidine, sympathomimetics:* urine alkalinization causes decreased renal clearance of these drugs and increased risk of toxicity. Monitor closely.
*Chlorpropamide, lithium, methotrexate, salicylates, tetracycline:* increased urine alkalinization causes increased renal clearance of these drugs and reduced effectiveness. Monitor closely.
*Enteric-coated drugs:* may be released prematurely in stomach. Avoid concomitant use.

#### CONTRAINDICATIONS
Contraindicated in patients with metabolic or respiratory alkalosis, in patients who are losing chlorides by

---

*Liquid form contains alcohol. **May contain tartrazine. †Canada only. ‡Australia only. ◊OTC.

vomiting or from continuous GI suction, in those receiving diuretics known to produce hypochloremic alkalosis; and in those with hypocalcemia in which alkalosis may produce tetany, hypertension, seizures, or CHF. Orally administered sodium bicarbonate is contraindicated in patients with acute ingestion of strong mineral acids.

**NURSING CONSIDERATIONS**
• Use with extreme caution in patients with CHF or other edematous or sodium-retaining conditions or renal insufficiency.
• **I.V. use:** May be added to other I.V. fluids. Sodium bicarbonate inactivates such catecholamines as norepinephrine and dopamine, and forms precipitate with calcium. Do not mix sodium bicarbonate with I.V. solutions of these agents, and flush I.V. line adequately.
• To avoid risk of alkalosis, obtain blood pH, $PaO_2$, $PaCO_2$, and serum electrolytes. Keep the doctor informed of serum laboratory results.
• If sodium bicarbonate is being used to produce an alkaline urine, monitor urine pH every 4 to 6 hours (should be above 7.0).
• **Alert:** Be aware that sodium bicarbonate is not routinely recommended for use in cardiac arrest because it may produce a paradoxical acidosis from $CO_2$ production. It should not be routinely administered during the early stages of resuscitation unless preexisting acidosis is clearly present. May be used at team leader's discretion after such interventions as defibrillation, cardiac compression, and administration of first-line drugs.

☑ **PATIENT TEACHING**
• Tell the patient not to take with milk. May cause hypercalcemia, alkalosis, and possibly renal calculi.
• Discourage use as an antacid. Offer

a nonabsorbable alternative antacid if it is to be used repeatedly.

---

# sodium lactate
*Pregnancy Risk Category: NR*

**HOW SUPPLIED**
*Injection:* ⅙ molar solution (167 mEq/L)
*Injection:* 5 mEq/ml

**ACTION**
Metabolized to sodium bicarbonate, producing buffering effect.

**ONSET, PEAK, DURATION**
Onset and serum levels peak right after infusion. Conversion of sodium lactate to bicarbonate requires 1 to 2 hours. Duration unknown.

**INDICATIONS & DOSAGE**
*Alkalinize urine –*
**Adults:** 30 ml of ⅙ molar solution/kg of body weight I.V., given in divided doses over 24 hours.
*Metabolic acidosis –*
**Adults:** ⅙ molar injection (167 mEq lactate/L I.V.); dosage depends on degree of bicarbonate deficit.

**ADVERSE REACTIONS**
**Other:** fever, infection or thrombophlebitis at injection site; with overdose – *metabolic alkalosis,* hypernatremia, hyperosmolarity.

**INTERACTIONS**
None significant.

**CONTRAINDICATIONS**
Contraindicated in patients with hypernatremia, lactic acidosis, or conditions in which sodium administration is detrimental.

**NURSING CONSIDERATIONS**
• Use with extreme caution in patients with metabolic or respiratory

---

*Reactions may be* common, uncommon, *life-threatening,* or COMMON AND LIFE-THREATENING.

alkalosis, severe hepatic or renal disease, shock, hypoxia, or beriberi.
- **I.V. use:** Add sodium lactate to other I.V. solutions, or give as an isotonic ⅙ molar solution. Drug is compatible with most common I.V. solutions.
- Do not mix with sodium bicarbonate; the drugs are incompatible.
- Monitor serum electrolyte levels to avoid alkalosis.

☑ **PATIENT TEACHING**
- Explain use and administration of drug to patient and family.
- Tell patient to report any unusual signs and symptoms.

---

## tromethamine
Tham

*Pregnancy Risk Category: C*

**HOW SUPPLIED**
*Injection:* 18 g/500 ml

**ACTION**
Combines with hydrogen ions and associated acid anions; resulting salts are excreted. Also has osmotic diuretic effect.

**ONSET, PEAK, DURATION**
Onset and peak are immediately after I.V. infusion. Duration unknown.

**INDICATIONS & DOSAGE**
*Metabolic acidosis associated with cardiac bypass surgery or with cardiac arrest –*
**Adults:** dosage depends on bicarbonate deficit. Calculate as follows: Each ml of 0.3 M tromethamine solution required = weight in kg × bicarbonate deficit (mEq/L). Additional therapy based on serial determinations of existing bicarbonate deficit.
**Children:** calculate dosage as above. Give slowly over 3 to 6 hours. Additional therapy based on degree of acidosis. Total 24-hour dosage should not exceed 33 to 40 ml/kg.

**ADVERSE REACTIONS**
**Respiratory:** *respiratory depression.*
**Other:** hypoglycemia, *hyperkalemia* (with decreased urine output), venospasm; I.V. thrombosis; inflammation, necrosis, and sloughing (if extravasation occurs); hemorrhagic hepatic necrosis.

**INTERACTIONS**
None significant.

**CONTRAINDICATIONS**
Contraindicated in patients with anuria, uremia, or chronic respiratory acidosis, or during pregnancy (except in acute, life-threatening situations).

**NURSING CONSIDERATIONS**
- Use cautiously in patients with renal disease and poor urine output. Monitor ECG and serum potassium levels.
- Make these determinations before, during, and after therapy: blood pH; carbon dioxide tension; bicarbonate, glucose, and electrolyte levels.
- **I.V. use:** Give slowly through 18G to 20G needle into largest antecubital vein, or by indwelling I.V. catheter.
- Be aware that drug should not be used longer than 1 day except in life-threatening situations.
- In patients with associated respiratory acidosis, have mechanical ventilation available.
- To prevent blood pH from rising above normal, be prepared to adjust dosage carefully, as ordered.
- If extravasation occurs, infiltrate area with 1% procaine and 150 units hyaluronidase, as ordered; may reduce vasospasm and dilute remaining drug locally.

☑ **PATIENT TEACHING**
- Explain use of drug to patient and family.
- Tell them to report reactions.

---

*Liquid form contains alcohol.   **May contain tartrazine.   †Canada only.   ‡Australia only.   ◇OTC.

**ferrous fumarate**
**ferrous gluconate**
**ferrous sulfate**
**ferrous sulfate, dried**
**iron dextran**
**polysaccharide iron complex**

### COMBINATION PRODUCTS
FERGON PLUS: ferrous gluconate 58 mg, vitamin B$_{12}$ ½ NF unit with intrinsic factor, and vitamin C 75 mg.
FEROCYL◊: ferrous fumarate 50 mg and docusate sodium 100 mg.
FERRO-DOCUSATE-T.R., FERRO-DOK TR, FERRO-DSS: ferrous fumarate 150 mg and docusate sodium 100 mg.
FERRO-SEQUELS◊: ferrous fumarate 50 mg and docusate sodium 100 mg.

---

### ferrous fumarate
Femiron◊, Feostat◊, Feostat Drops◊, Fumasorb◊, Fumerin◊, Hemocyte◊, Ircon◊, Nephro-Fer◊, Novofumar†, Palafer†, Palafer Pediatric Drops†, Span-FF◊

*Pregnancy Risk Category: A*

### HOW SUPPLIED
Each 100 mg of ferrous fumarate provides 33 mg of elemental iron.
*Tablets*◊: 63 mg, 195 mg, 200 mg, 300 mg, 324 mg, 325 mg, 350 mg
*Tablets (chewable)*: 100 mg◊
*Capsules (extended-release)*: 325 mg◊
*Oral suspension*: 100 mg/5 ml◊
*Drops*: 45 mg/0.6 ml◊

### ACTION
Provides elemental iron, an essential component in the formation of hemoglobin.

### ONSET, PEAK, DURATION
Onset occurs within 4 days. Peak effects occur in 7 to 10 days. Effects persist for 2 to 4 months.

### INDICATIONS & DOSAGE
*Iron deficiency –*
**Adults:** 200 mg P.O. t.i.d. or q.i.d.
**Children:** 3 mg/kg P.O. t.i.d., increased to 6 mg/kg P.O. t.i.d., as needed and tolerated.

### ADVERSE REACTIONS
**GI:** *nausea,* epigastric pain, vomiting, *constipation,* diarrhea, black stools, anorexia.
**Other:** suspension and drops may temporarily stain teeth.

### INTERACTIONS
*Antacids, cholestyramine resin, cimetidine, fluoroquinolones, levodopa, penicillamine, tetracycline, vitamin E:* decreased iron absorption. Separate doses by 2 to 4 hours.
*Chloramphenicol, vitamin C:* may increase iron absorption. Beneficial drug interaction.
*L-thyroxine:* decreased L-thyroxine absorption. Separate doses by at least 2 hours. Monitor thyroid function.
*Levodopa, methyldopa:* decreased absorption and efficacy of levodopa and methyldopa. Monitor for decreased effect of these agents.

### CONTRAINDICATIONS
Contraindicated in patients with primary hemochromatosis or hemosiderosis, in patients with hemolytic anemia unless iron deficiency anemia is also present, in those receiving repeated blood transfusions, and in patients with peptic ulcer disease, regional enteritis, or ulcerative colitis.

---

## NURSING CONSIDERATIONS
- Use cautiously on long-term basis.
- Keep in mind that GI upset may be related to dose. Between-meal doses are preferable, but can be given with some foods, although absorption may be decreased. Enteric-coated products reduce GI upset but also reduce amount of iron absorbed.
- Check for constipation; record color and amount of stools.
- Be aware that oral iron may turn stools black. Although this unabsorbed iron is harmless, it could mask the presence of melena.
- Monitor hemoglobin and hematocrit levels and reticulocyte count during therapy, as ordered.
- Know that combination products, such as Ferro-Sequels and Ferocyl, contain stool softeners, which help prevent constipation, a common adverse reaction.

### ☑ PATIENT TEACHING
- Tell patient to take tablets with juice (preferably orange juice) or water, but not with milk or antacids.
- To avoid staining teeth, tell patient to take suspension with straw and place drops at back of throat.
- Caution patient not to crush tablets, or allow the patient to chew extended-release iron preparations.
- If patient misses a dose, tell him to take it as soon as he remembers but not to double-dose.
- Advise patient to avoid certain foods that may impair oral iron absorption, including yogurt, cheese, eggs, milk, whole-grain breads and cereals, tea, and coffee.
- Inform parents that as little as three or four tablets can cause serious poisoning in children.

# ferrous gluconate
Fergon*◇, Ferralet◇, Ferralet Slow Release◇, Fertinic†, Novoferrogluc†, Simron◇

*Pregnancy Risk Category: A*

## HOW SUPPLIED
Each 100 mg of ferrous gluconate provides 11.6 mg of elemental iron.
*Tablets:* 300 mg◇, 320 mg◇, 325 mg◇
*Capsules:* 86 mg◇
*Elixir:* 300 mg/5 ml*◇

## ACTION
Provides elemental iron, an essential component in the formation of hemoglobin.

## ONSET, PEAK, DURATION
Onset occurs in 4 days. Peak effects occur in 7 to 10 days. Effects persist for 2 to 4 months.

## INDICATIONS & DOSAGE
*Iron deficiency –*
**Adults:** 300 to 325 mg P.O. q.i.d., increased to 650 mg q.i.d., as needed and tolerated.
**Children 2 years and over:** 8 mg/kg P.O. daily t.i.d., increased up to 16 mg P.O. t.i.d. as needed and tolerated.

## ADVERSE REACTIONS
**GI:** *nausea,* epigastric pain, vomiting, *constipation,* diarrhea, *black stools,* anorexia.
**Other:** elixir may temporarily stain teeth.

## INTERACTIONS
*Antacids, cholestyramine resin, cimetidine, fluoroquinolones, levodopa, penicillamine, tetracycline, vitamin E:* decreased iron absorption. Separate doses by at least 2 hours.
*Chloramphenicol, vitamin C:* may increase iron absorption. Beneficial drug interaction.
*L-thyroxine:* decreased L-thyroxine

absorption. Separate doses by at least 2 hours. Monitor thyroid function.

*Levodopa, methyldopa:* decreased absorption and efficacy of levodopa and methyldopa. Monitor for decreased effect of these agents.

## CONTRAINDICATIONS

Contraindicated in patients with peptic ulceration, regional enteritis, ulcerative colitis, hemosiderosis, and primary hemochromatosis; in patients with hemolytic anemia unless an iron deficiency anemia is also present; and in patients receiving repeated blood transfusions.

## NURSING CONSIDERATIONS

• Use cautiously on long-term basis.
• Keep in mind that GI upset may be related to dose. Between-meal doses are preferable, but can be given with some foods, although absorption may be decreased. Enteric-coated products reduce GI upset but also reduce amount of iron absorbed.
• Check for constipation; record color and amount of stools.
• Be aware that oral iron may turn stools black. This unabsorbed iron is harmless; however, it could mask melena.
• Monitor hemoglobin and hematocrit levels and reticulocyte count during therapy.

## ☑ PATIENT TEACHING

• Instruct patient to dilute liquid preparations in juice (preferably orange juice) or water, but not in milk or antacids. To promote absorption, tell patient to take tablets with orange juice.
• To avoid staining teeth, tell patient to take elixir with straw; the patient may take with water or fruit juice.
• If patient misses a dose, tell him to take it as soon as he remembers but not to double-dose.
• Advise patient to avoid certain

foods that may impair oral iron absorption, including yogurt, cheese, eggs, milk, whole-grain breads and cereals, tea, and coffee.
• Inform parents that as little as three or four tablets can cause serious iron poisoning in children.

---

## ferrous sulfate

Apo-Ferrous Sulfate†, Feosol*◊, Fer-In-Sol Drops*◊, Fer-In-Sol Syrup*◊, Fer-Iron Drops◊, Feritard‡, Fero-Grad†, Fero-Gradumet◊, Ferospace◊, Mol-Iron*◊

## ferrous sulfate, dried

Feosol◊, Fer-In-Sol◊, Ferra-TD◊, Ferralyn Lanacaps◊, Mol-Iron*◊, Novoferrosulfa†, PMS Ferrous Sulfate†, Slow-Fe◊

*Pregnancy Risk Category: A*

## HOW SUPPLIED

Ferrous sulfate is 20% elemental iron; dried and powdered, about 32% elemental iron.
*Tablets:* 195 mg◊, 300 mg◊, 324 mg◊; 200 mg (dried)
*Tablets (extended-release):* 159 mg (dried)◊, 525 mg
*Capsules:* 190 mg (dried), 250 mg◊
*Capsules (extended-release):* 150 mg (dried)◊, 159 mg (dried)◊
*Elixir:* 220 mg/5 ml*◊
*Syrup:* 90 mg/5 ml◊
*Solution:* 300 mg/5 ml
*Drops:* 125 mg/ml

## ACTION

Provides elemental iron, an essential component in the formation of hemoglobin.

## ONSET, PEAK, DURATION

Onset occurs within 4 days. Peak effects occur within 7 to 10 days. Effects persist for 2 to 4 months.

---

## INDICATIONS & DOSAGE
*Iron deficiency –*
**Adults:** 325 mg P.O. t.i.d. or q.i.d. Alternatively, 1 extended-release capsule (160 to 525 mg) P.O. b.i.d.
**Children:** 5 to 10 mg/kg P.O. t.i.d.

## ADVERSE REACTIONS
**GI:** *nausea,* epigastric pain, vomiting, *constipation, black stools,* diarrhea, anorexia.
**Other:** liquid forms may temporarily stain teeth.

## INTERACTIONS
*Antacids, cholestyramine resin, cimetidine, fluoroquinolones, levodopa, penicillamine, tetracycline, vitamin E:* decreased iron absorption. Separate doses if possible.
*Chloramphenicol, vitamin C:* may increase iron absorption. Beneficial drug interaction.
*L-thyroxine:* decreased L-thyroxine absorption. Separate doses by at least 2 hours. Monitor thyroid function.
*Levodopa, methyldopa:* decreased absorption and efficacy of levodopa and methyldopa. Monitor for decreased effect of these agents.

## CONTRAINDICATIONS
Contraindicated in patients with hemosiderosis and primary hemochromatosis; in those with hemolytic anemia unless iron deficiency anemia is also present; in those with peptic ulceration, ulcerative colitis, and regional enteritis; and in patients receiving repeated blood transfusions.

## NURSING CONSIDERATIONS
• Use cautiously on long-term basis.
• Keep in mind that GI upset may be related to dose. Between-meal doses are preferable, but can be given with some foods, although absorption may be decreased. Enteric-coated products reduce GI upset but also reduce amount of iron absorbed.

• Check for constipation; record color and amount of stools.
• Be aware that oral iron may turn stools black. Although this unabsorbed iron is harmless, it could mask melena.
• Monitor hemoglobin and hematocrit levels and reticulocyte count during therapy, as ordered.

## ☑ PATIENT TEACHING
• Tell patient to dilute liquid preparations in juice (preferably orange juice) or water, but not in milk or antacids. To promote iron absorption, tell patient to take tablets with orange juice.
• To avoid staining teeth, tell patient to take elixir with straw and place in back of throat.
• Instruct patient not to crush or chew extended-release preparations.
• If patient misses a dose, tell him to take it as soon as he remembers but not to double-dose.
• Advise patient to avoid certain foods that may impair oral iron absorption, including yogurt, cheese, eggs, milk, whole-grain breads and cereals, tea, and coffee.
• Inform parents that as little as three to four tablets can cause serious iron poisoning in children.

---

## iron dextran
Imferon†, InFeD
*Pregnancy Risk Category: NR*

## HOW SUPPLIED
1 ml iron dextran provides 50 mg elemental iron.
*Injection:* 50 mg elemental iron/ml

## ACTION
Provides elemental iron, an essential component in the formation of hemoglobin.

## ONSET, PEAK, DURATION
Not clearly defined.

## INDICATIONS & DOSAGE

*Iron deficiency anemia –*

**Adults and children:** I.M. or I.V. test dose required before administration. *I.M. (by Z-track method):* 0.5 ml test dose injected. If no reactions occur, daily dosage should ordinarily not exceed 0.5 ml (25 mg) for infants under 5 kg; 1 ml (50 mg) for children under 10 kg; 2 ml (100 mg) for heavier children and adults.

**I.V.:** 0.5 ml test dose injected over 30 seconds. If no reactions occur in 1 hour, remainder of therapeutic I.V. dose is given. Therapeutic dose repeated I.V. daily. Single dose should not exceed 100 mg. Give slowly (1 ml/minute).

## ADVERSE REACTIONS

**CNS:** headache, transitory paresthesia, arthralgia, myalgia, dizziness, malaise.
**CV:** *hypotensive reaction, peripheral vascular flushing with overly rapid I.V. administration.*
**GI:** nausea, anorexia.
**Respiratory:** *bronchospasm,* dyspnea.
**Skin:** rash, urticaria.
**Other:** *soreness and inflammation at I.M. injection site; brown skin discoloration at I.M. injection site; local phlebitis at I.V. injection site,* sterile abscess, necrosis, atrophy, fibrosis, *anaphylaxis,* delayed sensitivity reactions, fever, chills.

## INTERACTIONS

None significant.

## CONTRAINDICATIONS

Contraindicated in patients with hypersensitivity to the drug, in those with all anemias except iron deficiency anemia, and in those with acute infectious renal disease.

## NURSING CONSIDERATIONS

• Do not administer iron dextran concomitantly with oral iron preparations.
• Use with extreme caution in patients with serious hepatic impairment, rheumatoid arthritis, and other inflammatory diseases because these patients may be at higher risk for certain delays and reactions.
• Use cautiously in patients with a history of significant allergies or asthma.
• **I.V. use:** Check hospital policy before administering I.V.
• Keep in mind that I.M. or I.V. injections of iron are advisable only for patients for whom oral administration is impossible or ineffective. Use I.V. in the following situations: insufficient muscle mass for deep I.M. injection; impaired absorption from muscle due to stasis or edema; possibility of uncontrolled I.M. bleeding from trauma (as may occur in hemophilia); and with massive and prolonged parenteral therapy (as may be necessary in cases of chronic substantial blood loss).
• Upon completion of I.V. dose, flush the vein with 10 ml of 0.9% sodium chloride solution. The patient should rest 15 to 30 minutes after I.V. administration.
• For I.M. route, inject deeply into upper outer quadrant of buttock — never into arm or other exposed area — with a 2″ to 3″ 19G or 20G needle. Use Z-track method to avoid leakage into S.C. tissue and staining of skin.
• Minimize skin staining by using a separate needle to withdraw the drug from its container.
• Monitor the patient's vital signs for drug reactions, which range from pain, inflammation, and myalgia to hypotension, shock, and death.
• Monitor hemoglobin and hematocrit levels and reticulocyte count, as ordered.

---

Reactions may be *common,* uncommon, *life-threatening,* or COMMON AND LIFE-THREATENING.

## ☑ PATIENT TEACHING
• Advise the patient to avoid OTC vitamins that contain iron.
• Teach the patient symptoms of hypersensitivity or iron toxicity and to report them.

---

# polysaccharide iron complex
Hytinic, Niferex, Niferex-150, Nu-Iron, Nu-Iron-150

*Pregnancy Risk Category: NR*

## HOW SUPPLIED
*Capsules:* 150 mg
*Solution:* 100 mg/5 ml
*Tablets (film-coated):* 50 mg

## ACTION
Provides elemental iron, an essential component in the formation of hemoglobin.

## ONSET, PEAK, DURATION
Onset occurs within a few days. Peak reticulocyte effects occur in 5 to 10 days and hemoglobin concentrations rise after 2 to 4 weeks. Normal hemoglobin values are usually attained in 2 months unless blood loss continues.

## INDICATIONS & DOSAGE
*Treatment of uncomplicated iron deficiency anemia –*
**Adults and children 12 years and over:** 150 to 300 mg P.O. as capsules or tablets daily or 1 to 2 tsp of elixir P.O. daily.
**Children 6 to 12 years:** 150 mg to 300 mg P.O. as tablets or 1 tsp of elixir P.O. daily.
**Children 2 to 6 years:** ½ tsp P.O. daily.

## ADVERSE REACTIONS
Although nausea, constipation, black stools, and epigastric pain are common adverse reactions associated with iron therapy, few, if any, occur with polysaccharide iron complex.

## INTERACTIONS
*Antacids, cholestyramine resin, cimetidine, tetracycline, vitamin E:* decreased iron absorption. Separate doses by 2 to 4 hours.
*Chloramphenicol:* delayed response to iron therapy. Monitor patient.
*Fluoroquinolones, levodopa, methyldopa, penicillamine:* decreased GI absorption, possibly resulting in decreased serum levels or efficacy. Separate doses if possible.
*Levodopa, methyldopa:* decreased absorption and efficacy of levodopa and methyldopa. Monitor for decreased effect of these agents.
*Vitamin C:* may increase iron absorption, a beneficial drug interaction.

## CONTRAINDICATIONS
Contraindicated in patients with hypersensitivity to any component of the drug and in those with hemochromatosis and hemosiderosis.

## NURSING CONSIDERATIONS
• Check for constipation; record color and amount of stools.
• Know that oral iron may turn stools black. This unabsorbed iron is harmless; however, it may mask melena.
• Monitor hemoglobin and hematocrit values and reticulocyte count during therapy.

## ☑ PATIENT TEACHING
• Tell patient to take with juice (preferably orange juice) or water but not with milk or antacids.
• If patient misses a dose, tell him to take it as soon as he remembers but not to double-dose.
• Advise patient to avoid certain foods that may impair oral iron absorption, including yogurt, cheese, eggs, milk, whole-grain breads and cereals, tea, and coffee.
• Inform parents that as few as three tablets can cause serious iron poisoning in children.

---

*Liquid form contains alcohol.  **May contain tartrazine.  †Canada only.  ‡Australia only.  ◊OTC.

dalteparin sodium
enoxaparin sodium
heparin calcium
heparin sodium
warfarin sodium

**COMBINATION PRODUCTS**
None.

---

## dalteparin sodium
Fragmin

*Pregnancy Risk Category: B*

### HOW SUPPLIED
*Syringe:* 2,500 anti-factor Xa IU/0.2 ml

### ACTION
A low-molecular-weight heparin derivative that enhances the inhibition of factor Xa and thrombin by antithrombin.

### ONSET, PEAK, DURATION
Onset and duration unknown. Peak anti-factor Xa activity is obtained in about 4 hours.

### INDICATIONS & DOSAGE
*Prophylaxis against deep vein thrombosis in patients undergoing abdominal surgery who are at risk for thromboembolic complications –*
**Adults:** 2,500 IU S.C. daily, starting 1 to 2 hours prior to surgery and repeated once daily for 5 to 10 days postoperatively.

### ADVERSE REACTIONS
**Hematologic:** *thrombocytopenia.*
**Skin:** pruritus, rash, *hematoma at injection site,* pain or skin necrosis (rare) at injection site.
**Other:** hemorrhage, ecchymoses, bleeding complications, fever, *anaphylactoid reactions* (rare).

### INTERACTIONS
*Oral anticoagulants, antiplatelet agents:* May increase risk of bleeding. Use together cautiously.

### CONTRAINDICATIONS
Contraindicated in patients with hypersensitivity to the drug, heparin, or pork products; active major bleeding; or thrombocytopenia associated with positive in vitro tests for antiplatelet antibody in the presence of the drug.

### NURSING CONSIDERATIONS
● Use with extreme caution in patients with history of heparin-induced thrombocytopenia and in those at increased risk for hemorrhage, such as those with severe uncontrolled hypertension, bacterial endocarditis, congenital or acquired bleeding disorders, active ulceration and angiodysplastic GI disease, or hemorrhagic stroke or shortly after brain, spinal, or ophthalmologic surgery.
● Use with caution in patients with bleeding diathesis, thrombocytopenia, platelet defects, severe liver or kidney insufficiency, hypertensive or diabetic retinopathy, and recent GI bleeding.
● Know that patients who are candidates for dalteparin therapy are those who are at risk for deep vein thrombosis, including patients who are over age 40, obese, undergoing surgery under general anesthesia lasting longer than 30 minutes, or have additional risk factors (such as malignancy or a history of deep vein thrombosis or pulmonary embolism).
● Have patient assume a sitting or supine position when administering the drug. Give S.C. injection deeply. Injection sites include a U-shaped area around the navel, upper outer side of

---

Reactions may be *common,* uncommon, *life-threatening,* or **COMMON AND LIFE-THREATENING.**

thigh, and upper outer quadrangle of buttock. Rotate sites daily. When the area around the navel or the thigh is used, use thumb and forefinger to lift up a fold of skin while giving the injection. The entire length of the needle should be inserted at a 45- to 90-degree angle.

• Never administer the drug I.M.

• Do not mix with other injections or infusions unless specific compatibility data support such mixing.

• *Alert:* Be aware that drug is not interchangeable (unit for unit) with unfractionated heparin or other low-molecular-weight heparin.

• Know that periodic, routine CBCs (including platelet count) and fecal occult blood tests are recommended during the course of treatment. Patients do not require regular monitoring of PT or activated PTT.

• Monitor patient closely for thrombocytopenia.

• Be aware that the drug should be discontinued if a thromboembolic event occurs despite dalteparin prophylaxis.

### ☑ PATIENT TEACHING

• Instruct the patient and family to watch for and report signs of bleeding.

• Tell patient to avoid OTC drugs containing aspirin or other salicylates.

---

## enoxaparin sodium
Lovenox

*Pregnancy Risk Category: B*

### HOW SUPPLIED
*Injection:* 30 mg per 0.3 ml

### ACTION
A low-molecular weight heparin derivative that accelerates formation of antithrombin III-thrombin complex and deactivates thrombin, preventing conversion of fibrinogen to fibrin. En-

oxaparin has a higher anti-factor Xa-to anti-factor IIa-activity ratio.

### ONSET, PEAK, DURATION
Onset unknown. Peak effects occur 3 to 5 hours after S.C. injection. Effects persist up to 24 hours.

### INDICATIONS & DOSAGE
*To prevent pulmonary embolism and deep vein thrombosis after hip or knee replacement surgery —*
**Adults:** 30 mg S.C. b.i.d. for 7 to 10 days. Initial dose given as soon as possible after surgery, but no later than 24 hours postoperatively.

### ADVERSE REACTIONS
**CNS:** confusion.
**CV:** edema, peripheral edema.
**GI:** nausea.
**Hematologic:** hypochromic anemia, ***thrombocytopenia.***
**Other:** irritation, pain, hematoma, or erythema at the injection site; fever; pain; ***hemorrhage;*** ecchymoses; bleeding complications.

### INTERACTIONS
*Anticoagulants, antiplatelet agents:* increased risk of bleeding. Don't use together.

### CONTRAINDICATIONS
Contraindicated in patients with hypersensitivity to the drug or to heparin or pork products; in patients with active, major bleeding or thrombocytopenia; and in those who demonstrate antiplatelet antibodies in the presence of the drug.

### NURSING CONSIDERATIONS
• Use with extreme caution in patients with a history of heparin-induced thrombocytopenia.

• Use cautiously in patients with conditions that put them at increased risk for hemorrhage, such as bacterial endocarditis; congenital or acquired bleeding disorders; ulcer disease; an-

---

*Liquid form contains alcohol.   **May contain tartrazine.   †Canada only.   ‡Australia only.   ◊OTC.

giodysplastic GI disease; hemorrhagic stroke; or recent spinal, eye, or brain surgery.

• Draw blood to establish baseline coagulation parameters before therapy.

• Never administer the drug I.M.

• Don't massage after S.C. injection. Watch for signs of bleeding at site. Rotate sites and keep record.

• Avoid excessive I.M. injections of other drugs to prevent or minimize hematomas. If possible, don't give I.M. injections at all.

• Monitor platelet counts regularly. Patients with normal coagulation won't require close monitoring of PT or PTT.

• Regularly inspect the patient for bleeding gums, bruises on arms or legs, petechiae, nosebleeds, melena, tarry stools, hematuria, hematemesis.

• To treat severe overdose, give protamine sulfate (a heparin antagonist) by slow I.V. infusion at a concentration of 1% to equal the dosage of enoxaparin injected, as ordered.

☑ **PATIENT TEACHING**

• Instruct the patient and his family to watch for signs of bleeding and to notify the doctor immediately.

• Tell patient to avoid OTC drugs containing aspirin or other salicylates.

# heparin calcium
Calcilean†, Calciparine, Caprin‡, Uniparin-Ca‡

# heparin sodium
Hepalean†, Heparin Leo†, Heparin Lock Flush Solution (with Tubex), Hep-Lock, Liquaemin Sodium, Uniparin‡

*Pregnancy Risk Category: C*

## HOW SUPPLIED
Products are derived from beef lung or porcine intestinal mucosa.
**heparin calcium**
*Ampule:* 12,500 units/0.5 ml; 20,000 units/0.8 ml
*Syringe:* 5,000 units/0.2 ml
**heparin sodium**
*Carpuject:* 5,000 units/ml
*Disposable syringes:* 1,000 units/ml, 2,500 units/ml, 5,000 units/ml, 7,500 units/ml, 10,000 units/ml, 15,000 units/ml, 20,000 units/ml, 40,000 units/ml
*Premixed I.V. solutions:* 1,000 units in 500 ml of 0.9% sodium chloride solution; 2,000 units in 1,000 ml of 0.9% sodium chloride solution; 12,500 units in 250 ml of 0.45% sodium chloride solution; 25,000 units in 250 ml of 0.45% sodium chloride solution; 25,000 units in 500 ml of 0.45% sodium chloride solution; 10,000 units in 100 ml of $D_5W$; 12,500 units in 250 ml of $D_5W$; 25,000 units in 250 ml $D_5W$; 25,000 units in 500 ml $D_5W$; 20,000 units in 500 ml of $D_5W$
*Unit-dose ampules:* 1,000 units/ml, 5,000 units/ml, 10,000 units/ml
*Vials:* 1,000 units/ml, 2,500 units/ml, 5,000 units/ml, 7,500 units/ml, 10,000 units/ml, 15,000 units/ml, 20,000 units/ml, 40,000 units/ml
**heparin sodium flush**
*Disposable syringes:* 10 units/ml, 100 units/ml
*Vials:* 10 units/ml, 100 units/ml

## ACTION
Accelerates formation of antithrombin III-thrombin complex and deactivates thrombin, preventing conversion of fibrinogen to fibrin.

## ONSET, PEAK, DURATION
Onset occurs in 20 to 60 minutes after S.C. administration, immediately after I.V. injection. Plasma levels peak 2 to 4 hours after S.C. injection. Correlation between plasma level and drug effect is poor; heparin is rapidly cleared from plasma within ½ to 3 hours, but its duration of action is dose-dependent.

---

Reactions may be *common*, uncommon, *life-threatening*, or COMMON AND LIFE-THREATENING.

## INDICATIONS & DOSAGE

Heparin dosing is highly individualized, depending upon disease state, age, and renal and hepatic status.

*Deep vein thrombosis, MI—*
**Adults:** initially, 5,000 to 7,500 units I.V. push, then adjusted according to PTT and given I.V. q 4 hours (usually 4,000 to 5,000 units); or 5,000 to 7,500 units I.V. bolus, then 1,000 units/hour by I.V. infusion pump. Hourly rate adjusted 8 hours after bolus dose according to PTT.

*Pulmonary embolism; consumptive coagulopathy (such as disseminated intravascular coagulation)—*
**Adults:** initially, 7,500 to 10,000 units I.V. push, then adjusted according to PTT and given I.V. q 4 hours (usually 4,000 to 5,000 units); or 7,500 to 10,000 units I.V. bolus, then 1,000 units/hour by I.V. infusion pump. Hourly rate adjusted 8 hours after bolus dose according to PTT.

**Children:** initially, 50 units/kg I.V. drip. Maintenance dosage is 100 units/kg I.V. drip q 4 hours. Constant infusion: 20,000 units/m² daily. Dosages adjusted according to PTT.

*Prevention of embolism, venous thrombosis, pulmonary embolism, atrial fibrillation with embolism; postoperative deep vein thrombosis—*
**Adults:** 5,000 units S.C. q 12 hours. In surgical patients, first dose given 2 hours before procedure; followed with 5,000 units S.C. q 8 to 12 hours for 5 to 7 days or until patient can walk.

*Open-heart surgery—*
**Adults:** (total body perfusion) 150 to 300 units/kg continuous I.V infusion.

*Patency maintenance of I.V. indwelling catheters—*
**Adults:** 10 to 100 units I.V. flush. Use sufficient volume to fill the device. Not intended for therapeutic use.

## ADVERSE REACTIONS

**Hematologic:** *hemorrhage* (with excessive dosage), *overly prolonged clotting time,* **thrombocytopenia.**

**Other:** irritation; mild pain; hematoma; ulceration; cutaneous or subcutaneous necrosis; *"white clot" syndrome;* hypersensitivity reactions, including chills, fever, pruritus, rhinitis, urticaria, anaphylactoid reactions.

## INTERACTIONS

*Anticoagulants, oral:* increased additive anticoagulation. Monitor PT and PTT.

*Salicylates, other antiplatelet agents:* increased anticoagulant effect. Don't use together.

*Thrombolytics:* increased risk of hemorrhage. Monitor closely.

## CONTRAINDICATIONS

Contraindicated in patients hypersensitive to the drug. Conditionally contraindicated in patients with active bleeding; blood dyscrasia; or bleeding tendencies, such as hemophilia, thrombocytopenia, or hepatic disease with hypoprothrombinemia; suspected intracranial hemorrhage; suppurative thrombophlebitis; inaccessible ulcerative lesions (especially of GI tract) and open ulcerative wounds; extensive denudation of skin; ascorbic acid deficiency and other conditions that cause increased capillary permeability; during or after brain, eye, or spinal cord surgery; during spinal tap or spinal anesthesia; during continuous tube drainage of stomach or small intestine; in subacute bacterial endocarditis; shock; advanced renal disease; threatened abortion; severe hypertension.

Although heparin use is clearly hazardous in these conditions, its risks and its benefits must be evaluated.

## NURSING CONSIDERATIONS

● Use cautiously during menses; in patients with mild hepatic or renal disease, alcoholism, occupations with high risk of physical injury; immediately postpartum; and in patients with history of allergies, asthma, or GI ulcerations.

• Draw blood to establish baseline coagulation parameters before therapy.

• Know that when the patient requires anticoagulation during pregnancy, most clinicians use heparin.

• Keep in mind that drug requirements are higher in early phases of thrombogenic diseases and febrile states; lower when the patient's condition stabilizes.

• Be aware that elderly patients should usually start at lower doses.

• Check order and vial carefully. Heparin comes in various concentrations.

• Give low-dose injections sequentially between iliac crests in lower abdomen deep into S.C. fat. Inject drug S.C. slowly into fat pad. Leave needle in place for 10 seconds after injection; then withdraw needle. Don't massage after S.C. injection, and watch for signs of bleeding at injection site. Alternate sites every 12 hours—right for morning, left for evening.

• **I.V. use:** Administer I.V. using infusion pump to provide maximum safety because of long-term effect and irregular absorption when given S.C. Check constant I.V. infusions regularly, even when pumps are in good working order, to prevent overdosage or underdosage. Place notice above the patient's bed to inform I.V. team or laboratory personnel to apply pressure dressings after taking blood.

• During intermittent I.V. therapy, always draw blood ½ hour before next scheduled dose to avoid falsely elevated PTT. Blood for PTT may be drawn any time after 8 hours of initiation of continuous I.V. heparin therapy. Blood for PTT should never be drawn from the I.V. tubing of the heparin infusion or from the infused vein. Falsely elevated PTT will result. Always draw blood from the opposite arm.

• Don't skip a dose or "catch up" with an I.V. containing heparin. If I.V. runs out, restart it as soon as possible, and reschedule bolus dose immediately.

• Know that concentrated heparin solutions (greater than 100 units/ml) can irritate blood vessels.

• Never piggyback other drugs into an infusion line while the heparin infusion is running. Many antibiotics and other drugs deactivate heparin. Never mix another drug and heparin in the same syringe when giving a bolus.

• Avoid excessive I.M. injections of other drugs to prevent or minimize hematomas. If possible, don't give I.M. injections at all.

• Measure PTT carefully and regularly. Anticoagulation is present when PTT values are one and one-half to two times the control values.

• Monitor platelet count regularly. Thrombocytopenia caused by heparin may be associated with a type of arterial thrombosis known as "white clot" syndrome.

• Regularly inspect the patient for bleeding gums, bruises on arms or legs, petechiae, nosebleeds, melena, tarry stools, hematuria, hematemesis.

• **Alert:** To treat severe heparin calcium or heparin sodium overdose, use protamine sulfate, a heparin antagonist, as ordered. Dosage is based on the dose of heparin, its route of administration, and the time elapsed since it was given. As a general rule, 1 to 1.5 units of protamine/100 units of heparin is given if only a few minutes have elapsed; 0.5 to 0.75 mg protamine/100 units heparin if 30 to 60 minutes have elapsed, 0.25 to 0.375 mg protamine/100 units heparin if 2 hours or more have elapsed.

• Know that abrupt withdrawal may cause increased coagulability, and heparin therapy is usually followed by oral anticoagulants for prophylaxis.

---

Reactions may be *common,* uncommon, *life-threatening,* or **COMMON AND LIFE-THREATENING.**

## ☑ PATIENT TEACHING

• Instruct the patient and his family to watch for signs of bleeding and notify the doctor immediately.
• Tell the patient to avoid OTC medications containing aspirin, other salicylates, or drugs that may interact with heparin.

---

## warfarin sodium
Coumadin, Panwarfin, Sofarin, Warfilone Sodium†

*Pregnancy Risk Category: X*

### HOW SUPPLIED
*Tablets:* 1 mg, 2 mg, 2.5 mg, 4 mg, 5 mg, 7.5 mg, 10 mg

### ACTION
Inhibits vitamin K-dependent activation of clotting factors II, VII, IX, and X, formed in the liver.

### ONSET, PEAK, DURATION
Onset occurs in ½ to 3 days. Peak unknown. Effects persist for 2 to 5 days.

### INDICATIONS & DOSAGE
*Pulmonary embolism associated with deep vein thrombosis, M.I., rheumatic heart disease with heart valve damage, prosthetic heart valves, chronic atrial fibrillation –*
**Adults:** 10 to 15 mg P.O. for 2 to 4 days, then dosage based on daily PT. Usual maintenance dosage is 2 to 10 mg P.O. daily.

### ADVERSE REACTIONS
**GI:** anorexia, nausea, vomiting, cramps, *diarrhea,* mouth ulcerations, sore mouth.
**GU:** hematuria.
**Hematologic:** *hemorrhage* (with excessive dosage).
**Hepatic:** hepatitis, elevated liver function tests, jaundice.
**Skin:** dermatitis, urticaria, necrosis, gangrene, alopecia, *rash.*
**Other:** *fever.*

### INTERACTIONS
*Acetaminophen:* may increase bleeding with long-term (longer than 2 weeks) therapy with high doses (more than 2 g/day) of acetaminophen. Monitor very carefully.
*Allopurinol, amiodarone, anabolic steroids, cephalosporins, chloramphenicol, cimetidine, ciprofloxacin, clofibrate, danazol, diazoxide, diflunisal, disulfiram, erythromycin, ethacrynic acid, fenoprofen calcium, fluoroquinolones, glucagon, heparin, ibuprofen, influenza virus vaccine, isoniazid, ketoprofen, lovastatin, meclofenamate, methimazole, methylthiouracil, metronidazole, miconazole, nalidixic acid, neomycin (oral), pentoxifylline, propafenone, propoxyphene, propylthiouracil, quinidine, streptokinase, sulfinpyrazone, sulfonamides, sulindac, tamoxifen, tetracyclines, thiazides, thyroid drugs, tricyclic antidepressants, urokinase, vitamin E:* increased PT. Monitor the patient carefully for bleeding. Consider anticoagulant dosage reduction.
*Barbiturates, carbamazepine, corticosteroids, corticotropin, dicloxacillin, ethchlorvynol, griseofulvin, mercaptopurine, methaqualone, nafcillin, oral contraceptives containing estrogen, rifampin, spironolactone, sulcralfate, trazodone:* decreased PT with reduced anticoagulant effect. Monitor patient carefully.
*Chloral hydrate, glutethimide, sulfinpyrazone, triclofos sodium:* increased or decreased PT. Avoid use if possible, and monitor the patient carefully.
*Cholestyramine:* decreased response when administered too close together. Administer 6 hours after oral anticoagulants.
*Hydantoins:* increased serum levels of hydantoin. Monitor closely.
*Indomethacin, mefenamic acid, salicylates:* increased PT; ulcerogenic effects. Don't use together.
*Sulfonylureas (oral antidiabetic*

---

*Liquid form contains alcohol.   **May contain tartrazine.   †Canada only.   ‡Australia only.   ◇OTC.

*agents):* increased hypoglycemic response. Monitor blood glucose levels. *Foods or enteral products containing vitamin K:* may impair anticoagulation. Patient should maintain consistent daily intake of leafy green vegetables.

## CONTRAINDICATIONS

Contraindicated in pregnancy; in patients with bleeding or hemorrhagic tendencies, GI ulcerations, severe hepatic or renal disease, severe uncontrolled hypertension, subacute bacterial endocarditis, polycythemia vera, and vitamin K deficiency; and after recent eye, brain, or spinal cord surgery.

## NURSING CONSIDERATIONS

• Use cautiously in patients with diverticulitis, colitis, mild or moderate hypertension, mild or moderate hepatic or renal disease, with drainage tubes in any orifice; with regional or lumbar block anesthesia; or in any condition that increases risk of hemorrhage and during lactation.
• Draw blood to establish baseline coagulation parameters before therapy.
• Know that PT determinations are essential for proper control. Doctors typically try to maintain PT at one and one-half to two times normal; high incidence of bleeding when PT exceeds two and one-half times the control values.
• Give warfarin at the same time daily.
• Be aware that I.V. form may be obtained from manufacturer in the rare instances that oral therapy cannot be given. Follow manufacturer guidelines carefully regarding preparation and administration.
• Because onset of action is delayed, keep in mind that heparin sodium is often given during first few days of treatment. When heparin is being given simultaneously, blood for PT should not be drawn within 5 hours of intermittent I.V. heparin administration. However, blood for PT may be

drawn at any time during continuous heparin infusion.
• Regularly inspect the patient for bleeding gums, bruises on arms or legs, petechiae, nosebleeds, melena, tarry stools, hematuria, and hematemesis.
• Observe breast-feeding infants of patients on drug for unexpected bleeding.
• *Alert:* Withhold drug and call the doctor at once if fever or rash (signal severe adverse reactions) occurs.
• Be aware that half-life of warfarin's anticoagulant effect is 36 to 44 hours. Effect can be neutralized by vitamin K injections.
• Know that the drug is the best oral anticoagulant for the patient taking antacids or phenytoin.
• Know that elderly patients and patients with renal or hepatic failure are especially sensitive to warfarin effect.

## ☑ PATIENT TEACHING

• Stress importance of complying with prescribed dosage and follow-up appointments. The patient should carry a card that identifies him as a potential bleeder.
• Tell the patient and his family to watch for signs of bleeding and to call the doctor at once if they occur.
• Warn the patient to avoid OTC products containing aspirin, other salicylates, or drugs that may interact with warfarin.
• Tell the patient to notify the doctor if menses is heavier than usual; may require dosage adjustment.
• Tell the patient to use electric razor when shaving to avoid scratching skin and to use a soft toothbrush.
• Warn the patient to read food labels. Food and enteral feedings that contain vitamin K may impair anticoagulation.
• Tell the patient to eat a daily, consistent amount of leafy green vegetables, which contain vitamin K. Eating different amounts daily may alter anticoagulant effects.

# 67

# Blood derivatives

albumin 5%
albumin 25%
antihemophilic factor
anti-inhibitor coagulant complex
antithrombin III, human
factor IX (human)
factor IX complex
intravascular perfluorochemical
   emulsion
plasma protein fraction

**COMBINATION PRODUCTS**
None.

## albumin 5%
Albuminar 5%, Albutein 5%,
Buminate 5%, Plasbumin 5%

## albumin 25%
Albuminar 25%, Albutein 25%,
Buminate 25%, Plasbumin 25%

*Pregnancy Risk Category: C*

**HOW SUPPLIED**
**albumin 5%**
*Injection:* 50-ml, 250-ml, 500-ml,
1,000-ml vials
**albumin 25%**
*Injection:* 10-ml, 20-ml, 50-ml, 100-
ml vials

**ACTION**
Albumin 5% supplies colloid to the
blood and expands plasma volume.
Albumin 25% provides intravascular
oncotic pressure in a 5:1 ratio, causing
a fluid shift from interstitial spaces to
the circulation and slightly increasing
plasma protein concentration.

**ONSET, PEAK, DURATION**
Onset and peak occur immediately to
within 15 minutes if patient well hydrated. Duration of action depends on
the initial blood volume of the pa-

tient. If blood volume is reduced, volume expansion persists for many
hours; however, if blood volume is
normal, the effect lasts a shorter time.

**INDICATIONS & DOSAGE**
*Hypovolemic shock –*
**Adults:** initially, 500 to 750 ml 5%
solution by I.V. infusion, repeated
q 30 minutes, p.r.n. Alternatively,
100 to 200 ml I.V. of 25% solution,
repeated after 10 to 30 minutes, if
needed. Dosage varies with the patient's condition and response.
**Children:** 12 to 20 ml 5% solution/kg
by I.V. infusion, repeated in 15 to 30
minutes if response is not adequate.
Alternatively, 2.5 to 5 ml I.V. of 25%
solution/kg, repeated after 10 to 30
minutes if needed.
*Hypoproteinemia –*
**Adults:** 1,000 to 1,500 ml 5% solution by I.V. infusion daily, maximum
rate 5 to 10 ml/minute; or 25 to 100 g
25% solution by I.V. infusion daily,
maximum rate 2 ml/minute. Dosage
varies with the patient's condition and
response.
*Hyperbilirubinemia –*
**Infants:** 1 g albumin (4 ml 25%)/kg 1
to 2 hours before transfusion.

**ADVERSE REACTIONS**
**CNS:** headache.
**CV:** *vascular overload after rapid in-
fusion,* hypotension, tachycardia.
**GI:** increased salivation, nausea,
vomiting.
**Respiratory:** altered respiration, dys-
pnea, pulmonary edema.
**Skin:** urticaria, rash.
**Other:** chills, fever, back pain.

**INTERACTIONS**
None significant.

---

*Liquid form contains alcohol.  **May contain tartrazine.  †Canada only.  ‡Australia only.  ◇OTC.

## CONTRAINDICATIONS

Contraindicated in patients with hypersensitivity to the drug.

## NURSING CONSIDERATIONS

• Use with extreme caution in patients with hypertension, cardiac disease, severe pulmonary infection, severe chronic anemia, or hypoalbuminemia with peripheral edema.
• Make sure the patient is properly hydrated before infusion.
• Take care when preparing and administering drug to minimize waste. This product is expensive, and random supply shortages occur often.
• **I.V. use:** Avoid rapid I.V. infusion. Specific rate is individualized according to the patient's age, condition, and diagnosis. Know that 5% albumin is infused undiluted; 25% albumin may be infused undiluted or diluted with sterile water for injection, 0.9% sodium chloride solution, or $D_5W$ injection. Use solution promptly; contains no preservatives. Discard unused solution. Don't use cloudy solutions or those containing sediment. Solution should be clear amber color.
• **Alert:** Do not give more than 250 g in 48 hours.
• Watch for hemorrhage or shock after surgery or injury. Rapid rise in blood pressure may cause bleeding from sites that are not apparent at lower pressures.
• Monitor vital signs carefully.
• Watch for signs of vascular overload (heart failure or pulmonary edema).
• Monitor fluid intake and output and hemoglobin, hematocrit, serum protein, and electrolyte levels during therapy.
• Know that one volume of 25% albumin is equivalent to five volumes of 5% albumin in producing hemodilution and relative anemia.
• Follow storage instructions on bottle. Freezing may cause bottle to break.

## ☑ PATIENT TEACHING

• Explain to patient and family the use and administration of albumin.
• Tell patient to report adverse reactions promptly.

# antihemophilic factor (AHF)
Hemofil M, Humate-P, Hyate:C, Koate-HP, Koate-HS, Monoclate, Monoclate-P, Profilate OSD

*Pregnancy Risk Category: NR*

## HOW SUPPLIED

*Injection:* vials, with diluent. Units specified on label.

## ACTION

Directly replaces deficient clotting factor.

## ONSET, PEAK, DURATION

Onset immediate after I.V. administration. Time to peak effect is 1 to 2 hours after I.V. administration. Duration unknown.

## INDICATIONS & DOSAGE

*Spontaneous hemorrhage in patients with hemophilia A (factor VIII deficiency)* —
**Adults and children:** calculate dosage using this formula:

$$\text{AHF required (IU)} = \text{body weight (kg)} \times \text{desired factor VIII increase (\% of normal)} \times 0.5$$

To prevent spontaneous hemorrhage, the desired level of factor VIII is 5% of normal; for mild hemorrhage, 30% of normal; for moderate hemorrhage and minor surgery, 30% to 50% of normal; for severe hemorrhage, 80% to 100% of normal.
*Treatment of bleeding in patients with hemophilia A (factor VIII deficiency)* —
**Adults and children:** for minor hemorrhage into muscle and joints, 8 to 10 IU/kg I.V. q 8 to 12 hours for 1 or more days. For overt bleeding, an ini-

tial dose of 15 to 25 IU/kg I.V., followed by 8 to 15 IU/kg q 8 to 12 hours for 3 to 4 days. To treat massive bleeding or hemorrhage involving major organs, an initial dose of 40 to 50 IU/kg I.V., followed by 20 to 25 IU/kg I.V. q 8 to 12 hours.

*Prevention of bleeding in hemophilic patients requiring surgery* –
**Adults:** 25 to 30 IU/kg I.V. 1 hour before surgery, followed by one-half of the initial dosage 5 hours later. Dosage adjusted to achieve a level of AHF 80% to 100% of normal during surgery and maintained at 30% to 60% of normal for at least 10 to 14 days postoperatively.

## ADVERSE REACTIONS
**CV:** tightness in chest.
**GI:** nausea.
**Respiratory:** wheezing.
**Skin:** *urticaria.*
**Other:** *chills, fever,* hypersensitivity reactions, (stinging at injection site, fever, ***anaphylaxis***), risk of hepatitis B and HIV.

## INTERACTIONS
None significant.

## CONTRAINDICATIONS
Contraindicated in patients with hypersensitivity to murine (mouse) protein or to the drug.

## NURSING CONSIDERATIONS
• Use cautiously in neonates, infants, and patients with hepatic disease because of their susceptibility to hepatitis, which may be transmitted in antihemophilic factor.
• Monitor coagulation studies before therapy.
• As ordered, administer hepatitis B vaccine before administering antihemophilic factor.
• Refrigerate concentrate until ready to use. Warm concentrate and diluent bottles to room temperature before reconstituting. To mix drug, gently roll vial between hands.
• Use reconstituted solution within 3 hours. Store away from heat and do not refrigerate. Refrigeration after reconstitution may cause the active ingredient to precipitate. Don't shake or mix with other I.V. solutions.
• **I.V. use:** Take baseline pulse rate before I.V. administration. Use plastic syringe; drug may interact with glass syringe and bind to its surface. If pulse rate increases significantly, flow rate should be reduced or administration stopped.
• Do not use S.C. or I.M.
• Monitor vital signs regularly.
• Monitor coagulation studies frequently during therapy.
• Monitor the patient for allergic reactions.
• Be aware that some patients develop inhibitors to factor VIII, resulting in decreased response to the drug.
• Keep in mind that a new porcine product is now available for patients with congenital hemophilia A who have antibodies to human factor VIII:C.
• Keep in mind that risk of hepatitis, including non-A and non-B hepatitis, must be weighed against risk of the patient not receiving the drug.
• Because of the manufacturing process, be aware that the risk of HIV transmission is extremely low.

☑ **PATIENT TEACHING**
• Explain to patient and family the use and administration of antihemophilic factor.
• Tell patient to report adverse reactions promptly.

## anti-inhibitor coagulant complex
Autoplex T, Feiba VH Immuno
*Pregnancy Risk Category: C*

---

## HOW SUPPLIED
*Injection:* number of units of factor VIII correctional activity indicated on label of vial

## ACTION
Unknown. It has been suggested that efficacy may be related in part to the presence of the activated factors, which leads to more complete factor X activation in conjunction with tissue factor, phospholipid, and ionic calcium and allows the coagulation process to proceed beyond those stages where factor VIII is needed.

## ONSET, PEAK, DURATION
Onset occurs within 10 to 30 minutes. Peak and duration unknown.

## INDICATIONS & DOSAGE
*Prevention and control of hemorrhagic episodes in certain patients with hemophilia A who have developed inhibitor antibodies to antihemophilic factor; management of bleeding in patients with acquired hemophilia who have spontaneously acquired inhibitors to factor VIII —*
**Adults and children:** highly individualized and varies among manufacturers. For Autoplex T, 25 to 100 units/kg I.V., depending on the severity of hemorrhage. If no hemostatic improvement occurs within 6 hours after administration, dosage repeated. For Feiba VH Immuno, 50 to 100 units/kg I.V. q 6 or 12 hours until clear signs of improvement.

## ADVERSE REACTIONS
**CNS:** headache.
**CV:** changes in blood pressure, *acute MI, thromboembolic events.*
**GI:** nausea, vomiting.
**Hematologic:** *disseminated intravascular coagulation (DIC).*
**Skin:** flushing, rash, urticaria.
**Other:** fever, chills, hypersensitivity reactions, risk of hepatitis B and HIV.

## INTERACTIONS
*Antifibrinolytic agents:* may alter effects of anti-inhibitor coagulant complex. Do not use together.

## CONTRAINDICATIONS
Contraindicated in patients with signs of fibrinolysis, in those with DIC, and in those with a normal coagulation mechanism.

## NURSING CONSIDERATIONS
● Use with caution in patients with liver disease.
● As ordered, administer hepatitis B vaccine before administering drug.
● Keep epinephrine available to treat anaphylaxis.
● **I.V. use:** Warm the drug and diluent to room temperature prior to reconstitution. Reconstitute according to manufacturer's directions. Use the filter needle provided by the manufacturer to withdraw the reconstituted solution from the vial into the syringe; the filter needle should then be replaced with a sterile injection needle for administration. Administer as soon as possible. Autoplex T infusions should be completed within 1 hour after reconstitution; Feiba VH Immuno infusions, within 3 hours.
● The rate of administration should be individualized according to the patient's response. Autoplex T infusions may begin at a rate of 1 ml/minute; if well tolerated, the infusion rate may be increased gradually to 10 ml/minute. Feiba VH Immuno infusion rate should not exceed 2 units/kg.
● *Alert:* If flushing, lethargy, headache, transient chest discomfort, or changes in blood pressure or pulse rate develop because of a rapid rate of infusion, stop the drug and notify the doctor. Know that these symptoms usually disappear with cessation of the infusion. The infusion may then be resumed at a slower rate, as ordered.

---

Reactions may be *common,* uncommon, *life-threatening,* or **COMMON AND LIFE-THREATENING.**

- Monitor the patient closely for hypersensitivity reactions.
- Monitor vital signs regularly, and report significant changes to the doctor.
- Reassure patient that because of the manufacturing process, the risk of HIV transmission is extremely low.

☑ **PATIENT TEACHING**
- Explain to patient and family the use and administration of anti-inhibitor coagulant complex.
- Tell patient to report adverse reactions promptly.

---

## antithrombin III, human (AT-III, heparin cofactor I)
ATnativ, Thrombate III

*Pregnancy Risk Category: C*

### HOW SUPPLIED
*Injection:* 500 IU

### ACTION
Replaces deficient AT-III in patients with hereditary AT-III deficiency, normalizing coagulation inhibition and inhibiting thromboembolism formation. Also deactivates plasmin (to lesser extent than the clotting factor).

### ONSET, PEAK, DURATION
Onset immediate after I.V. administration. Peak unknown. Effects persist about 4 days.

### INDICATIONS & DOSAGE
*Thromboembolism associated with hereditary AT-III deficiency –*
**Adults and children:** initial dose is individualized to quantity required to increase AT-III activity to 120% of normal activity as determined 30 minutes after administration. Usual dose is 50 to 100 IU/minute I.V., not to exceed 100 IU/minute. Dose is calculated based on anticipated 1% increase in plasma AT-III activity pro-

duced by 1 IU/kg of body weight using the formula:

$$\text{Dose (Units)} = \frac{(\text{desired activity [\%]} - \text{baseline activity [\%]}) \times \text{weight (kg)}}{1\% \text{ (IU/kg)}}$$

Maintenance dosage is individualized to quantity required to increase AT-III activity to 80% of normal activity and is administered at 24-hour intervals.

To calculate subsequent dosages, multiply the desired AT-III activity (as percentage of normal) minus the baseline AT-III activity (as percentage of normal) by body weight (in kg). Divide by actual increase in AT-III activity (as percentage) produced by 1 IU/kg as determined 30 minutes after administration of initial dose.

Treatment is usually continued for 2 to 8 days but may be prolonged in pregnancy or when used with surgery or immobilization.

### ADVERSE REACTIONS
**CV:** vasodilation, lowered blood pressure.
**GU:** diuresis.

### INTERACTIONS
*Heparin:* increased anticoagulant effect of both drugs. Heparin dosage reduction may be necessary.

### CONTRAINDICATIONS
None known.

### NURSING CONSIDERATIONS
- Use with extreme caution in children and neonates because safety and efficacy have not been established.
- Use drug cautiously. It is prepared from pooled plasma from human donors and carries with it a minimal risk of transmission of viruses, including hepatitis and HIV.
- *Alert:* Because of the risk of neonatal thromboembolism (sometimes fatal) in children of parents with hereditary AT-III deficiency, anticipate ob-

---

*Liquid form contains alcohol. **May contain tartrazine. †Canada only. ‡Australia only. ◇OTC.

taining AT-III levels immediately after birth.

• **I.V. use:** Reconstitute using 10 ml of sterile water (provided), 0.9% sodium chloride solution, or $D_5W$. Do not shake vial. Dilute further in same diluent solution if desired.

• Obtain AT-III activity levels twice daily until the dosage requirement has stabilized, then daily immediately before dose. Functional assays are preferred because quantitative immunologic test results may be normal despite decreased AT-III activity.

• Monitor for dyspnea and increased blood pressure, which may occur if administration rate is too rapid.

• Keep in mind that 1 IU is equivalent to the quantity of endogenous AT-III present in 1 ml of normal human plasma.

• Keep in mind that heparin binds to AT-III lysine binding sites, resulting in increased efficacy of heparin.

• Know that drug is not recommended for long-term prophylaxis of thrombotic episodes.

• Store at 36° to 46° F (2° to 8° C).

☑ **PATIENT TEACHING**
• Explain to patient and parents the use and administration of antithrombin III, human.

• Instruct patient to report adverse reactions promptly.

---

### factor IX (human)
AlphaNine, AlphaNine SD, Mononine

### factor IX complex
Bebulin VH Immuno, Konyne-80, Profilnine Heat-Treated, Proplex T

*Pregnancy Risk Category: C*

**HOW SUPPLIED**
*Injection:* vials, with diluent. Units specified on label.

**ACTION**
Directly replaces deficient clotting factor.

**ONSET, PEAK, DURATION**
Onset immediate after I.V. administration. Time to peak effect is 10 to 30 minutes after I.V. administration. Duration unknown.

**INDICATIONS & DOSAGE**
*Factor IX deficiency (hemophilia B or Christmas disease), anticoagulant overdosage* —
**Adults and children:** units required = 0.8 to 1 × body weight in kg × percentage of desired increase of factor IX level. Give by slow I.V. infusion, rate not to exceed 3 ml/minute. Dosage is highly individualized, depending on degree of deficiency, level of factor IX desired, weight of the patient, and severity of bleeding.

**ADVERSE REACTIONS**
**CNS:** headache.
**CV:** *thromboembolic reactions, MI, disseminated intravascular coagulation, pulmonary embolism,* changes in blood pressure.
**GI:** nausea, vomiting.
**Skin:** urticaria.
**Other:** *transient fever, chills, flushing, tingling.*

**INTERACTIONS**
*Aminocaproic acid:* increased risk of thrombosis. Avoid concomitant use.

**CONTRAINDICATIONS**
Contraindicated in patients with hepatic disease in whom there is any suspicion of intravascular coagulation or fibrinolysis. Mononine is contraindicated in patients with hypersensitivity to murine (mouse) protein.

**NURSING CONSIDERATIONS**
• Use cautiously in neonates and infants because of susceptibility to hep-

atitis, which may be transmitted with factor IX complex.

• As ordered, administer hepatitis B vaccine before administering factor IX complex.

• Reconstitute with 20 ml of sterile water for injection for each vial of lyophilized drug. Keep refrigerated until ready to use; warm to room temperature before reconstituting. Use within 3 hours of reconstitution. Unstable in solution. Don't shake, refrigerate, or mix solution with other I.V. solutions. Store away from heat.

• **I.V. use:** Avoid rapid infusion. If tingling sensation, fever, chills, or headache develops, decrease flow rate and notify the doctor.

• Observe the patient for allergic reactions, and monitor vital signs regularly.

• Keep in mind that risk of hepatitis, including non-A and non-B hepatitis, must be weighed against risk of not receiving the drug.

• Because of the manufacturing process, be aware that the risk of HIV transmission is extremely low.

☑ **PATIENT TEACHING**
• Explain to family and patient the use and administration of factor IX.
• Tell patient to report adverse reactions promptly.

---

# intravascular perfluorochemical emulsion (IPE)
Fluosol

*Pregnancy Risk Category: B*

## HOW SUPPLIED
*Injection:* 20% emulsion; supplied in kit form with additive solutions (1 and 2) and materials to provide continuous oxygenation

## ACTION
An emulsion of synthetic perfluorochemicals that acts as an oxygen carrier.

## ONSET, PEAK, DURATION
Unknown.

## INDICATIONS & DOSAGE
*To prevent or decrease myocardial ischemia during percutaneous transluminal coronary angioplasty (PTCA) in patients at high risk for ischemic complications of angioplasty (including patients with a low baseline ejection fraction, patients with large areas of the myocardium at risk, patients with recent MI, and patients with unstable angina or refractory angina requiring hospitalization) –*
**Adults:** test dose of 0.5 ml is withdrawn from the prepared solution and injected into a peripheral vein. If no adverse reactions occur within 10 minutes, warmed, oxygenated emulsion may be administered by intracoronary injection at a rate of 60 to 90 ml/minute. Administered through the central lumen of an angioplasty balloon catheter without removing the guide wire. An angiographic power injector with a warming jacket is used.

## ADVERSE REACTIONS
**CV:** *ventricular tachycardia or fibrillation,* bradycardia, chest discomfort, hypotension.
**Respiratory:** dyspnea, increased respiratory rate, coughing.
**Skin:** mild pruritus.

## INTERACTIONS
*Anesthetics:* may prolong action of lipid-soluble anesthetics. Monitor the patient carefully.
*Hepatotoxic agents:* may enhance hepatotoxic effects of hepatotoxic agents. Monitor the patient closely.

---

## CONTRAINDICATIONS

Contraindicated in patients with hypersensitivity to any components of the compound and in those with functionally critical secondary stenosis in areas distal to the site of the lesion being treated.

## NURSING CONSIDERATIONS

• Use cautiously in asplenic patients because drug may accumulate.

• Know that breast-feeding is not recommended because drug is excreted in breast milk.

• Be aware that drug should be administered only by doctors familiar with PTCA. Follow institutional policy regarding emergency surgical procedures for coronary artery bypass graft surgery.

• **I.V. use:** Do not use an in-line filter when administering because it may damage the emulsion. Never administer any solution that shows evidence of emulsion separation.

• *Alert:* Oxygenate the emulsion. Do not add anything other than solutions 1 and 2 or carbogen gas (95% oxygen, 5% carbon dioxide) to the emulsion. Do not oxygenate with 100% oxygen because this will adversely affect the solution's final pH. Also warm to approximately 98.6° F (37° C) before administration. Infusion of solutions at room temperature has been associated with ventricular fibrillation.

• In the unlikely event that the patient reacts adversely to the test dose (1.2% of patients in clinical trials reacted), be prepared not to give the drug. Severe reactions can be managed with methylprednisolone or diphenhydramine.

• Anticipate allowing more than 4 minutes of perfusion time when used with an angiographic power injector reservoir of 260 ml and a flow rate of 60 ml/minute. Perfusion time should be limited by the patient's tolerance and the doctor's judgment.

• Because this drug reportedly accumulates in the body after repeated dosage, know that it should not be given more than once every 6 months.

• Store the container of intravascular perfluorochemical emulsion in the freezer (between 23° and -22° F [-5° and -30° C]). Do not use emulsions that appear to have partially thawed during storage. Use a warming cabinet or water bath set at 98.6° F to thaw the solution, not a microwave oven, because this may cause uneven heating of the solution. Allow at least 30 minutes for thawing of the solution. Do not refreeze thawed solutions, and use within 8 hours.

• Do not freeze the additive solutions (solutions 1 and 2); store at room temperature not exceeding 86° F (30° C).

☑ **PATIENT TEACHING**

• Explain to patient and family the use and administration of intravascular perfluorochemical emulsion.

• Tell patient to report adverse reactions promptly.

## plasma protein fraction
Plasmanate, Plasma-Plex, Plasmatein, Protenate

*Pregnancy Risk Category: C*

## HOW SUPPLIED

*Injection:* 5% solution in 50-ml, 250-ml, 500-ml vials

## ACTION

Supplies colloid to the blood and expands plasma volume.

## ONSET, PEAK, DURATION

Onset and serum levels peak immediately after I.V. infusion. Duration unknown.

## INDICATIONS & DOSAGE

*Shock* –

**Adults:** varies with the patient's condition and response, but usual dose is 250 to 500 ml I.V. (12.5 to 25 g protein), usually no faster than 10 ml/minute.

**Children:** 6.6 to 33 ml/kg (0.33 to 1.65 g/kg of protein) I.V., 5 to 10 ml/minute.

*Hypoproteinemia –*

**Adults:** 1,000 to 1,500 ml I.V. daily. Maximum infusion rate is 8 ml/minute.

## ADVERSE REACTIONS

**CNS:** headache.

**CV:** hypotension (after rapid infusion or intra-arterial administration); *vascular overload* (after rapid infusion); tachycardia.

**GI:** nausea, vomiting, hypersalivation.

**Respiratory:** dyspnea, pulmonary edema.

**Skin:** rash.

**Other:** flushing, chills, fever, back pain.

## INTERACTIONS

None significant.

## CONTRAINDICATIONS

Contraindicated in patients with severe anemia or heart failure and in those undergoing cardiac bypass.

## NURSING CONSIDERATIONS

• Use cautiously in patients with hepatic or renal failure, low cardiac reserve, and restricted sodium intake.

• **I.V. use:** Check expiration date before using. Don't use solutions that are cloudy, contain sediment, or have been frozen. Discard solutions in containers opened for more than 4 hours because it contains no preservatives.

• Know that solutions containing amino acids or alcohol may not be infused through the same I.V. line because the proteins may precipitate.

• If the patient is dehydrated, give additional fluids either P.O. or I.V., as ordered.

• Do not give more than 250 g or 5,000 ml in 48 hours.

• Monitor blood pressure. Be prepared to slow or stop infusion if hypotension suddenly occurs. Vital signs should return to normal gradually; monitor hourly.

• Watch for signs of vascular overload (heart failure or pulmonary edema).

• Monitor intake and output. Watch for and report decreased urine output.

• Keep in mind that drug contains 130 to 160 mEq sodium/liter.

☑ **PATIENT TEACHING**

• Explain to patient and family the use and administration of plasma protein fraction.

• Tell patient to report adverse reactions promptly.

---

*Liquid form contains alcohol.   **May contain tartrazine.   †Canada only.   ‡Australia only.   ◇OTC.

# 68

# Thrombolytic enzymes

alteplase
anistreplase
streptokinase
urokinase

**COMBINATION PRODUCTS**
None.

## alteplase (tissue plasminogen activator, recombinant; tPA)
Actilyse‡, Activase

*Pregnancy Risk Category: C*

### HOW SUPPLIED
*Injection:* 20-mg (11.6 million-IU), 50-mg (29 million-IU), 100 mg (58 million-IU) vials

### ACTION
Binds to fibrin in a thrombus, and locally converts plasminogen to plasmin, which initiates local fibrinolysis.

### ONSET, PEAK, DURATION
Onset immediate. Peak effects occur in about 45 minutes. Effects persist for about 4 hours.

### INDICATIONS & DOSAGE
*Lysis of thrombi obstructing coronary arteries in acute MI –*
**Adults:** 100 mg I.V. infusion over 3 hours as follows: 60 mg in the first hour, of which 6 to 10 mg is given as a bolus over the first 1 to 2 minutes. Then 20 mg/hour infusion for 2 hours. Smaller adults ( under 65 kg) should receive 1.25 mg/kg in a similar fashion (60% in the first hour, 10% as a bolus; then 20% of the total dose per hour for 2 hours).
*Management of acute massive pulmonary embolism –*
**Adults:** 100 mg I.V. infusion over 2

hours. Heparin begun at the end of the infusion when PTT or PT returns to twice normal or less.
Do not exceed 100-mg dose. Higher doses may increase risk of intracranial bleeding.

### ADVERSE REACTIONS
**CNS:** *cerebral hemorrhage,* fever.
**CV:** hypotension, arrhythmias, edema.
**GI:** nausea, vomiting.
**Hematologic:** *severe, spontaneous bleeding (cerebral, retroperitoneal, GU, GI).*
**Other:** bleeding at puncture sites, hypersensitivity reactions *(anaphylaxis).*

### INTERACTIONS
*Aspirin, coumarin anticoagulants, dipyridamole, heparin:* increased risk of bleeding. Monitor the patient carefully.

### CONTRAINDICATIONS
Contraindicated in patients with active internal bleeding, intracranial neoplasm, arteriovenous malformation, aneurysm, and severe uncontrolled hypertension. Also contraindicated in patients with a history of CVA, recent (within 2 months) intraspinal or intracranial trauma or surgery, or known bleeding diathesis.

### NURSING CONSIDERATIONS
• Use cautiously in patients with recent (within 10 days) major surgery; in pregnancy and first 10 days postpartum; organ biopsy; trauma (including cardiopulmonary resuscitation); GI or GU bleeding; cerebrovascular disease; hypertension (systolic pressure 180 mm Hg or higher or diastolic pressure 110 mm Hg or higher);

---

Reactions may be *common,* uncommon, *life-threatening,* or COMMON AND LIFE-THREATENING.

mitral stenosis, atrial fibrillation, or other condition that may lead to left heart thrombus; acute pericarditis or subacute bacterial endocarditis; septic thrombophlebitis; diabetic hemorrhagic retinopathy; in patients receiving anticoagulants; and in patients age 75 and older.

• Know that recanalization of occluded coronary arteries and improvement of heart function require initiation of treatment with alteplase as soon as possible after the onset of symptoms.

• **I.V. use:** Reconstitute drug with sterile water for injection (without preservatives) only. (Check manufacturer's labeling for specific information.) Do not use vial if the vacuum is not present. Reconstitute with a large-bore (18G) needle, directing the stream of sterile water at the lyophilized cake. Do not shake. Slight foaming is common, and solution should be clear or pale yellow.

• Keep in mind that drug may be administered as reconstituted (1 mg/ml) or diluted with an equal volume of 0.9% sodium chloride solution or $D_5W$ to make a 0.5 mg/ml solution. Adding other drugs to the infusion is not recommended.

• Reconstitute alteplase solution immediately before use, and administer it within 8 hours because it contains no preservatives. The drug may be temporarily stored at 35° to 86° F (2° to 30° C), but it is only stable for 8 hours at room temperature. Discard any unused solution.

• Be aware that heparin therapy is frequently initiated after treatment with alteplase to decrease the risk of rethrombosis.

• Have antiarrhythmics readily available, and carefully monitor ECG. Coronary thrombolysis is associated with arrhythmias induced by reperfusion of ischemic myocardium. Such arrhythmias do not differ from those commonly associated with MI.

• Avoid invasive procedures during thrombolytic therapy. Carefully monitor the patient for signs of internal bleeding, and frequently check all puncture sites. Bleeding is the most common adverse effect and may occur internally and at external puncture sites.

☑ **PATIENT TEACHING**
• Explain to patient and family use and administration of alteplase.
• Tell patient to report adverse reactions promptly.

---

### anistreplase (anisoylated plasminogen-streptokinase activator complex; APSAC)
Eminase

*Pregnancy Risk Category: C*

**HOW SUPPLIED**
*Injection:* 30 units-vial

**ACTION**
Anistreplase, derived from Lys-plasminogen and streptokinase, is formulated into a fibrinolytic enzyme plus activator complex with the activator temporarily blocked by an anisoyl group. The drug is activated in vivo by a nonenzymatic process that removes the anisoyl group. The active Lys-plasminogen-streptokinase activator complex is progressively formed in the bloodstream or within the thrombus.

**ONSET, PEAK, DURATION**
Onset immediate after I.V. administration. Peak effects occur in about 45 minutes. Effects persist for 6 hours to 2 days.

**INDICATIONS & DOSAGE**
*Lysis of coronary artery thrombi following acute MI—*
**Adults:** 30 units I.V. over 2 to 5 minutes. Administered by direct injection.

---

*Liquid form contains alcohol.  **May contain tartrazine.  †Canada only.  ‡Australia only.  ◇OTC.

## ADVERSE REACTIONS
**CNS:** *intracranial hemorrhage.*
**CV:** *arrhythmias, conduction disorders, hypotension.*
**EENT:** hemoptysis, gum or mouth hemorrhage.
**GI:** hemorrhage.
**GU:** hematuria.
**Hematologic:** *bleeding tendency,* eosinophilia.
**Skin:** hematoma, urticaria, pruritus, flushing, delayed (2 weeks after therapy) purpuric rash.
**Other:** bleeding at puncture sites, *anaphylaxis or anaphylactoid reactions (rare),* arthralgia.

## INTERACTIONS
*Heparin, oral anticoagulants, drugs that alter platelet function (including aspirin and dipyridamole):* may increase the risk of bleeding. Use together cautiously.

## CONTRAINDICATIONS
Contraindicated in patients with a history of severe allergic reaction to anistreplase or streptokinase; active internal bleeding, CVA, recent (within the past 2 months) intraspinal or intracranial surgery or trauma, aneurysm, arteriovenous malformation, intracranial neoplasm, uncontrolled hypertension, or known bleeding diathesis.

## NURSING CONSIDERATIONS
● Use cautiously in patients with recent (within 10 days) major surgery; trauma (including cardiopulmonary resuscitation); GI or GU bleeding; cerebrovascular disease; hypertension (systolic pressure 180 mm Hg or higher or diastolic pressure 110 mm Hg or higher); mitral stenosis, atrial fibrillation, or other conditions that may lead to left heart thrombus; acute pericarditis or subacute bacterial endocarditis; septic thrombophlebitis; diabetic hemorrhagic retinopathy; in pregnancy and first 10 days postpartum; in patients receiving anticoagulants; and in patients 75 years and older.
● **I.V. use:** Unlike other thrombolytics that must be infused, administer anistreplase by direct injection over 2 to 5 minutes.
● Reconstitute the drug by slowly adding 5 ml of sterile water for injection. Direct the stream against the side of the vial, not at the drug itself. Gently roll the vial to mix the dry powder and water. To avoid excessive foaming, don't shake the vial. The reconstituted solution should be colorless to pale yellow. Inspect for precipitate. If the drug is not administered within 30 minutes of reconstituting, discard the vial.
● Do not mix the drug with other medications; do not dilute the solution after reconstitution.
● Carefully monitor ECG during treatment. Be prepared to treat bradycardia or ventricular irritability. Thrombolytic therapy is associated with reperfusion arrhythmias that may signify successful thrombolysis. These arrhythmias are similar to those seen in the course of an acute MI and may include sinus bradycardia, accelerated idioventricular rhythm, ventricular tachycardia, or premature ventricular depolarizations.
● Carefully monitor the patient; avoid I.M. injections and nonessential handling or moving of patient. Bleeding is the most common adverse reaction and may occur internally and at external puncture sites.
● Be aware that heparin therapy is frequently initiated after treatment with anistreplase to decrease the risk of rethrombosis.
● Be aware that anistreplase is derived from human plasma. No cases of hepatitis or HIV infection have been reported to date. The manufacturing process is designed to purify

---

the plasma used in preparation of the drug.

● **Alert:** Keep in mind the efficacy of drug may be limited if antistreptokinase antibodies are present. Antibody levels may be elevated if more than 5 days has elapsed since previous treatment with anistreplase or streptokinase, or if the patient has had a recent streptococcal infection.

● Be aware that in vitro coagulation tests will be affected by the presence of anistreplase. This can be attenuated if blood samples are collected in the presence of aprotinin (150 to 200 units/ml).

☑ **PATIENT TEACHING**

● Explain to patient and family the use and administration of anistreplase.

● Tell patient to report adverse reactions promptly.

## streptokinase
Kabikinase, Streptase

*Pregnancy Risk Category: C*

### HOW SUPPLIED
*Injection:* 250,000 IU, 600,000 IU, 750,000 IU, 1,500,000 IU in vials for reconstitution

### ACTION
Activates plasminogen in two steps: Plasminogen and streptokinase form a complex that exposes the plasminogen-activating site; plasminogen is then converted to plasmin by cleavage of the peptide bond, leading to fibrinolysis.

### ONSET, PEAK, DURATION
Onset immediate after I.V. administration. Peak effects occur in 20 minutes to 2 hours. Effects persist for about 4 hours.

### INDICATIONS & DOSAGE
*Arteriovenous cannula occlusion –*
**Adults:** 250,000 IU in 2 ml I.V. solution by I.V. pump infusion into each occluded limb of the cannula over 25 to 35 minutes. Clamp off cannula for 2 hours. Then aspirate contents of cannula; flush with sodium chloride solution and reconnect.

*Venous thrombosis, pulmonary embolism, and arterial thrombosis and embolism –*
**Adults:** loading dose is 250,000 IU I.V. infusion over 30 minutes. Sustaining dose is 100,000 IU/hour I.V. infusion for 72 hours for deep vein thrombosis and 100,000 IU/hour over 24 to 72 hours by I.V. infusion pump for pulmonary embolism and arterial thrombosis or embolism.

*Lysis of coronary artery thrombi following acute MI –*
**Adults:** 140,000 units administered as a loading dose, followed by maintenance infusion. Loading dose is 20,000 IU via coronary catheter, followed by infusion of maintenance dose of 2,000 IU/minute over 60 minutes. Alternatively, may be administered as an I.V. infusion. Usual adult dose is 1.5 million IU infused over 60 minutes.

### ADVERSE REACTIONS
**CNS:** polyradiculoneuropathy, headache.
**CV:** reperfusion arrhythmias, *hypotension,* vasculitis.
**EENT:** periorbital edema.
**GI:** nausea.
**Hematologic:** *bleeding.*
**Respiratory:** minor breathing difficulty, *bronchospasm.*
**Skin:** urticaria, pruritus, flushing.
**Other:** phlebitis at injection site, hypersensitivity reactions *(anaphylaxis),* delayed hypersensitivity reactions (interstitial nephritis, serum sickness-like reactions), musculoskeletal pain, *angioedema, fever.*

---

*Liquid form contains alcohol. **May contain tartrazine. †Canada only. ‡Australia only. ◊OTC.

## INTERACTIONS

*Anticoagulants:* increased risk of bleeding. Monitor the patient closely.
*Antifibrinolytic agents:* streptokinase activity is inhibited and reversed by antifibrinolytic agents such as aminocaproic acid.
*Aspirin, dipyridamole, indomethacin, phenylbutazone, drugs affecting platelet activity:* increased risk of bleeding. Monitor patients closely. Combined therapy with low-dose aspirin (162.5 mg) or dipyridamole has improved acute and long-term results.

## CONTRAINDICATIONS

• Contraindicated in patients with ulcerative wounds, active internal bleeding, and recent CVA; recent trauma with possible internal injuries; visceral or intracranial malignant neoplasms; ulcerative colitis; diverticulitis; severe hypertension; acute or chronic hepatic or renal insufficiency; uncontrolled hypocoagulation; chronic pulmonary disease with cavitation; subacute bacterial endocarditis or rheumatic valvular disease; recent cerebral embolism, thrombosis, or hemorrhage.
• Also contraindicated within 10 days after intra-arterial diagnostic procedure or any surgery, including liver or kidney biopsy, lumbar puncture, thoracentesis, paracentesis, or extensive or multiple cutdowns.
• I.M. injections and other invasive procedures are contraindicated during streptokinase therapy.

## NURSING CONSIDERATIONS

• Use cautiously when treating arterial embolism that originates from left side of heart because of danger of cerebral infarction.
• Know that only doctors with wide experience in thrombotic disease management, where clinical and laboratory monitoring can be performed, should use streptokinase.
• Before using streptokinase to clear an occluded arteriovenous cannula, try flushing with heparinized sodium chloride solution, as ordered.
• Keep aminocaproic acid available to treat bleeding, and corticosteroids to treat allergic reactions.
• Have typed and crossmatched packed RBCs and whole blood ready to treat possible hemorrhage.
• Before initiating therapy, draw blood to determine PTT and PT. Rate of I.V. infusion depends on thrombin time and streptokinase resistance.
• To check for hypersensitivity reactions, give 100 IU intradermally as ordered; a wheal and flare response within 20 minutes means the patient is probably allergic. Monitor vital signs frequently.
• Be aware that if the patient has had either a recent streptococcal infection or recent treatment with streptokinase, a higher loading dose may be necessary.
• **I.V. use:** Reconstitute each vial with 5 ml of 0.9% sodium chloride solution for injection or D₅W solution. Further dilute to 45 ml (if necessary, total volume may be increased to 500 ml in a glass or 50 ml in a plastic container). Don't shake; roll gently to mix. Some flocculation may be present after reconstituting; discard if large amounts are present. Filter solution with 0.8-micron or larger filter. Use within 24 hours. Store powder at room temperature and refrigerate after reconstitution.
• Monitor the patient for excessive bleeding every 15 minutes for the 1st hour, every 30 minutes for the 2nd through 8th hours, then once every shift. If bleeding is evident, stop therapy and notify doctor. Know that pretreatment with heparin or drugs that affect platelets causes high risk of bleeding, but may improve long-term results. Monitor closely.
• Monitor pulses, color, and sensation of extremities every hour.
• Maintain the involved extremity in

straight alignment to prevent bleeding from the infusion site.

• Avoid unnecessary handling of patients; pad side rails. Bruising is more likely during therapy.

• Keep a laboratory flow sheet on the patient's chart to monitor PTT, PT, and hemoglobin and hematocrit levels.

• Keep venipuncture sites to a minimum; use pressure dressing on puncture sites for at least 15 minutes.

• *Alert:* Watch for signs of hypersensitivity. Notify the doctor immediately. Antihistamines or corticosteroids may be used to treat mild allergic reactions. If a severe reaction occurs, the infusion should be stopped immediately and the doctor notified.

• Be aware that heparin by continuous infusion is usually started within an hour after stopping streptokinase. Use infusion pump to administer heparin.

• Keep in mind that thrombolytic therapy in patients with acute MI may decrease infarct size, improve ventricular function, and decrease incidence of CHF. Streptokinase must be administered within 6 hours of the onset of symptoms for optimal effect.

☑ **PATIENT TEACHING**
• Explain to patient and family the use and administration of streptokinase.

• Tell patient to report adverse reactions promptly.

---

## urokinase
Abbokinase, Abbokinase Open-Cath, Ukidan‡

*Pregnancy Risk Category: B*

### HOW SUPPLIED
*Injection:* 5,000 units (IU) per unit-dose vial; 9,000 units (IU) per unit-dose vial; 250,000-IU vial

### ACTION
Activates plasminogen to plasmin by directly cleaving peptide bonds at two different sites, causing fibrolysis.

### ONSET, PEAK, DURATION
Onset immediate after I.V. administration. Peak effects occur in 20 minutes to 2 hours. Effects persist for about 4 hours.

### INDICATIONS & DOSAGE
*Lysis of acute massive pulmonary embolism and lysis of pulmonary embolism accompanied by unstable hemodynamics* –
**Adults:** for I.V. infusion *only* by constant infusion pump delivering total volume of 195 ml.
Priming dose: 4,400 IU/kg of urokinase-0.9% sodium chloride or $D_5W$ solution admixture, given over 10 minutes. Followed with 4,400 IU/kg at a rate of 15 ml/hour for 12 to 24 hours. Total volume should not exceed 200 ml. Therapy followed with continuous I.V. infusion of heparin, then oral anticoagulants.
*Coronary artery thrombosis* –
**Adults:** after a bolus dose of heparin ranging from 2,500 to 10,000 units, 6,000 IU/minute of urokinase is infused into the occluded artery for up to 2 hours. Average total dosage is 500,000 IU.
*Venous catheter occlusion* –
**Adults:** 5,000 IU instilled into occluded line and, after 5 minutes, is aspirated. Aspiration attempts repeated q 5 minutes for 30 minutes. If not patent after 30 minutes, the line is capped and urokinase left to work for 30 to 60 minutes before aspirating again. May require second instillation.

### ADVERSE REACTIONS
**CV:** reperfusion arrhythmias.
**Hematologic:** *bleeding.*
**Respiratory:** bronchospasm, minor breathing difficulties.

---

*Liquid form contains alcohol. **May contain tartrazine. †Canada only. ‡Australia only. ◇OTC.

**Other:** phlebitis at injection site, fever.

## INTERACTIONS
*Anticoagulants:* increased risk of bleeding. Monitor the patient closely. *Aspirin, dipyridamole, indomethacin, phenylbutazone, other drugs affecting platelet activity:* increased risk of bleeding.

## CONTRAINDICATIONS
• Contraindicated in patients with active internal bleeding, history of CVA, aneurysm, arteriovenous malformation, known bleeding diathesis, recent trauma with possible internal injuries, visceral or intracranial malignancy, pregnancy and first 10 days postpartum, ulcerative colitis, diverticulitis, severe hypertension, hemostatic defects including those secondary to severe hepatic or renal insufficiency, uncontrolled hypocoagulation, chronic pulmonary disease with cavitation, subacute bacterial endocarditis or rheumatic valvular disease, and recent cerebral embolism, thrombosis, or hemorrhage.
• Also contraindicated within 10 days after intra-arterial diagnostic procedure or any surgery (liver or kidney biopsy, lumbar puncture, thoracentesis, paracentesis, or extensive or multiple cutdowns) or within two months after intracranial or intraspinal surgery.
• I.M. injections and other invasive procedures are contraindicated during urokinase therapy.

## NURSING CONSIDERATIONS
• Have typed and crossmatched RBCs, whole blood, and aminocaproic acid available to treat bleeding, and corticosteroids to treat allergic reactions.
• **I.V. use:** Add 5 ml of sterile water for injection (without preservatives) to vial. Dilute further with 0.9% sodium chloride solution or $D_5W$ solution before infusion. The total volume of fluid administered should not exceed 200 ml. Don't use bacteriostatic water for injection to reconstitute; it contains preservatives. Urokinase solutions may be filtered through a 0.45-micron or smaller cellulose-membrane filter before administration.
• Monitor the patient for excessive bleeding every 15 minutes for the 1st hour; every 30 minutes for the 2nd through 8th hours; then once every shift. Pretreatment with drugs affecting platelets places patient at high risk of bleeding.
• Monitor pulses, color, and sensation of extremities every hour.
• Although the incidence of hypersensitivity reactions is low, watch for signs of this reaction.
• Keep a laboratory flow sheet on the patient's chart to monitor PTT, PT, and hemoglobin and hematocrit levels.
• Monitor vital signs.
• Keep venipuncture sites to a minimum; use pressure dressing on puncture sites for at least 15 minutes.
• Maintain the involved extremity in straight alignment to prevent bleeding from the infusion site.
• Avoid unnecessary handling of patients; pad side rails. Bruising is more likely during therapy.
• Be aware that heparin by continuous infusion is usually started within an hour after urokinase has been stopped to prevent recurrent thrombosis.

## ☑ PATIENT TEACHING
• Explain to patient and family the use and administration of urokinase.
• Instruct the patient to report adverse reactions promptly.

# 69

# Alkylating drugs

busulfan
carboplatin
carmustine
chlorambucil
cisplatin
cyclophosphamide
ifosfamide
lomustine
mechlorethamine hydrochloride
melphalan
streptozocin
thiotepa
uracil mustard

**COMBINATION PRODUCTS**
None.

---

## busulfan
Myleran

*Pregnancy Risk Category: D*

**HOW SUPPLIED**
*Tablets:* 2 mg

**ACTION**
Unknown. Thought to cross-link strands of cellular DNA and interferes with RNA transcription, causing an imbalance of growth that leads to cell death. Cell cycle-nonspecific.

**ONSET, PEAK, DURATION**
Onset of disease response occurs in 1 to 2 weeks. Peak and duration undefined.

**INDICATIONS & DOSAGE**
*Chronic myelocytic (granulocytic) leukemia –*
**Adults:** 4 to 8 mg P.O. daily, up to 12 mg P.O. daily, until WBC count falls to 15,000/mm³; drug stopped until WBC count rises to 50,000/mm³, and then resumed as before; or 4 to 8 mg P.O. daily until WBC count falls to

10,000 to 20,000/mm³; then daily dosage reduced as needed to maintain WBC count at this level (usually 1 to 3 mg daily).
**Children:** 0.06 to 0.12 mg/kg/day or 1.8 to 4.6 mg/m²/day P.O.; dosage adjusted to maintain WBC count at 20,000/mm³, but never less than 10,000/mm³.

**ADVERSE REACTIONS**
**CNS:** unusual tiredness or weakness, fatigue.
**GI:** cheilosis, dry mouth, anorexia.
**Hematologic:** leukopenia (WBC count falling after about 10 days and continuing to fall for 2 weeks after stopping drug), *thrombocytopenia, anemia, severe pancytopenia.*
**Respiratory:** *irreversible pulmonary fibrosis, (commonly called "busulfan lung").*
**Skin:** *transient hyperpigmentation,* rash, urticaria, anhidrosis.
**Other:** gynecomastia, alopecia, Addison-like wasting syndrome, profound hyperuricemia caused by increased cell lysis, cataracts, jaundice.

**INTERACTIONS**
*Anticoagulants, aspirin:* increased risk of bleeding. Avoid concomitant use.
*Thioguanine:* may cause hepatotoxicity, esophageal varices, or portal hypertension. Use together cautiously.

**CONTRAINDICATIONS**
Contraindicated in patients with chronic myelogenous leukemia, which is known to resist the drug.

**NURSING CONSIDERATIONS**
• Use cautiously in patients recently given other myelosuppressants or radiation treatment and in those with

---

depressed neutrophil or platelet count. Because high-dose therapy has been associated with seizures, use such therapy cautiously in patients with a history of head trauma or seizures or in patients receiving other drugs that lower the seizure threshold.

• Follow institutional policy regarding preparation and handling of drug. Label as a hazardous drug.

• Know that therapeutic effects are often accompanied by toxicity.

• To prevent bleeding, avoid all I.M. injections when platelet count is below 100,000/mm³.

• Monitor patient response (increased appetite and sense of well-being, decreased total WBC count, reduced size of spleen), which usually begins within 1 to 2 weeks.

• Monitor serum uric acid. To prevent hyperuricemia with resulting uric acid nephropathy, know that allopurinol may be ordered in addition to keeping patient adequately hydrated.

• Anticipate possible blood transfusion during treatment because of cumulative anemia.

• *Alert:* Be aware that pulmonary fibrosis may occur as late as 4 to 6 months after treatment with busulfan.

☑ **PATIENT TEACHING**
• Advise patient to watch for signs of infection (fever, sore throat, fatigue) and bleeding (easy bruising, nosebleeds, bleeding gums, melena). Tell patient to take temperature daily.

• Instruct patient to report symptoms of toxicity so dosage adjustments can be made. Persistent cough and progressive dyspnea with alveolar exudate, suggestive of pneumonia, may be the result of drug toxicity.

• Instruct patient to avoid any OTC product containing aspirin.

• Inform patient that drug may cause darkening of skin.

• Advise women of childbearing age to avoid becoming pregnant during therapy. Recommend patient consult with doctor before becoming pregnant.

• Warn breast-feeding patient to discontinue breast-feeding because of the possibility of infant toxicity.

## carboplatin
Paraplatin, Paraplatin-AQ†

*Pregnancy Risk Category: D*

**HOW SUPPLIED**
*Injection:* 50-mg, 150-mg, 450-mg vials

**ACTION**
Unknown. An alkylating agent that probably produces cross-linking of DNA strands. Cell cycle-nonspecific.

**ONSET, PEAK, DURATION**
Undefined.

**INDICATIONS & DOSAGE**
*Palliative treatment of ovarian cancer* —

**Adults:** 360 mg/m² I.V. on day 1 q 4 weeks; doses should not be repeated until platelet count exceeds 100,000/mm³ and neutrophil count exceeds 2,000/mm³. Subsequent doses are based on blood counts.
For patients with renal dysfunction: Patients with a creatinine clearance of 41 to 59 ml/minute should receive a starting dose of 250 mg/m²; patients with a creatinine clearance of 16 to 40 ml/minute should receive a starting dose of 200 mg/m². Recommended dosage adjustments are not available for patients with a creatinine clearance of 15 ml/minute or less.

**ADVERSE REACTIONS**
**CNS:** dizziness, confusion, peripheral neuropathy, ototoxicity, central neurotoxicity, paresthesia, *CVA.*
**CV:** *cardiac failure; embolism.*
**EENT:** visual disturbances; change in taste.

**GI:** constipation, diarrhea, *nausea, vomiting.*
**Hematologic:** **THROMBOCYTOPENIA,** *leukopenia, neutropenia, anemia,* **BONE MARROW SUPPRESSION.**
**Other:** alopecia; hypersensitivity reactions; *increased BUN, creatinine, AST, or alkaline phosphatase levels; pain; asthenia;* **anaphylaxis;** *decreased serum electrolyte levels.*

## INTERACTIONS
*Bone marrow suppressants (including radiation therapy):* increased hematologic toxicity. Monitor closely.
*Nephrotoxic agents:* enhanced nephrotoxicity of carboplatin. Use cautiously.

## CONTRAINDICATIONS
Contraindicated in patients with a history of hypersensitivity to cisplatin, platinum-containing compounds, or mannitol or with severe bone marrow suppression or bleeding.

## NURSING CONSIDERATIONS
• Determine serum electrolyte, creatinine, and BUN levels; CBC; and creatinine clearance before the first infusion and before each course of treatment.
• Follow institutional policy to reduce risks because preparation and administration of parenteral form of this drug is associated with mutagenic, teratogenic, and carcinogenic risks for personnel.
• Check ordered dose against laboratory test results carefully. Only one increase in dosage is recommended. Subsequent doses should not exceed 125% of starting dose.
• *Alert:* Have epinephrine, corticosteroids, and antihistamines available when administering carboplatin because anaphylactoid reactions may occur within minutes of administration.
• **I.V. use:** Reconstitute with $D_5W$, 0.9% sodium chloride solution, or

sterile water for injection to make a concentration of 10 mg/ml. Add 5 ml of diluent to the 50-mg vial, 15 ml of diluent to the 150-mg vial, or 45 ml of diluent to the 450-mg vial. It can then be further diluted for infusion with 0.9% sodium chloride solution or $D_5W$. A concentration as low as 0.5 mg/ml can be prepared. Give drug by continuous or intermittent infusion over at least 15 minutes.
• Do not use needles or I.V. administration sets containing aluminum to administer carboplatin; precipitation and loss of drug's potency may occur.
• Know that therapeutic effects are often accompanied by toxicity.
• To prevent bleeding, avoid all I.M. injections when platelet count is below 100,000/mm³.
• Monitor vital signs during infusion.
• Monitor CBC and platelet count frequently during therapy and, when indicated, until recovery. WBC and platelet count nadirs usually occur by day 21. Levels usually return to baseline by day 28. Know that dose should not be repeated unless platelet count exceeds 100,000/mm³.
• Administer antiemetic therapy as ordered. Carboplatin can produce severe vomiting.
• Anticipate possible blood transfusions during treatment because of cumulative anemia.
• Know that hydration or diuresis before or after treatment is not necessary.
• Keep in mind that bone marrow suppression may be more severe in patients with creatinine clearance below 60 ml/minute; dosage adjustments are recommended for such patients.
• Be aware that patients over age 65 are at greater risk for neurotoxicity.
• Store unopened vials at room temperature. Once reconstituted and diluted as directed, drug is stable at room temperature for 8 hours. Because the drug does not contain anti-

bacterial preservatives, discard unused drug after 8 hours.

• Advise patient to watch for signs of infection (fever, sore throat, fatigue) and bleeding (easy bruising, nose bleeds, bleeding gums, melena). Tell patient to take temperature daily.
• Instruct patient to avoid OTC products containing aspirin.
• Advise women of childbearing age to avoid becoming pregnant during therapy. Also recommend consulting with the doctor before becoming pregnant.
• Because of the possibility of infant toxicity, advise breast-feeding patient taking carboplatin to discontinue breast-feeding.

# carmustine (BCNU)
BiCNU

*Pregnancy Risk Category: D*

## HOW SUPPLIED
*Injection:* 100-mg vial (lyophilized), with a 3-ml vial of absolute alcohol supplied as a diluent

## ACTION
Inhibits enzymatic reactions involved with DNA synthesis, cross-links strands of cellular DNA, and interferes with RNA transcription, causing an imbalance of growth that leads to cell death. Cell cycle-nonspecific.

## ONSET, PEAK, DURATION
Undefined.

## INDICATIONS & DOSAGE
*Brain tumors, Hodgkin's disease, malignant lymphoma, and multiple myeloma—*
**Adults:** 75 to 100 mg/m² I.V. by slow infusion daily for 2 days; repeated q 6 weeks if platelet count is above 100,000/mm³ and WBC count is above 4,000/mm³. Dosage is reduced

by 30% when WBC count is 2,000 to 3,000/mm³ and platelet count is 25,000 to 75,000/mm³. Dosage is reduced by 50% when WBC count is less than 2,000/mm³ and platelet count is less than 25,000/mm³.

Alternative therapy: 150 to 200 mg/m² I.V. by slow infusion as a single dose, repeated q 6 weeks.

## ADVERSE REACTIONS
**CNS:** ataxia, drowsiness.
**EENT:** ocular toxicities.
**GI:** *nausea* beginning in 2 to 6 hours (can be severe), *vomiting.*
**GU:** nephrotoxicity, azotemia, *renal failure.*
**Hematologic:** *cumulative bone marrow suppression,* delayed 4 to 6 weeks, lasting 1 to 2 weeks; *leukopenia; thrombocytopenia; acute leukemia or bone marrow dysplasia* may occur after long-term use; anemia.
**Hepatic:** hepatotoxicity.
**Respiratory:** *pulmonary fibrosis.*
**Skin:** facial flushing, hyperpigmentation.
**Other:** *intense pain at infusion site from venous spasm;* possible hyperuricemia in lymphoma patients when rapid cell lysis occurs.

## INTERACTIONS
*Anticoagulants, aspirin:* increased risk of bleeding. Avoid concomitant use.
*Cimetidine:* may increase carmustine's bone marrow toxicity. Avoid combination if possible.

## CONTRAINDICATIONS
Contraindicated in patients with hypersensitivity to drug.

## NURSING CONSIDERATIONS
• Be aware that pulmonary toxicity appears to be dose-related. Obtain baseline pulmonary function tests as ordered before therapy.
• Follow institutional policy to reduce risks because preparation and admin-

---

Reactions may be *common,* uncommon, *life-threatening,* or COMMON AND LIFE-THREATENING.

istration of parenteral form of this drug is associated with carcinogenic, mutagenic, and teratogenic risks for personnel.

• To reduce nausea, give antiemetic before administering drug, as ordered.

• **I.V. use:** To reconstitute, dissolve 100 mg of carmustine in the 3 ml of absolute alcohol provided by the manufacturer. Dilute solution with 27 ml of sterile water for injection. Resultant solution contains 3.3 mg of carmustine/ml in 10% alcohol. Dilute in 0.9% sodium chloride solution or $D_5W$ for I.V. infusion. Give at least 250 ml over 1 to 2 hours. To reduce pain on infusion, dilute further or slow infusion rate.

• Discard drug if powder liquefies or appears oily (decomposition has occurred).

• Administer only in glass containers. Solution is unstable in plastic I.V. bags.

• Don't mix with other drugs during administration.

• Avoid contact with skin because carmustine will cause a brown stain. If drug comes into contact with skin, wash off thoroughly.

• Perform liver, renal function, and pulmonary function tests periodically, as ordered.

• Monitor CBC, as ordered.

• Monitor serum uric acid level, as ordered. To prevent hyperuricemia with resulting uric acid nephropathy, know that allopurinol may be used with adequate hydration.

• Be aware that therapeutic effects are often accompanied by toxicity.

• To prevent bleeding, avoid all I.M. injections when platelet count is below 100,000/mm³.

• Anticipate possible blood transfusions during treatment because of cumulative anemia.

• Store reconstituted solution in refrigerator for 48 hours or at room temperature for 8 hours. May decompose at temperatures above 80° F (26.6° C).

☑ **PATIENT TEACHING**
• Advise patient to watch for signs of infection (fever, sore throat, fatigue) and bleeding (easy bruising, nosebleeds, bleeding gums, melena). Tell patient to take temperature daily.
• Instruct patient to avoid any OTC product containing aspirin.
• Advise breast-feeding patient to discontinue breast-feeding during therapy because of possible infant toxicity.
• Advise women of childbearing age to avoid becoming pregnant during therapy. Recommend patient consult with doctor before becoming pregnant.

## chlorambucil
Leukeran

*Pregnancy Risk Category: D*

**HOW SUPPLIED**
*Tablets:* 2 mg

**ACTION**
Cross-links strands of cellular DNA and interferes with RNA transcription, causing an imbalance of growth that leads to cell death. Cell cycle-nonspecific.

**ONSET, PEAK, DURATION**
Clinical onset occurs within 3 to 4 weeks. Peak plasma concentration occurs in 1 hour. Duration undefined.

**INDICATIONS & DOSAGE**
*Chronic lymphocytic leukemia; malignant lymphomas including lymphosarcoma, giant follicular lymphoma, and Hodgkin's disease –*
**Adults:** 0.1 to 0.2 mg/kg P.O. daily for 3 to 6 weeks; then adjusted for maintenance (usually 4 to 10 mg daily).

## ADVERSE REACTIONS
**CNS:** *seizures,* peripheral neuropathy, tremor, muscle twitching, confusion, agitation, ataxia, flaccid paresis.
**GI:** *nausea, vomiting, stomatitis,* diarrhea.
**GU:** *azoospermia, infertility.*
**Hematologic:** *neutropenia,* delayed up to 3 weeks, lasting up to 10 days after last dose; *bone marrow suppression; thrombocytopenia; anemia;* myelosuppression (usually moderate, gradual, and rapidly reversible).
**Hepatic:** hepatotoxicity.
**Respiratory:** interstitial pneumonitis, *pulmonary fibrosis* (rare).
**Skin:** rash, hypersensitivity.
**Other:** allergic febrile reaction.

## INTERACTIONS
*Anticoagulants, aspirin:* increased risk of bleeding. Avoid concomitant use.

## CONTRAINDICATIONS
Contraindicated in patients with hypersensitivity or resistance to previous therapy. Patients hypersensitive to other alkylating agents may also be hypersensitive to chlorambucil.

## NURSING CONSIDERATIONS
● Use cautiously in patients with a history of head trauma or seizures or in patients receiving other drugs that lower the seizure threshold.
● Monitor CBC, as ordered.
● Monitor serum uric acid level, as ordered. To prevent hyperuricemia with resulting uric acid nephropathy, know that allopurinol may be used with adequate hydration.
● If WBC count falls below 2,000/mm³ or granulocyte count falls below 1,000/mm³, follow institutional policy for infection control in immunocompromised patients. Severe neutropenia is reversible up to cumulative dosage of 6.5 mg/kg in a single course.

● Be aware that therapeutic effects are often accompanied by toxicity.
● To prevent bleeding, avoid all I.M. injections when platelet count is below 100,000/mm³.
● Anticipate possible blood transfusions during treatment because of cumulative anemia.

## ☑ PATIENT TEACHING
● Advise patient to watch for signs of infection (fever, sore throat, fatigue) and bleeding (easy bruising, nosebleeds, bleeding gums, melena). Tell patient to take temperature daily.
● Instruct patient to avoid OTC products containing aspirin.
● Advise breast-feeding patient to discontinue breast-feeding during therapy because of possible infant toxicity.
● Advise women of childbearing age to avoid becoming pregnant during therapy and to notify doctor immediately if pregnancy is suspected.

---

# cisplatin (cis-platinum)
Platamine‡, Platinol, Platinol AQ

*Pregnancy Risk Category: D*

## HOW SUPPLIED
*Injection:* 0.5 mg/ml†, 1 mg/ml
*Powder for injection:* 10 mg, 50 mg

## ACTION
Unknown. Probably cross-links strands of cellular DNA and interferes with RNA transcription, causing an imbalance of growth that leads to cell death. Cell cycle-nonspecific.

## ONSET, PEAK, DURATION
Onset and peak undefined. Effects persist for several days after administration.

## INDICATIONS & DOSAGE
*Adjunctive therapy in metastatic testicular cancer –*
**Adults:** 20 mg/m² I.V. daily for 5

---

Reactions may be *common,* uncommon, *life-threatening,* or **COMMON AND LIFE-THREATENING.**

days. Repeated q 3 weeks for three cycles or longer.

*Adjunctive therapy in metastatic ovarian cancer—*

**Adults:** 100 mg/m$^2$ I.V.; repeated q 4 weeks. Or 75 to 100 mg/m$^2$ I.V. once q 4 weeks in combination with cyclophosphamide.

*Advanced bladder cancer—*

**Adults:** 50 to 70 mg/m$^2$ I.V. q 3 to 4 weeks. Patients who have received other antineoplastic agents or radiation therapy should receive 50 mg/m$^2$ q 4 weeks.

   *Note:* Prehydration and mannitol diuresis may reduce renal toxicity and ototoxicity significantly.

## ADVERSE REACTIONS

**CNS:** *peripheral neuritis,* loss of taste, *seizures.*

**EENT:** *tinnitus, hearing loss, ototoxicity,* vestibular toxicity.

**GI:** *nausea, vomiting* (beginning 1 to 4 hours after dose and lasting 24 hours).

**GU:** more prolonged and SEVERE RENAL TOXICITY with repeated courses of therapy.

**Hematologic:** MYELOSUPPRESSION; *leukopenia, thrombocytopenia, anemia;* nadirs in circulating platelet and WBC counts on days 18 to 23, with recovery by day 39.

**Other:** *anaphylactoid reaction, hypomagnesemia,* hypokalemia, hypocalcemia, hyponatremia, hypophosphatemia, hyperuricemia.

## INTERACTIONS

*Aminoglycoside antibiotics:* additive nephrotoxicity. Monitor renal function studies very carefully.

*Bumetanide, ethacrynic acid, furosemide:* additive ototoxicity. Avoid concomitant use.

*Phenytoin:* decreased serum phenytoin levels. Monitor serum levels.

## CONTRAINDICATIONS

Contraindicated in patients with hypersensitivity to the drug or to other platinum-containing compounds and in those with severe renal disease, hearing impairment, or myelosuppression.

## NURSING CONSIDERATIONS

• Monitor CBC, electrolyte levels (especially potassium and magnesium), platelet count, and renal function studies before initial and subsequent dosages, as ordered.

• To detect hearing loss, perform audiometry before initial dosage and subsequent courses, as ordered.

• Administer mannitol as 12.5-g I.V. bolus before starting cisplatin infusion, as ordered. Follow, if ordered, by infusion of mannitol at rate of up to 10 g/hour p.r.n. to maintain urine output during and 6 to 24 hours after cisplatin infusion.

• Hydrate patient with 0.9% sodium chloride solution before giving drug, as ordered. Maintain urine output of 100 ml/hour for 4 consecutive hours before therapy and for 24 hours after therapy.

• Follow institutional policy to reduce risks because preparation and administration of parenteral form of this drug is associated with carcinogenic, mutagenic, and teratogenic risks for personnel.

• **I.V. use:** Reconstitute powder using sterile water for injection. Add 10 ml to the 10-mg vial or 50 ml to the 50-mg vial to make a solution containing 1 mg/ml. If necessary, further dilute with dextrose 5% in 0.3% sodium chloride injection or dextrose 5% in 0.45% sodium chloride injection. Solutions are stable for 20 hours at room temperature. Don't refrigerate.

• Keep in mind that infusions are most stable in chloride-containing solutions (such as 0.9% sodium chloride, 0.45% sodium chloride, and 0.22% sodium chloride).

• Be aware that the manufacturer recommends administering the drug as an I.V. infusion in 2 liters of 0.9% sodium chloride solution with 37.5 g of mannitol over 6 to 8 hours.

• Do not use needles or I.V. administration sets that contain aluminum because it will displace the platinum, causing a loss of potency and formation of a black precipitate.

• Know that therapeutic effects are often accompanied by toxicity.

• Check current protocol. Some clinicians use I.V. sodium thiosulfate to minimize toxicity.

• Administer antiemetics, as ordered. Nausea and vomiting may be severe and protracted (up to 24 hours). Monitor intake and output. Continue I.V. hydration until patient can tolerate adequate oral intake.

• Keep in mind that ondansetron, granisetron, or high-dose metoclopramide has been used very effectively to treat and prevent nausea and vomiting. Some clinicians combine metoclopramide with dexamethasone and antihistamines, or ondansetron or granisetron with dexamethasone.

• Be alert that delayed-onset vomiting (3 to 5 days after treatment) has been reported. Patients may need prolonged antiemetic treatment.

• Know that renal toxicity is cumulative. Renal function must return to normal before next dose can be given.

• Know that dosage should not be repeated unless platelet count is over 100,000/mm³, WBC count is over 4,000/mm³, creatinine level is under 1.5 mg/dl, or BUN level is under 25 mg/dl.

• To prevent bleeding, avoid all I.M. injections when platelet counts are below 100,000/mm³.

• Anticipate possible blood transfusions during treatment because of cumulative anemia.

• To prevent hypokalemia, know that potassium chloride (10 to 20 mEq/L)

is frequently added to I.V. fluids before and after cisplatin therapy.

• **Alert:** Immediately administer epinephrine, corticosteroids, or antihistamines for anaphylactoid reactions, as ordered.

☑ **PATIENT TEACHING**
• Advise patient to watch for signs of infection (fever, sore throat, fatigue) and bleeding (easy bruising, nosebleeds, bleeding gums, melena). Tell patient to take temperature daily.

• Tell patient to report tinnitus or numbness in hands or feet immediately.

• Instruct patient to avoid any OTC products containing aspirin.

• Advise breast-feeding patient taking this drug to discontinue breast-feeding because of the possibility of infant toxicity.

• Advise women of childbearing age to avoid becoming pregnant during therapy. Also recommend consulting with doctor before becoming pregnant.

# cyclophosphamide
Cycoblastin‡, Cytoxan**, Cytoxan Lyophilized, Endoxan-Asta‡, Neosar, Procytox†

*Pregnancy Risk Category: D*

## HOW SUPPLIED
*Tablets:* 25 mg, 50 mg
*Injection:* 100-mg, 200-mg, 500-mg, 1-g, 2-g vials

## ACTION
Cross-links strands of cellular DNA and interferes with RNA transcription, causing an imbalance of growth that leads to cell death. Cell cycle-nonspecific.

## ONSET, PEAK, DURATION
Undefined.

---

## INDICATIONS & DOSAGE

*Breast, head, neck, prostate, lung, and ovarian cancers; Hodgkin's disease; chronic lymphocytic leukemia; chronic myelocytic leukemia; acute lymphoblastic leukemia; acute myelocytic leukemia; neuroblastoma; retinoblastoma; malignant lymphoma; multiple myeloma; mycosis fungoides; sarcoma –*

**Adults and children:** initially, 40 to 50 mg/kg I.V. in divided doses over 2 to 5 days. Alternatively, 10 to 15 mg/kg I.V. q 7 to 10 days, 3 to 5 mg/kg I.V. twice weekly, or 1 to 5 mg/kg P.O. daily, depending on patient tolerance. Subsequent dosages adjusted according to evidence of antitumor activity or leukopenia.

*"Minimal change" nephrotic syndrome in children –*
**Children:** 2.5 to 3 mg/kg P.O. daily for 60 to 90 days.

## ADVERSE REACTIONS

**CV:** *cardiotoxicity* (with very high doses and in combination with doxorubicin).
**GI:** anorexia, *nausea and vomiting* (beginning within 6 hours), abdominal pain, stomatitis, mucositis.
**GU:** HEMORRHAGIC CYSTITIS, fertility impairment.
**Hematologic:** *leukopenia,* nadir between days 8 to 15, recovery in 17 to 28 days; *thrombocytopenia; anemia.*
**Respiratory:** *pulmonary fibrosis* (high doses).
**Other:** *reversible alopecia, secondary malignant disease, anaphylaxis,* hypersensitivity reactions, hepatotoxicity.

## INTERACTIONS

*Barbiturates:* increased pharmacologic effect and enhanced cyclophosphamide toxicity due to induction of hepatic enzymes. Monitor patient closely.
*Cardiotoxic drugs:* additive adverse cardiac effects. Monitor for toxicity.

*Chloramphenicol, corticosteroids:* reduced activity of cyclophosphamide. Use cautiously.
*Digoxin:* may decrease serum digoxin levels. Monitor levels closely.
*Succinylcholine:* prolonged neuromuscular blockade. Don't use together.

## CONTRAINDICATIONS

Contraindicated in patients with hypersensitivity to the drug or with severe bone marrow suppression.

## NURSING CONSIDERATIONS

• Use cautiously in patients with leukopenia, thrombocytopenia, malignant cell infiltration of bone marrow, or hepatic or renal disease and in those who have recently undergone radiation therapy or chemotherapy.
• Follow institutional policy to reduce risks. Preparation and administration of parenteral form of this drug is associated with carcinogenic, mutagenic, and teratogenic risks for personnel.
• **I.V. use:** Reconstitute powder using sterile water for injection or bacteriostatic water for injection containing only parabens. For the nonlyophilized product, add 5 ml to the 100-mg vial, 10 ml to the 200-mg vial, 25 ml to the 500-mg vial, 50 ml to the 1-g vial, or 100 ml to the 2-g vial to produce a solution containing 20 mg/ml. Shake to dissolve; this may take up to 6 minutes, and it may be difficult to completely dissolve drug. Lyophilized preparation is much easier to reconstitute; check package insert for quantity of diluent needed to reconstitute drug.
• After reconstitution, administer as ordered by direct I.V. injection or infusion. For I.V. infusion, further dilute with D₅W, dextrose 5% in 0.9% sodium chloride injection, dextrose 5% in Ringer's injection, lactated Ringer's injection, sodium lactate injection, or 0.45% sodium chloride injection.

• Check reconstituted solution for small particles. Filter solution if necessary.

• Know that reconstituted solution is stable for 6 days refrigerated or 24 hours at room temperature. However, use stored solutions cautiously because the drug contains no preservatives.

• Don't give the drug at bedtime; infrequent urination during the night may increase the possibility of cystitis. If cystitis occurs, discontinue drug and notify doctor. Cystitis can occur months after therapy ceases. Mesna may be given to lower the incidence and severity of bladder toxicity.

• Monitor CBC and renal and liver function tests, as ordered.

• Monitor serum uric acid level, as ordered. To prevent hyperuricemia with resulting uric acid nephropathy, know that allopurinol may be used with adequate hydration.

• **Alert:** Monitor for cyclophosphamide toxicity if patient's corticosteroid therapy is discontinued.

• To prevent bleeding, avoid all I.M. injections when platelet count is below 100,000/mm³.

• Anticipate possible blood transfusions because of cumulative anemia.

• Know that therapeutic effects are often accompanied by toxicity.

☑ **PATIENT TEACHING**
• Warn patient that alopecia is likely to occur but that it is reversible.

• Advise patient to watch for signs of infection (fever, sore throat, fatigue) and bleeding (easy bruising, nosebleeds, bleeding gums, melena). Tell patient to take temperature daily.

• Instruct patient to avoid OTC products containing aspirin.

• To minimize the risk of hemorrhagic cystitis, encourage patient to void every 1 to 2 hours while awake and to drink at least 3 liters of fluid daily. If patient is taking oral form of drug, instruct him to avoid taking it at bedtime because infrequent urination increases risk of cystitis.

• Advise male and female patients to practice contraception while taking this drug and for 4 months after; drug is potentially teratogenic.

• Advise breast-feeding patient taking this drug to discontinue breast-feeding because of the possibility of infant toxicity.

• Advise women of childbearing age to avoid becoming pregnant during therapy. Also recommend consulting with doctor before becoming pregnant.

---

# ifosfamide
IFEX
*Pregnancy Risk Category: D*

**HOW SUPPLIED**
*Injection:* 1 g, 2 g†, 3 g†

**ACTION**
Cross-links strands of cellular DNA and interferes with RNA transcription, causing an imbalance of growth that leads to cell death. Cell cycle-nonspecific.

**ONSET, PEAK, DURATION**
Undefined.

**INDICATIONS & DOSAGE**
*Testicular cancer –*
**Adults:** 1.2 g/m²/day I.V. for 5 consecutive days. Treatment is repeated q 3 weeks or after the patient recovers from hematologic toxicity.

**ADVERSE REACTIONS**
**CNS:** *somnolence, confusion, **coma, seizures,** ataxia, hallucinations, depressive psychosis, dizziness, disorientation, cranial nerve dysfunction.*
**GI:** *nausea, vomiting.*
**GU:** *hemorrhagic cystitis, hematuria, nephrotoxicity.*
**Hematologic:** *leukopenia, **thrombocytopenia, myelosuppression.***

---

Reactions may be *common,* uncommon, *life-threatening,* or **COMMON AND LIFE-THREATENING.**

**Hepatic:** elevated liver enzyme levels, liver dysfunction.
**Other:** *alopecia, metabolic acidosis,* infection, phlebitis.

## INTERACTIONS

*Allopurinol:* may produce excessive ifosfamide effect by prolonging half-life. Monitor for enhanced toxicity.
*Anticoagulants, aspirin:* increased risk of bleeding. Avoid concomitant use.
*Barbiturates, chloral hydrate, phenytoin:* may increase ifosfamide toxicity by inducing hepatic enzymes that hasten the formation of toxic metabolites. Monitor patient closely.
*Corticosteroids:* may inhibit hepatic enzymes, reducing ifosfamide's effect. Monitor for enhanced ifosfamide toxicity if concurrent steroid dosage is suddenly reduced or discontinued.
*Myelosuppressants:* enhanced hematologic toxicity. Dosage adjustment may be necessary.

## CONTRAINDICATIONS

Contraindicated in patients with hypersensitivity to the drug and in those with severe bone marrow suppression.

## NURSING CONSIDERATIONS

● Use cautiously in patients with renal impairment or compromised bone marrow reserve as indicated by leukopenia, granulocytopenia, extensive bone marrow metastases, prior radiation therapy, or prior therapy with cytotoxic agents.
● Administer antiemetics, as ordered, before giving ifosfamide to help decrease nausea.
● Follow institutional policy to reduce risks. Preparation and administration of parenteral form of this drug is associated with carcinogenic, mutagenic, and teratogenic risks for personnel.
● **I.V. use:** Reconstitute each gram of drug with 20 ml of diluent to yield a solution of 50 mg/ml. Use sterile water for injection or bacteriostatic water for injection. Solutions may then be further diluted with sterile water, dextrose 2.5% or 5% in water, 0.45% or 0.9% sodium chloride for injection, 5% dextrose and 0.9% sodium chloride for injection, or lactated Ringer's injection.
● Infuse each dose over at least 30 minutes.
● As ordered, administer ifosfamide with a protecting agent (mesna) to prevent hemorrhagic cystitis. Obtain urinalysis before each dose. If microscopic hematuria is present, mesna must be given concomitantly with or before ifosfamide to prevent cystitis. (Dosage adjustments of mesna given concomitantly may be necessary.) Adequate fluid intake (2 liters/day, either P.O. or I.V.) is essential.
● Assess patients for mental status changes; dosage may have to be decreased.
● Know that ifosfamide and mesna are physically compatible and may be mixed in the same I.V. solution.
● Keep in mind that reconstituted solution is stable for 1 week at room temperature or 6 weeks if refrigerated. However, use solution within 6 hours if drug was reconstituted with sterile water without a preservative (such as benzyl alcohol or parabens).
● Don't give the drug at bedtime; infrequent voiding during the night may increase the possibility of cystitis. If cystitis develops, discontinue drug and notify doctor.
● Be aware that bladder irrigation with 0.9% sodium chloride solution may decrease the possibility of cystitis.
● Monitor CBC and renal and liver function tests, as ordered.
● To prevent bleeding, avoid all I.M. injections when platelet count is below 100,000/mm³.
● Anticipate possible blood transfusions because of cumulative anemia.

---

*Liquid form contains alcohol.   **May contain tartrazine.   †Canada only.   ‡Australia only.   ◊OTC.

☑ **PATIENT TEACHING**
• To minimize contact of ifosfamide and its metabolites with the bladder mucosa, remind patient to void frequently.
• Advise patient to watch for signs of infection (fever, sore throat, fatigue) and bleeding (easy bruising, nosebleeds, bleeding gums, melena). Tell patient to take temperature daily.
• Instruct patient to avoid OTC products containing aspirin.
• Advise breast-feeding patient to discontinue breast-feeding during therapy because of possible infant toxicity.
• Advise women of childbearing age to avoid becoming pregnant during therapy. Also recommend consulting with doctor before becoming pregnant.

# lomustine (CCNU)
CeeNU

*Pregnancy Risk Category: D*

## HOW SUPPLIED
*Capsules:* 10 mg, 40 mg, 100 mg, dose pack (two 10-mg, two 40-mg, two 100-mg capsules)

## ACTION
Cross-links strands of cellular DNA and interferes with RNA transcription, causing an imbalance of growth that leads to cell death. Cell cycle-nonspecific.

## ONSET, PEAK, DURATION
Undefined.

## INDICATIONS & DOSAGE
*Brain tumor, Hodgkin's disease* —
**Adults and children:** 100 to 130 mg/m² P.O. as a single dose q 6 weeks. Dosage reduced according to degree of bone marrow suppression. Repeat doses should not be given until WBC count is more than 4,000/mm³ and

platelet count is more than 100,000/mm³.

## ADVERSE REACTIONS
**CNS:** disorientation, lethargy, ataxia.
**GI:** *nausea, vomiting,* stomatitis.
**GU:** nephrotoxicity, progressive azotemia, *renal failure.*
**Hematologic:** *anemia, leukopenia,* delayed up to 6 weeks, lasting 1 to 2 weeks; thrombocytopenia, delayed up to 4 weeks, lasting 1 to 2 weeks; *bone marrow suppression,* delayed up to 4 to 6 weeks.
**Other:** hepatotoxicity, *secondary malignant disease,* pulmonary fibrosis, alopecia.

## INTERACTIONS
*Anticoagulants, aspirin:* increased risk of bleeding. Avoid concomitant use.

## CONTRAINDICATIONS
Contraindicated in patients with hypersensitivity to the drug.

## NURSING CONSIDERATIONS
• Use cautiously in patients with decreased platelet, WBC, or RBC counts and in those receiving other myelosuppressants.
• To avoid nausea, give antiemetic before administering, as ordered.
• Give 2 to 4 hours after meals; drug will be more completely absorbed if taken when the stomach is empty.
• Monitor CBC weekly, as ordered. Usually not administered more often than every 6 weeks; bone marrow toxicity is cumulative and delayed, usually occuring in 4 to 6 weeks after drug administration.
• Periodically monitor liver function tests, as ordered.
• To prevent bleeding, avoid all I.M. injections when platelet count is below 100,000/mm³.
• Anticipate possible blood transfusions because of cumulative anemia.

---

Reactions may be *common,* uncommon, *life-threatening,* or COMMON AND LIFE-THREATENING.

• Know that therapeutic effects are often accompanied by toxicity.

## ☑ PATIENT TEACHING
• Advise patient to watch for signs of infection (fever, sore throat, fatigue) and bleeding (easy bruising, nosebleeds, bleeding gums, melena). Tell patient to take temperature daily.
• Instruct patient to avoid OTC products containing aspirin.
• Advise breast-feeding patients to discontinue breast-feeding during therapy because of possible infant toxicity.
• Advise women of childbearing age to avoid becoming pregnant during therapy. Also recommend consulting with doctor before becoming pregnant.

---

## mechlorethamine hydrochloride (nitrogen mustard)
Mustargen

*Pregnancy Risk Category: D*

### HOW SUPPLIED
*Injection:* 10-mg vials

### ACTION
Cross-links strands of cellular DNA and interferes with RNA transcription, causing an imbalance of growth that leads to cell death. Cell cycle-nonspecific.

### ONSET, PEAK, DURATION
Onset occurs in seconds to minutes. Peak and duration undefined.

### INDICATIONS & DOSAGE
*Polycythemia vera, chronic lymphocytic leukemia, chronic myelocytic leukemia, malignant effusions (pericardial, peritoneal, pleural), mycosis fungoides, Hodgkin's disease, lymphosarcoma, bronchogenic cancer* –
**Adults:** 0.4 mg/kg or 10 mg/m² I.V. as a single dose or in divided doses of

0.1 to 0.2 mg/kg/day. Given through running I.V. infusion. Subsequent courses of therapy given when patient has recovered hematologically from previous course (usually 3 to 6 weeks).
*Malignant effusions* –
**Adults:** 0.2 to 0.4 mg/kg intracavitarily.

### ADVERSE REACTIONS
**CNS:** weakness, vertigo.
**EENT:** tinnitus; deafness with high doses.
**GI:** *nausea, vomiting,* and *anorexia* beginning within minutes, lasting 8 to 24 hours.
**Hematologic:** *thrombocytopenia,* lymphocytopenia, *agranulocytosis,* nadir of myelosuppression occurring by days 4 to 10 and lasting 10 to 21 days; mild anemia begins in 2 to 3 weeks.
**Skin:** rash, sloughing, severe irritation if drug extravasates or touches skin.
**Other:** *alopecia,* precipitation of herpes zoster, *anaphylaxis,* hyperuricemia; *thrombophlebitis,* amyloidosis, jaundice, menstrual irregularities, impaired spermatogenesis.

### INTERACTIONS
*Anticoagulants, aspirin:* increased risk of bleeding. Avoid concomitant use.

### CONTRAINDICATIONS
Contraindicated in patients with hypersensitivity to the drug and with known infectious diseases.

### NURSING CONSIDERATIONS
• Use cautiously in patients with severe anemia, depressed neutrophil or platelet count, or in those who have recently undergone radiation therapy or chemotherapy. Monitor CBC.
• Follow institutional policy to reduce risks. Preparation and administration of parenteral form of this drug is asso-

---

*Liquid form contains alcohol.   **May contain tartrazine.   †Canada only.   ‡Australia only.   ◇OTC.

ciated with carcinogenic, mutagenic, and teratogenic risks for personnel.
• Know that drug has been associated with severe nausea and vomiting. Premedicate with antiemetics as ordered.
• **I.V. use:** Reconstitute the drug using 10 ml of sterile water for injection or 0.9% sodium chloride injection. The resulting solution contains 1 mg/ml of mechlorethamine. Give by direct injection into a vein or into the tubing of a free-flowing I.V. solution.
• Prepare immediately before infusion. Very unstable solution. Visually inspect before using; use within 15 minutes, and discard unused solution.
• Do not use solutions that are discolored or contain particulate matter. Do not use vials that appear to contain droplets of water.
• Dispose of any equipment used in the preparation and administration of mechlorethamine properly and according to institutional policy. Neutralize unused solution with an equal volume of 5% sodium bicarbonate and 5% sodium thiosulfate.
• *Alert:* Make sure I.V. solution doesn't infiltrate. Mechlorethamine is a potent vesicant. If drug extravasates, apply cold compresses and infiltrate the area with isotonic sodium thiosulfate, as ordered.
• When given intracavitarily for sclerosing effect, dilute using up to 100 ml of 0.9% sodium chloride for injection. Turn patient from side to side every 15 minutes to 1 hour to distribute drug.
• Monitor serum uric acid level, as ordered. To prevent hyperuricemia with resulting uric acid nephropathy, know that mechlorethamine may be used with adequate hydration.
• Know that therapeutic effects are often accompanied by toxicity.
• Be aware that neurotoxicity increases with dose and patient age.
• To prevent bleeding, avoid all I.M. injections when platelet count is below 100,000/mm$^3$.

• Anticipate possible blood transfusions because of cumulative anemia.

☑ **PATIENT TEACHING**
• Advise patient to watch for signs of infection (fever, sore throat, fatigue) and bleeding (easy bruising, nosebleeds, bleeding gums, melena). Tell patient to take temperature daily.
• Instruct patient to avoid OTC products containing aspirin.
• Advise women of childbearing age to avoid becoming pregnant during therapy. Suggest consulting with doctor before becoming pregnant.
• Advise breast-feeding patient taking this drug to discontinue breastfeeding because of the possibility of infant toxicity.

# melphalan (L-phenylalanine mustard)
Alkeran

*Pregnancy Risk Category: D*

## HOW SUPPLIED
*Tablets (scored):* 2 mg
*Injection:* 50 mg

## ACTION
Cross-links strands of cellular DNA and interferes with RNA transcription, causing an imbalance of growth that leads to cell death. Cell cycle-nonspecific.

## ONSET, PEAK, DURATION
Undefined.

## INDICATIONS & DOSAGE
*Multiple myeloma—*
**Adults:** initially, 6 mg P.O. daily for 2 to 3 weeks; then drug is stopped for up to 4 weeks or until WBC and platelet counts stop dropping and begin to rise again; maintenance dosage of 2 mg daily then given. Alternative therapy: 0.15 mg/kg P.O. daily for 7 days, or 0.25 mg/kg for 4 days; repeated q 4 to 6 weeks.

Alternatively, administered I.V. to patients who can't tolerate oral therapy. 16 mg/m² given by infusion over 15 to 20 minutes at 2-week intervals for four doses. After patient has recovered from toxicity, drug given at 4-week intervals.

*Nonresectable advanced ovarian cancer—*
**Adults:** 0.2 mg/kg P.O. daily for 5 days. Repeated q 4 to 6 weeks, depending on bone marrow recovery.

## ADVERSE REACTIONS
**CV:** hypotension, tachycardia, edema.
**GI:** nausea, vomiting, diarrhea, oral ulceration.
**Hematologic:** *thrombocytopenia, leukopenia, bone marrow suppression,* hemolytic anemia.
**Respiratory:** *pneumonitis, pulmonary fibrosis,* dyspnea, bronchospasm.
**Skin:** pruritus, alopecia, urticaria.
**Other:** *anaphylaxis,* hypersensitivity, *anaphylaxis,* hepatotoxicity.

## INTERACTIONS
*Anticoagulants, aspirin:* increased risk of bleeding. Avoid concomitant use.
*Antigout agents:* decreased effectiveness. Dosage adjustments may be necessary.
*Bone marrow suppressants:* additive toxicity. Monitor closely.
*Vaccines:* decreased effectiveness of killed-virus vaccines and increased risk of toxicity from live-virus vaccines. Postpone routine immunization for at least 3 months after last dose of melphalan.

## CONTRAINDICATIONS
Contraindicated in patients with hypersensitivity to the drug and in those whose disease is known to be resistant to the drug. Patients hypersensitive to chlorambucil may have cross-sensitivity to melphalan.

## NURSING CONSIDERATIONS
• Be aware that drug is not recommended in patients with severe leukopenia, thrombocytopenia, or anemia or in those with chronic lymphocytic leukemia.
• Keep in mind that dosage may need to be reduced in patients with renal impairment.
• Know that melphalan is the drug of choice in combination with prednisone in patients with multiple myeloma.
• Follow institutional policy to reduce risks. Preparation and administration of parenteral form of the drug is associated with carcinogenic, mutagenic, and teratogenic risks for personnel.
• **I.V. use:** Because drug isn't stable in solution, reconstitute immediately before administering with the 10 ml of sterile diluent supplied by the manufacturer. Shake vigorously until a solution is clear. The resultant solution will contain 5 mg/ml of melphalan. Immediately dilute the required dose in 0.9% sodium chloride for injection. Final concentration shouldn't exceed 0.45 mg/ml. Give infusion over 15 to 20 minutes.
• Promptly dilute and administer; the reconstituted product begins to degrade within 30 minutes. After final dilution, nearly 1% of the drug degrades every 10 minutes. Don't refrigerate the reconstituted product because a precipitate will form.
• Give oral form on empty stomach. Food decreases drug absorption.
• Know that therapeutic effects are often accompanied by toxicity.
• Monitor serum uric acid level and CBC, as ordered.
• To prevent bleeding, avoid all I.M. injections when platelet count is below 100,000/mm³.
• Anticipate possible blood transfusions because of cumulative anemia.

## ☑ PATIENT TEACHING
• Advise patient to watch for signs of infection (fever, sore throat, fatigue)

---

*Liquid form contains alcohol. **May contain tartrazine. †Canada only. ‡Australia only. ◇OTC.

and bleeding (easy bruising, nose-bleeds, bleeding gums, melena). Tell patient to take temperature daily.
• Instruct patient to avoid OTC products containing aspirin.
• Advise women of childbearing age to avoid becoming pregnant during therapy. Suggest consulting with the doctor before becoming pregnant.
• Advise breast-feeding patient taking this drug to discontinue breastfeeding because of the possibility of infant toxicity.

---

## streptozocin
Zanosar

*Pregnancy Risk Category: C*

### HOW SUPPLIED
*Injection:* 1-g vials

### ACTION
Unknown. Probably cross-links strands of cellular DNA and interferes with RNA transcription, causing an imbalance of growth that leads to cell death. Cell cycle-nonspecific.

### ONSET, PEAK, DURATION
Undefined.

### INDICATIONS & DOSAGE
*Metastatic islet cell carcinoma of the pancreas –*
**Adults and children:** 500 mg/m$^2$ I.V. for 5 consecutive days q 6 weeks until maximum benefit or toxicity is observed. Alternatively, 1,000 mg/m$^2$ at weekly intervals for the first 2 weeks. Not to exceed a single dose of 1,500 mg/m$^2$.

### ADVERSE REACTIONS
**CNS:** confusion, lethargy, depression.
**GI:** *nausea, vomiting,* diarrhea.
**GU:** *renal toxicity* (evidenced by azotemia, glycosuria, and renal tubular acidosis), mild proteinuria.

**Hematologic:** *anemia, leukopenia, thrombocytopenia.*
**Hepatic:** elevated liver enzyme levels, jaundice, *liver dysfunction.*
**Other:** hyperglycemia, hypoglycemia, diabetes mellitus.

### INTERACTIONS
*Doxorubicin:* prolonged elimination half-life of doxorubicin. Dose of doxorubicin should be reduced.
*Other potentially nephrotoxic drugs, such as aminoglycosides:* increased risk of renal toxicity. Use cautiously.
*Phenytoin:* may decrease effectiveness of streptozocin in patients with pancreatic cancer. Monitor carefully.

### CONTRAINDICATIONS
None known.

### NURSING CONSIDERATIONS
• Use cautiously in patients with renal disease.
• Obtain renal function tests before therapy, as ordered.
• Follow institutional policy to reduce risks. Preparation and administration of parenteral form of this drug is associated with carcinogenic, mutagenic, and teratogenic risks for personnel.
• **I.V. use:** Reconstitute streptozocin powder with 9.5 ml of D$_5$W or 0.9% sodium chloride for injection. This will produce a pale gold solution. May be further diluted with D$_5$W or 0.9% sodium chloride for injection. Infuse over at least 15 minutes to minimize the risk of phlebitis.
• *Alert:* If extravasation occurs, stop infusion at once and notify doctor.
• Use within 12 hours of reconstitution. The product contains no preservatives and is not intended as a multiple-dose vial.
• Monitor renal function tests after each course of therapy, as ordered. Renal toxicity resulting from streptozocin therapy is dose-related and cumulative. Urinalysis; BUN, creatinine, and serum electrolyte levels; and creatinine

---

clearance should be obtained at least weekly during drug therapy. Weekly monitoring should continue for 4 weeks after each course.
• To minimize risk of renal toxicity, ensure adequate hydration using oral or parenteral fluids, as ordered.
• Test urine for protein and glucose levels each nursing shift. Mild proteinuria is one of the first signs of renal toxicity; notify the doctor, who may reduce the dosage.
• Monitor CBC and liver function studies at least weekly, as ordered.
• Make sure patients are being treated with an antiemetic. Nausea and vomiting occur in most patients.
• Know that therapeutic effects are often accompanied by toxicity.
• Store unopened and unreconstituted vials in the refrigerator.

☑ **PATIENT TEACHING**
• Advise patient to watch for signs of infection (fever, sore throat, fatigue) and bleeding (easy bruising, nosebleeds, bleeding gums, melena). Tell patient to take temperature daily.
• Advise breast-feeding patient taking this drug to discontinue breastfeeding because of the possibility of infant toxicity.

---

## thiotepa (TESPA, triethylenethiophosphoramide, TSPA)
Thiotepa

*Pregnancy Risk Category: NR*

### HOW SUPPLIED
*Injection:* 15-mg vials

### ACTION
Cross-links strands of cellular DNA and interferes with RNA transcription, causing an imbalance of growth that leads to cell death. Cell cyclenonspecific.

### ONSET, PEAK, DURATION
Undefined.

### INDICATIONS & DOSAGE
*Breast and ovarian cancers, lymphoma, Hodgkin's disease* –
**Adults and children over 12 years:** 0.3 to 0.4 mg/kg I.V. q 1 to 4 weeks or 0.2 mg/kg 4 to 5 days at intervals of 2 to 4 weeks.
*Bladder tumor* –
**Adults and children over 12 years:** 60 mg in 30 to 60 ml of water instilled in bladder for 2 hours once weekly for 4 weeks.
*Neoplastic effusions* –
**Adults and children over 12 years:** 0.6 to 0.8 mg/kg intracavitarily.

### ADVERSE REACTIONS
**CNS:** headache, dizziness, blurred vision, fatigue, weakness.
**EENT:** laryngeal edema, conjunctivitis.
**GI:** *nausea, vomiting,* abdominal pain, anorexia.
**GU:** amenorrhea, decreased spermatogenesis, dysuria, urine retention, hemorrhagic cystitis.
**Hematologic:** *leukopenia* begins within 5 to 10 days; *thrombocytopenia; neutropenia; anemia.*
**Respiratory:** asthma.
**Skin:** hives, rash, dermatitis.
**Other:** fever, alopecia, hypersensitivity, *anaphylactic shock.*

### INTERACTIONS
*Anticoagulants, aspirin:* increased risk of bleeding. Avoid concomitant use.

### CONTRAINDICATIONS
Contraindicated in patients with hypersensitivity to the drug and in those with severe bone marrow, hepatic, or renal dysfunction.

### NURSING CONSIDERATIONS
• Know that use in pregnancy is not recommended except in situations

---

*Liquid form contains alcohol. **May contain tartrazine. †Canada only. ‡Australia only. ◊OTC.

where the benefits outweigh the risk of teratogenicity involved.

• Use cautiously in patients with mild bone marrow suppression and renal or hepatic dysfunction.

• Follow institutional policy to minimize risks. Preparation and administration of parenteral form of this drug is linked with mutagenic, teratogenic, and carcinogenic risks to personnel.

• **I.V. use:** Reconstitute with 1.5 ml of sterile water for injection. Do not reconstitute with any other solution. Further dilute with 0.9% sodium chloride for injection, $D_5W$, dextrose 5% in 0.9% sodium chloride for injection, Ringer's injection, or lactated Ringer's injection. Solutions are stable for up to 5 days if refrigerated.

• Use local anesthetic at injection site, as ordered, if intense pain occurs.

• If pain occurs at insertion site, dilute the drug further or use a local anesthetic, as ordered, to reduce pain. Make sure drug does not infiltrate.

• Discard if solution appears grossly opaque or has a precipitate. Solutions should be clear to slightly opaque.

• For neoplastic effusions, mix drug with 2% procaine hydrochloride or epinephrine hydrochloride 1:1,000, as ordered.

• For bladder instillation: Dehydrate patients 8 to 10 hours before therapy. Instill drug into bladder by catheter; ask patients to retain solution for 2 hours. Know that volume may be reduced to 30 ml if discomfort is too great with 60 ml. Reposition patients every 15 minutes for maximum area contact.

• Monitor CBC weekly for at least 3 weeks after last dose, as ordered.

• Know that drug should be discontinued if WBC count is below 3,000/$mm^3$ or if platelet count is below 150,000/$mm^3$. If that occurs, notify doctor.

• Monitor serum uric acid levels, as ordered. To prevent hyperuricemia with resulting uric acid nephropathy,

know that allopurinol may be used with adequate hydration.

• Know that therapeutic effects are often accompanied by toxicity.

• To prevent bleeding, avoid all I.M. injections when platelet count is below 100,000/$mm^3$.

• Anticipate blood transfusions because of cumulative anemia.

• Be aware that GU adverse reactions are reversible in 6 to 8 months.

• Refrigerate and protect dry powder from direct sunlight to avoid possible drug breakdown.

☑ **PATIENT TEACHING**

• Advise patient to watch for signs of infection (fever, sore throat, fatigue) and bleeding (easy bruising, nosebleeds, bleeding gums, melena). Tell patient to take temperature daily. Tell patients to report even mild infections.

• Instruct patient to avoid OTC products containing aspirin.

• Advise breast-feeding patient to stop breast-feeding during therapy because of possible infant toxicity.

• Advise women of childbearing age to avoid becoming pregnant during therapy. Suggest consulting with doctor before becoming pregnant.

---

## uracil mustard
Uracil Mustard Capsules**
*Pregnancy Risk Category: NR*

**HOW SUPPLIED**
*Capsules:* 1 mg

**ACTION**
Cross-links strands of cellular DNA and interferes with RNA transcription, causing an imbalance of growth that leads to cell death. Cell cycle-nonspecific.

**ONSET, PEAK, DURATION**
Undefined.

---

Reactions may be *common,* uncommon, *life-threatening,* or COMMON AND LIFE-THREATENING.

## INDICATIONS & DOSAGE

*Chronic lymphocytic and myelocytic leukemia, Hodgkin's disease, malignant lymphoma of the histiocytic and lymphocytic types, reticulum cell sarcoma, mycosis fungoides, polycythemia vera* –

**Adults:** 0.15 mg/kg P.O. as a single dose weekly for 4 weeks. If response occurs, weekly administration may continue. Alternatively, 1 to 2 mg P.O. daily for 3 months or until desired response or toxicity; maintenance dosage is 1 mg daily for 3 of 4 weeks until optimum response or relapse; or 3 to 5 mg P.O. for 7 days, not to exceed total dosage of 0.5 mg/kg, then 1 mg daily until response, and then 1 mg daily for 3 of 4 weeks.
**Children:** 0.3 mg/kg P.O. as a single dose weekly for four weeks. If response occurs, weekly administration may continue.

## ADVERSE REACTIONS

**CNS:** irritability, nervousness, depression.
**GI:** *nausea, vomiting, diarrhea.*
**Hematologic:** bone marrow suppression, delayed 2 to 4 weeks; ***thrombocytopenia; leukopenia; anemia.***
**Skin:** pruritus, dermatitis.
**Other:** fertility impairment, hepatotoxicity, amenorrhea, azoospermia.

## INTERACTIONS

*Anticoagulants, aspirin:* increased risk of bleeding. Avoid concomitant use.

## CONTRAINDICATIONS

Contraindicated in patients with hypersensitivity to the drug and in those with aplastic anemia, thrombocytopenia, or leukopenia.

## NURSING CONSIDERATIONS

• Be aware that some commercially available capsules contain tartrazine dye, which may provoke hypersensitivity reactions in certain individuals.

This reaction is rare but is more likely to occur in aspirin-sensitive persons.
• Monitor platelet count. Check CBC once or twice weekly for 4 weeks; then 4 weeks after stopping drug, as ordered.
• Monitor serum uric acid level, as ordered. To prevent hyperuricemia and resulting uric acid nephropathy, know that allopurinol may be used with adequate hydration.
• Know that therapeutic effects are often accompanied by toxicity.
• To prevent bleeding, avoid all I.M. injections when platelet count is below 100,000/mm$^3$.
• Anticipate possible blood transfusions because of cumulative anemia.

## ☑ PATIENT TEACHING

• Instruct patient to take drug at bedtime to minimize nausea.
• Advise patient to watch for signs of infection (fever, sore throat, fatigue) and bleeding (easy bruising, nosebleeds, bleeding gums, melena). Tell patient to take temperature daily.
• Instruct patients to avoid OTC products containing aspirin.
• Advise breast-feeding patients to stop breast-feeding during therapy because of possible infant toxicity.
• Advise women of childbearing age to avoid becoming pregnant during therapy. Suggest consulting with doctor before becoming pregnant. Drug should not be used in pregnancy unless potential benefits outweigh potential risks.

---

\*Liquid form contains alcohol.   \*\*May contain tartrazine.   †Canada only.   ‡Australia only.   ◇OTC.

# 70

# Antimetabolites

cladribine
cytarabine
floxuridine
fludarabine phosphate
fluorouracil
hydroxyurea
mercaptopurine
methotrexate
methotrexate sodium
thioguanine

## COMBINATION PRODUCTS
None.

## cladribine (2-chlorodeoxyadenosine, CdA)
Leustatin

*Pregnancy Risk Category: D*

### HOW SUPPLIED
*Injection:* 1 mg/ml

### ACTION
Unknown. A purine nucleoside analogue that enters tumor cells, is phosphorylated by deoxycytidine kinase, and is subsequently converted into an active triphosphate deoxynucleotide. This metabolite probably impairs synthesis of new DNA, inhibits repair of existing DNA, and disrupts cellular metabolism.

### ONSET, PEAK, DURATION
Onset has a median time of approximately 4 months to response. Peak undefined. Median duration of response is greater than 8 months.

### INDICATIONS & DOSAGE
*Active hairy cell leukemia –*
**Adults:** 0.09 mg/kg daily by continuous I.V. infusion for 7 days.

### ADVERSE REACTIONS
**CNS:** *headache, fatigue,* dizziness, insomnia, asthenia.
**CV:** tachycardia, edema.
**EENT:** epistaxis.
**GI:** *nausea, decreased appetite, vomiting, diarrhea,* constipation, abdominal pain.
**GU:** acute renal insufficiency.
**Hematologic:** NEUTROPENIA, *anemia, thrombocytopenia.*
**Respiratory:** *abnormal breath or chest sounds, cough,* shortness of breath.
**Skin:** *rash, pruritus, erythema, purpura,* petechiae.
**Other:** *fever,* INFECTION, *local reaction at the injection site, chills, diaphoresis, malaise, trunk pain, myalgia, arthralgia,* hyperuricemia.

### INTERACTIONS
None significant.

### CONTRAINDICATIONS
Contraindicated in patients hypersensitive to the drug.

### NURSING CONSIDERATIONS
● Use cautiously in patients with renal or hepatic impairment.
● **I.V. use:** For a 24-hour infusion, add the calculated dose to a 500-ml infusion bag of 0.9% sodium chloride for injection. Once diluted, administer promptly or store in refrigerator for no more than 8 hours. Don't use solutions that contain dextrose because studies have shown increased degradation of the drug. Repeat preparation daily for 7 consecutive days.
● *Alert:* Because the drug product doesn't contain any bacteriostatic agents, use strict aseptic technique to prepare the daily admixture.
● Alternatively, prepare a 7-day infu-

sion solution, using bacteriostatic sodium chloride for injection, which contains 0.9% benzyl alcohol. Studies have shown acceptable physical and chemical stability using Pharmacia Deltec medication cassettes. First, pass the calculated amount of drug through a disposable 0.22-micron hydrophilic syringe filter into a sterile infusion reservoir. Next, add sufficient bacteriostatic sodium chloride injection to bring the total volume to 100 ml. Clamp off the line; then disconnect and discard the filter. If necessary, aseptically aspirate air bubbles from the reservoir using a new filter or a sterile vent filter assembly.

• Be aware that because the calculated dose dilutes the benzyl alcohol preservative, 7-day infusion solutions prepared for patients weighing more than 187 lb (85 kg) may have reduced preservative effectiveness.

• Because of the risk of hyperuricemia from tumor lysis, administer allopurinol, as ordered, during therapy.

• Monitor hematologic function closely, as ordered, especially during the first 4 to 8 weeks of therapy. Cladribine is a toxic drug, and some toxicity is expected during treatment. Severe bone marrow suppression, including neutropenia, anemia, and thrombocytopenia, has commonly been observed in patients treated with this drug; many patients also have preexisting hematologic impairment from their disease.

• Keep in mind that fever is common during the 1st month of therapy. In clinical trials, virtually all patients received parenteral antibiotics.

• To prevent bleeding, avoid all I.M. injections when platelet count is below 100,000/mm$^3$.

• Anticipate possible blood transfusions because of cumulative anemia.

• Refrigerate unopened vials at 36° to 46° F (2° to 8° C) and protect from light. Although freezing doesn't adversely affect the drug, a precipitate

may form; this will disappear if the drug is allowed to warm to room temperature gradually and the vial is vigorously shaken. Don't heat or microwave; don't refreeze.

☑ **PATIENT TEACHING**
• Advise patient to watch for signs of infection (fever, sore throat, fatigue) and bleeding (easy bruising, nosebleeds, bleeding gums, melena). Tell patient to take temperature daily.
• Advise women of childbearing age to avoid becoming pregnant because of the risk of fetal malformations.
• Advise breast-feeding patient to discontinue breast-feeding during therapy because of possible infant toxicity.

---

# cytarabine (ara-C, cytosine arabinoside)
Alexan‡, Cytosar†, Cytosar-U

*Pregnancy Risk Category: NR*

**HOW SUPPLIED**
*Injection:* 40-mg‡, 100-mg, 500-mg, 1-g, 2-g vials

**ACTION**
Inhibits DNA synthesis.

**ONSET, PEAK, DURATION**
Onset and duration undefined. Levels peak 20 to 60 minutes after S.C. injection.

**INDICATIONS & DOSAGE**
*Acute nonlymphocytic leukemia, acute lymphocytic leukemia, blast phase of chronic myelocytic leukemia –*
**Adults and children:** 100 mg/m$^2$ daily by continuous I.V. infusion or 100 mg/m$^2$ I.V. q 12 hours. Given for 7 days and repeated q 2 weeks. For maintenance, 1 mg/kg S.C. once or twice a week.
*Meningeal leukemia –*
**Adults and children:** highly variable from 5 mg/m$^2$ to 75 mg/m$^2$ intrathe-

cally. Frequency also varies from once a day for 4 days to once q 4 days. The most frequently used dosage is 30 mg/m², q 4 days until CSF fluid is normal.

## ADVERSE REACTIONS
**CNS:** neurotoxicity, malaise, dizziness, headache.
**EENT:** conjunctivitis.
**GI:** *nausea, vomiting,* diarrhea, anorexia, anal ulceration, abdominal pain; oral ulcers in 5 to 10 days; high dose given rapid I.V. may cause projectile vomiting.
**Hematologic:** *leukopenia,* with initial WBC count nadir 7 to 9 days after drug is stopped and a second (more severe) nadir 15 to 24 days after drug is stopped; anemia; reticulocytopenia; *thrombocytopenia,* with platelet count nadir occurring on day 10; *megaloblastosis.*
**Hepatic:** hepatotoxicity (usually mild and reversible), jaundice.
**Skin:** rash, pruritus.
**Other:** flulike syndrome, hyperuricemia, infection, fever, thrombophlebitis, myalgia, bone pain, *anaphylaxis,* renal dysfunction, edema.

## INTERACTIONS
*Digoxin:* may decrease serum digoxin levels. Monitor closely.

## CONTRAINDICATIONS
Contraindicated in patients hypersensitive to the drug.

## NURSING CONSIDERATIONS
• Use cautiously in patients with hepatic disease.
• To reduce nausea, give antiemetic before administering, as ordered. Nausea and vomiting are more frequent when large doses are administered rapidly by I.V. push. These reactions are less frequent when given by infusion.
• Follow institutional policy to reduce risks. Preparation and administration of parenteral form of this drug is associated with carcinogenic, mutagenic, and teratogenic risks for personnel.
• **I.V. use:** Reconstitute drug using the provided diluent, which is bacteriostatic water for injection containing benzyl alcohol. Avoid this diluent when preparing drug for neonates or for intrathecal use. Reconstitute 100-mg vial with 5 ml of diluent or 500-mg vial with 10 ml of diluent. Reconstituted solution is stable for 48 hours. Discard cloudy reconstituted solution.
• For I.V. infusion, further dilute using 0.9% sodium chloride for injection or $D_5W$.
• For intrathecal administration, use preservative-free 0.9% sodium chloride. Add 5 ml to the 100-mg vial or 10 ml to the 500-mg vial. Use immediately after reconstitution. Discard unused drug.
• Monitor fluid intake and output carefully. Maintain high fluid intake and give allopurinol, if ordered, to avoid urate nephropathy in leukemia induction therapy. Monitor serum uric acid level, as ordered.
• Monitor hepatic and renal function studies and CBC, as ordered.
• Know that therapy may be modified or stopped if granulocyte count is below 1,000/mm³ or if platelet count is below 50,000/mm³.
• Know that corticosteroid eyedrops are prescribed to prevent drug-induced keratitis.
• Provide diligent mouth care to help prevent stomatitis.
• **Alert:** Assess patients receiving high doses for neurotoxicity, which may first appear as nystagmus, but can progress to ataxia and cerebellar dysfunction.
• To prevent bleeding, avoid all I.M. injections when platelet count is below 100,000/mm³.
• Anticipate possible blood transfusions because of cumulative anemia.
• Know that therapeutic effects are often accompanied by toxicity.

---

## ☑ PATIENT TEACHING

• Advise patient to watch for signs of infection (fever, sore throat, fatigue) and bleeding (easy bruising, nosebleeds, bleeding gums, melena). Tell patients to take temperature daily.

• Advise breast-feeding patient to discontinue breast-feeding during therapy because of possible infant toxicity.

• Advise women of childbearing age to avoid becoming pregnant during therapy. Also recommend consulting with doctor before becoming pregnant. Drug may harm the fetus.

## floxuridine
FUDR

*Pregnancy Risk Category: D*

### HOW SUPPLIED
*Injection:* 500-mg vials (50 mg/ml in 10-ml vials or 100 mg/ml in 5-ml vials)

### ACTION
Inhibits DNA synthesis.

### ONSET, PEAK, DURATION
Undefined.

### INDICATIONS & DOSAGE
*GI adenocarcinoma metastatic to the liver* —

**Adults:** 0.1 to 0.6 mg/kg daily by intra-arterial infusion for 14 to 21 days or until toxicity occurs; or 0.4 to 0.6 mg/kg daily into hepatic artery.

### ADVERSE REACTIONS
**CNS:** cerebellar ataxia, malaise, weakness, headache, lethargy, disorientation, confusion, euphoria.
**CV:** myocardial ischemia, angina.
**EENT:** blurred vision, nystagmus, photophobia, epistaxis.
**GI:** *anorexia, stomatitis, nausea, vomiting, diarrhea, bleeding, enteritis,* GI ulceration.

**Hematologic:** *leukopenia, anemia, thrombocytopenia, agranulocytosis.*
**Skin:** *erythema,* dermatitis, pruritus, rash, alopecia, photosensitivity.
**Other:** thrombophlebitis, *anaphylaxis,* fever.

### INTERACTIONS
None significant.

### CONTRAINDICATIONS
Contraindicated in patients with poor nutritional state, bone marrow suppression, or serious infection.

### NURSING CONSIDERATIONS
• Use cautiously following high-dose pelvic radiation therapy or use of alkylating agents and in patients with impaired hepatic or renal function.

• Follow institutional policy to reduce risks. Preparation and administration of parenteral form of this drug is associated with carcinogenic, mutagenic, and teratogenic risks for personnel.

• Reconstitute with sterile water for injection. To prepare infusion, dilute in $D_5W$ or 0.9% sodium chloride solution.

• Refrigerated solution is stable for no more than 2 weeks.

• Use an infusion pump with intra-arterial infusions.

• Check line for bleeding, blockage, displacement, or leakage.

• Monitor fluid intake and output, CBC, and renal and hepatic function, as ordered.

• Know that use of antacid eases but won't prevent GI distress.

• Provide diligent mouth care to help prevent stomatitis.

• Be alert that severe skin and adverse GI reactions require stopping drug.

• Know that drug should be discontinued if WBC count falls below 3,500/mm³ or if platelet count falls below 100,000/mm³. If either occurs, notify doctor.

• To prevent bleeding, avoid all I.M.

---

injections when platelet count is below 100,000/mm$^3$.
• Anticipate possible blood transfusions because of cumulative anemia.

☑ **PATIENT TEACHING**
• Inform patient that therapeutic effect may be delayed 1 to 6 weeks.
• Advise patient to watch for signs of infection (fever, sore throat, fatigue) and bleeding (easy bruising, nosebleeds, bleeding gums, melena). Tell patient to take temperature daily.
• Advise breast-feeding patient to discontinue breast-feeding during therapy because of possible infant toxicity.
• Advise women of childbearing age to avoid becoming pregnant during therapy. Also recommend consulting with the doctor before becoming pregnant.

# fludarabine phosphate
Fludara

*Pregnancy Risk Category: D*

**HOW SUPPLIED**
*Powder for injection:* 50 mg

**ACTION**
Unknown. An antineoplastic antimetabolite that may have multifaceted actions. After conversion to its active metabolite, fludarabine interferes with DNA synthesis by inhibiting DNA polymerase alpha, ribonucleotide reductase, and DNA primase.

**ONSET, PEAK, DURATION**
Onset may occur within 7 to 21 hours. Peak and duration undefined.

**INDICATIONS & DOSAGE**
*B-cell chronic lymphocytic leukemia in patients who have either not responded or responded inadequately to at least one standard alkylating agent regimen* –
**Adults:** 25 mg/m$^2$ I.V. over 30 min-

utes for 5 consecutive days. Cycle repeated q 28 days.

**ADVERSE REACTIONS**
**CNS:** *fatigue, malaise, weakness, paresthesia,* peripheral neuropathy, headache, sleep disorder, depression, cerebellar syndrome, *CVA,* transient ischemic attack, agitation, *confusion; coma, death* (with very high doses).
**CV:** *edema,* angina, phlebitis, *arrhythmias, CHF,* supraventricular tachycardia, deep venous thrombosis, *aneurysm,* hemorrhage.
**EENT:** *visual disturbances,* hearing loss, delayed blindness (with high doses), sinusitis, pharyngitis, epistaxis.
**GI:** *nausea, vomiting, diarrhea,* constipation, *anorexia,* stomatitis, *GI bleeding,* esophagitis, mucositis.
**GU:** dysuria, *urinary infection* or hesitancy, proteinuria, hematuria, *renal failure.*
**Hematologic:** *myelosuppression.*
**Hepatic:** liver failure, cholelithiasis.
**Respiratory:** *cough, pneumonia, dyspnea, upper respiratory tract infection,* allergic pneumonitis, hemoptysis, hypoxia, bronchitis.
**Skin:** *rash,* pruritus, seborrhea.
**Other:** *fever, chills, infection, pain, myalgia,* tumor lysis syndrome, alopecia, *anaphylaxis,* diaphoresis, hypocalcemia, hyperkalemia, hyperglycemia, dehydration, hyperuricemia, hyperphosphatemia.

**INTERACTIONS**
*Other myelosuppressants:* increased toxicity. Avoid concomitant use.
*Pentostatin:* concurrent use increases risk of pulmonary toxicity. Avoid concomitant administration.

**CONTRAINDICATIONS**
Contraindicated in patients hypersensitive to the drug or its components.

**NURSING CONSIDERATIONS**
• Use cautiously in patients with renal insufficiency.

---

Reactions may be *common,* uncommon, *life-threatening,* or COMMON AND LIFE-THREATENING.

• Follow institutional policy to reduce risks. Preparation and administration of parenteral form of this drug is associated with mutagenic, teratogenic, and carcinogenic risks for personnel.

• **I.V. use:** To prepare solution, add 2 ml of sterile water for injection to the solid cake of fludarabine. Dissolution should occur within 15 seconds; each milliliter will contain 25 mg of drug. Dilute further in 100 or 125 ml of $D_5W$ or 0.9% sodium chloride for injection. Use within 8 hours of reconstitution.

• *Alert:* Monitor patients closely and expect modified dosage based on toxicity. Most toxic effects are dose-dependent. Advanced age, renal insufficiency, and bone marrow impairment may predispose patients to increased or excessive toxicity.

• Know that careful hematologic monitoring is required, especially of neutrophil and platelet counts. Bone marrow suppression can be severe.

• To prevent bleeding, avoid all I.M. injections when platelet count is below 100,00/mm³.

• Anticipate possible blood transfusions because of cumulative anemia.

• Know that optimal duration of therapy is not yet determined. Current recommendations suggest three additional cycles after achieving maximal response before discontinuing therapy.

• Store drug in refrigerator at 36° to 46° F (2° to 8° C).

☑ **PATIENT TEACHING**

• Advise patient to watch for signs of infection (fever, sore throat, fatigue) and bleeding (easy bruising, nosebleeds, bleeding gums, melena). Tell patient to take temperature daily.

• Advise women of childbearing age to avoid becoming pregnant during therapy. Also recommend consulting with doctor before becoming pregnant.

• Advise breast-feeding patient to

discontinue beast-feeding during therapy because of possible infant toxicity.

---

## fluorouracil
## (5-fluorouracil, 5-FU)
Adrucil, Efudex, Fluoroplex

*Pregnancy Risk Category: D*

**HOW SUPPLIED**
*Injection:* 50 mg/ml
*Cream:* 1%, 5%
*Topical solution:* 1%, 2%, 5%

**ACTION**
Inhibits DNA synthesis.

**ONSET, PEAK, DURATION**
Undefined.

**INDICATIONS & DOSAGE**
*Colon, rectal, breast, stomach, and pancreatic cancers –*
**Adults:** 12 mg/kg I.V. daily for 4 days; if no toxicity, dose increased to 6 mg/kg and given on the 6th, 8th, 10th, and 12th day; then a single weekly maintenance dose of 10 to 15 mg/kg I.V. begun after toxicity (if any) from initial course has subsided. (Dosages recommended based on actual body weight unless patient is obese or retaining fluid.) Maximum single recommended dose is 800 mg.
*Palliative treatment of advanced colorectal cancer –*
**Adults:** 425 mg/m² I.V. daily for 5 consecutive days. Given with 20 mg/m² of leucovorin I.V. Repeated at 4-week intervals for two additional courses; then repeated at intervals of 4 to 5 weeks if tolerated.
*Multiple actinic (solar) keratoses; superficial basal cell carcinoma –*
**Adults:** apply cream or topical solution b.i.d.

**ADVERSE REACTIONS**
**CNS:** acute cerebellar syndrome, confusion, disorientation, euphoria,

---

ataxia, headache, nystagmus, *weakness, malaise.*

**CV:** *myocardial ischemia, angina.*

**GI:** *stomatitis, GI ulcer* (may precede leukopenia), *nausea and vomiting* (in 30% to 50% of patients), *diarrhea, anorexia,* GI bleeding.

**Hematologic: *leukopenia, thrombocytopenia, agranulocytosis,*** anemia; WBC count nadir 9 to 14 days after first dose; platelet count nadir in 7 to 14 days.

**Skin:** *dermatitis; erythema; scaling; pruritus;* nail changes; pigmented palmar creases; erythematous, contact dermatitis, desquamative rash of hands and feet with long-term use ("hand-foot syndrome").

**Other:** *reversible alopecia in 5% to 20% of patients; pain, burning,* soreness, suppuration, swelling (with topical use), **anaphylaxis,** thrombophlebitis.

### INTERACTIONS

*Leucovorin calcium, prior treatment with alkylating agents:* increased toxicity of fluorouracil. Use with extreme caution.

### CONTRAINDICATIONS

Contraindicated in patients hypersensitive to the drug; patients who are in a poor nutritional state; patients with bone marrow suppression (WBC counts of 5,000/mm³ or less or platelet counts of 100,000/mm³ or less); patients with potentially serious infections; and in those who have had major surgery within the previous month.

### NURSING CONSIDERATIONS

• Use cautiously after high-dose pelvic radiation therapy or use of alkylating agents or in patients with impaired hepatic or renal function or widespread neoplastic infiltration of bone marrow.

• Follow institutional policy to reduce risks. Preparation and administration of parenteral form of this drug is associated with carcinogenic, mutagenic, and teratogenic risks for personnel.

• Give antiemetic, as ordered, before administering drug to reduce nausea.

• **I.V. use:** Know that drug may be administered by direct injection without dilution. For I.V. infusion, drug may be diluted with $D_5W$, sterile water for injection, or 0.9% sodium chloride for injection.

• Don't use cloudy solution. If crystals form, redissolve by warming.

• Use plastic I.V. containers for administering continuous infusions. Solution is more stable in plastic I.V. bags than in glass bottles.

• Don't refrigerate fluorouracil.

• Be aware that the manufacturer recommends using sodium hypochlorite 5% (household bleach) to inactivate the drug in the event of a spill.

• Apply topical form with caution near eyes, nose, and mouth.

• Avoid occlusive dressings with topical dressings because they increase the risk of inflammatory reactions in adjacent normal skin.

• Wash hands immediately after handling topical form of medication.

• Expect to use 1% topical concentration on the face. Higher concentrations are used for thicker-skinned areas or resistant lesions.

• Expect to use 5% topical strength for superficial basal cell carcinoma confirmed by biopsy.

• Be aware that ingestion and systemic absorption of topical form may cause leukopenia, thrombocytopenia, stomatitis, diarrhea, or GI ulceration, bleeding, and hemorrhage. Application to large ulcerated areas may cause systemic toxicity.

• Watch for stomatitis or diarrhea (signs of toxicity). May use topical oral anesthetic to soothe lesions, as ordered. Discontinue drug if diarrhea occurs and notify doctor.

• Encourage diligent oral hygiene to

prevent superinfection of denuded mucosa.

• Monitor WBC and platelet counts daily, as ordered. Watch for ecchymoses, petechiae, easy bruising, and anemia.

• Consider protective isolation measures if WBC count is less than 2,000/mm³.

• Monitor fluid intake and output, CBC, and renal and hepatic function tests, as ordered.

• Be aware that dermatologic adverse effects are reversible when drug is stopped.

• Be aware that therapeutic concentrations are not reached in CSF.

• To prevent bleeding, avoid all I.M. injections when platelet count is below 100,000/mm³.

• Anticipate possible blood transfusions because of cumulative anemia.

• **Alert:** Be alert that fluorouracil toxicity may be delayed for 1 to 3 weeks.

• Know that the drug is sometimes ordered as 5-fluorouracil or 5-FU. The numeral 5 is part of the drug name and should not be confused with dosage units.

☑ **PATIENT TEACHING**

• Warn patient that alopecia may occur, but that it's reversible.

• Caution patient to avoid prolonged exposure to sunlight or ultraviolet light when topical form is used.

• Tell patient to use highly protective sunblock to avoid inflammatory erythematous dermatitis. Long-term use of the drug is associated with erythematous, desquamative rash of the hands and feet. May be treated with pyridoxine (50 to 150 mg P.O. daily) for 5 to 7 days.

• Warn patient that topically treated area may be unsightly during therapy and for several weeks after therapy. Complete healing may take 1 or 2 months.

• Advise women of childbearing age to avoid becoming pregnant during therapy. Also recommend consulting with doctor before becoming pregnant.

• Advise breast-feeding patients to discontinue breast-feeding during therapy because of possible infant toxicity.

# hydroxyurea
Hydrea**

*Pregnancy Risk Category: NR*

**HOW SUPPLIED**
*Capsules:* 500 mg

**ACTION**
Unknown. Thought to inhibit DNA synthesis.

**ONSET, PEAK, DURATION**
Onset and duration unknown. Serum levels peak in 2 hours.

**INDICATIONS & DOSAGE**
*Melanoma; resistant chronic myelocytic leukemia; recurrent, metastatic, or inoperable ovarian cancer; head and neck cancers –*
**Adults:** 80 mg/kg P.O. as single dose q 3 days; or 20 to 30 mg/kg P.O. as a single daily dose.

**ADVERSE REACTIONS**
**CNS:** hallucinations, headache, dizziness, disorientation, *seizures,* malaise.
**GI:** *anorexia, nausea, vomiting, diarrhea,* stomatitis, constipation.
**GU:** increased BUN and serum creatinine levels.
**Hematologic:** *leukopenia, thrombocytopenia,* anemia, *megaloblastosis; dose-limiting and dose-related bone marrow suppression,* with rapid recovery.
**Skin:** rash, alopecia, erythema.
**Other:** fever, chills.

## INTERACTIONS
*Cytotoxic drugs, radiation therapy:*
enhanced toxicity of hydroxyurea.
Use together cautiously.

## CONTRAINDICATIONS
Contraindicated in patients hypersensitive to the drug and with marked bone marrow depression (leukopenia [less than 2,500/mm³ WBCs], thrombocytopenia [less than 100,000/mm³ platelets], or severe anemia).

## NURSING CONSIDERATIONS
• Use cautiously in patients with renal dysfunction.
• Routinely measure BUN, uric acid, and serum creatinine levels, as ordered.
• Monitor fluid intake and output; keep patients hydrated.
• To prevent bleeding, avoid all I.M. injections when platelet count is below 100,000/mm³.
• Anticipate possible blood transfusions because of cumulative anemia.
• Be aware that dosage modification may be required after chemotherapy or radiation therapy.
• Be aware that auditory and visual hallucinations and hematologic toxicity increase when decreased renal function exists.
• Know that the drug crosses blood-brain barrier.
• Be alert that concomitant radiation therapy may increase incidence or severity of GI distress or stomatitis.

## ☑ PATIENT TEACHING
• Tell patient who can't swallow capsules that he may empty contents into water and take immediately.
• Advise patient to watch for signs of infection (fever, sore throat, fatigue) and bleeding (easy bruising, nosebleeds, bleeding gums, melena). He should also take his temperature daily.
• Advise women of childbearing age to avoid becoming pregnant during therapy. Also recommend consulting with doctor before becoming pregnant.

# mercaptopurine (6-mercaptopurine, 6-MP)
Purinethol
*Pregnancy Risk Category: D*

## HOW SUPPLIED
*Tablets (scored):* 50 mg

## ACTION
Inhibits RNA and DNA synthesis.

## ONSET, PEAK, DURATION
Undefined.

## INDICATIONS & DOSAGE
*Acute myeloblastic leukemia, chronic myelocytic leukemia –*
**Adults:** 80 to 100 mg/m² (rounded to the nearest 25 mg) P.O. daily as a single dose up to 5 mg/kg/day.
**Children:** 70 mg/m² (rounded to the nearest 25 mg) P.O. daily.
*Acute lymphoblastic leukemia –*
**Children:** 70 mg/m² (rounded to the nearest 25 mg) P.O. daily.
Usual maintenance for adults and children: 1.5 to 2.5 mg/kg/day.

## ADVERSE REACTIONS
**GI:** *nausea, vomiting, and anorexia,* painful oral ulcers, diarrhea, pancreatitis, GI ulceration.
**Hematologic:** *leukopenia, thrombocytopenia, anemia* – all may persist several days after drug is stopped.
**Hepatic:** *jaundice,* hepatotoxicity.
**Skin:** rash, hyperpigmentation.
**Other:** hyperuricemia.

## INTERACTIONS
*Allopurinol:* slowed inactivation of mercaptopurine. Decrease mercaptopurine to one-quarter or one-third normal dose.
*Hepatotoxic drugs:* may enhance hepatotoxicity of mercaptopurine. Monitor for hepatotoxicity.

---

Reactions may be *common,* uncommon, *life-threatening,* or COMMON AND LIFE-THREATENING.

*Nondepolarizing neuromuscular blockers:* antagonized muscle relaxant effect. Notify the anesthesiologist that the patient is receiving mercaptopurine.

*Warfarin:* antagonized anticoagulant effect. Monitor P.T.

## CONTRAINDICATIONS

Contraindicated in patients whose disease has shown resistance to the drug.

## NURSING CONSIDERATIONS

• Be aware that dosage modifications may be required after chemotherapy or radiation therapy in patients with depressed neutrophil or platelet counts and in those with impaired hepatic or renal function.

• Be aware that drug is sometimes ordered as 6-mercaptopurine or 6-MP. The numeral 6 is part of drug name and does not signify number of dosage units.

• Monitor blood counts and serum transaminase, alkaline phosphatase, and bilirubin levels weekly during induction and monthly during maintenance, as ordered.

• Observe for signs of bleeding and infection.

• Monitor fluid intake and output. Encourage adequate fluid intake (3 liters daily).

• **Alert:** Watch for jaundice, clay-colored stools, and frothy dark urine. Hepatic dysfunction is reversible when drug is stopped. If hepatic tenderness occurs, drug should be stopped and doctor notified.

• Monitor serum uric acid level, as ordered. If allopurinol is ordered, use cautiously.

• To prevent bleeding, avoid all I.M. injections when platelet count is below 100,000/mm³.

• Anticipate possible blood transfusions because of cumulative anemia.

• Be alert that GI adverse reactions

are less common in children than in adults.

## ☑ PATIENT TEACHING

• Advise patient to watch for signs of infection (fever, sore throat, fatigue) and bleeding (easy bruising, nosebleeds, bleeding gums, melena). Tell patient to take temperature daily.

• Advise women of childbearing age to avoid becoming pregnant during therapy. Also recommend consulting with the doctor before becoming pregnant.

• Advise breast-feeding patients to discontinue breast-feeding during therapy because of possible infant toxicity.

---

## methotrexate

## methotrexate sodium
Folex , Folex PFS, Mexate-AQ, Rheumatrex

*Pregnancy Risk Category: X*

## HOW SUPPLIED
*Tablets (scored):* 2.5 mg
*Injection:* 20-mg, 25-mg, 50-mg, 100-mg, 250-mg vials, lyophilized powder, preservative-free; 25-mg/ml vials, preservative-free solution; 2.5-mg/ml, 25-mg/ml vials, lyophilized powder, preserved

## ACTION
Prevents reduction of folic acid to tetrahydrofolate by binding to dihydrofolate reductase.

## ONSET, PEAK, DURATION
Onset and duration undefined. Serum concentrations peak immediately after I.V. injection, within ½ to 1 hour after I.M. injection, or 1 to 2 hours after oral dose.

## INDICATIONS & DOSAGE
*Trophoblastic tumors (choriocarcinoma, hydatidiform mole)* —

---

*Liquid form contains alcohol.  **May contain tartrazine.  †Canada only.  ‡Australia only.  ◇OTC.

**Adults:** 15 to 30 mg P.O. or I.M. daily for 5 days. Repeated after 1 or more weeks, according to response or toxicity.

*Acute lymphocytic leukemia* –

**Adults and children:** 3.3 mg/m²/day P.O., I.M., or I.V. for 4 to 6 weeks or until remission occurs; then 20 to 30 mg/m² P.O. or I.M. twice weekly or 2.5 mg/kg I.V. q 14 days.

*Meningeal leukemia* –

**Adults and children:** 12 mg/m² or less (maximum 15 mg) intrathecally q 2 to 5 days until CSF is normal, then one additional dose.

*Burkitt's lymphoma (Stage I, II, or III)* –

**Adults:** 10 to 25 mg P.O. daily for 4 to 8 days with 1-week rest intervals.

*Lymphosarcoma (Stage III)* –

**Adults:** 0.625 to 2.5 mg/kg daily P.O., I.M., or I.V.

*Osteosarcoma* –

**Adults:** initially, 12 g/m² I.V. as 4-hour infusion. Subsequent doses 12 to 15 g/m² I.V. as 4-hour I.V. infusion given at 4th, 5th, 6th, 7th, 11th, 12th, 15th, 16th, 29th, 30th, 44th, 45th weeks after surgery. Given with leucovorin, 15 mg P.O., I.M., or I.V. q 6 hours for 10 doses, beginning 24 hours after start of methotrexate infusion.

*Mycosis fungoides* –

**Adults:** 2.5 to 10 mg P.O. daily, or 50 mg I.M. weekly, or 25 mg I.M. twice weekly.

*Psoriasis* –

**Adults:** 10 to 25 mg P.O., I.M., or I.V. as single weekly dose.

*Rheumatoid arthritis* –

**Adults:** initially, 7.5 mg P.O. weekly, either in a single dose or divided as 2.5 mg P.O. q 12 hours for three doses once a week. Dosage may be gradually increased to a maximum of 20 mg weekly.

## ADVERSE REACTIONS

**CNS:** *arachnoiditis* within hours of intrathecal use; subacute neurotoxic-ity, which may begin a few weeks later; *necrotizing demyelinating leukoencephalopathy* a few years later; malaise, fatigue, dizziness, headache, drowsiness, *seizures.*

**EENT:** pharyngitis, gingivitis, blurred vision.

**GI:** *stomatitis, diarrhea,* abdominal distress, anorexia, GI ulceration and bleeding, enteritis, *nausea, vomiting.*

**GU:** nephropathy, *tubular necrosis, renal failure,* hematuria, menstrual dysfunction, defective spermatogenesis, cystitis.

**Hematologic:** WBC and platelet count nadirs occurring on day 7; *anemia, leukopenia, thrombocytopenia* (all dose-related).

**Hepatic:** acute toxicity (elevated transaminase level), *chronic toxicity* (cirrhosis, *hepatic fibrosis*).

**Respiratory:** *pulmonary fibrosis; pulmonary interstitial infiltrates;* pneumonitis; dry, nonproductive cough.

**Skin:** *urticaria,* pruritus, hyperpigmentation, erythematous rashes, ecchymoses; psoriatic lesions (aggravated by exposure to sun), rash, photosensitivity.

**Other:** alopecia, osteoporosis (in children, with long-term use), fever, chills, reduced resistance to infection, septicemia, hyperuricemia, arthralgia, myalgia, diabetes, *sudden death.*

## INTERACTIONS

*Digoxin:* may decrease serum digoxin levels. Monitor closely.

*Folic acid derivatives:* antagonized methotrexate effect. Avoid concomitant use.

*NSAIDs, phenylbutazone, probenecid, salicylates, sulfonamides:* increased methotrexate toxicity; don't use together if possible.

*Phenytoin:* may decrease serum phenytoin levels. Monitor closely.

*Vaccines:* immunizations may be ineffective; risk of disseminated infection

---

with live-virus vaccines. Defer immunization, if possible.

## CONTRAINDICATIONS
Contraindicated in patients hypersensitive to the drug and during pregnancy or breast-feeding. It also is contraindicated in patients with psoriasis or rheumatoid arthritis who also have alcoholism, alcoholic liver, chronic liver disease, immunodeficiency syndromes, or preexisting blood dyscrasias.

## NURSING CONSIDERATIONS
• Use cautiously and at modified dosage in patients with impaired hepatic or renal function, bone marrow suppression, aplasia, leukopenia, thrombocytopenia, or anemia. Also use cautiously in patients with infection, peptic ulceration, and ulcerative colitis and in very young, elderly, or debilitated patients.
• Perform baseline pulmonary function tests, as ordered.
• Follow institutional policy to reduce risks. Preparation and administration of parenteral form of this drug is associated with carcinogenic, mutagenic, and teratogenic risks for personnel.
• **I.V. use:** Know that dilution of drug depends on product and that infusion guidelines vary, depending on dose. Check orders carefully, and follow product guidelines exactly.
• Reconstitute solutions without preservatives immediately before use, and discard any unused drug.
• Know that drug also may be used in combination regimens for a variety of cancers such as breast cancer, head and neck cancer, lymphoma, and lung cancer.
• Monitor pulmonary function tests periodically, as ordered, and fluid intake and output daily. Encourage fluid intake of 2 to 3 liters daily.
• Monitor serum uric acid level, as ordered.
• *Alert:* Alkalinize urine as ordered

by giving sodium bicarbonate tablets to prevent precipitation of drug, especially with high doses. Maintain urine pH at more than 6.5. Reduce dosage as ordered if BUN level reaches 20 to 30 mg/dl or creatinine level reaches 1.2 to 2 mg/dl. Stop drug if BUN level is greater than 30 mg/dl or creatinine level is greater than 2 mg/dl and notify doctor.
• Watch for increases in AST, ALT, and alkaline phosphatase levels, which may signal hepatic dysfunction.
• Watch for signs of bleeding (especially GI) and infection.
• Take temperature daily, and watch for cough, dyspnea, and cyanosis.
• To prevent bleeding, avoid all I.M. injections when platelet count is below 100,000/mm³.
• Anticipate blood transfusions because of cumulative anemia.
• Know that rash, redness, or ulcerations in mouth or adverse pulmonary reactions may signal serious complications. Therapy may be discontinued if ulcerative stomatitis or some other severe adverse GI reaction occurs, or if pulmonary toxicity is detected.
• Know that leucovorin rescue is necessary with high-dose (greater than 100 mg) protocols and is started 24 hours after beginning methotrexate therapy. Don't confuse with folic acid. This rescue technique is effective against systemic toxicity but does not interfere with the tumor cells' absorption of methotrexate.

## ☑ PATIENT TEACHING
• Advise patient to watch for signs of infection (fever, sore throat, fatigue) and bleeding (easy bruising, nosebleeds, bleeding gums, melena). Tell patient to take temperature daily.
• Teach and encourage diligent mouth care to reduce the risk of superinfection in the mouth.
• Tell patient to use highly protective sunblock when exposed to sunlight.

---

*Liquid form contains alcohol.   **May contain tartrazine.   †Canada only.   ‡Australia only.   ◇OTC.

• Advise patient not to discontinue leucovorin rescue if they experience severe nausea and vomiting. Parenteral leucovorin therapy may be necessary.
• Warn patient to avoid conception during and immediately after therapy because of possible abortion or congenital anomalies.
• Advise breast-feeding patient to discontinue breast-feeding during therapy because of possible infant toxicity.

---

## thioguanine (6-thioguanine, 6-TG)
Lanvis†

*Pregnancy Risk Category: D*

### HOW SUPPLIED
*Tablets (scored):* 40 mg

### ACTION
Inhibits purine synthesis.

### ONSET, PEAK, DURATION
Undefined.

### INDICATIONS & DOSAGE
*Acute nonlymphocytic leukemia, chronic myelogenous leukemia –*
**Adults and children:** initially, 2 mg/kg P.O. daily (usually calculated to nearest 20 mg). If necessary, dose is then increased gradually to 3 mg/kg/day as tolerated.

### ADVERSE REACTIONS
**GI:** nausea, vomiting, stomatitis, diarrhea, anorexia.
**Hematologic:** *leukopenia, anemia, thrombocytopenia* (occurs slowly over 2 to 4 weeks).
**Hepatic:** *hepatotoxicity,* jaundice.
**Other:** hyperuricemia.

### INTERACTIONS
*Myelosuppressants:* increased risk of toxicity, especially myelosuppression,

bleeding, and hepatotoxicity. Use together cautiously.

### CONTRAINDICATIONS
Contraindicated in patients whose disease has shown resistance to the drug.

### NURSING CONSIDERATIONS
• Use cautiously and with dosage modification in patients with renal or hepatic dysfunction.
• Monitor CBC daily during induction and then weekly during maintenance therapy, as ordered.
• Monitor serum uric acid level, as ordered.
• Watch for jaundice; may be reversible if drug is stopped promptly. Stop drug if hepatotoxicity or hepatic tenderness occurs.
• To prevent bleeding, avoid all I.M. injections when platelet count is below 100,000/mm³.
• Anticipate possible blood transfusions because of cumulative anemia.
• Know that drug is sometimes ordered as 6-thioguanine. The numeral 6 is part of drug name and does not signify dosage units.

### ☑ PATIENT TEACHING
• Advise patient to watch for signs of infection (fever, sore throat, fatigue) and bleeding (easy bruising, nosebleeds, bleeding gums, melena). Tell patient to take temperature daily.
• Advise women of childbearing age to avoid becoming pregnant during therapy. Also recommend consulting with doctor before becoming pregnant.
• Advise breast-feeding patient to discontinue breast-feeding during therapy because of possible infant toxicity.

---

# 71

# Antibiotic antineoplastic drugs

bleomycin sulfate
dactinomycin
daunorubicin hydrochloride
doxorubicin hydrochloride
idarubicin hydrochloride
mitomycin
pentostatin
plicamycin

**COMBINATION PRODUCTS**
None.

---

## bleomycin sulfate
Blenoxane

*Pregnancy Risk Category: NR*

---

**HOW SUPPLIED**
*Injection:* 15-unit vials

**ACTION**
Unknown. Thought to inhibit DNA synthesis and cause scission of single- and double-stranded DNA.

**ONSET, PEAK, DURATION**
Undefined.

**INDICATIONS & DOSAGE**
Dosage and indications may vary. Check the treatment protocol with the doctor.
*Squamous cell carcinoma (head and neck, skin, penis, cervix, and vulva), lymphosarcoma, reticulum cell carcinoma, testicular carcinoma –*
**Adults:** 10 to 20 units/m$^2$ I.V., I.M., or S.C. one or two times weekly to total of 300 to 400 units.
*Hodgkin's disease –*
**Adults:** 10 to 20 units/m$^2$ I.V., I.M., or S.C. one or two times weekly. After 50% response, maintenance dosage is 1 unit I.M. or I.V. daily or 5 units I.M. or I.V. weekly.

**ADVERSE REACTIONS**
**GI:** *stomatitis, anorexia, nausea, vomiting,* diarrhea.
**Respiratory:** pulmonary toxicity such as PNEUMONITIS, *pulmonary fibrosis.*
**Skin:** *erythema, hyperpigmentation, acne, rash, striae, skin tenderness, pruritus.*
**Other:** *reversible alopecia, chills,* weight loss, fever.

**INTERACTIONS**
*Digitalis glycosides:* decreased serum digoxin levels. Monitor closely.
*Phenytoin:* decreased serum phenytoin levels. Monitor closely.

**CONTRAINDICATIONS**
Contraindicated in patients hypersensitive to the drug.

**NURSING CONSIDERATIONS**
• Use cautiously in patients with renal or pulmonary impairment.
• Obtain pulmonary function tests as ordered. Drug should be stopped if tests show a marked decline.
• Follow institutional policy to reduce risks. Preparation and administration of parenteral form of this drug is associated with carcinogenic, mutagenic, and teratogenic risks for personnel.
• **I.V. use:** Reconstitute drug with 5 ml or more of D$_5$W or 0.9% sodium chloride for injection. For I.V. infusion, dilute with 50 to 100 ml of D$_5$W or 0.9% sodium chloride for injection.
• For I.M. use, dilute drug in 1 to 5 ml of sterile water for injection, bacteriostatic water for injection, 0.9% sodium chloride for injection, or D$_5$W.
• Monitor injection site for irritation.
• **Alert:** Adverse pulmonary reactions are common in patients over age 70.

---

*Liquid form contains alcohol. **May contain tartrazine. †Canada only. ‡Australia only. ◇OTC.

Pulmonary fibrosis is fatal in 1% of patients, especially when cumulative dosage exceeds 400 units.
• Monitor chest X-ray, as ordered, and listen to lungs regularly.
• Monitor for fever, which may be treated with antipyretics. This reaction usually occurs within 3 to 6 hours of administration.
• Watch for hypersensitivity reactions, which may be delayed for several hours, especially in patients with lymphoma (test dose of 1 to 2 units should be given before first two doses in these patients. If no reaction occurs, regular dosage is followed).
• Don't use adhesive dressings on skin.
• Refrigerate unopened vials containing dry powder. Refrigerated, reconstituted solution is stable for 4 weeks; at room temperature, for 2 weeks. Bleomycin may adsorb to plastic I.V. bags. For prolonged stability, use glass containers.

☑ **PATIENT TEACHING**
• Warn patient that alopecia may occur, but that it's usually reversible.
• Tell patient to report adverse reactions promptly and to take infection-control and bleeding precautions.

---

## dactinomycin (actinomycin D)
Cosmegen
*Pregnancy Risk Category: C*

### HOW SUPPLIED
*Injection:* 500 mcg-vial

### ACTION
Unknown. May interfere with DNA-dependent RNA synthesis by intercalation.

### ONSET, PEAK, DURATION
Undefined.

### INDICATIONS & DOSAGE
Dosage and indications vary. Check treatment protocol with the doctor.
*Sarcoma, trophoblastic tumors in women, testicular cancer* –
**Adults:** 500 mcg/m² (0.5 mg) I.V. daily for 5 days. Maximum dosage is 15 mcg/kg or 400 to 600 mcg/m²/day for 5 days. After bone marrow recovery, course may be repeated.
*Wilms' tumor, rhabdomyosarcoma, Ewing's sarcoma* –
**Children:** 10 to 15 mcg/kg or 450 mcg/m²/day I.V. for 5 days. Maximum dosage is 500 mcg/day. Or 2.5 mg/m² I.V. in equally divided daily doses over 7 days. After bone marrow recovery, course may be repeated.

### ADVERSE REACTIONS
**GI:** *anorexia, nausea, vomiting,* abdominal pain, diarrhea, *stomatitis,* ulceration, proctitis.
**Hematologic:** *anemia, leukopenia, thrombocytopenia, pancytopenia, aplastic anemia, agranulocytosis.*
**Hepatic:** *hepatotoxicity.*
**Skin:** *erythema;* desquamation; *hyperpigmentation of skin, especially in previously irradiated areas; acnelike eruptions (reversible).*
**Other:** phlebitis and severe damage to soft tissue at injection site, reversible alopecia, malaise, fatigue, lethargy, fever, myalgia, hypocalcemia, *death.*

### INTERACTIONS
*Bone marrow suppressants:* additive toxicity. Monitor closely.
*Vitamin K derivatives:* decreased effectiveness. Monitor closely.

### CONTRAINDICATIONS
Contraindicated in patients with chickenpox or herpes zoster.

### NURSING CONSIDERATIONS
• To reduce nausea, give antiemetic before drug, as ordered.
• Follow institutional policy to reduce risks. Preparation and administration

---

Reactions may be *common,* uncommon, *life-threatening,* or COMMON AND LIFE-THREATENING.

of parenteral form of this drug is associated with carcinogenic, mutagenic, and teratogenic risks for personnel.
- **I.V. use:** Use only sterile water (without preservatives) as diluent for reconstitution. Add 1.1 ml to vial to yield gold-colored solution containing 0.5 mg/ml. Give by direct injection into a vein or through tubing of a free-flowing I.V. solution of 0.9% sodium chloride for injection or D₅W.
- For I.V. infusion, dilute with up to 50 ml of D₅W or 0.9% sodium chloride for injection; infuse over 15 minutes.
- Administer through a running I.V. line with good blood return. If infiltration occurs, apply cold compresses to area and notify doctor.
- If skin contact occurs, irrigate with water for at least 15 minutes.
- *Alert:* Be aware that dosage must be reduced in patients who have recently been treated with, or who will receive concomitant treatment with, radiation therapy or other chemotherapy drugs.
- In the event of a spill, use a solution of trisodium phosphate 5% to inactivate the drug.
- Monitor CBC and platelet counts and renal and hepatic functions, as ordered.
- Monitor for stomatitis, diarrhea, leukopenia, or thrombocytopenia.
- Discard unused solutions.

☑ **PATIENT TEACHING**
- Advise patient to watch for signs of infection (fever, sore throat, fatigue) and bleeding (easy bruising, nosebleeds, bleeding gums, melena) and to take temperature daily.
- Tell patient that alopecia may occur, but that it's usually reversible.

## daunorubicin hydrochloride
Cerubidin‡, Cerubidine
*Pregnancy Risk Category: D*

**HOW SUPPLIED**
*Injection:* 20 mg-vial

**ACTION**
Unknown. May interfere with DNA-dependent RNA synthesis by intercalation.

**ONSET, PEAK, DURATION**
Undefined.

**INDICATIONS & DOSAGE**
Dosage and indications vary. Check treatment protocol with the doctor.
*Remission induction in acute nonlymphocytic (myelogenous, monocytic, erythroid) leukemia –*
**Adults:** in combination, 30 to 45 mg/m²/day I.V. on days 1, 2, and 3 of the first course and on days 1 and 2 of subsequent courses with cytarabine infusions.
*Remission induction in acute lymphocytic leukemia –*
**Adults:** 45 mg/m²/day I.V. on days 1, 2, and 3.
**Children 2 years and older:** 25 mg/m² I.V. on day 1 every week, for up to 6 weeks, if needed.
**Children under 2 years:** 0.5 mg/m² (1 mg/kg) I.V. on day 1 every week, for up to 6 weeks, if needed.

**ADVERSE REACTIONS**
**CV:** *irreversible cardiomyopathy* (dose-related), ECG changes.
**GI:** *nausea, vomiting,* diarrhea.
**GU:** red urine (transient).
**Hematologic:** *bone marrow suppression* (lowest blood counts 10 to 14 days after administration).
**Hepatic:** *hepatotoxicity.*
**Skin:** rash.
**Other:** *severe cellulitis or tissue sloughing if drug extravasates, alopecia,* fever, chills, hyperuricemia.

**INTERACTIONS**
*Dexamethasone, heparin:* don't mix. May form a precipitate.

*Doxorubicin:* additive cardiotoxicity. Monitor closely.
*Hepatotoxic drugs:* increased risk of additive hepatotoxicity. Monitor closely.

## CONTRAINDICATIONS
None reported.

## NURSING CONSIDERATIONS
• Use cautiously in patients with myelosuppression or impaired cardiac, renal, or hepatic function.
• Know that cardiac function studies (including ECG) should be performed before treatment and then periodically throughout therapy.
• Follow institutional policy to reduce risks. Preparation and administration of parenteral form of this drug is associated with carcinogenic, mutagenic, and teratogenic risks for personnel.
• **I.V. use:** Reconstitute drug using 4 ml of sterile water for injection to produce a 5 mg/ml solution.
• Withdraw the desired dose into a syringe containing 10 to 15 ml of 0.9% sodium chloride for injection. Inject into the tubing of a free-flowing I.V. solution of $D_5W$ or 0.9% sodium chloride for injection over 2 to 3 minutes. Alternatively, dilute in 50 ml of 0.9% sodium chloride for injection, and infuse over 10 to 15 minutes, or dilute in 100 ml, and infuse over 30 to 45 minutes.
• Inject into tubing of free-flowing I.V. line. If extravasation occurs, discontinue I.V. infusion immediately, apply ice to area for 24 to 48 hours, and notify doctor.
• Never give drug I.M. or S.C.
• Be aware that cumulative dosage is limited to 500 to 600 mg/m² (450 mg/m² when patients are also receiving or have received cyclophosphamide or radiation therapy to cardiac area).
• Know that therapeutic effects are often accompanied by toxicity.
• Monitor CBC and hepatic function tests, as ordered; monitor ECG every month during therapy.
• Monitor pulse rate closely. Light resting pulse rate is a sign of cardiac adverse reactions. Notify the doctor if this occurs.
• *Alert:* Stop drug immediately and notify doctor if signs of CHF or cardiomyopathy develop.
• Monitor for nausea and vomiting which may be very severe and may last 24 to 48 hours.
• Anticipate the need for blood transfusions to combat anemia.
• Know that reddish color is similar to that of doxorubicin. Take care to avoid confusing the two drugs.
• Optimally, use within 8 hours of preparation. Reconstituted solution is stable for 24 hours at room temperature or 48 hours if refrigerated.

## ☑ PATIENT TEACHING
• Advise patient to watch for signs of infection (fever, sore throat, fatigue) and bleeding (easy bruising, nosebleeds, bleeding gums, melena) and to take temperature daily.
• Advise patient that red urine for 1 to 2 days is normal and does not indicate the presence of blood in urine.
• Advise patient that alopecia may occur, but that it's usually reversible.
• Advise women of childbearing age to avoid becoming pregnant during therapy and to consult with doctor before becoming pregnant.

---

# doxorubicin hydrochloride
Adriamycin‡, Adriamycin PFS, Adriamycin RDF, Rubex

*Pregnancy Risk Category: NR*

## HOW SUPPLIED
*Injection (preservative-free):* 2 mg/ml
*Powder for injection:* 10-mg, 20-mg, 50-mg, 100-mg, 150-mg vials

---

## ACTION
Unknown. May interfere with DNA-dependent RNA synthesis by intercalation.

## ONSET, PEAK, DURATION
Undefined.

## INDICATIONS & DOSAGE
Dosage and indications vary. Check treatment protocol with the doctor.
*Bladder, breast, lung, ovarian, stomach, testicular, and thyroid cancers; Hodgkin's disease; acute lymphoblastic and myeloblastic leukemia; Wilms' tumor; neuroblastoma; lymphoma; sarcoma* –
**Adults:** 60 to 75 mg/m$^2$ I.V. as single dose q 3 weeks; or 30 mg/m$^2$ I.V. in single daily dose, days 1 to 3 of 4-week cycle. Alternatively, 20 mg/m$^2$ I.V. once weekly. Maximum cumulative dosage is 550 mg/m$^2$.

## ADVERSE REACTIONS
**CV:** cardiac depression, seen in such ECG changes as sinus tachycardia, T-wave flattening, ST-segment depression, voltage reduction; *arrhythmias; acute left ventricular failure; irreversible cardiomyopathy.*
**EENT:** conjunctivititis.
**GI:** *nausea, vomiting,* diarrhea, *stomatitis,* esophagitis, anorexia.
**GU:** red urine (transient).
**Hematologic:** *leukopenia* during days 10 to 15 with recovery by day 21; *thrombocytopenia;* MYELOSUPPRESSION.
**Skin:** urticaria, facial flushing.
**Other:** *severe cellulitis or tissue sloughing* (if drug extravasates); hyperuricemia; *complete alopecia within 3 to 4 weeks* (hair may regrow 2 to 5 months after drug is stopped); fever; chills; *anaphylaxis.*

## INTERACTIONS
*Aminophylline, cephalothin, dexamethasone, fluorouracil, heparin, hy-drocortisone:* may form a precipitate. Don't mix together.
*Digoxin:* may decrease serum digoxin levels. Monitor closely.
*Streptozocin:* increased and prolonged blood levels. Dosage may have to be adjusted.

## CONTRAINDICATIONS
Contraindicated in patients with marked myelosuppression induced by previous treatment with other antitumor agents or by radiotherapy and in patients who have received lifetime cumulative dosage of 550 mg/m$^2$.

## NURSING CONSIDERATIONS
• Know that cardiac function studies (including ECG) should be performed before treatment and then periodically throughout therapy. Be aware that dexrazoxane may be administered concomitantly with doxorubicin if the accumulated dose of doxorubicin has reached 300 mg/m$^2$.
• Premedicate with antiemetic, as ordered, to reduce nausea.
• Follow institutional policy to reduce risks. Preparation and administration of parenteral form of this drug is associated with carcinogenic, mutagenic, and teratogenic risks for personnel.
• **I.V. use:** Reconstitute using preservative-free 0.9% sodium chloride for injection. Add 5 ml to the 10-mg vial, 10 ml to the 20-mg vial, or 25 ml to the 50-mg vial. Shake vial and allow drug to dissolve; final concentration will be 2 mg/ml. Give by direct injection into the tubing of a free-flowing I.V. solution containing D$_5$W or 0.9% sodium chloride for injection.
• Don't place I.V. line over joints or in extremities with poor venous or lymphatic drainage. If extravasation occurs, discontinue I.V. infusion immediately, apply ice to area for 24 to 48 hours, and notify doctor. Monitor area closely because extravasation may be progressive. Early consulta-

---

tion with a plastic surgeon may be advisable.

• If vein streaking occurs, slow administration rate. However, if welts occur, stop administration and report this to the doctor.

• If skin or mucosal contact occurs, immediately wash with soap and water.

• In the event of a leak or spill, inactivate drug with 5% sodium hypochlorite solution (household bleach).

• Never give this drug I.M. or S.C.

• Know that dosage modification may be required in patients with myelosuppression and in those with impaired cardiac or hepatic function, and in elderly patients.

• Be prepared to decrease dosage if serum bilirubin level rises: 50% of the dosage should be given when bilirubin is 1.2 to 3 mg/100 ml; 25% when it's greater than 3 mg/100 ml.

• Monitor CBC and hepatic function tests, as ordered; monitor ECG monthly during therapy.

• Be prepared to stop drug or slow rate of infusion if tachycardia develops and notify the doctor.

• *Alert:* If signs of CHF develop, stop the drug and notify the doctor. In many instances, CHF can be prevented by limiting cumulative dosage to 550 mg/m$^2$ (400 mg/m$^2$ when patients are also receiving or have received cyclophosphamide or radiation therapy to cardiac area).

• Know that reddish color is similar to that of daunorubicin. Take care to avoid confusing the two drugs.

• Keep in mind that esophagitis is very common in patients who have also received radiation therapy.

• Know that refrigerated, reconstituted solution is stable for 48 hours; at room temperature, it's stable for 24 hours.

☑ **PATIENT TEACHING**
• Advise patient to watch for signs of infection (fever, sore throat, fatigue) and bleeding (easy bruising, nosebleeds, bleeding gums, melena) and to take temperature daily.

• Advise patient that orange to red urine for 1 to 2 days is normal and does not indicate presence of blood.

• Warn patient that alopecia may occur, but that it's usually reversible.

# idarubicin hydrochloride
Idamycin

*Pregnancy Risk Category: D*

**HOW SUPPLIED**
*Powder for injection:* 5 mg, 10 mg

**ACTION**
Unknown Probably inhibits nucleic acid synthesis by intercalation and interacts with the enzyme topoisomerase II. It is highly lipophilic, which results in an increased rate of cellular uptake.

**ONSET, PEAK, DURATION**
Onset and duration undefined. Intracellular drug levels peak within a few minutes after injection.

**INDICATIONS & DOSAGE**
Dosage and indications vary. Check treatment protocol with the doctor.
*Acute myeloid leukemia, including FAB (French-American-British) classifications M1 through M7, in combination with other approved antileukemic agents —*
**Adults:** 12 mg/m$^2$/day for 3 days by slow I.V. injection (over 10 to 15 minutes) in combination with 100 mg/m$^2$/day of cytarabine for 7 days by continuous I.V. infusion; or as a 25 mg/m$^2$ bolus (cytarabine), followed by 200 mg/m$^2$/day (cytarabine) for 5 days by continuous infusion.

A second course may be administered if needed. If patients experience severe mucositis, administration is delayed until recovery is complete and dosage reduced by 25%. Dosage should also be reduced in patients with hepatic or renal impairment. Idarubicin should not be given if bilirubin level is above 5 mg/dl.

## ADVERSE REACTIONS
**CNS:** *headache, changed mental status,* peripheral neuropathy, *seizures.*
**CV:** *CHF,* atrial fibrillation, chest pain, *MI,* asymptomatic decline in left ventricular ejection fraction, *myocardial insufficiency, arrhythmias,* HEMORRHAGE, *myocardial toxicity.*
**GI:** *nausea, vomiting, cramps, diarrhea, mucositis, severe enterocolitis with perforation* (rare).
**GU:** decreased renal function.
**Hematologic:** *myelosuppression.*
**Hepatic:** changes in hepatic function.
**Skin:** *rash, urticaria, bullous erythrodermatous rash on palms and soles,* hives at injection site, erythema at previously irradiated sites, tissue necrosis at injection site (if extravasation occurs).
**Other:** INFECTION, *alopecia, fever,* hyperuricemia, hypersensitivity reactions.

## INTERACTIONS
*Alkaline solutions, heparin:* incompatibility. Idarubicin should not be mixed with other drugs unless specific compatibility data is available.

## CONTRAINDICATIONS
None reported.

## NURSING CONSIDERATIONS
• Use with extreme caution in patients with bone marrow suppression induced by previous drug therapy or radiotherapy or in patients with hepatic or renal function impairment.
• Take preventive measures (including adequate hydration) before starting treatment. Hyperuricemia may result from rapid lysis of leukemic cells. Allopurinol may be ordered.
• Assess patient for systemic infection and ensure that it's controlled before therapy begins.
• Give antiemetics, as ordered, to prevent or treat nausea and vomiting.
• Follow institutional policy to reduce risks. Preparation and administration of parenteral form of this drug is associated with carcinogenic, mutagenic, and teratogenic risks for personnel.
• **I.V. use:** Reconstitute to a final concentration of 1 mg/ml using 0.9% sodium chloride for injection without preservatives. Add 5 ml to the 5-mg vial or 10 ml to the 10-ml vial. Do *not* use bacteriostatic sodium chloride. Vial is under negative pressure.
• Administer over 10 to 15 minutes into a free-flowing I.V. infusion of 0.9% sodium chloride or 5% dextrose solution running into a large vein.
• Drug is a vesicant. If extravasation occurs, discontinue infusion immediately and notify doctor. Treat with intermittent ice packs — for ½ hour immediately, and then for ½ hour four times daily for 4 days.
• Know that reconstituted solutions are stable for 3 days (72 hours) at room temperature (59° to 86° F [15° to 30° C]); 7 days if refrigerated. Label any unused solutions with CHEMO-THERAPY HAZARD label.
• Monitor hepatic and renal function tests and CBC frequently, as ordered.
• To prevent bleeding, avoid all I.M. injections when platelet count is below 100,000/mm³.
• Anticipate the need for blood transfusions to combat anemia.
• Notify doctor if signs or symptoms of CHF occur.

## ☑ PATIENT TEACHING
• Instruct patient to recognize signs and symptoms of extravasation and to call the doctor or nurse if these occur.
• Warn patient to watch for signs of infection (fever, sore throat, fatigue) and bleeding (easy bruising, nosebleeds, bleeding gums, melena).
• Advise patient that red urine for

---

several days is normal and does not indicate presence of blood.

• Advise women of childbearing age to avoid becoming pregnant during therapy and to consult with doctor before becoming pregnant.

## mitomycin (mitomycin-C)
Mutamycin

*Pregnancy Risk Category: NR*

### HOW SUPPLIED
*Injection:* 5-mg, 20-mg, 40-mg vials

### ACTION
Acts like an alkylating agent, cross-linking strands of DNA. This causes an imbalance of cell growth, leading to cell death.

### ONSET, PEAK, DURATION
Undefined.

### INDICATIONS & DOSAGE
Dosage and indications vary. Check treatment protocol with the doctor.
*Disseminated adenocarcinoma of stomach or pancreas* –
**Adults:** 20 mg/m² as a I.V. single dose. Cycle repeated after 6 to 8 weeks when WBC and platelet counts have returned to normal.

### ADVERSE REACTIONS
**CNS:** headache, neurologic abnormalities, confusion, drowsiness, fatigue.
**GI:** *nausea, vomiting, anorexia, diarrhea.*
**Hematologic: THROMBOCYTOPENIA, LEUKOPENIA** (may be delayed up to 8 weeks and may be cumulative with successive doses).
**Respiratory:** *interstitial pneumonitis,* pulmonary edema, dyspnea, nonproductive cough, adult respiratory distress syndrome.
**Other:** desquamation, induration, pruritus, *pain at injection site; septicemia;* cellulitis, ulceration, slough-

ing with extravasation; *reversible alopecia; fever; microangiopathic hemolytic anemia, characterized by thrombocytopenia, renal failure, and hypertension;* blurred vision, pain.

### INTERACTIONS
*Vinca alkaloids:* may cause acute respiratory distress when administered concomitantly. Monitor closely.

### CONTRAINDICATIONS
Contraindicated in patients hypersensitive to the drug and in those with thrombocytopenia, coagulation disorders, or an increase in bleeding tendency due to other causes.

### NURSING CONSIDERATIONS
• Follow institutional policy to reduce risks. Preparation and administration of parenteral form of this drug is associated with mutagenic, teratogenic, and carcinogenic risks to personnel.
• **I.V. use:** Using sterile water for injection, reconstitute the 5-mg vials with 10 ml, the 20-mg vials with 40 ml, and the 40-mg vials with 80 ml.
• For infusion, dilute with 0.9% sodium chloride for injection, D₅W, or sodium lactate for injection. After dilution, drug is stable for 3 hours in D₅W, 12 hours in 0.9% sodium chloride for injection, and 24 hours in sodium lactate for injection at room temperature.
• Avoid extravasation. Stop infusion immediately if extravasation occurs because of the potential for severe ulceration and necrosis, and notify doctor.
• Never give this drug I.M. or S.C.
• Continue CBC and blood studies, as ordered, at least 7 weeks after therapy is stopped.
• To prevent bleeding, avoid all I.M. injections when platelet count is below 100,000/mm³.
• Anticipate the need for blood transfusions to combat anemia.

---

Reactions may be *common,* uncommon, *life-threatening,* or **COMMON AND LIFE-THREATENING.**

• Monitor renal function tests, as ordered.

### ☑ PATIENT TEACHING
• Warn patient to watch for signs of infection (fever, sore throat, fatigue) and bleeding (easy bruising, nosebleeds, bleeding gums, melena). Tell patient to take temperature daily.
• Warn patient that alopecia may occur, but that it's usually reversible.

---

## pentostatin (2'-deoxycoformycin)
Nipent

*Pregnancy Risk Category: D*

### HOW SUPPLIED
*Powder for injection:* 10 mg-vial

### ACTION
Inhibits the enzyme adenosine deaminase (ADA), causing an increase in intracellular levels of deoxyadenosine triphosphate. This leads to cell damage and death. Because the greatest activity of ADA is in cells of the lymphoid system (especially malignant T cells), pentostatin is useful in treating leukemias.

### ONSET, PEAK, DURATION
Undefined.

### INDICATIONS & DOSAGE
*Alpha-interferon-refractory hairy-cell leukemia—*
**Adults:** 4 mg/m² I.V. every other week.

### ADVERSE REACTIONS
**CNS:** *headache, neurologic symptoms, anxiety, confusion, depression, dizziness, insomnia, nervousness, paresthesia, somnolence, abnormal thinking, fatigue.*
**CV:** *arrhythmias, abnormal ECG, thrombophlebitis, peripheral edema, hemorrhage.*
**EENT:** *abnormal vision, conjunctivitis, ear pain, eye pain, epistaxis, pharyngitis, rhinitis, sinusitis.*
**GI:** *nausea, vomiting, anorexia, diarrhea, constipation, flatulence, stomatitis.*
**GU:** *hematuria, dysuria, increased BUN and creatinine levels.*
**Hematologic:** *myelosuppression,* LEUKOPENIA, *anemia, thrombocytopenia, lymphadenopathy.*
**Hepatic:** *elevated liver enzyme levels.*
**Respiratory:** *cough, bronchitis, dyspnea, lung edema, pneumonia.*
**Skin:** *ecchymosis, petechiae, rash, eczema, dry skin, herpes simplex or zoster, maculopapular rash, vesiculobullous rash, pruritus, seborrhea, discoloration, diaphoresis.*
**Other:** *fever,* INFECTION, *pain, hypersensitivity reactions, chills, sepsis,* DEATH, NEOPLASM, *chest pain, abdominal pain, back pain, flulike syndrome, asthenia, malaise, myalgia, arthralgia, weight loss.*

### INTERACTIONS
*Cytarabine or vidarabine:* increased incidence or severity of adverse effects associated with either drug. Avoid concomitant use.
*Fludarabine:* risk of severe or fatal pulmonary toxicity. Don't use together.

### CONTRAINDICATIONS
Contraindicated in patients hypersensitive to the drug.

### NURSING CONSIDERATIONS
• Use cautiously and only under the supervision of a doctor qualified and experienced in the use of chemotherapeutic agents. Adverse reactions after pentostatin therapy are common.
• Know that use in patients with renal damage (creatinine clearance of 60 ml/minute or less) should be avoided.
• Make sure patients are adequately hydrated before therapy. Administer 500 to 1,000 ml of D₅W in 0.45% so-

---

dium chloride solution, as ordered, for hydration.

• Follow institutional policy to reduce risks. Preparation and administration of parenteral form of this drug is associated with mutagenic, teratogenic, and carcinogenic risks to personnel.

• **I.V. use:** Add 5 ml of sterile water for injection to the vial containing pentostatin powder for injection. Mix thoroughly to make a solution of 2 mg/ml. Drug may be administered by I.V. bolus injection or diluted further in 25 or 50 ml of D₅W or 0.9% sodium chloride for injection and infused over 20 to 30 minutes.

• Use reconstituted solution within 8 hours; it contains no preservatives.

• Treat all spills and waste products with 5% sodium hypochlorite (household bleach).

• Give an additional 500 ml of D₅W, as ordered, for hydration after drug is administered.

• Know that the optimal duration of therapy is unknown. Current recommendations suggest two additional courses of therapy after a complete response. If a partial response is not evident after 6 months of therapy, drug will be discontinued. If a partial response is evident, drug will be continued for another 6 months.

• *Alert:* Withhold or discontinue drug in patients with evidence of CNS toxicity, a severe rash, or an active infection, and notify the doctor. Drug may be resumed when the infection clears.

• Temporarily withhold drug if the absolute neutrophil count falls below 200/mm³ and the pretreatment level was over 500/mm³, and notify the doctor. No recommendations exist regarding dosage adjustments in patients with anemia, neutropenia, or thrombocytopenia.

• Be aware that drug should be used only in patients who have hairy-cell leukemia refractory to alpha-interferon. This is defined as disease that progresses after a minimum of 3 months of treatment with alpha-interferon or disease that does not exhibit a response after 6 months of therapy.

### ☑ PATIENT TEACHING

• Advise patient to watch for signs of infection (fever, sore throat, fatigue) and bleeding (easy bruising, nosebleeds, bleeding gums, melena) and to take temperature daily.

• Advise women of childbearing age to avoid becoming pregnant during therapy and to consult with doctor before becoming pregnant.

## plicamycin (mithramycin)
Mithracin

*Pregnancy Risk Category: X*

**HOW SUPPLIED**
*Injection:* 2.5-mg vials

**ACTION**
Unknown. Thought to form a complex with DNA, thus inhibiting RNA synthesis. Also inhibits osteocytic activity, blocking calcium and phosphorus resorption from bone.

**ONSET, PEAK, DURATION**
Onset occurs in 1 to 2 days. Effects peak 3 days after single dose and persist for 7 to 10 days.

**INDICATIONS & DOSAGE**
Dosage and indications vary. Check treatment protocol with the doctor.
*Hypercalcemia associated with advanced malignant disease –*
**Adults:** 15 to 25 mcg/kg/day I.V. for 3 to 4 days. Dosage repeated at weekly intervals until desired response is obtained.
*Testicular cancer –*
**Adults:** 25 to 30 mcg/kg/day I.V. for 8 to 10 days or until toxicity occurs.

**ADVERSE REACTIONS**
**CNS:** drowsiness, weakness, lethargy, headache, malaise.

---

Reactions may be *common,* uncommon, *life-threatening,* or COMMON AND LIFE-THREATENING.

**GI:** *nausea, vomiting,* anorexia, diarrhea, stomatitis.

**GU:** increased BUN and serum creatinine levels.

**Hematologic:** *leukopenia, thrombocytopenia; bleeding syndrome* (from epistaxis to generalized hemorrhage); *facial flushing.*

**Hepatic:** *elevated liver enzymes levels,* hepatotoxicity.

**Skin:** facial flushing, rash.

**Other:** *decreased serum calcium,* potassium, and phosphorus levels; irritation, *death,* fever, cellulitis with extravasation.

## INTERACTIONS
None significant.

## CONTRAINDICATIONS
Contraindicated in patients with thrombocytopenia, bone marrow suppression, or coagulation and bleeding disorders and in women who are or who may become pregnant.

## NURSING CONSIDERATIONS
• Use with extreme caution in patients with significant renal or hepatic impairment.

• Obtain baseline platelet count and PT before therapy, as ordered.

• To reduce nausea, give antiemetic before administering, as ordered.

• Follow institutional policy to reduce risks. Preparation and administration of parenteral form of this drug is associated with carcinogenic, mutagenic, and teratogenic risks for personnel.

• **I.V. use:** To prepare solution, add 4.9 ml of sterile water for injection to vial and shake to dissolve. Then dilute for I.V infusion in 1,000 ml of D$_5$W or 0.9% sodium chloride. Administer by infusion over 4 to 6 hours. Discard unused drug.

• Be aware that slow infusion reduces nausea that develops with I.V. push.

• Avoid extravasation. Plicamycin is a vesicant. If I.V. solution infiltrates,
stop immediately, notify doctor, and use ice packs. Restart I.V. line.

• Avoid contact with skin or mucous membranes.

• Monitor platelet count and PT during therapy, as ordered. Discontinue drug if WBC count is less than 4,000/mm$^3$, if platelet count falls to less than 150,000/mm$^3$, or if PT is prolonged more than 4 seconds longer than control, and notify doctor.

• **Alert:** Know that facial flushing is an early indicator of bleeding.

• To prevent bleeding, avoid all I.M. injections when platelet count is below 100,000/mm$^3$.

• Anticipate the need for blood transfusions to combat anemia.

• Monitor lactate dehydrogenase, AST, ALT, alkaline phosphatase, BUN, creatinine, potassium, calcium, and phosphorus levels, as ordered.

• Monitor patients for tetany, carpopedal spasm, Chvostek's sign, and muscle cramps; check serum calcium level. Precipitous drop in calcium level is possible.

• Store lyophilized powder in refrigerator and protect from light.

• Be aware that patients receiving drug for treatment testicular cancer may require calcium supplementation.

## ☑ PATIENT TEACHING
• Advise patient to watch for signs of infection (fever, sore throat, fatigue) and bleeding (easy bruising, nosebleeds, bleeding gums, melena) and to take temperature daily.

• Advise women of childbearing age to avoid becoming pregnant during therapy and to consult with doctor before becoming pregnant.

---

anastrozole
bicalutamide
diethylstilbestrol
(See Chapter 55, ESTROGENS AND
PROGESTINS)
estramustine phosphate sodium
flutamide
goserelin acetate
leuprolide acetate
megestrol acetate
tamoxifen citrate
testolactone

**COMBINATION PRODUCTS**
None.

▼ *NEW DRUG*

## anastrozole
Arimidex
*Pregnancy Risk Category: D*

**HOW SUPPLIED**
*Tablets:* 1 mg

**ACTION**
A potent, selective nonsteroidal aromatase inhibitor that significantly lowers serum estradiol concentrations, thereby inhibiting stimulation of breast cancer cell growth in postmenopausal women.

**ONSET, PEAK, DURATION**
Unknown.

**INDICATIONS & DOSAGE**
*Treatment of advanced breast cancer in postmenopausal women with disease progression after tamoxifen therapy —*
**Adults:** 1 mg P.O. daily.

**ADVERSE REACTIONS**
CNS: *headache,* dizziness, depression, paresthesia.
CV: chest pain, edema.

GI: *nausea,* vomiting, diarrhea, constipation, abdominal pain, anorexia, dry mouth, weight gain, increased appetite.
GU: vaginal hemorrhage, vaginal dryness.
Respiratory: dyspnea, increased cough, pharyngitis.
Skin: *hot flushes,* rash, sweating.
Other: *asthenia, pain, back pain,* bone pain, peripheral edema, pelvic pain, thromboembolic disease.

**INTERACTIONS**
None.

**CONTRAINDICATIONS**
None known.

**NURSING CONSIDERATIONS**
• Use cautiously in breast-feeding women.
• Know that pregnancy must be ruled out before treatment.
• Be aware that drug should be administered under the supervision of a qualified doctor experienced in the use of anticancer drugs.

☑ **PATIENT TEACHING**
• Instruct the patient to report adverse reactions.
• Stress the importance of follow-up care.

▼ *NEW DRUG*

## bicalutamide
Casodex
*Pregnancy Risk Category: X*

**HOW SUPPLIED**
*Tablets:* 50 mg

---

Reactions may be *common,* uncommon, *life-threatening,* or COMMON AND LIFE-THREATENING.

## ACTION
A nonsteroidal antiandrogen that binds to cytosol androgen receptors in target tissue.

## ONSET, PEAK, DURATION
Unknown.

## INDICATIONS & DOSAGE
*Adjunct therapy for treatment of advanced prostate cancer –*
**Adults:** 50 mg P.O. once daily in morning or evening.

## ADVERSE REACTIONS
**CNS:** headache, dizziness, paresthesia, insomnia.
**CV:** *hot flashes,* hypertension, chest pain, peripheral edema.
**GI:** *constipation, nausea, diarrhea,* abdominal pain, flatulence, increased liver enzymes, vomiting, weight loss.
**GU:** nocturia, hematuria, urinary tract infection, impotence, gynecomastia, urinary incontinence.
**Hematologic:** hypochromic anemia, iron deficiency anemia.
**Respiratory:** dyspnea.
**Skin:** rash, sweating.
**Other:** *general pain, back pain, pelvic pain, asthenia, infection,* flu syndrome, hyperglycemia, bone pain.

## INTERACTIONS
*Coumarin anticoagulants:* displacement of these drugs from their protein-binding sites. Monitor prothrombin times closely, and know that the anticoagulant dose may need adjustment.

## CONTRAINDICATIONS
Contraindicated in patients with hypersensitivity to the drug or any component.

## NURSING CONSIDERATIONS
● Use cautiously in patients with moderate-to-severe hepatic impairment (drug is extensively metabolized by the liver).

● Bicalutamide is used in combination with a luteinizing hormone-releasing hormone analogue. Treatment should be started at the same time for both drugs.
● Give drug at same time each day.
● Regularly monitor serum prostate specific antigen (PSA) levels, as ordered. PSA levels help in assessing response to therapy. Report elevated levels to the doctor, who should evaluate the patient to determine disease progression.
● Monitor liver function studies, as ordered. When a patient develops jaundice or exhibits laboratory evidence of liver injury in the absence of liver metastases, drug should be discontinued. Abnormalities are usually reversible on discontinuation.

## ☑ PATIENT TEACHING
● Tell the patient to take drug at the same time each day, without regard to meals.
● Urge him not to stop drug therapy without consulting the doctor.

# estramustine phosphate sodium
Emcyt, Estracyst‡
*Pregnancy Risk Category: NR*

## HOW SUPPLIED
*Capsules:* 140 mg

## ACTION
Unknown. A combination of estrogen and an alkylating agent; probably acts by its ability to bind selectively to a protein present in the prostate gland.

## ONSET, PEAK, DURATION
Unknown.

## INDICATIONS & DOSAGE
*Palliative treatment of metastatic or progressive prostate cancer –*
**Adults:** 10 to 16 mg/kg P.O. in three or four divided doses. Usual dosage is

14 mg/kg daily. Therapy continued for up to 3 months and, if successful, maintained as long as the patient responds.

## ADVERSE REACTIONS
**CNS:** lethargy, insomnia, headache, anxiety.
**CV:** *MI,* sodium and fluid retention, thrombophlebitis, *CHF, stroke.*
**GI:** *nausea, vomiting,* diarrhea, anorexia, flatulence, GI bleeding, thirst.
**Hematologic:** *leukopenia, thrombocytopenia.*
**Respiratory:** *edema, pulmonary embolism,* dyspnea.
**Skin:** rash, pruritus, dry skin, flushing.
**Other:** *painful gynecomastia and breast tenderness,* thinning of hair, leg cramps, chest pain.

## INTERACTIONS
*Calcium-rich foods (milk and dairy products) and calcium containing drugs such as antacids:* impaired absorption of estramustine. Do not administer at same time.

## CONTRAINDICATIONS
Contraindicated in patients hypersensitive to estradiol and nitrogen mustard. Also contraindicated in those with active thrombophlebitis or thromboembolic disorders, except when the actual tumor mass is the cause of the thromboembolic phenomenon.

## NURSING CONSIDERATIONS
• Use cautiously in patients with history of thrombophlebitis or thromboembolic disorders and cerebrovascular or coronary artery disease. Monitor weight regularly in these patients. Estramustine may exaggerate preexisting peripheral edema or CHF.
• Also use cautiously in patients with impaired liver function.
• Be aware that each 140-mg capsule contains 12.5 mg of sodium.

• Monitor blood pressure and blood glucose periodically throughout therapy. Drug may increase blood pressure and decrease blood glucose.
• Keep in mind that estramustine is a combination of estrogen estradiol and a nitrogen mustard, shown to be effective in patients refractory to estrogen therapy alone.
• Be aware that patients may continue therapy as long as response is favorable. Some patients have taken the drug for more than 3 years.
• Store capsules in refrigerator.

### ☑ PATIENT TEACHING
• Tell patient to take this drug on an empty stomach (2 hours before or 1 hour after meals) and to avoid taking with milk or dairy products.
• Because of the possibility of mutagenic effects, advise patient and partner to use contraception if woman is of childbearing age.

---

# flutamide
Euflex†, Eulexin

*Pregnancy Risk Category: D*

## HOW SUPPLIED
*Capsules:* 125 mg, 250 mg†

## ACTION
Inhibits androgen uptake or prevents binding of androgens in nucleus of cells within target tissues.

## ONSET, PEAK, DURATION
Onset and duration unknown. Plasma levels peak 2 hours after dose.

## INDICATIONS & DOSAGE
*Metastatic prostate cancer (stage $D_2$) in combination with luteinizing hormone-releasing hormone analogues such as leuprolide acetate –*
**Adults:** 250 mg P.O. q 8 hours.

## ADVERSE REACTIONS
**CNS:** *drowsiness, confusion, depression, anxiety, nervousness.*
**CV:** peripheral edema, hypertension.
**GI:** *diarrhea, nausea, vomiting.*
**GU:** *impotence, loss of libido.*
**Hematologic:** anemia, leukopenia, ***thrombocytopenia,*** hemolytic anemia.
**Hepatic:** elevated liver enzyme levels, hepatitis.
**Skin:** rash, photosensitivity.
**Other:** *hot flashes,* gynecomastia.

## INTERACTIONS
None significant.

## CONTRAINDICATIONS
Contraindicated in patients hypersensitive to the drug.

## NURSING CONSIDERATIONS
• Monitor liver function tests periodically, as ordered.
• Know that flutamide must be taken continuously with the agent used for medical castration (such as leuprolide acetate) to allow the full benefit of therapy. Leuprolide suppresses testosterone production while flutamide inhibits testosterone action at the cellular level. Together, they can impair the growth of androgen-responsive tumors.

## ☑ PATIENT TEACHING
• Advise patient not to discontinue drug therapy without consulting the doctor.
• Instruct patient to report adverse reactions promptly.

---

## goserelin acetate
Zoladex

*Pregnancy Risk Category: X*

## HOW SUPPLIED
*Implants:* 3.6 mg

## ACTION
A luteinizing hormone-releasing hormone (LHRH) analogue that acts on the pituitary to decrease the release of follicle-stimulating hormone and luteinizing hormone, resulting in dramatically lowered serum levels of sex hormones.

## ONSET, PEAK, DURATION
Onset occurs in 2 to 4 weeks. Serum levels peak after 12 to 15 days. Suppression of hormone production to castration levels persists throughout therapy.

## INDICATIONS & DOSAGE
*Palliative treatment of advanced prostate cancer; endometriosis –*
**Adults:** 1 implant S.C. q 28 days into the upper abdominal wall. For endometriosis, maximum duration of therapy is 6 months.

## ADVERSE REACTIONS
**CNS:** lethargy, pain (worsened in the first 30 days), dizziness, *insomnia,* anxiety, *depression, headache,* chills, *emotional lability.*
**CV:** edema, ***CHF, arrhythmias,*** *peripheral edema,* ***CVA,*** hypertension, ***MI,*** peripheral vascular disorder, chest pain.
**GI:** nausea, vomiting, diarrhea, constipation, ulcer, anorexia, abdominal pain.
**GU:** impotence, *sexual dysfunction, lower urinary tract symptoms,* renal insufficiency, urinary obstruction, *vaginitis,* urinary tract infection, amenorrhea.
**Hematologic:** anemia.
**Respiratory:** COPD, upper respiratory infection.
**Skin:** rash, *diaphoresis, acne, seborrhea,* hirsutism.
**Other:** *hot flashes,* gout, hyperglycemia, weight increase, breast swelling and tenderness, *changes in breast size, pain, changes in libido, asthenia, infection,* breast pain, back pain.

---

**INTERACTIONS**
None significant.

**CONTRAINDICATIONS**
Contraindicated in patients with hypersensitivity to LHRH, LHRH agonist analogues, or to goserelin acetate. Also contraindicated during pregnancy or breast-feeding.

**NURSING CONSIDERATIONS**
• Because use of the drug is associated with a loss of bone mineral density in women, use cautiously in patients with other risk factors for osteoporosis, such as family history of osteoporosis, chronic alcohol or tobacco abuse, or the use of drugs such as corticosteroids or anticonvulsants that affect bone density.
• Before administering to female patients, rule out pregnancy.
• Administer drug into the upper abdominal wall using aseptic technique. After cleaning the area with an alcohol swab (and injecting a local anesthetic), stretch the patient's skin with one hand while grasping the barrel of the syringe with the other. Insert the needle into the subcutaneous fat; then change direction of the needle so that it parallels the abdominal wall. The needle should then be pushed in until the hub touches the patient's skin; then withdrawn about 1 cm (this creates a gap for the drug to be injected) before depressing the plunger completely.
• To avoid the need for a new syringe and injection site, do not aspirate after inserting the needle.
• **Alert:** Know that the implant comes in a preloaded syringe. If the package is damaged, do not use the syringe. Make sure that the drug is visible in the translucent chamber of the syringe.
• When used for prostate cancer, be aware that LHRH analogues such as goserelin may initially cause a worsening of prostatic cancer symptoms because the drug initially increases testosterone serum levels. A few patients may experience increased bone pain. Rarely, disease exacerbation (either spinal cord compression or ureteral obstruction) has occurred.

☑ **PATIENT TEACHING**
• Advise patient to report every 28 days for a new implant. A delay of a couple of days is permissible.
• Tell women to use a nonhormonal form of contraception during treatment. Caution patient about the significant risks to the fetus should pregnancy occur.
• Tell patient to call the doctor if menstruation persists or if breakthrough bleeding occurs. Menstruation should stop during treatment.
• After therapy ends, inform patient that she may experience a delayed return of menses. Persistent amenorrhea is rare.

---

## leuprolide acetate
Lucrin‡, Lupron, Lupron Depot, Lupron Depot-Ped

*Pregnancy Risk Category: X*

**HOW SUPPLIED**
*Injection:* 1 mg/0.2 ml (5 mg/ml) in 2.8-ml multiple-dose vials
*Depot injection:* 3.75 mg/ml, 7.5 mg/ml, 11.5 mg/ml, 15 mg/ml

**ACTION**
Initially stimulates but then inhibits the release of follicle-stimulating hormone and luteinizing hormone, resulting in testosterone suppression.

**ONSET, PEAK, DURATION**
Testosterone concentrations decline to castrate levels within 2 to 4 weeks. Time to peak effect for amenorrhea usually occurs after 1 to 2 months of therapy. Normal pituitary-gonadal system function is usually restored within 4 to 12 weeks after therapy is

---

Reactions may be *common*, uncommon, *life-threatening*, or **COMMON AND LIFE-THREATENING**.

withdrawn. Cyclic bleeding in females usually returns within 60 to 90 days after therapy is withdrawn.

## INDICATIONS & DOSAGE
*Advanced prostate cancer –*
**Adults:** 1 mg S.C. daily. Alternatively, 7.5 mg I.M. (depot injection) monthly.
*Endometriosis –*
**Adults:** 3.75 mg I.M (depot injection only) as a single injection once a month for up to 6 months.
*Central precocious puberty –*
**Children:** initially, 0.3 mg/kg (minimum 7.5 mg) I.M. (depot injection only) as a single injection q 4 weeks. Dosage may be increased in increments of 3.75 mg q 4 weeks, if needed. Therapy should be discontinued before female child reaches age 11 and before male child reaches age 12.

## ADVERSE REACTIONS
**CNS:** *dizziness, depression, headache, pain,* insomnia.
**CV:** arrhythmias, angina, *MI, peripheral edema, ECG changes,* hypertension, murmur.
**GI:** *nausea, vomiting,* anorexia, constipation.
**GU:** *impotence, vaginitis,* urinary frequency, hematuria, urinary tract infection, gynecomastia.
**Hepatic:** elevated liver enzyme levels.
**Respiratory:** dyspnea, sinus congestion, pulmonary fibrosis.
**Other:** transient bone pain during first week of treatment, *hot flashes,* skin reactions at injection site, *androgen-like effects,* joint disorder, myalgia, neuromuscular disorder, *weight gain or loss,* anemia, dermatitis, *asthenia.*

## INTERACTIONS
None significant.

## CONTRAINDICATIONS
Contraindicated in patients hypersensitive to the drug or other gonadotropin-releasing hormone analogues, during pregnancy or lactation, and in women with undiagnosed vaginal bleeding.

## NURSING CONSIDERATIONS
• Use cautiously in patients hypersensitive to benzyl alcohol.
• Never administer by I.V. injection.
• Know that once-monthly depot injection should be administered under medical supervision. Use supplied diluent to reconstitute drug. Draw 1 ml into a syringe with a 22G needle (extra diluent is provided and should be discarded). Inject into vial; then shake well. Suspension will appear milky. Although the suspension is stable for 24 hours after reconstitution, it contains no bacteriostatic agent. Use immediately.
• Be aware that response to the treatment of central precocious puberty should be monitored q 1 to 2 months after the start of therapy with a GnRH stimulation test and sex steroid levels. Measurement of bone age for advancement should be done q 6 to 12 months.
• Know that drug use may cause an increase in the signs and symptoms being treated during first few weeks of therapy.

## ☑ PATIENT TEACHING
• Prior to starting a child on treatment of central precocious puberty, ensure that parents understand the importance of continuous therapy.
• Carefully instruct patient who will self-administer S.C. injection about proper administration techniques and advise them to use only the syringes provided by the manufacturer.
• Advise patient that if another syringe must be substituted, a low-dose insulin syringe (U-100, 0.5 ml) may be an appropriate choice but that nee-

---

*Liquid form contains alcohol.   **May contain tartrazine.   †Canada only.   ‡Australia only.   ◊OTC.

dle gauge should not be smaller than 22G.

• Advise patient to store the drug at room temperature, protected from light and sources of heat.

• Reassure patient with history of undesirable effects from other endocrine therapies that leuprolide is much easier to tolerate.

• Reassure patient that these effects are transient and will disappear after about 1 week. Worsening of prostate cancer symptoms or central precocious puberty symptoms may occur initially.

---

## megestrol acetate
Megace, Megostat‡

*Pregnancy Risk Category: D*

### HOW SUPPLIED
*Tablets:* 20 mg, 40 mg
*Oral suspension:* 40 mg/ml

### ACTION
A progestin that changes the tumor's hormonal environment and alters the neoplastic process. Mechanism responsible for appetite stimulation is unknown.

### ONSET, PEAK, DURATION
Unknown.

### INDICATIONS & DOSAGE
*Breast cancer –*
**Adults:** 40 mg P.O. q.i.d.
*Endometrial cancer –*
**Adults:** 40 to 320 mg P.O. daily in divided doses.
*Treatment of anorexia, cachexia, or unexplained significant weight loss in patients with AIDS –*
**Adults:** 800 mg P.O. (oral suspension) daily in divided doses.

### ADVERSE REACTIONS
**CV:** thrombophlebitis.
**GI:** nausea, vomiting.

**GU:** breakthrough menstrual bleeding.
**Respiratory:** *pulmonary embolism,* dyspnea.
**Skin:** rash.
**Other:** weight gain, increased appetite, carpal tunnel syndrome, alopecia, hyperglycemia.

### INTERACTIONS
None significant.

### CONTRAINDICATIONS
Contraindicated in patients hypersensitive to the drug and during pregnancy.

### NURSING CONSIDERATIONS
• Use cautiously in patients with history of thrombophlebitis.
• Know that megestrol is a relatively nontoxic drug with a low incidence of adverse effects.
• Be aware that 2 months is an adequate trial when treating patients with cancer.

### ☑ PATIENT TEACHING
• Inform patient that therapeutic response isn't immediate.
• Advise breast-feeding patient to discontinue breast-feeding during therapy because of possible infant toxicity.

---

## tamoxifen citrate
Alpha-Tamoxifen†, Nolvadex, Nolvadex-D†‡, Novo-Tamoxifen†, Tamofen†, Tamone†, Tamoplex†

*Pregnancy Risk Category: D*

### HOW SUPPLIED
*Tablets:* 10 mg, 20 mg
*Tablets (enteric-coated)†:* 10 mg, 20 mg

### ACTION
Exact antineoplastic action is unknown; acts as an estrogen antagonist.

---

### ONSET, PEAK, DURATION
Onset occurs in 4 to 10 weeks, but may take several months. Peak unknown. Estrogen antagonism may persist for several weeks after drug is discontinued.

### INDICATIONS & DOSAGE
*Advanced premenopausal and postmenopausal breast cancers* –
**Adults:** 10 to 20 mg P.O. b.i.d.

### ADVERSE REACTIONS
**GI:** *nausea, vomiting, diarrhea.*
**GU:** *vaginal discharge* and bleeding, *irregular menses, increased BUN, amenorrhea.*
**Hematologic:** transient fall in WBC or platelet counts, leukopenia, ***thrombocytopenia.***
**Skin:** *skin changes.*
**Other:** temporary bone or tumor pain, *hot flashes,* brief exacerbation of pain from osseous metastases, *weight gain or loss, fluid retention.*

### INTERACTIONS
*Coumarin-type anticoagulants:* may cause significant increase in anticoagulant effect. Monitor patient and PT closely.

### CONTRAINDICATIONS
Contraindicated in patients hypersensitive to the drug.

### NURSING CONSIDERATIONS
• Use cautiously in patients with existing leukopenia or thrombocytopenia. Monitor CBC closely in these patients, as ordered.
• Monitor serum lipid levels, as ordered, during long-term therapy in patients with preexisting hyperlipidemia.
• Monitor serum calcium levels, as ordered. Drug may compound hypercalcemia related to bone metastases during initiation of therapy.
• Know that the drug acts as an "antiestrogen." Best results have been reported in patients with positive estrogen receptors.
• Be aware that adverse reactions are usually minor and well tolerated.

### ☑ PATIENT TEACHING
• Tell patient taking enteric-coated tablets (Nolvadex-D†‡) to swallow the tablets whole without crushing or chewing. Tell her not to take antacids within 2 hours of a dose.
• Reassure patient that acute exacerbation of bone pain during tamoxifen therapy usually indicates drug will produce good response. Use analgesic to relieve pain.
• Strongly encourage a woman who's taking or has taken tamoxifen to have regular gynecologic examinations because of increased risk of uterine cancer associated with its use.
• Advise patient to use barrier form of contraception because short-term therapy induces ovulation in premenopausal women.
• Advise women of childbearing age to avoid becoming pregnant during therapy. Also recommend consulting with doctor before becoming pregnant.

---

## testolactone
Teslac
Controlled Substance Schedule III
*Pregnancy Risk Category: C*

### HOW SUPPLIED
*Tablets:* 50 mg

### ACTION
Exact antineoplastic action is unknown. An androgen that probably changes the tumor's hormonal environment and alters the neoplastic process.

### ONSET, PEAK, DURATION
Onset occurs in 6 to 12 weeks. Peak and duration unknown.

---

## INDICATIONS & DOSAGE

*Advanced postmenopausal breast cancer; advanced premenopausal breast cancer in women whose ovarian function has been terminated –*
**Women:** 250 mg P.O. q.i.d.

## ADVERSE REACTIONS

**CNS:** paresthesia, peripheral neuropathy.
**CV:** increased blood pressure, edema.
**GI:** nausea, vomiting, diarrhea, anorexia, glossitis.
**Other:** alopecia, erythema.

## INTERACTIONS

*Oral anticoagulants:* increased pharmacologic effects. Monitor patient and PT carefully.

## CONTRAINDICATIONS

Contraindicated in patients hypersensitive to the drug and in males with breast cancer.

## NURSING CONSIDERATIONS

• Monitor fluid and electrolyte levels, especially calcium level.
• Force fluids to aid calcium excretion and encourage exercise to prevent hypercalcemia. Immobilized patients are prone to hypercalcemia.
• Know that higher-than-recommended doses do not increase incidence of remission.

## ☑ PATIENT TEACHING

• Inform patient that therapeutic response isn't immediate. Three months is an adequate trial for this drug.
• Tell patient to notify doctor if numbness or tingling occurs in fingers, toes, or face.

---

Reactions may be *common,* uncommon, *life-threatening,* or **COMMON AND LIFE-THREATENING.**

altretamine
asparaginase
bacillus Calmette-Guérin (BCG),
   live intravesical
dacarbazine
etoposide
mitotane
mitoxantrone hydrochloride
paclitaxel
pegaspargase
porfimer sodium
procarbazine hydrochloride
teniposide
tretinoin
vinblastine sulfate
vincristine sulfate
vinorelbine tartrate

**COMBINATION PRODUCTS**
None.

---

## altretamine
## (hexamethylmelamine; HMM)
Hexalen

*Pregnancy Risk Category: D*

---

**HOW SUPPLIED**
*Capsules:* 50 mg

**ACTION**
Unknown. Structurally similar to tri-
ethylenemelamine, but not an alkylating agent. Metabolism is important
for antitumor activity.

**ONSET, PEAK, DURATION**
Onset and duration undefined. Plasma
levels peak in ½ to 3 hours.

**INDICATIONS & DOSAGE**
*Palliative treatment of persistent or re-
current ovarian cancer after first-line
therapy with cisplatin or alkylating
agent-based combination therapy –*

**Adults:** 260 mg/m² P.O. daily in four
divided doses with meals and h.s. for
14 or 21 consecutive days in a 28-day
cycle.

**ADVERSE REACTIONS**
**CNS:** *peripheral neuropathy,* ataxia,
paresthesia, fatigue, *seizures,* dizziness, vertigo.
**GI:** *nausea and vomiting,* anorexia.
**Hematologic:** *leukopenia, thrombocytopenia,* anemia.
**Skin:** erythematous maculopapular
eczema.
**Other:** increased serum creatinine
and BUN levels, alopecia.

**INTERACTIONS**
*Cimetidine:* may increase half-life of
altretamine. Monitor for toxicity.
*MAO inhibitors:* severe orthostatic
hypotension. Avoid concomitant use.

**CONTRAINDICATIONS**
Contraindicated in patients hypersensitive to the drug and in those with
preexisting severe bone marrow suppression or severe neurologic toxicity.

**NURSING CONSIDERATIONS**
● Obtain baseline CBC and platelet
count, as ordered, before each course
of therapy, and monitor monthly.
● Perform a careful neurologic assessment before each course of therapy.
● Know that continuous high-dose
daily treatment is associated with a
higher incidence of mild to moderate
neurotoxicity. It appears to be reversible when therapy is discontinued.
● **Alert:** Be prepared to discontinue
drug temporarily for at least 14 days if
laboratory tests show a platelet count
below 75,000/mm³, WBC count below 2,000/mm³, or granulocyte count

---

*Liquid form contains alcohol. **May contain tartrazine. †Canada only. ‡Australia only. ◊OTC.

below 1,000/mm³. Also discontinue temporarily, as ordered, if patients experience severe GI distress that is unresponsive to symptomatic treatment or develop signs of progressive neuropathy. Drug should be discontinued, as ordered, if neurologic symptoms fail to stabilize.
• Continuous daily use of this drug is associated with nausea and vomiting, which is usually treatable with antiemetics. If nausea and vomiting is severe, dosage reduction or temporary discontinuation may be necessary.

### ☑ PATIENT TEACHING
• Tell patient to take drug with meals to minimize nausea and vomiting.
• Tell patient to watch for signs of infection (fever, sore throat, fatigue) and bleeding (easy bruising, nosebleeds, bleeding gums, melena) and to take temperature daily.
• Advise patient to use contraception; drug may harm fetus.

---

## asparaginase
### (L-asparaginase)
Elspar, Kidrolase†

*Pregnancy Risk Category: C*

### HOW SUPPLIED
*Injection:* 10,000-unit vial

### ACTION
Destroys the amino acid asparagine, which is needed for protein synthesis in acute lymphocytic leukemia. This leads to death of the leukemic cell.

### ONSET, PEAK, DURATION
Onset almost immediate. Time to peak plasma concentration is almost immediate after I.V. administration; 4 to 24 hours after I.M. administration. Effects persist for 23 to 33 days after withdrawal of therapy.

### INDICATIONS & DOSAGE
*Acute lymphocytic leukemia (in combination with other drugs)* –
**Adults and children:** 1,000 IU/kg I.V. daily for 10 days, injected over 30 minutes or by slow I.V. push; or 6,000 IU/m² I.M. at intervals specified in protocol.
*Sole induction agent for acute lymphocytic leukemia* –
**Adults:** 200 IU/kg I.V. daily for 28 days.

### ADVERSE REACTIONS
**CNS:** confusion, drowsiness, depression, hallucinations, *intracranial hemorrhage,* fatigue, *coma,* agitation, headache, lethargy, somnolence.
**GI:** *vomiting, anorexia, nausea,* cramps, weight loss.
**GU:** azotemia, *renal failure,* glycosuria, polyuria.
**Hematologic:** *anemia, hypofibrinogenemia,* depression of other clotting factors, *leukopenia.*
**Hepatic:** elevated AST and ALT levels, *hepatotoxicity.*
**Skin:** *rash, urticaria,* hypersensitivity reactions.
**Other:** HEMORRHAGIC PANCREATITIS AND ANAPHYLAXIS, chills, *death, fatal hyperthermia,* fever, *hyperglycemia.*

### INTERACTIONS
*Methotrexate:* decreased methotrexate effectiveness. Avoid concomitant use.
*Prednisone, vincristine:* increased toxicity. Monitor patient closely.

### CONTRAINDICATIONS
Contraindicated in patients with pancreatitis or history of pancreatitis and previous hypersensitivity unless desensitized.

### NURSING CONSIDERATIONS
• Use cautiously in patients with preexisting hepatic dysfunction. Because of the unpredictability of adverse re-

---

actions, drug should be given in hospital setting with close supervision.
• Monitor baseline blood and urine glucose levels before therapy.
• Be aware that allopurinol should be started before therapy begins to help prevent uric acid nephropathy.
• *Alert:* Know that risk of hypersensitivity increases with repeated dosages. Patients may be desensitized, but this doesn't rule out risk of allergic reactions. Routine administration of a 2-IU I.V. test dose may identify high-risk patients.
• Know that drug should not be used as sole agent to induce remission unless combination therapy is inappropriate. Not recommended for maintenance therapy.
• Follow institutional policy to reduce risks. Preparation and administration of parenteral form of this drug is associated with carcinogenic, mutagenic, and teratogenic risks for personnel.
• **I.V. use:** Give I.V. injection over 30 minutes through a running infusion of 0.9% sodium chloride solution or 5% dextrose solution.
• For I.M. injection, limit dose at single injection site to 2 ml.
• Reconstitute with 2 to 5 ml of either sterile water for injection or sodium chloride for injection.
• Don't use cloudy solutions.
• If drug contacts skin or mucous membranes, wash with copious amounts of water for at least 15 minutes.
• Refrigerate unopened dry powder. Reconstituted solution is stable for 8 hours if refrigerated.
• Keep epinephrine, diphenhydramine, and I.V. corticosteroids available for treating anaphylaxis.
• Monitor CBC and bone marrow function tests, as ordered.
• Obtain serum amylase level determinations, as ordered, to check pancreatic status. If elevated, asparaginase should be discontinued.
• Help prevent occurrence of tumor

lysis which can result in uric acid nephropathy by increasing fluid intake.
• Monitor blood and urine glucose during therapy. Watch for signs of hyperglycemia, such as polydipsia, polyphagia, and polyuria.
• Know that drug may affect clotting factors, leading to thrombosis or, more commonly, severe bleeding. Monitor patient and bleeding studies closely.
• Because of vomiting, administer parenteral fluids, as ordered, for 24 hours or until oral fluids are tolerated.
• Know that some patients may develop hypersensitivity to asparaginase, derived from cultures of *Escherichia coli. Erwinia* asparaginase, derived from cultures of *Erwinia carotovora,* has been used in these patients without cross-sensitivity.

☑ **PATIENT TEACHING**
• Tell patient to watch for signs of infection (fever, sore throat, fatigue) and bleeding (easy bruising, nosebleeds, bleeding gums, melena) and to take temperature daily.
• Stress importance of maintaining an adequate fluid intake to help prevent hyperuricemia. If adverse GI reactions prevent patient from drinking fluids, tell patient to notify doctor.

---

# bacillus Calmette-Guérin (BCG), live intravesical
ImmuCyst†, TheraCys, TICE BCG

*Pregnancy Risk Category: C*

## HOW SUPPLIED
**TheraCys**
*Suspension (freeze-dried) for bladder instillation:* 27 mg/vial
**TICE BCG**
*Suspension (freeze-dried) for bladder instillation:* about 50 mg/ampule

## ACTION
Unknown. Instillation of the live bacterial suspension causes a local in-

flammatory response. Local infiltration of histiocytes and leukocytes is followed by a decrease in superficial tumors within the bladder.

## ONSET, PEAK, DURATION
Undefined.

## INDICATIONS & DOSAGE
*In situ carcinoma of the urinary bladder (primary and relapsed)* –
**Adults:** three reconstituted and diluted vials administered intravesically once weekly for 6 weeks (induction), followed by additional treatments at 3, 6, 12, 18, and 24 months (TheraCys); or, one bladder instillation (one ampule suspended in 50 ml of sterile, preservative-free sodium chloride solution) once weekly for 6 weeks, and then once monthly for 6 to 12 months (TICE BCG).

## ADVERSE REACTIONS
**GI:** *nausea, vomiting, anorexia,* diarrhea.
**GU:** *dysuria, urinary frequency, hematuria, cystitis, urinary urgency,* nocturia, urinary incontinence, *urinary tract infection,* cramps, pain, decreased bladder capacity, renal toxicity, genital pain.
**Hematologic:** *anemia,* leukopenia.
**Hepatic:** elevated liver enzyme levels.
**Other:** hypersensitivity reaction, *malaise, fever, chills,* myalgia, arthralgia, ***disseminated mycobacterial infection.***

## INTERACTIONS
*Antibiotics:* may attenuate the response to BCG intravesical. Avoid concomitant use.
*Bone marrow suppressants, immunosuppressants, and radiation therapy:* may impair the response to BCG intravesical by decreasing the immune response; may also increase the risk of osteomyelitis or disseminated BCG infection. Avoid concomitant use.

## CONTRAINDICATIONS
Contraindicated in immunocompromised patients, in those receiving immunosuppressive therapy, and in those with urinary tract infection or fever of unknown origin. If fever is caused by infection, the drug should be withheld until patient recovers.

## NURSING CONSIDERATIONS
• Determine patient's reactivity to tuberculin before therapy. Tuberculin sensitivity may be rendered positive by BCG intravesical treatment.
• Know that this drug should not be handled by a caregiver with a known immunologic deficiency.
• Be aware that BCG intravesical should not be administered within 7 to 14 days of transurethral resection or biopsy. Fatal disseminated BCG infection has occurred after traumatic catheterization.
• To administer TheraCys, reconstitute only with 1 ml of provided diluent per vial just before use. Do not remove rubber stopper to prepare solution. Use immediately. Add contents of three reconstituted vials to 50 ml of sterile, preservative-free sodium chloride solution (final volume, 53 ml). Instill a urethral catheter into bladder under aseptic conditions, drain bladder, and then infuse 53 ml of prepared solution by gravity feed. Remove catheter and properly dispose of unused drug.
• To administer TICE BCG, use thermosetting plastic or sterile glass containers and syringes. Draw 1 ml of sterile, preservative-free sodium chloride solution into a 3-ml syringe. Add to one ampule of drug; gently expel back into ampule three times to ensure thorough mixing. Use immediately. Dispense cloudy suspension into top end of a catheter-tipped syringe that contains 49 ml of sodium chloride solution. Gently rotate syringe. Properly dispose of unused drug.

---

Reactions may be *common,* uncommon, ***life-threatening,*** or **COMMON AND LIFE-THREATENING.**

• Handle drug and material used for instillation as infectious material because it contains live, attenuated mycobacteria. Dispose of associated equipment (syringes, catheters, and containers) as biohazardous waste.

• Use strict aseptic technique to administer the drug to minimize trauma to the GU tract and to prevent introducing other contaminants.

• If there is evidence of traumatic catheterization, do not administer the drug and alert doctor. Subsequent treatment may resume after 1 week as if no interruption occurred.

• Carefully monitor patient's urinary status because the drug causes an inflammatory response in the bladder.

• Closely monitor patients for evidence of systemic BCG infection. BCG infections are rarely detected by positive cultures. Know that therapy should be withheld if systemic infection is suspected (short-term high fever above 103° F [39.4° C] or persistent fever above 101° F [38.3° C] for longer than 2 days or with severe malaise). Contact an infectious disease specialist for initiation of fast-acting antituberculosis therapy, as ordered.

• Know that drug is not used as an immunizing agent to prevent cancer or tuberculosis; drug should not be confused with BCG vaccine.

• Keep in mind that drug has the potential to cause hypersensitivity. Manage symptomatically.

• Be aware that patients with a small bladder capacity may experience increased local irritation with the usual dose of BCG intravesical.

• Be prepared to treat bladder irritation symptomatically with phenazopyridine, acetaminophen, and propantheline, as ordered. Systemic hypersensitivity can be treated with diphenhydramine. In order to minimize the risk of systemic infection, some clinicians give isoniazid for 3 days starting on the first day of treatment.

☑ **PATIENT TEACHING**
• Tell patient to retain the drug in the bladder for 2 hours after instillation (if possible). For the first hour, have patient lie 15 minutes prone, 15 minutes supine, and 15 minutes on each side; the second hour may be spent in the sitting position.

• Tell patient to sit when voiding.

• Instruct patient to disinfect urine for 6 hours after instillation of drug. Tell him to pour undiluted household bleach (5% sodium hypochlorite solution) in equal volume to voided urine into the toilet and wait 15 minutes before flushing.

• Tell patient to notify doctor if symptoms worsen or if any of the following symptoms develops: blood in the urine, fever and chills, frequent urge to urinate, painful urination, nausea, vomiting, joint pain, or rash.

• *Alert:* Caution patient that a cough that develops after therapy could indicate a life-threatening BCG infection. Tell him to report it immediately.

## dacarbazine (DTIC)
DTIC†, DTIC-Dome
*Pregnancy Risk Category: C*

**HOW SUPPLIED**
*Injection:* 100-mg, 200-mg vials

**ACTION**
Unknown. Probably cross-links strands of cellular DNA and interferes with RNA transcription, causing an imbalance of growth that leads to cell death. Cell cycle-nonspecific.

**ONSET, PEAK, DURATION**
Undefined.

**INDICATIONS & DOSAGE**
*Metastatic malignant melanoma –*
**Adults:** 2 to 4.5 mg/kg I.V. daily for 10 days; then repeated q 4 weeks as tolerated. Or 250 mg/m² I.V. daily for 5 days, repeated at 3-week intervals.

*Hodgkin's disease –*
**Adults:** 150 mg/m² I.V. daily (in combination with other agents) for 5 days, repeated q 4 weeks; or 375 mg/m² on the first day of a combination regimen, repeated q 15 days.

## ADVERSE REACTIONS
**GI:** *severe nausea and vomiting, anorexia.*
**Hematologic:** *leukopenia and thrombocytopenia.*
**Hepatic:** transient increase in liver enzyme levels, *hepatotoxicity* (rare).
**Skin:** phototoxicity, rash, facial flushing.
**Other:** *flulike syndrome* (fever, malaise; myalgia, beginning 7 days after treatment ends and lasts possibly 7 to 21 days), alopecia, *anaphylaxis;* severe pain if I.V. solution infiltrates or if solution is too concentrated; tissue damage; facial paresthesia.

## INTERACTIONS
*Anticoagulants, aspirin:* increased risk of bleeding. Avoid concomitant use.
*Bone marrow suppressants:* additive toxicity. Monitor closely.
*Phenobarbital, phenytoin, other drugs that induce hepatic metabolism:* enhanced dacarbazine activation and risk of toxicity. Monitor closely.

## CONTRAINDICATIONS
Contraindicated in patients hypersensitive to the drug.

## NURSING CONSIDERATIONS
• Use cautiously if bone marrow function is impaired.
• Administer antiemetics, as ordered, before giving dacarbazine. Nausea and vomiting may sometimes subside after several doses.
• Follow institutional policy to reduce risks. Preparation and administration of parenteral form of this drug is associated with carcinogenic, mutagenic, and teratogenic risks for personnel.

• **I.V. use:** Reconstitute drug using sterile water for injection. Add 9.9 ml to the 100-mg vial or 19.7 ml to the 200-mg vial. The resulting solution will be colorless to clear yellow. For infusion, further dilute by using up to 250 ml of 0.9% sodium chloride solution or D₅W; infuse over 30 minutes.
• May dilute further or slow infusion rate to decrease pain at insertion site.
• Avoid extravasation during infusion. If I.V. solution infiltrates, discontinue immediately, apply ice to area for 24 to 48 hours, and notify doctor.
• Keep in mind that reconstituted solutions are stable for 8 hours at room temperature and normal lighting conditions, or up to 3 days if refrigerated. Diluted solutions are stable for 8 hours at normal room temperature and light, or up to 24 hours if refrigerated. If solutions turn pink, decomposition has occurred; discard drug.
• Discard refrigerated solution after 72 hours and room temperature solution after 8 hours.
• To prevent bleeding, avoid all I.M. injections when platelet count is below 100,000/mm³.
• Anticipate the need for blood transfusions to combat anemia.
• Know that therapeutic effects are often accompanied by toxicity. Monitor CBC and platelet count.
• For Hodgkin's disease, be aware that drug is usually given with bleomycin, vinblastine, and doxorubicin.

### ☑ PATIENT TEACHING
• Tell patient to watch for signs of infection (fever, sore throat, fatigue) and bleeding (easy bruising, nosebleeds, bleeding gums, melena) and to take temperature daily.
• Instruct patient to avoid OTC products containing aspirin.
• Advise patient to avoid sunlight and sunlamps for first 2 days after treatment.
• Reassure patient that flulike syn-

drome may be treated with mild antipyretics, such as acetaminophen.

## etoposide (VP-16)
VePesid

*Pregnancy Risk Category: D*

### HOW SUPPLIED
*Capsules:* 50 mg
*Injection:* 100 mg/5 ml

### ACTION
Unknown. It is thought to damage DNA and inhibit DNA synthesis. Appears to be cell-cycle specific.

### ONSET, PEAK, DURATION
Undefined.

### INDICATIONS & DOSAGE
*Testicular cancer –*
**Adults:** 50 to 100 mg/m² P.O. or I.V. on 5 consecutive days q 3 to 4 weeks; or 100 mg/m² on days 1, 3, and 5 q 3 to 4 weeks.
*Small-cell carcinoma of the lung –*
**Adults:** 35 mg/m²/day I.V. for 4 days; 50 mg/m²/day I.V. for 5 days. Oral dosage is two times the I.V. dose, rounded to the nearest 50 mg.

### ADVERSE REACTIONS
**CNS:** peripheral neuropathy.
**CV:** hypotension (from too-rapid infusion).
**GI:** *nausea and vomiting, anorexia, diarrhea,* abdominal pain, *stomatitis.*
**Hematologic:** *anemia,* **myelosuppression** (dose-limiting), LEUKOPENIA, THROMBOCYTOPENIA.
**Other:** *reversible alopecia,* **anaphylaxis** (rare), phlebitis at injection site (infrequent).

### INTERACTIONS
*Warfarin:* may further prolong PT. Monitor closely.

### CONTRAINDICATIONS
Contraindicated in patients hypersensitive to the drug.

### NURSING CONSIDERATIONS
• Use cautiously in patients who have had cytotoxic or radiation therapy.
• Obtain baseline blood pressure prior to therapy.
• Have diphenhydramine, hydrocortisone, epinephrine, and emergency equipment available to establish an airway in case of anaphylaxis.
• Follow institutional policy to reduce risks. Preparation and administration of parenteral form of this drug is associated with carcinogenic, mutagenic, and teratogenic risks for personnel.
• **I.V. use:** Give drug by slow I.V. infusion (over at least 30 minutes) to prevent severe hypotension.
• Dilute the drug for infusion in either D₅W or 0.9% sodium chloride solution to a concentration of 0.2 or 0.4 mg/ml. Higher concentrations may crystallize.
• Do not administer through a membrane-type in-line filter because the diluent may dissolve it.
• Know that solutions diluted to 0.2 mg/ml are stable for 96 hours at room temperature in plastic or glass unprotected from light; solutions diluted to 0.4 mg/ml are stable for 48 hours under the same conditions.
• Store capsules in refrigerator.
• *Alert:* Monitor blood pressure every 30 minutes during infusion. If systolic pressure falls below 90 mm Hg, stop infusion and notify the doctor.
• Monitor CBC, as ordered. Observe for signs of bone marrow suppression.
• Observe oral cavity for signs of ulceration.
• To prevent bleeding, avoid all I.M. injections when platelet count is below 100,000/mm³.
• Anticipate the need for blood transfusion to combat anemia.
• Know that etoposide has caused

complete remissions in small-cell lung cancer and testicular cancer.

### ☑ PATIENT TEACHING
• Tell patient to watch for signs of infection (fever, sore throat, fatigue) and bleeding (easy bruising, nosebleeds, bleeding gums, melena) and to take temperature daily.
• Inform patient of need for frequent blood pressure readings during I.V. administration.

---

## mitotane
Lysodren

*Pregnancy Risk Category: C*

### HOW SUPPLIED
*Tablets (scored):* 500 mg

### ACTION
Unknown. May suppress function of adrenocortical tissue and hinder extra-adrenal metabolism of cortisol.

### ONSET, PEAK, DURATION
Steroid levels decrease within 2 to 3 days; tumor response, within 6 months. Levels peak 3 to 5 hours after dose. Duration undefined.

### INDICATIONS & DOSAGE
*Inoperable adrenocortical cancer —*
**Adults:** initially, 2 to 6 g P.O. daily in divided doses t.i.d. or q.i.d.; increased to 9 to 10 g P.O. daily, in divided doses t.i.d. or q.i.d. Dosage is adjusted until maximum tolerated dosage is achieved (varies from 2 to 16 g/day but is usually 8 to 10 g/day).

### ADVERSE REACTIONS
**CNS:** *depression, somnolence, lethargy, vertigo;* brain damage and dysfunction in long-term, high-dose therapy.
**CV:** hypertension.
**EENT:** visual disturbances.
**GI:** *severe nausea, vomiting, diarrhea, anorexia.*

**GU:** hemorrhagic cystitis.
**Skin:** dermatitis, *maculopapular rash.*
**Other:** increased serum cholesterol level, adrenal insufficiency.

### INTERACTIONS
*Warfarin:* increased metabolism, which may require higher warfarin doses. Monitor PT closely.

### CONTRAINDICATIONS
Contraindicated in patients hypersensitive to the drug. Be aware that drug should not be used in patients in shock or who have suffered trauma.

### NURSING CONSIDERATIONS
• Use cautiously in patients with hepatic disease.
• To reduce nausea, give antiemetic before mitotane, as ordered.
• Monitor effectiveness according to reduction in pain, weakness, and anorexia.
• Assess and record behavioral and neurologic signs daily. Prolonged therapy has been associated with significant neurologic impairment.
• Be aware that use of corticosteroids may avoid acute adrenocorticoid insufficiency and is usually required. Glucocorticoid dosage should be increased in periods of physiologic stress such as infection or trauma.
• Because drug distributes mostly to body fat, know that obese patients may need higher dosage and may have longer-lasting adverse reactions.
• Keep in mind that an adequate therapeutic trial is at least 3 months, but treatment can continue if clinical benefits are observed.

### ☑ PATIENT TEACHING
• Warn ambulatory patient to avoid activities that require alertness and good motor coordination until CNS effects of the drug are known.
• Instruct patient to notify doctor if severe adverse GI or skin reactions

---

Reactions may be *common,* uncommon, ***life-threatening,*** or COMMON AND LIFE-THREATENING.

occur because dosage adjustment may be needed.

## mitoxantrone hydrochloride
Novantrone

*Pregnancy Risk Category: D*

### HOW SUPPLIED
*Injection:* 2 mg/ml in 10-ml, 12.5-ml, 15-ml vials

### ACTION
Not fully understood; probably cell-cycle nonspecific. Reacts with DNA, producing cytotoxic effect.

### ONSET, PEAK, DURATION
Undefined.

### INDICATIONS & DOSAGE
*Combination initial therapy for acute nonlymphocytic leukemia –*
**Adults:** induction begins with 12 mg/m$^2$ I.V. daily on days 1 through 3, in combination with 100 mg/m$^2$ daily of cytarabine on days 1 through 7. A second induction may be given if response is not adequate. Maintenance therapy: 12 mg/m$^2$ on days 1 and 2, in combination with cytarabine on days 1 through 5.

### ADVERSE REACTIONS
**CNS:** *seizures,* headache.
**CV:** *CHF, arrhythmias,* tachycardia.
**EENT:** conjunctivitis.
**GI:** *bleeding, abdominal pain, diarrhea, nausea, mucositis, vomiting, stomatitis.*
**GU:** *renal failure.*
**Hematologic:** *myelosuppression.*
**Hepatic:** jaundice.
**Respiratory:** *dyspnea, cough.*
**Skin:** *petechiae, ecchymoses.*
**Other:** *alopecia,* hyperuricemia, *sepsis, fungal infections, fever.*

### INTERACTIONS
*Heparin:* physically incompatible. Do not mix together.

### CONTRAINDICATIONS
Contraindicated in patients hypersensitive to mitoxantrone.

### NURSING CONSIDERATIONS
● Use cautiously in patients with prior exposure to anthracyclines or other cardiotoxic drugs.
● Be aware that patients with significant myelosuppression should not receive mitoxantrone unless the benefits outweigh the risks.
● Follow institutional policy to minimize risks. Preparation and administration of parenteral form is associated with mutagenic, teratogenic, and carcinogenic risks to personnel.
● **I.V. use:** Dilute dose (available as an aqueous solution of 2 mg/ml in volumes of 10, 12.5, and 15 ml) in at least 50 ml of 0.9% sodium chloride injection or D$_5$W injection. Administer by direct injection into a free-flowing I.V. line of 0.9% sodium chloride or D$_5$W injection over at least 3 minutes. Mixing with other drugs is not recommended.
● If drug extravasates, discontinue infusion immediately and notify doctor.
● Be prepared to administer allopurinol, as ordered. Uric acid nephropathy can be avoided by hydrating the patient before and during therapy.
● Closely monitor hematologic and laboratory chemistry parameters.
● To prevent bleeding, avoid all I.M. injections if platelet count falls below 100,000/mm$^3$.
● Anticipate the need for blood transfusion to combat anemia.
● Be aware that left ventricular ejection fraction should be monitored.
● Be prepared to treat infections with antibiotics, as ordered.
● If severe nonhematologic toxicity occurs during the first course, know

---

that the second course should be delayed until patient recovers.
• Store undiluted solution at room temperature. Diluted mixture is stable for 7 days at room temperature.

### ☑ PATIENT TEACHING
• Inform patient that urine may appear blue-green within 24 hours after administration and some bluish discoloration of the sclera may occur. These effects are not harmful.
• Advise patient to watch for signs of bleeding and infection.
• Advise women of childbearing age to avoid pregnancy during therapy. Also recommend consulting doctor before becoming pregnant.

---

## paclitaxel
Taxol
*Pregnancy Risk Category: D*

### HOW SUPPLIED
*Injection:* 30 mg/5 ml

### ACTION
Prevents depolymerization of cellular microtubules, thus inhibiting the normal reorganization of the microtubule network necessary for mitosis and other vital cellular functions.

### ONSET, PEAK, DURATION
Undefined.

### INDICATIONS & DOSAGE
*Metastatic ovarian cancer after failure of first-line or subsequent chemotherapy* –
**Adults:** 135 mg/m² or 175 mg/m² I.V. over 3 hours q 3 weeks.
*Breast cancer after failure of combination chemotherapy for metastatic disease or relapse within 6 months of adjuvant chemotherapy* –
**Adults:** 175 mg/m² I.V. over 3 hours every 3 weeks.

### ADVERSE REACTIONS
**CNS:** *peripheral neuropathy.*
**CV:** *bradycardia, hypotension, abnormal ECG.*
**GI:** *nausea, vomiting, diarrhea, mucositis.*
**Hematologic:** NEUTROPENIA, LEUKOPENIA, THROMBOCYTOPENIA, anemia, *bleeding.*
**Hepatic:** *elevated liver enzyme levels.*
**Other:** *hypersensitivity reactions (anaphylaxis), alopecia, myalgia, arthralgia, phlebitis, cellulitis at injection site, infections.*

### INTERACTIONS
*Cisplatin:* possible additive myelosuppressive effects. Use together cautiously.
*Ketoconazole:* inhibited paclitaxel metabolism. Use together cautiously.

### CONTRAINDICATIONS
Contraindicated in patients hypersensitive to the drug or to polyoxyethylated castor oil, a vehicle used in drug solution, and in patients with baseline neutrophil counts below 1,500/mm³.

### NURSING CONSIDERATIONS
• Use cautiously in patients who have received radiation therapy because they may display more frequent or more severe myelosuppression.
• To reduce the incidence or severity of hypersensitivity, anticipate pretreating patients with corticosteroids, such as dexamethasone, and antihistamines, as ordered. Both histamine-1 receptor antagonists, such as diphenhydramine, and histamine-2 receptor antagonists, such as cimetidine or ranitidine, may be used. Severe hypersensitivity reactions have occurred in as many as 2% of patients treated in early clinical trials.
• Follow institutional protocol for the safe handling, preparation, and administration of chemotherapeutic drugs. Preparation and administration of parenteral form of this drug is asso-

---

ciated with carcinogenic, mutagenic, and teratogenic risks for personnel. Mark all waste materials with CHEMOTHERAPY HAZARD labels.

• **I.V. use:** Dilute concentrate before infusion. Compatible solutions include 0.9% sodium chloride injection, $D_5W$, 5% dextrose in 0.9% sodium chloride injection, and 5% dextrose in Ringer's lactate injection. Dilute to a final concentration of 0.3 to 1.2 mg/ml. Diluted solutions are stable for 27 hours at room temperature.

• Prepare and store infusion solutions in glass containers. The undiluted concentrate shouldn't contact polyvinylchloride I.V. bags or tubing. Store diluted solution in glass or polypropylene bottles, or use polypropylene or polyolefin bags. Administer through polyethylene-lined administration sets, and use an in-line 0.22-micron filter.

• Take care to avoid extravasation.

• Continuously monitor patients for 30 minutes after initiating the infusion. Continue close monitoring throughout the infusion.

• Frequently monitor blood counts during therapy. Bone marrow toxicity is the most common and dose-limiting toxicity. Packed RBC or platelet transfusions may be necessary in severe cases. Institute bleeding precautions as appropriate.

• Avoid all I.M. injections when platelet count is below 100,000/mm³.

• If patient develops significant cardiac conduction abnormalities, initiate appropriate therapy and continuous cardiac monitoring during therapy and subsequent infusions.

☑ **PATIENT TEACHING**
• Tell patient to watch for signs of infection (fever, sore throat, fatigue) and bleeding (easy bruising, nosebleeds, bleeding gums, melena), and to take temperature daily.

• Teach patient the signs and symptoms of peripheral neuropathy, such as a tingling or burning sensation or numbness in the extremities, and advise her to report these symptoms immediately. Although mild symptoms are common, severe symptoms occur infrequently. Dosage reduction may be necessary.

• Warn patient that alopecia is common (up to 82% of patients).

• Advise women of childbearing age to avoid becoming pregnant during therapy and to consult with doctor before becoming pregnant.

---

## pegaspargase
(PEG-L-asparaginase)
Oncaspar
*Pregnancy Risk Category: C*

**HOW SUPPLIED**
*Injection:* 750 IU/ml

**ACTION**
A modified version of the enzyme L-asparaginase that exerts its cytotoxic activity by inactivating the amino acid asparagine. Asparagine is required by tumor cells to synthesize proteins. Because the tumor cells cannot synthesize their own asparagine, protein synthesis and, eventually, synthesis of DNA and RNA is inhibited.

**ONSET, PEAK, DURATION**
Undefined.

**INDICATIONS & DOSAGE**
*Acute lymphoblastic leukemia (ALL) in patients who require L-asparaginase but have developed hypersensitivity to the native forms of L-asparaginase* —
**Adults and children with body surface area (BSA) of at least 0.6 m²:** 2,500 IU/m² I.M. or I.V. q 14 days.
**Children with BSA less than 0.6 m²:** 82.5 IU/kg I.M. or I.V. q 14 days.

---

## ADVERSE REACTIONS

**CNS:** seizures, headache, paresthesia, *status epilepticus,* somnolence, coma, mental status changes, dizziness, emotional lability, mood changes, parkinsonism, confusion, disorientation, fatigue.

**CV:** hypotension, tachycardia, chest pain, subacute bacterial endocarditis, hypertension.

**EENT:** epistaxis.

**Endocrine:** hyperglycemia, hypoglycemia.

**GI:** nausea, vomiting, abdominal pain, anorexia, diarrhea, constipation, indigestion, flatulence, GI pain, mucositis, *pancreatitis (sometimes fulminant and fatal),* increased serum amylase and lipase levels, severe colitis.

**GU:** increased BUN level, increased creatinine level, increased urinary frequency, hematuria, severe hemorrhagic cystitis, renal dysfunction, renal failure.

**Hematologic:** *thrombosis;* prolonged PTs, prolonged PTTs, decreased antithrombin III; disseminated intravascular coagulation; decreased fibrinogen; hemolytic anemia; *leukopenia; pancytopenia; agranulocytosis; thrombocytopenia;* increased thromboplastin; easy bruising; ecchymoses; *hemorrhage* (may be fatal).

**Hepatic:** jaundice, abnormal liver function test results, bilirubinemia, increased ALT and AST, ascites, hypoalbuminemia, fatty changes in liver, *liver failure.*

**Metabolic:** hyperuricemia, hyponatremia, uric acid nephropathy, hypoproteinemia, proteinuria, weight loss, metabolic acidosis, increased blood ammonia level, hyperglycemia, hypoglycemia.

**Musculoskeletal:** arthralgia, myalgia, musculoskeletal pain, joint stiffness, cramps.

**Respiratory:** cough, *severe bronchospasm,* upper respiratory tract infection.

**Skin:** itching, alopecia, fever blister, purpura, hand whiteness, fungal changes, nail whiteness and ridging, erythema simplex, petechial rash, injection pain or reaction, localized edema.

**Other:** hypersensitivity reactions, including *anaphylaxis,* rash, erythema, edema, pain, fever, chills, urticaria, dyspnea, or bronchospasm; pain in extremities; peripheral edema; malaise; night sweats; mouth tenderness; infection; *sepsis, septic shock.*

## INTERACTIONS

*Aspirin, dipyridamole, heparin, NSAIDs, warfarin:* imbalances in coagulation factors may occur, predisposing the patient to bleeding or thrombosis. Use together cautiously.

*Methotrexate:* during the period of its inhibition of protein synthesis and cell replication, pegaspargase may interfere with the action of such drugs as methotrexate, which require cell replication for their lethal effects. Monitor for decreased effectiveness.

*Protein-bound drugs:* depletion of serum proteins by pegaspargase may increase toxicity of other drugs that bind to proteins. Monitor for toxicity. Pegaspargase also may interfere with enzymatic detoxification of other drugs, particularly in the liver. Administer concomitantly with caution.

## CONTRAINDICATIONS

Contraindicated in patients with pancreatitis or a history of pancreatitis; in those who have had significant hemorrhagic events associated with prior L-asparaginase therapy; and in those with previous serious allergic reactions, such as generalized urticaria, bronchospasm, laryngeal edema, hypotension, or other unacceptable adverse reactions to pegaspargase.

## NURSING CONSIDERATIONS

• Use cautiously in pregnant patients and in patients with liver dysfunction.

---

Reactions may be *common,* uncommon, *life-threatening,* or COMMON AND LIFE-THREATENING.

• Know that pegaspargase should be used as the sole induction agent only when a combined regimen that uses other chemotherapeutic agents is inappropriate because of toxicity or other specific patient-related factors, or in patients refractory to other therapy.

• Be aware that I.M. route is preferred because it has the lowest incidence of hepatotoxicity, coagulopathy, and GI and renal disorders.

• Do not administer if drug has been frozen. Although there may not be a change in the appearance of the drug, pegaspargase's activity is destroyed after freezing. Obtain new dose from pharmacist.

• Avoid excessive agitation; do *not* shake. Keep refrigerated at 36° to 46° F (2° to 8° C). Do not use if cloudy or if precipitate is present. Do not use if stored at room temperature for more than 48 hours. Do not freeze. Discard unused portions. Use only one dose per vial; do not reenter the vial.

• The drug may be a contact irritant, and the solution must be handled and administered with care. Gloves are recommended. Inhalation of vapors and contact with skin or mucous membranes, especially those of the eyes, must be avoided. In case of contact, wash with copious amounts of water for at least 15 minutes.

• When administering I.M., limit the volume administered at a single injection site to 2 ml. If the volume to be administered is greater than 2 ml, use multiple injection sites.

• When administered I.V., give over a period of 1 to 2 hours in 100 ml of 0.9% sodium chloride or dextrose 5% injection through an infusion that is already running.

• *Alert:* Monitor patient closely for hypersensitivity reactions. Hypersensitivity reactions, including life-threatening anaphylaxis, may occur during therapy, especially in patients with known hypersensitivity to the other forms of L-asparaginase. As a routine precaution, keep patients under observation for 1 hour and have resuscitation equipment and other agents necessary to treat anaphylaxis (such as epinephrine, oxygen, and I.V. steroids) readily available. Know that moderate to life-threatening hypersensitivity reactions require discontinuation of L-asparaginase.

• As a guide to the effects of therapy, monitor the patient's peripheral blood count and bone marrow, as ordered. A fall in circulating lymphoblasts is often noted after initiating therapy. This may be accompanied by a marked rise in serum uric acid levels.

• Obtain frequent serum amylase determinations, as ordered, to detect pancreatitis. Monitor patient's blood glucose during therapy to detect hyperglycemia.

• Monitor patient for liver dysfunction when pegaspargase is used in conjunction with hepatotoxic chemotherapeutic agents.

• Be aware that pegaspargase may affect a number of plasma proteins; therefore, monitoring of fibrinogen, PT, and PTT may be indicated. Question doctor if not ordered.

### ☑ PATIENT TEACHING

• Inform the patient of the possibility of hypersensitivity reactions and the importance of alerting the staff immediately if any occur.

• Instruct patient not to take any other drugs, including OTC preparations, until approved by the doctor because the risk of bleeding is higher when pegaspargase is given concomitantly with certain drugs, such as aspirin, or because it may increase the toxicity of other medications.

• Instruct the patient to report signs and symptoms of infection (fever, chills, and malaise); drug may have immunosuppressant activity.

---

*Liquid form contains alcohol.   **May contain tartrazine.   †Canada only.   ‡Australia only.   ◇OTC.

▼ *NEW DRUG*

## porfimer sodium
Photofrin

*Pregnancy Risk Category: C*

### HOW SUPPLIED
*Injection:* 75 mg/vial

### ACTION
A photosensitizing drug that damages cancer cells through propagation of radical reactions. Tumor death also occurs through ischemic necrosis secondary to vascular occlusion that appears to be partly mediated by release of thromboxane $A_2$. Cytotoxic and antitumor actions of porfimer depend on light and oxygen.

### ONSET, PEAK, DURATION
Unknown.

### INDICATIONS & DOSAGE
*Palliative treatment for patients with completely obstructing esophageal cancer or for those with partially obstructing esophageal cancer who cannot be treated with laser therapy—*
**Adults:** 2 mg/kg I.V. for 3 to 5 minutes (first stage of therapy), followed by illumination with laser light 40 to 50 hours later (second stage). A total of three courses (each course consisting of both stages) may be given, separated by at least 30 days.

### ADVERSE REACTIONS
**CNS:** anxiety, confusion, *insomnia.*
**CV:** hypotension, hypertension, cardiac failure, atrial fibrillation, tachycardia.
**GI:** *constipation, abdominal pain, nausea, vomiting,* diarrhea, dyspepsia, dysphagia, eructation, esophageal edema, esophageal tumor bleeding, esophageal stricture, esophagitis, hematemesis, melena, anorexia.
**GU:** urinary tract infection.
**Hematologic:** *anemia.*
**Respiratory:** coughing, *dyspnea,*

*pharyngitis, pleural effusion, pneumonia,* respiratory insufficiency, tracheoesophageal fistula.
**Skin:** *photosensitivity.*
**Other:** *back or chest pain,* asthenia, substantial or general pain, edema, fever, surgical complication, dehydration, weight loss, moniliasis.

### INTERACTIONS
*Other photosensitizing drugs (tetracyclines, sulfonamides, phenothiazines, sulfonylurea hypoglycemic agents, thiazide diuretics, griseofulvin):* may increase photosensitivity reaction. Use together cautiously.

### CONTRAINDICATIONS
Contraindicated in patients with porphyria, tracheoesophageal or bronchoesophageal fistula, tumor eroding into major blood vessel, or hypersensitivity to porphyrins.

### NURSING CONSIDERATIONS
• Women receiving porfimer must not breast-feed because it isn't known whether this drug is excreted in human milk.
• Safety and efficacy in children have not been established.
• Before each course of treatment, patients should be evaluated for a tracheoesophageal or bronchoesophageal fistula.
• **I.V. use:** Reconstitute each vial of porfimer with 31.8 ml of 5% dextrose solution or 0.9% sodium chloride solution for injection, resulting in final concentration of 2.5 mg/ml. Shake until dissolved. Do not mix porfimer with other drugs in same solution. Reconstituted drug is opaque. Inspect carefully for particulate and discoloration before administration. Protect reconstituted drug from bright light, and use immediately.
• Take precautions to prevent extravasation at injection site. If it occurs, protect the area from light.
• Don't allow drug to contact eyes or

---

Reactions may be *common,* uncommon, *life-threatening,* or **COMMON AND LIFE-THREATENING.**

skin during preparation or administration. Protect an exposed person from bright light.
• Know that the patient must receive 630 nm wavelength laser light therapy 40 to 50 hours after porfimer injection for drug to be effective. A second laser light treatment (but not a second injection) may be given as early as 96 hours or as late as 120 hours after injection. Before a second treatment, the residual tumor should be debrided; be aware that vigorous debridement may cause tumor bleeding. Monitor patient closely.
• Know that inflammation of treatment area may cause substernal chest pain. Notify the doctor if this occurs; pain may be sufficiently intense to warrant short-term use of opiate analgesics.
• Monitor CBC regularly to detect anemia. Drug and laser therapy may cause tumor bleeding.

☑ **PATIENT TEACHING**
• Instruct patient to avoid direct sunlight and bright indoor light for 30 days after injection, but tell him to expose skin to ambient indoor light. After 30 days, he should expose a small area of skin (not face) to sunlight for 10 minutes. If he doesn't develop a photosensitivity reaction (erythema, edema, blistering) within 24 hours, he can gradually resume outdoor activities while exercising caution. If photosensitivity occurs, he should avoid sunlight and bright indoor light for 2 weeks before retesting.
• Urge patient traveling to an area with stronger sun to retest his photosensitivity level.
• Warn patient that ultraviolet sunscreens do not protect against photosensitivity.
• Advise patient to wear dark sunglasses with an average white light transmittance of less than 4% when outdoors.
• Advise female patients of childbearing age to use an effective contraceptive and to notify the doctor of suspected pregnancy.

---

# procarbazine hydrochloride
Matulane, Natulan†

*Pregnancy Risk Category: D*

---

**HOW SUPPLIED**
*Capsules:* 50 mg

**ACTION**
Unknown. Thought to inhibit DNA, RNA, and protein synthesis.

**ONSET, PEAK, DURATION**
Unknown.

**INDICATIONS & DOSAGE**
Dosage and indications vary. Check treatment protocol with the doctor.
*Adjunct treatment of Hodgkin's disease (stages III and IV), other cancers using MOPP (nitrogen mustard, vincristine, procarbazine, prednisone) regimen –*
**Adults:** 2 to 4 mg/kg P.O. daily in a single dose or divided doses for the 1st week. Then, 4 to 6 mg/kg/day until WBC count falls below 4,000/mm³ or platelet count falls below 100,000/mm³. After bone marrow recovers, maintenance dosage of 1 to 2 mg/kg/day resumed. For the MOPP regimen, 100 mg/m²/day P.O. for 14 days.
**Children:** 50 mg/m² P.O. daily for 1st week; then 100 mg/m² until response or toxicity occurs. Maintenance dosage is 50 mg/m² P.O. daily after bone marrow recovery.

**ADVERSE REACTIONS**
**CNS:** nervousness, depression, headache, dizziness, *coma,* insomnia, nightmares, paresthesia, neuropathy, *hallucinations,* confusion, *seizures.*
**CV:** hypotension, tachycardia, syncope.
**EENT:** retinal hemorrhage, nystagmus, photophobia.

---

*Liquid form contains alcohol.  **May contain tartrazine.  †Canada only.  ‡Australia only.  ◇OTC.

**GI:** *nausea, vomiting,* anorexia, stomatitis, dry mouth, dysphagia, diarrhea, constipation.
**GU:** hematuria, urinary frequency, nocturia.
**Hematologic:** *bleeding tendency, thrombocytopenia, leukopenia, anemia,* hemolytic anemia.
**Respiratory:** *pleural effusion,* pneumonitis.
**Skin:** dermatitis, pruritus, rash.
**Other:** reversible alopecia, gynecomastia.

## INTERACTIONS
*CNS depressants:* additive depressant effects. Avoid concomitant use.
*Digoxin:* may decrease serum digoxin levels. Monitor closely.
*Drugs and foods high in tyramine (Chianti wine, cheese), local anesthetics, sympathomimetics, tricyclic antidepressants:* possible tremor, palpitations, increased blood pressure. Monitor closely.
*Ethanol:* mild disulfiram-like reaction. Warn patients not to drink alcoholic beverages.

## CONTRAINDICATIONS
Contraindicated in patients hypersensitive to the drug and in those with inadequate bone marrow reserve as shown by bone marrow aspiration.

## NURSING CONSIDERATIONS
• Use cautiously in patients with impaired hepatic or renal function.
• Monitor CBC and platelet counts, as ordered.
• To prevent bleeding, avoid all I.M. injections when platelet count is below 100,000/mm³.
• Anticipate the need for blood transfusions to combat anemia.
• Be prepared to discontinue drug if patient becomes confused or if paresthesia or other neuropathies develop. Notify doctor.

## ✓ PATIENT TEACHING
• To decrease nausea and vomiting, advise patient to take drug at bedtime and in divided doses.
• Tell patient to watch for signs of infection (fever, sore throat, fatigue) and bleeding (easy bruising, nosebleeds, bleeding gums, melena) and to take temperature daily.
• Warn patient to avoid alcohol while taking this drug. Urge him to stop medication and check with the doctor immediately if he experiences a disulfiram-like reaction (chest pains, rapid or irregular heartbeat, severe headache, stiff neck).
• Instruct patient not to eat foods high in tyramine.
• Warn patient to avoid hazardous activities that require alertness and good motor coordination until the CNS effects are known.
• Advise women of childbearing age to avoid becoming pregnant during therapy and to consult with doctor before becoming pregnant.

---

# teniposide (VM-26)
Vumon

*Pregnancy Risk Category: D*

## HOW SUPPLIED
*Injection:* 10 mg/ml

## ACTION
A phase-specific cytotoxic drug that acts in the late S or early $G_2$ phase of the cell cycle, thus preventing cells from entering mitosis.

## ONSET, PEAK, DURATION
Undefined.

## INDICATIONS & DOSAGE
*Refractory childhood acute lymphoblastic leukemia –*
**Children:** optimum dosage hasn't been established. In clinical trials, dosages ranged from 165 to 250 mg/m² I.V. once or twice weekly for 4 to 6

weeks. Usually used in combination with other agents.

## ADVERSE REACTIONS
**CV:** hypotension from rapid infusion.
**GI:** *nausea and vomiting, mucositis, diarrhea.*
**Hematologic:** MYELOSUPPRESSION (dose-limiting), LEUKOPENIA, NEUTROPENIA, THROMBOCYTOPENIA, *anemia.*
**Other:** alopecia (rare), *anaphylaxis* (rare), rash, *infection,* bleeding, hypersensitivity reactions (chills, fever, urticaria, tachycardia, *bronchospasm,* dyspnea, hypotension, flushing); *phlebitis and extravasation* (at injection site).

## INTERACTIONS
*Heparin:* physical incompatibility. Don't mix together.

## CONTRAINDICATIONS
Contraindicated in patients hypersensitive to the drug or to polyoxyethylated castor oil, an injection vehicle.

## NURSING CONSIDERATIONS
• Be aware that some clinicians may decide to use this drug despite a patient's history of hypersensitivity because the therapeutic benefits outweigh its risks. Such patients should be treated with antihistamines and corticosteroids before the infusion begins and should be closely watched during drug administration.
• Obtain baseline blood counts, renal and hepatic function tests, as ordered.
• Monitor blood pressure before therapy.
• Have on hand diphenhydramine, hydrocortisone, epinephrine, and emergency equipment to establish an airway in case of anaphylaxis.
• Follow institutional policy to reduce risks. Preparation and administration of parenteral form of this drug is associated with carcinogenic, mutagenic, and teratogenic risks for personnel.

• **I.V. use:** Dilute drug in either $D_5W$ or 0.9% sodium chloride injection to a final concentration of 0.1, 0.2, 0.4, or 1 mg/ml. Don't agitate vigorously; precipitation of drug may occur. Discard cloudy solutions. Prepare and store the drug in glass containers. Infuse over 45 to 90 minutes to prevent hypotension.
• Don't mix with other drugs or solutions.
• Ensure careful placement of the I.V. catheter. Extravasation can result in local tissue necrosis or sloughing.
• Don't administer through a membrane-type in-line filter because the diluent may dissolve it.
• Monitor blood counts and renal and hepatic function tests, as ordered.
• Monitor blood pressure every 30minutes during infusion. If systolic blood pressure falls below 90 mm Hg, stop infusion and notify the doctor.
• Keep in mind that solutions containing 0.5 to 1 mg/ml are stable for 4 hours; those containing 0.1 to 0.2 mg/ml are stable for 6 hours at room temperature.

## ☑ PATIENT TEACHING
• Tell patient to report signs and symptoms of infection (fever, sore throat, fatigue) and bleeding (easy bruising, nosebleeds, bleeding gums, melena) and to take temperature daily.
• Advise women of childbearing age to avoid becoming pregnant during therapy and to consult with doctor before becoming pregnant.

▼ *NEW DRUG*

# tretinoin
Vesanoid
*Pregnancy Risk Category: D*

## HOW SUPPLIED
*Capsules:* 10 mg

## ACTION
Unknown.

## ONSET, PEAK, DURATION
Onset and duration unknown. Peak levels occur in 1 to 2 hours.

## INDICATIONS & DOSAGE
*Induction of remission in patients with acute promyelocytic leukemia (APL), French-American-British (FAB) classification M3 (including M3 variant), when anthracycline chemotherapy is contraindicated or unsuccessful —*
**Adults and children 1 year and older:** 45 mg/m²/day P.O. in two evenly divided doses. Therapy should be discontinued 30 days after complete remission is documented or after 90 days of treatment, whichever occurs first.

## ADVERSE REACTIONS
**CNS:** *headache,* cerebral hemorrhage, dizziness, *paresthesia, anxiety, insomnia, depression, confusion,* **cerebral hemorrhage,** intracranial hypertension, agitation, hallucination, abnormal gait, agnosia, aphasia, asterixis, cerebellar edema, cerebellar disorders, **convulsions, coma,** CNS depression, dysarthria, encephalopathy, facial paralysis, hemiplegia, hyporeflexia, hypotaxia, no light reflex neurologic reaction, spinal cord disorder, tremor, leg weakness, unconsciousness, dementia, forgetfulness, somnolence, slow speech.
**CV:** *chest discomfort, arrhythmias, hypotension, hypertension, phlebitis, edema, cardiac failure,* **cardiac arrest, myocardial infarction,** enlarged heart, heart murmur, ischemia, stroke, myocarditis, pericarditis, secondary cardiomyopathy.
**EENT:** *ear fullness,* hearing loss, *visual disturbances, ocular disorders.*
**GI:** *GI hemorrhage, nausea, vomiting, anorexia, abdominal pain, gastrointestinal disorders, diarrhea, constipation, dyspepsia, abdominal distention,* hepatosplenomegaly, hepatitis, ulcer, unspecified liver disorder, *weight gain or loss.*

**GU:** *renal insufficiency,* dysuria, **acute renal failure,** micturition frequency, renal tubular necrosis, enlarged prostate.
**Hematologic:** leukocytosis, *hemorrhage, disseminated intravascular coagulation.*
**Respiratory:** *pneumonia, upper respiratory tract disorders, dyspnea, respiratory insufficiency, pleural effusion, rales, expiratory wheezing,* lower respiratory tract disorders, pulmonary infiltrate, bronchial asthma, pulmonary edema, laryngeal edema, unspecified pulmonary disease, pulmonary hypertension.
**Skin:** *flushing, skin mucous membrane dryness, pruritis, decreased sweating, alopecia, skin changes.*
**Other:** *fever, infections, malaise, shivering, peripheral edema, pain, injection site reactions, myalgia, bone pain, mucositis,* flank pain, cellulitis, facial edema, fluid imbalance, pallor, lymph disorder, acidosis, hypothermia, ascites, bone inflammation, hypercholesterolemia, hypertriglyceridemia, elevated liver function studies.

## INTERACTIONS
None.

## CONTRAINDICATIONS
Contraindicated in patients with hypersensitivity to retinoids or parabens, used as preservatives in gelatin capsule.

## NURSING CONSIDERATIONS
• Drug is not recommended for use in pregnant or breast-feeding women.
• Because patients with APL are at high risk and can have severe reactions, tretinoin should be administered under supervision of a doctor with experience in managing such patients and in a facility with services sufficient to monitor drug tolerance and protect and maintain a patient compromised by toxicity.
• About 25% of patients in clinical

---

Reactions may be *common,* uncommon, *life-threatening,* or **COMMON AND LIFE-THREATENING.**

trials experienced Retinoic Acid-APL Syndrome, characterized by fever, dyspnea, weight gain, radiographic pulmonary infiltrates, and pleural or pericardial effusions. Notify doctor immediately if any of these appears, because the syndrome has occasionally been accompanied by impaired myocardial contractility and episodic hypotension with or without concomitant leukocytosis. Some patients have died from progressive hypoxemia and multiorgan failure. The syndrome generally occurs during the first month of therapy. Prompt treatment with high-dose steroids appears to reduce morbidity and mortality.

• Monitor CBC and platelet counts regularly. Patients with high WBC counts at diagnosis are at increased risk for further, rapid elevations. Rapidly evolving leukocytosis is associated with a higher risk of life-threatening complications.

• Monitor the patient (especially a child) for pseudotumor cerebri. Early signs and symptoms include papilledema, headache, nausea, vomiting, and visual disturbances. Notify the doctor immediately if any occurs.

• Monitor cholesterol and triglyceride levels and liver function studies. Notify the doctor of abnormalities.

• Maintain infection control and bleeding precautions, and provide prompt treatment, as ordered.

• Ensure that pregnancy testing and contraception counseling are repeated monthly throughout therapy.

### ☑ PATIENT TEACHING
• Explain infection control and bleeding precautions. Tell the patient to notify the doctor of signs and symptoms of infection (fever, sore throat, fatigue) or bleeding (easy bruising, nosebleeds, bleeding gums, melena) and to take temperature daily.

• Inform a female patient that a pregnancy test is required 1 week before therapy begins and that therapy will be delayed, if possible, until a negative result is obtained.

• Instruct a female patient to use contraception during therapy and for 1 month after discontinuation, even with a history of infertility or menopause, unless a hysterectomy has been performed. Tell her to use two methods of contraception simultaneously, unless abstinence is the chosen method, and to notify the doctor immediately of suspected pregnancy.

---

## vinblastine sulfate (VLB)
Alkaban-AQ, Velban, Velbe†‡, Velsar

*Pregnancy Risk Category: NR*

### HOW SUPPLIED
*Injection:* 10-mg vials (lyophilized powder), 1 mg/ml in 10-ml vials

### ACTION
Arrests mitosis in metaphase, blocking cell division.

### ONSET, PEAK, DURATION
Undefined.

### INDICATIONS & DOSAGE
*Breast or testicular cancer, Hodgkin's disease and malignant lymphoma, choriocarcinoma, lymphosarcoma, mycosis fungoides, Kaposi's sarcoma, histiocytosis* –
**Adults:** 0.1 mg/kg or 3.7 mg/m² I.V. weekly or q 2 weeks. May be increased to maximum dosage of 0.5 mg/kg or 18.5 mg/m² I.V. weekly according to response. Dosage should not be repeated if WBC count is less than 4,000/mm³.
**Children:** initial dose, 2.5 mg/m² I.V. Dosage increased by 1.25 mg/m² until WBC count is below 3,000/mm³ or tumor response is seen. Maximum dosage is 12.5 mg/m² I.V. weekly.

---

## ADVERSE REACTIONS
**CNS:** depression, *paresthesia, peripheral neuropathy and neuritis, numbness, loss of deep tendon reflexes, muscle pain and weakness,* **seizures,** *CVA,* headache.
**CV:** hypertension, *MI.*
**EENT:** pharyngitis.
**GI:** *nausea, vomiting,* ulcer, bleeding, *constipation, ileus, anorexia,* diarrhea, *weight loss,* abdominal pain, *stomatitis.*
**Hematologic:** *anemia, leukopenia* (nadir occurs days 4 to 10 and lasts another 7 to 14 days), ***thrombocytopenia.***
**Respiratory:** *acute bronchospasm,* shortness of breath.
**Skin:** vesiculation.
**Other:** reversible alopecia, *irritation, phlebitis,* cellulitis, necrosis with extravasation.

## INTERACTIONS
*Mitomycin:* increased risk of bronchospasm and shortness of breath. Monitor patient's respiratory status.
*Phenytoin:* decreased plasma phenytoin levels. Monitor closely.

## CONTRAINDICATIONS
Contraindicated in patients with severe leukopenia or bacterial infection.

## NURSING CONSIDERATIONS
• Use cautiously in patients with hepatic dysfunction.
• To reduce nausea, give antiemetic before drug, as ordered.
• Follow institutional policy to reduce risks. Preparation and administration of parenteral form of this drug is associated with carcinogenic, mutagenic, and teratogenic risks for personnel.
• **I.V. use:** Inject directly into vein or tubing of running I.V. line over 1 minute. May also be given in 50 ml of D$_5$W or 0.9% sodium chloride solution infused over 15 minutes. If extravasation occurs, stop infusion immediately and notify doctor. The manufacturer recommends that moderate heat be applied to area of leakage. Local injection of hyaluronidase may help disperse drug, as ordered. Some clinicians prefer to apply ice packs on and off every 2 hours for 24 hours, with local injection of hydrocortisone or 0.9% sodium chloride.
• Reconstitute 10-mg vial with 10 ml of sodium chloride injection or sterile water. This yields 1 mg/ml. Refrigerate reconstituted solution. Discard after 30 days.
• Do not administer into a limb with compromised circulation.
• ***Alert:*** After administering, monitor for development of life-threatening acute bronchospasm. If this occurs, notify the doctor immediately. Reaction is most likely to occur in patients who are also receiving mitomycin.
• Monitor patient for stomatitis. Be prepared to stop drug if stomatitis occurs and notify doctor.
• Assess bowel activity. Give laxatives as needed and ordered. May use stool softeners prophylactically.
• Know that dosage should not be repeated more frequently than every 7 days or severe leukopenia will occur.
• Assess for numbness and tingling in hands and feet. Assess gait for early evidence of footdrop.
• Take care to avoid confusing vinblastine with vincristine or vindesine.
• Know that the drug is less neurotoxic than vincristine.
• Anticipate a decrease in dosage by 50% if bilirubin levels are greater than 3 mg/100 ml.

## ☑ PATIENT TEACHING
• Tell patient to report signs and symptoms of infection (fever, sore throat, fatigue) and bleeding (easy bruising, nosebleeds, bleeding gums, melena) and to take temperature daily.
• Warn patient that alopecia may occur, but explain that it's usually reversible.

---

Reactions may be *common,* uncommon, ***life-threatening,*** or **COMMON AND LIFE-THREATENING.**

# vincristine sulfate
Oncovin, Vincasar PFS

*Pregnancy Risk Category: D*

## HOW SUPPLIED
*Injection:* 1 mg/ml in 1-ml, 2-ml, 5-ml multiple-dose vials; 1 mg/ml in 1-ml, 2-ml preservative-free vials

## ACTION
Arrests mitosis in metaphase, blocking cell division.

## ONSET, PEAK, DURATION
Undefined.

## INDICATIONS & DOSAGE
*Acute lymphoblastic and other leukemias, Hodgkin's disease, malignant lymphoma, neuroblastoma, rhabdomyosarcoma, Wilms' tumor* –
**Adults:** 1.4 mg/m$^2$ I.V. weekly. Maximum weekly dosage is 2 mg.
**Children over 10 kg:** 2 mg/m$^2$ I.V. weekly.
**Children 10 kg and under:** initially, 0.05 mg/kg I.V. weekly. Maximum single dose is 2 mg.

## ADVERSE REACTIONS
**CNS:** *peripheral neuropathy,* sensory loss, *loss of deep tendon reflexes, paresthesia, wristdrop and footdrop, seizures, coma,* headache, ataxia, cranial nerve palsies, *jaw pain,* hoarseness, vocal cord paralysis, visual disturbances), *muscle weakness and cramps* – some neurotoxicities may be permanent.
**CV:** hypotension.
**EENT:** diplopia, optic and extraocular neuropathy, ptosis.
**GI:** diarrhea, *constipation, cramps,* ileus that mimics surgical abdomen, paralytic ileus, *nausea, vomiting,* anorexia, weight loss, dysphagia, *intestinal necrosis, stomatitis.*
**GU:** urine retention, SIADH, dysuria, acute uric acid neuropathy, polyuria.

**Hematologic:** anemia, *leukopenia, thrombocytopenia.*
**Respiratory:** *acute bronchospasm,* dyspnea.
**Other:** *reversible alopecia,* fever, severe local reaction with extravasation, *phlebitis,* cellulitis at injection site, hyponatremia.

## INTERACTIONS
*Asparaginase:* decreased hepatic clearance of vincristine. Monitor for toxicity.
*Calcium channel blockers:* enhanced vincristine accumulation in cells.
*Digoxin:* decreased digoxin effects. Monitor serum digoxin level.
*Mitomycin:* possibly increased frequency of bronchospasm and acute pulmonary reactions. Monitor patient's respiratory status.

## CONTRAINDICATIONS
Contraindicated in patients who are hypersensitive to the drug or who have the demyelinating form of Charcot-Marie-Tooth syndrome. Do not give to patients who are concurrently receiving radiation therapy through ports that include the liver.

## NURSING CONSIDERATIONS
• Use cautiously in patients with hepatic dysfunction, neuromuscular disease, or infection.
• Follow institutional policy to reduce risks. Preparation and administration of parenteral form of this drug is associated with carcinogenic, mutagenic, and teratogenic risks for personnel.
• **I.V. use:** Inject directly into vein or tubing of running I.V. line slowly over 1 minute. May also be given in 50 ml of D$_5$W or 0.9% sodium chloride solution infused over 15 minutes. If drug extravasates, stop infusion immediately and notify doctor. Apply heat on and off every 2 hours for 24 hours. Administer 150 units hyaluronidase, as ordered, to area of infiltrate.
• Don't administer 5-mg vials to one

patient as a single dose. The 5-mg vials are for multiple-dose use only.

• **Alert:** After administering, monitor for development of life-threatening acute bronchospasm. If this occurs, notify the doctor immediately. This reaction is most likely to occur in those also receiving mitomycin.

• Monitor for hyperuricemia, especially in patients with leukemia or lymphoma. Maintain hydration and administer allopurinol, as ordered, to prevent uric acid nephropathy. Monitor for toxicity.

• Monitor fluid intake and output. Fluid restriction may be necessary if SIADH develops.

• Because of the risk of neurotoxicity, know that drug should not be given more than once a week. Children are more resistant to neurotoxicity than adults. Neurotoxicity is dose-related and usually reversible.

• Check for depression of Achilles tendon reflex, numbness, tingling, footdrop or wristdrop, difficulty in walking, ataxia, and slapping gait. Also check ability to walk on heels. Support patients when walking.

• Monitor bowel function. Give stool softener or laxative, as ordered, or water before dosing. Constipation may be an early sign of neurotoxicity.

• Take care to avoid confusing vincristine with vinblastine or vindesine.

• Know that all vials (1-mg, 2-mg, 5-mg) contain 1 mg/ml solution and should be refrigerated.

☑ **PATIENT TEACHING**
• Tell patient to report signs and symptoms of infection (fever, sore throat, fatigue) and bleeding (easy bruising, nosebleeds, bleeding gums, melena) and to take temperature daily.

• Warn patient that alopecia may occur, but explain that it's usually reversible.

• Advise women of childbearing age to avoid becoming pregnant during therapy and to consult with doctor before becoming pregnant.

---

# vinorelbine tartrate
Navelbine

*Pregnancy Risk Category: D*

## HOW SUPPLIED
*Injection:* 10 mg/ml, 50 mg/5 ml

## ACTION
A semisynthetic vinca alkaloid that exerts its antineoplastic effect by disrupting microtubule assembly, which, in turn, disrupts spindle formation and prevents mitosis.

## ONSET, PEAK, DURATION
Undefined.

## INDICATIONS & DOSAGE
*Alone or as adjunct therapy with cisplatin for first-line treatment of ambulatory patients with nonresectable advanced non-small-cell lung cancer (NSCLC); alone or with cisplatin in stage IV of NSCLC; with cisplatin in stage III of NSCLC –*
**Adults:** 30 mg/m² I.V. weekly. In combination treatment, same dosage used along with 120 mg/m² of cisplatin, given on days 1 and 29, then q 6 weeks.

## ADVERSE REACTIONS
**GI:** *nausea, vomiting, anorexia, diarrhea, constipation, stomatitis.*
**Hematologic:** *bone marrow suppression (agranulocytosis, LEUKOPENIA, thrombocytopenia, anemia).*
**Hepatic:** *abnormal liver function test results, bilirubinemia.*
**Respiratory:** dyspnea.
**Skin:** *alopecia,* rash, *injection pain or reaction.*
**Other:** *peripheral neuropathy, asthenia,* jaw pain, *fatigue,* myalgia, SIADH, chest pain, arthralgia.

---

## INTERACTIONS

*Cisplatin:* increased risk of bone marrow suppression when used concomitantly with cisplatin. Monitor patient's hematologic status closely.

*Mitomycin:* may cause pulmonary reactions. Monitor patient's respiratory status closely.

## CONTRAINDICATIONS

Contraindicated in patients with pretreatment granulocyte counts less than 1,000 cells/mm$^3$.

## NURSING CONSIDERATIONS

• Use with extreme caution in patients whose bone marrow may have been compromised by previous exposure to radiation therapy or chemotherapy or whose bone marrow is still recovering from chemotherapy.

• Use cautiously in patients with hepatic impairment.

• Check patient's granulocyte count before administration. The count should be equal to or greater than 1,000 cells/mm$^3$ for drug to be administered. Withhold drug and notify doctor if count is less.

• Know that vinorelbine must be diluted before administration to a concentration of 1.5/ml to 3 mg/ml with D5W or 0.9% sodium chloride solution in a syringe. Alternatively, dilute to a concentration of 0.5 mg/ml to 2 mg/ml in an I.V. bag. Administer the drug I.V. over 6 to 10 minutes into the side port of a free-flowing I.V. line that is closest to the I.V. bag, followed by flushing with at least 75 to 125 ml of D$_5$W or 0.9% sodium chloride solution.

• Avoid extravasation when administering vinorelbine because drug can cause considerable irritation, localized tissue necrosis, and thrombophlebitis. If extravasation occurs, drug administration should be stopped immediately and any remaining dosage portion injected into a different vein.

• Be aware that dosage adjustments are made according to hematologic toxicity or hepatic insufficiency, whichever results in the lower dosage. Expect dosage reduction of 50% if granulocyte count falls below 1,500 cells/mm$^3$ but is greater than 1,000 cells/mm$^3$. If three consecutive doses are skipped because of agranulocytosis, further vinorelbine therapy should not be given.

• Know that the drug may be a contact irritant, and the solution must be handled and administered with care. Gloves are recommended. Inhalation of vapors and contact with skin or mucous membranes, especially those of the eyes, must be avoided. In case of contact, wash with copious amounts of water for at least 15 minutes.

• Monitor patient closely for hypersensitivity reactions.

• As a guide to the effects of therapy, monitor patient's peripheral blood count and bone marrow, as ordered.

## ☑ PATIENT TEACHING

• Instruct patient not to take any other drugs, including OTC preparations, until approved by the doctor.

• Tell patient to report signs and symptoms of infection (fever, sore throat, fatigue) and bleeding (easy bruising, nosebleeds, bleeding gums, melena) and to take temperature daily.

---

*Liquid form contains alcohol.   **May contain tartrazine.   †Canada only.   ‡Australia only.   ◇OTC.

# 74

# Immunosuppressants

azathioprine
cyclosporine
levamisole hydrochloride
lymphocyte immune globulin
muromonab-CD3
mycophenolate mofetil
tacrolimus

## COMBINATION PRODUCTS
None.

---

## azathioprine
Imuran, Thioprine‡
*Pregnancy Risk Category: D*

### HOW SUPPLIED
*Tablets:* 50 mg
*Injection:* 100 mg

### ACTION
Unknown.

### ONSET, PEAK, DURATION
Onset occurs in 4 to 8 weeks. Serum levels peak in 1 to 2 hours. Clinical effects may persist for several days after the drug is discontinued.

### INDICATIONS & DOSAGE
*Immunosuppression in kidney transplantation* –
**Adults and children:** initially, 3 to 5 mg/kg P.O. or I.V. daily, usually beginning on the day of transplantation. Maintained at 1 to 3 mg/kg daily (dosage varies considerably according to patient response).
*Severe, refractory rheumatoid arthritis* –
**Adults:** initially, 1 mg/kg P.O. as a single dose or divided into two doses. If patient response is not satisfactory after 6 to 8 weeks, dosage may be increased by 0.5 mg/kg daily (up to a

maximum of 2.5 mg/kg daily) at 4-week intervals.

### ADVERSE REACTIONS
**GI:** *nausea, vomiting, pancreatitis,* steatorrhea, diarrhea, abdominal pain.
**Hematologic:** LEUKOPENIA *bone marrow suppression,* anemia, *pancytopenia, thrombocytopenia, immunosuppression* (possibly profound).
**Hepatic:** *hepatotoxicity,* jaundice.
**Skin:** rash.
**Other:** arthralgia, alopecia, *infections,* fever, myalgia, *increased risk of neoplasia.*

### INTERACTIONS
*Allopurinol:* impaired inactivation of azathioprine. Decrease azathioprine dose to one-quarter or one-third normal dose.
*Angiotensin converting enzyme inhibitors:* combination may cause severe leukopenia. Monitor patient closely.
*Nondepolarizing neuromuscular blockers:* azathioprine may reverse the neuromuscular blockade.
*Vaccines:* decreased immune response. Postpone routine immunization.

### CONTRAINDICATIONS
Contraindicated in patients hypersensitive to the drug.

### NURSING CONSIDERATIONS
• Use cautiously in patients with hepatic or renal dysfunction.
• Administer drug after meals to minimize adverse GI effects.
• **I.V. use:** Reconstitute 100-mg vial with 10 ml of sterile water for injection. Visually inspect for particles before giving. Drug may be administered by direct I.V. injection or further

---

diluted in 0.9% sodium chloride for injection or D$_5$W and infused over 30 to 60 minutes. Use only for patients unable to tolerate oral medications.
• To prevent bleeding, avoid all I.M. injections when platelet count is below 100,000/mm³.
• Monitor hemoglobin and WBC and platelet counts at least once monthly, as ordered, more often at beginning of treatment. Notify doctor if counts drop suddenly or become dangerously low. The drug may need to be temporarily withheld.
• Watch for early signs of hepatotoxicity: clay-colored stools, dark urine, pruritus, and yellow skin and sclera; and for increased alkaline phosphatase, bilirubin, AST, and ALT levels.
• Be aware that therapeutic response usually occurs within 8 weeks.
• Keep in mind that the benefits must be weighed against the risk with systemic viral infections, such as chickenpox and herpes zoster.
• Be aware that patients with rheumatoid arthritis previously treated with aklylating agents, such as cyclophosphamide, chlorambucil, melphalan, or others may have a prohibitive risk of neoplasia if treated with the drug.
• Know that drug should not be used for treating rheumatoid arthritis in pregnant women.

☑ **PATIENT TEACHING**
• Warn patient to report even mild infections (colds, fever, sore throat, and malaise) because drug is a potent immunosuppressant.
• Instruct patient to avoid conception during therapy and for 4 months after stopping therapy.
• Warn patient that some thinning of hair is possible.
• Tell patient taking this drug for refractory rheumatoid arthritis that it may take up to 12 weeks to be effective.

# cyclosporine (cyclosporin)
Sandimmun‡, Sandimmune
*Pregnancy Risk Category: C*

**HOW SUPPLIED**
*Oral solution:* 100 mg/ml
*Injection:* 50 mg/ml
*Capsules:* 25 mg, 50 mg, 100 mg

**ACTION**
Unknown. Thought to inhibit the proliferation and function of T lymphocytes.

**ONSET, PEAK, DURATION**
Onset and duration unknown. Serum levels peak within 3½ hours after oral dose.

**INDICATIONS & DOSAGE**
*Prophylaxis of organ rejection in kidney, liver, or heart transplantation –*
**Adults and children:** 15 mg/kg P.O. 4 to 12 hours before transplantation and continued daily postoperatively for 1 to 2 weeks. Then dosage reduced by 5% each week to maintenance level of 5 to 10 mg/kg/day. Alternatively, 5 to 6 mg/kg I.V. concentrate 4 to 12 hours before transplantation. Postoperatively, dosage repeated daily until patients can tolerate oral forms.

**ADVERSE REACTIONS**
**CNS:** *tremor, headache, seizures,* confusion, paresthesia.
**CV:** *hypertension.*
**EENT:** *gum hyperplasia,* oral thrush, sinusitis.
**GI:** *nausea, vomiting,* diarrhea, abdominal discomfort.
**GU: NEPHROTOXICITY.**
**Hematologic:** anemia, *leukopenia, thrombocytopenia,* hemolytic anemia.
**Hepatic:** *hepatotoxicity.*
**Skin:** acne, flushing.
**Other:** increased low-density lipoprotein levels, *infections, hirsutism, anaphylaxis,* gynecomastia.

---

*Liquid form contains alcohol.   **May contain tartrazine.   †Canada only.   ‡Australia only.   ◊OTC.

## INTERACTIONS

*Acyclovir, aminoglycosides, ampho-tericin B, co-trimoxazole, melphalan, NSAIDs:* increased risk of nephrotoxicity. Avoid concomitant use.

*Azathioprine, corticosteroids, cyclophosphamide, verapamil:* increased immunosuppression. Monitor closely.

*Carbamazepine, isoniazid, phenobarbital, phenytoin, rifampin:* possible decreased immunosuppressant effect. Know that cyclosporine dosage may need to be increased.

*Cimetidine, diltiazem, erythromycin, fluconazole, imipenem-cilastatin, ketoconazole, metoclopramide, methylprednisone, nicardipine, predniso-lone:* may increase blood levels of cyclosporine. Monitor for increased toxicity.

*Vaccines:* decreased immune response. Postpone routine immunization.

## CONTRAINDICATIONS

Contraindicated in patients hypersensitive to the drug or to polyoxyethylated castor oil (found in injectable form).

## NURSING CONSIDERATIONS

● Measure oral solution doses carefully in an oral syringe. To increase palatability, mix with whole milk, chocolate milk, or fruit juice. Use a glass container to minimize adherence to container walls.

● Give dosage once daily in the morning.

● **I.V. use:** Administer cyclosporine I.V. concentrate at one-third the oral dose and dilute before use. Dilute each milliliter of the concentrate in 20 to 100 ml of D₅W or 0.9% sodium chloride for injection. Dilute immediately before administration; infuse over 2 to 6 hours. Usually reserved for patients who cannot tolerate oral medications.

● Always give cyclosporine concomitantly with adrenal corticosteroids as ordered.

● Monitor cyclosporine blood levels at regular intervals. Absorption of cyclosporine oral solution can be erratic.

● Monitor BUN and serum creatinine levels. Cyclosporine may cause nephrotoxicity. Nephrotoxicity may develop 2 to 3 months after transplant surgery, possibly requiring dosage reduction. Promptly report to the doctor any signs or symptoms that suggest the development of nephrotoxicity.

● Know that doctor must differentiate between transplanted kidney rejection and cyclosporine-induced nephrotoxicity.

● Monitor liver function tests, as ordered, for hepatotoxicity, which usually occurs during first month after transplant.

## ☑ PATIENT TEACHING

● Encourage patient to take drug at same time each day, and teach him how to measure dosage and mask taste of oral solution, if prescribed.

● Advise patient to take with meals if drug causes nausea. Anorexia, nausea, and vomiting are usually transient and most frequently occur at the start of therapy.

● Stress to patient that therapy should not be stopped without the doctor's approval.

● To prevent thrush, instruct patient to swish and swallow nystatin four times daily.

● Recommend use of mechanical contraceptive measures such as diaphragm or condom while receiving cyclosporine therapy. Advise female patient not to use oral contraceptives.

## levamisole hydrochloride
Ergamisol

*Pregnancy Risk Category: C*

---

## HOW SUPPLIED
*Tablets:* 50 mg (base)

## ACTION
Unknown. It appears to restore depressed immune function and may potentiate the actions of monocytes and macrophages and enhance T-cell responses.

## ONSET, PEAK, DURATION
Onset and duration unknown. Plasma levels peak in 1½ to 2 hours.

## INDICATIONS & DOSAGE
*Adjuvant treatment of Dukes' stage C colon cancer (with fluorouracil) after surgical resection –*
**Adults:** 50 mg P.O. q 8 hours for 3 days, beginning no sooner than 7 days and no later than 30 days after surgery, provided that the patient is out of the hospital, ambulating, and maintaining normal oral nutrition; has well-healed wounds; and has recovered from any postoperative complications. Fluorouracil (450 mg/m²/day I.V.) is given for 5 days with a 3-day course of levamisole starting 21 to 34 days after surgery.

Maintenance dosage is 50 mg P.O. q 8 hours for 3 days q 2 weeks for 1 year. Given in conjunction with fluorouracil maintenance therapy (450 mg/m²day by rapid I.V. push once a week, beginning 28 days after the initial 5-day course) for 1 year.

## ADVERSE REACTIONS
**CNS:** *dizziness, headache, paresthesia, somnolence, depression, nervousness, insomnia, anxiety, fatigue, fever.*
**CV:** *chest pain, edema.*
**EENT:** *blurred vision, conjunctivitis, stomatitis, dysgeusia, altered sense of smell.*
**GI:** *nausea, diarrhea, vomiting, anorexia, abdominal pain, constipation, flatulence, dyspepsia.*

**Hematologic:** *agranulocytosis, leukopenia, thrombocytopenia,* anemia.
**Skin:** *dermatitis, exfoliative dermatitis, pruritus, urticaria.*
**Other:** hyperbilirubinemia, rigors, *alopecia, infection, arthralgia, myalgia.*

## INTERACTIONS
*Ethanol:* may precipitate a disulfiram-like reaction. Avoid concomitant use.
*Phenytoin:* plasma levels may be elevated when administered with levamisole and fluorouracil. Monitor phenytoin plasma levels.

## CONTRAINDICATIONS
Contraindicated in patients hypersensitive to the drug.

## NURSING CONSIDERATIONS
• *Alert:* Use cautiously and with close hematologic monitoring because agranulocytosis, which is sometimes fatal, may occur. Neutropenia is usually reversible when therapy is discontinued.
• Obtain baseline CBC with differential, platelet count, and electrolyte levels, and liver function studies, as ordered, immediately before starting therapy.
• Be aware that if levamisole therapy begins 7 to 20 days after surgery, fluorouracil should be started with the second course of levamisole therapy. It should begin no sooner than 21 days and no later than 35 days after surgery. If levamisole is deferred until 21 to 30 days after surgery, fluorouracil therapy should begin with the first course of levamisole.
• Know that dosage modifications are based on hematologic parameters. If WBC count is 2,500/mm³ to 3,500/mm³, don't administer fluorouracil as ordered until WBC count is above 3,500/mm³. When fluorouracil is restarted, reduce dosage by 20% as ordered. If WBC count stays below 2,500/mm³ for over 10 days after flu-

orouracil is withdrawn, discontinue levamisole, as ordered.
• Know that recommended doses should not be exceeded. Higher doses are associated with greater incidence of agranulocytosis.
• Obtain CBC with differential and platelet count at weekly intervals, as ordered, before treatment with fluorouracil. Obtain electrolyte levels and liver function studies every 3 months for 1 year, as ordered.
• If platelet count is below 100,000/mm³, know that therapy with both fluorouracil and levamisole should be discontinued and doctor notified.

### ☑ PATIENT TEACHING
• Tell patient to promptly report the development of stomatitis or diarrhea. If either of these reactions occur during the initial course of fluorouracil therapy, drug is discontinued and then weekly fluorouracil therapy is begun 28 days after the start of the initial course. If stomatitis or diarrhea develops during the weekly doses of fluorouracil, fluorouracil therapy is deferred until these symptoms subside. Then fluorouracil therapy is started at reduced dosages (decrease dose by 20%).
• Advise patient to immediately report any flulike symptoms, such as fever and chills.

---

## lymphocyte immune globulin (antithymocyte globulin [equine], ATG)
Atgam
*Pregnancy Risk Category: C*

### HOW SUPPLIED
*Injection:* 50 mg of equine IgG/ml in 5-ml ampules

### ACTION
Unknown. Inhibits cell-mediated immune responses by either altering T-cell function or eliminating antigen-reactive T cells.

### ONSET, PEAK, DURATION
Onset and duration unknown. Plasma levels peak after 5 days.

### INDICATIONS & DOSAGE
*Prevention of acute renal allograft rejection –*
**Adults and children:** 15 mg/kg I.V. daily for 14 days, followed by alternate-day dosing for 14 days; the first dose should be given within 24 hours of transplantation.
*Treatment of acute renal allograft rejection –*
**Adults and children:** 10 to 15 mg/kg I.V. daily for 14 days. Additional alternate-day therapy up to a total of 21 doses can be given. Therapy should be initiated when rejection is diagnosed.
*Aplastic anemia –*
**Adults:** 10 to 20 mg/kg I.V daily for 8 to 14 days. Additional alternative-day therapy up to a total of 21 doses can be administered.

### ADVERSE REACTIONS
**CNS:** malaise, *seizures,* headache.
**CV:** *hypotension, chest pain,* thrombophlebitis, tachycardia, edema, iliac vein obstruction, renal artery stenosis.
**EENT:** *laryngospasm.*
**GI:** *nausea, vomiting, diarrhea,* hiccups, epigastric pain, abdominal distention, stomatitis.
**Hematologic:** LEUKOPENIA, THRMOBOCYTOPENIA, *hemolysis, aplastic anemia.*
**Hepatic:** elevated liver enzyme level.
**Respiratory:** *dyspnea, pulmonary edema.*
**Skin:** *rash, pruritus, urticaria.*
**Other:** *febrile reactions,* serum sickness, *anaphylaxis, infections, arthralgia,* night sweats, lymphadenopathy, hyperglycemia, *chills, myalgia, arthralgia.*

---

Reactions may be *common,* uncommon, *life-threatening,* or COMMON AND LIFE-THREATENING.

## INTERACTIONS
*Muromonab-CD3:* increased risk of infection. Monitor closely.

## CONTRAINDICATIONS
Contraindicated in patients hypersensitive to the drug. An intradermal skin test is recommended at least 1 hour before the first dose. Marked local swelling or erythema larger than 10 mm indicates an increased potential for severe systemic reaction, such as anaphylaxis. Severe reactions to the skin test, such as hypotension, tachycardia, dyspnea, generalized rash, or anaphylaxis, usually preclude further administration of the drug.

## NURSING CONSIDERATIONS
• Use cautiously in patients receiving additional immunosuppressive therapy (such as corticosteroids or azathioprine) because of the increased potential for infection. Do not dilute ATG concentrate with dextrose solutions or solutions with a low salt concentration because a precipitate may form. The proteins in ATG can be denatured by air. ATG is unstable in acidic solutions.
• **I.V. use:** Dilute concentrated drug for injection before administration. Dilute the required dose in 250 to 1,000 ml of 0.45% or 0.9% sodium chloride solution. The final concentration of drug should not exceed 1 mg/ml. When adding ATG to the infusion solution, make sure the container is inverted so that the drug does not contact air inside the container. Gently rotate or swirl the container to mix contents; do not shake because this may cause excessive foaming or denature the drug protein. Infuse with an in-line filter with a pore size of 0.2 to 1 micron over no less than 4 hours (most institutions infuse over 4 to 8 hours).
• Do not use solutions that are more than 12 hours old, including actual infusion time.

• Refrigerate at 35° to 47° F (2° to 8° C). ATG concentrate is heat-sensitive. Do not freeze.
• Monitor for signs of infection.

### ☑ PATIENT TEACHING
• Instruct patient to report adverse drug reactions promptly, especially signs of infection (fever, sore throat, fatigue).
• Tell patient to alert nurse immediately if discomfort occurs at I.V. insertion site because drug can cause a chemical phlebitis.

---

# muromonab-CD3
Orthoclone OKT3
*Pregnancy Risk Category: C*

## HOW SUPPLIED
*Injection:* 1 mg/1 ml in 5-ml ampules

## ACTION
Muromonab-CD3 is an immunoglobulin G antibody that reacts in the T-lymphocyte membrane with a molecule (CD3) needed for antigen recognition. This drug depletes the blood of CD3$^+$ T cells, which leads to restoration of allograft function and reversal of rejection.

## ONSET, PEAK, DURATION
Onset almost immediate. Peak unknown. Number of circulating CD3$^+$ T cells returns to pretreatment levels within 1 week after drug is withdrawn.

## INDICATIONS & DOSAGE
*Acute allograft rejection in renal transplant patients; in steroid-resistant hepatic or cardiac allograft rejection –*
**Adults:** 5 mg I.V. bolus once daily for 10 to 14 days.

## ADVERSE REACTIONS
**CNS:** *tremor, headache, seizures, encephalopathy, cerebral edema.*

---

*Liquid form contains alcohol. **May contain tartrazine. †Canada only. ‡Australia only. ◊OTC.

**CV:** *chest pain, tachycardia,* hypertension.
**GI:** *nausea, vomiting, diarrhea.*
**Respiratory:** *severe pulmonary edema, dyspnea, wheezing.*
**Other:** *fever, chills, tremors,* **INFECTION,** *anaphylaxis,* increased serum creatinine, *cytokine release syndrome* (from flulike symptoms to shock), *aseptic meningitis, risk of neoplasia.*

## INTERACTIONS
*Immunosuppressants:* increased risk of infection. Monitor closely.
*Indomethacin:* increased muromonab-CD3 levels with encephalopathy and other CNS effects. Monitor patient closely.
*Live virus vaccines:* may potentiate replication and increase effects of virus vaccine.

## CONTRAINDICATIONS
Contraindicated in pregnancy and lactation. Also contraindicated in patients with hypersensitivity to the drug or to any other product of murine (mouse) origin; who have antimurine antibody titers equal to or greater than 1:1,000; who have fluid overload, as evidenced by chest X-ray or a weight gain greater than 3% within the week before treatment; or who have history of seizures or are predisposed to seizures.

## NURSING CONSIDERATIONS
• Obtain chest X-ray within 24 hours before starting drug treatment, as ordered.
• Assess patients for signs of fluid overload before treatment.
• Keep in mind that treatment should begin in a facility that is equipped and staffed for cardiopulmonary resuscitation and where patients can be monitored closely.
• Be alert that most adverse reactions develop within ½ to 6 hours after the first dose.
• Administer an antipyretic, as or-

dered, before giving the drug to help lower incidence of expected pyrexia and chills. Corticosteroids may also be administered, as ordered, before first injection to help decrease the incidence of adverse reactions. Methylprednisolone sodium succinate (1 mg/kg) before injection, followed by hydrocortisone sodium succinate (100 mg) 30 minutes after injection, have been recommended to alleviate the severity of the first-dose reaction.
• Be aware that muromonab-CD3 is a monoclonal antibody preparation. Patients develop antibodies to this preparation that can lead to loss of effectiveness and more severe adverse reactions if a second course of therapy is attempted. Therefore, experts believe that this drug should be used for only a single course of treatment.
• **I.V. use:** Draw solution into a syringe through a low protein-binding 0.2- or 0.22-micron filter. Discard filter and attach needle for I.V. bolus injection.
• Do not add or infuse other drugs simultaneously through the same I.V. line. If the same I.V. line is used for sequential infusion of other drugs, flush with saline before and after infusion of muromonab-CD3.

## ☑ PATIENT TEACHING
• Inform patient of expected adverse reactions.
• Reassure him that reactions will be less severe as treatment progresses.

▼ *NEW DRUG*

# mycophenolate mofetil
CellCept
*Pregnancy Risk Category: C*

## HOW SUPPLIED
*Capsules:* 250 mg

## ACTION
Inhibits proliferative response of T-and B-lymphocytes, suppresses anti-

body formation by B-lymphocytes, and may inhibit recruitment of leukocytes into sites of inflammation and graft rejection.

## ONSET, PEAK, DURATION
Onset and duration unknown. Peak levels occur in 30 to 75 minutes.

## INDICATIONS & DOSAGE
*Prophylaxis of organ rejection in patients receiving allogenic renal transplants —*

**Adults:** 1 g P.O. b.i.d. within 72 hours after transplantation, in combination with corticosteroids and cyclosporine.

## ADVERSE REACTIONS
**CNS:** *tremor,* insomnia, dizziness, *headache.*
**CV:** *chest pain, hypertension, edema.*
**GI:** *diarrhea, constipation, nausea, dyspepsia, vomiting, oral moniliasis, abdominal pain.*
**GU:** *urinary tract infection, hematuria,* kidney tubular necrosis.
**Hematologic:** *anemia, leukopenia,* **THROMBOCYTOPENIA,** hypochromic anemia, leukocytosis.
**Metabolic:** *hypercholesteremia, hypophosphatemia, hypokalemia,* hyperkalemia, hyperglycemia.
**Respiratory:** *dyspnea, cough,* pharyngitis, bronchitis, pneumonia.
**Skin:** *acne,* rash.
**Other:** *pain, fever, infection, sepsis, asthenia, back pain.*

## INTERACTIONS
*Acyclovir, ganciclovir:* increased risk of toxicity for both drugs. Monitor patient closely.
*Antacids with magnesium and aluminum hydroxides:* decreased absorption of mycophenolate. Separate dosages.
*Cholestyramine:* may interfere with enterohepatic recirculation, reducing mycophenolate bioavailability. Avoid concurrent use.

*Oral contraceptives:* may affect efficacy of oral contraceptives.

## CONTRAINDICATIONS
Contraindicated in patients with hypersensitivity to the drug, mycophenolic acid, or any drug component.

## NURSING CONSIDERATIONS
• Drug is not recommended for use in pregnant patients (unless benefits outweigh risks to fetus) or in breast-feeding women.
• Use cautiously in patients with gastrointestinal disorders.
• Safety of drug has not been established in children.
• Doses greater than 1 g b.i.d. should be avoided after immediate posttransplant period in patients with severe chronic renal impairment.
• Because of potential teratogenic effects, do not open or crush capsule. Avoid inhaling the powder in the capsule or having it contact skin or mucous membranes. If such contact occurs, wash thoroughly with soap and water, and rinse eyes with plain water.
• Monitor CBC regularly, as ordered. If neutropenia develops, notify the doctor, who may interrupt therapy, reduce the dose, order diagnostic tests, or give additional treatment.

## ☑ PATIENT TEACHING
• Warn patient not to open or crush capsules but to swallow them whole, on an empty stomach.
• Stress the importance of not interrupting or stopping therapy without first consulting the doctor.
• Inform female patient that a pregnancy test is required 1 week before therapy begins.
• Instruct female patient to use contraception during therapy and for 6 weeks after discontinuation, even with a history of infertility, unless a hysterectomy has been performed. Tell her to use two methods of contraception simultaneously, unless absti-

nence is the chosen method, and to notify the doctor immediately of suspected pregnancy.

# tacrolimus
Prograf

Pregnancy Risk Category: C

## HOW SUPPLIED
*Capsules:* 1 mg, 5 mg
*Injection:* 5 mg/ml

## ACTION
Precise mechanism unknown. Inhibits T-lymphocyte activation, which results in immunosuppression.

## ONSET, PEAK, DURATION
Onset and duration unknown. Serum levels peak in 1.5 to 3.5 hours.

## INDICATIONS & DOSAGE
*Prophylaxis of organ rejection in allogenic liver transplantation—*
**Adults:** 0.05 to 0.1 mg/kg/day I.V. as a continuous infusion administered no sooner than 6 hours after transplantation. Oral therapy should be substituted as soon as possible, with the first oral dose given 8 to 12 hours after discontinuing the I.V. infusion. The recommended initial oral dosage is 0.15 to 0.3 mg/kg/day P.O. in two divided doses q 12 hours. Dosage should be titrated according to clinical response.
**Children:** initially, 0.1 mg/kg/day I.V., followed by 0.3 mg/kg/day P.O. on a schedule similar to that for adults, adjusted as needed.

## ADVERSE REACTIONS
**CNS:** *headache, tremor, insomnia, paresthesia.*
**CV:** *hypertension, peripheral edema.*
**GI:** *diarrhea, nausea, constipation, abnormal liver function test, anorexia, vomiting, abdominal pain.*
**GU:** *abnormal renal function, in-*creased creatinine or BUN levels, urinary tract infection, oliguria.*
**Hematologic:** *anemia, leukocytosis,* **THROMBOCYTOPENIA**
**Metabolic:** *hyperkalemia, hypokalemia, hyperglycemia, hypomagnesemia.*
**Respiratory:** *pleural effusion, atelectasis, dyspnea.*
**Skin:** *pruritus, rash.*
**Other:** *pain, fever, asthenia, back pain, ascites,* **anaphylaxis.**

## INTERACTIONS
*Bromocriptine, cimetidine, clarithromycin, clotrimazole, cyclosporine, danazol, diltiazem, erythromycin, fluconazole, itraconazole, ketoconazole, methylprednisolone, metoclopramide, nicardipine, verapamil:* may increase tacrolimus levels. Monitor for adverse effects.
*Carbamazepine, phenobarbital, phenytoin, rifabutin, rifampin:* may decrease tacrolimus levels. Monitor effectiveness of tacrolimus.
*Cyclosporine:* increased risk of excess nephrotoxicity. Do not administer together.
*Immunosuppressants (except adrenal corticosteroids):* may oversuppress the immune system. Monitor patient closely, especially during times of stress.
*Inducers of cytochrome P-450 enzyme system:* may increase tacrolimus metabolism and decrease plasma levels. Dosage adjustment may be needed.
*Inhibitors of cytochrome P-450 enzyme system:* may decrease tacrolimus metabolism and increase plasma levels. Dosage adjustment may be needed.
*Nephrotoxic drugs, such as aminoglycosides, amphotericin B, cisplatin, cyclosporine:* may cause additive or synergistic effects. Monitor closely.
*Viral vaccines:* tacrolimus may interfere with the immune response to live virus vaccines.

---

Reactions may be *common*, uncommon, *life-threatening*, or **COMMON AND LIFE-THREATENING.**

## CONTRAINDICATIONS

Contraindicated in patients with hypersensitivity to the drug. The I.V. form is contraindicated in those who are hypersensitive to castor oil derivatives.

## NURSING CONSIDERATIONS

• *Alert:* Know that because of the risk of anaphylaxis, injection should be used only in patients who cannot take the oral form.

• Keep epinephrine 1:1,000 available to treat anaphylaxis.

• Be aware that children with normal renal and hepatic function may require higher dosages than adults.

• Also be aware that patients with hepatic or renal dysfunction should receive the lowest dosage possible.

• Expect to administer adrenal corticosteroids concomitantly with this drug.

• **I.V. use:** Dilute drug with 0.9% sodium chloride for injection or 5% dextrose injection to a concentration between 0.004 mg/ml and 0.02 mg/ml prior to use. Diluted infusion solution should be stored for no more than 24 hours in glass or polyethylene containers. The drug should not be stored in a polyvinyl chloride container because of decreased stability and the potential for extraction of phthalates.

• Monitor the patient continuously during the first 30 minutes of I.V. administration and frequently thereafter for signs and symptoms of anaphylaxis.

• Monitor the patient for signs of neurotoxicity and nephrotoxicity, especially in a patient receiving a high dosage or having renal dysfunction.

• Monitor the patient for signs and symptoms of hyperkalemia, and obtain serum potassium levels regularly, as ordered. Know that potassium-sparing diuretics should be avoided during tacrolimus therapy.

• Monitor the patient's blood glucose level regularly, as ordered, and the patient for signs and symptoms of hyperglycemia. Be aware that treatment of hyperglycemia may be necessary.

• Be aware that patients receiving this drug are at increased risk for infections, lymphomas, and other malignant diseases.

• Know that other immunosuppressants (except for adrenal corticosteroids) should not be used during tacrolimus therapy.

## ☑ PATIENT TEACHING

• Instruct the patient to check with the doctor before taking any other medication during tacrolimus therapy.

• Tell the patient to report adverse reactions promptly.

---

# 75

# Vaccines and toxoids

BCG vaccine
cholera vaccine
diphtheria and tetanus toxoids, adsorbed
diphtheria and tetanus toxoids and pertussis vaccine
diphtheria and tetanus toxoids and acellular pertussis vaccine
*Haemophilus* b conjugate vaccines
hepatitis A vaccine, inactivated
hepatitis B vaccine, recombinant
influenza virus vaccine, 1995-1996 trivalent types A & B (purified surface antigen)
influenza virus vaccine, 1995-1996 trivalent types A & B (split or purified split virus)
influenza virus vaccine, 1995-1996 trivalent types A & B (whole virion)
Japanese encephalitis virus vaccine, inactivated
measles, mumps, and rubella virus vaccine, live
measles (rubeola) and rubella virus vaccine, live attenuated
measles (rubeola) virus vaccine, live attenuated
meningococcal polysaccharide vaccine
mumps virus vaccine, live
plague vaccine
pneumococcal vaccine, polyvalent
poliovirus vaccine, live, oral, trivalent
poliovirus vaccine, inactivated
rabies vaccine, adsorbed
rabies vaccine, human diploid cell
rubella and mumps virus vaccine, live
rubella virus vaccine, live attenuated
tetanus toxoid, adsorbed
tetanus toxoid, fluid
typhoid vaccine
typhoid vaccine, oral
typhoid Vi polysaccharide vaccine
varicella virus vaccine
yellow fever vaccine

## COMBINATION PRODUCTS
TETRAMUNE: 10 mcg purified *Haemophilus* b saccharide and approximately 25 mcg CRM$_{197}$ protein, 12.5 Lf ( limit flocculation) units inactivated diphtheria, 5 Lf units inactivated tetanus, and 4 protective units pertussis/0.5 ml.

## BCG vaccine
*Pregnancy Risk Category: C*

**HOW SUPPLIED**
*Percutaneous vaccine:* 1 to $8 \times 10^8$ CFU/vial (Tice strain)

**ACTION**
A live, attenuated bacterial vaccine prepared from *Mycobacterium bovis* that promotes active immunity to tuberculosis (TB).

**ONSET, PEAK, DURATION**
Unknown.

**INDICATIONS & DOSAGE**
*TB exposure –*
**Adults and children 1 month and over:** 0.2 to 0.3 ml (percutaneous vaccine) applied to cleaned skin followed by application of multiple-puncture disk.
**Infants less than 1 month:** dosage reduced by one-half by using 2 ml of sterile water without preservatives when reconstituting.

Reactions may be *common*, uncommon, *life-threatening*, or COMMON AND LIFE-THREATENING.

## ADVERSE REACTIONS
**Systemic:** osteomyelitis, lymphadenopathy, allergic reaction.

## INTERACTIONS
*Immunosuppressants:* may reduce response to BCG vaccine. Avoid if possible.
*Isoniazid, rifampin, streptomycin:* inhibited multiplication of BCG. Avoid using together.

## CONTRAINDICATIONS
Contraindicated in patients with hypogammaglobulinemia, in the presence of a positive tuberculin reaction (when meant for use as immunoprophylactic after exposure to TB) in immunosuppressed patients, in those with fresh smallpox vaccinations, in those who have suffered burns, and in patients receiving corticosteroid therapy. Patients should avoid this vaccine during pregnancy.

## NURSING CONSIDERATIONS
● Use cautiously in patients with chronic skin disease. Inject in area of healthy skin only.
● Obtain history of allergies and reaction to immunization.
● Keep epinephrine 1:1,000 available to treat anaphylaxis.
● Do not shake vial after reconstitution. Use within 2 hours.
● Keep in mind that recommended injection site is over the insertion point of deltoid muscle.
● Don't administer to febrile children.
● Know that expected lesion forms in 7 to 14 days. Papules reach a maximum diameter of 3 mm, then fade.
● Allow at least 6 to 8 weeks between BCG and live virus vaccines; administer killed virus vaccines 7 days before or 10 days after BCG, as ordered.
● Know that vaccine is of no value as immunoprophylactic in patients with positive tuberculin test.
● Destroy live vaccine by autoclaving or treating with formaldehyde solution before disposal.

## ☑ PATIENT TEACHING
● Advise patient to have tuberculin skin test 2 to 3 months after BCG vaccination.
● Tell patient to report unusual signs and symptoms after vaccination.

# cholera vaccine
*Pregnancy Risk Category: C*

## HOW SUPPLIED
*Injection:* suspension of killed *Vibrio cholerae* (each milliliter contains 8 units of Inaba and Ogawa serotypes) in 1.5-ml and 20-ml vials

## ACTION
Promotes active immunity to cholera.

## ONSET, PEAK, DURATION
Although onset and peak are not precisely known, most patients develop immunity after second dose. Effects persist for 3 to 6 months.

## INDICATIONS & DOSAGE
*Primary immunization for persons traveling to areas where cholera is endemic or epidemic –*
**Adults and children over 10 years:** two doses of 0.5 ml I.M. or S.C., 1 week to 1 month apart, before traveling in cholera area. Booster is 0.5 ml q 6 months as needed.
**Children 6 months to 4 years:** 0.2 ml I.M. or S.C. Boosters of same dose should be given q 6 months as needed.
**Children 5 to 10 years:** 0.3 ml I.M. or S.C. Boosters of same dose should be given q 6 months as needed.

## ADVERSE REACTIONS
**Systemic:** malaise, fever, headache.
**Other:** *erythema, swelling, pain, induration at injection site.*

---

*Liquid form contains alcohol.  **May contain tartrazine.  †Canada only.  ‡Australia only.  ◊OTC.

## INTERACTIONS
*Plague, typhoid, or other vaccines with systemic adverse reactions:* enhanced toxicity. Don't use together.
*Yellow fever vaccine:* simultaneous administration may interfere with immune response to both vaccines. Administer 3 weeks apart.

## CONTRAINDICATIONS
Contraindicated in those with acute illness or a history of severe systemic reaction or allergic response to vaccine.

## NURSING CONSIDERATIONS
• Obtain history of allergies and reaction to immunization.
• Keep epinephrine 1:1,000 available to treat anaphylaxis.
• Shake vial vigorously before withdrawing each dose.
• Do not administer I.M. to persons with thrombocytopenia or any coagulation disorder that would contraindicate I.M. injection.
• Administer I.M. in deltoid muscle in adults and children over 3 years.
• Keep in mind that I.M. and S.C. routes give higher levels of protection. May be given intradermally (preferably into the inner surface of the forearm) to adults and children over 5 years, but the volume of injection is limited to 0.2 ml.
• Know that vaccine is about 50% effective in reducing clinical illness incidence for 3 to 6 months.

☑ **PATIENT TEACHING**
• Advise patients that pain, induration, and swelling are common at the injection site for 24 to 48 hours.
• Tell travelers to avoid food and water that may be contaminated.

---

## diphtheria and tetanus toxoids, adsorbed
*Pregnancy Risk Category: C*

## HOW SUPPLIED
Available in pediatric (DT) and adult (Td) strengths
*Injection (for pediatric use):* diphtheria toxoid 6.6 Lf (limit flocculation) units and tetanus toxoid 5 Lf units per 0.5 ml; diphtheria toxoid 7.5 Lf units and tetanus toxoid 7.5 Lf units per 0.5 ml; diphtheria toxoid 10 Lf units and tetanus toxoid 5 Lf units per 0.5 ml; diphtheria toxoid 12.5 Lf units and tetanus toxoid 5 Lf units per 0.5 ml; diphtheria toxoid 15 Lf units and tetanus toxoid 10 Lf units per 0.5 ml
*Injection (for adult use):* diphtheria toxoid 2 Lf units and tetanus toxoid 2 Lf units per 0.5 ml; diphtheria toxoid 2 Lf units and tetanus toxoid 5 Lf units per 0.5 ml; diphtheria toxoid 2 Lf units and tetanus toxoid 10 Lf units per 0.5 ml

## ACTION
Promotes immunity to diphtheria and tetanus by inducing production of antitoxins.

## ONSET, PEAK, DURATION
Onset and peak unknown. Effects persist for 10 years.

## INDICATIONS & DOSAGE
*Primary immunization* –
**Adults and children 7 years or over:** adult strength; 0.5 ml I.M. 4 to 8 weeks apart for two doses and a third dose 6 to 12 months after the second dose. Booster is 0.5 ml I.M. q 10 years.
**Infants 6 weeks to 1 year:** pediatric strength; 0.5 ml I.M. at least 4 weeks apart for three doses. Give booster dose 6 to 12 months after third injection.
**Children 1 to 6 years:** use pediatric strength; 0.5 ml I.M. at least 4 weeks apart for two doses. Give booster dosage 6 to 12 months after the second injection. If the final immunizing dose is given after the seventh birthday, use the adult strength.

---

Reactions may be *common,* uncommon, *life-threatening,* or **COMMON AND LIFE-THREATENING.**

## ADVERSE REACTIONS
Systemic: *anaphylaxis,* chills, fever, malaise, headache, tachycardia, hypotension.
Other: *pain, stinging, edema, erythema, induration at injection site,* flushing, urticaria, pruritus.

## INTERACTIONS
None significant.

## CONTRAINDICATIONS
Contraindicated in immunosuppressed patients and in those receiving radiation or corticosteroid therapy. Vaccination should be deferred in patients with respiratory illness and during polio outbreaks; also deferred in those with acute illness except during emergency. When polio is a risk, single antigen is used. Know that in children under 6 years, use only when diphtheria, tetanus, and pertussis combination is contraindicated because of pertussis component.

## NURSING CONSIDERATIONS
• Obtain history of allergies and reaction to immunization.
• Before injection, verify strength (pediatric or adult) of toxoid used.
• Keep epinephrine 1:1,000 available to treat anaphylaxis.
• Give in site not recently used for vaccines or toxoids.
• Know that drug is not used to treat an acute diphtheria infection.

## ☑ PATIENT TEACHING
• Advise patient that local reactions such as pain and pruritus are common at the injection site.
• Review primary immunization schedule with patient or parents, and stress importance of compliance with subsequent injections.

# diphtheria and tetanus toxoids and pertussis vaccine (DTP, DPT)
DTwP, Tri-Immunol

# diphtheria and tetanus toxoids and acellular pertussis vaccine
Acel-Imune, Tripedia

## HOW SUPPLIED
**whole-cell vaccine**
*Injection:* 6.5 Lf (limit flocculation) units inactivated diphtheria, 5 Lf units inactivated tetanus, and 4 protective units pertussis per 0.5 ml, in 2.5, 5, and 7.5-ml vials; 10 Lf units inactivated diphtheria, 5.5 Lf units inactivated tetanus, and 4 protective units pertussis per 0.5 ml in 5 ml vials (DTwP); 12.5 Lf units inactivated diphtheria, 5 Lf units inactivated tetanus, and 4 protective units pertussis per 0.5 ml, in 7.5-ml vials (Tri-Immunol)
**acellular vaccine**
*Injection:* 5 Lf units inactivated diphtheria, 5 Lf units inactivated tetanus, and 300 hemagglutinating units of acellular pertussis vaccine per 0.5 ml; 66.7 Lf units inactivated diphtheria, 5 Lf units inactivated tetanus, and 46.8 pertussis antigens per 0.5 ml

## ACTION
Promotes active immunity to diphtheria, tetanus, and pertussis (DTP) by inducing production of antitoxins and antibodies.

## ONSET, PEAK, DURATION
Onset and peak unknown. Effects persist for 10 years.

## INDICATIONS & DOSAGE
*Primary immunization –*
**Children 6 weeks to 6 years:** 0.5 ml I.M. 4 to 8 weeks apart for three doses and a fourth dose 1 year later. Booster is 0.5 ml I.M. when starting

---

school unless 4th dose in series was administered after child's fourth birthday; then, a booster is not necessary at time of school entrance.

Not advised for adults or children over 6 years.

The acellular vaccine may be used only for the fourth or fifth dose in children 15 months (Tripedia) or 17 months (Acel-Imune) to 7 years who have been immunized with three or four doses of the whole-cell vaccine.

## ADVERSE REACTIONS
**Systemic:** *seizures, encephalopathy, anaphylaxis, shock,* peripheral neuropathy, thrombocytopenic purpura. **Other:** *soreness, redness,* expected nodule remaining several weeks at injection site, *fever,* hypersensitivity reactions, urticaria.

## INTERACTIONS
*Immunosuppressants:* may reduce response to DPT vaccine. Avoid if possible.

## CONTRAINDICATIONS
Contraindicated in immunosuppressed patients, in those on corticosteroid therapy, and in those with a history of seizures. Vaccination should be deferred in patients with acute febrile illness. Children with preexisting neurologic disorders should not receive pertussis component. Also, children who exhibit neurologic signs after DPT injection shouldn't receive pertussis component in any succeeding injections. Diphtheria and tetanus toxoids (called DT) should be given instead.

## NURSING CONSIDERATIONS
• Obtain history of allergies and reaction to immunization.
• Keep epinephrine 1:1,000 available to treat anaphylaxis.
• Shake before using. Refrigerate.
• Administer only by deep I.M. injec-

tion, preferably in thigh or deltoid muscle. Don't give S.C.
• Keep in mind that DPT injection may be given at same time as trivalent oral polio vaccine.
• Know that acellular vaccine may be associated with a lower incidence of local pain and fever.
• Know that vaccine is not used for active infection.

☑ **PATIENT TEACHING**
• Make sure parents know the risks and benefits of this vaccine before it is administered.
• Tell parents to report systemic reactions promptly; remind them that local reactions are common.

---

# *Haemophilus* b conjugate vaccines

## *Haemophilus* b conjugate vaccine, diphtheria CRM₁₉₇ protein conjugate (HbOC)
HibTITER

## *Haemophilus* b conjugate vaccine, diphtheria toxoid conjugate (PRP-D)
ProHIBiT

## *Haemophilus* b conjugate vaccine, meningococcal protein conjugate (PRP-OMP)
PedvaxHIB

## HOW SUPPLIED
*Haemophilus* b conjugate vaccine, diphtheria CRM₁₉₇ protein conjugate
*Injection:* 10 mcg of purified *Haemophilus* b saccharide and approximately 25 mcg CRM₁₉₇ protein per 0.5 ml
*Haemophilus* b conjugate vaccine, diphtheria toxoid conjugate
*Injection:* 25 mcg of *Haemophilus influenzae* type B (HIB) capsular poly-

saccharide and 18 mcg of diphtheria toxoid protein per 0.5 ml

**Haemophilus b conjugate vaccine, meningococcal protein conjugate**

*Powder for injection:* 15 mcg of *Haemophilus* b PRP, 250 mcg *Neisseria meningitidis* OMPC per dose

## ACTION

Promotes active immunity to HIB; is a polymer of ribose, ribitol, and phosphate (PRP) and is covalently linked to highly antigenic substances, enabling the vaccine to promote an immune response in infants.

## ONSET, PEAK, DURATION

Unknown.

## INDICATIONS & DOSAGE

*Immunization against HIB infection—conjugate vaccine, diphtheria CRM$_{197}$ protein conjugate*

**Infants:** 0.5 ml I.M. at age 2 months. Repeated at 4 months and 6 months. A booster dose is required at age 15 months.

**Previously unvaccinated infants 2 to 6 months:** 0.5 ml I.M. Repeated in 2 months and again in 4 months for a total of three doses. Booster dose given at age 15 months.

**Previously unvaccinated infants 7 to 11 months:** 0.5 ml I.M. Repeated in 2 months, for a total of two doses. Booster dose given at age 15 months (but no sooner than 2 months after the last vaccination).

**Previously unvaccinated infants 12 to 14 months:** 0.5 ml I.M. Booster dose given at age 15 months (but no sooner than 2 months after the first vaccination).

**Previously unvaccinated children 15 months to 5 years:** 0.5 ml I.M. A booster dose is not required.

*Conjugate vaccine, diphtheria toxoid conjugate*

**Previously unvaccinated children 15 months to 5 years:** 0.5 ml I.M. A booster dose is not required. Not recommended for use in children under age 15 months.

*Conjugate vaccine, diphoid toxoid conjugate*

**Children 15 months to 5 years:** single dose of 0.5 ml I.M.

*conjugate vaccine, meningococcal protein conjugate*

**Infants:** 0.5 ml I.M. at age 2 months. Repeated at 4 months. Booster dose is required at age 12 months.

**Previously unvaccinated infants 2 to 6 months:** 0.5 ml I.M. Repeated in 2 months. Booster dose given at age 12 months.

**Previously unvaccinated infants 7 to 11 months:** 0.5 ml I.M. Repeated in 2 months. Booster dose given at 15 months (but no sooner than 2 months after the last vaccination).

**Previously unvaccinated infants 12 to 14 months:** 0.5 ml I.M. Booster dose given at age 15 months (but no sooner than 2 months after the first vaccination).

**Previously unvaccinated children 15 months to 5 years:** 0.5 ml I.M. A booster dose is not required.

## ADVERSE REACTIONS

**Systemic:** *anaphylaxis,* fever.
**Other:** *erythema, pain at injection site,* diarrhea, vomiting, crying.

## INTERACTIONS

*Immunosuppressants:* may suppress antibody response to HIB vaccine. Know that immunization may need to be deferred.

## CONTRAINDICATIONS

Contraindicated in patients with acute illness.

## NURSING CONSIDERATIONS

• Keep epinephrine 1:1,000 available in case of anaphylaxis.
• Don't administer intradermally or I.V. Must administer I.M.
• Administer into anterolateral aspect of the upper thigh in small children.

---

*Liquid form contains alcohol.   **May contain tartrazine.   †Canada only.   ‡Australia only.   ◇OTC.

Injections may be made into the deltoid muscle of larger children if sufficient muscle mass is present.

• Know that vaccine is not routinely given to adults or children over 5 years unless they are at high risk for infection (including patients with chronic conditions such as functional asplenia, splenectomy, Hodgkin's disease, or sickle cell anemia).

• *Alert:* Don't administer to febrile children.

• Know that immunization against HIB infection is recommended for children with HIV infections. The usual immunization schedule should be followed in these children.

• This vaccine and DPT may be given simultaneously. A combination product is commercially available.

• Know that diphtheria toxoid conjugate vaccine (ProHIBiT) is not recommended in children under 15 months.

• HIB is an important cause of meningitis in infants and preschool children.

• Keep in mind that this vaccine protects against HIB only and will not protect children against any other microorganisms that cause meningitis.

• Know that children vaccinated with nonconjugated vaccine (no longer available in the United States) need not be routinely revaccinated if the primary immunization occurred at 24 months. However, if the first vaccination occurred at 18 to 23 months, revaccinate the child with conjugate vaccine, as ordered, provided at least 2 months have elapsed.

### ☑ PATIENT TEACHING
• Warn patient or parents that pain may occur at injection site.

• Tell patient or parents to notify doctor if adverse reactions persist or become severe.

# hepatitis A vaccine, inactivated
Havrix

*Pregnancy Risk Category: C*

## HOW SUPPLIED
*Injection:* 360 ELISA units (EL.U.)/ 0.5 ml; 1,440 EL.U./1 ml

## ACTION
Promotes active immunity to hepatitis A virus.

## ONSET, PEAK, DURATION
In clinical studies, 80% to 98% of adults vaccinated were seroconverted by day 15 and 96% were seroconverted in 1 month. When a booster was given 6 months after the first dose, 100% of patients were seropositive 1 month later. In clinical studies of children receiving the drug, 99% of those vaccinated were seroconverted following two doses. When a booster (third) dose was administered 6 months after the first dose, 100% of the children were seropositive 1 month later. Effects persist for at least 6 months. Duration beyond 6 months has not been established.

## INDICATIONS & DOSAGE
*Active immunization against hepatitis A virus —*

**Adults:** 1,440 EL.U./1 ml I.M. as a single dose. For booster dose, 1,440 EL. U./1 ml I.M. given 6 to 12 months after initial dosage. Booster dose is recommended to ensure the highest antibody titer.

**Children 2 to 18 years:** two doses consisting of 360 EL.U./0.5 ml I.M. given 1 month apart. For booster dose, 360 EL.U./0.5 ml I.M. given 6 to 12 months after initial dosage. Booster dose is recommended to ensure the highest antibody titer.

---

Reactions may be *common,* uncommon, *life-threatening,* or COMMON AND LIFE-THREATENING.

## ADVERSE REACTIONS

**CNS:** episode of hypertonia, insomnia, photophobia, vertigo, *headache*.
**GI:** *anorexia, nausea,* abdominal pain, diarrhea, dysgeusia, vomiting.
**Musculoskeletal:** arthralgia, elevation of creatine phosphokinase level, myalgia.
**Respiratory:** pharyngitis, other upper respiratory tract infections.
**Skin:** pruritus, rash, urticaria, *induration, redness, swelling,* hematoma, *injection site soreness.*
**Other:** *fatigue, fever, malaise,* lymphadenopathy, ***anaphylaxis.***

## INTERACTIONS

None significant.

## CONTRAINDICATIONS

Contraindicated in patients with hypersensitivity to any component of the vaccine.

## NURSING CONSIDERATIONS

• Use with caution in patients with thrombocytopenia or bleeding disorders and in those who are taking an anticoagulant because bleeding may occur following an I.M. injection.
• As with any vaccine, administration of hepatitis A vaccine should be delayed, if possible, in patients with any febrile illness.
• Keep epinephrine available to treat an anaphylactoid reaction.
• Be aware that if vaccine is administered to immunosuppressed persons or persons receiving immunosuppressants, the expected immune response may not be obtained.
• Know that persons who should receive the vaccine include people traveling to or living in areas of higher endemicity for hepatitis A (Africa, Asia [except Japan], the Mediterranean basin, Eastern Europe, the Middle East, Central and South America, Mexico, and parts of the Caribbean), military personnel, native peoples of Alaska and the Americas, persons engaging in high-risk sexual activity, and users of illegal injectable drugs. Certain institutional workers, employees of child day-care centers, laboratory workers who handle live hepatitis A virus, and handlers of primate animals also may benefit.
• **I.M. use:** Shake vial or syringe well before withdrawal and use. After it has been agitated thoroughly, the vaccine is an opaque white suspension. Discard if it appears otherwise. No dilution or reconstitution is necessary.
• Administer as an I.M. injection into the deltoid region in adults. It should not be administered in the gluteal region; such injections may result in suboptimal response. Never inject I.V., S.C., or intradermally.
• Be aware that hepatitis A vaccine will not prevent infection in persons who have an unrecognized hepatitis A infection at the time of vaccination.

## ☑ PATIENT TEACHING

• Inform the patient that the vaccine will not prevent hepatitis caused by other agents, such as hepatitis B virus, hepatitis C virus, hepatitis E virus, and other pathogens known to infect the liver.
• Warn the patient about local adverse reactions. Tell patient to report persistent or severe reactions promptly.

---

# hepatitis B vaccine, recombinant

Engerix-B, Recombivax HB
*Pregnancy Risk Category: C*

## HOW SUPPLIED

*Injection:* 2.5 mcg hepatitis B surface antigen (HBs)Ag/0.5ml (Recombivax HB, pediatric formulation); 5 mcg HBsAg/0.5 ml (Recombivax HB, adolescent/high-risk infant formulation); 10 mcg HBsAg/0.5 ml (Engerix-B, adolescent/pediatric formulation); 10 mcg HBsAg/ml (Recombivax HB, adult formulation); 20 mcg HBsAg/ml (Engerix-B, adult formulation); 40 mcg HBsAg/ml (Recombivax HB dialysis formulation)

**ACTION**
Promotes active immunity to hepatitis B.

**ONSET, PEAK, DURATION**
Not fully defined.

**INDICATIONS & DOSAGE**
*Immunization against infection from all known subtypes of hepatitis B virus (HBV); primary preexposure prophylaxis against HBV; or postexposure prophylaxis (when given with hepatitis B immune globulin) –*
*Engerix-B*
**Adults:** initially, 20 mcg (1-ml adult formulation) is given I.M., followed by a second dose of 20 mcg I.M. 30 days later. A third dose of 20 mcg I.M. is given 6 months after the initial dose.
**Adults undergoing dialysis or receiving immunosuppressants:** initially, 40 mcg I.M. (divided into two 20-mcg doses and administered at different sites). Followed with a second dose of 40 mcg I.M. in 30 days, and a final dose of 40 mcg I.M. 6 months after the initial dose.
   *Note:* Certain populations (neonates born to infected mothers, persons recently exposed to the virus, and travelers to high-risk areas) may receive the vaccine on an abbreviated schedule, with the initial dose followed by a second dose in 1 month, and the third dose after 2 months. For prolonged maintenance of protective antibody titers, a booster dose is recommended 12 months after the initial dose.
**Adolescents 11 to 20 years of age:** initially, 10 mcg (0.5-ml adolescent/pediatric formulation) I.M., followed by a second dose of 10 mcg I.M. 30 days later. A third dose of 10 mcg

I.M. is given 6 months after the initial dose. Alternatively, 20 mcg (1-ml adult formulation) is given I.M., followed by a second dose of 20 mcg I.M. 30 days later. A third dose of 20 mcg I.M. is given 6 months after the initial dose.
**Neonates and children up to 11 years:** initially, 10 mcg (0.5-ml pediatric formulation) I.M., followed by a second dose of 10 mcg I.M. 30 days later. A third dose of 10 mcg I.M. is given 6 months after the initial dose.
*Recombivax HB*
**Adults:** initially, 10 mcg (1-ml adult formulation) I.M., followed by a second dose of 10 mcg I.M. 30 days later. A third dose of 10 mcg is given I.M. 6 months after the initial dose.
**Adults undergoing dialysis:** initially, 40 mcg I.M. (use dialysis formulation, which contains 40 mcg/ml). Followed with a second dose of 40 mcg I.M. in 30 days, and a final dose of 40 mcg I.M. 6 months after the initial dose.
**Children 11 to 20 years:** initially, 5 mcg (0.5-ml adolescent/high-risk infant formulation) I.M., followed by a second dose of 5 mcg I.M. 30 days later. A third dose of 5 mcg is given I.M. 6 months after the initial dose.
**Children 1 to 11 years:** initially, 2.5 mcg (0.5-ml pediatric formulation) I.M., followed by a second dose of 2.5 mcg I.M. 30 days later. A third dose of 2.5 mcg I.M. is given 6 months after the initial dose.
**Infants born of HBsAg-negative mothers:** initially, 2.5 mcg (0.5 ml pediatric formulation) I.M., followed by a second dose of 0.5 mcg 30 days later. A third dose of 0.5 mcg is given I.M. 6 months after the initial dose.
**Infants born of HBsAg-positive mothers:** initially, 5 mcg (0.5-ml adolescent/high-risk infant formulation) I.M., followed by a second dose of 5 mcg I.M. 30 days later. A third dose of 5 mcg is given I.M. 6 months after the initial dose.

---

Reactions may be *common*, uncommon, *life-threatening*, or COMMON AND LIFE-THREATENING.

## ADVERSE REACTIONS
**Systemic:** headache, dizziness, nausea, insomnia, paresthesia, neuropathy, pharyngitis, anorexia, diarrhea, arthralgia, vomiting, slight fever, transient malaise, flulike symptoms, myalgia.
**Other:** local inflammation at injection site, *injection site soreness.*

## INTERACTIONS
None significant.

## CONTRAINDICATIONS
Contraindicated in patients hypersensitive to yeast; recombinant vaccines are derived from yeast cultures.

## NURSING CONSIDERATIONS
• Use cautiously in patients with serious, active infections or compromised cardiac or pulmonary status and in those for whom a febrile or systemic reaction could pose a risk.
• Know that the American Academy of Pediatrics recommends hepatitis B vaccination for all neonates and encourages immunization for adolescents when resources allow.
• Although anaphylaxis has not been reported, always keep epinephrine available when giving this vaccine to counteract possible reaction.
• Thoroughly agitate vial just before administration to restore suspension.
• Give adults and adolescents the vaccine in the deltoid muscle; give infants and young children the vaccine in the anterolateral aspect of the thigh. Never administer I.V.
• Administer S.C. in persons at risk for hemorrhage, such as hemophiliacs. Otherwise, do not use this route; it may lead to an increased incidence or severity of local reactions.
• Keep in mind that certain health care personnel (especially those working with dialysis patients, in blood banks, in emergency medicine, with selected patients and patient contacts, or among populations in which the in-fection is endemic [native peoples of Alaska, Indo-Chinese, and Haitian refugees]), certain military personnel, morticians and embalmers, sexually active homosexual men, prostitutes, prisoners, and users of illegal injectable drugs are at increased risk for infection and should be considered for the vaccine.
• Be aware that recombinant hepatitis B vaccine is not made with any human plasma products.
• Refrigerate both opened and unopened vials. Don't freeze.

☑ **PATIENT TEACHING**
• Warn patient or parents about local adverse reactions. Tell patient to report persistent or severe reactions promptly.
• Review immunization schedule with patient or parents, and stress importance of completing series.

---

## influenza virus vaccine, 1995-1996 trivalent types A & B (purified surface antigen)
Fluvirin

## influenza virus vaccine, 1995-1996 trivalent types A & B (split or purified split virus)
Fluogen, Flu-Shield, Fluzone

## influenza virus vaccine, 1995-1996 trivalent types A & B (whole virion)
Fluzone (Whole)

*Pregnancy Risk Category: C*

---

## HOW SUPPLIED
*Injection:* 15 mcg A/Texas/36/91-like (H1N1), 15 mcg A/Johannesburg/33/94-like (H3N2), and 15 mcg B/Beijing/184/93-like hemagglutinin antigens per 0.5 ml

---

*Liquid form contains alcohol. **May contain tartrazine. †Canada only. ‡Australia only. ◇OTC.

## ACTION
Promotes immunity to influenza by inducing production of antibodies.

## ONSET, PEAK, DURATION
Although onset and peak not precisely known, most patients develop immunity in 2 to 4 weeks. Immunity declines following vaccination, possibly within 6 months.

## INDICATIONS & DOSAGE
*Influenza prophylaxis* –
**Adults and children 12 years and over:** 0.5 ml whole virus, split virus, or purified split virus I.M. Only one dose is required.
**Children 9 to 12 years:** 0.5 ml split virus or purified split virus I.M. Only one dose is required.
**Children 3 to 9 years:** 0.5 ml split virus or purified split virus I.M. Repeated in 4 weeks unless child has been previously vaccinated.
**Children 6 to 36 months:** 0.25 ml split virus or purified split virus I.M. Repeated in 4 weeks unless child has been previously vaccinated.

## ADVERSE REACTIONS
**Systemic:** *anaphylaxis,* fever, malaise, myalgia.
**Other:** erythema, induration, and *soreness at injection site.*
   Fever and malaise reactions occur most often in children and in others not exposed to influenza viruses. Severe reactions in adults are rare.

## INTERACTIONS
*Theophylline, warfarin:* clearance may be impaired.

## CONTRAINDICATIONS
Contraindicated in patients with hypersensitivity to eggs. Vaccination should be deferred in patients with acute respiratory or other active infection.

## NURSING CONSIDERATIONS
• Use cautiously in patients with a history of sulfite allergy.
• Obtain history of allergies, especially to eggs, and reaction to immunization.
• Keep epinephrine 1:1,000 available to treat anaphylaxis.
• Note that the combination of antigens used to create influenza vaccine changes annually even though some antigens may be the same as previous years. Do not use leftover supplies to immunize patients for the current flu season.
• Thoroughly agitate vial just before administration to restore suspension.
• Give injections for adults and older children in deltoid muscle; for infants and children under 3 years, give in anterolateral aspect of thigh.
• Ideally, vaccinations should be performed in November because outbreaks of influenza generally don't occur until December. The vaccine should not be given too early in the season because antibody titers may begin to decline before the flu season.
• Know that children 12 years and under should be given their second dose in December, if possible.
• Vaccines may be given to both children and adults throughout the flu season, even as late as April.
• Know that doctor may not give children pertussis vaccine within 3 days of influenza virus vaccine. However, the American Academy of Pediatrics recommends that influenza vaccine can be administered simultaneously (but at a different site and with a different syringe) with other routine vaccinations in children.
• Know that this vaccine is considered safe in pregnant patients. Vaccination shouldn't be postponed, regardless of the stage of pregnancy, in patients who have high-risk conditions and who will be in the first trimester of pregnancy when flu season begins.

---

Reactions may be *common,* uncommon, *life-threatening,* or COMMON AND LIFE-THREATENING.

• Keep in mind that immunodeficient patients may receive two doses 1 month apart; however, there is little evidence that booster doses improve the immunogenic response to the vaccine. Know that chemoprophylaxis with amantadine may be helpful.

• Know that vaccine is strongly recommended for anyone over 6 months; for patients with chronic disease, metabolic disorders, or medical conditions that put them at risk for complications from influenza; for health care workers, especially doctors, nurses, employees of nursing homes, volunteer workers, and other personnel in both hospital and outpatient settings; and for household members who may contact persons at high risk for medical complications of influenza. Also recommended for anyone who wishes to reduce the chance of infection.

• Keep in mind that allergic reactions, which usually occur immediately, are extremely rare.

• Be alert that paralysis associated with Guillain-Barré syndrome is rare, and has only been associated with the 1976 vaccine.

• Remember that although there is little information regarding influenza in persons with HIV, it is recommended that these patients receive the vaccine. Patients with advanced disease may exhibit a low response; there is no evidence that a booster dose will improve the immune response.

### ☑ PATIENT TEACHING

• Advise patient about the risks of vaccination as compared with risk of influenza and its complications.

• Ensure that patient understands that annual vaccination with the current vaccine is necessary because immunity to influenza decreases in the year after the injection.

• Ensure that patient understands that the vaccine cannot cause influenza. Fever, malaise, and myalgia may begin 6 to 12 hours after vaccination and

persist 1 to 2 days. Such systemic reactions are not common.

---

# Japanese encephalitis virus vaccine, inactivated
JE-VAX
*Pregnancy Risk Category: C*

### HOW SUPPLIED
*Injection:* 1-ml, 10-ml vials

### ACTION
Provides active immunity against Japanese encephalitis (JE), a mosquito-borne arboviral flavivirus infection that's the leading cause of viral encephalitis in Asia.

### ONSET, PEAK, DURATION
Not clearly defined. An immune response is thought to occur within 10 days. Duration of protection is thought to be at least 2 years in persons receiving three doses.

### INDICATIONS & DOSAGE
*Active immunization against JE –*
**Primary immunization schedule**
**Adults and children 3 years and over:** 1 ml S.C. on days 0, 7, and 30.
**Children 1 to 3 years:** 0.5 ml S.C. on days 0, 7, and 30.
*Booster doses*
**Adults and children 3 years and over:** 1 ml S.C. q 2 years.
**Children 1 to 3 years:** 0.5 ml S.C. q 2 years.

### ADVERSE REACTIONS
**Systemic:** *headache; dizziness; nausea; vomiting; abdominal pain; **respiratory distress; anaphylaxis;** rash;* generalized urticaria; *fever; malaise; chills; myalgia;* angioedema of the face, oropharynx, extremities, or lips. **Other:** *local tenderness and swelling at injection site.*

### INTERACTIONS
None significant.

---

## CONTRAINDICATIONS

Contraindicated in patients hypersensitive to the drug or to thimerosal, a preservative, and in patients who exhibited severe adverse reactions, such as generalized urticaria or angioedema, to a prior dose of the vaccine. Because the vaccine is derived from mouse brain, its use is contraindicated in patients hypersensitive to substances of murine or neural origin.

## NURSING CONSIDERATIONS

- Use cautiously in pregnant or breast-feeding patients, elderly patients, and those with a history of urticaria after vaccines, drugs, or insect stings. Advanced age may be a risk factor for developing symptomatic illness after JE infection. JE acquired during pregnancy can cause intrauterine infection and fetal death.
- Use vaccine to provide protection against JE in persons planning to travel or reside in areas where the virus is endemic. It's not indicated for all persons traveling to or residing in Asia. For most travelers to Asia, the risk for acquiring JE is extremely low. Contact the Centers for Disease Control and Prevention at (404) 332-4555 for current travel advisories.
- Keep epinephrine 1:1,000 and other resuscitation equipment and drugs available to treat anaphylaxis and other adverse reactions.
- To prepare vaccine for injection, use supplied diluent (sterile water for injection). Add 1.3 ml of diluent to the single-dose vial and 11 ml of diluent to the 10-dose vial. Shake vial thoroughly to ensure dissolution of vaccine. After reconstitution, refrigerate vaccine (36° to 46° F [2° to 8° C]) for up to 8 hours.
- Follow the recommended three-dose schedule for best results. Be aware that when time constraints prohibit the use of this schedule, an abbreviated schedule with injections on days 0, 7, and 14 may be used.
- Know that when it isn't possible to follow usual dose schedule, a two-dose regimen with injections on days 0 and 7 may be used. Antibodies will be induced in about 80% of patients with this schedule. A two-dose regimen should not be used unless circumstances are unusual.
- Monitor patients closely for 30 minutes after injection.
- Be aware that reactions to the first dose have occurred a median of 12 hours after injection (88% happened within 3 days). The delay between the second dose and adverse effects was usually longer, with a median of 3 days and some effects not seen for 2 weeks. Some patients exhibited adverse reactions to the second or third dose, even when the first or second dose was well tolerated.

## ☑ PATIENT TEACHING

- Warn patient about the possibility of delayed generalized urticaria or delayed angioedema of the extremities, face, oropharynx or (especially) the lips. Generalized urticaria or angioedema may occur within minutes of vaccination. Most reactions occur within 48 hours. However, reactions that may be related to the vaccine have occurred as late as 17 days after the injection.
- Because of the possibility of delayed reactions, advise patient to remain in areas where medical care is available for 10 days after injection. Caution against international travel during this time. Advise patient to seek medical assistance as soon as any reaction appears.
- Encourage patient and parents to report adverse effects after vaccination. Health care providers should report these adverse effects to the U.S. Department of Health and Human Services Vaccine Adverse Event Reporting System (VAERS). Contact VAERS at (800) 822-7967 for infor-

---

Reactions may be *common,* uncommon, *life-threatening,* or **COMMON AND LIFE-THREATENING.**

mation about the system and reporting forms.
• Teach patient about precautions that may limit exposure to mosquito bites, such as using insect repellents, wearing protective clothing, and avoiding outdoor activities, especially in the evening.

---

## measles, mumps, and rubella virus vaccine, live
M-M-R II

*Pregnancy Risk Category: C*

### HOW SUPPLIED
*Injection:* single-dose vial containing not less than 1,000 TCID$_{50}$ (tissue culture infective doses) of attenuated measles virus derived from Enders' attenuated Edmonston strain (grown in chick embryo culture), 20,000 TCID$_{50}$ of the Jeryl Lynn (B level) mumps strain (grown in chick embryo culture), and 1,000 TCID$_{50}$ of the Wistar RA 27/3 strain of rubella virus (propagated in human diploid cell culture) per 0.5-ml dose

### ACTION
Promotes immunity to measles, mumps, and rubella virus by inducing production of antibodies.

### ONSET, PEAK, DURATION
Although onset and peak are not precisely known, most patients develop immunity in 2 to 6 weeks. Effects have been shown to persist up to 11 years without decline.

### INDICATIONS & DOSAGE
*Routine vaccination –*
**Children:** one vial S.C. A two-dose schedule is recommended, with the first dose given at 15 months (12 months in high-risk areas) and the second dose given either at 4 to 6 years or at 11 or 12 years.

### ADVERSE REACTIONS
**Systemic:** urticaria, rash, fever, regional lymphadenopathy, diarrhea, *anaphylaxis.*
**Other:** erythema at injection site.

### INTERACTIONS
*Immune serum globulin, plasma, whole blood:* antibodies in serum may interfere with immune response. Don't use vaccine within 3 months of transfusion.

### CONTRAINDICATIONS
Contraindicated in immunosuppressed patients; in those with cancer, blood dyscrasia, gamma globulin disorders, fever, active untreated tuberculosis, or anaphylactic or anaphylactoid reactions to neomycin or eggs; in those receiving corticosteroid or radiation therapy; and in pregnant patients.

### NURSING CONSIDERATIONS
• Obtain history of allergies, especially anaphylactic reactions to antibiotics, or reaction to immunization.
• Keep epinephrine 1:1,000 available to treat anaphylaxis.
• Inject into outer aspect of upper arm. Don't give I.V.
• Use only diluent supplied. Discard 8 hours after reconstituting.
• Refrigerate; protect from light. Solution may be used if red, pink, or yellow, but must be clear.
• Know that incidence of adverse effects is low (0.5% to 4%).
• Treat fever with antipyretics, such as acetaminophen.
• Be aware that presence of maternal antibodies may prevent response in children under 12 months.
• Keep in mind that the Immunization Practices Advisory Committee recommends that colleges and other post-high school educational institutions, as well as medical institutions employing health care providers, obtain documentation of the receipt of two

---

doses of vaccine after age 1 (or other proof of immunity, such as infection, documented by a doctor). Combined measles, mumps, and rubella vaccine is preferred.
• *Alert:* The Centers for Disease Control and Prevention recommends that, during a measles outbreak in a health care facility, susceptible personnel exposed to the measles virus (whether or not they received measles vaccine or immunoglobulin) avoid patient contact for days 5 through 21 after such exposure. If they become ill, they should avoid patient contact for at least 7 days after developing rash.
• Clinical trials indicate that vitamin A supplementation reduces morbidity and mortality in children with measles. In these studies, 100,000 to 400,000 IU daily have been used.

### ☑ PATIENT TEACHING
• Warn parents about adverse reactions associated with the vaccine.
• Review immunization schedule with parents, and stress importance of receiving second injection at the appropriate time to maintain immunization.

## measles (rubeola) and rubella virus vaccine, live attenuated
M-R-Vax II

*Pregnancy Risk Category: C*

### HOW SUPPLIED
*Injection:* single-dose vial containing not less than 1,000 TCID$_{50}$ (tissue culture infective doses) per 0.5 ml of attenuated measles virus derived from Enders' attenuated Edmonston strain (grown in chick embryo culture); 1,000 TCID$_{50}$ of the Wistar RA 27/3 strain of rubella virus

### ACTION
Promotes immunity to measles and rubella virus by inducing production of antibodies.

### ONSET, PEAK, DURATION
Although onset and peak are not clearly defined, immunity for most patients occurs in 2 to 6 weeks. Effects have been shown to persist up to 11 years without decline.

### INDICATIONS & DOSAGE
*Immunization –*
**Adults and children 15 months and older:** 0.5 ml (1,000 units) S.C.

### ADVERSE REACTIONS
**Systemic:** rash, fever, lymphadenopathy, *anaphylaxis.*

### INTERACTIONS
*Immune serum globulin, plasma, whole blood:* antibodies in serum may interfere with immune response. Don't use vaccine within 3 months of transfusion.
*Tuberculin skin test:* may temporarily decrease response to test. Defer skin testing.

### CONTRAINDICATIONS
Contraindicated in immunosuppressed patients; in those with cancer, blood dyscrasia, gamma globulin disorders, fever, active untreated tuberculosis or anaphylactic or anaphylactoid reactions to eggs or neomycin; in those receiving corticosteroid or radiation therapy; and in pregnant patients.

### NURSING CONSIDERATIONS
• Obtain history of allergies, especially anaphylactic reactions to antibiotics.
• Keep epinephrine 1:1,000 available to treat anaphylaxis.
• Use only diluent supplied. Discard 8 hours after reconstituting.
• Inject into outer upper arm. Don't inject I.V.
• Store in refrigerator and protect from light. Solution may be used if red, pink, or yellow, but must be clear (with no precipitation).

Reactions may be *common,* uncommon, *life-threatening,* or COMMON AND LIFE-THREATENING.

- **Alert:** Vaccine should not be given within 1 month of other live virus vaccines, except oral poliovirus vaccine. Immunization should be deferred in patients with acute illness.
- Allow at least 3 weeks between BCG and rubella vaccines.

### ☑ PATIENT TEACHING
- Warn patient or parents about adverse reactions associated with vaccine.
- Inform patient or parents that immunization does not require more than 1 injection.

---

## measles (rubeola) virus vaccine, live attenuated
Attenuvax

*Pregnancy Risk Category: C*

### HOW SUPPLIED
*Injection:* single-dose vial containing not less than 1,000 TCID$_{50}$ (tissue culture infective doses) of attenuated measles virus derived from Enders' attenuated Edmonston strain (grown in chick embryo culture)

### ACTION
Promotes immunity to measles virus by inducing production of antibodies.

### ONSET, PEAK, DURATION
Although exact onset and peak unknown, most patients develop immunity within 2 to 6 weeks. Vaccine-induced antibody levels have been shown to persist for at least 13 years without substantial decline.

### INDICATIONS & DOSAGE
*Immunization* –
**Adults and children age 15 months or over:** 0.5 ml (1,000 units) S.C. A two-dose schedule is recommended, with the first dose given at age 15 months (age 12 months in high-risk areas) and the second dose given at age 4 to 6 or 11 to 12 years of age.

*Measles outbreak control* –
**Children:** if cases occur in children under age 1, children should be vaccinated as young as age 6 months. All students and siblings should be revaccinated if they are without documentation of measles immunity.
**Adults:** school personnel born in or after 1957 should be revaccinated if they are without proof of measles immunity. If the outbreak is in a medical facility, all workers born in or after 1957 should be revaccinated if they are without proof of immunity. Revaccination should be considered for persons born before 1957 as well.

### ADVERSE REACTIONS
**Systemic:** febrile seizures in susceptible children, anorexia, leukopenia, fever, rash, lymphadenopathy, *anaphylaxis.*
**Other:** erythema, swelling, and tenderness at injection site.

### INTERACTIONS
*Immune serum globulin, plasma, whole blood:* antibodies in serum may interfere with immune response. Don't use vaccine within 3 months of transfusion.
*Tuberculin skin test:* may temporarily decrease response to test. Defer skin testing.

### CONTRAINDICATIONS
Contraindicated in immunosuppressed patients; in those with cancer, blood dyscrasia, gamma globulin disorders, fever, active untreated tuberculosis, or anaphylactic or anaphylactoid reactions to neomycin or eggs; in those receiving corticosteroid or radiation therapy; and in pregnant patients.

### NURSING CONSIDERATIONS
- Obtain history of allergies, especially anaphylactic reactions to antibiotics, or reaction to immunization. Immunization should be deferred in

---

patients with acute illness or after administration of blood or plasma.

• Keep epinephrine 1:1,000 available to treat anaphylaxis.

• Use only diluent supplied. Discard 8 hours after reconstituting.

• Do not give I.V.

• Refrigerate and protect from light. Reconstituted solution is clear yellow with no precipitation. Do not use if discolored.

• Know that vaccine may be given with oral poliovirus vaccine.

• Keep in mind that the Immunization Practices Advisory Committee recommends that colleges and other post-high school educational institutions, as well as medical institutions employing health care providers, obtain documentation of the receipt of two doses of vaccine after age 1 (or other proof of immunity, such as infection, documented by a doctor). Combined measles, mumps, and rubella vaccine is preferred.

• *Alert:* The Centers for Disease Control and Prevention recommends that, during a measles outbreak in a health care facility, susceptible personnel exposed to the measles virus (whether or not they received measles vaccine or immune globulin) avoid patient contact for days 5 through 21 after such exposure. If they become ill, they should avoid patient contact for at least 7 days after developing rash.

• Know that if attenuated measles vaccine is administered immediately after exposure to the disease, some protection may be provided. This level of protection is significantly increased if the vaccine is administered even a few days before exposure.

☑ **PATIENT TEACHING**

• Warn patient about adverse reactions associated with vaccine.

• Review immunization schedule with patient or parents and stress importance of receiving second injection at appropriate time.

• Stress the importance of avoiding pregnancy for 3 months after vaccination. Offer to provide contraception information.

# meningococcal polysaccharide vaccine
Menomune-A/C/Y/W-135

*Pregnancy Risk Category: C*

## HOW SUPPLIED
*Injection:* 1-dose, 10-dose, and 50-dose vials with vial of diluent

## ACTION
Promotes active immunity to meningitis.

## ONSET, PEAK, DURATION
Although exact onset and peak unknown, most patients develop immunity in 10 to 14 days. Antibody titers decline within 3 years.

## INDICATIONS & DOSAGE
*Meningococcal meningitis prophylaxis –*
**Adults and children 2 years and older:** 0.5 ml S.C.

## ADVERSE REACTIONS
**Systemic:** headache, malaise, chills, fever, muscle cramps, *anaphylaxis.*
**Other:** *pain, tenderness, erythema, induration* (at injection site).

## INTERACTIONS
None significant.

## CONTRAINDICATIONS
Contraindicated in immunosuppressed and pregnant patients and patients with hypersensitivity to thimerosal. Vaccination should be deferred in patients with acute illness.

## NURSING CONSIDERATIONS
• Obtain history of allergies and reaction to immunization.

- Keep epinephrine 1:1,000 available to treat anaphylaxis.
- Do not give I.V.
- Know that vaccine may be given with other immunizations.
- Know that routine vaccination is not recommended. Vaccine should be reserved for individuals at risk. These are individuals who live or are traveling to epidemic or highly endemic areas, household or institutional contacts of meningococcal disease as an adjunct to appropriate antibiotic chemoprophylaxis, medical and laboratory personnel at risk of exposure to meningococcal disease, presence of terminal complement component deficiency, and patients with anatomic or functional asplenia.
- Be aware that some clinicians will revaccinate children if they are at high risk and if they previously received vaccine before age 4 years.

### ☑ PATIENT TEACHING
- Warn patient or parents about adverse reactions associated with vaccine.
- Stress to patient the importance of avoiding pregnancy for 3 months after vaccination. Offer to provide contraception information.

---

## mumps virus vaccine, live
Mumpsvax

*Pregnancy Risk Category: C*

### HOW SUPPLIED
*Injection:* single-dose vial containing not less than 20,000 TCID$_{50}$ (tissue culture infective doses) of attenuated mumps virus derived from Jeryl Lynn mumps strain (grown in chick embryo culture) per 0.5 ml and vial of diluent; single-dose vial containing not less than 5,000 TCID50 (tissue culture infective doses) of the U.S. Reference Mumps Virus in each 0.5ml†

### ACTION
Promotes active immunity to mumps.

### ONSET, PEAK, DURATION
Although exact onset and peak unknown, most patients develop immunity in 2 to 3 weeks. Effects persist for at least 20 years; probably lifelong.

### INDICATIONS & DOSAGE
*Immunization –*
**Adults and children 1 year and older:** 0.5 ml (5,000 units) S.C.

### ADVERSE REACTIONS
**CNS:** *febrile seizures* (rare).
**Other:** *slight fever,* rash, malaise, mild allergic reactions, mild lymph adenopathy, diarrhea, injection-site reaction.

### INTERACTIONS
*Immune serum globulin, plasma, whole blood:* antibodies in serum may interfere with immune response. Don't use vaccine within 3 months of transfusion.
*Tuberculin skin test:* may temporarily decrease response to test. Defer skin testing.

### CONTRAINDICATIONS
Contraindicated in immunosuppressed patients; in those with cancer, blood dyscrasia, gamma globulin disorders, fever, untreated active tuberculosis, or anaphylactic or anaphylactoid reactions to neomycin or eggs; in those receiving corticosteroid or radiation therapy; and in pregnant patients.

### NURSING CONSIDERATIONS
- Obtain history of allergies, especially anaphylactic reactions to antibiotics, and reaction to immunization. Defer in patients with acute or febrile illness and for 3 months after transfusions or treatment with immune serum globulin.

---

*Liquid form contains alcohol.   **May contain tartrazine.   †Canada only.   ‡Australia only.   ◊OTC.

- Keep epinephrine 1:1,000 available to treat anaphylaxis.
- Use only diluent supplied. Discard 8 hours after reconstituting.
- Do not give I.V.
- Refrigerate and protect from light. Reconstituted solution is clear yellow; do not use if discolored.
- Treat fever with antipyretics.
- Do not give this vaccine less than 1 month before or after immunization with other live virus vaccines; however, Attenuvax, Meruvax, or monovalent or trivalent live, oral poliovirus vaccine may be administered simultaneously.
- Know that vaccine is not recommended for infants under 12 months because retained maternal mumps antibodies may interfere with the immune response.
- Do not use for delayed hypersensitivity (allergy) skin testing. Use mumps skin-test antigen, a killed viral product.

☑ **PATIENT TEACHING**
- Warn patient or parents about adverse reactions associated with vaccine.
- Stress to patient the importance of avoiding pregnancy for 3 months after vaccination. Offer to provide contraception information.

## plague vaccine

*Pregnancy Risk Category: C*

### HOW SUPPLIED
*Injection:* 1.8 to 2.2 billion killed plague bacilli (*Yersinia pestis*)/ml in 20-ml vials

### ACTION
Promotes active immunity to plague caused by *Y. pestis*.

### ONSET, PEAK, DURATION
Onset and peak unknown. Effects persist for 6 to 12 months.

### INDICATIONS & DOSAGE
*Primary immunization and booster –*
**Adults and children 11 years and older:** 1 ml I.M., followed by 0.2 ml in 4 to 12 weeks, then 0.2 ml 3 to 6 months after the second dose. Booster is 0.1 to 0.2 ml q 6 months while in plague area.
**Children under 1 year:** ⅕ adult primary or booster dose.
**Children 1 to 4 years:** ⅖ adult primary or booster dose.
**Children 5 to 10 years:** ⅗ adult primary or booster dose.

### ADVERSE REACTIONS
**Systemic:** headache, malaise, *slight fever, lymphadenopathy,* **anaphylaxis,** arthralgia, myalgia, nausea, vomiting, leukocytosis.
**Other:** swelling, *induration, and erythema at injection site.*

### INTERACTIONS
*Cholera, typhoid vaccine:* increased risk of adverse effects. Don't give at the same time.

### CONTRAINDICATIONS
Contraindicated in immunosuppressed or pregnant patients and in those hypersensitive to beef, soy, casein, phenol, or formaldehyde. Patients who have had severe local or systemic reactions to plague vaccine should not be revaccinated. Also contraindicated in patients with severe thrombocytopenia or any coagulation disorder that would contraindicate I.M. injections.

### NURSING CONSIDERATIONS
- Obtain history of allergies and reaction to immunization. Know that immunization should be deferred in patients with respiratory infection.
- Keep epinephrine 1:1,000 available to treat anaphylaxis.
- Inject into the deltoid area, the preferred site.
- Recommended for all laboratory

and field personnel working with *Yersinia pestis*.

• Warn patient or parents about adverse reactions associated with vaccine.
• Caution women of childbearing age to notify doctor of suspected pregnancy before administration.

---

## pneumococcal vaccine, polyvalent
Pneumovax 23, Pnu-Imune 23

*Pregnancy Risk Category: C*

### HOW SUPPLIED
*Injection:* 25 mcg each of 23 polysaccharide isolates/0.5 ml

### ACTION
Promotes active immunity to infections caused by *Streptococcus pneumoniae*.

### ONSET, PEAK, DURATION
Onset occurs in 2 to 3 weeks. Peak unknown. Effects persist for 5 to 10 years in most patients.

### INDICATIONS & DOSAGE
*Pneumococcal immunization –*
**Adults and children 2 years and older:** 0.5 ml I.M. or S.C.
Not recommended for children under 2 years.

### ADVERSE REACTIONS
**Systemic:** *anaphylaxis, slight fever,* myalgia, rash, arthralgia.
**Other:** *soreness at injection site;* severe local reaction associated with revaccination within 3 years.

### INTERACTIONS
None significant.

### CONTRAINDICATIONS
Contraindicated in patients hypersensitive to the drug or its components (phenol). Also contraindicated in patients with Hodgkin's disease who have received extensive chemotherapy or nodal irradiation.

### NURSING CONSIDERATIONS
• Check immunization history to avoid revaccination within 3 years.
• Obtain history of allergies and reaction to immunization. Eggs and egg protein are not used during the manufacture of the vaccine; contains phenol as a preservative.
• Keep epinephrine 1:1,000 available to treat anaphylaxis.
• Inject in deltoid or midlateral thigh. Don't inject I.V.
• When splenectomy is being considered, know that vaccine should be given at least 2 weeks before procedure to ensure adequate antibody response. This vaccine may be less effective in splenectomized patients.
• Vaccine protects against 23 pneumococcal types, accounting for 90% of pneumococcal disease.
• Know that the vaccine may be administered to children 2 years of age and over to prevent pneumococcal otitis media although the Center for Disease Control does not recommend otitis media as indicator for this vaccine.
• Vaccine is recommended for all adults over 65 years.
• Be aware that simultaneous administration with influenza virus vaccine is safe and effective.
• Keep refrigerated. Reconstitution or dilution not necessary.

• Warn patient about adverse reactions associated with this vaccine.
• Tell patient to treat fever with mild antipyretics.

---

# poliovirus vaccine, live, oral, trivalent (TOPV)
Orimune

# poliovirus vaccine, inactivated (IPV)
IPOL, Poliovax

*Pregnancy Risk Category: C*

## HOW SUPPLIED
*Oral vaccine:* mixture of three live viruses (types 1, 2, and 3), grown in monkey kidney tissue culture, in 0.5-ml single-dose Dispettes
*Inactivated virus vaccine injection:* mixture of three types of poliovirus (types 1, 2, and 3) grown in tissue culture. IPOL uses monkey kidney cultures; Poliovax uses human diploid cell cultures.

## ACTION
Promotes immunity to poliomyelitis by inducing humoral antibodies and antibodies in the lymphatic tissue.

## ONSET, PEAK, DURATION
An antibody response usually occurs within 7 to 10 days with TOPV; unknown with IPV. Peak effects occur in 21 days with TOPV; unknown for IPV. Duration is thought to last for years.

## INDICATIONS & DOSAGE
*Poliovirus immunization –*
**Children and nonimmunized adults:** 0.5 ml P.O. (TOPV), followed by a second dose of 0.5 ml in 6 to 8 weeks. A third 0.5-ml dose is given 6 to 12 months after second dose. A reinforcing dose of 0.5 ml should be given before entry to school.
**Infants:** 0.5 ml P.O. at 2 months, 4 months, and 18 months.
*Poliovirus immunization in persons who cannot receive TOPV –*
**Adults:** 0.5 ml S.C., followed by a second dose in 4 to 8 weeks. A third dose is given in 6 to 12 months.
**Children:** 0.5 ml S.C. at 2 months and 4 months. A third dose is given at 15 to 18 months. A reinforcing dose of 0.5 ml S.C. should be given before entry into school.

## ADVERSE REACTIONS
**Systemic:** *poliomyelitis, fever,* sleepiness, crying, decreased appetite, hypersensitivity reactions.
**Other:** erythema, induration, *pain* (at injection site).

## INTERACTIONS
*Immune serum globulin, plasma, whole blood:* antibodies in serum may interfere with immune response. Don't use vaccine within 3 months of transfusion.
*Tuberculin skin test:* may suppress response to skin test. Don't test for 6 weeks.

## CONTRAINDICATIONS
Oral vaccine is contraindicated in immunosuppressed patients; in those with cancer or immunoglobulin abnormalities; and in those receiving radiation, antimetabolite, alkylating agent, or corticosteroid therapy. These patients should receive IPV. Injectable vaccine is contraindicated in patients hypersensitive to neomycin, streptomycin, or polymixin B.

## NURSING CONSIDERATIONS
• Use with caution in siblings of child with known immunodeficiency syndrome. IPV is the preferred form.
• Obtain history of allergies and reaction to immunization.
• Do not administer oral form of vaccine parenterally.
• Keep frozen until used. Once thawed, if unopened, may refrigerate up to 30 days; if opened, up to 7 days. Thaw before administration.
• Know that color change from pink to yellow has no effect on efficacy of

the vaccine. Yellow color is caused by storage at low temperatures.
- **Alert:** Know that parenteral form should be administered to immunodeficient patients or those with altered immune status because they may be at risk for developing the disease if live virus vaccine is administered.
- Oral vaccine should be deferred in patients with vomiting or diarrhea. Both forms of vaccine should be deferred in patients with acute illness.
- Do not administer to neonates under 6 weeks.
- Be aware that the highest risk of poliovirus infection occurs after the first dose of the oral vaccine.
- Know that adults at high risk for exposure who have completed a primary course may receive another dose.
- Keep in mind that vaccine is not effective in modifying or preventing existing or incubating poliomyelitis.

☑ **PATIENT TEACHING**
- Make sure parents know the risks and benefits of this vaccine before it's administered.
- Warn patient or parents about adverse reactions associated with this vaccine.

## rabies vaccine, adsorbed

*Pregnancy Risk Category: C*

**HOW SUPPLIED**
*Injection:* single dose 1-ml vial

**ACTION**
Promotes active immunity to rabies.

**ONSET, PEAK, DURATION**
Onset unknown. Antibody levels peak within 2 weeks after the last of the three doses. Duration unknown, although at 9 to 12 months after immunization, 97% of patients continue to have antibody titers at or above a level of 0.1 IU (which is considered by the Centers for Disease Control and Prevention as the minimal acceptable antibody titer for complete rabies virus neutralization).

**INDICATIONS & DOSAGE**
*Preexposure prophylaxis rabies immunization for persons in high-risk groups—*
**Adults and children:** 1 ml I.M. at 0, 7, and 21 or 28 days for a total of three injections. Patients at increased risk for rabies should be checked q 6 months and given a booster vaccination, 1 ml I.M, as needed, to maintain adequate serum titer.
*Postexposure rabies prophylaxis—*
**Adults and children not previously vaccinated against rabies:** 20 IU/kg doses of human rabies immune globulin (HRIG) I.M. and five 1-ml injections of rabies vaccine adsorbed I.M. given on days 0, 3, 7, 14, and 28.
**Adults and children previously vaccinated against rabies:** two 1-ml injections of rabies vaccine adsorbed given I.M. given on days 1 and 3. HRIG should not be given.

**ADVERSE REACTIONS**
**Systemic:** *headache, nausea, slight fever, fatigue,* reaction resembling serum sickness, *abdominal pain, myalgia, dizziness.*
**Other:** *anaphylaxis; transient pain, erythema, swelling or itching at injection site;* aching of the injected muscle, mild inflammatory reaction at injection site.

**INTERACTIONS**
*Antimalarial drugs, corticosteroids, immunosuppressants:* decreased response to rabies vaccine. Avoid concomitant use.

**CONTRAINDICATIONS**
Contraindicated in patients who have experienced life-threatening allergic reactions to previous injections of this vaccine or to components of this vaccine, including thimerosal.

---

*Liquid form contains alcohol.   **May contain tartrazine.   †Canada only.   ‡Australia only.   ◇OTC.

## NURSING CONSIDERATIONS

• Use with caution in patients with a history of non-life-threatening allergic reactions to previous injections of the vaccine, in patients with hypersensitivity to monkey-derived proteins, and in children.

• Keep epinephrine 1:1,000 available to treat an anaphylactoid reaction.

• Administer as an I.M. injection into the deltoid region in adults and older children. For younger children, the midanterolateral aspect of the thigh also is acceptable. Know that this vaccine is not for use by the intradermal route. Take care not to inject the vaccine near a peripheral nerve or into adipose or subcutaneous tissue.

• Know that the vaccine is normally a light pink color because of the presence of phenol red in the suspension.

• Know that preexposure immunization should be delayed in persons with an acute illness.

• *Alert:* If patient experiences a serious adverse reaction to the vaccine, report the reaction promptly to the manufacturer: Michigan Department of Public Health, 517-335-8050 during working hours or 517-335-9030 at other times.

## ☑ PATIENT TEACHING

• Inform patient about adverse reactions associated with this vaccine and importance of alerting doctor so any serious adverse reaction can be reported.

• Caution patient not to perform hazardous activities if dizziness occurs.

---

# rabies vaccine, human diploid cell (HDCV)

Imovax, Imovax I.D.

*Pregnancy Risk Category: C*

## HOW SUPPLIED

*Intradermal injection:* 0.25 IU rabies antigen/dose
*I.M. injection:* 2.5 IU of rabies antigen/ml, in single-dose vial with diluent

## ACTION

Promotes active immunity to rabies.

## ONSET, PEAK, DURATION

Onset occurs within 1 week. Antibody levels peak after 1 to 2 months. Effects persist for 2 or more years.

## INDICATIONS & DOSAGE

*Postexposure antirabies immunization—*

**Adults and children:** five 1-ml doses of HDCV I.M. (for example, in the deltoid region). First dose given as soon as possible after exposure; an additional dose given on each of days 3, 7, 14, and 28 after first dose. If no antibody response after this primary series occurs, a booster dose is recommended.

*Preexposure prophylaxis immunization for persons in high-risk groups—*

**Adults and children:** three 1-ml injections administered I.M. First dose given on day 0 (the first day of therapy), second dose on day 7, and third dose on either day 21 or 28. Alternatively, 0.1 ml intradermally on the same dosage schedule.

## ADVERSE REACTIONS

**Systemic:** *headache,* dizziness, *nausea,* abdominal pain, diarrhea, muscle aches, *fever,* **anaphylaxis,** *serum sickness, fatigue.*

**Other:** *pain, erythema, swelling, or itching at injection site.*

## INTERACTIONS

*Antimalarial drugs, corticosteroids, immunosuppressants:* decreased response to rabies vaccine. Avoid concomitant use.

## CONTRAINDICATIONS

No contraindications reported for persons after exposure. An acute febrile

---

Reactions may be *common,* uncommon, *life-threatening,* or **COMMON AND LIFE-THREATENING.**

illness contraindicates use of vaccine for persons previously exposed.

## NURSING CONSIDERATIONS
• Use cautiously in patients with a history of hypersensitivity.
• Keep epinephrine 1:1,000 available to treat anaphylaxis.
• *Alert:* Do not use intradermal route for postexposure rabies vaccination.
• Know that the alternative regimen of 0.1-ml doses is only for preexposure prophylaxis. For postexposure prophylaxis, only use the 1-ml doses.
• Be aware that the Centers for Disease Control and Prevention recommends a booster dose with Imovax for all persons who may have been exposed to rabies since October 15, 1984 and who have received postexposure prophylaxis with Wyvac, unless acceptable titers were proven.
• Be prepared to stop corticosteroid therapy during immunizing period unless therapy is essential for the treatment of other conditions.
• Keep in mind that some patients who receive booster doses experience serum sickness-like hypersensitivity reactions. These reactions usually respond to antihistamines.

☑ **PATIENT TEACHING**
• Inform patient about adverse reactions associated with vaccine. Tell patient to report persistent or severe reactions to doctor.
• Stress importance of receiving booster, if appropriate for patient.

## rubella and mumps virus vaccine, live
Biavax II

*Pregnancy Risk Category: C*

## HOW SUPPLIED
*Injection:* single-dose vial containing not less than 1,000 TCID$_{50}$ (tissue culture infective doses) of the Wistar RA 27/3 rubella virus (propagated in hu-man diploid cell culture) and not less than 20,000 TCID$_{50}$ of the Jeryl Lynn mumps strain (grown in chick embryo cell culture)

## ACTION
Promotes immunity to rubella and mumps by inducing antibody production.

## ONSET, PEAK, DURATION
Although onset and peak unknown, most people acquire immunity in 2 to 6 weeks. Effects persist for 10 years or longer.

## INDICATIONS & DOSAGE
*Measles and mumps immunization –*
**Adults and children 1 year and older:** 0.5 ml (1,000 units) S.C.

## ADVERSE REACTIONS
**Systemic:** polyneuritis, rash, thrombocytopenic purpura, urticaria, fever, diarrhea, arthritis, arthralgia, *anaphylaxis,* lymphadenopathy.
**Other:** pain, erythema, induration (at injection site).

## INTERACTIONS
*Immune serum globulin, plasma, whole blood:* antibodies in serum may interfere with immune response. Don't give vaccine within 3 months of transfusion.
*Tuberculin skin test:* may temporarily decrease response to test. Defer skin testing.

## CONTRAINDICATIONS
Contraindicated in pregnant or immunosuppressed patients; in those with cancer, blood dyscrasia, gamma globulin disorders, fever, or active untreated tuberculosis; history of anaphylaxis or anaphylactoid reactions to neomycin or eggs; and in those receiving corticosteroid (except those receiving corticosteroids as replacement therapy) or radiation therapy.

---

*Liquid form contains alcohol.  **May contain tartrazine.  †Canada only.  ‡Australia only.  ◊OTC.

## NURSING CONSIDERATIONS
• Obtain history of allergies, especially anaphylactic reaction to antibiotics, and reaction to immunization.
• Keep epinephrine 1:1,000 available to treat anaphylaxis.
• Know that in patients with acute illness and after administration of immune serum globulin, blood, or plasma, the vaccination should be deferred.
• Use only diluent supplied. Discard 8 hours after reconstituting.
• Inject into outer upper arm. Don't inject I.V.
• Allow an interval of at least 3 weeks between BCG and rubella vaccines.
• Refrigerate and protect from light. Reconstituted solution is clear yellow; don't use if discolored.

### ☑ PATIENT TEACHING
• Inform patient about adverse reactions associated with vaccine.
• Stress to patients the importance of avoiding pregnancy for 3 months after vaccination. Offer to provide contraception information.

---

## rubella virus vaccine, live attenuated (RA 27/3)
Meruvax II

*Pregnancy Risk Category: C*

### HOW SUPPLIED
*Injection:* single-dose vial containing not less than 1,000 TCID$_{50}$ (tissue culture infective doses) of the Wistar RA 27/3 strain of rubella virus (propagated in human diploid cell culture)

### ACTION
Promotes immunity to rubella by inducing production of antibodies.

### ONSET, PEAK, DURATION
Although the precise onset and peak unknown, most patients develop immunity in 2 to 6 weeks. Effects persist for 10 years or longer.

### INDICATIONS & DOSAGE
*Measles immunization* –
**Adults and children 1 year and older:** 0.5 ml (1,000 units) S.C.

### ADVERSE REACTIONS
**Systemic:** polyneuritis, rash, thrombocytopenic purpura, urticaria, arthralgia, malaise, headache, sore throat, fever, arthritis, *anaphylaxis*, lymphadenopathy.
**Other:** pain, erythema, induration (at injection site).

### INTERACTIONS
*Immune serum globulin, plasma, whole blood:* antibodies in serum may interfere with immune response. Don't use vaccine within 3 months of transfusion. Immune serum globulin may be given 2 weeks before vaccine.
*Tuberculin skin test:* may temporarily decrease response to test. Defer skin testing.

### CONTRAINDICATIONS
Contraindicated in pregnant or immunosuppressed patients; in those with cancer, blood dyscrasia, gamma globulin disorders, fever, or active untreated tuberculosis; in those with a history of hypersensitivity to neomycin; and in patients receiving corticosteroid (except those receiving corticosteroids as replacement therapy) or radiation therapy.

### NURSING CONSIDERATIONS
• Obtain history of allergies and reaction to immunization.
• Keep epinephrine 1:1,000 available to treat anaphylaxis.
• Immunization should be deferred in patients with acute illness and after administration of human immune serum globulin, blood, or plasma.
• Use only diluent supplied. Discard 8 hours after reconstituting.

---

Reactions may be *common*, uncommon, *life-threatening*, or COMMON AND LIFE-THREATENING.

• Inject into outer upper arm. Don't inject I.V.
• Refrigerate and protect from light. Reconstituted solution is clear yellow; don't use if discolored.
• Allow at least 3 weeks between BCG and rubella vaccines.

☑ **PATIENT TEACHING**
• Inform patient about adverse reactions associated with vaccine.
• Stress to patient the importance of avoiding pregnancy for 3 months after vaccination. Offer to provide contraception information.

---

## tetanus toxoid, adsorbed

## tetanus toxoid, fluid

*Pregnancy Risk Category: C*

### HOW SUPPLIED
**tetanus toxoid, adsorbed**
*Injection:* 5 to 10 Lf (limit flocculation) units of inactivated tetanus/0.5-ml dose, in 0.5-ml syringes and 5-ml vials
**tetanus toxoid, fluid**
*Injection:* 4 to 5 Lf units of inactivated tetanus/0.5-ml dose, in 0.5-ml syringes and 7.5-ml vials

### ACTION
Promotes immunity to tetanus by inducing antitoxin production.

### ONSET, PEAK, DURATION
Although exact onset and peak unknown, most patients possess immunity after two doses. Effects unknown but may persist for 10 years or more.

### INDICATIONS & DOSAGE
*Primary immunization –*
**Adults and children 6 years and over:** 0.5 ml (adsorbed) I.M. 4 to 8 weeks apart for two doses; then third dose 6 to 12 months after the second. Alternatively, 0.5 ml (fluid) I.M. or S.C. 4 to 8 weeks apart for three doses; then fourth dose of 0.5 ml 6 to 12 months after third dose.
**Children 6 weeks to 6 years:** 0.5 ml (adsorbed) I.M. at ages 2, 4, and 6 months. A fourth dose is given at age 15 to 18 months. A fifth dose is given at age 4 to 6 years, just before entry into school, if indicated.
*Booster doses –*
**Adults:** 0.5 ml I.M. at 10-year intervals.

### ADVERSE REACTIONS
**Systemic:** tachycardia, hypotension, urticaria, pruritus, slight fever, chills, malaise, aches and pains, flushing, *anaphylaxis.*
**Other:** erythema, induration, nodule (at injection site).

### INTERACTIONS
*Chloramphenicol:* may interfere with response to tetanus toxoid.

### CONTRAINDICATIONS
Contraindicated in immunosuppressed patients and in those with immunoglobulin abnormalities or severe hypersensitivity or neurologic reactions to the toxoid or any ingredient in it, such as thimerosal. Also contraindicated in patients with thrombocytopenia or any coagulation disorder that would contraindicate I.M. injection unless the potential benefits outweigh the risks. Vaccination should be deferred in patients with acute illness and during polio outbreaks, except in emergencies.

### NURSING CONSIDERATIONS
• Use cautiously (adsorbed form) in infants or children with cerebral damage, neurologic disorders, or a history of febrile seizures.
• Obtain history of allergies and reaction to immunization.
• Determine date of last tetanus immunization.
• Keep epinephrine 1:1,000 available to treat anaphylaxis.

---

*Liquid form contains alcohol. **May contain tartrazine. †Canada only. ‡Australia only. ◇OTC.

• Know that vaccine is used for prevention, not treatment, of tetanus infections.
• Do not confuse this drug with tetanus immune globulin, human.
• Be aware that adsorbed form produces longer duration of immunity. Fluid form provides quicker booster effect in patients actively immunized previously.

☑ **PATIENT TEACHING**
• Advise patient to avoid use of hot or cold compresses at injection site; this may increase severity of local reaction.
• Instruct patient to report persistent or severe adverse reactions.

---

## typhoid vaccine

### typhoid vaccine, oral
Vivotif Berna Vaccine

*Pregnancy Risk Category: C*

### HOW SUPPLIED
*Injection:* suspension of killed Ty-2 strain of *Salmonella typhi;* 8 units/ml in 5-ml, 10-ml, and 20-ml vials
*Capsules (enteric-coated):* 2 to 6 × $10^9$ colony-forming units of viable *Salmonella typhi* Ty$^{21}$a and 5 to 50 × $10^9$ bacterial cells of nonviable Ty$^{21}$a$^2$

### ACTION
Provides active immunity to typhoid fever.

### ONSET, PEAK, DURATION
Immunity occurs at end of primary immunity immunization. Peak unknown. Effects persist for 3 to 5 years.

### INDICATIONS & DOSAGE
*Primary immunization –*
**Adults:** one capsule (oral vaccine) on alternate days taken 1 hour before meals for four doses. Protocol repeated as booster q 5 years.

**Adults and children over 10 years:** 0.5 ml S.C. (injection); repeated in 4 weeks. Protocol repeated as booster q 3 years.
**Children 6 months to 10 years:** 0.25 ml S.C. (injection); repeated in 4 weeks. Protocol repeated as booster q 3 years.

### ADVERSE REACTIONS
**CNS:** headache.
**GI:** nausea, abdominal cramps, vomiting.
**Skin:** rash, urticaria, swelling, pain, inflammation (at injection site).
**Other:** *fever,* malaise, *anaphylaxis,* myalgia.

### INTERACTIONS
*Sulfonamides, other antibiotics:* may impair antibody response. Don't use together.

### CONTRAINDICATIONS
Contraindicated in immunosuppressed patients and in patients with hypersensitivity to the vaccine. Vaccination should be deferred in patients with acute illness.

### NURSING CONSIDERATIONS
• Obtain history of allergies and reaction to immunization.
• Treat fever with antipyretics.
• Keep epinephrine 1:1,000 available to treat anaphylaxis.
• Shake thoroughly before withdrawing from vial.
• Do not give parenteral form intradermally.
• Refrigerate oral vaccine at 35.5° to 50° F (2° to 10° C).

☑ **PATIENT TEACHING**
• When administering oral vaccine, ensure that patient understands the importance of taking all four doses and following the alternate-day regimen.
• Tell patient to take oral vaccine with cold or lukewarm water and not to

---

chew or crush enteric-coated capsules.

• Inform patient about adverse reactions associated with vaccine.

---

## typhoid Vi polysaccharide vaccine
Typhim Vi

*Pregnancy Risk Category: C*

### HOW SUPPLIED
*Injection:* 0.5-ml syringe, 20-dose vial, 50-dose vial

### ACTION
Promotes active immunity to typhoid fever.

### ONSET, PEAK, DURATION
Unknown.

### INDICATIONS & DOSAGE
*Active immunization against typhoid fever—*
**Adults and children 2 years and older:** 0.5 ml I.M. as a single dose. Reimmunization every 2 years with 0.5 ml I.M. as a single dose, if needed.

### ADVERSE REACTIONS
**CNS:** *headache.*
**GI:** nausea, vomiting, abdominal cramps.
**Skin:** *pain or tenderness, induration, erythema* (at injection site), rash, urticaria.
**Other:** *malaise,* myalgia, fever.

### INTERACTIONS
None significant.

### CONTRAINDICATIONS
Contraindicated in patients with hypersensitivity to any component of the vaccine. The vaccine should not be used to treat a patient with typhoid fever or given to a patient who is a chronic typhoid carrier.

### NURSING CONSIDERATIONS
• Use with caution in patients with thrombocytopenia or a bleeding disorder and those who are taking an anticoagulant because bleeding may occur following an I.M. injection in these individuals.

• As with any vaccine, administration should be delayed, if possible, in patients with any febrile illness.

• Although anaphylaxis is rare, keep epinephrine available to treat an anaphylactoid reaction.

• Be aware that if vaccine is administered to immunosuppressed persons or those receiving immunosuppressants, the expected immune response may not be obtained.

• Know that persons who should receive the vaccine include people traveling to or living in areas of higher endemicity for typhoid fever.

• **I.M. use:** Administer as an I.M. injection into the deltoid region in adults and into the deltoid or vastus lateralis in children. It should not be administered in the gluteal region or areas where there may be a nerve trunk. Never inject I.V.

### ☑ PATIENT TEACHING
• Advise the patient to take all necessary precautions to avoid contact with or ingestion of contaminated food and water.

• Inform the patient that immunization should be given at least 2 weeks prior to expected exposure. Although an optimal reimmunization schedule has not been established, recommended reimmunization consists of a single dose for U.S. travelers every 2 years if exposure to typhoid fever is possible.

• Inform the patient about the adverse reactions associated with vaccine.

---

## varicella virus vaccine
Varivax

*Pregnancy Risk Category: C*

### HOW SUPPLIED
*Injection:* single dose vial containing 1350 PFV of Oka/Merck varicella virus (live)

### ACTION
Prevents chickenpox by inducing the production of antibodies to varicella-zoster virus.

### ONSET, PEAK, DURATION
Although the precise onset and peak unknown, most patients develop immunity in 4 to 6 weeks. Effects persist for at least 2 years.

### INDICATIONS & DOSAGE
*Prevention of varicella-zoster (chickenpox) infections –*
**Adults and children 13 years and over:** 0.5 ml S.C. followed by a second 0.5 ml dose 4 to 8 weeks later.
**Children 1 to 12 years:** 0.5 ml S.C.

### ADVERSE REACTIONS
**Other:** *fever, injection site reactions (swelling, redness, pain, rash),* varicella-like rash.

### INTERACTIONS
*Blood products, immune globulin:* may inactivate vaccine. Defer vaccination for at least 5 months following blood or plasma transfusions or administration of immune globulin or varicella-zoster immune globulin.
*Immunosuppressants:* risk of severe reactions to live-virus vaccines. Postpone routine vaccination.
*Salicylates:* Reye's syndrome has been reported. Avoid use of salicylates for 6 weeks after varicella infections.

### CONTRAINDICATIONS
Contraindicated in patients hypersensitive to the drug; in those with history of anaphylactoid reaction to neomycin, blood dyscrasia, leukemia, lymphomas, neoplasms affecting bone marrow or lymphatic system, primary and acquired immunosuppressive states, active untreated tuberculosis, or any febrile respiratory illness or other active febrile infection; and in pregnant patients.

### NURSING CONSIDERATIONS
• To reconstitute the vaccine, first withdraw 0.7 ml of diluent into the syringe to be used for reconstitution. Inject all the diluent in the syringe into the vial of lyophilized vaccine, and gently agitate to mix thoroughly. Administer immediately after reconstitution. Discard if not used within 30 minutes.
• Have epinephrine available for potential anaphylaxis reaction.
• Vaccine has been safely and effectively used in combination with measles, mumps, and rubella vaccine.
• Know that in clinical trials, the vaccine was less effective in adults as compared with children.
• Be aware studies are under way to determine the incidence of herpes zoster, which may occur following a latent period.
• *Alert:* Know that the vaccine contains a live attenuated virus. There is some evidence that children who develop a rash may be capable of transmitting the virus.
• A Safety Study protocol program is available for children and adolescents (ages 12 to 17 years) with acute lymphocytic leukemia. Doctors can enroll patients in this program by contacting Biopharm Clinical Services at (215) 283-0897.

### ☑ PATIENT TEACHING
• Inform patients or parents of adverse reactions associated with vaccine.
• Caution women of childbearing age

to notify doctor of suspected pregnancy before administration.

## yellow fever vaccine
YF-Vax

*Pregnancy Risk Category: C*

### HOW SUPPLIED
*Injection:* live, attenuated 17D yellow fever virus in 1- and 5-dose vials, with diluent; supplied only to designated yellow fever vaccination centers authorized to issue yellow fever vaccination certificates

### ACTION
Provides active immunity to yellow fever.

### ONSET, PEAK, DURATION
Effective immunity occurs in 7 to 10 days. Peak occurs within 28 days of vaccination. Immunity lasts more than 10 years and may persist for life.

### INDICATIONS & DOSAGE
*Primary vaccination –*
**Adults and children 9 months and over:** 0.5 ml deep S.C.; booster is 0.5 ml S.C. q 10 years.

### ADVERSE REACTIONS
**Systemic:** *anaphylaxis, fever, malaise,* myalgia, headache.
**Other:** mild swelling, pain (at injection site).

### INTERACTIONS
*Cholera vaccine:* concurrent administration may interfere with immune response to both yellow fever and cholera vaccines. Administer 3 weeks apart.
*Immunosuppressants:* may increase viral replication and the development of infection with yellow fever virus. Immunization should be deferred until immunosuppressant is discontinued.

### CONTRAINDICATIONS
Contraindicated in immunosuppressed patients; in those with cancer, gamma globulin deficiency, or hypersensitivity to chickens or eggs; or in those receiving corticosteroid or radiation therapy. Also contraindicated during pregnancy and in infants under 9 months, except in high-risk areas. Information regarding these areas can be obtained from the Centers for Disease Control and Prevention, Division of Vector-Borne Infectious Diseases, at (303) 221-6400.

### NURSING CONSIDERATIONS
• Obtain history of allergies, especially to chicken or eggs, and reaction to immunization.
• Keep epinephrine 1:1,000 available to treat anaphylaxis.
• Reconstitute with sodium chloride injection that contains no preservatives (they decrease potency).
• Keep frozen. Don't use unless shipping case contains some dry ice on arrival. Avoid vigorous shaking; carefully swirl mixture until suspension is uniform. Use within 1 hour after reconstituting. Discard remainder.
• Yellow fever vaccine should not be given within 1 month of other live virus vaccines; may be given concurrently with hepatitis B vaccine.

### ☑ PATIENT TEACHING
• Inform patient about adverse reactions associated with vaccine.
• Caution women of childbearing age to notify doctor of suspected pregnancy before administration.

---

*Liquid form contains alcohol. **May contain tartrazine. †Canada only. ‡Australia only. ◇OTC.

# 76

## Antitoxins and antivenins

black widow spider antivenin
Crotalidae antivenin, polyvalent
diphtheria antitoxin, equine
*Micrurus fulvius* antivenin

**COMBINATION PRODUCTS**
None.

## black widow spider antivenin
Antivenin *(Latrodectus mactans)*
*Pregnancy Risk Category: C*

**HOW SUPPLIED**
*Injection:* combination package — one vial of antivenin (6,000-unit vial), one 2.5-ml vial of diluent (sterile water for injection), and one 1-ml vial of normal equine (horse) serum (1:10 dilution) for sensitivity testing

**ACTION**
Unknown.

**ONSET, PEAK, DURATION**
Unknown.

**INDICATIONS & DOSAGE**
*Black widow spider bite —*
**Adults and children:** 2.5 ml I.M. in anterolateral thigh. Second dose may be needed. In severe cases, antivenin may be given I.V.

**ADVERSE REACTIONS**
**Systemic:** hypersensitivity reactions, *anaphylaxis, neurotoxicity.*

**INTERACTIONS**
None significant.

**CONTRAINDICATIONS**
Contraindicated in patients hypersensitive to the drug when desensitization is not feasible.

**NURSING CONSIDERATIONS**
• Immobilize patient; splint the bitten limb to prevent spread of venom.
• Obtain history of allergies, especially to horses, and reaction to immunization. Have epinephrine 1:1,000 available in case of anaphylaxis.
• For best results, know that antivenin should be given as soon as possible.
• Test for sensitivity before giving the drug, as ordered. Use 0.2 ml of a 1:10 dilution in 0.9% sodium chloride solution.
• **Alert:** Give I.M. dosage in anterolateral thigh so that a tourniquet may be applied if a systemic reaction occurs.
• **I.V. use:** Dilute antivenin in 10 to 50 ml of 0.9% sodium chloride solution and infuse over 15 minutes.
• Watch the patient for 2 to 3 days. Venom is neurotoxic and may cause respiratory paralysis and seizures.

☑ **PATIENT TEACHING**
• Explain to patient and family how drug will be administered.
• Instruct patient to report adverse reactions promptly.

## Crotalidae antivenin, polyvalent
*Pregnancy Risk Category: NR*

**HOW SUPPLIED**
*Injection:* combination package — one vial of lyophilized serum, one vial of diluent (10 ml of bacteriostatic water for injection), and one 1-ml vial of normal horse serum (diluted 1:10) for sensitivity testing

**ACTION**
Neutralizes and binds venom of snakes of the species crotalids (pit vi-

---

Reactions may be *common,* uncommon, *life-threatening,* or COMMON AND LIFE-THREATENING.

pers), including rattlesnakes, water moccasins, and copperheads.

## ONSET, PEAK, DURATION
Unknown.

## INDICATIONS & DOSAGE
*Crotalid (rattlesnake) bites* –
**Adults and children:** initially, 20 to 150 ml I.V., depending on severity of bite and patient response. If large amount of venom, more than 150 ml may be given I.V. directly into superficial vein. Subsequent doses based on patient's response; may need another 10 to 50 ml if swelling progresses, if systemic symptoms increase, or if new manifestations appear.

## ADVERSE REACTIONS
**Systemic:** *hypersensitivity reactions, anaphylaxis, serum sickness,* lymphadenopathy, arthralgia, fever.
**Other:** pain, erythema, urticaria.

## INTERACTIONS
*Antihistamines:* enhanced toxicity of crotaline venoms. Don't use together.

## CONTRAINDICATIONS
Contraindicated in patients hypersensitive to the drug.

## NURSING CONSIDERATIONS
• Use cautiously. Studies indicate that 60% of patients treated with this antivenin develop hypersensitivity.
• Immobilize the patient immediately. Splint the bitten extremity.
• Obtain history of allergies, especially to horses, and reaction to immunization. Have epinephrine 1:1,000 ready in case of hypersensitivity reaction.
• *Alert:* Type and crossmatch blood as soon as possible; hemolysis from venom prevents accurate crossmatching.
• For best results, antivenin should be administered as soon as possible.
• Test for sensitivity before giving drug. Give 0.02 to 0.03 ml of a 1:10 dilution in 0.9% sodium chloride solution intradermally. Read results after 5 to 10 minutes. Watch carefully for delayed allergic reaction or relapse.
• Be aware that children, who have less resistance and less body fluid to dilute venom, may need twice the adult dose.
• Give corticosteroids as prescribed. If a large number of vials are administered, serum sickness may result.
• Discard unused portion.

## ☑ PATIENT TEACHING
• Explain to patient and family that a test dose will be given first to check for sensitivity to the drug.
• Instruct patient to report adverse reactions promptly.

---

# diphtheria antitoxin, equine
*Pregnancy Risk Category: NR*

## HOW SUPPLIED
*Injection:* not less than 500 units/ml in 10,000-unit and 20,000-unit vials

## ACTION
Unknown.

## ONSET, PEAK, DURATION
Unknown.

## INDICATIONS & DOSAGE
*Diphtheria prevention* –
**Adults and children:** 5,000 to 10,000 units I.M.
*Diphtheria treatment* –
**Adults and children:** 20,000 to 80,000 units or more slow I.V. Additional doses may be given in 24 hours. I.M. route may be used in mild cases.

## ADVERSE REACTIONS
**Systemic:** hypersensitivity reactions, *anaphylaxis,* serum sickness (urticaria, pruritus, fever, malaise, arthralgia) may occur in 7 to 12 days.
**Other:** pain, erythema, urticaria.

## INTERACTIONS
None significant.

---

*Liquid form contains alcohol. **May contain tartrazine. †Canada only. ‡Australia only. ◇OTC.

**CONTRAINDICATIONS**
Contraindicated in patients hypersensitive to the drug.

**NURSING CONSIDERATIONS**
• Obtain history of allergies, especially to horses, and reaction to immunization. Have epinephrine 1:1,000 ready in case of hypersensitivity reaction. Antitoxin should be used with extreme caution in patients with history of allergic disorders.
• Test for sensitivity before giving the drug, as ordered.
• *Alert:* If patient has symptoms of diphtheria (sore throat, fever, tonsillar membrane), therapy should be started immediately, without waiting for culture reports.
• For storage, refrigerate antitoxin at 35.6° to 50° F (2° to 10° C). Before administering, warm to 90° to 95° F (32.2° to 35° C), never higher.

☑ **PATIENT TEACHING**
• Explain to patient and family that a test dose will be given first to check for sensitivity to the drug.
• Tell patient to report adverse reactions promptly.

---

## *Micrurus fulvius* antivenin

*Pregnancy Risk Category: NR*

**HOW SUPPLIED**
*Injection:* combination package with 10 ml of diluent

**ACTION**
Neutralizes and binds coral snake venom.

**ONSET, PEAK, DURATION**
Unknown.

**INDICATIONS & DOSAGE**
*Eastern and Texas coral snake bite –*
**Adults and children:** 30 to 50 ml (3 to 5 vials) slow I.V. through running I.V. of 0.9% sodium chloride solution. First

1 to 2 ml given over 3 to 5 minutes, and signs of allergic reaction watched for. If no signs develop, injection is continued. 100 ml or more may be needed.
   Not effective for Sonoran or Arizona coral snake bites.

**ADVERSE REACTIONS**
**Systemic:** hypersensitivity reactions, *anaphylaxis,* fever, arthralgia, lymphadenopathy.
**Other:** pain, erythema, urticaria.

**INTERACTIONS**
None significant.

**CONTRAINDICATIONS**
Contraindicated in patients hypersensitive to the drug.

**NURSING CONSIDERATIONS**
• Immobilize the patient and splint bitten limb to prevent spread of venom.
• Obtain accurate patient history of allergies, especially to horses, and reaction to immunization. Make sure epinephrine 1:1,000 is available in case of hypersensitivity reaction.
• Test for sensitivity before giving the drug, as ordered.
• Antivenin should be given as soon as possible (before onset of neurotoxic signs); asymptomatic patients should be treated because systemic signs usually develop later.
• Watch the patient carefully for 24 hours. Venom is neurotoxic and may cause respiratory paralysis.

☑ **PATIENT TEACHING**
• Explain to patient and family that a test dose will be given first to check for sensitivity to the drug.
• Tell patient to report adverse reactions promptly.

---

cytomegalovirus immune
    globulin, intravenous
hepatitis B immune globulin,
    human
immune globulin intramuscular
immune globulin intravenous
rabies immune globulin, human
respiratory syncytial virus
    immune globulin intravenous,
    human
Rh₀(D) immune globulin, human
Rh₀(D) immune globulin
    intravenous, human
tetanus immune globulin, human
varicella-zoster immune globulin

**COMBINATION PRODUCTS**
None.

---

## cytomegalovirus immune globulin (human), intravenous (CMV-IGIV)
CytoGam

*Pregnancy Risk Category: C*

### HOW SUPPLIED
*Powder for injection:* 2.5 g with 50 ml sterile water diluent

### ACTION
Provides passive immunity by supplying a relatively high concentration of immunoglobulin (Ig) G antibodies against CMV. Increasing these antibody levels in CMV-exposed patients may attenuate or reduce the incidence of serious CMV disease.

### ONSET, PEAK, DURATION
Unknown.

### INDICATIONS & DOSAGE
*To attenuate primary CMV disease in seronegative kidney transplant recipi-*ents who receive a kidney from a CMV seropositive donor—
**Adults:** administered I.V. based on time after transplantation:
  —within 72 hours: 150 mg/kg
  —2 weeks after: 100 mg/kg
  —4 weeks after: 100 mg/kg
  —6 weeks after: 100 mg/kg
  —8 weeks after: 100 mg/kg
  —12 weeks after: 50 mg/kg
  —16 weeks after: 50 mg/kg.
 Initial dose given at 15 mg/kg/hour. Increased to 30 mg/kg/hour after 30 minutes if no untoward reactions occur, then to 60 mg/kg/hour after another 30 minutes if no reactions occur. Volume should not exceed 75 ml/hour. Subsequent doses may be given at 15 mg/kg/hour for 15 minutes, increasing q 15 minutes in a stepwise fashion to 60 mg/kg/hour.

### ADVERSE REACTIONS
**Systemic:** hypotension, nausea, vomiting, wheezing, ***anaphylaxis.***
**Other:** flushing, chills, muscle cramps, back pain, fever.

### INTERACTIONS
*Live virus vaccines:* may interfere with the immune response to live virus vaccines. Vaccination should be deferred for at least 3 months.

### CONTRAINDICATIONS
Contraindicated in patients with sensitivity to other human Ig preparations or with selective IgA deficiency.

### NURSING CONSIDERATIONS
● Obtain vital signs before therapy.
● **I.V. use:** Reconstitute as follows: Remove tab portion of vial cap and clean rubber stopper with 70% alcohol or equivalent. Add 50 ml of sterile water for injection. To avoid foaming,

---

*Liquid form contains alcohol.  **May contain tartrazine.  †Canada only.  ‡Australia only.  ◇OTC.

do not shake vial. After adding water, release residual vacuum in vial to hasten dissolution. Rotate vial gently to wet all undissolved powder. Allow powder to dissolve for 30 minutes before administration. Inspect vial for clarity and particles.
• If possible, administer through a separate I.V. line, using a constant infusion pump. Filters are unnecessary. If unable to administer through separate line, piggyback into preexisting line of sodium chloride injection or one of the following dextrose solutions with or without sodium chloride: dextrose 2.5% in water, D₅W, dextrose 10% in water, or dextrose 20% in water. Do not dilute more than 1:2 with any of the above solutions.
• Begin infusion within 6 hours of reconstitution; finish within 12 hours.
• Monitor the patient's vital signs closely midinfusion, postinfusion, and before any increase in infusion rate.
• *Alert:* If anaphylaxis or drop in blood pressure occurs, discontinue infusion, notify the doctor, and be prepared to administer CPR and such drugs as diphenhydramine and epinephrine.
• Refrigerate powder for injection at 36° to 46° F (2° to 8° C). Do not store reconstituted drug.

☑ **PATIENT TEACHING**
• Review the drug therapy regimen with patient, and stress importance of compliance in follow-up visits.
• Instruct patient to report adverse reactions promptly.

---

# hepatitis B immune globulin, human
H-BIG, Hep-B-Gammagee, HyperHep

*Pregnancy Risk Category: C*

## HOW SUPPLIED
*Injection:* 1-ml, 4-ml, 5-ml vials

## ACTION
Provides passive immunity to hepatitis B.

## ONSET, PEAK, DURATION
Onset occurs in 1 to 6 days. Peak levels occur 3 to 11 days after I.M. administration. Protective for 2 months or more.

## INDICATIONS & DOSAGE
*Hepatitis B exposure in high-risk patients –*
**Adults and children:** 0.06 ml/kg I.M. within 7 days after exposure. Dosage repeated 28 days after exposure if patient refuses hepatitis B vaccine.
**Neonates born to patients who test positive for hepatitis B surface antigen (HBsAg):** 0.5 ml within 12 hours of birth.

## ADVERSE REACTIONS
**Systemic:** *anaphylaxis,* urticaria, angioedema.
**Other:** pain and tenderness at the injection site.

## INTERACTIONS
*Live virus vaccines:* may interfere with response to live virus vaccines. Defer routine immunization for 3 months.

## CONTRAINDICATIONS
Contraindicated in patients with a history of anaphylactic reactions to immune serum.

## NURSING CONSIDERATIONS
• Obtain history of allergies and reaction to immunizations. Make sure epinephrine 1:1,000 is available in case of anaphylaxis.
• Inject into anterolateral aspect of thigh or deltoid muscle areas in older children and adults; inject into anterolateral aspect of thigh for neonates and children under 3 years.
• For postexposure prophylaxis (for

example, needle stick, direct contact), know that drug is usually given with hepatitis B vaccine.

☑ **PATIENT TEACHING**
● Inform patient that pain and tenderness may occur at injection site.
● Tell patient to report any signs of hypersensitivity immediately.

## immune globulin intramuscular (IGIM, IG, gamma globulin)
Gamastan, Gammar

## immune globulin intravenous (IGIV)
Gamimune N, Gammagard S/D, Gammar-IV, Iveegam, Sandoglobulin, Venoglobulin-I

*Pregnancy Risk Category: C*

### HOW SUPPLIED
**immune globulin intramuscular**
*Injection:* 2-ml, 10-ml vials
**immune globulin intravenous**
*Injection:* 5% in 10-ml, 50-ml, 100-ml vials (Gamimune N)
*Powder for injection:* 50 mg protein/ml in 0.5-g, 2.5-g, 5-g, 10-g vials (Gammagard); 2.5-g vials (Gammar-IV); 500-mg and 1-g vials (Iveegam); 1-g, 3-g, 6-g vials (Sandoglobulin); 2.5-g, 5-g vials (Venoglobulin-I)

### ACTION
Provides passive immunity by increasing antibody titer. The primary component is IgG.

### ONSET, PEAK, DURATION
Onset and peak occur immediately after I.V. administration; peak occurs 2 to 5 days after I.M. injection. Duration unknown.

### INDICATIONS & DOSAGE
*Agammaglobulinemia or hypogammaglobulinemia –*

**Adults:** 30 to 50 ml I.M. monthly. Alternatively, 100 to 200 mg/kg I.V. (Gamimune N) monthly. Infused at 0.01 to 0.02 ml/kg/minute for 30 minutes. If no discomfort, rate increased to maximum of 0.08 ml/kg/minute. For Sandoglobulin, 200 mg/kg I.V. monthly. Infused at 0.5 to 1 ml/minute. After 15 to 30 minutes, infusion rate increased to 1.5 to 2.5 ml/minute.
**Children:** 20 to 40 ml I.M. monthly.
*Hepatitis A exposure –*
**Adults and children:** 0.02 ml/kg I.M. as soon as possible after exposure. Up to 0.06 ml/kg may be given q 4 to 6 months if exposure will be 3 months or longer.
*Modification or prevention of measles –*
**Adults and children:** 0.25 ml/kg I.M. within 6 days after exposure.
*Measles exposure in immunocompromised child –*
**Children:** 0.5 ml/kg I.M. within 6 days after exposure.
*Prophylaxis in primary immunodeficiencies –*
**Adults and children:** 100 to 200 mg/kg by I.V. infusion monthly (Gamimune only). Infusion rate is 0.01 to 0.02 ml/kg/minute for 30 minutes. If no discomfort occurs, rate increased to maximum of 0.08 ml/kg/minute.
*Idiopathic thrombocytopenic purpura –*
**Adults:** 0.4 g/kg Gamimune N or Sandoglobulin I.V. for 5 consecutive days or 1,000 mg/kg Gammagard. Additional doses may be given based on response. Up to three doses given (every other day) if necessary. Or, Venoglobulin-I 500 mg/kg daily for 2 to 7 days.

### ADVERSE REACTIONS
**Systemic:** headache, urticaria, malaise, fever, *anaphylaxis,* nausea, vomiting, chills, dyspnea, chest pain, hip pain, faintness, chest tightness, shortness of breath.

---

*Liquid form contains alcohol. **May contain tartrazine. †Canada only. ‡Australia only. ◊OTC.

**Other:** pain, erythema, muscle stiffness at injection site.

## INTERACTIONS
*Live virus vaccines:* Don't give within 3 months after administration of immune globulin.

## CONTRAINDICATIONS
Contraindicated in patients hypersensitive to the drug.

## NURSING CONSIDERATIONS
• Obtain history of allergies and reaction to immunizations. Make sure epinephrine 1:1,000 is available in case of anaphylaxis.
• **I.V. use:** Be aware that I.V. products are not interchangeable. Gammagard requires a filter, which is supplied by the manufacturer.
• Know that most adverse effects are related to a rapid infusion rate.
• When giving I.M., use gluteal region. Doses over 10 ml should be divided and injected into several muscle sites to reduce pain and discomfort.
• Know that immune globulin should not be given for prophylaxis against hepatitis A if 6 weeks or more have elapsed since exposure or after onset of clinical illness.

### ☑ PATIENT TEACHING
• Explain to patient and family how drug will be administered.
• Tell patient that local reactions may occur at injection site. Instruct him to notify doctor promptly if adverse reactions persist or become severe.

---

## rabies immune globulin, human
Hyperab, Imogam

*Pregnancy Risk Category: C*

## HOW SUPPLIED
*Injection:* 150 IU/ml in 2-ml, 10-ml vials

## ACTION
Provides passive immunity to rabies.

## ONSET, PEAK, DURATION
Although onset and peak are not closely defined, an adequate titer of passive antibody is present 24 hours after injection. Exact duration unknown, but it is short.

## INDICATIONS & DOSAGE
*Rabies exposure –*
**Adults and children:** 20 IU/kg I.M. at time of first dose of rabies vaccine. Half of dose is used to infiltrate wound area; the remainder is given I.M.

## ADVERSE REACTIONS
**Systemic:** slight fever, *anaphylaxis, angioedema, rash, nephrotic syndrome.*
**Other:** pain, redness, induration at injection site.

## INTERACTIONS
*Corticosteroids and immunosuppressants:* interferes with response. Avoid during postexposure immunization period.
*Live virus vaccines (measles, mumps, rubella, or polio):* interferes with response to vaccine. Delay immunization if possible.

## CONTRAINDICATIONS
None known.

## NURSING CONSIDERATIONS
• Use with caution in patients with history of prior systemic allergic reactions following the administration of human immunoglobulin preparations or in patients known to be hypersensitive to thimerosal or who have immunoglobulin A deficiency.
• Obtain history of animal bites, allergies, and reaction to immunizations. Have epinephrine 1:1,000 available to treat anaphylaxis.
• Ask patients when last tetanus im-

---

Reactions may be *common,* uncommon, *life-threatening,* or **COMMON AND LIFE-THREATENING.**

munization was received; many doctors order a booster at this time.
• Use only with rabies vaccine and immediate local treatment of wound. Don't give rabies vaccine and rabies immune globulin in same syringe or at same site. Give regardless of time between exposure and start of therapy.
• Don't administer live-virus vaccines within 3 months of rabies immune globulin.
• Don't administer more than 5 ml I.M. at one injection site; divide I.M. doses greater than 5 ml, and administer at different sites.
• Know that this immune serum provides passive immunity. Do not confuse this drug with rabies vaccine, which is a suspension of attenuated or killed microorganisms used to confer active immunity. The two drugs are often given together prophylactically after exposure to rabid animals.

☑ **PATIENT TEACHING**
• Inform patient that local reactions may occur at injection site. Instruct him to notify doctor promptly if reactions persist or become severe.
• Tell patient that a tetanus shot may also be necessary.

▼ *NEW DRUG*

## respiratory syncytial virus immune globulin intravenous, human
Respigam

*Pregnancy Risk Category: C*

### HOW SUPPLIED
*Injection:* 50 mg ± 10 mg/ml in a 50-ml single-use vial

### ACTION
Provides passive immunity to respiratory syncytial virus (RSV).

### ONSET, PEAK, DURATION
Unknown, although antibodies persist for at least 1 month.

### INDICATIONS & DOSAGE
*Prevention of serious lower respiratory tract infections caused by RSV in children with bronchopulmonary dysplasia (BPD) or history of premature birth –*
**Premature infants and children under 2 years:** Single infusion monthly. Give 1.5 ml/kg/hour I.V. for 15 minutes; then, if clinical condition allows a higher rate, increase to 3 ml/kg/hour for 15 minutes and then to a maximum of 6 ml/kg/hour until infusion ends. Maximum recommended total dosage per monthly infusion is 750 mg/kg.

### ADVERSE REACTIONS
**CNS:** dizziness, anxiety.
**CV:** fluid overload, tachycardia, hypertension, palpitations, chest tightness.
**GI:** vomiting, diarrhea, gastroenteritis, abdominal cramps.
**Respiratory:** respiratory distress, wheezing, rales, hypoxia, tachypnea, dyspnea.
**Skin:** rash, flushing, pruritus.
**Other:** fever, injection site inflammation, overdose effect, myalgia, arthralgia, hypersensitivity reactions including anaphylaxis.

### INTERACTIONS
*Live-virus vaccines, such as mumps, rubella, and especially measles:* may interfere with response. If such vaccines are given during or within 10 months after RSV-IGIV, be aware that reimmunization is recommended, if appropriate.

### CONTRAINDICATIONS
Contraindicated in patients with history of severe hypersensitivity to drug or other human immunoglobulin.

### NURSING CONSIDERATIONS
• Know that children with fluid overload should not receive drug.
• Safety and efficacy of drug have not been established in children with congenital heart disease (CHD). In clini-

cal trials, children with CHD, especially those with right to left shunts, had an increased frequency of cardiac surgery and severe, life-threatening adverse reactions.

• Know that first dose should be given before RSV season begins and that subsequent doses should be given monthly throughout the RSV season to maintain protection. Children with RSV should continue to receive monthly doses for duration of RSV season.

• **I.V. use:** Drug does not contain a preservative. Single-use vial should be entered only once, and the infusion should begin within 6 hours and be completed within 12 hours after vial is entered. Do not use if solution is turbid. Administer through I.V. line using a constant infusion pump. Predilution of drug before infusion is not recommended. Although filters are not necessary for the infusion, an in-line filter with a pore size larger than 15 micrometers may be used. Give the drug separately from other drugs.

• Adhere to infusion rate guidelines; most adverse reactions may be related to the rate used. In especially ill children with BPD, slower rates may be indicated.

• Assess cardiopulmonary status and vital signs before beginning the infusion, before each rate increase, and every 30 minutes thereafter until 30 minutes after completion of the infusion.

• Monitor closely for signs of fluid overload. Children with BPD may be more prone to this condition. Report increases in heart rate, respiratory rate, retractions, or rales. Have a loop diuretic, such as furosemide or bumetanide, available.

• **Alert:** If patient develops hypotension, anaphylaxis, or severe allergic reaction, stop infusion and administer epinephrine (1:1000), as ordered.

• Know that patients with selective IgA deficiency can develop antibodies to IgA and have anaphylactic or allergic reactions to subsequent administration of blood products containing IgA, including RSV-IGIV. Monitor these patients closely during subsequent RSV-IGIV administration.

☑ **PATIENT TEACHING**
• Explain to parents the importance of their child receiving drug monthly throughout the RSV season, even if already infected.

• Tell parents how drug is administered and which adverse reactions are associated with administration. Instruct parents to report adverse reactions promptly.

# Rh₀(D) immune globulin, human

Gamulin Rh, HypRho-D, HypRho D-MiniDose, MICRhoGAM, Mini-Gamulin Rh, RhoGAM

# Rh₀(D) immune globulin intravenous, human

WinRho SD

*Pregnancy Risk Category: C*

## HOW SUPPLIED
**Rh₀(D) immune globulin, human**
*Injection:* 300 mcg of Rh₀(D) immune globulin/vial (standard dose); 50 mcg of Rh₀(D) immune globulin/vial (microdose)
**Rh₀(D) immune globulin I.V., human**
*Injection:* 120 mcg, 300 mcg

## ACTION
Suppresses the active antibody response and formation of anti-Rh₀(D) in Rh₀(D)-negative, Dᵘ-negative persons, exposed to Rh-positive blood.

## ONSET, PEAK, DURATION
Unknown.

---

## INDICATIONS & DOSAGE
*Rh$_o$(D) immune globulin, human*
*Rh exposure –*
**Adults (after abortion, miscarriage, ectopic pregnancy; or postpartum):** transfusion unit or blood bank determines fetal packed RBC volume entering patient's blood; then one vial I.M. is given if fetal packed RBC volume is less than 15 ml. More than one vial I.M. may be required if large fetomaternal hemorrhage occurs; must be given within 72 hours after delivery or miscarriage.
*Transfusion accidents –*
**Adults and children:** consult blood bank or transfusion unit at once; must be given within 72 hours.
*After postabortion or miscarriage to prevent Rh antibody formation –*
**Adults:** consult transfusion unit or blood bank. One microdose vial will suppress immune reaction to 2.5 ml Rh$_o$(D)-positive RBCs. Ideally, should be given within 3 hours, but may be given up to 72 hours after abortion or miscarriage.
*Rh$_o$(D) immune globulin I.V., human*
*Rh exposure –*
**Adults (after abortion, aminocentesis [after 34 weeks gestation], or any other manipulation late in pregnancy [after 34 weeks gestation] associated with increased risk of Rh isoimmunization):** 120 mcg I.M. or I.V.; must be given within 72 hours after delivery, miscarriage, or manipulation.
*Pregnancy –*
**Adults:** 300 mcg (WinRho SD) I.M. or I.V. at 28 weeks gestation. If administered early in the pregnancy, additional doses should be given at 12-week intervals to maintain adequate levels of passively acquired anti-Rh antibodies. Then, within 72 hours of delivery, 120 mcg should be given I.M. or I.V. If 72 hours have elapsed, drug should be given as soon as possible, up to 28 days.
*Transfusion accidents –*

**Adults:** 600 mcg I.V q 8 hours or 1200 mcg I.M. q 12 hours until total dose administered. Total dose depends on volume of packed red blood cells or whole blood infused.
*Immune thrombocytopenic purpura (ITP) –*
**Adults:** initially 50 mcg/kg I.V. If hemoglobin is less than 10 g/dl, initial dose is reduced to 25 to 40 mcg/kg. Initial dose may be administered as a single dose or divided into two doses and administered on separate days. Then, 25 to 60 mcg/kg I.V. may be administered, as needed, to elevate platelet counts with specific dosage that's determined individually.

## ADVERSE REACTIONS
**Systemic:** slight fever.
**Other:** discomfort at injection site.

## INTERACTIONS
*Live virus vaccines:* may interfere with response. Delay immunization if possible.

## CONTRAINDICATIONS
Contraindicated in Rh$_o$(D)-positive or D$^u$-positive patients and those previously immunized to Rh$_o$(D) blood factor. Also contraindicated in patients with anaphylactic or severe systemic reaction to human globulin.

## NURSING CONSIDERATIONS
• Use extreme caution when administering drug to patients with IgA deficiency. Because of risk of the patient developing IgA antibodies and having an anaphylactic reaction, the doctor must weigh the potential benefits of treatment against the potential for hypersensitivity reactions.
• Obtain history of allergies and reaction to immunization. Be sure epinephrine 1:1,000 is available in case of anaphylaxis.
• **Alert:** Immediately after delivery, send a sample of neonate's cord blood to laboratory for typing and cross-

matching. Confirm if mother is $Rh_o(D)$-negative and $D^u$-negative. Administer drug to mother as ordered only if infant is $Rh_o(D)$-positive or $D^u$-positive.

• **I.V. use:** Reconstitute *only* with 0.9% sodium chloride solution. Do *not* administer with other products.

• Keep in mind that this immune serum provides passive immunity to the patient exposed to $Rh_o$-positive fetal blood during pregnancy. Prevents formation of maternal antibodies (active immunity), which would endanger future $Rh_o$-positive pregnancies.

• Know that vaccination with live virus vaccines should be deferred for 3 months after administration of $Rh_o(D)$ immune globulin.

• Know that MICRhoGAM is recommended for every patient undergoing abortion or miscarriage up to 12 weeks' gestation unless she is $Rh_o(D)$-positive or $D^u$-positive or has Rh antibodies, or unless the father or fetus is Rh-negative.

• Refrigerate at 36° to 46° F (2° to 8° C) and use within 4 hours of reconstitution. Discard unused drug.

☑ **PATIENT TEACHING**

• Explain to patient how drug protects future $Rh_o$-positive fetuses, if used because of pregnancy or explain to patient drug use in condition indicated.

• Warn patient about adverse reactions associated with drug.

## tetanus immune globulin, human
Homo-Tet, Hu-Tet, Hyper-Tet

*Pregnancy Risk Category: C*

### HOW SUPPLIED
*Injection:* 250-unit vial or syringe

### ACTION
Provides passive immunity to tetanus.

### ONSET, PEAK, DURATION
Onset unknown. Peak levels occur 2 to 3 days after I.M. injection. Protection lasts about 4 weeks.

### INDICATIONS & DOSAGE
*Tetanus exposure —*
**Adults and children:** 250 units I.M.
*Tetanus treatment —*
**Adults and children:** single doses of 3,000 to 6,000 units I.M. have been used. Optimal dosage schedules have not been established.

### ADVERSE REACTIONS
**Systemic:** slight fever, hypersensitivity reactions, *anaphylaxis,* angioedema, nephrotic syndrome.
**Other:** pain, stiffness, erythema at injection site.

### INTERACTIONS
None significant.

### CONTRAINDICATIONS
Contraindicated in patients with thrombocytopenia or any coagulation disorder that would contraindicate I.M. injection unless potential benefits outweigh the risks.

### NURSING CONSIDERATIONS
• Obtain history of injury, tetanus immunizations, last tetanus toxoid injection, allergies, and reaction to immunizations. Have epinephrine 1:1,000 available to treat hypersensitivity reaction.

• Know that tetanus immune globulin is used only if wound is more than 24 hours old or patient has had fewer than two tetanus toxoid injections.

• Thoroughly clean wound and remove all foreign matter.

• Inject into deltoid muscle for adults and children 3 years and over and into anterolateral aspect of the thigh in neonates and children under 3 years.

• Do not confuse this drug with tetanus toxoid. Tetanus immune globulin is not a substitute for tetanus toxoid, which

should be given at the same time to produce active immunization. Don't give at same site as toxoid.
• Be aware that antibodies remain at effective levels for about 4 weeks, which is several times the duration of antitoxin-induced antibodies. This protects patients for the incubation period of most tetanus cases.

☑ **PATIENT TEACHING**
• Warn patient about local adverse reactions associated with drug.
• Instruct patient to report serious adverse reactions promptly.

---

### varicella-zoster immune globulin (VZIG)
*Pregnancy Risk Category: NR*

#### HOW SUPPLIED
*Injection:* 10% to 18% solution of the globulin fraction of human plasma containing 125 units of varicella-zoster virus antibody (volume is about 1.25 ml)

#### ACTION
Provides passive immunity to varicella-zoster virus.

#### ONSET, PEAK, DURATION
Unknown, although antibodies persist for at least 1 month.

#### INDICATIONS & DOSAGE
*Passive immunization of susceptible immunodeficient patients after exposure to varicella (chickenpox or herpes zoster) –*
**Adults and children over 40 kg:** 625 units I.M.
**Children 30.1 to 40 kg:** 500 units I.M.
**Children 20.1 to 30 kg:** 375 units I.M.
**Children 10.1 to 20 kg:** 250 units I.M.
**Children to 10 kg:** 125 units I.M.

#### ADVERSE REACTIONS
**Systemic:** GI distress, malaise, headache, respiratory distress, ***anaphylaxis***.
**Other:** discomfort at injection site, rash.

#### INTERACTIONS
*Live virus vaccines:* may interfere with response. Defer vaccination for 3 months after administration of VZIG.

#### CONTRAINDICATIONS
Contraindicated in those with history of severe reaction to human immune serum globulin or thrombocytopenia.

#### NURSING CONSIDERATIONS
• Obtain accurate patient history of allergies and reaction to immunization. Make sure epinephrine 1:1,000 is available in case of anaphylaxis.
• For maximum benefit, administer as soon as possible after presumed exposure. May be of benefit when given as late as 96 hours after exposure.
• Administer only by deep I.M. injection into a large muscle mass such as the gluteal muscle. Never administer I.V.
• Refrigerate vial.
• Although usually restricted to children under 15 years, be aware that VZIG may be administered to adolescents and adults if necessary.
• VZIG is not recommended for nonimmunosuppressed patients.
• Be alert that drug is not commercially distributed. Available only from 20 regional U.S. distribution centers. These centers will distribute to Canada and overseas. Contact the Massachusetts Public Health Biologic Laboratories or The Centers for Disease Control and Prevention for more information.

☑ **PATIENT TEACHING**
• Warn patient about local adverse reactions associated with drug.
• Instruct patient to report serious adverse reactions to doctor promptly.

---

*Liquid form contains alcohol.  **May contain tartrazine.  †Canada only.  ‡Australia only.  ◇OTC.

# 78

## Biological response modifiers

aldesleukin
epoetin alfa
filgrastim
interferon alfa-2a, recombinant
interferon alfa-2b, recombinant
interferon alfa-n3
interferon beta-1b, recombinant
interferon gamma-1b
sargramostim

**COMBINATION PRODUCTS**
None.

---

## aldesleukin (interleukin-2, IL-2)
Proleukin

*Pregnancy Risk Category: C*

### HOW SUPPLIED
*Powder for injection:* 22 million IU/vial

### ACTION
Unknown, although stimulation of an immunologic host reaction to the tumor may be involved.

### ONSET, PEAK, DURATION
Unknown, although tumor regression may continue up to 12 months following initiation of therapy.

### INDICATIONS & DOSAGE
*Metastatic renal cell carcinoma* –
**Adults:** 600,000 IU/kg (0.037 mg/kg) I.V. q 8 hours for 5 days (total of 14 doses). After a 9-day rest, the sequence is repeated for another 14 doses. Repeat courses may be given after a rest period of at least 7 weeks.

### ADVERSE REACTIONS
**CNS:** *headache, mental status changes, dizziness, sensory dysfunction, special senses disorders, syncope, motor dysfunction, coma,* fatigue.
**CV:** *hypotension, sinus tachycardia, arrhythmias, bradycardia, PVCs, premature atrial contractions, myocardial ischemia, MI, CHF, cardiac arrest,* myocarditis, endocarditis, *CVA,* pericardial effusion, thrombosis, *capillary leak syndrome (CLS).*
**EENT:** conjunctivitis.
**GI:** *nausea, vomiting, diarrhea, stomatitis, anorexia, bleeding, dyspepsia, constipation.*
**GU:** *oliguria, anuria, proteinuria, hematuria, dysuria,* urine retention, urinary frequency.
**Hematologic:** *anemia, THRMOBOCYTOPENIA, LEUKOPENIA, coagulation disorders,* leukocytosis, eosinophilia.
**Hepatic:** *jaundice;* ascites; hepatomegaly; *elevated bilirubin, serum transaminase, alkaline phosphatase levels.*
**Respiratory:** *pulmonary congestion, dyspnea, pulmonary edema, respiratory failure, pleural effusion, apnea, pneumothorax,* tachypnea.
**Skin:** *pruritus, erythema, rash, dryness, exfoliative dermatitis,* purpura, alopecia, petechiae.
**Other:** *elevated BUN and serum creatinine levels; hypomagnesemia; acidosis; hypocalcemia; hypophosphatemia; hypokalemia; hyperuricemia; hypoalbuminemia;* hypoproteinemia; hyponatremia; hyperkalemia; arthralgia; myalgia; *fever; chills; abdominal, chest, or back pain; weakness; malaise;* edema; *infections of catheter tip, urinary tract, or injection site; phlebitis; SEPSIS; weight gain;* weight loss.

### INTERACTIONS
*Antihypertensives:* increased risk of hypotension. Monitor closely.
*Cardiotoxic, hepatotoxic, myelotoxic,*

---

Reactions may be *common*, uncommon, *life-threatening*, or COMMON AND LIFE-THREATENING.

*or nephrotoxic drugs:* enhanced toxicity. Avoid concomitant use.
*Corticosteroids:* decreased antitumor effectiveness of aldesleukin. Avoid concomitant use.
*Psychotropic agents:* unpredictable interaction. Because aldesleukin can alter CNS function, use together cautiously.

**CONTRAINDICATIONS**
Contraindicated in patients hypersensitive to the drug or any component of the formulation and in patients with abnormal cardiac (thallium) stress test or pulmonary function tests or organ allografts. Retreatment is contraindicated in patients who experience any of the following adverse effects: pericardial tamponade; disturbances in cardiac rhythm that were uncontrolled or unresponsive to intervention; sustained ventricular tachycardia (five beats or more); chest pain accompanied by ECG changes, indicating MI or angina pectoris; renal dysfunction requiring dialysis for 72 hours or more; coma or toxic psychosis lasting 48 hours or more; seizures that were repetitive or difficult to control; ischemia or perforation of the bowel; GI bleeding requiring surgery.

**NURSING CONSIDERATIONS**
• This drug should not be used unless the patient has had definitive tests documenting normal cardiac and pulmonary function. Use with extreme caution in patients with normal test results if they have a history of cardiac or pulmonary disease and in patients with a history of seizure disorders.
• Use cautiously and with close clinical monitoring because severe adverse effects usually accompany therapy at the recommended dosage.
• Use cautiously in patients who require large volumes of fluid (such as patients with hypercalcemia).

• Know that drug should be administered only in a hospital under the direction of a doctor experienced in the use of chemotherapeutic agents. An intensive care facility and intensive care or cardiopulmonary specialists must be available.
• Monitor hematologic tests, including CBC, differential, and platelet counts; serum electrolyte levels; and renal and liver function tests, and obtain chest X-ray before therapy, as ordered. Repeat daily during therapy.
• Treat patients with bacterial infections before therapy, as ordered.
• **I.V. use:** To avoid altering the pharmacologic properties of the drug, reconstitute and dilute carefully, and follow manufacturer's recommendations. Do not mix with other drugs or albumin.
• Reconstitute the vial containing 22 million IU (1.3 mg) with 1.2 ml of sterile water for injection. Do not use bacteriostatic water or 0.9% sodium chloride for injection; these diluents increase aggregation of drug. Direct the stream at the sides of the vial and gently swirl to reconstitute. Do not shake. The reconstituted solution will have a concentration of 18 million IU (1.1 mg)/ml. It should be particle-free and colorless to slightly yellow.
• Add the ordered dose of reconstituted drug to 50 ml of $D_5W$ and infuse over 15 minutes. Do not use an in-line filter. Plastic infusion bags are preferred because they provide consistent drug delivery.
• Discard unused portion. Vials are for single-dose use and contain no preservatives.
• Refrigerate powder for injection or reconstituted solutions. Return drug to room temperature before administering to patients. After reconstitution and dilution, administer within 48 hours.
• Be prepared to adjust dosage of other drugs as ordered to compensate for renal and hepatic impairment oc-

---

*Liquid form contains alcohol. **May contain tartrazine. †Canada only. ‡Australia only. ◇OTC.

curring during treatment. Know that dosage is modified by withholding a dose or interrupting therapy rather than by reducing the dose, as ordered.

• Withhold dose and notify doctor if patient develops moderate to severe lethargy or somnolence; continued administration can result in coma.

• Administer packed RBCs or platelets, as ordered. Severe anemia or thrombocytopenia may occur.

• **Alert:** Know that this drug has been associated with CLS, a condition caused by the loss of vascular tone, in which plasma proteins and fluids escape into the extravascular space. Mean arterial blood pressure begins to drop within 2 to 12 hours of treatment; edema and effusions may be severe, and death can result from hypoperfusion of major organs. Other conditions that accompany CLS include arrhythmias, MI, angina, mental status changes, renal insufficiency, respiratory distress or failure, and GI bleeding or infarction.

• Therapy is associated with impaired neutrophil function, which can lead to disseminated infection. Many studies employed prophylactic antibiotic therapy with oxacillin, nafcillin, ciprofloxacin, or vancomycin; check protocol and administer antibiotics, as ordered. Monitor for infection.

• Know that patients should be neurologically stable with a negative computed tomography scan for CNS metastases. Drug may exacerbate symptoms in patients with unrecognized or undiagnosed CNS metastases.

### ☑ PATIENT TEACHING
• Explain administration schedule to patient and caregivers, and stress importance of compliance.
• Instruct patient to report adverse reactions promptly.

## epoetin alfa (erythropoietin)
Epogen, Procrit

*Pregnancy Risk Category: C*

### HOW SUPPLIED
*Injection:* 2,000 units/ml, 3,000 units/ml, 4,000 units/ml, 10,000 units/ml

### ACTION
Mimics the effects of erythropoietin, a naturally occurring hormone produced by the kidneys. Epoetin alfa is one of the factors controlling the rate of RBC production. It acts on the erythroid tissues in the bone marrow, stimulating mitotic activity of erythroid progenitor cells and early precursor cells. It functions as a growth factor and as a differentiating factor, enhancing rate of RBC production.

### ONSET, PEAK, DURATION
Increase in reticulocyte count occurs within 7 to 10 days; RBC count, hematocrit, and hemoglobin increase in 2 to 6 weeks. Serum levels peak immediately after I.V. infusion or within 4 to 24 hours after S.C. administration. Hematocrit level may begin to decrease about 2 weeks after discontinuation.

### INDICATIONS & DOSAGE
*Anemia due to reduced production of endogenous erythropoietin caused by end-stage renal disease –*
**Adults:** dosage is individualized. Starting dose is 50 to 100 units/kg I.V. three times weekly. (Nondialysis patients with chronic renal failure or patients receiving continuous peritoneal dialysis may receive the drug by S.C. injection or I.V.) Dosage is reduced when target hematocrit level is reached or if the hematocrit rises more than 4 points in any 2-week period. Dosage is increased if hematocrit does not increase by 5 to 6 points

---

after 8 weeks of therapy. Maintenance dosage is highly individualized.

*Adjunctive treatment of HIV-infected patients with anemia secondary to zidovudine therapy –*

**Adults:** 100 units/kg I.V. or S.C. three times weekly for 8 weeks or until target hemoglobin level is reached. If response is not satisfactory after 8 weeks, dose may be increased by 50 to 100 units/kg I.V. or S.C. three times weekly. After 4 to 8 weeks, dosage may be further increased in increments of 50 to 100 units/kg three times weekly, up to a maximum of 300 units/kg I.V. or S.C. three times weekly.

*Anemia secondary to cancer chemotherapy –*

**Adults:** 150 units/kg S.C. three times weekly for 8 weeks or until target hemoglobin level is reached. If response is not satisfactory after 8 weeks, dosage may be increased up to 300 units/kg S.C. three times weekly.

## ADVERSE REACTIONS

**CNS:** *headache,* **seizures,** *paresthesia, fatigue,* dizziness.
**CV:** *hypertension, edema.*
**GI:** *nausea, vomiting, diarrhea.*
**Respiratory:** *cough, shortness of breath.*
**Skin:** *rash,* urticaria.
**Other:** increased clotting of arteriovenous grafts, *pyrexia, arthralgia, cough, injection site reactions, asthenia.*

## INTERACTIONS
None significant.

## CONTRAINDICATIONS
Contraindicated in patients with uncontrolled hypertension, hypersensitivity to mammalian cell-derived products or albumin (human).

## NURSING CONSIDERATIONS
• Monitor blood pressure before therapy. Up to 80% of patients with chronic renal failure have hypertension. Blood pressure may rise, especially when the hematocrit level is increasing in the early part of therapy.

• **I.V. use:** Give by direct injection without dilution. Solution contains no preservatives. Discard unused portion. Do not mix with other drugs.

• When used in HIV-infected patients, be prepared to individualize dosage based on response, as ordered. Dosage recommendations are for patients with endogenous erythropoietin levels of 500 units/L or less and cumulative zidovudine doses of 4.2 g/week or less.

• Be aware that patients treated with epoetin alfa may require additional heparin to prevent clotting during dialysis treatments.

• Monitor blood count, as ordered. Hematocrit level may rise and cause excessive clotting.

• Institute diet restrictions or drug therapy to control blood pressure. Reduce dosage in patients who exhibit a rapid rise in hematocrit (more than 4 points in any 2-week period), as ordered, to prevent hypertension.

• Know that the patient's response to epoetin alfa depends on the amount of endogenous erythropoietin in the plasma. Patients with levels of 500 units/L or more usually have transfusion-dependent anemia and will probably not respond to the drug. Those with levels below 500 units/L usually respond well.

• Keep in mind that patients with end-stage renal disease may experience an improved appetite and enhanced well-being as a result of increased hematocrit level.

## ☑ PATIENT TEACHING
• After injection (usually within 2 hours), inform patient that pain or discomfort in limbs (long bones) and pelvis and coldness and sweating are not uncommon. Symptoms may per-

---

*Liquid form contains alcohol. **May contain tartrazine. †Canada only. ‡Australia only. ◇OTC.

sist up to 12 hours and then disappear.

• Advise patient that blood specimens will be drawn weekly for blood counts and that dosage adjustments may be made based on the results.

• Advise patient to avoid driving or operating heavy machinery during initiation of therapy. A relationship between excessively rapid hematocrit rise and seizures may exist.

# filgrastim (granulocyte colony-stimulating factor; G-CSF)
Neupogen

*Pregnancy Risk Category: C*

## HOW SUPPLIED
*Injection:* 300 mcg/ml

## ACTION
A glycoprotein that stimulates proliferation and differentiation of hematopoietic cells. Filgrastim is specific for neutrophils.

## ONSET, PEAK, DURATION
Onset occurs in 5 to 60 minutes. Serum levels peak in 24 hours. Effects decline by 50% in first 24 hours after drug is discontinued, and absolute neutrophil count returns to pretreatment levels within 1 to 7 days.

## INDICATIONS & DOSAGE
*To decrease incidence of infection in patients with nonmyeloid malignant disease receiving myelosuppressive antineoplastic agents –*
**Adults and children:** 5 mcg/kg/day I.V. or S.C. as a single dose given no sooner than 24 hours after cytotoxic chemotherpy. Doses may be increased in increments of 5 mcg/kg for each chemotherapy cycle depending on the duration and severity of the nadir of the absolute neutrophil count (ANC).
*To decrease incidence of infection in patients with nonmyeloid malignant disease receiving myelosuppressive antineoplastic agents followed by bone marrow transplantation –*
**Adults and children:** 10 mcg/kg/day I.V. or S.C. at least 24 hours after cytotoxic chemotherapy and bone marrow infusion. Subsequent dosages adjusted according to the neutrophil response.
*Congenital neutropenia –*
**Adults:** 6 mcg/kg S.C. b.i.d. Dosage adjusted according to patient's response.
*Idiopathic or cyclic neutropenia –*
**Adults:** 5 mcg/kg S.C. daily. Dosage adjusted according to patient's response.

## ADVERSE REACTIONS
**CNS:** headache, weakness.
**CV:** *MI,* arrhythmias, chest pain.
**GI:** *nausea, vomiting, diarrhea, mucositis,* stomatitis, constipation.
**Hematologic:** *thrombocytopenia,* leukocytosis.
**Respiratory:** dyspnea, cough.
**Skin:** *alopecia,* rash, cutaneous vasculitis.
**Other:** *skeletal pain, fever, fatigue, hypersensitivity reactions.*

## INTERACTIONS
*Chemotherapeutic agents:* rapidly dividing myeloid cells are potentially sensitive to cytotoxic agents. Do not use concomitantly.

## CONTRAINDICATIONS
Contraindicated in patients hypersensitive to proteins derived from *Escherichia coli* or to the drug or its components.

## NURSING CONSIDERATIONS
• Obtain baseline CBC and platelet count before therapy, as ordered.
• **I.V. use:** Dilute in 50 to 100 ml of $D_5W$ and give by intermittent infusion over 15 to 60 minutes or continuous infusion over 24 hours. If the final concentration of the drug is going to

be 2 to 15 mcg/ml, add albumin at a concentration of 2 mg/ml (0.2%) to minimize binding of the drug to plastic containers or tubing.
• Once a dose is withdrawn, do not reenter vial. Discard unused portion. Vials are for single-dose use and contain no preservatives.
• Refrigerate at 36° to 46° F (2° to 8° C). Do not freeze; avoid shaking. Store at room temperature for a maximum of 6 hours; discard after 6 hours.
• Obtain CBC and platelet count twice weekly during therapy, as ordered. Patients who receive this drug may potentially receive high doses of chemotherapy, which may increase the risk of toxicities.
• Be aware that a transiently increased neutrophil count is common 1 or 2 days after initiation of therapy. Give daily for up to 2 weeks or until the ANC has returned to 10,000/mm$^3$ after the expected chemotherapy-induced neutrophil nadir, as ordered.

☑ **PATIENT TEACHING**
• If patient will be self-administering the drug, teach him how to administer it and how to dispose of used needles, syringes, drug containers, and unused medicine.
• Instruct patient to report persistent or serious adverse reactions promptly.

## interferon alfa-2a, recombinant (rIFN-A)
Roferon-A

*Pregnancy Risk Category: C*

### HOW SUPPLIED
*Injection:* 3 million IU/vial; 18 and 36 million IU/multiple-dose vial

### ACTION
Unknown. Appears to involve direct antiproliferative action against tumor cells or viral cells to inhibit replication and modulation of host immune response by enhancing the phagocytic activity of macrophages and by augmenting specific cytotoxicity of lymphocytes for target cells.

### ONSET, PEAK, DURATION
Onset unknown. Peak levels occur 3.8 hours after I.M. administration or 7.3 hours after S.C. administration. Duration unknown.

### INDICATIONS & DOSAGE
*Hairy-cell leukemia –*
**Adults:** for induction, 3 million units S.C. or I.M. daily for 16 to 24 weeks. For maintenance, 3 million units S.C. or I.M. three times a week.
*AIDS-related Kaposi's sarcoma –*
**Adults:** for induction, 36 million units S.C. or I.M. daily for 10 to 12 weeks. For maintenance, 36 million units S.C. or I.M. three times a week.

### ADVERSE REACTIONS
**CNS:** *dizziness, confusion,* paresthesia, numbness, lethargy, *depression, decreased mental status,* forgetfulness, *coma,* nervousness, insomnia, sedation, apathy, anxiety, irritability, fatigue, vertigo, gait disturbances, incoordination.
**CV:** hypotension, chest pain, arrhythmias, palpitations, syncope, *CHF,* hypertension, edema, *MI.*
**EENT:** *dryness or inflammation of the oropharynx,* rhinorrhea, sinusitis, conjunctivitis, earache, eye irritation.
**GI:** *anorexia, nausea, diarrhea, vomiting,* abdominal fullness, *abdominal pain,* flatulence, constipation, hypermotility, gastric distress, *weight loss, change in taste.*
**GU:** transient impotence.
**Hematologic:** *leukopenia,* mild *thrombocytopenia.*
**Hepatic:** *hepatitis.*
**Respiratory:** *cough, dyspnea.*
**Skin:** *rash, dryness, pruritus, partial alopecia,* urticaria, flushing.
**Other:** inflammation at injection site (rare), *flulike syndrome (fever, fatigue, myalgia, headache, chills, ar-*

---

*Liquid form contains alcohol. **May contain tartrazine. †Canada only. ‡Australia only. ◊OTC.

thralgia), diaphoresis, excessive salivation, cyanosis, night sweats, hot flashes.

## INTERACTIONS

*Aminophylline, theophylline:* may reduce theophylline clearance. Monitor serum levels.

*CNS depressants:* enhanced CNS effects. Avoid concomitant use.

*Live virus vaccine:* increased risk of adverse reactions and decreased antibody response. Don't use together.

## CONTRAINDICATIONS

Contraindicated in patients hypersensitive to the drug or to murine (mouse) immunoglobulin.

## NURSING CONSIDERATIONS

• Use cautiously in patients with severe hepatic or renal function impairment, seizure disorders, compromised CNS function, cardiac disease, or myelosuppression.
• Obtain allergy history. Drug contains phenol as a preservative and serum albumin as a stabilizer.
• Use S.C. administration route in patients whose platelet count is below 50,000/mm³.
• Administer at bedtime to minimize daytime drowsiness.
• Make sure patients are well hydrated, especially during initial stages of treatment.
• At the beginning of therapy, assess patients for flulike symptoms, which tend to diminish with continued therapy. Premedicate with acetaminophen to minimize symptoms.
• Monitor blood studies, as ordered. Interferons may decrease hemoglobin and hematocrit levels, WBC count, platelet count, and neutrophil count; increase PT and PTT; and increase serum levels of AST, ALT, lactate dehydrogenase, alkaline phosphatase, calcium, phosphorus, and fasting glucose, which are dose-related and reversible. Recovery occurs within several days or weeks after withdrawal of drug.
• Monitor for CNS adverse reactions, such as decreased mental status and dizziness, during therapy.
• For patients who develop thrombocytopenia, exercise extreme care in performing invasive procedures; inspect injection site and skin frequently for signs of bruising; limit frequency of I.M. injections; test urine, emesis fluid, stool, and secretions for occult blood.
• Keep in mind that severe adverse reactions may require dosage reduction to one-half or discontinuation of therapy until reactions subside.
• Know that different brands of interferon may not be equivalent and may require different dosage.
• ***Alert:*** Neurotoxicity and cardiotoxicity are more common in elderly patients, especially those with underlying CNS or cardiac impairment.
• Be alert that use with blood dyscrasia-causing medications, bone marrow suppressant, or radiation therapy may increase bone marrow suppressant effects. Dosage reduction may be required.
• Refrigerate the drug.

## ☑ PATIENT TEACHING

• Advise patient that laboratory tests will be performed before and periodically during therapy. Tests include a CBC with differential, platelet count, blood chemistry and electrolyte studies, liver function tests, and, if he has a preexisting cardiac disorder or advanced stages of cancer, ECGs.
• Instruct patient in proper oral hygiene during treatment because the bone marrow suppressant effects of interferon may lead to microbial infection, delayed healing, and gingival bleeding. This drug may also decrease salivary flow.
• Emphasize need to follow the doctor's instructions about taking and re-

---

Reactions may be *common,* uncommon, ***life-threatening,*** or **COMMON AND LIFE-THREATENING.**

cording temperature and how and when to take acetaminophen.

• Advise patient to check with the doctor for instructions after missing a dose.

• Tell patient that drug may cause temporary loss of some hair, which should return when drug is withdrawn.

• If patient will be self-administering drug, teach him how to prepare and administer it and how to dispose of used needles, syringes, containers, and unused medication.

• Warn patient not to have any immunization without the doctor's approval and to avoid contact with persons who have taken oral polio vaccine. Concurrent use with a live virus vaccine may potentiate replication of vaccine virus, increase adverse reactions, and decrease patient's antibody response. The patient is at increased risk for infection during therapy.

## interferon alfa-2b, recombinant (IFN-alpha 2)
Intron A

*Pregnancy Risk Category: C*

### HOW SUPPLIED
*Injection:* 3 million IU/vial with diluent, 5 million IU/vial with diluent, 10 million IU/vial with diluent, 18 million IU/vial with diluent, 25 million IU/vial with diluent, 50 million IU/vial with diluent

### ACTION
Unknown. Appears to involve direct antiproliferative action against tumor cells or viral cells to inhibit replication, and modulation of host immune response by enhancing the phagocytic activity of macrophages and by augmenting specific cytotoxicity of lymphocytes for target cells.

### ONSET, PEAK, DURATION
Onset and duration unknown. Serum levels peak in 3 to 12 hours.

### INDICATIONS & DOSAGE
*Hairy-cell leukemia* –
**Adults:** 2 million units/m² I.M. or S.C., three times a week.
*Condylomata acuminata (genital or venereal warts)* –
**Adults:** 1 million units for each lesion intralesionally three times a week for 3 weeks.
*AIDS-related Kaposi's sarcoma* –
**Adults:** 30 million units/m² S.C. or I.M. three times a week.
*Chronic hepatitis B* –
**Adults:** 30 to 35 units weekly I.M. or S.C., administered either as 5 million units daily or 10 million units three times a week for 16 weeks.
*Chronic hepatitis non A, non B/C (NANB/C)* –
**Adults:** 3 million units I.M. or S.C. three times a week.

### ADVERSE REACTIONS
**CNS:** *dizziness, confusion, paresthesia,* lethargy, *depression, difficulty in thinking or concentrating, insomnia,* anxiety, *fatigue, hypoesthesia, amnesia,* nervousness, *somnolence,* weakness, *malaise.*
**CV:** hypotension, *chest pain.*
**EENT:** visual disturbances, hearing disorders, pharyngitis, *nasal congestion, sinusitis,* rhinitis, stye.
**GI:** *anorexia, nausea, diarrhea, vomiting,* abdominal pain, *dyspepsia,* constipation, loose stools, eructation, *dry mouth,* dysgeusia, stomatitis, gingivitis.
**GU:** transient impotence, gynecomastia.
**Hematologic:** *leukopenia,* anemia, *thrombocytopenia.*
**Respiratory:** *dyspnea, coughing.*
**Skin:** *rash, dryness, pruritus, alopecia,* moniliasis, flushing, dermatitis.
**Other:** *flulike symptoms (fever, fatigue, headache, chills, muscle*

---

*Liquid form contains alcohol.  **May contain tartrazine.  †Canada only.  ‡Australia only.  ◊OTC.

aches), arthralgia, asthenia, rigors, back pain, increased diaphoresis.

## INTERACTIONS
*Aminophylline, theophylline:* may reduce theophylline clearance. Monitor serum concentrations.

*CNS depressants:* enhanced CNS effects. Avoid concomitant use.

*Live virus vaccines:* risk of enhanced adverse reactions to vaccine or decreased antibody response. Postpone immunization.

*Zidovudine:* may be synergistic adverse effects (higher incidence of neutropenia). Carefully monitor WBC count.

## CONTRAINDICATIONS
Contraindicated in patients hypersensitive to the drug.

## NURSING CONSIDERATIONS
• Use cautiously in patients with a history of CV disease, pulmonary disease, diabetes mellitus, coagulation disorders, and severe myelosuppression.

• Use S.C. administration route in patients whose platelet count is below 50,000/mm$^3$.

• Administer at bedtime to minimize daytime drowsiness.

• When administering interferon for condylomata acuminata, use only 10-million-IU vial because dilution of other strengths required for intralesional use results in a hypertonic solution. Do not reconstitute 10-million-IU vial with more than 1 ml of diluent. Use tuberculin or similar syringe and 25G to 30G needle. Do not inject too deeply beneath lesion or too superficially. As many as five lesions can be treated at one time. To ease discomfort, administer in evening with acetaminophen.

• Make sure patients are well hydrated, especially during initial treatment.

• At the beginning of treatment, monitor most patients for flulike symptoms, which tend to diminish with continued therapy. Premedicate with acetaminophen to minimize flulike symptoms.

• Monitor blood studies, as ordered. Interferons may decrease hemoglobin and hematocrit levels, WBC count, platelet count, and neutrophil count; increase PT and PTT; and increase serum levels of AST, ALT, lactate dehydrogenase, alkaline phosphatase, calcium, phosphorus, and fasting glucose, which are dose-related and reversible. Recovery occurs within several days or weeks after interferon withdrawal.

• Periodically monitor for adverse CNS reactions, such as decreased mental status and dizziness, during therapy.

• For patients who develop thrombocytopenia: exercise extreme care in performing invasive procedures; inspect injection site and skin frequently for signs of bruising; limit frequency of I.M. injections; test urine, emesis fluid, stool, and secretions for occult blood.

• Keep in mind that severe adverse reactions may require dosage reduction to one-half or discontinuation of therapy until reactions subside.

• *Alert:* Be aware that neurotoxicity and cardiotoxicity are more common in elderly patients, especially those with underlying CNS or cardiac impairment.

• Be alert that use with blood dyscrasia-causing medications, bone marrow suppressants, or radiation therapy may increase bone marrow suppressant effects. Dosage reduction may be required.

• Refrigerate the drug.

• Keep in mind that maximum response usually occurs 4 to 8 weeks after initiation of therapy. If results are not satisfactory after 12 to 16 weeks, a second course may be instituted. Patients with 6 to 10 condylomata may

---

Reactions may be *common,* uncommon, *life-threatening,* or COMMON AND LIFE-THREATENING.

receive a second course of treatment; patients with more than 10 condylomata may receive additional courses.

☑ **PATIENT TEACHING**
• Advise patient to avoid contact with persons with viral illness and those who have recently taken oral polio vaccine. The patient is at increased risk for infection during therapy.
• Advise patient that laboratory tests will be performed before and periodically during therapy. Tests include a CBC with differential, platelet count, blood chemistry and electrolyte studies, liver function tests, and, if he has a preexisting cardiac disorder or advanced stages of cancer, ECGs.
• Instruct patient in proper oral hygiene during treatment because the bone marrow suppressant effects of interferon may lead to microbial infection, delayed healing, and gingival bleeding. This drug may also decrease salivary flow.
• Advise patient to check with the doctor for instructions after missing a dose.
• Emphasize need to follow the doctor's instructions about taking and recording temperature and how and when to take acetaminophen.
• If patient will be self-administering drug, teach him how to prepare the injection and how to use a disposable syringe. Give him information on drug stability.
• Tell patient drug may cause temporary loss of some hair, which should return when drug is withdrawn.

---

**interferon alfa-n3**
Alferon N

*Pregnancy Risk Category: C*

**HOW SUPPLIED**
*Injection:* 5 million units/ml in 1-ml vials

**ACTION**
A naturally occurring antiviral agent derived from human leukocytes. It attaches to membrane receptors and causes cellular changes, including increased protein synthesis.

**ONSET, PEAK, DURATION**
Unknown.

**INDICATIONS & DOSAGE**
*Condylomata acuminata (genital or venereal warts)* –
**Adults:** 0.05 ml for each wart by intralesional injection. Treatment usually continues twice weekly for up to 8 weeks. Dosage should not exceed 0.5 ml (2.5 million units) per session.

**ADVERSE REACTIONS**
**CNS:** dizziness, light-headedness, insomnia, depression.
**CV:** hypotension.
**GI:** dyspepsia, heartburn, vomiting, nausea, diarrhea.
**Other:** *acute hypersensitivity reactions with mild to moderate flulike syndrome (myalgia, fever, chills, fatigue, headache), arthralgia, back pain, malaise, soreness at injection site, chest pains.*

**INTERACTIONS**
None significant.

**CONTRAINDICATIONS**
Contraindicated in patients hypersensitive to interferon alfa and in those with a history of anaphylactic reactions to murine (mouse) immunoglobulin, egg protein, or neomycin.

**NURSING CONSIDERATIONS**
• Use cautiously in patients with debilitating illnesses (uncontrolled CHF, unstable angina, severe pulmonary disease, coagulation disorders, seizure disorders, severe myelosuppression, or diabetes mellitus with ketoacidosis) because of the association of interferon with a flulike syndrome.

---

*Liquid form contains alcohol.  **May contain tartrazine.  †Canada only.  ‡Australia only.  ◇OTC.

• Although anaphylaxis hasn't been reported, be prepared to treat acute hypersensitivity reactions.
• Inject each lesion at the base of the wart, using a 30G needle.
• Administer acetaminophen for flu-like symptoms.

☑ **PATIENT TEACHING**
• Teach patient how to recognize symptoms of hypersensitivity: urticaria, tightness of the chest, wheezing, shortness of breath. Tell him to report such symptoms immediately.
• Explain to patient that warts will continue to disappear after completion of 8 weeks of therapy and discontinuation of drug.

# interferon beta-1b, recombinant
Betaseron
*Pregnancy Risk Category: C*

## HOW SUPPLIED
*Powder for injection:* 9.6 million IU (0.3 mg)

## ACTION
A naturally occurring antiviral and immunoregulatory agent derived from human fibroblasts. It attaches to membrane receptors and causes cellular changes, including increased protein synthesis.

## ONSET, PEAK, DURATION
Unknown.

## INDICATIONS & DOSAGE
*To reduce the frequency of exacerbations in patients with relapsing-remitting multiple sclerosis –*
**Adults:** 8 million IU (0.25 mg) S.C. every other day.

## ADVERSE REACTIONS
**CNS:** depression, anxiety, emotional lability, depersonalization, *suicidal tendencies,* confusion, somnolence, hypertonia, asthenia, migraine, *seizures, headache,* dizziness.
**CV:** palpitations, hypertension, tachycardia, peripheral vascular disorder, hemorrhage.
**EENT:** laryngitis, *sinusitis, conjunctivitis,* abnormal vision.
**GI:** *diarrhea, constipation, abdominal pain, vomiting.*
**GU:** *menstrual disorders (bleeding or spotting, early or delayed menses, fewer days of menstrual flow, menorrhagia).*
**Hematologic:** *decreased WBC and absolute neutrophil counts.*
**Respiratory:** *dyspnea.*
**Other:** *flulike symptoms (fever, chills, malaise, myalgia, diaphoresis),* elevated ALT levels, *elevated bilirubin levels,* breast pain, *pelvic pain; inflammation, pain, and necrosis at injection site, lymphadenopathy, pain,* generalized edema, *myasthenia, diaphoresis,* alopecia.

## INTERACTIONS
None significant.

## CONTRAINDICATIONS
Contraindicated in patients hypersensitive to interferon beta or human albumin.

## NURSING CONSIDERATIONS
• Use cautiously in women of childbearing age. Inconclusive evidence exists about the drug's teratogenic effects, but it may be an abortifacient.
• To reconstitute, inject 1.2 ml of the supplied diluent (0.54% sodium chloride injection) into the vial and gently swirl to dissolve drug. Do not shake. Reconstituted solution will contain 8 million IU (0.25 mg)/ml. Discard vials that contain particulate material or discolored solution.
• Inject immediately after preparation.
• Rotate injection sites to minimize local reactions.
• Refrigerate the drug or reconsti-

tuted product (up to 3 hours) at 36° to 46° F (2° to 8° C). Do not freeze.

☑ **PATIENT TEACHING**
• Warn patient of childbearing age about dangers to the fetus. If a patient becomes pregnant during therapy, tell her to notify the doctor and stop taking the drug.
• Teach the patient how to self-administer S.C. injections, including solution preparation, use of aseptic technique, rotation of injection sites, and equipment disposal. Periodically reevaluate the patient's technique.
• Advise patient to take this drug at bedtime to minimize the mild flulike symptoms that commonly occur.

---

## interferon gamma-1b
Actimmune

*Pregnancy Risk Category: C*

**HOW SUPPLIED**
*Injection:* 100 mcg (3 million units)/vial

**ACTION**
Acts as an interleukin-type lymphokine. It has potent phagocyte-activating properties and enhances the oxidative metabolism of tissue macrophages.

**ONSET, PEAK, DURATION**
Onset and duration unknown. Peak levels occur within 7 hours after S.C. use.

**INDICATIONS & DOSAGE**
*Chronic granulomatous disease –*
**Adults with a body surface area > 0.5 m²:** 50 mcg/m² (1.5 million units/m²) S.C. three times weekly, preferably h.s. The preferred injection site is the deltoid or anterior thigh muscle.
**Adults with a body surface area ≤ 0.5 m²:** 1.5 mcg/kg/dose three times weekly.

**ADVERSE REACTIONS**
**CNS:** *fatigue,* decreased mental status, gait disturbance, dizziness.
**GI:** *nausea, vomiting, diarrhea,* abdominal pain.
**Hematologic:** neutropenia, *thrombocytopenia.*
**Metabolic:** elevated liver enzyme levels (at high doses).
**Skin:** *rash, erythema or tenderness at the injection site.*
**Other:** flulike syndrome (headache, fever, chills, myalgia, arthralgia), weight loss, back pain, proteinuria.

**INTERACTIONS**
*Myelosuppressive agents:* possible additive myelosuppression. Monitor closely.
*Zidovudine:* increased plasma levels of zidovudine. Dosage adjustments are necessary when used concurrently.

**CONTRAINDICATIONS**
Contraindicated in patients hypersensitive to the drug or to genetically engineered products derived from *Escherichia coli.*

**NURSING CONSIDERATIONS**
• Use cautiously in patients with cardiac disease, including arrhythmias, ischemia, or CHF. The flulike syndrome commonly seen at high doses of the drug can exacerbate these conditions.
• Use cautiously in patients with compromised CNS function or seizure disorders. CNS adverse reactions that may occur at high doses of the drug can exacerbate these conditions.
• Use myelosuppressive agents together with caution.
• Premedicate with acetaminophen to minimize symptoms at the beginning of therapy. Flulike symptoms tend to diminish with continued therapy.
• Discard unused portion. Each vial

---

*Liquid form contains alcohol.  **May contain tartrazine.  †Canada only.  ‡Australia only.  ◊OTC.

is for single-dose use only and does not contain a preservative.
- Refrigerate drug immediately. Vials must be stored at 36° to 46° F (2° to 8° C); do not freeze. Do not shake the vial; avoid excessive agitation. Discard vials that have been left at room temperature for more than 12 hours.

☑ **PATIENT TEACHING**
- If patient will be self-administering drug, teach him how to administer it and how to dispose of used needles, syringes, containers, and unused medication.
- Instruct patient how to manage flu-like symptoms that commonly occur.

# sargramostim (granulocyte-macrophage colony-stimulating factor, GM-CSF)
Leukine, Prokine

*Pregnancy Risk Category: C*

## HOW SUPPLIED
*Powder for injection:* 250 mcg, 500 mcg

## ACTION
A glycoprotein containing 127 amino acids manufactured by recombinant DNA technology in a yeast expression system. It differs from the natural human granulocyte-macrophage colony-stimulating factor by substitution of leucine for arginine at position 23. The carbohydrate moiety may also be different. Sargramostim induces cellular responses by binding to specific receptors on cell surfaces of target cells.

## ONSET, PEAK, DURATION
Onset occurs within 30 minutes. Peak levels occur in 2 hours. Duration unknown.

## INDICATIONS & DOSAGE
*Acceleration of hematopoietic reconstitution after autologous bone marrow transplantation in patients with malignant lymphoma or acute lymphoblastic leukemia or during autologous bone marrow transplantation in patients with Hodgkin's disease*–
**Adults:** 250 mcg/m$^2$ daily for 21 consecutive days given as a 2-hour I.V. infusion beginning 2 to 4 hours after bone marrow transplantation.
*Bone marrow transplantation failure or engraftment delay*–
**Adults:** 250 mcg/m$^2$/day for 14 days as a 2-hour I.V. infusion. Dose may be repeated after 7 days of no therapy. If engraftment still has not occurred, a third course of 500 mcg/m$^2$/day I.V. for 14 days may be tried after another 7 days of no therapy.

## ADVERSE REACTIONS
**CNS:** *malaise, CNS disorders, asthenia.*
**CV:** *blood dyscrasias, edema,* hemorrhage, supraventricular arrhythmia, pericardial effusion.
**GI:** *nausea, vomiting, diarrhea, anorexia, hemorrhage, GI disorders, stomatitis.*
**GU:** *urinary tract disorder,* abnormal kidney function.
**Hepatic:** *liver damage.*
**Respiratory:** *dyspnea, lung disorders,* pleural effusion.
**Skin:** *alopecia, rash.*
**Other:** *fever, mucous membrane disorder, peripheral edema, sepsis.*

## INTERACTIONS
*Corticosteroids, lithium:* may potentiate myeloproliferative effects of sargramostim. Use cautiously.

## CONTRAINDICATIONS
Contraindicated in patients with excessive leukemic myeloid blasts in bone marrow or peripheral blood and in those with hypersensitivity to the

---

Reactions may be *common,* uncommon, *life-threatening,* or COMMON AND LIFE-THREATENING.

drug or any of its components or to yeast-derived products.

## NURSING CONSIDERATIONS

• Use cautiously in patients with pre-existing cardiac disease, hypoxia, preexisting fluid retention, pulmonary infiltrates, CHF, or impaired renal or hepatic function because these conditions may be exacerbated.

• **I.V. use:** Reconstitute with 1 ml of sterile water for injection. Direct stream of sterile water against side of vial and *gently swirl* contents to minimize foaming. Avoid excessive or vigorous agitation or shaking. Dilute in 0.9% sodium chloride solution. If final concentration is below 10 mcg/ml, add human albumin at a final concentration of 0.1% to the sodium chloride solution *before* adding sargramostim to prevent adsorption to components of the delivery system. For a final concentration of 0.1% human albumin, add 1 mg human albumin/1 ml sodium chloride. Administer as soon as possible after mixing and no later than 6 hours after reconstituting.

• Discard any unused portion. Vials are for single-dose use and contain no preservatives. Do not reenter the vial.

• Don't add other medications to infusion solution because no data exist regarding solution compatibility and stability.

• Refrigerate the sterile powder, reconstituted solution, and diluted solution for injection. Don't freeze or shake. Don't use after expiration date.

• Anticipate reducing dose by half or temporarily discontinue if severe adverse reactions occur and notify doctor. Therapy may be resumed when reactions abate. Transient rashes and local reactions at the injection site may occur; no serious allergic or anaphylactic reactions have been reported.

• Do not administer within 24 hours of last dose of chemotherapy or within 12 hours of last dose of radiotherapy because rapidly dividing progenitor cells may be sensitive to these cytotoxic therapies and drug would be ineffective.

• Monitor CBC with differential, including examination for presence of blast cells biweekly, as ordered. Stimulation of marrow precursors may result in rapid rise of WBC count. If blast cells appear or increase to 10% or more of the WBC count or if progression of the underlying disease occurs, know that therapy should be discontinued. If the absolute neutrophil count is above 20,000/$mm^3$ or if platelet count is above 50,000/$mm^3$, know that drug is temporarily discontinued or dose is reduced by half.

• Keep in mind that blood counts return to normal or baseline levels within 3 to 7 days after stopping treatment.

• Know that drug effect may be limited in patients who have received extensive radiotherapy to hematopoietic sites for treatment of primary disease in the abdomen or chest or who have been exposed to multiple agents (alkylating, anthracycline antibiotics, antimetabolites) before autologous bone marrow transplantation.

• Be aware that sargramostim is effective in accelerating myeloid recovery in patients receiving bone marrow purged from monoclonal antibodies.

• Keep in mind that the drug can act as a growth factor for any tumor type, particularly myeloid malignant disease.

## ☑ PATIENT TEACHING

• Review administration schedule with patient and caregivers, and address their concerns.

• Instruct patient to report adverse reactions promptly.

---

*Liquid form contains alcohol.   **May contain tartrazine.   †Canada only.   ‡Australia only.   OTC.

# 79

## Ophthalmic anti-infectives

bacitracin
chloramphenicol
ciprofloxacin hydrochloride
erythromycin
gentamicin sulfate
idoxuridine
natamycin
norfloxacin
ofloxacin 0.3%
polymyxin B sulfate
silver nitrate 1%
sulfacetamide sodium 10%
sulfacetamide sodium 15%
sulfacetamide sodium 30%
sulfisoxazole diolamine
tobramycin
trifluridine
vidarabine

### COMBINATION PRODUCTS

BLEPHAMIDE S.O.P. STERILE OPHTHALMIC OINTMENT: sulfacetamide sodium 10% and prednisolone acetate 0.2%.

CETAPRED OINTMENT: sulfacetamide sodium 10% and prednisolone acetate 0.25%.

CHLOROMYCETIN-HYDROCORTISONE OPHTHALMIC: chloramphenicol 0.25% and hydrocortisone acetate 0.5% (as the prepared solution).

CORTISPORIN OPHTHALMIC OINTMENT: polymyxin B sulfate 10,000 units, bacitracin zinc 400 units, neomycin sulfate 0.35%, and hydrocortisone 1%.

CORTISPORIN OPHTHALMIC SUSPENSION: polymyxin B sulfate 10,000 units, neomycin sulfate 0.35%, and hydrocortisone 1%.

ISOPTO CETAPRED: sulfacetamide sodium 10% and prednisolone acetate 0.25%.

MAXITROL OINTMENT/OPHTHALMIC SUSPENSION: dexamethasone 0.1%, neomycin sulfate 0.35%, and polymyxin B sulfate 10,000 units.

METIMYD OPHTHALMIC OINTMENT/SUSPENSION: sulfacetamide sodium 10% and prednisolone acetate 0.5%.

MYCITRACIN OPHTHALMIC OINTMENT: polymyxin B sulfate 5,000 units, neomycin sulfate 3.5 mg, and bacitracin 500 units.

NEOSPORIN OPHTHALMIC: polymyxin B sulfate 10,000 units, neomycin sulfate 1.75 mg, and gramicidin 0.025 mg.

NEOSPORIN OPHTHALMIC OINTMENT: polymyxin B sulfate 10,000 units, neomycin sulfate 3.5 mg, and bacitracin zinc 400 units/g.

NEOTAL: polymyxin B sulfate 5,000 units, neomycin sulfate 5 mg, and bacitracin zinc 400 units.

OPHTHOCORT: chloramphenicol 1.0%, polymyxin B sulfate 10,000 units, and hydrocortisone acetate 0.5%.

OPTIMYD: prednisolone phosphate 0.5% and sulfacetamide sodium 10%.

POLYSPORIN OPHTHALMIC OINTMENT: polymyxin B sulfate 10,000 units and bacitracin zinc 500 units.

POLYTRIM OPHTHALMIC: trimethoprim sulfate 1 mg and polymyxin B sulfate 10,000 units/ml.

PRED G: prednisolone acetate 0.6%, gentamicin sulfate equivalent to gentamicin base 0.3%, chlorobutanol 0.5%, petrolatum, white petrolatum, mineral oil, and lanolin alcohol.

STATROL: neomycin sulfate 3.5 mg and polymyxin B sulfate 10,000 units.

TOBRADEX: dexamethasone 0.1%, tobramycin 0.3%, chlorobutanol 0.5%, mineral oil, and white petrolatum.

VASOCIDIN OPHTHALMIC OINTMENT: sulfacetamide sodium 10%,

---

prednisolone acetate 0.5%, and phenylephrine hydrochloride 0.125%.
VASOCIDIN OPHTHALMIC SOLUTION: sulfacetamide sodium 10% and prednisolone phosphate 0.25%.
VASOSULF: sulfacetamide sodium 15% and phenylephrine hydrochloride 0.125%.

## bacitracin

*Pregnancy Risk Category: NR*

### HOW SUPPLIED
*Ophthalmic ointment:* 500 units/g

### ACTION
Inhibits protein synthesis. Bactericidal or bacteriostatic, depending on concentration and infection.

### ONSET, PEAK, DURATION
Unknown. Systemic absorption is negligible.

### INDICATIONS & DOSAGE
*Surface bacterial infections involving conjunctiva and cornea –*
**Adults and children:** small amount of ointment applied into conjunctival sac one or more times daily or p.r.n. until favorable response is observed.

### ADVERSE REACTIONS
**EENT:** slowed corneal wound healing, temporary visual haze.
**Other:** overgrowth of nonsusceptible organisms.

### INTERACTIONS
*Heavy metals (for example, silver nitrate):* inactivation of bacitracin. Don't use together.

### CONTRAINDICATIONS
Contraindicated in hypersensitive and atopic patients.

### NURSING CONSIDERATIONS
• Ophthalmic ointment may be stored at room temperature.

• Clean eye area of excessive exudate before application.

### ☑ PATIENT TEACHING
• Teach patient how to apply; tell him only a small amount of ointment is needed and that it may cause blurred vision. Advise patient to wash hands before and after administering and not to touch tip of tube to eye or surrounding tissue.
• Advise patient to watch for and report signs of sensitivity (itching lids, swelling, or constant burning).
• Tell patient not to share medication, washcloths, or towels with family members and to notify doctor if anyone develops same symptoms.
• Stress importance of compliance with recommended therapy.

## chloramphenicol

AK-Chlor, Chloromycetin Ophthalmic, Chloroptic, Chloroptic S.O.P., Chlorsig‡, Fenicol†, Isopto Fenicol†, Ophthoclor Ophthalmic, Pentamycetin†, Sopamycetin†

*Pregnancy Risk Category: NR*

### HOW SUPPLIED
*Ophthalmic ointment:* 1%
*Ophthalmic solution:* 0.5%
*Powder for ophthalmic solution:* 25 mg

### ACTION
Inhibits protein synthesis. Bacteriostatic or bactericidal, depending on concentration.

### ONSET, PEAK, DURATION
Unknown. Systemic absorption occurs, but has not been characterized; higher levels occur with ophthalmic ointment.

### INDICATIONS & DOSAGE
*Surface bacterial infection involving conjunctiva or cornea –*
**Adults and children:** 1 or 2 drops of solution instilled in eye q 3 to 6 hours

---

*Liquid form contains alcohol.   **May contain tartrazine.   †Canada only.   ‡Australia only.   ◇OTC.

or more frequently, if necessary. Or, a small amount of ointment applied to lower conjunctival sac q 3 to 6 hours or more frequently, if necessary. Continued for at least 48 hours after eye appears normal.

## ADVERSE REACTIONS
**EENT:** optic atrophy in children, stinging or burning of eye after instillation, blurred vision (with ointment). **Hematologic:** *bone marrow hypoplasia with prolonged use, aplastic anemia.*
**Skin:** dermatitis.
**Other:** overgrowth of nonsusceptible organisms; hypersensitivity reactions, including itching and burning eye, angioedema.

## INTERACTIONS
None significant.

## CONTRAINDICATIONS
Contraindicated in patients hypersensitive to the drug.

## NURSING CONSIDERATIONS
• If chloramphenicol drops are to be given every hour and then tapered, follow order closely to ensure adequate anterior chamber levels.
• Reconstitute powder for ophthalmic solution with supplied diluent. Use 5 ml of diluent to make a 0.5% solution, 10 ml of diluent to make a 0.25% solution, or 15 ml to make a 0.16% solution.
• Store in tightly closed, light-resistant container.
• If patients have more than a superficial infection, anticipate using systemic therapy as well.

## ☑ PATIENT TEACHING
• Teach patient how to instill drops or apply ointment. Advise him to wash hands before and after administering ointment or solution, and warn him not to touch tip of applicator to eye or surrounding tissue.
• Tell patient to clean eye area of excessive exudate before application.
• Instruct patient to apply light finger pressure on lacrimal sac for 1 minute after drops are instilled.
• Tell patient not to share medication, washcloths, or towels with family members and to notify doctor if anyone develops same symptoms.
• Tell patient to watch for and report signs of sensitivity (itching lids, swelling, or constant burning).
• Tell patient to notify the doctor if no improvement occurs in 3 days.
• Stress importance of compliance with recommended therapy.

---

# ciprofloxacin hydrochloride
Ciloxan

*Pregnancy Risk Category: C*

## HOW SUPPLIED
*Ophthalmic solution:* 0.3% (base) in 2.5- and 5-ml containers

## ACTION
Inhibits bacterial DNA gyrase, an enzyme necessary for bacterial replication. Bacteriostatic or bactericidal, depending on concentration.

## ONSET, PEAK, DURATION
Unknown. Systemic absorption is negligible.

## INDICATIONS & DOSAGE
*Corneal ulcers caused by* Pseudomonas aeruginosa, Staphylococcus aureus, S. epidermidis, Streptococcus pneumoniae, *and possibly* Serratia marcescens *and* Streptococcus viridans—
**Adults and children over 12 years:** 2 drops in the affected eye q 15 minutes for the first 6 hours; then 2 drops q 30 minutes for the remainder of the first day. On day 2, 2 drops hourly. On days 3 to 14, 2 drops q 4 hours.
*Bacterial conjunctivitis caused by* Staphylococcus aureus *and* S. epider-

midis *and possibly* Streptococcus pneumoniae —
**Adults and children over 12 years:** 1 or 2 drops into the conjunctival sac of the affected eye q 2 hours while awake for the first 2 days. Then 1 or 2 drops q 4 hours while awake for the next 5 days.

## ADVERSE REACTIONS
**EENT:** *local burning or discomfort, white crystalline precipitate* (in the superficial portion of the corneal defect in patients with corneal ulcers), *margin crusting, crystals or scales, foreign body sensation, itching, conjunctival hyperemia,* bad or bitter taste in mouth, corneal staining, allergic reactions, keratopathy, lid edema, tearing, photophobia, decreased vision.
**GI:** nausea.

## INTERACTIONS
None significant.

## CONTRAINDICATIONS
Contraindicated in patients with a history of hypersensitivity to ciprofloxacin or other fluoroquinolone antibiotics.

## NURSING CONSIDERATIONS
• Be aware that it's unknown if drug is excreted in breast milk after application to the eye; however, systemically administered ciprofloxacin has been detected in human milk. Use caution.
• *Alert:* Discontinue drug at the first sign of hypersensitivity reactions, such as rash, and notify doctor. Serious hypersensitivity reactions, including anaphylaxis, have occurred in patients receiving systemic fluoroquinolone therapy.
• If corneal epithelium is still compromised after 14 days of treatment, continue therapy, as ordered.
• Institute appropriate therapy if superinfection occurs. Prolonged use may result in overgrowth of nonsusceptible organisms, including fungi.

## ☑ PATIENT TEACHING
• Tell patient to clean eye area of excessive exudate before instilling.
• Teach patient how to instill drops. Advise him to wash hands before and after administering solution and not to touch tip of dropper to eye or surrounding tissues.
• Instruct patient to apply light finger pressure on lacrimal sac for 1 minute after drops are instilled.
• Tell patient not to share medication, washcloths, or towels with family members and to notify doctor if anyone develops same symptoms.
• Stress importance of compliance with recommended therapy.

# erythromycin
Ilotycin Ophthalmic Ointment

*Pregnancy Risk Category: NR*

## HOW SUPPLIED
*Ophthalmic ointment:* 0.5%

## ACTION
Inhibits protein synthesis. Bacteriostatic, but may be bactericidal in high concentrations or against highly susceptible organisms.

## ONSET, PEAK, DURATION
Unknown. Systemic absorption is negligible.

## INDICATIONS & DOSAGE
*Acute and chronic conjunctivitis, trachoma, other eye infections —*
**Adults and children:** 1 cm in length applied directly to the infected eye up to six times daily, depending on severity of infection.
*Prophylaxis of ophthalmia neonatorum due to* Neisseria gonorrhoeae *or* Chlamydia trachomatis —
**Neonates:** a ribbon of ointment approximately 1 cm long applied in the lower conjunctival sac of each eye shortly after birth.

---

## ADVERSE REACTIONS
**EENT:** slowed corneal wound healing, blurred vision.
**Skin:** urticaria, dermatitis.
**Other:** overgrowth of nonsusceptible organisms with long-term use; hypersensitivity reactions, including itching and burning eyes.

## INTERACTIONS
None significant.

## CONTRAINDICATIONS
Contraindicated in patients hypersensitive to the drug.

## NURSING CONSIDERATIONS
• For prophylaxis of ophthalmia neonatorum, ointment should be applied no later than 1 hour after birth. Used in neonates born either by vaginal delivery or by cesarean section. Gently massage the eyelids for 1 minute to spread the ointment.
• Be aware that drug has a limited antibacterial spectrum.
• To be used only when sensitivity studies show it is effective against infecting organisms. Not for use in infections of unknown etiology.
• Store at room temperature in tightly closed, light-resistant container.

## ☑ PATIENT TEACHING
• Tell patient to clean eye area of excessive exudate before application.
• Teach patient how to apply. Advise him to wash hands before and after administering ointment, and warn him not to touch tip of applicator to eye or surrounding tissue.
• Instruct patient to apply light finger pressure on lacrimal sac for 1 minute after administering.
• Warn patient that ointment may cause blurred vision.
• Advise patient to watch for and report signs of sensitivity (itching lids, swelling, or constant burning).
• Tell patient not to share medication, washcloths, or towels with family members and to notify doctor if anyone develops same symptoms.
• Stress importance of compliance with recommended therapy.

---

# gentamicin sulfate
Garamycin Ophthalmic, Genoptic, Gentacidin, Gentak, Ocu-Gent

*Pregnancy Risk Category: C*

## HOW SUPPLIED
*Ophthalmic ointment:* 0.3% (base)
*Ophthalmic solution:* 0.3% (base)

## ACTION
Unknown. Thought to inhibit protein synthesis and is usually bactericidal.

## ONSET, PEAK, DURATION
Unknown. Only small amounts of the drug are absorbed systemically.

## INDICATIONS & DOSAGE
*External ocular infections (conjunctivitis, keratoconjunctivitis, corneal ulcers, blepharitis, blepharoconjunctivitis, meibomianitis, and dacryocystitis) caused by susceptible organisms, especially* Pseudomonas aeruginosa, Proteus, Klebsiella pneumoniae, Escherichia coli, *and other gram-negative organisms*—
**Adults and children:** 1 to 2 drops instilled in eye q 4 hours. In severe infections, up to 2 drops q hour. Alternatively, ointment applied to lower conjunctival sac b.i.d. or t.i.d.

## ADVERSE REACTIONS
**EENT:** burning, stinging, or blurred vision (with ointment), transient irritation (from solution), conjunctival hyperemia.
**Other:** hypersensitivity reactions; overgrowth of nonsusceptible organisms with long-term use.
  Systemic absorption from excessive use may cause systemic toxicities.

---

Reactions may be *common,* uncommon, *life-threatening,* or **COMMON AND LIFE-THREATENING.**

## INTERACTIONS
None significant.

## CONTRAINDICATIONS
Contraindicated in patients hypersensitive to the drug.

## NURSING CONSIDERATIONS
• Use cautiously in patients with history of sensitivity to aminoglycosides because cross-sensitivity may occur.
• Have culture taken before giving drug. Therapy may begin before culture results are known.
• If ophthalmic gentamicin is given concomitantly with systemic gentamicin, monitor serum gentamicin levels.
• Know that solution is not for injection into the conjunctiva or anterior chamber of the eye.
• Store away from heat.

## ☑ PATIENT TEACHING
• Tell patient to clean eye area of excessive exudate before instilling.
• Teach patient how to instill drops or apply ointment. Advise him to wash hands before and after administering ointment or solution and not to touch tip of dropper or tube to eye or surrounding tissues.
• Instruct patient to apply light finger pressure on lacrimal sac for 1 minute after drops are instilled.
• Tell patient to watch for and report signs of sensitivity (itching lids, swelling, or constant burning).
• Tell patient not to share medication, washcloths, or towels with family members and to notify doctor if anyone develops same symptoms.
• **Alert:** Stress importance of following recommended therapy. *Pseudomonas* infections can cause complete vision loss within 24 hours if infection is not controlled.

# idoxuridine (IDU)
Herplex, Stoxil

*Pregnancy Risk Category: NR*

## HOW SUPPLIED
*Ophthalmic ointment:* 0.5%
*Ophthalmic solution:* 0.1%

## ACTION
Interferes with DNA synthesis.

## ONSET, PEAK, DURATION
Unknown. Systemic absorption is unlikely.

## INDICATIONS & DOSAGE
*Herpes simplex keratitis –*
**Adults and children:** 1 drop of solution instilled into conjunctival sac q hour during day and q 2 hours at night, or 1 cm strip of ointment applied to conjunctival sac q 4 hours or 5 times daily, with last dose h.s.

## ADVERSE REACTIONS
**EENT:** temporary visual haze; blurred vision (with ointment); irritation, pain, burning, or inflammation of eye; mild edema of eyelid or cornea; photophobia; small punctate defects in corneal epithelium; corneal ulceration; slowed corneal wound healing (with ointment).
**Other:** hypersensitivity reactions.

## INTERACTIONS
*Boric acid:* precipitate formation; increased risk of ocular toxicity. Avoid concomitant use.

## CONTRAINDICATIONS
Contraindicated in patients with hypersensitivity to the drug.

## NURSING CONSIDERATIONS
• Do not mix idoxuridine with other topical eye medications.
• Keep in mind that drug is not for long-term use. Therapy should not continue longer than 21 days.

• Keep idoxuridine 0.1% solution in a tightly closed, light-resistant container at room temperature.

### ☑ PATIENT TEACHING

• Advise patient not to use old solution; causes ocular burning and has no antiviral activity.
• Tell patient to clean eye area of excessive exudate before application.
• Teach patient how to instill drops or apply ointment. Advise him to wash hands before and after administering, and warn him not to touch tip of dropper to eye or surrounding tissue.
• Instruct patient to apply light finger pressure on lacrimal sac for 1 minute after drops are instilled.
• Advise patient to watch for and report signs of sensitivity (itching lids, swelling, or constant burning).
• Also instruct patient to notify his doctor if symptoms do not diminish in 7 days; drug will need to be discontinued and alternative therapy begun.
• Tell patient not to share medication, washcloths, or towels with family members and to notify doctor if anyone develops same symptoms.
• Tell patient to minimize photophobia by wearing sunglasses and avoiding prolonged exposure to sunlight.
• Stress importance of compliance with recommended therapy.

## natamycin
Natacyn

*Pregnancy Risk Category: NR*

### HOW SUPPLIED
*Ophthalmic suspension:* 5%

### ACTION
Increases fungal cell-membrane permeability.

### ONSET, PEAK, DURATION
Unknown.

### INDICATIONS & DOSAGE
*Fungal keratitis –*
**Adults:** initially, 1 drop instilled in conjunctival sac q 1 to 2 hours. After 3 to 4 days, dosage reduced to 1 drop six to eight times daily.
*Blepharitis or fungal conjunctivitis –*
**Adults:** 1 drop instilled q 4 to 6 hours.

### ADVERSE REACTIONS
**EENT:** ocular edema, hyperemia, conjunctival chemosis.

### INTERACTIONS
None significant.

### CONTRAINDICATIONS
Contraindicated in patients hypersensitive to the drug.

### NURSING CONSIDERATIONS
• Administer drug as ordered for 14 to 21 days or until active disease subsides. Be prepared to reduce dosage gradually at 4- to 7-day intervals, as ordered, to ensure that organism has been eliminated. If infection does not improve within 7 to 10 days of therapy, clinical and laboratory reevaluation is recommended.
• Shake well before use. Refrigerate or store at room temperature.
• Drug is the only antifungal available as ophthalmic preparation.

### ☑ PATIENT TEACHING
• Tell patient to clean eye area of excessive exudate before application.
• Teach patient how to instill drops. Advise him to wash hands before and after administering solution and not to touch tip of dropper to eye or surrounding tissue.
• Instruct patient to apply light finger pressure on lacrimal sac for 1 minute after drops are instilled.
• Tell patient not to share medication, washcloths, or towels with family members and to notify doctor if anyone develops same symptoms.

---

Reactions may be *common,* uncommon, *life-threatening,* or COMMON AND LIFE-THREATENING.

• Stress importance of compliance with recommended therapy.

## norfloxacin
Chibroxin

*Pregnancy Risk Category: C*

### HOW SUPPLIED
*Ophthalmic solution:* 0.3% in 5-ml containers

### ACTION
Inhibits bacterial DNA gyrase, an enzyme necessary for bacterial replication. Bacteriostatic or bactericidal, depending on concentration.

### ONSET, PEAK, DURATION
Unknown. Systemic absorption is negligible.

### INDICATIONS & DOSAGE
*Conjunctivitis caused by susceptible strains of bacteria –*
**Adults and children 1 year and over:** 1 or 2 drops in the affected eye q.i.d. for up to 7 days. If condition warrants, 2 drops may be applied q 2 hours during the waking hours of the first day of treatment.

### ADVERSE REACTIONS
**EENT:** local burning or discomfort, itching, chemosis, photophobia, conjunctival hyperemia, white crystallin precipitates, lid margin crusting, bad or bitter taste in mouth, nausea, hypersensitivity reactions.
**GI:** nausea.

### INTERACTIONS
*Caffeine, cyclosporine, theophylline:* impaired metabolism of these drugs with systemic norfloxacin. It's unknown if ophthalmic norfloxacin will have this effect. Monitor closely.
*Oral anticoagulants:* enhanced activity with systemic norfloxacin. It's unknown if ophthalmic norfloxacin will have this effect. Monitor closely.

### CONTRAINDICATIONS
Contraindicated in patients with a history of hypersensitivity to norfloxacin or other fluoroquinolone antibiotics. Drug shouldn't be injected into eye.

### NURSING CONSIDERATIONS
• Be aware that drug is indicated for treating conjunctivitis when caused by susceptible bacteria. Known susceptible strains include *Acinetobacter calcoaceticus, Aeromonas hydrophila, Haemophilus influenzae, Proteus mirabilis, Serratia marcescens, Staphylococcus aureus, S. epidermidis, S. warnerii,* and *Streptococcus pneumoniae.*
• *Alert:* Discontinue drug at the first sign of hypersensitivity, such as rash, and notify doctor. Serious hypersensitivity reactions, including anaphylaxis, have occurred in patients receiving systemic fluoroquinolone therapy.
• Institute appropriate therapy if superinfection occurs. Prolonged use may result in overgrowth of nonsusceptible organisms, including fungi.
• Know that although systemically administered fluoroquinolones have been shown to cause arthropathy in young animals, ophthalmic norfloxacin has not produced this adverse effect.

### ☑ PATIENT TEACHING
• Tell patient to clean eye area of excessive exudate before application.
• Teach patient how to instill drops. Advise him to wash hands before and after administering and not to touch the tip of the tube or dropper to eye or surrounding tissue.
• Tell patient not to share medication, washcloths, or towels with family members and to notify doctor if anyone develops same symptoms.
• Stress the importance of compliance with recommended therapy.

---

# ofloxacin 0.3%
Ocuflox

*Pregnancy Risk Category: C*

## HOW SUPPLIED
*Ophthalmic solution:* 0.3%

## ACTION
Bactericidal; inhibits bacterial DNA gyrase, an enzyme necessary for bacterial replication.

## ONSET, PEAK, DURATION
Unknown.

## INDICATIONS & DOSAGE
*Conjunctivitis caused by* Staphylococcus aureus, S. epidermidis, Streptococcus pneumoniae, Enterobacter cloacae, Haemophilus influenzae, Proteus mirabilis, *and* Pseudomonas aeruginosa —
**Adults and children older than 1 year:** 1 to 2 drops in the conjunctival sac q 2 to 4 hours daily, while awake, for the first 2 days and then four times daily for up to 5 additional days.

## ADVERSE REACTIONS
**CNS:** dizziness (rare).
**EENT:** *transient ocular burning or discomfort,* stinging, redness, itching, photophobia, lacrimation, eye dryness.

## INTERACTIONS
None significant.

## CONTRAINDICATIONS
Contraindicated in patients with history of hypersensitivity to ofloxacin, to other fluoroquinolones, or to any of the components of this drug; and in breast-feeding women.

## NURSING CONSIDERATIONS
• **Alert:** Know that the drug should not be injected into the conjunctiva or introduced directly into the anterior chamber of the eye.

• Be aware that drug should be discontinued if improvement does not occur within 7 days. Prolonged use may result in overgrowth of nonsusceptible organisms, including fungi.

## ☑ PATIENT TEACHING
• If an allergic reaction occurs, tell patient to discontinue the drug and call the doctor. Serious acute hypersensitivity reactions may require emergency treatment.
• Teach patient how to instill drops. Advise him to wash hands before and after instilling solution, and warn him not to touch tip of the dropper to eye or surrounding tissue.
• Advise patient to apply light finger pressure on lacrimal sac for 1 minute after drug instillation.
• Stress the importance of compliance with recommended therapy.
• Warn patient not to use leftover medication for a new eye infection.
• Remind patients to discard drug when no longer needed.

---

# polymyxin B sulfate

*Pregnancy Risk Category: NR*

## HOW SUPPLIED
*Ophthalmic sterile powder for solution:* 500,000-unit vials to be reconstituted to 20 to 50 ml

## ACTION
Bactericidal. Alters the osmotic barrier of the bacteria cell membrane.

## ONSET, PEAK, DURATION
Unknown. Systemic absorption is negligible.

## INDICATIONS & DOSAGE
*Used alone or in combination with other agents to treat superficial eye infections involving the conjunctiva and cornea resulting from infection with* Pseudomonas *or other gram-negative organism —*

---

Reactions may be *common,* uncommon, *life-threatening,* or **COMMON AND LIFE-THREATENING.**

**Adults and children:** 1 to 3 drops of 0.1% to 0.25% (10,000 to 25,000 units/ml) instilled q hour. Interval increased according to patient response; or up to 10,000 units subconjunctivally daily. Not to exceed 2 million units daily.

**ADVERSE REACTIONS**
**EENT:** eye irritation, conjunctivitis.
**Other:** overgrowth of nonsusceptible organisms, hypersensitivity reactions (local burning, itching).

**INTERACTIONS**
None significant.

**CONTRAINDICATIONS**
Contraindicated in patients hypersensitive to the drug.

**NURSING CONSIDERATIONS**
• Reconstitute carefully to ensure correct drug concentration in solution.
• Know that drug is often used in combination with neomycin sulfate.
• Be aware that drug is one of the most effective antibiotics against gram-negative organisms, especially *Pseudomonas.*
• In severe, life-threatening *Pseudomonas* infections, know that polymyxin B may be used as an ocular irrigant.

☑ **PATIENT TEACHING**
• Tell patient to clean eye area of excessive exudate before application.
• Teach patient how to instill drops . Advise him to wash hands before and after administering solution, and warn him not to touch tip of dropper to eye or surrounding tissue.
• Instruct patient to apply light finger pressure on lacrimal sac for 1 minute after drops are instilled.
• Advise patient to watch for and report signs of sensitivity (itching lids, swelling, or constant burning).
• Tell patient not to share medication, washcloths, or towels with family

members and to notify doctor if anyone develops same symptoms.
• Stress importance of compliance with recommended therapy.

---

**silver nitrate 1%**
*Pregnancy Risk Category: NR*

**HOW SUPPLIED**
*Ophthalmic solution:* 1%

**ACTION**
Causes protein denaturation, which prevents gonorrheal ophthalmia neonatorum. Bacteriostatic, germicidal, astringent, caustic, and escharotic.

**ONSET, PEAK, DURATION**
Unknown. Systemic absorption is negligible.

**INDICATIONS & DOSAGE**
*Prevention of gonorrheal ophthalmia neonatorum –*
**Neonates:** clean eyelids thoroughly; 2 drops of 1% solution instilled into the lower conjunctival sac of each eye at the angle of the nasal bridge and eyes, preferably immediately after delivery but no later than 1 hour after delivery.

**ADVERSE REACTIONS**
**EENT:** periorbital edema, temporary staining of lids and surrounding tissue, *conjunctivitis.*

**INTERACTIONS**
*Bacitracin:* inactivation of silver nitrate. Don't use together.
*Sulfonamides:* Incompatible with silver preparations. Don't use together.

**CONTRAINDICATIONS**
None known.

**NURSING CONSIDERATIONS**
• Always wash hands before instilling solution.
• Apply within 1 hour of birth, as ordered. Used in neonates born either

---

*Liquid form contains alcohol. **May contain tartrazine. †Canada only. ‡Australia only. ◇OTC.

by vaginal delivery or by cesarean section.
• Be aware that instillation may be delayed slightly to allow neonate to bond with mother.
• Don't use repeatedly.
• Don't irrigate eyes after instillation.
• Never use concentrations greater than 1% in the eye.
• If a concentrated solution is accidentally used in eye, promptly irrigate with 0.9% sodium chloride solution to prevent severe eye irritation or blindness.
• Handle carefully. Solution may stain skin and utensils.
• Know that prophylaxis against gonococcal ophthalmia neonatorum is legally required for neonates in most states. Because of a high incidence of conjunctivitis (more than 90%), many clinicians prefer antibiotic ointments, such as erythromycin, as an alternative.
• Store wax ampules away from light and heat. Do not freeze or use when cold.

☑ **PATIENT TEACHING**
• Inform parents of need for drug and explain how it is administered.
• Answer questions and address their concerns.

---

## sulfacetamide sodium 10%
Bleph-10 Liquifilm Ophthalmic, Cetamide Ophthalmic, Ocu-Sul-10, Sodium Sulamyd 10% Ophthalmic, Sulf-10 Ophthalmic

## sulfacetamide sodium 15%
Isopto Cetamide Ophthalmic, Ocu-Sul-15

## sulfacetamide sodium 30%
Ocu-Sul-30, Sodium Sulamyd 30% Ophthalmic

*Pregnancy Risk Category: NR*

---

**HOW SUPPLIED**
*Ophthalmic ointment:* 10%
*Ophthalmic solution:* 10%, 15%, 30%

**ACTION**
Bacteriostatic although, in high concentrations, may be bactericidal. Prevents uptake of PABA, a metabolite of bacterial folic acid synthesis.

**ONSET, PEAK, DURATION**
Unknown. Systemic absorption is negligible.

**INDICATIONS & DOSAGE**
*Inclusion conjunctivitis, corneal ulcers, trachoma, chlamydial infection* –
**Adults and children:** 1 to 2 drops of 10% solution instilled into lower conjunctival sac q 2 to 3 hours during day, less often at night; or 1 to 2 drops of 15% solution instilled into lower conjunctival sac q 1 to 2 hours initially. Interval increased as condition responds; or 1 drop of 30% solution instilled into lower conjunctival sac q 2 hours. 1.25 to 2.5 cm 10% ointment applied into conjunctival sac q.i.d. and h.s. Ointment may be used at night along with drops during the day.

**ADVERSE REACTIONS**
**EENT:** slowed corneal wound healing (ointment), pain (on instillation of eyedrops), headache or brow pain, photophobia, periorbital edema.
**Other:** hypersensitivity reactions (including itching or burning), overgrowth of nonsusceptible organisms, *Stevens-Johnson syndrome.*

**INTERACTIONS**
*Gentamicin (ophthalmic):* in vitro antagonism. Avoid using together.
*Local anesthetics (procaine, tetracaine), PABA derivatives:* decreased sulfacetamide sodium action. Wait ½ to 1 hour after instilling anesthetic or

---

PABA derivative before instilling sulfacetamide.
*Silver preparations:* precipitate formation. Avoid using together.

### CONTRAINDICATIONS
• Contraindicated in patients hypersensitive to sulfonamides. Not recommended for children under 2 months.

### NURSING CONSIDERATIONS
• Keep in mind that drug has been replaced by other antibiotics for treating major ocular infections; still used for minor ocular infections.
• Be aware that drug is often used with oral tetracycline in treating trachoma and inclusion conjunctivitis.
• Store in tightly closed, light-resistant container away from heat.

### ☑ PATIENT TEACHING
• Tell patient to clean eye area of excessive exudate before instilling.
• Teach patient how to instill drops or apply ointment. Advise him to wash hands before and after administering ointment or solution and not to touch tip of dropper to eye or surrounding tissues.
• Instruct patient to apply light finger pressure on lacrimal sac for 1 minute after drops are instilled.
• Warn patient that eyedrops burn slightly.
• Advise patient to watch for and report signs of sensitivity (itching lids, swelling, or constant burning).
• Tell patient to wait at least 5 minutes before administering other eyedrops.
• Warn patient that solution may stain clothing.
• Tell patient to minimize photophobia by wearing sunglasses and avoiding prolonged exposure to sunlight.
• Advise patient not to use discolored solution.
• Tell patient not to share eye medication, washcloths, or towels with family members. If anyone develops the

same symptoms, the doctor should be notified.
• Stress importance of compliance with recommended therapy.

---

## sulfisoxazole diolamine
Gantrisin Ophthalmic Solution

*Pregnancy Risk Category: C*

### HOW SUPPLIED
*Ophthalmic solution:* 4%

### ACTION
Inhibits bacterial synthesis of dihydrofolic acid by competing with PABA, thus exerting a bacteriostatic effect.

### ONSET, PEAK, DURATION
Unknown.

### INDICATIONS & DOSAGE
*Conjunctivitis, corneal ulcers, and other superficial ocular infections; adjunct in systemic sulfonamide therapy of trachoma* −
**Adults and children:** 2 to 3 drops instilled in the conjunctival sac three or more times daily.

### ADVERSE REACTIONS
**CNS:** *headache.*
**EENT:** *ocular irritation, itching, chemosis, periorbital edema.*
**Other:** ***Stevens-Johnson syndrome,*** overgrowth of nonsusceptible organisms.

### INTERACTIONS
*Gentamicin sulfate:* antagonism may occur. Do not administer together.
*Silver-containing preparations:* incompatible. Do not administer together.

### CONTRAINDICATIONS
Contraindicated in patients with hypersensitivity to this drug or other sulfonamides, in infants under age 2

---

*Liquid form contains alcohol.   **May contain tartrazine.   †Canada only.   ‡Australia only.   ◊OTC.

months, during pregnancy at full term, and in breast-feeding women.

## NURSING CONSIDERATIONS
• Use with caution in patients with severe dry eye.
• Drug should be discarded when patient's infection is eliminated.

## ☑ PATIENT TEACHING
• Teach patient how to instill drops. Advise him to wash hands before and after instilling solution, and warn him not to touch tip of the dropper to the eye or surrounding tissue.
• Advise patient to apply light finger pressure on lacrimal sac for 1 minute after drug instillation.
• Stress the importance of compliance with recommended therapy.
• Warn patient not to use leftover medication for a new eye infection.

---

# tobramycin
Tobrex

*Pregnancy Risk Category: B*

## HOW SUPPLIED
*Ophthalmic ointment:* 0.3%
*Ophthalmic solution:* 0.3%

## ACTION
Unknown. Thought to inhibit protein synthesis. Usually bactericidal.

## ONSET, PEAK, DURATION
Unknown. Systemic absorption is negligible.

## INDICATIONS & DOSAGE
*External ocular infections caused by susceptible bacteria –*
**Adults and children:** in mild to moderate infections, 1 or 2 drops instilled into the affected eye q 4 hours, or a thin strip of ointment applied q 8 to 12 hours. In severe infections, 2 drops instilled into the infected eye q 30 to 60 minutes until condition improves; then frequency reduced. Or, a thin strip of ointment applied q 3 to 4 hours until improvement; then frequency reduced.

## ADVERSE REACTIONS
**EENT:** burning or stinging on instillation, lid itching or swelling, conjunctival erythema, blurred vision (with ointment).
**Other:** hypersensitivity reactions, overgrowth of nonsusceptible organisms.

## INTERACTIONS
None significant.

## CONTRAINDICATIONS
Contraindicated in patients hypersensitive to the drug.

## NURSING CONSIDERATIONS
• When two different ophthalmic solutions are used, allow at least 5 minutes before instillation.
• *Alert:* Know that tobramycin ophthalmic solution is not for injection and should not be injected into the conjunctiva or directly into the anterior chamber of the eye.
• If topical ocular tobramycin is administered concomitantly with systemic tobramycin, carefully monitor serum levels.
• Stop drug and notify the doctor if patient develops symptoms of tobramycin overdose (keratitis, erythema, increased lacrimation, edema, and lid itching).
• Know that prolonged use may result in overgrowth of nonsusceptible organisms, including fungi.
• Be aware that drug is often used to combat gram-negative organisms that are resistant to gentamicin.

## ☑ PATIENT TEACHING
• Tell patient to clean eye area of excessive exudate before application.
• Teach patient how to instill drops or apply ointment. Advise him to wash hands before and after administering

---

ointment or solution and to avoid touching tip of dropper to eye or surrounding tissue.
• Instruct patient to apply light finger pressure on lacrimal sac for 1 minute after drops are instilled.
• Advise patient to watch for signs of sensitivity, such as itching lids, swelling, or constant burning. Tell patient who develops these signs to discontinue drug and notify the doctor immediately.
• Tell patient not to share medication, washcloths, or towels with family members and to notify doctor if anyone develops same symptoms.
• Stress importance of compliance with recommended therapy.

## trifluridine
Viroptic Ophthalmic Solution 1%

*Pregnancy Risk Category: C*

### HOW SUPPLIED
*Ophthalmic solution:* 1%

### ACTION
Unknown. Thought to interfere with DNA synthesis.

### ONSET, PEAK, DURATION
Unknown.

### INDICATIONS & DOSAGE
*Primary keratoconjunctivitis and recurrent epithelial keratitis caused by herpes simplex virus, types I and II—*
**Adults:** 1 drop of solution into the affected eye q 2 hours while patient is awake to a maximum of 9 drops daily until corneal ulcer reepithelialization occurs; then 1 drop q 4 hours (minimum 5 drops daily) for an additional 7 days.

### ADVERSE REACTIONS
**EENT:** *stinging on instillation,* edema of eyelids, increased intraocular pressure, epithelial keratopathy, superfi-

cial punctate keratopathy, stromal edema, irritation, keratitis sicca.
**Other:** hypersensitivity reactions.

### INTERACTIONS
None significant.

### CONTRAINDICATIONS
Contraindicated in patients hypersensitive to the drug.

### NURSING CONSIDERATIONS
• Be aware that doctor should consider another form of therapy if improvement doesn't occur after 7 days' treatment or complete reepithelialization after 14 days' treatment. Know that trifluridine should not be used for more than 21 days continuously due to potential ocular toxicity.
• Watch for signs of increased intraocular pressure.
• Continue trifluridine for several days after steroid therapy, as ordered.
• Know that drug is prescribed only for those patients with clinical diagnosis of herpetic keratitis and keratoconjuncitvitis.
• Be aware that drug is more effective than vidarabine or idoxuridine with fewer adverse reactions.
• Keep refrigerated. Do not use if past the expiration date.

### ☑ PATIENT TEACHING
• Tell patient to clean eye area of excessive exudate before application.
• Teach patient how to instill drops. Advise him to wash hands before and after administering, and warn him not to touch tip of dropper to eye or surrounding tissue.
• Instruct patient to apply light finger pressure on lacrimal sac for 1 minute after drops are instilled.
• Reassure patient that mild local irritation of the conjunctiva and cornea that occurs when solution is instilled is usually temporary.
• Tell patient not to share eye medications, washcloths, or towels with fam-

ily members. If anyone develops the same symptoms, the doctor should be notified.
● Stress importance of complying with recommended therapy.

## vidarabine
Vira-A

*Pregnancy Risk Category: C*

### HOW SUPPLIED
*Ophthalmic ointment:* 3% in 3.5-g tube (equivalent to 2.8% vidarabine)

### ACTION
Unknown. Thought to interfere with DNA synthesis.

### ONSET, PEAK, DURATION
Unknown. Systemic absorption is negligible.

### INDICATIONS & DOSAGE
*Acute keratoconjunctivitis, superficial keratitis, and recurrent epithelial keratitis caused by herpes simplex types I and II*—
**Adults and children:** 1 cm of ointment applied into lower conjunctival sac five times daily at 3-hour intervals.

### ADVERSE REACTIONS
**EENT:** temporary burning, itching, mild irritation, pain, lacrimation, foreign body sensation, conjunctival injection, punctal occlusion, sensitivity, superficial punctate keratitis, photophobia.
**Other:** hypersensitivity reactions.

### INTERACTIONS
None significant.

### CONTRAINDICATIONS
Contraindicated in patients hypersensitive to the drug.

### NURSING CONSIDERATIONS
● Use cautiously and with close monitoring with steroids. Vidarabine continued for several days after steroid therapy.
● Be aware that drug is not effective against RNA virus, adenoviral ocular infections, or bacterial, fungal, or chlamydial infections.
● Store in tightly closed, light-resistant container.

### ☑ PATIENT TEACHING
● Warn patient not to exceed recommended frequency or duration of dosage. Not for long-term use. Treatment should not exceed 21 days, or 3 to 5 days after healing.
● Tell patient to clean eye area of excessive exudate before application.
● Teach patient how to apply. Advise him to wash hands before and after administering ointment and to avoid touching tip of tube to eye or surrounding tissue.
● Instruct patient to apply light finger pressure on lacrimal sac for 1 minute after drops are instilled.
● Explain to patient that the ointment may produce a temporary visual haze.
● Advise patient to watch for signs of sensitivity, such as itching lids, swelling, or constant burning. Tell patient who develops such signs to stop drug and notify the doctor immediately.
● Tell patient to minimize photophobia by wearing sunglasses and avoiding prolonged exposure to sunlight.
● Tell patient not to share eye medication, washcloths, or towels with family members. If anyone develops the same symptoms, the doctor should be notified.
● Stress importance of complying with recommended therapy.

---

Reactions may be *common,* uncommon, *life-threatening,* or COMMON AND LIFE-THREATENING.

dexamethasone
dexamethasone sodium
  phosphate
diclofenac sodium 0.1%
fluorometholone
flurbiprofen sodium
ketorolac tromethamine
medrysone
prednisolone acetate
  (suspension)
prednisolone sodium phosphate
  (solution)
rimexolone
suprofen

## COMBINATION PRODUCTS
Corticosteroids for ophthalmic use are commonly combined with antibiotics and sulfonamides. See Chapter 79, OPHTHALMIC ANTI-INFECTIVES.

# dexamethasone
Maxidex Ophthalmic Suspension

# dexamethasone sodium phosphate
Decadron Phosphate Ophthalmic, Maxidex Ophthalmic

*Pregnancy Risk Category: C*

## HOW SUPPLIED
**dexamethasone**
*Ophthalmic suspension:* 0.1%
**dexamethasone sodium phosphate**
*Ophthalmic ointment:* 0.05%
*Ophthalmic solution:* 0.1%

## ACTION
Unknown. Thought to decrease the infiltration of WBCs at the site of inflammation.

## ONSET, PEAK, DURATION
Unknown.

## INDICATIONS & DOSAGE
*Uveitis; iridocyclitis; inflammatory conditions of eyelids, conjunctiva, cornea, anterior segment of globe; corneal injury from chemical or thermal burns, or penetration of foreign bodies; allergic conjunctivitis; suppression of graft rejection after keratoplasty –*
**Adults and children:** 1 to 2 drops of suspension or solution instilled or 1.25 to 2.5 cm of ointment applied into conjunctival sac. In severe disease, drops may be used hourly, tapering to discontinuation as condition improves. In mild conditions, drops may be used up to four to six times daily or ointment applied t.i.d. or q.i.d. As condition improves, dosage tapered to b.i.d., then once daily. Treatment may extend from a few days to several weeks.

## ADVERSE REACTIONS
**EENT:** increased intraocular pressure; thinning of cornea, interference with corneal wound healing, increased susceptibility to viral or fungal corneal infection, corneal ulceration; with excessive or long-term use — glaucoma exacerbation, cataracts, defects in visual acuity and visual field, optic nerve damage; mild blurred vision; burning, stinging, or redness of eyes; watery eyes, discharge, discomfort, ocular pain, foreign body sensation.
**Other:** systemic effects and adrenal suppression with excessive or long-term use.

## INTERACTIONS
None significant.

---

*Liquid form contains alcohol.  **May contain tartrazine.  †Canada only.  ‡Australia only.  ◇OTC.

## CONTRAINDICATIONS

Contraindicated in patients with acute superficial herpes simplex (dendritic keratitis), vaccinia, varicella, or other fungal or viral diseases of cornea and conjunctiva; ocular tuberculosis; or any acute, purulent, untreated infection of the eye.

## NURSING CONSIDERATIONS

• Use cautiously in patients with corneal abrasions that may be infected (especially with herpes).
• Use cautiously in patients with glaucoma (any form), because intraocular pressure may increase. Glaucoma medications may need to be increased to compensate.
• Drug is not for long-term use.
• Watch for corneal ulceration; may require stopping drug.
• Be aware that corneal viral and fungal infections may be exacerbated by steroid application.

## ☑ PATIENT TEACHING

• Tell patient to shake suspension well before use.
• Teach patient how to instill drops or apply ointment. Advise him to wash hands before and after administering ointment or solution, and warn him not to touch tip of dropper to eye or surrounding tissue.
• Tell patient to apply light finger pressure on lacrimal sac for 1 minute after instillation.
• Advise patient that he may use eye pad with ointment.
• Warn patient not to use leftover medication for a new eye inflammation; may cause serious problems.
• *Alert:* Warn patient to call the doctor immediately and to stop drug if visual acuity changes or visual field diminishes.
• Tell patient not to share medication, washcloths, or towels with family members and to notify doctor if anyone develops symptoms.

• Stress the importance of compliance with recommended therapy.

---

## diclofenac sodium 0.1%
Voltaren Ophthalmic
*Pregnancy Risk Category: B*

## HOW SUPPLIED
*Ophthalmic solution:* 0.1%

## ACTION
Unknown. Thought to inhibit the enzyme cyclooxygenase, which is essential in the biosynthesis of prostaglandins; prostaglandins may be mediators of certain kinds of intraocular inflammation.

## ONSET, PEAK, DURATION
Unknown.

## INDICATIONS & DOSAGE
*Postoperative inflammation following removal of cataract –*
**Adults:** 1 drop in the conjunctival sac q.i.d., beginning 24 hours after surgery and continuing throughout the first 2 weeks of the postoperative period.

## ADVERSE REACTIONS
**EENT:** *transient stinging and burning, increased intraocular pressure, keratitis,* anterior chamber reaction, ocular allergy.
**Systemic:** nausea, vomiting, viral infection.

## INTERACTIONS
None significant.

## CONTRAINDICATIONS
Contraindicated in patients with hypersensitivity to any component of the drug and in those wearing soft contact lenses. Because of the known effects of prostaglandin-inhibiting drugs on the fetal CV system (closure of the ductus arteriosus), the use of this

---

Reactions may be *common,* uncommon, *life-threatening,* or COMMON AND LIFE-THREATENING.

drug during late pregnancy should be avoided.

## NURSING CONSIDERATIONS
• Use cautiously in patients with hypersensitivity to acetylsalicylic acid, phenylacetic acid derivatives, and other NSAIDs; the potential for cross-sensitivity exists. It should also be used cautiously in surgical patients with known bleeding tendencies and in those receiving medications that may prolong bleeding time.
• Drug may slow or delay healing.
• Most cases of increased intraocular pressure have occurred postoperatively and before drug administration.

## ☑ PATIENT TEACHING
• Teach patient how to instill drops. Advise him to wash hands before and after instilling solution, and warn him not to touch tip of the dropper to eye or surrounding tissue.
• Advise patient to apply light finger pressure on lacrimal sac for 1 minute after drug instillation.
• Stress the importance of compliance with recommended therapy.
• Warn patient not to use leftover medication for a new eye inflammation.
• Remind patient to discard drug when no longer needed.

---

## fluorometholone
Flarex, FML Forte, FML Liquifilm Ophthalmic, FML S.O.P.

*Pregnancy Risk Category: C*

## HOW SUPPLIED
*Ophthalmic ointment:* 0.1%
*Ophthalmic suspension:* 0.1%, 0.25%

## ACTION
Unknown. Thought to decrease the infiltration of WBCs at inflammation site.

## ONSET, PEAK, DURATION
Unknown.

## INDICATIONS & DOSAGE
*Inflammatory and allergic conditions of cornea, conjunctiva, sclera, anterior uvea —*
**Adults and children:** 1 to 2 drops instilled in conjunctival sac b.i.d. to q.i.d. May be given q hour during first 1 to 2 days if needed. Alternatively, 1.25-cm ribbon of ointment applied to conjunctival sac q 4 hours, decreased to one to three times a day as inflammation subsides.

## ADVERSE REACTIONS
**EENT:** increased intraocular pressure, thinning of cornea, interference with corneal wound healing, corneal ulceration, increased susceptibility to viral or fungal corneal infections; with excessive or long-term use — glaucoma exacerbation, discharge, discomfort, ocular pain, foreign body sensation, cataracts, decreased visual acuity, diminished visual field, optic nerve damage.
**Other:** systemic effects and adrenal suppression in excessive or long-term use.

## INTERACTIONS
None significant.

## CONTRAINDICATIONS
Contraindicated in patients with vaccinia, varicella, acute superficial herpes simplex (dendritic keratitis), or other fungal or viral eye diseases; ocular tuberculosis; or any acute, purulent, untreated eye infection.

## NURSING CONSIDERATIONS
• Use cautiously in patients with corneal abrasions that may be contaminated (especially with herpes).
• Safety and efficacy in children under age 2 have not been established.
• Drug is not for long-term use.
• Shake well before using.

---

• Be aware that drug is less likely to cause increased intraocular pressure with long-term use than other ophthalmic anti-inflammatory drugs (except medrysone).
• Store in tightly covered, light-resistant container.

☑ **PATIENT TEACHING**
• Teach patient how to instill drops or apply ointment. Advise him to wash hands before and after administering ointment or solution, and warn him not to touch tip of dropper to eye or surrounding tissue.
• Advise patient to apply light finger pressure on lacrimal sac for 1 minute after instillation.
• Advise patient to call the doctor immediately and to stop drug if visual acuity decreases or visual field diminishes.
• Warn patient not to use leftover medication for a new eye inflammation; may cause serious problems.
• Tell patient not to share eye medication, washcloths, or towels with family members. If anyone develops similar symptoms, the doctor should be notified.

## flurbiprofen sodium
Ocufen Liquifilm

*Pregnancy Risk Category: B*

**HOW SUPPLIED**
*Ophthalmic solution:* 0.03%

**ACTION**
Unknown. An NSAID that's thought to inhibit the cyclooxygenase enzyme essential in the biosynthesis of prostaglandin.

**ONSET, PEAK, DURATION**
Unknown.

**INDICATIONS & DOSAGE**
*Inhibition of intraoperative miosis* —
**Adults:** 1 drop instilled into the affected eye approximately every ½ hour, beginning 2 hours before and continuing during surgery. A total of 4 drops is given.

**ADVERSE REACTIONS**
**EENT:** transient burning and stinging on instillation, ocular irritation.

**INTERACTIONS**
*Acetylcholine, carbachol:* may be rendered ineffective. Avoid concomitant use.
*Anticoagulants:* increased risk of bleeding if significant systemic absorption occurs. Monitor closely.

**CONTRAINDICATIONS**
Contraindicated in patients with hypersensitivity to the drug.

**NURSING CONSIDERATIONS**
• Use cautiously in patients who may be allergic to aspirin and other NSAIDs.
• Use cautiously in patients with bleeding tendencies and those who are receiving medications that may prolong clotting times.
• Be aware that wound healing may be delayed.

☑ **PATIENT TEACHING**
• Advise patient to alert the doctor immediately if visual acuity decreases or visual field diminishes.
• Urge him to take drug as prescribed.

## ketorolac tromethamine
Acular

*Pregnancy Risk Category: C*

**HOW SUPPLIED**
*Ophthalmic solution:* 0.5%

**ACTION**
Unknown. An NSAID that is thought to inhibit the action of cyclooxygenase, an enzyme responsible for prosta-

glandin synthesis. Prostaglandins mediate the inflammatory response and also cause miosis.

**ONSET, PEAK, DURATION**
Unknown. Systemic absorption is negligible.

**INDICATIONS & DOSAGE**
*Relief of ocular itching caused by seasonal allergic conjunctivitis –*
**Adults:** 1 drop into the conjunctival sac instilled in each eye q.i.d.

**ADVERSE REACTIONS**
**EENT:** *transient stinging and burning on instillation,* superficial keratitis, superficial ocular infections, ocular irritation.
**Other:** hypersensitivity reactions.

**INTERACTIONS**
None significant.

**CONTRAINDICATIONS**
Contraindicated in patients hypersensitive to any component of the formulation and in wearers of soft contact lenses.

**NURSING CONSIDERATIONS**
• Use cautiously in patients hypersensitive to other NSAIDs or aspirin and in patients with bleeding disorders.
• Store drug away from heat in a dark, tightly closed container and protect from freezing.

☑ **PATIENT TEACHING**
• Teach patient how to instill drops. Advise him to wash hands before and after instilling solution, and warn him not to touch tip of dropper to eye or surrounding tissue.
• Advise patient to apply light finger pressure on lacrimal sac for 1 minute after instillation.
• Remind patient to discard drug when it's no longer needed.
• Stress the importance of compliance with recommended therapy.

# medrysone
HMS Liquifilm Ophthalmic
*Pregnancy Risk Category: C*

**HOW SUPPLIED**
*Ophthalmic suspension:* 1%

**ACTION**
Unknown. Thought to decrease the infiltration of WBCs at the site of inflammation.

**ONSET, PEAK, DURATION**
Unknown. Although systemic absorption occurs, plasma levels are very low and systemic effects are negligible.

**INDICATIONS & DOSAGE**
*Allergic conjunctivitis, vernal conjunctivitis, episcleritis, ophthalmic epinephrine sensitivity reaction –*
**Adults and children:** 1 drop instilled into conjunctival sac q 4 hours. May use q hour during first 1 to 2 days if needed.

**ADVERSE REACTIONS**
**EENT:** thinning of cornea, interference with corneal wound healing, increased susceptibility to viral or fungal corneal infection, corneal ulceration; with excessive or long-term use – discharge, discomfort, ocular pain, foreign body sensation, glaucoma exacerbation, cataracts, visual acuity and visual field defects, optic nerve damage.
**Other:** systemic effects and adrenal suppression with excessive or long-term use.

**INTERACTIONS**
None significant.

**CONTRAINDICATIONS**
Contraindicated in patients with vaccinia, varicella, acute superficial herpes simplex (dendritic keratitis), viral diseases of conjunctiva and cor-

---

*Liquid form contains alcohol. **May contain tartrazine. †Canada only. ‡Australia only. ◊OTC.

nea, ocular tuberculosis, fungal or viral eye diseases, iritis, uveitis, or any acute, purulent, untreated eye infection.

**NURSING CONSIDERATIONS**
• Use cautiously in patients with corneal abrasions that may be contaminated (especially with herpes).
• Using leftover medication for a new eye inflammation may cause serious problems.

☑ **PATIENT TEACHING**
• Teach patient how to instill drops. Advise him to wash hands before and after instilling solution, and warn him not to touch tip of dropper to eye or surrounding tissue.
• Tell patient to shake well before using. Don't freeze.
• Advise patient to apply light finger pressure on lacrimal sac for 1 minute after instillation.
• Tell patient not to share medication, washcloths, or towels with family members and to notify doctor if anyone develops symptoms.
• Stress the importance of compliance with recommended therapy.

---

# prednisolone acetate (suspension)
Econopred Ophthalmic, Econopred Plus Ophthalmic, Ocu-Pred-A, Pred-Forte, Pred Mild Ophthalmic

# prednisolone sodium phosphate (solution)
AK-Pred, Hydeltrasol Ophthalmic, Inflamase Forte, Inflamase Ophthalmic, Ocu-Pred, Predsol Eye Drops‡

*Pregnancy Risk Category: C*

**HOW SUPPLIED**
**prednisolone acetate**
*Ophthalmic suspension:* 0.12%, 0.125%, 1%

**prednisolone sodium phosphate**
*Ophthalmic solution:* 0.125%, 1%

**ACTION**
Unknown. Thought to decrease the infiltration of WBCs at the site of inflammation.

**ONSET, PEAK, DURATION**
Unknown. Although systemic absorption occurs, plasma levels are very low and systemic effects are negligible.

**INDICATIONS & DOSAGE**
*Inflammation of palpebral and bulbar conjunctiva, cornea, and anterior segment of globe –*
**Adults and children:** 1 to 2 drops instilled into eye. In severe conditions, may be used hourly, tapering to discontinuation as inflammation subsides. In mild conditions, may be used up to six times daily.

**ADVERSE REACTIONS**
**EENT:** increased intraocular pressure; thinning of cornea, interference with corneal wound healing, increased susceptibility to viral or fungal corneal infection, corneal ulceration; with excessive or long-term use – discharge, discomfort, foreign body sensation, glaucoma exacerbation, cataracts, visual acuity and visual field defects, optic nerve damage.
**Other:** systemic effects and adrenal suppression with excessive or long-term use.

**INTERACTIONS**
None significant.

**CONTRAINDICATIONS**
Contraindicated in patients with acute, untreated, purulent ocular infections; acute superficial herpes simplex (dendritic keratitis); vaccinia, varicella, or other viral or fungal eye diseases; or ocular tuberculosis.

---

Reactions may be *common*, uncommon, *life-threatening*, or COMMON AND LIFE-THREATENING.

## NURSING CONSIDERATIONS
• Use cautiously in patients with corneal abrasions that may be contaminated (especially with herpes).
• Shake suspension and check dosage before administering to ensure using the correct strength. Store in tightly covered container.

### ☑ PATIENT TEACHING
• Teach patient how to instill drops. Advise him to wash hands before and after applying, and warn him not to touch tip of dropper to eye or surrounding area.
• Advise patient to apply light finger pressure on lacrimal sac for 1 minute after instillation.
• Tell patient on long-term therapy to have frequent tonometric examinations.
• Warn patient not to use leftover medication for a new eye inflammation; may cause serious problems.
• Tell patient not to share eye medication, washcloths, or towels with family members. If anyone develops similar symptoms, the doctor should be notified.
• Stress the importance of compliance with recommended therapy.

## rimexolone
Vexol 1% Ophthalmic Suspension

*Pregnancy Risk Category: C*

### HOW SUPPLIED
*Ophthalmic suspension:* 1%

### ACTION
Exact mechanism unknown. A corticosteroid, it inhibits edema, cellular infiltration, capillary dilation, fibroblastic proliferation, and deposition of collagen and scar formation associated with inflammation.

### ONSET, PEAK, DURATION
Unknown.

## INDICATIONS & DOSAGE
*Postoperative inflammation following ocular surgery –*
**Adults:** 1 to 2 drops instilled into the conjunctival sac q.i.d., beginning 24 hours after surgery and continuing throughout the first 2 weeks of the postoperative period.
*Anterior uveitis –*
**Adults:** 1 to 2 drops in the conjunctival sac q hour during waking hours for the first week, 1 drop q 2 hours during waking hours of the second week, and then tapered until uveitis is resolved.

### ADVERSE REACTIONS
**EENT:** *blurred vision, ocular discharge, ocular pain or discomfort, increased intraocular pressure, foreign-body sensation, ocular hyperemia, ocular pruritus,* sticky sensation, increased fibrin formation, eye dryness, conjunctival edema, corneal staining, keratitis, lacrimation, photophobia, edema, irritation, corneal ulcer, brow pain, crusting at margin of eyelid, corneal edema, infiltrate, corneal erosion.
**Other:** headache, hypotension, rhinitis, pharyngitis, taste perversion.

### INTERACTIONS
None significant.

### CONTRAINDICATIONS
Contraindicated in patients with hypersensitivity to any component of the drug. Also contraindicated in those with epithelial herpes simplex keratitis, vaccinia, varicella, and most other viral diseases of the cornea and conjunctiva; mycobacterial infection of the eye; and fungal disease of the eye or acute purulent untreated infections that may be masked or enhanced by the presence of a steroid.

### NURSING CONSIDERATIONS
• Monitor patient's blood pressure throughout therapy.

---

*Liquid form contains alcohol. **May contain tartrazine. †Canada only. ‡Australia only. ◇OTC.

• Never use leftover medication for a new eye inflammation.

### ☑ PATIENT TEACHING
• Teach patient how to instill drops. Advise him to shake the dispenser well before using. Also advise him to wash hands before and after instilling suspension, and warn him not to touch tip of the dropper to eye or surrounding tissue.
• Advise patient to apply light finger pressure on lacrimal sac for 1 minute after drug instillation.
• Stress the importance of compliance with recommended therapy.
• Remind patient to discard drug when no longer needed.
• Advise patient to have intraocular pressure checked frequently.

---

## suprofen
Profenal

*Pregnancy Risk Category: C*

### HOW SUPPLIED
*Ophthalmic solution:* 1%

### ACTION
Unknown. An NSAID that inhibits the action of cyclooxygenase, an enzyme responsible for the synthesis of prostaglandins. Prostaglandins mediate the inflammatory response and also cause miosis.

### ONSET, PEAK, DURATION
Unknown. Systemic absorption is negligible.

### INDICATIONS & DOSAGE
*Inhibition of intraoperative miosis –*
**Adults:** 2 drops instilled into the conjunctival sac q 4 hours the day before surgery. On the day of surgery, 2 drops instilled 3 hours, 2 hours, and 1 hour before surgery.

### ADVERSE REACTIONS
**EENT:** *transient stinging and burning on instillation,* discomfort, itching, redness, iritis, pain, chemosis, photophobia, irritation, punctate epithelial staining.
**Other:** hypersensitivity reactions.

### INTERACTIONS
*Acetylcholine, carbachol:* may be ineffective in patients treated with suprofen.

### CONTRAINDICATIONS
Contraindicated in patients hypersensitive to any component of the formulation and in patients with epithelial herpes simplex keratitis.

### NURSING CONSIDERATIONS
• Use cautiously in patients hypersensitive to other NSAIDs or aspirin.
• Use cautiously in patients with bleeding disorders.
• **Alert:** Drug may be absorbed into breast milk following topical ocular administration. It is recommended that breast-feeding be discontinued during administration.

### ☑ PATIENT TEACHING
• Teach patient how to instill drops. Advise him to wash hands before and after administering solution and not to touch tip of dropper to eye or surrounding tissues.
• Tell patient to apply light finger pressure on lacrimal sac for 1 minute after drops are instilled.
• Tell him to store drug away from heat in a dark, tightly closed container and to protect drug from freezing.
• Remind patient to discard drug when it's no longer needed.
• Stress importance of compliance with recommended therapy.

---

**acetylcholine chloride**
**carbachol (intraocular)**
**carbachol (topical)**
**demecarium bromide**
**echothiophate iodide**
**isoflurophate**
**physostigmine sulfate**
**pilocarpine**
**pilocarpine hydrochloride**
**pilocarpine nitrate**

## COMBINATION PRODUCTS

E-PILO: epinephrine bitartrate 1% and pilocarpine hydrochloride 1%, 2%, 3%, 4%, or 6%.
ISOPTO P-ES: pilocarpine hydrochloride 2% and physostigmine salicylate 0.25%.
$P_1E_1$, $P_2E_1$, $P_3E_1$, $P_4E_1$, $P_6E_1$: epinephrine bitartrate 1% and pilocarpine hydrochloride 1%, 2%, 3%, 4%, or 6%.

## acetylcholine chloride
Miochol

*Pregnancy Risk Category: NR*

### HOW SUPPLIED
*Ophthalmic injection:* 1%

### ACTION
A cholinergic that causes contraction of the sphincter muscles of the iris, resulting in miosis, and that produces ciliary spasm, deepening of the anterior chamber, and vasodilation of conjunctival vessels of the outflow tract.

### ONSET, PEAK, DURATION
Onset occurs within seconds. Peak unknown. Effects persist for about 10 minutes.

### INDICATIONS & DOSAGE
*Anterior segment surgery –*
**Adults and children:** before or after securing sutures, the doctor gently instills 0.5 to 2 ml into anterior chamber.

### ADVERSE REACTIONS
**CV:** bradycardia, hypotension.
**EENT:** corneal edema, clouding, or decompensation.
**Respiratory:** breathing difficulties.
**Other:** flushing, diaphoresis.

### INTERACTIONS
None significant.

### CONTRAINDICATIONS
Contraindicated in patients with hypersensitivity to the drug or any of its components.

### NURSING CONSIDERATIONS
● Reconstitute immediately before using, shaking vial gently until clear solution is obtained.
● Discard any unused solution.
● Don't gas-sterilize vial. Ethylene oxide may produce formic acid.

### ☑ PATIENT TEACHING
● Inform patient about need for drug during surgical procedure, and answer any questions and address concerns.
● Instruct patient to report breathing difficulties immediately.

## carbachol (intraocular)
Miostat

## carbachol (topical)
Isopto Carbachol

*Pregnancy Risk Category: NR*

### HOW SUPPLIED
*Intraocular injection:* 0.01%
*Topical ophthalmic solution:* 0.75%, 1.5%, 2.25%, 3%

---

*Liquid form contains alcohol.  **May contain tartrazine.  †Canada only.  ‡Australia only.  ◇OTC.

## ACTION
A cholinergic that causes contraction of the sphincter muscles of the iris, resulting in miosis, and that produces ciliary spasm, deepening of the anterior chamber, and vasodilation of conjunctival vessels of the outflow tract.

## ONSET, PEAK, DURATION
Onset occurs in 10 to 20 minutes. Peak effect occurs 4 hours after topical application, 2 to 5 minutes after intraocular injection. Effects persist about 8 hours after topical application, 24 hours after intraocular injection.

## INDICATIONS & DOSAGE
*To produce pupillary miosis in ocular surgery –*
**Adults:** before or after securing sutures, the doctor gently instills 0.5 ml (intraocular form) into anterior chamber.
*Open-angle glaucoma –*
**Adults:** 1 to 2 drops instilled (topical form) q 4 to 8 hours.

## ADVERSE REACTIONS
**CNS:** headache, syncope.
**CV:** arrhythmia, hypotension.
**EENT:** spasm of eye accommodation, conjunctival vasodilation, eye and brow pain, transient stinging and burning, corneal clouding, bullous keratopathy, salivation.
**GI:** abdominal cramps, diarrhea.
**GU:** urinary urgency.
**Respiratory:** asthma.
**Other:** diaphoresis, flushing.

## INTERACTIONS
*Pilocarpine:* additive effect. Use together cautiously.

## CONTRAINDICATIONS
Contraindicated in patients with hypersensitivity to drug or in patients where cholinergic effects such as constriction are undesirable (for example, acute iritis, some forms of secondary glaucoma, pupillary block glaucoma, or acute inflammatory disease of the anterior chamber).

## NURSING CONSIDERATIONS
● Use cautiously in patients with acute heart failure, bronchial asthma, peptic ulcer, hyperthyroidism, GI spasm, Parkinson's disease, and urinary tract obstruction.
● In case of toxicity, give atropine parenterally as ordered.
● The drug is used in open-angle glaucoma, especially when patients are resistant or allergic to pilocarpine hydrochloride or nitrate.
● *Alert:* Keep in mind that patients with dark eyes (hazel or brown irises) may require stronger solutions or more frequent instillation because eye pigment may absorb the drug.
● If tolerance to the drug develops, know that the doctor may switch to another miotic for a short time.

## ☑ PATIENT TEACHING
● Teach patient how to instill. Advise him to wash hands before and after and to apply light finger-pressure on lacrimal sac for 1 minute after drops are instilled. Warn him not to exceed recommended dosage.
● Warn patient to avoid hazardous activities, such as operating machinery or driving, until temporary blurring subsides. Reassure patient that blurred vision usually diminishes with prolonged use.
● Tell glaucoma patient that long-term use may be necessary. Stress compliance. Tell him to remain under medical supervision for periodic tonometric readings.

## demecarium bromide
Humorsol

*Pregnancy Risk Category: X*

## HOW SUPPLIED
*Ophthalmic solution:* 0.125%, 0.25%

---

Reactions may be *common,* uncommon, *life-threatening,* or COMMON AND LIFE-THREATENING.

## ACTION

An anticholinesterase drug that inhibits the enzymatic destruction of acetylcholine by inactivating cholinesterase, leaving acetylcholine free to act on the effector cells of the iridic sphincter and ciliary muscles, causing pupillary constriction and spasm of accommodation.

## ONSET, PEAK, DURATION

Onset occurs in 15 to 60 minutes. Miotic effect peaks within 2 hours; intraocular pressure (IOP) reduction occurs within 24 hours. Miosis persists for 3 to 10 days; IOP reduction, about 9 days.

## INDICATIONS & DOSAGE

*Acute angle-closure glaucoma after iridectomy, primary open-angle glaucoma* –
**Adults:** 1 drop instilled once or twice daily.
*Treatment of convergent strabismus (uncomplicated)* –
**Adults:** 1 drop instilled daily for 2 to 3 weeks, then reduced to 1 drop q 2 days for 3 to 4 weeks. After reevaluation, 1 drop instilled once or twice weekly to once q 2 days as determined by the patient's condition. Reevaluated q 4 to 12 weeks; dosage adjusted as needed. Discontinued after 4 months if dosage required is 1 drop q 2 days.
*Diagnosis of convergent strabismus* –
**Adults:** 1 drop instilled daily for 2 weeks, then 1 drop q 2 days for 2 to 4 weeks.

## ADVERSE REACTIONS

**CNS:** brow ache, unusual fatigue or weakness, headache.
**CV:** bradycardia, palpitations.
**EENT:** retinal detachment, iris cysts, conjunctival thickening, lens opacities, paradoxical increase in IOP, *lac-*

*rimation,* obstruction of nasolacrimal canals; eye pain, burning, redness, stinging and irritation; twitching eyelids; *blurred vision;* visual disturbances.
**GI:** nausea, vomiting, diarrhea, abdominal cramps or pain.
**GU:** loss of bladder control.

## INTERACTIONS

*Anticholinergics, antimyasthenics, other cholinesterase inhibitors:* potential for additive toxicity. Monitor closely.
*Carbamate or organophosphate-type insecticides (parathion, malathion):* increased risk of systemic effects through respiratory tract or skin. Warn patients to protect themselves.
*Cocaine:* increased risk of cocaine toxicity; anticholinesterase effects may last weeks or months. Avoid concomitant use.
*Epinephrine:* additive effect, resulting in better control and lower dosages of both drugs.
*Local anesthetics, ophthalmic tetracaine:* increased risk of systemic toxicity and prolonged ocular anesthetic effect. Monitor closely.
*Ophthalmic adrenocorticoids:* increased IOP and decreased antiglaucoma effectiveness. Avoid concomitant use.
*Ophthalmic belladonna alkaloids, cyclopentolate:* may antagonize miotic effects. Avoid concomitant use.
*Succinylcholine:* enhanced neuromuscular blockade, possible CV collapse and prolonged respiratory depression or apnea may occur for several weeks or months after demecarium is discontinued. Advise the anesthesiologist that the patient has received demecarium.

## CONTRAINDICATIONS

Contraindicated in patients with hypersensitivity to drug, acute angle-closure glaucoma before iridectomy, and other forms of glaucoma (except for primary open-angle glaucoma).

## NURSING CONSIDERATIONS
• Use with extreme caution, if at all, in patients with history or risk of retinal detachment, marked vagotonia, bronchial asthma, spastic GI conditions, urinary tract obstruction, peptic ulcer, severe bradycardia, hypotension, hypertension, hyperthyroidism, acute cardiac failure, recent MI, epilepsy, marked vasomotor instability, or parkinsonism.
• Use with caution in patients with corneal abrasion.
• Administer phenylephrine concurrently, as ordered, to reduce incidence of iris cyst formation.
• If tolerance to the drug develops after prolonged use, know that the doctor may switch to another miotic for a short time.
• Know that toxicity is cumulative; toxic systemic symptoms may not appear for weeks or months after start of therapy. Atropine sulfate S.C., I.M., or I.V. is antidote of choice.

## ☑ PATIENT TEACHING
• Teach patient how to instill demecarium. Advise him to wash hands before and after instilling drug, to avoid touching applicator tip to any surface, and to remove excess solution around eyes with clean tissue and without touching eye. Warn him not to exceed recommended dosage.
• If dose is missed, instruct patient not to double dose. If schedule is every other day, tell patient to instill as soon as possible if remembered same day; if remembered later, tell him not to instill until next day, then skip a day and resume regular schedule. If schedule is once a day, tell patient to instill as soon as possible. If not remembered until next day, tell him to skip missed dose and resume schedule. If schedule is more than once daily, tell patient to instill as soon as

possible. If close to time for next dose, tell him to skip missed dose and resume regular schedule.
• Tell patient that regular medical supervision is required to check ocular pressure.
• Advise patient to carry medical identification card at all times during therapy.

---

## echothiophate iodide (ecotiopate iodide)
Phospholine Iodide

*Pregnancy Risk Category: NR*

### HOW SUPPLIED
*Ophthalmic powder for solution:* for reconstitution to make 0.03%, 0.06%, 0.125%, and 0.25% solutions

### ACTION
An anticholinesterase drug that inhibits the enzymatic destruction of acetylcholine by inactivating cholinesterase, leaving acetylcholine free to act on the effector cells of the iridic sphincter and ciliary muscles, causing pupillary constriction and spasm of accommodation.

### ONSET, PEAK, DURATION
Miosis occurs in 10 to 30 minutes; intraocular pressure (IOP) reduction, 4 to 8 hours. Miotic effect peaks within 30 minutes; IOP reduction occurs within 24 hours. Effects persist for several days to 4 weeks.

### INDICATIONS & DOSAGE
*Primary open-angle glaucoma, conditions obstructing aqueous outflow —*
**Adults and children:** 1 drop of 0.03% to 0.125% solution instilled into conjunctival sac daily. Maximum dosage is 1 drop b.i.d. Lowest possible dosage used for continuous control of IOP.
*Diagnosis of convergent strabismus —*
**Adults:** 1 drop of 0.125% solution instilled daily h.s. for 2 to 3 weeks.

---

*Treatment of convergent strabismus –*
**Adults:** initially, 1 drop of 0.125% solution instilled into each eye daily h.s. for 2 to 3 weeks. Dosage decreased to 1 drop of 0.125% solution every other day or 1 drop of 0.06% solution daily. The 0.03% solution may be used instead for some patients.

## ADVERSE REACTIONS
**CNS:** fatigue, muscle weakness, paresthesia, headache.
**CV:** bradycardia, hypotension.
**EENT:** ciliary spasm or spasm of eye accommodation, ciliary or circumcorneal injection, nonreversible cataract formation (time- and dose-related), reversible iris cysts, pupillary block, blurred or dimmed vision, eye or brow pain, twitching of eyelids, hyperemia, photophobia, lens opacities, lacrimation, retinal detachment.
**GI:** diarrhea, nausea, vomiting, abdominal pain, intestinal cramps, salivation.
**GU:** frequent urination.
**Respiratory:** *bronchoconstriction.*
**Other:** diaphoresis, flushing.

## INTERACTIONS
*Anticholinergics, ophthalmic belladonna alkaloids (such as atropine), cyclopentolate:* antagonized miotic effects. Avoid concomitant use.
*Cocaine:* increased risk of cocaine toxicity. Avoid concomitant use.
*Local anesthetics, ophthalmic tetracaine:* increased rate of systemic toxicity and prolonged ocular anesthesia. Monitor closely.
*Ophthalmic adrenocorticoids:* increased intraocular pressure and decreased antiglaucoma effectiveness. Avoid concomitant use.
*Other cholinesterase inhibitors, organophosphate insecticides (parathion, malathion):* possible additive effect causing systemic effects. Warn patients exposed to insecticides to protect themselves.

*Succinylcholine:* respiratory and CV collapse. Don't use together.
*Systemic anticholinesterase agents for myasthenia gravis, pilocarpine:* effects may be additive. Monitor patients for signs of toxicity.

## CONTRAINDICATIONS
Contraindicated in patients with hypersensitivity to drug or iodine, acute angle-closure glaucoma before iridectomy, and other forms of glaucoma (except for primary open-angle glaucoma).

## NURSING CONSIDERATIONS
● Use with extreme caution, if at all, in patients with seizure disorders, vasomotor instability, parkinsonism, bronchial asthma, spastic GI conditions, urinary tract obstruction, peptic ulcer, severe bradycardia or hypotension, vascular hypertension, MI, or history or risk of retinal detachment.
● Use with caution in patients with corneal abrasion.
● Reconstitute powder, using only diluent provided to avoid contamination. Discard refrigerated, reconstituted solution after 6 months; solution stored at room temperature, after 1 month.
● Stop drug, as ordered, at least 2 weeks preoperatively if succinylcholine is to be used in surgery.
● Know that toxicity is cumulative; toxic systemic symptoms may not appear for weeks or months after start of therapy. Atropine sulfate S.C., I.M., or I.V. is antidote of choice.

## ☑ PATIENT TEACHING
● Advise patient to carry medical identification card at all times during therapy. Drug is a potent, long-acting, and irreversible.
● Teach patient how to instill drug. Advise him to wash hands before and after instilling drug, to avoid touching applicator tip to any surface and to ap-

---

*Liquid form contains alcohol. **May contain tartrazine. †Canada only. ‡Australia only. ◇OTC.

ply light finger pressure on lacrimal sac for 1 minute after instillation.
• Tell patient to instill drug at bedtime because it causes transient blurred vision. Warn him that transient brow pain or dimmed or blurred vision is common at first but usually disappears within 5 to 10 days.
• Warn patient to report salivation, diarrhea, profuse diaphoresis, urinary incontinence, or muscle weakness to the doctor.
• Tell patient to remain under constant medical supervision and not to exceed recommended dosage.

## isoflurophate
Floropryl

*Pregnancy Risk Category: X*

### HOW SUPPLIED
*Ophthalmic ointment:* 0.025%

### ACTION
An anticholinesterase drug that inhibits the enzymatic destruction of acetylcholine by inactivating cholinesterase, leaving acetylcholine free to act on the effector cells of the iridic sphincter and ciliary muscles, causing pupillary constriction and spasm of accommodation.

### ONSET, PEAK, DURATION
Unknown.

### INDICATIONS & DOSAGE
*Glaucoma* –
**Adults:** 0.5-cm ribbon of ointment applied to conjunctiva q 8 to 72 hours.
*Diagnosis of convergent strabismus (uncomplicated)* –
**Adults:** 0.5-cm ribbon of ointment applied to conjunctiva h.s. for 2 weeks.
*Treatment of convergent strabismus* –
**Adults:** 0.5-cm ribbon of ointment applied to each eye h.s. for 2 weeks, then once every 2 to 7 days, depending on the patient's condition, for 2

months. If the patient cannot be maintained on a dosage interval of at least 48 hours, the drug should be discontinued.

### ADVERSE REACTIONS
**CNS:** headache, brow ache, unusual fatigue or weakness.
**CV:** slow or irregular heartbeat.
**EENT:** retinal detachment, iris cysts, conjunctival thickening, lens opacities, obstruction of nasolacrimal canals, paradoxical increase in intraocular pressure (IOP); *eye burning,* redness, pain, stinging or irritation; *twitching of eyelids; blurred vision;* visual disturbances.
**GI:** nausea, vomiting, diarrhea, abdominal cramps or pain.
**GU:** loss of bladder control.
**Other:** diaphoresis, flushing.

### INTERACTIONS
*Anticholinergics, antimyasthenics, other cholinesterase inhibitors:* potential for additive toxicity. Monitor closely.
*Carbamate or organophosphate-type insecticides (parathion, malathion):* increased risk of systemic effects through respiratory tract or skin. Warn patients to protect themselves.
*Cocaine:* increased risk of cocaine toxicity; anticholinesterase effects may last weeks or months. Avoid concomitant use.
*Epinephrine:* additive effect, resulting in better control and lower dosages of both drugs.
*Local anesthetics, ophthalmic tetracaine:* increased risk of systemic toxicity, prolonged ocular anesthesia. Monitor closely.
*Ophthalmic adrenocorticoids:* increased IOP and decreased antiglaucoma effectiveness. Avoid concomitant use.
*Ophthalmic belladonna alkaloids, cyclopentolate:* may antagonize miotic effects. Avoid concomitant use.
*Ophthalmic physostigmine:* may

---

Reactions may be *common,* uncommon, ***life-threatening,*** or **COMMON AND LIFE-THREATENING.**

shorten duration of action. Avoid concomitant use.

*Succinylcholine:* enhanced neuromuscular blockade, possible CV collapse, prolonged respiratory depression, or apnea may occur for several weeks or months after demecarium is discontinued. Advise the anesthesiologist that the patient has received demecarium.

## CONTRAINDICATIONS

Contraindicated in patients with hypersensitivity to drug or acute angle-closure glaucoma before iridectomy.

## NURSING CONSIDERATIONS

• Use with extreme caution, if at all, in patients with bronchial asthma, pronounced bradycardia and hypotension, seizure disorders, spastic GI disturbances, Parkinson's disease, marked vagotonia, MI, or history of retinal detachment.

• Use with caution in patients with corneal abrasion.

• Administer phenylephrine concurrently, as ordered, to reduce incidence of iris cyst formation.

• If tolerance to the drug develops after prolonged use, know that the doctor may switch to another miotic for a short time.

• Know that toxicity is cumulative; toxic systemic symptoms may not appear for weeks or months after therapy is discontinued. Atropine sulfate S.C., I.M., or I.V. is antidote of choice.

## ☑ PATIENT TEACHING

• Teach patient how to apply drug. Advise him to wash hands before and after application, to avoid touching applicator tip to any surface and to wipe tip with clean tissue. Warn him not to exceed recommended dosage.

• If dose is missed, instruct patient not to double dose. If schedule is every other day, tell patient to apply as soon as possible if remembered same

day; if remembered later, tell him not to apply until next day, then skip a day and resume regular schedule. If schedule is once a day, tell patient to apply as soon as possible. If not remembered until next day, tell him to skip missed dose and resume schedule. If schedule is more than once daily, tell him to apply as soon as possible. If close to time for next dose, tell patient to skip missed dose and resume regular schedule.

• Tell patient that regular medical supervision is required to check ocular pressure.

• Advise patient to carry medical identification card at all times during therapy.

## physostigmine sulfate
Eserine Sulfate

*Pregnancy Risk Category: NR*

### HOW SUPPLIED
*Ophthalmic ointment:* 0.25%

### ACTION
Causes contraction of iris sphincter muscles resulting in miosis, and contraction of ciliary muscle, increasing outflow of aqueous humor and decreasing intraocular pressure.

### ONSET, PEAK, DURATION
Onset occurs within 30 minutes. Peak unknown. Effects persist for 12 to 48 hours.

### INDICATIONS & DOSAGE
*Open-angle glaucoma—*
**Adults and children:** 1 to 2 drops of solution instilled 2 to 4 times daily or a thin strip of ointment applied once daily to t.i.d.

### ADVERSE REACTIONS
**CNS:** headache, weakness.
**CV:** slow or irregular heartbeat.
**EENT:** blurred vision, eye pain, burning, redness, stinging, eye irrita-

---

*Liquid form contains alcohol.  **May contain tartrazine.  †Canada only.  ‡Australia only.  ◇OTC.

tion, twitching of eyelids, watering of eyes.
**GI:** nausea, vomiting, diarrhea.
**GU:** loss of bladder control.
**Other:** diaphoresis, muscle weakness, shortness of breath.

## INTERACTIONS
*Echothiophate, isoflurophate:* duration of action may be shortened. Monitor closely.
*Ophthalmic belladonna alkaloids:* may antagonize miotic actions. Avoid concomitant use.

## CONTRAINDICATIONS
Contraindicated in patients with intolerance to physostigmine, active uveitis, or corneal injury.

## NURSING CONSIDERATIONS
• Be aware that ointment may be used at night because of its longer duration of action.
• If tolerance to the drug develops, know that the doctor may switch to another miotic for a short time.

## ☑ PATIENT TEACHING
• Teach patient how to instill drug. Advise him to wash hands before and after instilling and to avoid touching applicator tip to any surface.
• Warn him not to exceed recommended dosage.

## pilocarpine
Ocusert Pilo

## pilocarpine hydrochloride
Adsorbocarpine, Isopto Carpine, Miocarpine†, Ocusert Pilo, Pilocar, Pilocel, Pilomiotin, Pilopine HS, Pilopt‡

## pilocarpine nitrate
Ocusert Pilo, Pilagan, P.V. Carpine Liquifilm

*Pregnancy Risk Category: NR*

## HOW SUPPLIED
**pilocarpine**
*Extended-release insert:* 20 mcg/hour, 40 mcg/hour for 7 days
**pilocarpine hydrochloride**
*Ophthalmic solution:* 0.25%, 0.5%, 1%, 2%, 3%, 4%, 5%, 6%, 8%, 10%
*Ophthalmic gel:* 4%
**pilocarpine nitrate**
*Ophthalmic solution:* 1%, 2%, 4%

## ACTION
A cholinergic that causes contraction of iris sphincter muscles, resulting in miosis and that produces ciliary spasm, deepening of the anterior chamber, and vasodilation of conjunctival vessels of the outflow tract.

## ONSET, PEAK, DURATION
Onset of miosis occurs within 10 to 30 minutes; intraocular pressure (IOP) reduction, within 60 minutes. Miotic effect peaks within 30 minutes; IOP reduction occurs within 75 minutes. Miosis effects persist up to 8 hours; IOP reduction, 4 to 14 hours with topical solution, up to 24 hours with gel, and up to 7 days with extended-release ocular system.

## INDICATIONS & DOSAGE
*Primary open-angle glaucoma—*
**Adults and children:** 1 to 2 drops instilled q 4 to 12 hours or 1-cm ribbon of 4% gel (Pilopine HS) applied h.s. Alternatively, one Ocusert Pilo system (20 or 40 mcg/hour) applied q 7 days.
*Emergency treatment of acute angle-closure glaucoma—*
**Adults and children:** 1 drop of 2% solution instilled q 5 to 10 minutes for three to six doses, followed by 1 drop q 1 to 3 hours until pressure is controlled.
*Preoperative and postopertive intraocular tension; mydriasis caused by mydriatic or cycloplegic agents—*
**Adults and children:** 1 to 2 drops instilled three to four times daily or 1-

cm ribbon of 4% gel (Pilopine HS) applied h.s.

## ADVERSE REACTIONS
**CV:** hypertension, tachycardia.
**EENT:** periorbital or supraorbital headache, *myopia,* ciliary spasm, *blurred vision,* conjunctival irritation, transient stinging and burning, keratitis, lens opacity, retinal detachment, lacrimation, changes in visual field, *brow pain.*
**GI:** nausea, vomiting, diarrhea, salivation.
**Respiratory:** *bronchoconstriction, pulmonary edema.*
**Other:** hypersensitivity reactions, diaphoresis.

## INTERACTIONS
*Carbachol, echothiophate:* additive effect. Don't use together.
*Ophthalmic belladonna alkaloids (such as atropine and scopolamine), cyclopentolate:* decreased pilocarpine antiglaucoma effectiveness and blocked mydriatic effects of these agents. Avoid concomitant use.
*Phenylephrine:* decreased dilation by phenylephrine. Don't use together.

## CONTRAINDICATIONS
Contraindicated in patients with hypersensitivity to drug or when cholinergic effects such as constriction are undesirable (for example, acute iritis, some forms of secondary glaucoma, pupillary block glaucoma, acute inflammatory disease of the anterior chamber).

## NURSING CONSIDERATIONS
● Use cautiously in patients with acute cardiac failure, bronchial asthma, peptic ulcer, hyperthyroidism, GI spasm, urinary tract obstruction, and Parkinson's disease.
● *Alert:* Keep in mind that patients with dark eyes may require stonger solutions.

## ☑ PATIENT TEACHING
● Instruct patient to apply gel at bedtime because it will blur vision. Warn him to avoid hazardous activities, such as operating machinery or driving, until temporary blurring subsides.
● Teach patient how to instill pilocarpine. Advise him to wash hands before and after instilling drug and to apply light finger pressure on lacrimal sac for 1 minute after drops are instilled. Warn patient not to touch applicator tip to eye or surrounding tissue.
● If the Ocusert Pilo system falls out of the eye during sleep, tell patient to wash hands, rinse the insert in cool tap water, and reposition it in the eye. Also tell him not to use a deformed insert.
● Warn patient that transient brow pain and myopia are common at first but usually disappear within 10 to 14 days.

---

atropine sulfate
cyclopentolate hydrochloride
epinephrine hydrochloride
epinephryl borate
homatropine hydrobromide
phenylephrine hydrochloride
scopolamine hydrobromide
tropicamide

## COMBINATION PRODUCTS
CYCLOMYDRIL OPHTHALMIC: cyclopentolate hydrochloride 0.2% and
phenylephrine hydrochloride 1%.
MUROCOLL-2: scopolamine hydrobromide 0.3% and phenylephrine hydrochloride 10%.

## atropine sulfate
Atropisol, Atropt‡, BufOpto
Atropine, Isopto Atropine

*Pregnancy Risk Category: C*

### HOW SUPPLIED
*Ophthalmic ointment:* 0.5%, 1%
*Ophthalmic solution:* 0.5%, 1%, 2%

### ACTION
A potent mydriatic and cycloplegic
whose anticholinergic action leaves
the pupil under unopposed adrenergic
influence, causing it to dilate.

### ONSET, PEAK, DURATION
Onset unknown. Mydriatic effect
peaks within 30 to 40 minutes; cycloplegic, within 1 to 3 hours. Effects of
mydriasis persist for 7 to 12 days; of
cycloplegia, 6 to 12 days.

### INDICATIONS & DOSAGE
*Acute iritis; uveitis* –
**Adults:** 1 to 2 drops instilled into the
eyes up to four times daily or a small
strip of ointment applied to the conjunctival sac up to three times daily.

**Children:** 1 to 2 drops of 0.5% solution instilled into the eyes up to three
times daily or a small strip of ointment applied to the conjunctival sac
up to three times daily.
*Cycloplegic refraction* –
**Adults:** 1 to 2 drops of 1% solution
instilled 1 hour before refraction.
**Children:** 1 to 2 drops of 0.5% solution instilled in each eye b.i.d. for 1
to 3 days before eye examination and
1 hour before refraction.

### ADVERSE REACTIONS
**CNS:** confusion, somnolence, headache.
**CV:** tachycardia.
**EENT:** ocular congestion with long-
term use, conjunctivitis, contact dermatitis of eye, ocular edema, *blurred
vision,* eye dryness, photophobia, increased intraocular pressure (IOP),
transient stinging and burning, irritation, hyperemia, blurred vision.
**GI:** dry mouth, abdominal distention
in infants.
**Skin:** dryness.

### INTERACTIONS
None significant.

### CONTRAINDICATIONS
Contraindicated in patients with glaucoma, hypersensitivity to drug or belladonna alkaloids, or who have adhesions between the iris and lens. Atropine should not be used during the
first 3 months of life because of the
possible association between cycloplegia produced and development of
amblyopia.

### NURSING CONSIDERATIONS
• Use cautiously in elderly patients
and in those where increased IOP may
be encountered.

• **Alert:** Treat drops and ointment as poison (not for internal use); signs of poisoning are disorientation and confusion. Antidote of choice is physostigmine salicylate I.V. or I.M.

• Watch for signs of glaucoma: increased intraocular pressure, ocular pain, headache, progressive blurring of vision. If present, notify the doctor

#### ☑ PATIENT TEACHING

• Teach patient how to instill atropine. Advise him to wash hands before and after instilling drug and to apply light finger pressure on lacrimal sac for 1 minute after instillation. Warn him not to touch tip of dropper or tube to eye or surrounding tissue.

• Warn patient to avoid hazardous activities, such as operating machinery or driving, until temporary blurring subsides.

• Advise patient to ease photophobia by wearing dark glasses.

---

### cyclopentolate hydrochloride

AK-Pentolate, Cyclogyl

*Pregnancy Risk Category: NR*

#### HOW SUPPLIED

*Ophthalmic solution:* 0.5%, 1%, 2%

#### ACTION

A potent mydriatic and cycloplegic whose anticholinergic action leaves the pupil under unopposed adrenergic influence, causing it to dilate.

#### ONSET, PEAK, DURATION

Onset rapid. Mydriatic effect peaks within 30 to 60 minutes; cycloplegic, within 25 to 75 minutes. Effects of mydriasis persist for 1 day; of cycloplegia, 0.25 to 1 day.

#### INDICATIONS & DOSAGE

*Diagnostic procedures requiring mydriasis and cycloplegia* –
**Adults:** 1 or 2 drops of 0.5%, 1%, or 2% solution instilled into the eyes followed by 1 or 2 drops in 5 to 10 minutes, if needed.

**Children:** 1 drop of 0.5%, 1%, or 2% solution instilled into each eye, followed in 5 to 10 minutes with 1 drop 0.5% or 1% solution, if necessary.

#### ADVERSE REACTIONS

**CNS:** irritability, confusion, somnolence, hallucinations, ataxia, *seizures,* behavioral disturbances in children.
**CV:** tachycardia.
**EENT:** eye burning on instillation, blurred vision, eye dryness, *photophobia,* ocular congestion, contact dermatitis in eye, conjunctivitis, increased intraocular pressure (IOP), transient stinging and burning, irritation, hyperemia.
**GU:** urine retention.
**Skin:** dryness.

#### INTERACTIONS

*Carbachol, pilocarpine:* may counteract mydriatic effect. Avoid concomitant use.
*Long-acting cholinergic antiglaucoma agents:* miotic actions may be inhibited. Avoid concomitant use.

#### CONTRAINDICATIONS

Contraindicated in patients with glaucoma, hypersensitivity to drug or belladonna alkaloids, or who have adhesions between the iris and lens.

#### NURSING CONSIDERATIONS

• Use with extreme caution in infants and young children.
• Use cautiously in elderly patients and others where increased IOP may be encountered.
• Know that drug is superior to homatropine hydrobromide, and has a shorter duration of action. Physostigmine is antidote of choice.

---

*Liquid form contains alcohol. **May contain tartrazine. †Canada only. ‡Australia only. ◊OTC.

## ☑ PATIENT TEACHING
• Teach patient how to instill drug. Advise him to wash hands before and after instilling drug and to apply light finger pressure on lacrimal sac for 1 minute after drops are instilled. Warn him not to touch tip of dropper to eye or surrounding tissue and that drug will burn when instilled.
• Warn patient to avoid hazardous activities, such as operating machinery or driving, until temporary blurring subsides.
• Advise patient to ease photophobia by wearing dark glasses.

# epinephrine hydrochloride
Epifrin, Glaucon

# epinephryl borate
Epinal, Eppy/N

*Pregnancy Risk Category: C*

## HOW SUPPLIED
**epinephrine hydrochloride**
*Ophthalmic solution:* 0.1%, 0.25%, 0.5%, 1%, 2%
**epinephryl borate**
*Ophthalmic solution:* 0.5%, 1%, 2%

## ACTION
An adrenergic that dilates the pupil by contracting the dilator muscle.

## ONSET, PEAK, DURATION
Onset of mydriasis occurs within a few minutes; of intraocular pressure (IOP) reduction, within 1 hour. IOP reduction peaks within 4 to 8 hours. Effects of mydriasis persist for several hours; of IOP reduction, 12 to 24 hours.

## INDICATIONS & DOSAGE
*Open-angle glaucoma –*
**Adults:** 1 or 2 drops of 1 or 2% solution once or twice daily. Dosage adjusted according to tonometric readings. The frequency of instillation

may vary from once every 2 to 4 days to four times daily.
*During ocular surgery –*
**Adults:** 1 or more drops of 0.1% hydrochloride solution up to three times.

## ADVERSE REACTIONS
**CNS:** brow ache, headache, lightheadedness.
**CV:** palpitations, tachycardia, arrhythmia, hypertension.
**EENT:** corneal or conjunctival pigmentation or corneal edema in longterm use; follicular hypertrophy; chemosis; conjunctivitis; iritis; hyperemic conjunctiva; maculopapular rash; eye stinging, burning, and tearing on instillation; eye pain; allergic lid reaction; ocular irritation.

## INTERACTIONS
*Cyclopropane, halogenated hydrocarbons:* arrhythmias, tachycardia. Use together cautiously, if at all.
*Digitalis glycosides:* increased risk of arrhythmias. Monitor closely.
*Local or systemic sympathomimetics:* additive toxic effects. Avoid concomitant use.
*MAO inhibitors:* exaggerated adrenergic effects. Adjust dose of epinephrine carefully.
*Topical miotics, beta-adrenergic blockers, osmotic agents, systemic carbonic anhydrase inhibitors:* additive lowering of IOP. Use together cautiously.
*Tricyclic antidepressants, antihistamines (diphenhydramine, dexchlorpheniramine):* potentiated cardiac effects of epinephrine. Monitor closely.

## CONTRAINDICATIONS
Contraindicated in patients with angle-closure glaucoma or when nature of the glaucoma has not been established and in patients with hypersensitivity to the drug, organic mental syndrome, or cardiac dilation and coronary insufficiency.

---

### NURSING CONSIDERATIONS
• Use cautiously in elderly patients and in those with diabetes mellitus, hypertension, Parkinson's disease, hyperthyroidism, aphakia (eye without lens), cardiac disease, cerebral arteriosclerosis, or bronchial asthma.
• Be aware that drug can also can be injected into anterior chamber to produce rapid mydriasis during cataract removal or can be used to control local bleeding during surgery.
• **Alert:** Don't substitute one salt if another one is ordered; epinephrine salts are not interchangeable.
• Monitor blood pressure and other vital signs.

### ☑ PATIENT TEACHING
• Teach patient how to instill drug. Advise him to wash hands before and after instilling drug and to apply light finger pressure on lacrimal sac for 1 minute after drops are instilled. Warn him not to touch tip of dropper to eye or surrounding tissue.
• Advise patient not to use while wearing soft contact lenses because discoloration of lenses may occur.
• Tell patient not to use darkened solution.

---

## homatropine hydrobromide
Homatrine, Homatropine, Isopto Homatropine

*Pregnancy Risk Category: C*

### HOW SUPPLIED
*Ophthalmic solution:* 2%, 5%

### ACTION
Anticholinergic action leaves the pupil under unopposed adrenergic influence, causing it to dilate.

### ONSET, PEAK, DURATION
Onset rapid. Mydriatic effect peaks within 40 to 60 minutes; cycloplegic, within 30 to 60 minutes. Effects of mydriasis persist for 1 to 3 days; of cycloplegia, 1 to 3 days.

### INDICATIONS & DOSAGE
*Cycloplegic refraction –*
**Adults and children:** 1 to 2 drops instilled into the eyes; if needed, repeated in 5 to 10 minutes for two or three doses.
*Uveitis –*
**Adults and children:** 1 to 2 drops instilled into the eyes q 3 to 4 hours.
   *Note:* Use only 2% solution with children. Patients with heavily pigmented irises may require larger doses.

### ADVERSE REACTIONS
**CNS:** confusion, somnolence, headache.
**CV:** tachycardia.
**EENT:** eye irritation, *blurred vision, photophobia,* increased intraocular pressure (IOP), transient stinging and burning, conjunctivitis, vascular congestion, edema.
**GI:** dry mouth.
**Skin:** dryness, rash.

### INTERACTIONS
None significant.

### CONTRAINDICATIONS
Contraindicated in patients with hypersensitivity to the drug or to other belladonna alkaloids, such as atropine, and in those with glaucoma or who have adhesions between the iris and lens.

### NURSING CONSIDERATIONS
• Use cautiously in elderly patients and others where increased IOP may be encountered.
• **Alert:** Be aware that homatropine is similar to atropine but weaker, with a shorter duration of action. May produce symptoms of atropine poisoning, such as severe dryness of mouth or tachycardia.

---

*Liquid form contains alcohol. **May contain tartrazine. †Canada only. ‡Australia only. ◇OTC.

## ☑ PATIENT TEACHING

● Teach patient how to instill drug. Advise him to wash hands before and after instilling drug and to apply light finger pressure on lacrimal sac for 1 minute after drops are instilled. Warn him not to touch tip of dropper to eye or surrounding tissue.

● Warn patient to avoid hazardous activities, such as operating machinery or driving, until temporary blurring subsides.

● Advise patient to ease photophobia by wearing dark glasses.

---

## phenylephrine hydrochloride

AK-Dilate, AK-Nefrin Ophthalmic◇, I-Phrine 2.5%, Isopto Frin◇, Mydfrin, Neo-Synephrine, Prefrin Liquifilm

*Pregnancy Risk Category: C*

### HOW SUPPLIED

*Ophthalmic solution:* 0.12%◇, 2.5%, 10%

### ACTION

An adrenergic that dilates the pupil by contracting the dilator muscle.

### ONSET, PEAK, DURATION

Onset is rapid. Mydriatic effect peaks within 15 to 60 minutes after using the 2.5% solution; 10 to 90 minutes after using the 10% solution. Effects of 2.5% solution persist for about 3 hours; of 10% solution, 3 to 7 hours.

### INDICATIONS & DOSAGE

*Mydriasis without cycloplegia –*
**Adults and children:** 1 or 2 drops of 2.5% or 10% solution instilled before examination. May be repeated in 10 to 60 minutes, if needed.
*Mydriasis and vasoconstriction –*
**Adults and adolescents:** 1 or 2 drops of 2.5% or 10% solution
**Children:** 1 drop of 2.5% solution.
*Chronic mydriasis –*

**Adults and adolescents:** 1 drop of 2.5% or 10% solution instilled b.i.d. or t.i.d.
**Children:** 1 drop of 2.5% solution instilled b.i.d. or t.i.d.
*Posterior synechia (adhesion of iris) –*
**Adults and children:** 1 drop of 10% solution.

Do not use 10% concentration in infants.

### ADVERSE REACTIONS

**CNS:** brow ache, headache.
**CV:** *hypertension* (with 10% solution), tachycardia, palpitations, *PVCs, MI.*
**EENT:** transient eye burning or stinging on instillation, blurred vision, increased intraocular pressure, keratitis, lacrimation, reactive hyperemia of eye, allergic conjunctivitis, rebound miosis.
**Skin:** pallor, dermatitis.
**Other:** trembling, diaphoresis.

### INTERACTIONS

*Guanethidine:* increased mydriatic and pressor effects of phenylephrine. Use together cautiously.
*Levodopa (systemic):* reduced mydriatic effect of phenylephrine. Use together cautiously.
*MAO inhibitors, beta blockers:* may cause arrhythmias because of increased pressor effect. Use together cautiously.
*Topically applied atropine, cyclopentolate, homatropine, scopolamine:* may increase dilation of pupil. Use together cautiously.
*Tricyclic antidepressants:* potentiated cardiac effects of epinephrine. Use together cautiously.

### CONTRAINDICATIONS

Contraindicated in patients with hypersensitivity to drug or angle-closure glaucoma and in those who wear soft contact lenses.

---

Reactions may be *common,* uncommon, *life-threatening,* or **COMMON AND LIFE-THREATENING.**

## NURSING CONSIDERATIONS
• Use cautiously in patients with marked hypertension, cardiac disorders, advanced arteriosclerotic changes, Type I diabetes, or hyperthyroidism; in children of low body weight; and in elderly patients.
• Know that systemic adverse reactions are least likely with 2.5% solution and greatest with 10% solution.

## ☑ PATIENT TEACHING
• Teach patient how to instill drug. Advise him to wash hands before and after instilling drug and to apply light finger pressure on lacrimal sac for 1 minute after drops are instilled. Warn him not to touch tip of dropper to eye or surrounding tissue.
• Warn patient not to exceed recommended dosage because systemic effects can result. Monitor blood pressure and pulse rate.
• Advise patient to contact the doctor if condition persists longer than 12 hours after discontinuation of the drug.
• Warn patient to avoid hazardous activities, such as operating machinery or driving, until temporary blurring subsides.
• Advise patient to ease photophobia by wearing dark glasses.
• Tell patient not to use brown solutions or solutions that contain precipitate.

---

## scopolamine hydrobromide
Isopto Hyoscine

*Pregnancy Risk Category: NR*

### HOW SUPPLIED
*Ophthalmic solution:* 0.25%

### ACTION
Anticholinergic action leaves the pupil under unopposed adrenergic influence, causing it to dilate.

## ONSET, PEAK, DURATION
Onset is rapid. Mydriatic effect peaks within 15 to 30 minutes; cycloplegic effect, within 30 to 45 minutes. Effects persist up to 1 week.

## INDICATIONS & DOSAGE
*Cycloplegic refraction* –
**Adults:** 1 to 2 drops of 0.25% solution 1 hour before refraction.
**Children:** 1 drop of 0.25% solution b.i.d. for 2 days before refraction.
*Iritis, uveitis* –
**Adults:** 1 to 2 drops of 0.25% solution once daily, b.i.d., or t.i.d.
**Children:** 1 drop once daily to t.i.d.

## ADVERSE REACTIONS
**CNS:** confusion, delirium, somnolence, acute psychotic reactions, headache, hallucinations.
**CV:** tachycardia.
**EENT:** ocular congestion with prolonged use, conjunctivitis, *blurred vision,* eye dryness, increased intraocular pressure, *photophobia,* transient stinging and burning, edema.
**GI:** dry mouth.
**Skin:** dryness, contact dermatitis.

## INTERACTIONS
None significant.

## CONTRAINDICATIONS
Contraindicated in patients with shallow anterior chamber and angle-closure glaucoma or hypersensitivity to the drug.

## NURSING CONSIDERATIONS
• Use with extreme caution (if at all) in infants and small children.
• Use cautiously in patients with cardiac disease and in elderly patients.
• Observe patients closely for adverse CNS effects (such as disorientation and delirium).
• Know that scopolamine may be used in patients sensitive to atropine because it's faster acting and has a

---

shorter duration of action and fewer adverse reactions.

☑ **PATIENT TEACHING**
● Teach patient how to instill drug. Advise him to wash hands before and after instilling drug and to apply light finger pressure on lacrimal sac for 1 minute after drops are instilled. Warn him to avoid touching tip of dropper to eye or surrounding tissue.
● Warn patient to avoid hazardous activities, such as operating machinery or driving, until temporary blurring subsides.
● Advise patient to ease photophobia by wearing dark glasses.

---

# tropicamide
Mydriacyl, Tropicacyl
*Pregnancy Risk Category: NR*

## HOW SUPPLIED
*Ophthalmic solution:* 0.5%, 1%

## ACTION
The shortest-acting cycloplegic available, whose anticholinergic action leaves the pupil under unopposed adrenergic influence, causing it to dilate.

## ONSET, PEAK, DURATION
Onset rapid. Mydriatic effect peaks within 20 to 40 minutes; cycloplegic effect, within 20 to 35 minutes. Effects persist up to 7 hours.

## INDICATIONS & DOSAGE
*Cycloplegic refraction –*
**Adults:** 1 drop of 1% solution; repeated in 5 minutes. If needed, additional drop in 20 to 30 minutes.
**Children:** 1 drop of 0.5% or 1% solution; repeated in 5 minutes, if needed.
*Fundus examinations –*
**Adults and children:** 1 to 2 drops of 0.5% solution in each eye 15 to 20 minutes before examination; instilla-

tion may be repeated q 30 minutes as needed.

## ADVERSE REACTIONS
**CNS:** confusion, somnolence, hallucinations, behavioral disturbances in children.
**EENT:** *transient eye stinging on instillation,* increased intraocular pressure, hyperemia, irritation, conjunctivitis, edema, *blurred vision, photophobia; dry throat.*
**GI:** dry mouth.
**Skin:** dryness.

## INTERACTIONS
None significant.

## CONTRAINDICATIONS
Contraindicated in patients with shallow anterior chamber and angle-closure glaucoma or hypersensitivity to drug.

## NURSING CONSIDERATIONS
● Use cautiously in elderly patients.
● Know that tropicamide's mydriatic effect is greater than its cycloplegic effect.

☑ **PATIENT TEACHING**
● Teach patient how to instill drug. Advise him to wash hands before and after instilling drug and to apply light finger pressure on lacrimal sac for 1 minute after drops are instilled. Warn him not to touch tip of dropper to eye or surrounding tissue.
● Warn patient that drug causes transient stinging.
● Warn patient to avoid hazardous activities, such as operating machinery or driving, until temporary blurring subsides.
● Advise patient to ease photophobia by wearing dark glasses.

---

# 83

# Ophthalmic vasoconstrictors

**naphazoline hydrochloride**
**oxymetazoline hydrochloride**
**tetrahydrozoline hydrochloride**

## COMBINATION PRODUCTS

ALBALON-A LIQUIFILM: naphazoline hydrochloride 0.05% and antazoline phosphate 0.5%.
BLEPHAMIDE LIQUIFILM SUSPENSION: phenylephrine hydrochloride 0.12%, sulfacetamide sodium 10%, and prednisolone acetate 0.2%.
PREFRIN-A: phenylephrine hydrochloride 0.12%, pyrilamine maleate 0.1%, and antipyrine 0.1%.
VASOCIDIN OPHTHALMIC OINTMENT: phenylephrine hydrochloride 0.125%, sulfacetamide sodium 10%, and prednisolone acetate 0.5%.
VASOCIDIN OPHTHALMIC SOLUTION: phenylephrine hydrochloride 0.125%, sulfacetamide sodium 10%, and prednisolone sodium phosphate 0.25%.
VASOCON-A OPHTHALMIC SOLUTION: naphazoline hydrochloride 0.05% and antazoline phosphate 0.5%.
ZINCFRIN◇: phenylephrine hydrochloride 0.12% and zinc sulfate 0.25%.

## naphazoline hydrochloride

AK-Con, Albalon Liquifilm, Allerest◇, Clear Eyes◇, Degest 2◇, Estivin II, Naphcon◇, Naphcon Forte, Optazine‡, Vasoclear◇, Vasocon Regular

*Pregnancy Risk Category: C*

## HOW SUPPLIED

*Ophthalmic solution:* 0.012%◇, 0.02%◇, 0.03%◇, 0.1%

## ACTION

Unknown. Thought to cause vasoconstriction by local adrenergic action on the blood vessels of the conjunctiva.

## ONSET, PEAK, DURATION

Local vasoconstriction usually occurs within 10 minutes. Peak unknown. Effects persist for 2 to 6 hours.

## INDICATIONS & DOSAGE

*Ocular congestion, irritation, itching—*
**Adults:** 1 to 3 drops of 0.1% solution instilled q 3 to 4 hours or 1 to 2 drops of 0.012% to 0.03% solution up to q.i.d.

## ADVERSE REACTIONS

**CNS:** headache, dizziness, nervousness, weakness.
**EENT:** transient eye stinging, pupillary dilation, eye irritation, photophobia, blurred vision, increased intraocular pressure, keratitis, lacrimation.
**GI:** nausea.
**Other:** diaphoresis.

## INTERACTIONS

*Tricyclic antidepressants, MAO inhibitors:* hypertensive crisis if naphazoline is systemically absorbed. Use together cautiously.

## CONTRAINDICATIONS

Contraindicated in patients with hypersensitivity to any of drug's ingredients and in patients with acute angle-closure glaucoma. Use of 0.1% solution is contraindicated in children.

## NURSING CONSIDERATIONS

• Use cautiously in patients with hyperthyroidism, cardiac disease, hypertension, or diabetes mellitus.

---

*Liquid form contains alcohol. **May contain tartrazine. †Canada only. ‡Australia only. ◇OTC.

• Know that drug is most widely used ocular decongestant.
• Be aware that drug can produce marked sedation and coma in children, especially infants.
• Store in tightly closed container.

### ☑ PATIENT TEACHING
• Teach patient how to instill drug. Advise him to wash hands before and after instilling drug and to apply light finger pressure on lacrimal sac for 1 minute after drops are instilled. Warn him not to touch tip of dropper to eye or surrounding tissue.
• Warn patient not to exceed recommended dosage. Rebound congestion and conjunctivitis may occur with frequent or prolonged use.
• Tell patient to notify the doctor if photophobia, blurred vision, pain, or lid edema develops.
• Instruct patient not to use OTC preparations longer than 72 hours without consulting a doctor.

---

## oxymetazoline hydrochloride
OcuClear◊, Visine L.R.◊

*Pregnancy Risk Category: C*

### HOW SUPPLIED
*Ophthalmic solution:* 0.025%

### ACTION
A direct-acting sympathomimetic amine that acts on alpha-adrenergic receptors in the arterioles of the conjunctiva to produce vasoconstriction, resulting in decreased conjunctival congestion.

### ONSET, PEAK, DURATION
Onset occurs within 5 minutes. Peak unknown. Effects persist for approximately 6 hours.

### INDICATIONS & DOSAGE
*Relief of eye redness due to minor eye irritations —*

**Adults and children 6 years and over:** 1 to 2 drops in the conjunctival sac two to four times daily (spaced at least 6 hours apart).

### ADVERSE REACTIONS
**CNS:** headache, light-headedness, nervousness, insomnia.
**CV:** palpitations, tachycardia, irregular heartbeat.
**EENT:** *transient stinging upon initial instillation,* blurred vision, reactive hyperemia with excessive dosage or prolonged use, keratitis, lacrimation, increase in intraocular pressure.
**Other:** trembling.

### INTERACTIONS
*Tricyclic antidepressants, maprotiline:* if significant systemic absorption of oxymetazoline occurs, concurrent use may potentiate the pressor effect of oxymetazoline.

### CONTRAINDICATIONS
Contraindicated in patients hypersensitive to any component of the drug and in those with angle-closure glaucoma.

### NURSING CONSIDERATIONS
• Use cautiously in patients with hyperthyroidism, cardiac disease, hypertension, and eye disease, infection, or injury.
• Don't use if solution has become cloudy or changes color.

### ☑ PATIENT TEACHING
• Teach patient how to instill drops. Advise him to wash hands before and after instilling solution, and warn him not to touch tip of dropper to eye or surrounding tissue.
• Advise patient to apply light finger pressure on lacrimal sac for 1 minute after drug instillation.
• Advise patient to stop the drug and see a doctor if eye pain occurs, if vision changes, or if redness or irrita-

---

Reactions may be *common,* uncommon, ***life-threatening,*** or **COMMON AND LIFE-THREATENING.**

tion continues, worsens, or lasts for more than 72 hours.

# tetrahydrozoline hydrochloride
Murine Plus◇, Optigene◇, Soothe◇, Tetrasine◇, Visine◇

*Pregnancy Risk Category: C*

## HOW SUPPLIED
*Ophthalmic solution:* 0.05%◇

## ACTION
Unknown. Thought to cause vasoconstriction by local adrenergic action on the blood vessels of the conjunctiva.

## ONSET, PEAK, DURATION
Onset occurs within a few minutes. Peak unknown. Effects persist for 4 to 8 hours.

## INDICATIONS & DOSAGE
*Conjunctival congestion, irritation, and allergic conditions –*
**Adults and children over 2 years:** 1 to 2 drops of 0.05% solution instilled up to four times daily or as directed by the doctor.

## ADVERSE REACTIONS
**CNS:** headache, drowsiness, insomnia, dizziness, tremor.
**CV:** *cardiac arrhythmias.*
**EENT:** transient eye stinging, pupillary dilation, increased intraocular pressure, keratitis, lacrimation, eye irritation.

## INTERACTIONS
*Guanethidine, MAO inhibitors, tricyclic antidepressants:* hypertensive crisis if tetrahydrozoline is systemically absorbed. Don't use together.

## CONTRAINDICATIONS
Contraindicated in patients hypersensitive to the drug or any of its components, and in those with angle-closure glaucoma or other serious eye diseases.

## NURSING CONSIDERATIONS
• Use cautiously in patients with hyperthyroidism, heart disease, hypertension, or diabetes mellitus.
• Rebound congestion may occur with frequent or prolonged use.

## ☑ PATIENT TEACHING
• Teach patient how to instill drug. Advise him to wash hands before and after instilling drug and to apply light finger pressure on lacrimal sac for 1 minute after drops are instilled. Warn him not to touch tip of dropper to eye or surrounding tissue.
• Warn patient not to exceed recommended dosage.
• Tell patient to stop drug and notify the doctor if redness or irritation persists or increases or if no relief occurs within 2 days.
• Caution patient not to share eye medications with others.

---

*Liquid form contains alcohol.   **May contain tartrazine.   †Canada only.   ‡Australia only.   ◇OTC.

# 84

# Miscellaneous ophthalmics

apraclonidine hydrochloride
betaxolol hydrochloride
botulinum toxin type A
carteolol hydrochloride
dapiprazole hydrochloride
dipivefrin
dorzolamide hydrochloride
fluorescein sodium
isosorbide
levobunolol hydrochloride
levocabastine hydrochloride
lodoxamide tromethamine
metipranolol hydrochloride
sodium chloride, hypertonic
timolol maleate

## COMBINATION PRODUCTS

FLURESS: fluorescein sodium 0.25%
and benoxinate hydrochloride 0.4%.

---

## apraclonidine hydrochloride

Iopidine

*Pregnancy Risk Category: C*

### HOW SUPPLIED

*Ophthalmic solution:* 0.5%, 1%

### ACTION

Unknown; an alpha-adrenergic agonist that reduces intraocular pressure (IOP), possibly by decreasing production of aqueous humor.

### ONSET, PEAK, DURATION

Onset occurs within 1 hour. Peak effect occurs within 3 to 5 hours. Effects persist at least 12 hours.

### INDICATIONS & DOSAGE

*Prevention or control of IOP elevation before and after ocular laser surgery –*
**Adults:** 1 drop of 1% solution instilled 1 hour before initiation of laser surgery on the anterior segment, followed by 1 drop immediately after surgery.
*Short-term adjunct therapy in patients who require additional IOP reduction –*
**Adults:** 1 or 2 drops of 0.5% solution instilled into affected eyes t.i.d.

### ADVERSE REACTIONS

**CNS:** insomnia, irritability, dream disturbances, headache, irritability, paresthesia.
**CV:** bradycardia, vasovagal attack, palpitations, hypotension, orthostatic hypotension.
**EENT:** upper eyelid elevation, conjunctival blanching and microhemorrhage, mydriasis, eye burning or discomfort, foreign body sensation in eye, eye dryness and *itching, hyperemia,* conjunctivitis, blurred vision, nasal burning or dryness, or increased pharyngeal secretions.
**GI:** abdominal pain, discomfort, diarrhea, vomiting, taste disturbances, dry mouth.
**Skin:** pruritus not associated with rash, sweaty palms.
**Other:** body heat sensation, decreased libido, extremity pain or numbness, allergic response.

### INTERACTIONS

*Topical pilocarpine or beta-adrenergic blockers:* additive effects in lowering IOP. Use together cautiously.

### CONTRAINDICATIONS

Contraindicated in patients hypersensitive to apraclonidine or clonidine.

### NURSING CONSIDERATIONS

● Use cautiously in patients with severe cardiac disease including hypertension or history of vasovagal attack.

---

Reactions may be *common,* uncommon, *life-threatening,* or COMMON AND LIFE-THREATENING.

- Closely monitor patients who tend to develop exaggerated decreases in IOP after drug therapy.
- Observe patients closely for vasovagal attack during laser surgery.
- Closely monitor patients with severe systemic disease, including hypertension, even though drug's systemic effects (altered heart rate and blood pressure) are uncommon after usual dose.

☑ **PATIENT TEACHING**
- Teach patient how to instill 0.5% solution. Advise him to wash hands before and after instilling drug and to apply light finger pressure on lacrimal sac for 1 minute after instillation.
- Warn patient not to touch tip of dropper to eye or surrounding tissue.
- Tell patient to separate intervals between each ophthalmic product instillation by at least 5 minutes to avoid washing away the previous dose.
- Encourage patient to comply with the three-times-daily dosage regimen.

---

**betaxolol hydrochloride**
Betoptic

*Pregnancy Risk Category: C*

**HOW SUPPLIED**
*Ophthalmic solution:* 0.5%
*Ophthalmic suspension:* 0.25%

**ACTION**
Unknown, although as a cardioselective beta blocker it reduces formation and possibly increases outflow of aqueous humor.

**ONSET, PEAK, DURATION**
Onset occurs in ½ to 1 hour. Intraocular pressure (IOP) reduction peaks after a single dose within about 2 hours. Effects persist for 12 or more hours.

**INDICATIONS & DOSAGE**
*Chronic open-angle glaucoma and ocular hypertension –*
**Adults:** 1 or 2 drops of 0.5% solution or 0.25% suspension b.i.d.

**ADVERSE REACTIONS**
**CNS:** insomnia, depressive neurosis.
**EENT:** *eye stinging on instillation causing brief discomfort,* photophobia, erythema, itching, keratitis, occasional tearing.

**INTERACTIONS**
*Calcium channel blockers:* AV conduction disturbances, ventricular failure, and hypotension if significant systemic absorption occurs. Monitor closely.
*Cocaine:* may inhibit betaxolol's effects. Avoid concomitant use.
*Digitalis glycosides:* excessive bradycardia; patients may require ECG monitoring if significant systemic absorption occurs.
*Inhalation hydrocarbon anesthetics:* prolonged severe hypotension if significant systemic absorption occurs. Tell the anesthesiologist that the patient is receiving ophthalmic betaxolol.
*Ophthalmic epinephrine, dipivefrin:* may produce mydriasis. Use together cautiously.
*Oral antidiabetic agents, insulin:* risk of hypoglycemia or hyperglycemia if significant systemic absorption occurs. Dosage adjustments of antidiabetic agents or hypoglycemic medication may be necessary.
*Phenothiazines:* additive hypotensive effects; increased risk of adverse effects if significant systemic absorption occurs. Monitor closely.
*Reserpine:* excessive beta blockade. Monitor closely.
*Systemic beta blockers:* additive effects. Monitor closely.

---

## CONTRAINDICATIONS

Contraindicated in patients with hypersensitivity to drug, sinus bradycardia, greater-than-first-degree AV block, cardiogenic shock, or overt heart failure.

## NURSING CONSIDERATIONS

• Use cautiously in patients with restricted pulmonary function, diabetes mellitus, hyperthyroidism, or a history of heart failure.
• Keep in mind that some patients may need a few weeks' treatment to stabilize IOP-lowering response. Determine IOP after 4 weeks of treatment.

## ☑ PATIENT TEACHING

• Teach patient how to instill drug. Advise him to wash hands before and after instilling drug and to apply light finger pressure on lacrimal sac for 1 minute after instillation. Warn him not to touch tip of dropper to eye or surrounding tissue. He should shake suspension well before instilling.
• Encourage patient to comply with twice-daily dosage regimen.
• Advise patient to ease photophobia by wearing dark glasses.

---

# botulinum toxin type A

Botox

*Pregnancy Risk Category: C*

## HOW SUPPLIED

*Powder for injection:* 100-unit vial

## ACTION

A protein that produces a neuromuscular paralysis by binding to acetylcholine receptors on the motor endplate and that may inhibit the release of acetylcholine from presynaptic nerve endings.

## ONSET, PEAK, DURATION

Onset occurs in 1 or 2 days after injection. Peak occurs within 1 to 2 weeks. Effects persist for 2 to 6 weeks.

## INDICATIONS & DOSAGE

*Strabismus –*
**Adults and children 12 years and over:** injections should be made only by doctors familiar with the technique, which involves surgical exposure of the region as well as electromyographic guidance of the injection needle.

Dosage varies with the degree of deviation (lower doses are used for small deviations). For vertical muscles and for horizontal strabismus of less than 20 prism diopters, the usual dosage is 1.25 to 2.5 units injected into any one muscle. For horizontal strabismus of 20 to 50 prism diopters, dosage is 2.5 to 5 units into any one muscle. For persistent (greater than 1 month's duration) palsy of the sixth cranial nerve, dosage is 1.25 to 2.5 units into the medial rectus muscle.

Subsequent injections for recurrent or residual strabismus should not be made until 7 to 14 days after the initial dose and unless substantial function has returned to the injected and adjacent muscles. Dosage may be increased up to twice the initial dose for patients experiencing incomplete paralysis; subsequent doses in patients with adequate response should not be increased. The maximum single dose for any one muscle is 25 units.

*Blepharospasm –*
**Adults:** initially, 1.25 to 2.5 units injected into the medial and lateral pretarsal orbicularis oculi of the upper lid and into the lateral pretarsal orbicularis oculi of the lower lid. Effects should be apparent within 3 days and peak within 1 to 2 weeks. Dosage may be doubled if inadequate paralysis is achieved; however, exceeding 5 units per site produces no apparent benefit. Each treatment lasts about 3 months and can be repeated indefinitely.

---

Reactions may be *common,* uncommon, *life-threatening,* or COMMON AND LIFE-THREATENING.

Cumulative dosage should not exceed 200 units/month.

## ADVERSE REACTIONS
**EENT:** *ptosis, vertical deviation* (after treatment of strabismus), *eye irritation, photophobia* (after treatment of blepharospasm), *swelling of eyelid.*
**Skin:** diffuse rash, ecchymoses.

## INTERACTIONS
*Aminoglycoside antibiotics, other drugs that interfere with neuromuscular transmission:* may potentiate effect of botulinum toxin. Use caution when administered concomitantly.

## CONTRAINDICATIONS
Contraindicated in patients hypersensitive to the drug or any of its components.

## NURSING CONSIDERATIONS
• Reconstitute the drug with preservative-free 0.9% sodium chloride solution. The vacuum in the vial should be noticeable when reconstituting. Inject the diluent into the vial gently because severe agitation can denature the protein.

• Keep in mind reconstituting with 1 ml of 0.9% sodium chloride solution produces a concentration of 10 units/0.1 ml; adding 2 ml yields 5 units/0.1 ml. Adding more diluent (such as 4 ml to produce 2.5 units/0.1 ml or 8 ml to yield 1.25 units/0.1 ml) or using different injection volumes may also be used to adjust dosage.

• Reconstituted drug should be clear, colorless, and free of particulate matter. Record the date and time of reconstitution. Keep reconstituted drug in the refrigerator until use. Drug should be administered within 4 hours of removal from the freezer.

• Prepare the injection by drawing slightly more volume than needed into a sterile 1-ml syringe. Expel air bubbles in the barrel of the syringe and attach an electromyographic injection needle (if treating strabismus), such as a 1½″, 27G needle. Expel leftover drug into an appropriate waste container while checking for leakage around the needle. Be sure to use a new needle and syringe for each injection.

• **Alert:** Have epinephrine available in case of an anaphylactic reaction.

• Apply several drops of an ocular decongestant and a topical anesthetic as ordered before treating strabismus.

• Freeze at or below 23° F ( − 5° C).

## ☑ PATIENT TEACHING
• Explain use and how drug is administered to patient and family. Answer questions and address concerns.

• Inform patient about the adverse reactions associated with drug. Instruct him to report persistent or severe adverse reactions promptly.

---

# carteolol hydrochloride
Ocupress Ophthalmic Solution, 1%

*Pregnancy Risk Category: C*

## HOW SUPPLIED
*Ophthalmic solution:* 1%

## ACTION
A nonselective beta-adrenergic blocking agent that reduces intraocular pressure, although the exact mechanism of action has not been definitely demonstrated.

## ONSET, PEAK, DURATION
Unknown.

## INDICATIONS & DOSAGE
*Chronic open-angle glaucoma, intraocular hypertension –*
**Adults:** 1 drop in the conjunctival sac of the affected eye b.i.d.

## ADVERSE REACTIONS
**EENT:** *transient eye irritation, burning, tearing, conjunctival hyperemia,*

ocular edema, blurred and cloudy vision, photophobia, decreased night vision, ptosis, blepharoconjunctivitis, abnormal corneal staining, corneal sensitivity.
**Systemic:** bradycardia, hypotension, arrhythmias, palpitations, dyspnea, asthenia, headache, dizziness, insomnia, sinusitis, taste perversion.

## INTERACTIONS
*Oral beta-adrenergic blockers, catecholamine-depleting agents (such as reserpine):* may cause additive effects and the development of hypotension or bradycardia. Monitor patient closely.

## CONTRAINDICATIONS
Contraindicated in patients hypersensitive to any component of the drug and in those with bronchial asthma, severe COPD, sinus bradycardia, second- or third-degree AV block, overt cardiac failure, or cardiogenic shock.

## NURSING CONSIDERATIONS
• Use with caution in patients with nonallergic bronchospastic disease, diabetes mellitus, hyperthyroidism, hypersensitivity to other beta-adrenergic agents, or decreased pulmonary function and in breast-feeding patients.
• **Alert:** Discontinue drug at the first sign of cardiac failure and notify the doctor.
• Be aware that when the drug is used to reduce elevated intraocular pressure in angle-closure glaucoma, it should be used in combination with a miotic and should not be used alone.

## ☑ PATIENT TEACHING
• Tell patient that if more than one topical ophthalmic drug is being used, the drugs should be administered at least 10 minutes apart.
• Teach patient how to instill drops. Advise him to wash hands before and after instilling solution, and warn him

not to touch tip of the dropper to eye or surrounding tissue.
• Also teach patient to keep bottle tightly closed when not in use and to protect it from light.
• Tell patient that drug is a beta-adrenergic blocker and, although it is administered topically, it has the potential to be absorbed systemically. Advise patient to apply light finger pressure on lacrimal sac for 1 minute after drug instillation to minimize systemic absorption.
• Also tell patient that the same types of adverse reactions that are attributable to beta-adrenergic agent therapy may occur with topical administration. If signs of serious adverse reactions or hypersensitivity occur, tell the patient to discontinue the drug and notify the doctor immediately.
• Advise patient to ease photophobia by wearing dark glasses.
• Stress the importance of compliance with recommended therapy.

---

# dapiprazole hydrochloride
Rēv-Eyes

*Pregnancy Risk Category: B*

## HOW SUPPLIED
*Ophthalmic powder:* 25 mg-vial with 5 ml diluent and dropper supplied

## ACTION
Blocks alpha-adrenergic receptors in smooth muscle, producing miosis through an effect on the dilator muscle of the iris.

## ONSET, PEAK, DURATION
Onset rapid. Peak and duration unknown.

## INDICATIONS & DOSAGE
*Mydriasis* —
**Adults:** 2 drops instilled into the conjunctiva of each eye, followed in 5 minutes by another 2 drops.

---

## ADVERSE REACTIONS
**CNS:** *headache, brow ache.*
**EENT:** *conjunctival injection lasting 20 minutes, eye burning on instillation, ptosis, lid erythema, lid edema, chemosis, eye itching or dryness, punctate keratitis, corneal edema, photophobia, blurry vision, dryness of eye, tearing.*

## INTERACTIONS
None significant.

## CONTRAINDICATIONS
Contraindicated in patients hypersensitive to the drug or any of its components; when pupil constriction is undesirable, as in acute iritis; to reduce intraocular pressure; and to treat open-angle glaucoma.

## NURSING CONSIDERATIONS
• To prepare, remove and discard aluminum seals and rubber stoppers from both drug and diluent vials. Pour diluent into drug vial, and attach dropper assembly. Shake vial to ensure mixing.
• To avoid contamination, do not touch dropper to any surface.
• Be aware that drug should not be used in same patient more than once per week.
• Be aware that eye color can affect the rate of pupillary constriction, but not the final pupil size.
• Store at room temperature for 21 days. Discard any discolored solution.

## ☑ PATIENT TEACHING
• Explain use and administration of drug to patient and family.
• Warn patient about adverse reactions associated with drug.

## dipivefrin
Propine

*Pregnancy Risk Category: B*

## HOW SUPPLIED
*Ophthalmic solution:* 0.1%

## ACTION
A prodrug of epinephrine, dipivefrin is converted to epinephrine in the eye. The liberated epinephrine appears to decrease aqueous production and increase aqueous outflow.

## ONSET, PEAK, DURATION
Onset occurs within 30 minutes. Peak effect occurs within 1 hour. Effects persist for 12 hours or more.

## INDICATIONS & DOSAGE
*Intraocular pressure (IOP) reduction in chronic open-angle glaucoma —*
**Adults:** for initial glaucoma therapy, 1 drop of 0.1% solution q 12 hours. Adjustments in dosage then made based on patient response as determined by tonometric readings.

## ADVERSE REACTIONS
**CV:** tachycardia, hypertension, arrhythmias.
**EENT:** eye burning or stinging, conjunctival injection, conjunctivitis, mydriasis, allergic reaction, photophobia.

## INTERACTIONS
*Digitalis glycosides, inhalation hydrocarbon anesthetics, tricyclic antidepressants:* increased risk of adverse cardiac effects if significant systemic absorption occurs. Monitor closely.
*Ophthalmic beta blockers, osmotic agents, systemically administered carbonic anhydrase inhibitors:* additive lowering of IOP. Use together cautiously. Monitor for potential adverse effects.
*Systemic sympathomimetics:* possible additive effects if significant systemic absorption occurs. Monitor closely.

## CONTRAINDICATIONS
Contraindicated in patients with angle-closure glaucoma or hypersensitivity to drug.

## NURSING CONSIDERATIONS
• Use cautiously in patients with aphakia or CV disease, history of hypersensitivity to epinephrine, and asthma.
• Be aware that drug is often used concomitantly with other antiglaucoma drugs.
• Know that drug may have fewer adverse reactions than conventional epinephrine therapy.

## ☑ PATIENT TEACHING
• Teach patient how to instill dipivefrin. Advise him to wash hands before and after instilling drug and to avoid touching tip of dropper to eye or surrounding tissue.
• Instruct patient to report persistent or serious adverse reactions promptly.

---

## dorzolamide hydrochloride
Trusopt

*Pregnancy Risk Category: C*

## HOW SUPPLIED
*Ophthalmic solution: 2%*

## ACTION
Inhibits carbonic anhydrase in the ciliary processes of the eye, which decreases aqueous humor secretion, presumably by slowing the formation of bicarbonate ions with a subsequent reduction in sodium and fluid transport. The result is a reduction in intraocular pressure (IOP).

## ONSET, PEAK, DURATION
Unknown.

## INDICATIONS & DOSAGE
*Treatment of increased IOP in patients with ocular hypertension or open-angle glaucoma –*

**Adults:** 1 drop in the conjunctival sac of the affected eye t.i.d.

## ADVERSE REACTIONS
**EENT:** *ocular burning, stinging, or discomfort; superficial punctate keratitis; ocular allergic reaction; blurred vision; lacrimation; dryness; photophobia;* iridocyclitis.
**Systemic:** *bitter taste,* headache, nausea, asthenia, fatigue, rash, urolithiasis.

## INTERACTIONS
*Oral carbonic anhydrase inhibitors:* may cause additive effects. Do not administer concomitantly.

## CONTRAINDICATIONS
Contraindicated in patients hypersensitive to any component of the drug and in those with renal impairment.

## NURSING CONSIDERATIONS
• Use with caution in patients with hepatic impairment.
• If more than one topical ophthalmic drug is being used, the drugs should be administered at least 10 minutes apart.

## ☑ PATIENT TEACHING
• Teach patient how to instill drops. Advise him to wash hands before and after instilling solution, and warn him not to touch tip of the dropper to eye or surrounding tissue.
• Tell patient that the drug is a sulfonamide and, although it is administered topically, it can be absorbed systemically. Advise patient to apply light finger pressure on lacrimal sac for 1 minute after drug instillation to minimize systemic absorption.
• Tell patient that the same types of adverse reactions that are attributable to sulfonamides may occur with topical administration. If signs of serious adverse reactions or hypersensitivity occur, tell the patient to discontinue

---

Reactions may be *common,* uncommon, *life-threatening,* or COMMON AND LIFE-THREATENING.

the drug and notify the doctor immediately.

• Advise patient to discontinue the drug and notify the doctor if any ocular reactions, particularly conjunctivitis and eyelid reactions, occur.

• Tell patient not to wear soft contact lenses while using this drug.

• Stress the importance of compliance with recommended therapy.

## fluorescein sodium
Fluorescite, Fluor-I-Strip, Fluor-I-Strip A.T., Ful-Glo, Funduscein Injections

*Pregnancy Risk Category: C*

### HOW SUPPLIED
*Ophthalmic solution:* 2%
*Ophthalmic strips:* 0.6 mg, 1 mg, 9 mg
*Parenteral injection:* 10%, 25%

### ACTION
A water-soluble dye that produces an intense green fluorescence in alkaline solution (pH 5.0 or less) or a bright yellow one when viewed under cobalt blue illumination.

### ONSET, PEAK, DURATION
Onset immediate. Peak and duration unknown.

### INDICATIONS & DOSAGE
*Diagnostic in corneal abrasions and foreign bodies; fitting hard contact lenses; lacrimal patency; fundus photography; applanation tonometry* –
**Adults and children:** 1 or 2 drops of 2% solution followed by irrigation; or strip moistened with sterile water, then conjunctiva or fornix touched with moistened tip, and eye flushed with irrigating solution. Patient should blink several times after application.
*Retinal angiography* –
**Adults:** 5 ml of 10% solution (500

mg) or 3 ml of 25% solution (750 mg) rapidly injected into antecubital vein.
**Children:** 0.077 ml of 10% solution (7.7 mg/kg body weight) or 0.044 ml of 25% solution (7.5 mg/kg body weight) rapidly injected into antecubital vein.

### ADVERSE REACTIONS
Topical use:
**EENT:** eye stinging or burning, yellow tears.
I.V. use:
**CNS:** headache, dizziness, syncope, *seizures.*
**CV:** hypotension, *shock, cardiac arrest, thrombophlebitis.*
**GI:** nausea, vomiting, GI distress.
**GU:** bright yellow urine (persists for 24 to 36 hours).
**Respiratory:** transient dyspnea, bronchospasm.
**Skin:** yellow skin discoloration (fades in 6 to 12 hours), urticaria, pruritus.
**Other:** hypersensitivity reactions, including urticaria and *anaphylaxis;* extravasation at injection site; fever; angioedema.

### INTERACTIONS
None significant.

### CONTRAINDICATIONS
Contraindicated in patients with hypersensitivity to drug; do not use with soft contact lenses (lenses may become discolored).

### NURSING CONSIDERATIONS
• Use cautiously in patients with history of allergy or bronchial asthma.
• Always use aseptic technique. Easily contaminated by *Pseudomonas aeruginosa.*
• **I.V. use:** Keep an antihistamine, epinephrine, and oxygen available when giving parenterally. Avoid extravasation during injection.
• Use topical anesthetic as ordered before instilling to relieve burning and irritation.

---

• Never instill dye while patients are wearing soft contact lenses; fluorescein will ruin them.
• Be aware that defects appear green under normal light or bright yellow under cobalt blue illumination. Foreign bodies are surrounded by a green ring. Similar lesions of the conjunctiva are delineated in orange-yellow.
• Don't freeze; store below 80° F (26.7° C).

☑ **PATIENT TEACHING**
• Warn patient that urine will be bright yellow after injection and that routine urinalysis will be abnormal within 1 hour after injection.
• Tell patient to report persistent or serious adverse reactions promptly.

---

## isosorbide
Ismotic
*Pregnancy Risk Category: B*

**HOW SUPPLIED**
*Oral solution:* 45% (100 g/225 ml) in 220-ml containers

**ACTION**
Acts as an osmotic agent by promoting redistribution of water and thereby producing diuresis.

**ONSET, PEAK, DURATION**
Onset occurs within 30 minutes. Peak effects occur in 1 to 1½ hours. Duration unknown.

**INDICATIONS & DOSAGE**
*Short-term reduction of intraocular pressure (IOP) caused by glaucoma –*
**Adults:** initially, 1.5 g/kg P.O. Usual dosage range is 1 to 3 g/kg.

**ADVERSE REACTIONS**
**CNS:** vertigo, light-headedness, lethargy, headache, confusion, disorientation, irritability, syncope, dizziness.
**GI:** gastric discomfort, nausea, vomiting.

**Other:** hypernatremia, hyperosmolality, thirst.

**INTERACTIONS**
None significant.

**CONTRAINDICATIONS**
Contraindicated in patients with anuria caused by severe renal disease, severe dehydration, acute pulmonary edema, and hemorrhagic glaucoma.

**NURSING CONSIDERATIONS**
• Know that additional doses should be used cautiously, especially in patients with diseases associated with sodium retention, such as CHF.
• To improve palatability, pour medication over cracked ice and tell patients to sip it.
• Monitor patients closely for 5 to 10 minutes after administration for adverse effects.
• Keep in mind that isosorbide is especially useful for rapid reduction of IOP. May be used to interrupt acute attack of glaucoma before laser surgery.
• In patients with diseases associated with sodium retention, carefully monitor fluid and electrolyte balance.

☑ **PATIENT TEACHING**
• Tell patient that this drug may induce thirst.
• Caution patient not to perform hazardous activities if adverse CNS reactions occur.

---

## levobunolol hydrochloride
Betagan
*Pregnancy Risk Category: C*

**HOW SUPPLIED**
*Ophthalmic solution:* 0.25%, 0.5%

**ACTION**
Unknown. A nonselective beta blocker that is thought to reduce for-

---

mation and possibly increase outflow of aqueous humor.

### ONSET, PEAK, DURATION
Onset occurs within 1 hour. Intraocular pressure (IOP) reduction peaks within 2 to 6 hours after a single dose. Effects persist up to 24 hours.

### INDICATIONS & DOSAGE
*Chronic open-angle glaucoma and ocular hypertension –*
**Adults:** 1 to 2 drops once daily or b.i.d.

### ADVERSE REACTIONS
**CNS:** headache, depression, insomnia.
**CV:** slight reduction in resting heart rate.
**EENT:** *transient eye stinging and burning,* tearing, erythema, itching, keratitis, corneal punctate staining, photophobia; decreased corneal sensitivity with long-term use.
**GI:** nausea.
**Skin:** urticaria.
**Other:** evidence of beta blockade and systemic absorption *(hypotension, bradycardia, syncope,* **asthmatic attacks in patients with a history of asthma,** and **CHF**).

### INTERACTIONS
*Propranolol, metoprolol, and other oral beta-adrenergic blockers:* increased ocular and systemic effects. Use together cautiously.
*Reserpine and other catecholamine-depleting drugs:* enhanced hypotensive and bradycardiac effects. Monitor closely.
*Topical miotics, dipivefrin, epinephrine; systemically administered carbonic anhydrase inhibitors:* additive lowered IOP. Use together cautiously.

### CONTRAINDICATIONS
Contraindicated in patients with hypersensitivity to drug, bronchial asthma, history of bronchial asthma or severe COPD, sinus bradycardia, second- or third-degree AV block, cardiac failure, and cardiogenic shock.

### NURSING CONSIDERATIONS
• Use cautiously in patients with chronic bronchitis and emphysema, diabetes mellitus, hyperthyroidism, and myasthenia gravis.
• Avoid letting dropper touch the patient's eye or surrounding tissue.

### ☑ PATIENT TEACHING
• Teach patient how to instill levobunolol. Advise him to wash hands before and after instilling drug and to apply light finger pressure on lacrimal sac for 1 minute after drops are instilled.
• Warn patient not to touch dropper to eye or surrounding tissue.

---

## levocabastine hydrochloride
Livostin

*Pregnancy Risk Category: C*

### HOW SUPPLIED
*Ophthalmic suspension:* 0.05%

### ACTION
Selectively blocks ophthalmic histamine $H_1$ receptors.

### ONSET, PEAK, DURATION
Unknown.

### INDICATIONS & DOSAGE
*Temporary relief of seasonal allergic conjunctivitis –*
**Adults and children 12 years and over:** 1 drop q.i.d. for up to 2 weeks.

### ADVERSE REACTIONS
**CNS:** headache, fatigue, somnolence.
**EENT:** *transient eye discomfort upon instillation (burning, stinging), eye discharge,* dryness, pain, or redness;

---

lacrimation; eyelid edema; visual disturbances; pharyngitis.
**GI:** dry mouth, nausea.
**Respiratory:** cough, dyspnea.
**Skin:** rash.

## INTERACTIONS
None significant.

## CONTRAINDICATIONS
Contraindicated in patients hypersensitive to the drug or any of its components and while soft contacts are worn.

## NURSING CONSIDERATIONS
• Know that drug is for ophthalmic use only; it should never be injected.

## ☑ PATIENT TEACHING
• Teach patient how to instill levocabastine. Advise him to wash hands before and after instilling drug and to avoid touching tip of dropper to eye or surrounding tissue. He should shake suspension well before instilling.
• Warn patient that he may experience transient discomfort or burning upon instillation. Tell him to contact the doctor if pain persists.
• Tell patient not to wear soft contact lenses during therapy.
• Tell patient to store drug at room temperature and to avoid freezing. He should not use a discolored solution.

---

## lodoxamide tromethamine
Alomide

*Pregnancy Risk Category: B*

### HOW SUPPLIED
*Ophthalmic solution:* 0.1%

### ACTION
Stabilizes mast cells and prevents the release of inflammation mediators.

### ONSET, PEAK, DURATION
Unknown.

## INDICATIONS & DOSAGE
*Vernal conjunctivitis, vernal keratoconjunctivitis, vernal keratitis* —
**Adults and children 2 years and over:** 1 to 2 drops in affected eye q.i.d. for up to 3 months.

## ADVERSE REACTIONS
**CNS:** headache, dizziness, somnolence.
**EENT:** *transient eye discomfort upon instillation (burning, stinging);* anterior chamber cells; blepharitis; blurred vision; chemosis; corneal erosion, ulcer, or abrasion; crystalline deposits; epitheliopathy; sensation of foreign body, stickiness, or warmth; hyperemia; keratitis; keratopathy; ocular edema, discharge, swelling, fatigue, itching, or allergy; pruritus; scales on eyelids or eyelash; tearing; dry nose.
**GI:** nausea, stomach discomfort.
**Skin:** rash, heat sensation.

## INTERACTIONS
None significant.

## CONTRAINDICATIONS
Contraindicated in patients hypersensitive to the drug or any of its components.

## NURSING CONSIDERATIONS
• Know that drug is for ophthalmic use only; it should never be injected.
• Check expiration date before using.

## ☑ PATIENT TEACHING
• Teach patient how to instill lodoxamide. Advise him to wash hands before and after instilling drug and to avoid touching tip of dropper to eye or surrounding tissue.
• Tell him to contact the doctor if discomfort or burning persists upon instillation.
• Advise patient not to wear soft contact lenses during therapy.

---

# metipranolol hydrochloride
OptiPranolol

*Pregnancy Risk Category: C*

## HOW SUPPLIED
*Ophthalmic solution:* 0.3% in 5- or 10-ml dropper bottles

## ACTION
Unknown. A noncardioselective beta-adrenergic blocker that appears to reduce aqueous production and to reduce elevated and normal intraocular pressure (IOP), with or without glaucoma, with little or no effect on pupil size or accommodation. IOP above 24 mm Hg is reduced an average of 20% to 26%.

## ONSET, PEAK, DURATION
Onset occurs within 30 minutes. Peak effect occurs within about 2 hours. Effects persist about 12 to 24 hours.

## INDICATIONS & DOSAGE
*IOP reduction in ocular conditions, including ocular hypertension and chronic open-angle glaucoma —*
**Adults:** 1 drop into affected eye b.i.d. If IOP is not at a satisfactory level, concomitant therapy to lower it may be instituted.

## ADVERSE REACTIONS
**CNS:** headache, anxiety, dizziness, depression, somnolence, nervousness, asthenia, brow ache.
**CV:** hypertension, *MI*, atrial fibrillation, angina, palpitation, bradycardia.
**EENT:** transient local eye discomfort, tearing, conjunctivitis, eyelid dermatitis, blurred vision, blepharitis, abnormal vision, photophobia, eye edema, rhinitis, epistaxis.
**GI:** nausea.
**Respiratory:** dyspnea, bronchitis, cough.
**Skin:** rash.
**Other:** hypersensitivity reactions, myalgia.

## INTERACTIONS
*Calcium channel blockers, digitalis glycosides, quinidine:* increased risk of adverse cardiac effects if significant amount of drug is systemically absorbed. Use together cautiously.
*Fentanyl, general anesthetics:* excessive hypotension. Monitor closely.
*Metoprolol tartrate, propranolol, other oral beta-adrenergic blockers:* increased ocular and systemic effects. Use together cautiously.
*Reserpine and other catecholamine-depleting drugs:* enhanced hypotensive and bradycardia-induced effects. Avoid concurrent use.

## CONTRAINDICATIONS
Contraindicated in patients hypersensitive to the drug or any of its components and in patients with bronchial asthma, history of bronchial asthma or severe COPD, sinus bradycardia, second- or third-degree AV block, cardiac failure, and cardiogenic shock.

## NURSING CONSIDERATIONS
• Use cautiously in patients with non-allergic bronchospasm, chronic bronchitis, emphysema, diabetes mellitus (especially in those subject to spontaneous hypoglycemia), hyperthyroidism, or cerebrovascular insufficiency.
• Anticipate using pilocarpine, other miotics, or systemic carbonic anhydrase inhibitors concomitantly if IOP is not adequately controlled.
• Check expiration date on bottle before use. Do not use if eyedrops have changed color.
• Be aware that a slight increase in outflow facility has been demonstrated with metipranolol. Like other noncardioselective beta-adrenergic blockers, metipranolol does not have significant local anesthetic (membrane-stabilizing) actions or intrinsic sympathomimetic activity.

---

*Liquid form contains alcohol. **May contain tartrazine. †Canada only. ‡Australia only. ◊OTC.

☑ **PATIENT TEACHING**
• Teach patient how to instill metipranolol. Instruct him to first wash hands thoroughly and then tilt head back or lie down and gaze upward. Tell patient to gently grasp lower eyelid below eyelashes and pull eyelid away from eye to form a pouch. Then have him place dropper directly over eye, avoiding contact with eye or any surface; look up just before applying drop; and look down for several seconds after instillation and slowly release eyelid.
• Tell patient to close eyes gently for 1 to 2 minutes and to apply gentle pressure to inside corner of eye at bridge of nose to retard draining of solution from intended area. Warn him not to rub eye or rinse dropper.

---

## sodium chloride, hypertonic
Adsorbonac Ophthalmic Solution, Muro-128 Ointment, Sodium Chloride Ointment 5%

*Pregnancy Risk Category: NR*

### HOW SUPPLIED
*Ophthalmic ointment:* 5%
*Ophthalmic solution:* 2%, 5%

### ACTION
An osmotic agent that removes excess fluid from the cornea.

### ONSET, PEAK, DURATION
Unknown.

### INDICATIONS & DOSAGE
*Temporary relief of corneal edema –*
**Adults and children:** 1 to 2 drops q 3 to 4 hours, or ointment applied h.s.

### ADVERSE REACTIONS
**EENT:** slight eye stinging.
**Other:** hypersensitivity reactions.

### INTERACTIONS
None significant.

### CONTRAINDICATIONS
Contraindicated in patients hypersensitive to the drug or any of its components.

### NURSING CONSIDERATIONS
• Know that ophthalmic solution is for topical use only; never inject.
• Check expiration date before using.

☑ **PATIENT TEACHING**
• Teach patient how to instill drug. Advise him to wash hands before and after instilling drug and to apply light finger pressure on lacrimal sac for 1 minute after drops are instilled. Warn patient not to touch dropper to eye or surrounding tissue.
• Tell patient to prevent caking on dropper bottle tip by putting a few drops of sterile irrigation solution inside bottle cap.
• Warn patient that ointment may cause blurred vision.
• If patient experiences severe headache, pain, rapid change in vision, acute redness of eyes, sudden appearance of floating spots, pain on exposure to light, or double vision, tell him to discontinue the drug and notify doctor.
• Advise patient to store drug in tightly closed container.

---

## timolol maleate
Timoptic Solution, Timoptic-XE

*Pregnancy Risk Category: C*

### HOW SUPPLIED
*Ophthalmic solution:* 0.25%, 0.5%
*Ophthalmic gel:* 0.25%, 0.5%

### ACTION
Unknown. A beta blocker that is thought to reduce aqueous formation and possibly increase aqueous outflow.

---

Reactions may be *common,* uncommon, *life-threatening,* or COMMON AND LIFE-THREATENING.

## ONSET, PEAK, DURATION
Onset occurs within 30 minutes. Peak effects occur within 1 to 2 hours. Effects persist for 12 to 24 hours.

## INDICATIONS & DOSAGE
*Chronic open-angle, secondary, and aphakic glaucomas; ocular hypertension –*
**Adults:** initially, 1 drop of 0.25% solution in each affected eye b.i.d.; maintenance dosage is 1 drop daily. If no response, 1 drop of 0.5% solution in each affected eye b.i.d. If intraocular pressure (IOP) is controlled, dosage reduced to 1 drop daily. Alternatively, 1 drop of gel in each affected eye once daily.

## ADVERSE REACTIONS
**CNS:** depression, fatigue, dizziness, lethargy, hallucinations, confusion.
**CV:** slight reduction in resting heart rate, arrhythmia, *CVA, cardiac arrest,* heart block, palpitations.
**EENT:** minor eye irritation, decreased corneal sensitivity with long-term use, conjunctivitis, blepharitis, keratitis, visual disturbances, diplopia, ptosis.
**Other:** *evidence of beta blockade and systemic absorption (hypotension, bradycardia, syncope, asthmatic attacks in patients with a history of asthma,* and *CHF).*

## INTERACTIONS
*Calcium channel blockers, digitalis glycosides, quinidine:* increased risk of adverse cardiac effects if significant amounts of timolol are systemically absorbed. Use together cautiously.
*Fentanyl, general anesthetics:* excessive hypotension. Monitor closely.
*Metoprolol tartrate, propranolol, other oral beta-adrenergic blockers:* increased ocular and systemic effects. Use together cautiously.
*Reserpine and other catecholamine-depleting drugs:* enhanced hypoten-sive and bradycardia-induced effects. Avoid concurrent use.

## CONTRAINDICATIONS
Contraindicated in patients hypersensitive to the drug and in patients with bronchial asthma, history of bronchial asthma or severe COPD, sinus bradycardia, second- or third-degree AV block, cardiac failure, and cardiogenic shock.

## NURSING CONSIDERATIONS
● Use cautiously in patients with non-allergic bronchospasm, chronic bronchitis, emphysema, diabetes mellitus, hyperthyroidism, or cerebrovascular insufficiency.
● Administer other ophthamic agents at least 10 minutes before administering gel form of drug.
● Monitor diabetic patients carefully. Systemic beta-blocking effects can mask some signs of hypoglycemia in diabetic patients.
● Be aware that some patients may need a few weeks' treatment to stabilize pressure-lowering response. Determine IOP after 4 weeks of treatment.
● Know that the drug can be used safely in patients with glaucoma who wear conventional hard contact lenses.

## ☑ PATIENT TEACHING
● Teach patient how to instill timolol. Advise him to wash hands before and after instilling drug and to apply light finger pressure on lacrimal sac for 1 minute after drops are instilled. Warn patient not to touch dropper to eye or surrounding tissue.
● Instruct patient using gel form of drug to invert the container and shake once before each use. Also tell him to administer other ophthalmic agents at least 10 minutes before administering the gel drop.

**acetic acid**
**boric acid**
**carbamide peroxide**
**chloramphenicol**
**triethanolamine polypeptide**
   **oleate-condensate**

## COMBINATION PRODUCTS
BOROFAIR OTIC: acetic acid 2% and aluminum acetate 2%.

---

## acetic acid
Domeboro Otic, VoSol Otic

*Pregnancy Risk Category: NR*

### HOW SUPPLIED
*Otic solution:* 2% acetic acid in aluminum acetate solution (Domeboro Otic), 2% acetic acid with 3% propylene glycol diacetate (VoSol Otic)

### ACTION
Inhibits or destroys bacteria in the ear canal.

### ONSET, PEAK, DURATION
Unknown.

### INDICATIONS & DOSAGE
*External ear canal infection –*
**Adults and children:** 4 to 6 drops into ear canal t.i.d. or q.i.d.; or insert saturated wick for first 24 hours, then continue with instillations.
*Prophylaxis of swimmer's ear –*
**Adults and children:** 2 drops in each ear b.i.d.

### ADVERSE REACTIONS
**EENT:** ear irritation or itching.
**Skin:** urticaria.
**Other:** overgrowth of nonsusceptible organisms.

### INTERACTIONS
None significant.

### CONTRAINDICATIONS
Contraindicated in patients with perforated eardrum.

### NURSING CONSIDERATIONS
• Reculture any persistent drainage.
• Be aware that drug has anti-infective, anti-inflammatory, and antipruritic effects. *Pseudomonas aeruginosa* is particularly sensitive to this drug.

### ☑ PATIENT TEACHING
• Instruct patient or caregiver how to administer drug.
• Warn patient to avoid touching ear with dropper to prevent reinfection.

---

## boric acid
Aurocaine 2◊, Auro-Dri◊, Dri/Ear◊, Ear-Dry◊

*Pregnancy Risk Category: NR*

### HOW SUPPLIED
*Otic solution:* 2.75% boric acid in isopropyl alcohol

### ACTION
Weak bacteriostatic that inhibits or destroys bacteria in the ear canal; also is a fungistatic agent.

### ONSET, PEAK, DURATION
Unknown.

### INDICATIONS & DOSAGE
*External ear canal infection –*
**Adults and children:** 3 to 6 drops into ear canal; plug with cotton. Repeated t.i.d. or q.i.d.

---

Reactions may be *common,* uncommon, *life-threatening,* or COMMON AND LIFE-THREATENING.

**ADVERSE REACTIONS**
**EENT:** ear irritation or itching.
**Skin:** urticaria.
**Other:** overgrowth of nonsusceptible organisms.

**INTERACTIONS**
None significant.

**CONTRAINDICATIONS**
Contraindicated in patients with a perforated eardrum or excoriated membranes in ear.

**NURSING CONSIDERATIONS**
• Watch for signs of superinfection (continual pain, inflammation, fever).

☑ **PATIENT TEACHING**
• Instruct patient or caregiver how to administer drug.
• Warn patient to avoid touching ear with dropper to prevent reinfection.
• Tell patient using cotton plug to always moisten with medication.

---

## carbamide peroxide
Debrox◇

*Pregnancy Risk Category: NR*

**HOW SUPPLIED**
*Otic solution:* 6.5% carbamide in glycerin or glycerin and propylene glycol

**ACTION**
A ceruminolytic that emulsifies and disperses accumulated cerumen.

**ONSET, PEAK, DURATION**
Onset and peak unknown. Duration is 15 to 30 minutes.

**INDICATIONS & DOSAGE**
*Impacted cerumen* –
**Adults and children:** 5 to 10 drops into ear canal b.i.d. for up to 4 days. Allow solution to remain in ear canal for 15 to 30 minutes; remove with warm water.

**ADVERSE REACTIONS**
None reported.

**INTERACTIONS**
None significant.

**CONTRAINDICATIONS**
Contraindicated in patients with a perforated eardrum.

**NURSING CONSIDERATIONS**
• Use in children under 12 years only under a doctor's direction.

☑ **PATIENT TEACHING**
• Instruct patient or caregiver how to administer drug.
• Warn patient to avoid touching ear with dropper to prevent reinfection.
• Tell patient to flush ear gently with warm water, using a rubber bulb syringe.
• Tell patient to call the doctor if redness, pain, or swelling persists.

---

## chloramphenicol
Chloromycetin Otic, Sopamycetin†

*Pregnancy Risk Category: NR*

**HOW SUPPLIED**
*Otic solution:* 0.5%

**ACTION**
Inhibits or destroys bacteria in the ear canal.

**ONSET, PEAK, DURATION**
Unknown.

**INDICATIONS & DOSAGE**
*External ear canal infection* –
**Adults and children:** 2 to 3 drops into ear canal t.i.d.

**ADVERSE REACTIONS**
**EENT:** ear itching or burning.
**Skin:** pruritus, urticaria.
**Other:** overgrowth of nonsusceptible organisms, burning, bone marrow hypoplasia, *aplastic anemia.*

---

*Liquid form contains alcohol.  **May contain tartrazine.  †Canada only.  ‡Australia only.  ◇OTC.

**INTERACTIONS**
None significant.

**CONTRAINDICATIONS**
Contraindicated in patients with a perforated eardrum.

**NURSING CONSIDERATIONS**
• Obtain history of use and reaction to drug.
• Watch for signs of superinfection (continued pain, inflammation, fever). Avoid prolonged use.
• Reculture any persistent drainage.
• Watch for signs of sore throat (early sign of toxicity).

☑ **PATIENT TEACHING**
• Instruct patient or caregiver how to administer drug.
• Warn patient to avoid touching ear with dropper to avoid reinfection.

---

**triethanolamine polypeptide oleate-condensate**
Cerumenex

*Pregnancy Risk Category: NR*

**HOW SUPPLIED**
*Otic solution:* 10% in 6-ml, 12-ml bottles with droppers

**ACTION**
A ceruminolytic that emulsifies and disperses accumulated cerumen.

**ONSET, PEAK, DURATION**
Onset and peak unknown. Duration is 15 to 30 minutes.

**INDICATIONS & DOSAGE**
*Impacted cerumen –*
**Adults and children:** fill ear canal with solution and insert cotton plug. After 15 to 30 minutes, flush ear with warm water.

**ADVERSE REACTIONS**
**EENT:** ear erythema or itching.
**Skin:** severe eczema.

**INTERACTIONS**
None significant.

**CONTRAINDICATIONS**
Contraindicated in perforated eardrum, otitis media, and otitis externa.

**NURSING CONSIDERATIONS**
• *Alert:* If hypersensitivity is suspected, anticipate patch test by placing 1 drop of drug on inner forearm; cover with small bandage. Read results in 24 hours. If any reaction (redness, swelling) occurs, know that drug should not be used.

☑ **PATIENT TEACHING**
• Teach patient how to apply the drug. He should moisten cotton plug with medication before insertion, leave cotton in place for a maximum of 30 minutes, and flush ear gently with warm water, using a rubber bulb syringe.
• Tell patient not to use drops more often than prescribed.
• Warn patient that this medication is for use only in the ears.
• Advise patient to discontinue the drug if adverse reactions occur and to contact the doctor immediately.
• Tell patient to keep container tightly closed and away from moisture.

---

Reactions may be *common,* uncommon, *life-threatening,* or **COMMON AND LIFE-THREATENING.**

beclomethasone dipropionate
budesonide
dexamethasone sodium
  phosphate
ephedrine sulfate
epinephrine hydrochloride
flunisolide
fluticasone propionate
naphazoline hydrochloride
oxymetazoline hydrochloride
phenylephrine hydrochloride
tetrahydrozoline hydrochloride
triamcinolone acetonide
xylometazoline hydrochloride

### COMBINATION PRODUCTS
4-WAY NASAL SPRAY◊: phenylephrine hydrochloride 0.5%, naphazoline
hydrochloride 0.05%, and pyrilamine
maleate 0.2%.

---

## beclomethasone dipropionate
Beconase AQ Nasal Spray,
Beconase Nasal Inhaler,
Vancenase AQ Nasal Spray,
Vancenase Nasal Inhaler

*Pregnancy Risk Category: C*

### HOW SUPPLIED
*Nasal aerosol:* 42 mcg/metered spray,
50 mcg/metered spray‡
*Nasal spray:* 42 mcg/metered spray,
50 mcg/metered spray‡

### ACTION
A corticosteroid that decreases nasal
inflammation, mainly by stabilizing
leukocyte lysosomal membranes.

### ONSET, PEAK, DURATION
Onset occurs within 5 to 7 days. Time
to maximal benefit is up to 3 weeks
for some patients. Duration unknown.

### INDICATIONS & DOSAGE
*Relief of symptoms of seasonal or pe-
rennial rhinitis; prevention of recurrence of nasal polyps after surgical removal—*
**Adults and children over 12 years:**
usual dosage is 1 or 2 sprays in each
nostril, b.i.d., t.i.d., or q.i.d.

### ADVERSE REACTIONS
**CNS:** headache.
**EENT:** *mild transient nasal burning
and stinging,* nasal congestion, sneezing, burning, stinging, dryness, epistaxis, nasopharyngeal fungal infections.

### INTERACTIONS
None significant.

### CONTRAINDICATIONS
Contraindicated in patients hypersensitive to the drug and in patients experiencing status asthmaticus or other
acute episodes of asthma.

### NURSING CONSIDERATIONS
• Use cautiously, if at all, in patients
with active or quiescent respiratory
tract tubercular infections or untreated fungal, bacterial, or systemic
viral or ocular herpes simplex infections. Also use cautiously in patients
who have recently had nasal septal ulcers, nasal surgery, or trauma.
• Observe the patient for fungal infections.
• Be aware that beclomethasone is not
effective for acute exacerbations of
rhinitis. Decongestants or antihistamines may be needed.

### ☑ PATIENT TEACHING
• To instill, instruct the patient to
shake the container before using; to
blow nose to clear nasal passages; and

---

*Liquid form contains alcohol. **May contain tartrazine. †Canada only. ‡Australia only. ◊OTC.

to tilt head slightly forward and insert nozzle into nostril, pointing away from septum. Tell him to hold the other nostril closed and then to inspire gently and spray. Next, have him shake the container again and repeat in the other nostril.

• Advise the patient to pump the nasal spray three or four times before the first use, and once or twice before first use each day. The cap and nosepiece of the activator should be cleaned in warm water every day, then allowed to air-dry.

• Advise the patient to use drug regularly, as prescribed, because its effectiveness depends on regular use.

• Explain that the drug's therapeutic effects, unlike those of decongestants, are not immediate. Most patients achieve benefit within a few days, but some may require 2 to 3 weeks.

• Warn the patient not to exceed recommended dosages because of the risk of hypothalamic-pituitary-adrenal function suppression.

• Tell the patient to notify the doctor if symptoms don't improve within 3 weeks or if nasal irritation persists.

• Teach the patient good nasal and oral hygiene.

---

## budesonide
Rhinocort

*Pregnancy Risk Category: C*

### HOW SUPPLIED
*Nasal spray:* 32 mcg/metered spray (7-g canister)

### ACTION
Unknown. A corticosteroid that probably decreases nasal inflammation, mainly by inhibiting the activities of specific cells and the mediators involved in the allergic response.

### ONSET, PEAK, DURATION
Not clearly defined.

### INDICATIONS & DOSAGE
*Symptoms of seasonal or perennial allergic rhinitis –*
**Adults and children 6 years and older:** 2 sprays in each nostril in the morning and evening or 4 sprays in each nostril in the morning. Maintenance dosage should be the fewest number of sprays needed to control symptoms.

### ADVERSE REACTIONS
**CNS:** nervousness.
**EENT:** *nasal irritation, epistaxis, pharyngitis,* reduced sense of smell, nasal pain, hoarseness.
**GI:** bad taste, dry mouth, dyspepsia, nausea.
**Respiratory:** *cough,* moniliasis, wheezing, dyspnea.
**Skin:** facial edema, rash, pruritus, contact dermatitis.
**Other:** myalgia, hypersensitivity reactions.

### INTERACTIONS
None significant.

### CONTRAINDICATIONS
Contraindicated in patients hypersensitive to the drug or any of its components and in those who have had recent septal ulcers, nasal surgery, or nasal trauma until total healing has occurred.

### NURSING CONSIDERATIONS
• Use cautiously in patients with tuberculous infections; untreated fungal, bacterial, or systemic viral infections; or ocular herpes simplex.

### ☑ PATIENT TEACHING
• To instill, instruct the patient to shake the container before using; to blow nose to clear nasal passages; and to tilt head slightly forward and insert nozzle into nostril, pointing away from septum. Tell him to hold the other nostril closed and then to inspire gently and spray. Next, have him

---

*Reactions may be* common, uncommon, *life-threatening,* or COMMON AND LIFE-THREATENING.

shake container again and repeat in the other nostril.

• Instruct the patient that the product should be used by one person only to prevent the spread of infection.

• Advise the patient not to break, incinerate, or store canister in extreme heat; contents under pressure.

• Warn the patient not to exceed prescribed dosage or use for long periods of time because of the risk of hypothalamic-pituitary-adrenal axis suppression.

• Tell the patient to contact the doctor if symptoms do not improve in 3 weeks or if condition worsens.

• Teach the patient good nasal and oral hygiene.

## dexamethasone sodium phosphate
Dexacort Phosphate Turbinaire
*Pregnancy Risk Category: C*

### HOW SUPPLIED
*Nasal aerosol:* 84 mcg/metered spray, 170 doses/12.6 g canister

### ACTION
Decreases nasal inflammation, mainly by stabilizing leukocyte lysosomal membranes.

### ONSET, PEAK, DURATION
Not clearly defined.

### INDICATIONS & DOSAGE
*Allergic or inflammatory conditions, nasal polyps –*
**Adults:** 2 sprays in each nostril b.i.d. or t.i.d. Maximum dosage is 12 sprays daily.
**Children 6 to 12 years:** 1 or 2 sprays in each nostril b.i.d. Maximum 8 sprays daily.

Each spray delivers 0.1 mg dexamethasone sodium phosphate equal to 0.084 mg dexamethasone.

### ADVERSE REACTIONS
**EENT:** nasal irritation, dryness, rebound nasal congestion.
**Other:** hypersensitivity reactions, systemic effects with prolonged use (pituitary-adrenal suppression, sodium retention, *CHF,* hypertension, peptic ulceration, ecchymoses, petechiae, masking of infection).

### INTERACTIONS
None significant.

### CONTRAINDICATIONS
Contraindicated in patients with hypersensitivity to drug or in patients with systemic fungal infections, tuberculosis, viral and fungal nasal conditions, or ocular herpes simplex.

### NURSING CONSIDERATIONS
• Use cautiously in patients with diabetes mellitus, peptic ulcer, ulcerative colitis, abscess or other pyrogenic infection, diverticulitis, fresh intestinal anastomosis, renal insufficiency, hypertension, osteoporosis, and myasthenia gravis.

• Frequently monitor blood pressure and serum potassium level. Hypertension and hypokalemia can occur with systemic absorption.

• Monitor for fluid retention which can occur from systemic absorption.

• Be prepared to gradually reduce dosage as nasal condition improves.

• Notify the doctor if you suspect underlying bacterial infection that should be controlled with anti-infectives.

• Know that irritation or sensitivity may require stopping drug.

### ☑ PATIENT TEACHING
• To instill, instruct the patient to shake the container before using; to blow nose to clear nasal passages; and to tilt head slightly forward and insert nozzle into nostril, pointing away from septum. Tell him to hold the other nostril closed and then to inspire

gently and spray. Next, have him shake container again and repeat in the other nostril.
• Teach the patient good nasal and oral hygiene.
• Warn the patient that product should be used by only one person to prevent spread of infection.
• Warn the patient to avoid prolonged use because of the risk of hypothalamic-pituitary-adrenal-axis suppression.
• Advise the patient to contact the doctor if he experiences fever, joint or muscle aches, or extreme tiredness.
• Advise the patient not to break, incinerate, or store canister in extreme heat; contents under pressure.

## ephedrine sulfate
Vicks Vatronol Nose Drops◇

*Pregnancy Risk Category: NR*

### HOW SUPPLIED
*Nasal solution:* 0.5%◇

### ACTION
Causes local vasoconstriction of dilated arterioles, reducing blood flow and nasal congestion.

### ONSET, PEAK, DURATION
Unknown.

### INDICATIONS & DOSAGE
*Nasal congestion –*
**Adults and children:** 2 to 3 drops of 0.5% solution into each nostril. Used no more frequently than q 4 hours.

### ADVERSE REACTIONS
**CNS:** nervousness, excitation.
**CV:** *tachycardia.*
**EENT:** rebound nasal congestion with long-term or excessive use, mucosal irritation.

### INTERACTIONS
*MAO inhibitors:* hypertensive crisis if ephedrine is absorbed. Don't use together.

### CONTRAINDICATIONS
Contraindicated in patients with angle-closure glaucoma, psychoneurosis, angina pectoris, substantial organic heart disease, cardiovascular disease, and hypersensitivity to the drug or other sympathomimetics.

### NURSING CONSIDERATIONS
• Use cautiously in patients with hyperthyroidism, hypertension, diabetes mellitus, or prostatic hyperplasia.

### ☑ PATIENT TEACHING
• Teach patient how to instill nose-drops.
• Instruct patient that product should be used by only one person to prevent spread of infection.
• Tell patient not to exceed recommended dosage and to use only when needed.

## epinephrine hydrochloride
Adrenalin Chloride

*Pregnancy Risk Category: NR*

### HOW SUPPLIED
*Nasal solution:* 0.1%

### ACTION
Causes local vasoconstriction of dilated arterioles, reducing blood flow and nasal congestion.

### ONSET, PEAK, DURATION
Onset occurs within 1 minute. Peak and duration unknown.

### INDICATIONS & DOSAGE
*Nasal congestion, local superficial bleeding –*
**Adults and children:** instill 1 or 2 drops of solution.

---

Reactions may be *common,* uncommon, *life-threatening,* or **COMMON AND LIFE-THREATENING.**

## ADVERSE REACTIONS
**CNS:** nervousness, excitation.
**CV:** *tachycardia.*
**EENT:** rebound nasal congestion, slight sting upon application.

## INTERACTIONS
None significant.

## CONTRAINDICATIONS
Contraindicated in patients with hypersensitivity to the drug.

## NURSING CONSIDERATIONS
• Use cautiously in patients with hyperthyroidism, coronary artery disease, hypertension, or diabetes mellitus.

## ☑ PATIENT TEACHING
• Teach patient how to instill nosedrops.
• Instruct patient that product should be used by only one person to prevent spread of infection.
• Tell patient not to exceed recommended dosage and to use only when needed.

---

## flunisolide
Nasalide, Rhinalar Nasal Mist‡
*Pregnancy Risk Category: C*

### HOW SUPPLIED
*Nasal inhalant:* 25 mcg/metered spray, 200 doses/bottle‡
*Nasal solution:* 0.25 mg/ml in pump spray bottle

### ACTION
Decreases nasal inflammation, mainly by stabilizing leukocyte lysosomal membranes by unknown mechanism.

### ONSET, PEAK, DURATION
Unknown.

## INDICATIONS & DOSAGE
*Symptoms of seasonal or perennial rhinitis –*
**Adults:** starting dose is 2 sprays (50 mcg) in each nostril b.i.d. Total daily dosage is 200 mcg. If necessary, dosage may be increased to 2 sprays in each nostril t.i.d. Maximum total daily dosage is 8 sprays in each nostril (400 mcg daily).
**Children 6 to 14 years:** starting dose is 1 spray (25 mcg) in each nostril t.i.d. or 2 sprays (50 mcg) in each nostril b.i.d. Total daily dosage is 150 to 200 mcg. Maximum total daily dosage is 4 sprays in each nostril (200 mcg daily).

## ADVERSE REACTIONS
**CNS:** headache.
**EENT:** *mild, transient nasal burning and stinging,* nasal congestion, nasopharyngeal fungal infection, burning, stinging, dryness, sneezing, epistaxis, watery eyes.
**GI:** nausea, vomiting.

## INTERACTIONS
None significant.

## CONTRAINDICATIONS
Contraindicated in patients hypersensitive to the drug. Also, drug should not be used in the presence of untreated localized infection involving nasal mucosa.

## NURSING CONSIDERATIONS
• Use cautiously, if at all, in patients with active or quiescent respiratory tract tubercular infections or in untreated fungal, bacterial, or systemic viral or ocular herpes simplex infections. Also use cautiously in patients who have recently had nasal septal ulcers, nasal surgery, or nasal trauma.
• Be aware that flunisolide is not effective for acute exacerbations of rhinitis. Decongestants or antihistamines may be needed.

---

*Liquid form contains alcohol. **May contain tartrazine. †Canada only. ‡Australia only. ◊OTC.

• To instill, instruct patient to shake the container before using; to blow nose to clear nasal passages; and to tilt head slightly forward and insert nozzle into nostril, pointing away from septum. Tell him to hold the other nostril closed, and then to inspire gently and spray. Next, have him shake container again and repeat in the other nostril. Tell patient to clean nosepiece with warm water if it becomes clogged.
• Explain that the drug's therapeutic effects, unlike those of decongestants, are not immediate. Most patients achieve benefit within a few days, but some may require 2 to 3 weeks.
• Advise patient to use drug regularly, as prescribed, because its effectiveness depends on regular use.
• Warn patient not to exceed recommended dosage to avoid suppression of hypothalamic-pituitary-adrenal function.
• Tell patient to stop drug and notify the doctor if symptoms don't diminish within 3 weeks or if nasal irritation persists.

---

# fluticasone propionate
Flonase

*Pregnancy Risk Category: C*

## HOW SUPPLIED
*Nasal spray:* 50 mcg/metered spray (9-g, 15-g bottles)

## ACTION
Decreases nasal inflammation, mainly by stabilizing leukocyte lysosomal membranes via unknown mechanism.

## ONSET, PEAK, DURATION
Unknown.

## INDICATIONS & DOSAGE
*Seasonal and perennial allergic rhinitis —*

**Adults and children 12 years and older:** initially, two sprays (50 mcg each spray) in each nostril once daily. Alternatively, one spray in each nostril b.i.d. After a few days, dosage may be reduced to one spray in each nostril daily. Maximum daily dosage should not exceed two sprays in each nostril.

## ADVERSE REACTIONS
**CNS:** headache.
**EENT:** epistaxis, nasal burning, blood in nasal mucus, pharyngitis, nasal irritation.

## INTERACTIONS
None reported.

## CONTRAINDICATIONS
Contraindicated in patients with hypersensitivity to drug or any component.

## NURSING CONSIDERATIONS
• Use cautiously, if at all, in patients with active or quiescent tuberculous infections; untreated fungal, bacterial, or systemic viral infections; or ocular herpes simplex. Also use cautiously in patients already receiving systemic corticosteroids (because of the increased likelihood of hypothalamic-pituitary-adrenal suppression) and in breast-feeding women.
• Drug should not be used in patients with recent nasal septal ulcers, nasal surgery, or nasal trauma until healing has occurred.
• Although they rarely occur, monitor for signs of immediate hypersensitivity reactions or contact dermatitis after intranasal administration.

☑ PATIENT TEACHING
• Urge patient to read patient instruction sheet before using drug for first time.
• Explain how to instill drug. Tell patient to shake container before use; to blow nose to clear nasal passages; and

---

to tilt head slightly forward and insert nozzle into nostril, pointing away from the septum. Tell him to hold the other nostril closed and then to inspire gently and spray. Next, have patient shake container again and repeat this procedure in the other nostril.

• Stress importance of adhering to a schedule for instillation because drug effectiveness depends on regular use. Caution patient not to exceed recommended dose; doing so may lead to hypercorticism, suppression of HPA function, or suppression of growth in children or teenagers.

• Tell patient to notify the doctor if symptoms do not improve or condition worsens.

• Warn patient to avoid exposure to chickenpox and measles and, if exposed, to obtain medical advice.

• Instruct patient to watch for and report signs and symptoms of nasal infection.

## naphazoline hydrochloride
Privine◇

*Pregnancy Risk Category: NR*

### HOW SUPPLIED
*Nasal drops:* 0.05% solution
*Nasal spray:* 0.05% solution

### ACTION
Causes local vasoconstriction of dilated arterioles, reducing blood flow and nasal congestion.

### ONSET, PEAK, DURATION
Onset occurs within 10 minutes. Peak unknown. Effects persist 2 to 6 hours.

### INDICATIONS & DOSAGE
*Nasal congestion –*
**Adults and children 12 years and older:** 2 drops or sprays instilled in each nostril q 3 to 4 hours.
**Children 6 to 12 years:** 1 to 2 drops or sprays instilled in each nostril q 3

to 6 hours, p.r.n. Not to be used longer than 3 to 5 days.

### ADVERSE REACTIONS
**EENT:** rebound nasal congestion with excessive or long-term use, sneezing, stinging, dryness of mucosa.
**Other:** systemic effects in children after excessive or long-term use, marked sedation.

### INTERACTIONS
None significant.

### CONTRAINDICATIONS
Contraindicated in patients with hypersensitivity to drug.

### NURSING CONSIDERATIONS
• Use cautiously in patients with hyperthyroidism, heart disease, hypertension, or diabetes mellitus.

### ☑ PATIENT TEACHING
• Teach patient how to use drug. For nasal drops, instruct patient to tilt head back as far as possible, instill drops, then lean head forward while inhaling and to repeat procedure for other nostril. For nasal spray, instruct him to hold spray container and head upright. Tell patient not to shake the container.

• Tell patient that product should be used by only one person to prevent spread of infection.

• Warn patient not to exceed recommended dosage.

• Tell patient to contact the doctor if nasal congestion persists after 5 days.

# oxymetazoline hydrochloride

Afrin◇, Afrin Children's Strength Nose Drops◇, Allerest 12-Hour Nasal◇, Chlorphed-LA◇, Coricidin Nasal Mist◇, Dristan Long Lasting◇, Drixine Nasal‡, Duramist Plus◇, Duration◇, 4-Way Long-Acting Nasal, Genasal Spray◇, Neo-Synephrine 12 Hour◇, Nostrilla◇, NTZ Long Acting Nasal◇, Sinarest 12-Hour◇, Sinex Long-Acting◇, Twice-A-Day Nasal◇

*Pregnancy Risk Category: NR*

## HOW SUPPLIED
*Nasal solution:* 0.025%◇, 0.05%◇

## ACTION
Unknown. Thought to cause local vasoconstriction of dilated arterioles, reducing blood flow and nasal congestion.

## ONSET, PEAK, DURATION
Onset occurs in 5 to 10 minutes. Peak effect occurs within 6 hours. Effects persist less than 12 hours.

## INDICATIONS & DOSAGE
*Nasal congestion—*
**Adults and children 6 years and over:** 2 to 3 drops or sprays of 0.05% solution in each nostril b.i.d.
**Children 2 to 6 years:** 2 to 3 drops of 0.025% solution in each nostril b.i.d. Use no longer than 3 to 5 days.

## ADVERSE REACTIONS
**CNS:** headache, drowsiness, dizziness, insomnia, possible sedation.
**CV:** palpitations, *CV collapse,* hypertension.
**EENT:** rebound nasal congestion or irritation with excessive or long-term use, dryness of nose and throat, increased nasal discharge, stinging, sneezing.

**Other:** systemic effects in children with excessive or long-term use.

## INTERACTIONS
None significant.

## CONTRAINDICATIONS
Contraindicated in patients with hypersensitivity to drug.

## NURSING CONSIDERATIONS
● Use cautiously in patients with hyperthyroidism, cardiac disease, hypertension, or diabetes mellitus.

## ☑ PATIENT TEACHING
● Teach patient how to apply oxymetazoline. Tell him to hold head upright to minimize swallowing of medication, then sniff spray briskly.
● Tell patient that product should be used by only one person to prevent spread of infection.
● Tell patient not to exceed recommended dosage and to use only when needed.
● *Alert:* Warn patient that excessive use may cause bradycardia, hypotension, dizziness, and weakness.

# phenylephrine hydrochloride

Alconefrin 12◇, Alconefrin 25◇, Alconefrin 50◇, Doktors◇, Duration◇, Neo-Synephrine◇, Nostril◇, Rhinall◇, Rhinall-10◇, Sinex◇, St. Joseph Measured Dose Nasal Decongestant◇

*Pregnancy Risk Category: NR*

## HOW SUPPLIED
*Nasal jelly:* 0.5%
*Nasal solution:* 0.125%, 0.16%, 0.2%, 0.25%, 0.5%, 1%

## ACTION
Causes local vasoconstriction of dilated arterioles, reducing blood flow and nasal congestion.

---

Reactions may be *common,* uncommon, *life-threatening,* or COMMON AND LIFE-THREATENING.

## ONSET, PEAK, DURATION
Onset is rapid. Peak unknown. Effects persist for ½ to 4 hours.

## INDICATIONS & DOSAGE
*Nasal congestion –*
**Adults and children 12 years and over:** 2 to 3 drops or 1 to 2 sprays instilled in each nostril or small amount of jelly to nasal mucosa q 4 hours, p.r.n.
**Children 6 to 12 years:** 2 to 3 drops or 1 to 2 sprays of a 0.25% solution instilled in each nostril.
**Children under 6 years:** 2 to 3 drops of 0.125% solution q 4 hours, p.r.n.

## ADVERSE REACTIONS
**CNS:** headache, tremor, dizziness, nervousness.
**CV:** *palpitations, tachycardia, PVCs,* hypertension, pallor.
**EENT:** transient burning or stinging, dryness of nasal mucosa, rebound nasal congestion with continued use.
**GI:** nausea.

## INTERACTIONS
None significant.

## CONTRAINDICATIONS
Contraindicated in patients with hypersensitivity to drug.

## NURSING CONSIDERATIONS
• Use cautiously in patients with hyperthyroidism, marked hypertension, Type I diabetes mellitus, cardiac disease, or advanced arteriosclerotic changes; in children of low body weight; and in elderly patients.

## ☑ PATIENT TEACHING
• Teach patient how to apply phenylephrine. Tell him to hold head upright to minimize swallowing of medication, then to sniff spray briskly.
• Tell patient that product should be used by only one person to prevent spread of infection.
• Tell patient not to exceed recommended dosage and to use only when needed.
• Advise patient to contact the doctor if symptoms persist beyond 3 days.

---

# tetrahydrozoline hydrochloride
Tyzine Drops, Tyzine Pediatric Drops
*Pregnancy Risk Category: C*

## HOW SUPPLIED
*Nasal solution:* 0.05%, 0.1%

## ACTION
Unknown. Thought to cause local vasoconstriction of dilated arterioles, reducing blood flow and nasal congestion.

## ONSET, PEAK, DURATION
Onset occurs within a few minutes. Peak unknown. Effects persist for 4 to 8 hours.

## INDICATIONS & DOSAGE
*Nasal congestion –*
**Adults and children over 6 years:** 2 to 4 drops of 0.1% solution or spray into each nostril q 4 to 6 hours, p.r.n.
**Children 2 to 6 years:** 2 to 3 drops of 0.05% solution into each nostril q 4 to 6 hours, p.r.n.

## ADVERSE REACTIONS
**EENT:** transient burning, stinging; sneezing, rebound nasal congestion with excessive or long-term use.

## INTERACTIONS
None significant.

## CONTRAINDICATIONS
Contraindicated in patients with hypersensitivity to drug and in those with angle-closure glaucoma or other serious eye diseases. Also contraindicated in children under 2 years. The 0.1% solution is contraindicated in children under 6 years.

---

*Liquid form contains alcohol. **May contain tartrazine. †Canada only. ‡Australia only. ◇OTC.

## NURSING CONSIDERATIONS
• Use cautiously in patients with hyperthyroidism, hypertension, and diabetes mellitus.

## ☑ PATIENT TEACHING
• Teach patient how to apply tetrahydrozoline. Tell him to hold head upright to minimize swallowing of medication, then sniff spray briskly.
• Instruct patient that product should be used by only one person to prevent spread of infection.
• Tell patient not to exceed recommended dosage and to use only as needed for 3 to 5 days.

---

## triamcinolone acetonide
Nasacort

*Pregnancy Risk Category: C*

## HOW SUPPLIED
*Nasal aerosol:* 55 mcg/metered spray

## ACTION
Unknown. A glucocorticoid with anti-inflammatory properties.

## ONSET, PEAK, DURATION
A decrease in symptoms may occur within 12 hours after therapy is started. Effects peak within 3 to 4 days and may last for several days after drug is discontinued.

## INDICATIONS & DOSAGE
*Relief of symptoms of seasonal or perennial allergic rhinitis* –
**Adults and children 12 years and over:** initially, 2 sprays (110 mcg) in each nostril once daily. Increased as needed up to 440 mcg daily either as once-daily dosage or in divided doses up to four times daily. After desired effect is obtained, dosage decreased, if possible, to as little as one spray (55 mcg) in each nostril daily.

## ADVERSE REACTIONS
**EENT:** *nasal irritation,* dry mucous membranes, nasal and sinus congestion, irritation, burning, stinging, throat discomfort, sneezing, epistaxis.
**Other:** *headache.*

## INTERACTIONS
None significant.

## CONTRAINDICATIONS
Contraindicated in patients hypersensitive to any component of the drug.

## NURSING CONSIDERATIONS
• Use with extreme caution, if at all, in patients with active or quiescent tuberculosis infection of the respiratory tract and in patients with untreated fungal, bacterial, or systemic viral infection or ocular herpes simplex.
• Use cautiously in patients who are already receiving systemic corticosteroids because of the increased likelihood of hypothalamic-pituitary-adrenal suppression compared with a therapeutic dosage of either one alone. Also use cautiously in patients with recent nasal septal ulcers, nasal surgery, or trauma because of the inhibitory effect on wound healing. Also use with caution in breast-feeding women.
• *Alert:* Be aware that when excessive doses are used, signs and symptoms of hyperadrenocorticism and adrenal suppression may occur; the drug should be discontinued slowly.

## ☑ PATIENT TEACHING
• Urge the patient to read the patient-instruction sheet contained in each package before using drug for the first time.
• To instill, instruct the patient to shake the container before using; to blow nose to clear nasal passages; and to tilt head slightly forward and insert nozzle into nostril, pointing away from the septum. Tell him to hold the

other nostril closed and then to inspire gently and spray. Next, have the patient shake container again and repeat this procedure in the other nostril.
• Tell the patient to discard the canister after 100 actuations.
• Stress the importance of using the drug on a regular schedule because its effectiveness depends on regular use. However, caution the patient not to exceed the dosage prescribed because serious adverse reactions may occur.
• Tell the patient to notify the doctor if symptoms do not diminish within 2 to 3 weeks or if condition worsens.
• Warn the patient to avoid exposure to chickenpox or measles and, if exposed to either, to obtain medical advice.
• Instruct the patient to watch for signs and symptoms of nasal infection. If symptoms occur, tell the patient to notify the doctor because the drug may need to be discontinued and appropriate local therapy given.
• Advise the patient not to break canister, to incinerate canister, or to store canister in extreme heat; contents are under pressure and may explode.

---

# xylometazoline hydrochloride
4-Way Long Acting, Neo-Synephrine II, Otrivin, Sine-Off Nasal Spray, Sinex-L.A.

*Pregnancy Risk Category: NR*

## HOW SUPPLIED
*Nasal solution:* 0.05%, 0.1%

## ACTION
Unknown. Thought to cause local vasoconstriction of dilated arterioles, reducing blood flow and nasal congestion.

## ONSET, PEAK, DURATION
Onset occurs in 5 to 10 minutes. Peak unknown. Effects persist for 5 to 6 hours.

## INDICATIONS & DOSAGE
*Nasal congestion* –
**Adults and children 12 years and over:** 2 to 3 drops or sprays of 0.1% solution in each nostril q 8 to 10 hours.
**Children 2 to 12 years:** 2 to 3 drops of 0.05% solution in each nostril q 8 to 10 hours.
**Children 6 months to 2 years:** 1 drop of 0.05% solution instilled into each nostril q 6 hours, p.r.n.

## ADVERSE REACTIONS
**EENT:** transient burning, stinging; dryness or ulceration of nasal mucosa; sneezing; rebound nasal congestion or irritation with excessive or long-term use.

## INTERACTIONS
None significant.

## CONTRAINDICATIONS
Contraindicated in patients with hypersensitivity to drug or angle-closure glaucoma.

## NURSING CONSIDERATIONS
• Use cautiously in patients with hyperthyroidism, cardiac disease, hypertension, diabetes mellitus, and advanced arteriosclerosis.

## ☑ PATIENT TEACHING
• Teach patient how to apply xylometazoline. Have patient hold head upright to minimize swallowing of medication, then sniff spray briskly.
• Tell patient that product should be used by only one person to prevent spread of infection.
• Tell patient not to exceed recommended dose and to use only as needed for 3 to 5 days.

---

# 87

## Local anti-infectives

acyclovir
amphotericin B
azelaic acid cream
bacitracin
butoconazole nitrate
chloramphenicol
ciclopirox olamine
clindamycin phosphate
clotrimazole
econazole nitrate
erythromycin
gentamicin sulfate
gentian violet
ketoconazole
mafenide acetate
metronidazole (topical)
miconazole nitrate
mupirocin
naftifine
neomycin sulfate
nitrofurazone
nystatin
oxiconazole nitrate
podofilox
silver sulfadiazine
sulconazole nitrate
terbinafine hydrochloride
terconazole
tetracycline hydrochloride
tioconazole
tolnaftate

### COMBINATION PRODUCTS
BENZAMYCIN GEL: erythromycin 3% and benzoyl peroxide 5%.
LANABIOTIC◊: polymyxin B sulfate 5,000 units, neomycin sulfate 5 mg, bacitracin 500 units, and lidocaine 40 mg/g.
LOTRISONE CREAM: clotrimazole 1% and betamethasone dipropionate 0.05%.
MYCITRACIN OINTMENT◊: polymyxin B sulfate 5,000 units, bacitracin 500 units, and neomycin sulfate 3.5 mg/g.

MYCOLOG II CREAM, OINTMENT: triamcinolone acetonide 0.1% and nystatin 100,000 units/g.
NEO-CORTEF OINTMENT: hydrocortisone acetate 1% and neomycin sulfate 0.5%.
NEODECADRON CREAM: dexamethasone phosphate 0.1% and neomycin sulfate 0.5%.
NEOSPORIN CREAM†◊: polymyxin B sulfate 10,000 units and neomycin sulfate 5 mg.
NEOSPORIN OINTMENT◊: polymyxin B sulfate 5,000 units, bacitracin zinc 400 units, and neomycin sulfate 5 mg/g.
POLYSPORIN OINTMENT◊: polymyxin B sulfate 10,000 units and bacitracin zinc 500 units/g.
VIOFORM-HYDROCORTISONE MILD CREAM: iodochlorhydroxyquin 3% and hydrocortisone 0.5%.

---

### acyclovir
Zovirax

*Pregnancy Risk Category: C*

**HOW SUPPLIED**
*Ointment:* 5%

**ACTION**
Inhibits herpes simplex and varicella-zoster viral DNA synthesis by inhibiting viral DNA polymerase action.

**ONSET, PEAK, DURATION**
Not applicable.

**INDICATIONS & DOSAGE**
*Initial herpes genitalis; limited, non-life-threatening mucocutaneous herpes simplex virus infections in immunocompromised patients—*
**Adults and children:** cover all lesions q 3 hours six times daily for 7

days. Although dosage will vary depending on the total lesion area, use about a ½" ribbon of ointment on each 4" square of surface area.

## ADVERSE REACTIONS
**Skin:** transient burning and stinging, rash, pruritus, vulvitis.

## INTERACTIONS
None significant.

## CONTRAINDICATIONS
Contraindicated in patients with hypersensitivity or chemical intolerance to the drug.

## NURSING CONSIDERATIONS
• As ordered, start therapy as early as possible after onset of symptoms.
• Apply with a finger cot or rubber glove to prevent autoinoculation of other body sites and transmission of infection to other persons.
• Know that the drug is for cutaneous use only; don't apply to the eye.

## ☑ PATIENT TEACHING
• Teach the patient that virus transmission can occur during treatment.
• Emphasize importance of compliance for successful therapy.

---

# amphotericin B
Fungizone

*Pregnancy Risk Category: B*

## HOW SUPPLIED
*Cream:* 3%
*Lotion:* 3%
*Ointment:* 3%

## ACTION
Usually fungistatic; binds to sterols in the fungal cell membrane, resulting in increased membrane permeability and subsequent cell leakage.

## ONSET, PEAK, DURATION
Not applicable.

## INDICATIONS & DOSAGE
*Cutaneous or mucocutaneous candidal infections –*
**Adults and children:** apply liberally b.i.d. to q.i.d. for 1 to 3 weeks; interdigital lesions and paronychias treated for 2 to 4 weeks, and onychomycoses for several months because relapses are common.

## ADVERSE REACTIONS
**Skin:** possible dryness, contact sensitivity, erythema, burning, pruritus.

## INTERACTIONS
None significant.

## CONTRAINDICATIONS
Contraindicated in patients hypersensitive to the drug.

## NURSING CONSIDERATIONS
• Clean area before applying.
• Report local irritation. Cream may dry skin; ointment may irritate if applied to moist, hairy areas.
• Avoid using occlusive dressings.
• Be aware that cream or lotion is preferred for such areas as groin folds, armpit, and neck creases.
• Stop drug if irritation or hypersensitivity occurs, and notify doctor.
• Store at room temperature.

## ☑ PATIENT TEACHING
• Tell patient to use drug for full treatment period, even if condition has improved.
• Inform patient that cream discolors skin slightly when rubbed in; lotion or ointment may stain nail lesions but not skin if thoroughly rubbed in.
• Tell patient that fabric discoloration caused by cream or lotion can be removed by washing; discoloration by ointment, by cleaning fluid.

---

*Liquid form contains alcohol. **May contain tartrazine. †Canada only. ‡Australia only. ◊OTC.

▼ *NEW DRUG*

## azelaic acid cream
Azelex 20%
*Pregnancy Risk Category: B*

**HOW SUPPLIED**
Cream: 20%

**ACTION**
Unknown. May inhibit microbial cellular protein synthesis.

**ONSET, PEAK, DURATION**
Not applicable.

**INDICATIONS & DOSAGE**
*Mild to moderate inflammatory acne vulgaris –*
**Adults:** Apply a thin film and gently but thoroughly massage into affected areas b.i.d, in morning and evening.

**ADVERSE REACTIONS**
**Skin:** pruritus, burning, stinging, tingling.

**INTERACTIONS**
None reported.

**CONTRAINDICATIONS**
Contraindicated in patients with hypersensitivity to any drug component.

**NURSING CONSIDERATIONS**
• Monitor the patient for early signs of hypopigmentation, especially a patient with dark complexion.
• If sensitivity or severe irritation occurs, notify the doctor, who may discontinue drug and order appropriate treatment.

☑ **PATIENT TEACHING**
• Instruct the patient to wash and pat dry affected areas before applying drug and to wash hands well after application. Warn him not to apply occlusive dressings or wrappings to affected areas.

• Warn him that skin irritation may occur when drug is applied to broken or inflamed skin, usually at start of therapy. Tell him to notify the doctor if irritation persists.
• Advise him to keep drug away from mouth, eyes, and other mucous membranes. If contact occurs, tell him to rinse thoroughly with water and consult a doctor if irritation persists.
• Advise him to report abnormal changes in skin color.
• Urge him to use drug for the full treatment period.

## bacitracin
Baciguent◊, Bacitin†
*Pregnancy Risk Category: NR*

**HOW SUPPLIED**
*Ointment:* 500 units/g

**ACTION**
Bactericidal or bacteriostatic, depending on organism and concentration of drug; inhibits bacterial cell wall synthesis.

**ONSET, PEAK, DURATION**
Not applicable.

**INDICATIONS & DOSAGE**
*Topical infections, impetigo, abrasions, cuts, and minor burns or wounds –*
**Adults and children:** apply thin film b.i.d., t.i.d., or p.r.n., depending on severity of condition.

**ADVERSE REACTIONS**
**Skin:** stinging, rashes, other allergic reactions; pruritus, burning, swelling of lips or face.
**Systemic:** *possible systemic adverse reactions when used over large areas for prolonged periods, including potential nephrotoxicity and ototoxicity; hypersensitivity reactions;* tightness in chest, hypotension.

---

Reactions may be *common,* uncommon, *life-threatening,* or COMMON AND LIFE-THREATENING.

## INTERACTIONS
None significant.

## CONTRAINDICATIONS
Contraindicated in patients hypersensitive to the drug and in atopic patients.

## NURSING CONSIDERATIONS
• Clean area before applying, especially if crusted or suppurative.
• Anticipate alternative treatment for burns that cover more than 20% of body surface, especially if the patient suffers impaired renal function.
• Prolonged use may result in overgrowth of nonsusceptible organisms, particularly *Candida* species.

### ☑ PATIENT TEACHING
• If no improvement occurs or condition worsens, tell the patient to stop using and notify the doctor.
• Instruct patient to report systemic and skin adverse reactions that persist or are severe.

---

## butoconazole nitrate
Femstat

*Pregnancy Risk Category: C*

## HOW SUPPLIED
*Vaginal cream:* 2% with applicators supplied

## ACTION
Unknown. Thought to control or destroy fungus by disrupting cell membrane permeability, causing osmotic instability.

## ONSET, PEAK, DURATION
Unknown.

## INDICATIONS & DOSAGE
*Vulvovaginal mycotic infections caused by* Candida *species –*
**Adults:** for nonpregnant patient, 1 applicatorful intravaginally h.s. for 3 days. If needed, treat for another 3 days. For pregnant patient during second or third trimester, 1 applicatorful intravaginally h.s. for 6 days.

## ADVERSE REACTIONS
**GU:** vulvovaginal burning and itching, soreness, and swelling.
**Skin:** finger itching.

## INTERACTIONS
None significant.

## CONTRAINDICATIONS
Contraindicated in patients hypersensitive to the drug.

## NURSING CONSIDERATIONS
• Confirm diagnosis by smears or cultures, as ordered.
• Know that drug should be used in the first trimester of pregnancy only when the potential benefits outweigh the possible risks to the fetus.
• Drug may be used with oral contraceptive and antibiotic therapy.

### ☑ PATIENT TEACHING
• Teach the patient how to apply drug, and tell her not to use tampons during treatment.
• Advise the patient to keep affected area cool and dry, wear loose-fitting cotton clothing, avoid feminine hygiene sprays, wash daily with unscented soap, dry thoroughly with clean towel, and prevent reinfection by wiping perineum from front to back.
• Tell the patient's sexual partner to wear a condom during intercourse until treatment is complete. He should consult the doctor if he experiences penile itching, redness, or discomfort.

---

## chloramphenicol
Chloromycetin

*Pregnancy Risk Category: NR*

## HOW SUPPLIED
*Cream:* 1%

---

## ACTION
Usually bacteriostatic but may be bactericidal in high concentrations; inhibits bacterial protein synthesis.

## ONSET, PEAK, DURATION
Not applicable.

## INDICATIONS & DOSAGE
*Superficial skin infections caused by susceptible bacteria –*
**Adults and children:** after cleaning skin, apply t.i.d. or q.i.d.

## ADVERSE REACTIONS
**Skin:** possible contact sensitivity; burning, urticaria, pruritus, angioedema in hypersensitive patients.

## INTERACTIONS
None significant.

## CONTRAINDICATIONS
Contraindicated in patients hypersensitive to the drug or any components of the formulation.

## NURSING CONSIDERATIONS
• Be aware that prolonged use may result in overgrowth of fungi or other nonsusceptible organisms.
• Know that topical use of this drug should be supplemented by appropriate systemic medication for all but very superficial infections.
• Discontinue if hypersensitivity reactions develop, and notify the doctor.

## ☑ PATIENT TEACHING
• Tell the patient to avoid prolonged or frequent intermittent use. Systemically administered chloramphenicol has been linked to serious adverse reactions and toxicity.
• If no improvement occurs or if condition worsens, advise patient to discontinue drug and notify the doctor.
• Tell the patient to continue using for full treatment period prescribed.

# ciclopirox olamine
Loprox

*Pregnancy Risk Category: B*

## HOW SUPPLIED
*Cream:* 1%
*Lotion:* 1%

## ACTION
Unknown. Thought to deplete essential fungal intracellular substrates by blocking amino acid transport and altering cell membrane integrity.

## ONSET, PEAK, DURATION
Not applicable.

## INDICATIONS & DOSAGE
*Tinea pedis, cruris, corporis, and versicolor; cutaneous candidiasis –*
**Adults and children over 10 years:** massage gently into the affected and surrounding areas b.i.d., in the morning and evening for 2 to 4 weeks.

## ADVERSE REACTIONS
**Skin:** pruritus, burning, irritation, redness.

## INTERACTIONS
None significant.

## CONTRAINDICATIONS
Contraindicated in patients hypersensitive to the drug.

## NURSING CONSIDERATIONS
• Don't use occlusive dressings.
• Avoid drug contact with eyes.

## ☑ PATIENT TEACHING
• Reassure patient that hypopigmentation from tinea versicolor will resolve gradually.
• If hypersensitivity reaction occurs, advise patient to discontinue treatment and notify the doctor.
• Tell patient to continue using drug for prescribed period even if symptoms have improved.

---

Reactions may be *common*, uncommon, *life-threatening*, or **COMMON AND LIFE-THREATENING**.

- Tell patient to call doctor if no improvement occurs in 4 weeks.

## clindamycin phosphate
Cleocin T Gel, Lotion, Solution;
Cleocin Vaginal Cream

*Pregnancy Risk Category: B*

### HOW SUPPLIED
*Gel:* 1%
*Lotion:* 1%
*Topical solution:* 1%
*Vaginal cream:* 2%

### ACTION
Bacteriostatic or bactericidal, based on drug concentration and susceptibility of organism; suppresses growth of susceptible organisms in sebaceous glands by blocking protein synthesis.

### ONSET, PEAK, DURATION
Not applicable for gel, lotion, or solution. Unknown for vaginal cream.

### INDICATIONS & DOSAGE
*Inflammatory acne vulgaris, grades II and III –*
**Adults and adolescents:** apply to skin b.i.d., morning and evening.
*Bacterial vaginosis –*
**Adults:** 1 applicatorful intravaginally h.s. for 7 consecutive days.

### ADVERSE REACTIONS
**GI:** upset, diarrhea, bloody diarrhea, abdominal pain, colitis (including pseudomembranous colitis).
**GU:** *cervicitis or vaginitis,* Candida albicans overgrowth, *vulvar irritation.*
**Skin:** *dryness,* rash, *redness,* pruritus, swelling, irritation, contact dermatitis, burning.

### INTERACTIONS
*Abrasive or medicated soaps or cleansers; acne preparations or other preparations containing peeling agents (benzoyl peroxide, resorcinol, sali-* *cylic acid, sulfur, tretinoin); alcohol-containing products (after-shave, cosmetics, perfumed toiletries, shaving creams or lotions); astringent soaps or cosmetics; isotretinoin; medicated cosmetics or cover-ups:* potential cumulative dryness, resulting in excessive skin irritation. Use cautiously.

### CONTRAINDICATIONS
Contraindicated in patients hypersensitive to the drug; in those with a history of ulcerative colitis, regional enteritis, or antibiotic-associated colitis; and in those with a history of atopic reactions.

### NURSING CONSIDERATIONS
- For treating acne, know that drug may be used concurrently with tretinoin or benzoyl peroxide as well as systemic antibiotics.
- Know that drug can cause excessive dryness.

### ☑ PATIENT TEACHING
- Tell the patient to wash area with warm water and soap, rinse, and pat dry and to wait 30 minutes after washing or shaving to apply.
- Warn the patient to avoid too-frequent washing of area. Tell him to cover entire affected area but to avoid contact with eyes, nose, mouth, and other mucous membranes.
- Tell the patient to use only as prescribed.
- Tell the patient to dab, not roll, applicator-tipped bottle. If tip becomes dry, he should invert bottle and depress tip several times to moisten.
- Warn the patient not to smoke while applying topical solution.
- When used intravaginally, make sure the patient knows how to use applicators that come with the drug.
- If diarrhea occurs, tell the patient to check with the doctor or pharmacist before using antidiarrheal medication because it may worsen the condition.

# clotrimazole
Canesten†, Gyne-Lotrimin◊,
Lotrimin, Mycelex, Mycelex-7◊,
Mycelex-G, Mycelex-OTC◊

*Pregnancy Risk Category: B*

## HOW SUPPLIED
*Lozenges:* 1%
*Cream:* 1%
*Topical lotion:* 1%
*Topical solution:* 1%
*Vaginal cream:* 1%◊
*Vaginal tablets:* 100 mg◊, 500 mg
*Combination pack:* vaginal inserts
100 mg and vulvar cream 1%◊

## ACTION
Fungistatic but may be fungicidal, depending on concentration. Alters fungal cell wall permeability and produces osmotic instability.

## ONSET, PEAK, DURATION
For lozenges, onset and peak unknown; effects persist for 3 hours. Not
applicable for other forms.

## INDICATIONS & DOSAGE
*Superficial fungal infections (tinea
pedis, tinea cruris, tinea corporis, or
tinea versicolor; candidiasis)* –
**Adults and children:** apply thinly
and massage into affected and surrounding area, morning and evening,
for 2 to 8 weeks.
*Vulvovaginal candidiasis* –
**Adults:** two 100-mg vaginal tablets
inserted daily h.s. for 3 consecutive
days, or one 500-mg vaginal tablet
daily h.s. for 3 days; or 1 applicatorful
vaginal cream daily h.s. for 7 to 14
days.
*Oropharyngeal candidiasis treat-
ment* –
**Adults and children:** dissolve lozenge over 15 to 30 minutes in mouth
five times daily for 14 consecutive
days.
*Prevention of oropharyngeal candidi-
asis in patients immunocompromised*

by such conditions as chemotherapy,
radiotherapy, or steroid therapy in the
treatment of leukemia, solid tumors,
or renal transplantation –
**Adults and children:** dissolve lozenge over 15 to 30 minutes in mouth
three times daily for duration of chemotherapy or until steroid is reduced
to maintenance levels.

## ADVERSE REACTIONS
**GI:** nausea and vomiting (with lozenges), lower abdominal cramps.
**GU:** *mild vaginal burning or irritation*
(with vaginal use), cramping, urinary
frequency.
**Skin:** blistering, *erythema,* edema,
blistering, pruritus, burning, stinging,
peeling, urticaria, skin fissures, general irritation.

## INTERACTIONS
None significant.

## CONTRAINDICATIONS
Contraindicated in patients hypersensitive to the drug. Also contraindicated for ophthalmic use.

## NURSING CONSIDERATIONS
• Clean area before applying.
• Watch for and report irritation or
sensitivity; discontinue if irritation
occurs and notify doctor.
• Know that improvement usually
demonstrated within a week; if no improvement occurs in 4 weeks, diagnosis should be reviewed.
• When compliance is a problem, be
aware that mild to moderate vaginal
candidiasis may be treated with a single 500-mg tablet.

## ☑ PATIENT TEACHING
• Reassure the patient that hypopigmentation from tinea versicolor will
resolve gradually.
• Warn the patient not to use occlusive wrappings or dressings.
• Ensure that the patient understands
that frequent or persistent yeast infec-

---

Reactions may be *common,* uncommon, *life-threatening,* or COMMON AND LIFE-THREATENING.

tions may be a symptom of a more serious medical problem such as AIDS.
• Warn the patient that topical preparation may stain clothing.
• Emphasize the need to continue treatment for full course.

---

## econazole nitrate
Ecostatin†, Spectazole

*Pregnancy Risk Category: C*

**HOW SUPPLIED**
*Cream:* 1%

**ACTION**
Fungistatic; may be fungicidal, depending on concentration. Alters fungal cell wall permeability and promotes osmotic instability.

**ONSET, PEAK, DURATION**
Not applicable.

**INDICATIONS & DOSAGE**
*Tinea pedis, tinea cruris, tinea corporis and tinea versicolor; cutaneous candidiasis –*
**Adults and children:** rub into affected areas once daily for at least 2 weeks.
*Cutaneous candidiasis –*
**Adults and children:** rub into affected areas b.i.d.

**ADVERSE REACTIONS**
**Skin:** burning, pruritus, stinging, erythema.

**INTERACTIONS**
*Topical corticosteroids:* may inhibit antifungal effect.

**CONTRAINDICATIONS**
Contraindicated in patients hypersensitive to the drug.

**NURSING CONSIDERATIONS**
• Clean affected area before applying.
• Don't use occlusive dressings.

---

☑ **PATIENT TEACHING**
• Tell patient to use drug for entire treatment period, even if symptoms improve. Instruct him to notify the doctor if no improvement occurs after 2 weeks (tinea cruris, tinea corporis, and tinea versicolor) or 4 weeks (tinea pedis).
• Reassure patient that hypopigmentation from tinea versicolor will resolve gradually.
• If condition persists or worsens or if irritation occurs, tell patient to stop use and call doctor.
• Warn that drug may stain clothing.

---

## erythromycin
Akne-mycin, A/T/S, Del-Mycin, Emgel, Erycette, EryDerm, EryGel, Ery-Sol†, ETS†, Sans-Acne†, Staticin, T-Stat†

*Pregnancy Risk Category: B*

**HOW SUPPLIED**
*Ointment:* 2%
*Topical gel:* 2%
*Topical solution:* 1.5%\*, 2%\*
*Pledgets:* 2%

**ACTION**
Usually bacteriostatic but may be bactericidal in high concentrations or against highly susceptible organisms. Disrupts protein synthesis in susceptible bacteria.

**ONSET, PEAK, DURATION**
Not applicable.

**INDICATIONS & DOSAGE**
*Inflammatory acne vulgaris –*
**Adults and children:** apply to affected areas b.i.d.

**ADVERSE REACTIONS**
**Skin:** sensitivity reactions, erythema, burning, *dryness, pruritus,* irritation, peeling, oily skin.

---

## INTERACTIONS

*Abrasive or medicated soaps or cleansers; acne preparations or other preparations containing peeling agents (benzoyl peroxide, resorcinol, salicylic acid, sulfur, tretinoin); alcohol-containing products (after-shave, cosmetics, perfumed toiletries, shaving creams or lotions); astringent soaps or cosmetics; isotretinoin; medicated cosmetics or cover-ups:* may cause cumulative dryness, resulting in excessive skin irritation. Use cautiously.

## CONTRAINDICATIONS

Contraindicated in patients hypersensitive to the drug.

## NURSING CONSIDERATIONS

• Wash, rinse, and dry affected areas before application.
• Know that prolonged use may be necessary when treating acne vulgaris; such use may result in overgrowth of nonsusceptible organisms.

## ☑ PATIENT TEACHING

• Advise patient not to use near eyes, nose, mouth, or other mucous membranes.
• If no improvement occurs or if condition worsens, tell patient to stop using and notify the doctor.

---

## gentamicin sulfate
Garamycin, G-Myticin

*Pregnancy Risk Category: NR*

### HOW SUPPLIED
*Cream:* 0.1%
*Ointment:* 0.1%

### ACTION
A bactericidal agent that disrupts bacterial protein synthesis by binding to ribosomes although its exact mechanism is unknown.

### ONSET, PEAK, DURATION
Not applicable.

## INDICATIONS & DOSAGE

*Superficial infections of the skin caused by susceptible bacteria —*
**Adults and children over 1 year:** rub in small amount gently t.i.d. or q.i.d., with or without gauze dressing.

## ADVERSE REACTIONS

**Skin:** minor skin irritation, possible photosensitivity, allergic contact dermatitis.

## INTERACTIONS
None significant.

## CONTRAINDICATIONS

Contraindicated in patients hypersensitive to the drug or in those who may exhibit cross-sensitivity with other aminoglycosides, such as neomycin.

## NURSING CONSIDERATIONS

• *Alert:* Avoid use on large skin lesions or over a wide area because of possible systemic toxic effects.
• Know that use should be restricted to selected patients; widespread use may lead to resistant organisms.
• Prolonged use may result in overgrowth of nonsusceptible organisms.

## ☑ PATIENT TEACHING

• Tell patient to clean affected area before applying. Have him remove crusts before application for impetigo contagiosa to enhance absorption.
• Tell patient to store in cool place.
• If no improvement occurs or if condition worsens, tell patient to stop using and notify the doctor.

---

## gentian violet (methylrosaniline chloride, crystal violet)
Genapax

*Pregnancy Risk Category: NR*

### HOW SUPPLIED
*Topical solution:* 1%◦, 2%◦
*Tampons:* 5 mg

---

## ACTION
Unknown, although drug has fungistatic and antibacterial activity.

## ONSET, PEAK, DURATION
Not applicable.

## INDICATIONS & DOSAGE
*Superficial skin infections –*
**Adults and children:** apply with swab b.i.d.
*Vaginal fungal infections –*
**Adults:** 1 tampon inserted for 3 to 4 hours daily or b.i.d. for 12 days. For resistant infections, an additional tampon inserted h.s.

## ADVERSE REACTIONS
**Skin:** *permanent discoloration if applied to granulation tissue;* irritation or ulceration of mucous membranes.

## INTERACTIONS
None significant.

## CONTRAINDICATIONS
Contraindicated in patients hypersensitive to the drug.

## NURSING CONSIDERATIONS
• Tattooing of the skin may occur if applied to granulation tissue.
• **Alert:** Toxicity has occurred after ingestion or with excessive use.

## ☑ PATIENT TEACHING
• Instruct patient to apply carefully to avoid undue staining.
• Tell patient to keep affected area clean, dry, and exposed to air to prevent spread of infection.
• Instruct patient not to use on ulcerative facial lesions and not to use occlusive dressings.
• Inform patient that drug will stain skin and clothing.

# ketoconazole
Nizoral

*Pregnancy Risk Category: C*

## HOW SUPPLIED
*Cream:* 2%
*Shampoo:* 2%

## ACTION
Unknown. An imidazole that probably inhibits yeast growth by altering the permeability of the cell membrane.

## ONSET, PEAK, DURATION
Not applicable.

## INDICATIONS & DOSAGE
*Tinea corporis, tinea cruris, tinea pedis, and tinea versicolor caused by susceptible organisms; seborrheic dermatitis; cutaneous candidiasis –*
**Adults:** cover the affected and immediate surrounding area once daily for at least 2 weeks; for seborrheic dermatitis, apply b.i.d. for 4 weeks. When using shampoo, wet hair, lather, and massage for 1 minute. Rinse and repeat, but leave drug on scalp for 3 minutes before rinsing. Shampoo twice weekly for 4 weeks, with at least 3 days between shampoos.

## ADVERSE REACTIONS
**Skin:** severe irritation, pruritus, stinging.

## INTERACTIONS
None significant.

## CONTRAINDICATIONS
Contraindicated in patients hypersensitive to the drug.

## NURSING CONSIDERATIONS
• Be aware that most patients show improvement soon after treatment begins.
• Keep in mind that treatment of tinea cruris or tinea corporis should con-

---

*Liquid form contains alcohol.   **May contain tartrazine.   †Canada only.   ‡Australia only.   ◊OTC.

tinue for at least 2 weeks to reduce the possibility of recurrence.

### ☑ PATIENT TEACHING
• Tell patient to discontinue drug and notify doctor if hypersensitivity reaction occurs.
• Advise patient to check with the doctor if condition worsens; drug may have to be discontinued and diagnosis redetermined.

---

## mafenide acetate
Sulfamylon

*Pregnancy Risk Category: C*

### HOW SUPPLIED
*Cream:* 8.5%

### ACTION
Unknown, although it interferes with bacterial cellular metabolism.

### ONSET, PEAK, DURATION
Not applicable.

### INDICATIONS & DOSAGE
*Adjunctive treatment of second- and third-degree burns to prevent infection caused by susceptible organisms (especially* Pseudomonas aeruginosa)—
**Adults and children:** apply 1/16″ thickness of cream daily or b.i.d. to clean, debrided wounds. Reapply p.r.n. to keep burned area covered.

### ADVERSE REACTIONS
**Hematologic:** eosinophilia.
**Respiratory:** tachypnea.
**Skin:** pain, *burning sensation,* rash, pruritus, swelling, urticaria, blisters, erythema.
**Other:** *metabolic acidosis,* facial edema.

### INTERACTIONS
None significant.

### CONTRAINDICATIONS
None known.

### NURSING CONSIDERATIONS
• Use cautiously in patients with acute renal failure and in those with known hypersensitivity to the drug or to sulfonamides.
• Clean area before applying, bathing patient daily, if possible.
• Use sterile gloves and instruments when applying cream to minimize risk of further wound contamination.
• Keep burn areas medicated at all times.
• *Alert:* Closely monitor acid-base balance, especially in patients with pulmonary and renal dysfunction. If acidosis occurs, discontinue use for 24 to 48 hours and notify doctor.
• Be aware that sometimes it is difficult to distinguish between adverse reactions and effects of severe burn.

### ☑ PATIENT TEACHING
• Tell patient purpose of drug and importance of keeping burned areas covered with the drug at all times. Tell patient to alert nurse if drug rubs off in any area visible to patient.
• Tell patient to report adverse reactions, especially pain or burning when drug is applied; these symptoms may indicate allergy. Tell patient to notify doctor if pain is severe or prolonged; treatment may need to be temporarily stopped.

---

## metronidazole (topical)
MetroGel, MetroGel-Vaginal

*Pregnancy Risk Category: B*

### HOW SUPPLIED
*Topical gel:* 0.75%
*Vaginal gel:* 0.75%

### ACTION
Unknown; may cause bactericidal effect by interacting with bacterial DNA. Active against many anaerobic gram-negative bacilli, anaerobic gram-positive cocci, *Gardnerella vaginalis,* and *Campylobacter fetus.*

---

Reactions may be *common,* uncommon, *life-threatening,* or COMMON AND LIFE-THREATENING.

## ONSET, PEAK, DURATION
Not applicable for topical gel. Onset and duration unknown for vaginal gel; peak effects occur in 6 to 12 hours after intravaginal use.

## INDICATIONS & DOSAGE
*Acne rosacea –*
**Adults:** apply a thin film to affected area b.i.d., morning and evening. Frequency and duration of therapy is adjusted after response is seen.
*Bacterial vaginosis –*
**Adults:** 1 applicatorful b.i.d., morning and evening, for 5 days.

## ADVERSE REACTIONS
*Topical gel*
**EENT:** lacrimation (if drug applied around the eyes).
*Vaginal form*
**CNS:** dizziness, light-headedness, headache.
**GI:** cramps, pain, nausea, diarrhea, constipation, metallic or bad taste in mouth.
**GU:** *cervicitis, vaginitis.*
**Skin:** rash, *transient redness, dryness, mild burning, stinging.*
**Other:** overgrowth of nonsusceptible organisms, decreased appetite.

## INTERACTIONS
*Oral anticoagulants:* may potentiate anticoagulant effect. Monitor the patient for potential adverse reactions.

## CONTRAINDICATIONS
Contraindicated in patients hypersensitive to drug or its ingredients (such as parabens) and other nitromidazole derivatives.

## NURSING CONSIDERATIONS
• Use cautiously in patients with history or evidence of blood dyscrasia; chemically related compounds are associated with blood dyscrasia.
• Use vaginal gel cautiously in patients with history of CNS diseases; a theoretical risk of seizures and peripheral neuropathy exist because these adverse reactions are associated with the oral form.
• Topical metronidazole therapy has not been linked with the adverse effects observed with parenteral or oral metronidazole therapy (including disulfiram-like reactions after alcohol ingestion). However, some drug may be absorbed after topical use.

## ☑ PATIENT TEACHING
• Instruct the patient using topical gel to avoid use of drug around the eyes. Also advise the patient to clean area thoroughly before use, but wait 15 to 20 minutes after cleaning the skin before applying drug to minimize risk of local irritation. Cosmetics may be used after applying drug.
• If local reactions occur, advise the patient to apply less frequently or to discontinue and contact the doctor.

# miconazole nitrate
Micatin◊, Monistat-Derm Cream and Lotion, Monistat 3 Vaginal Suppository, Monistat 7 Vaginal Cream◊, Monistat 7 Vaginal Suppository◊

*Pregnancy Risk Category: C*

## HOW SUPPLIED
*Cream:* 2%◊
*Powder:* 2%◊
*Spray:* 2%◊
*Vaginal cream:* 2%◊
*Vaginal suppositories:* 100 mg◊, 200 mg

## ACTION
A fungicidal imidazole that disrupts fungal cell membrane permeability.

## ONSET, PEAK, DURATION
Not applicable for spray or cream form. Onset, peak, and duration unknown for suppositories.

---

## INDICATIONS & DOSAGE

*Tinea pedis, tinea cruris, tinea corporis; cutaneous candidiasis (moniliasis); common dermatophyte infections –*

**Adults and children:** apply or spray sparingly b.i.d. for 2 to 4 weeks.

*Tinea versicolor –*

**Adults and children:** apply sparingly once daily for 2 weeks.

*Vulvovaginal candidiasis –*

**Adults:** 1 applicatorful or 100 mg suppository (Monistat 7) inserted intravaginally h.s. for 7 days; course repeated if necessary. Alternatively, 200 mg suppository (Monistat 3) intravaginally h.s. for 3 days.

## ADVERSE REACTIONS

**CNS:** headache.

**GU:** vulvovaginal burning, pruritus, or irritation with vaginal cream; pelvic cramps.

**Skin:** irritation, burning, maceration, allergic contact dermatitis.

## INTERACTIONS

None significant.

## CONTRAINDICATIONS

Contraindicated in patients hypersensitive to the drug.

## NURSING CONSIDERATIONS

• Know that concurrent use of intravaginal forms and certain latex products, such as vaginal contraceptive diaphragms, are not recommended because of possible interaction.

• Don't use occlusive dressings.

## ☑ PATIENT TEACHING

• Advise patient that drug is for perineal or intravaginal use only. Keep out of eyes.

• Ensure that patient understands that frequent or persistent yeast infections may be a symptom of a more serious medical problem such as AIDS.

• Tell patient to cautiously insert intravaginal forms high into the vagina with applicator provided.

• Tell patient drug may stain clothing.

• Warn patient to discontinue if sensitivity or chemical irritation occurs.

• Tell patient to continue using for full treatment period prescribed.

---

# mupirocin
Bactroban

*Pregnancy Risk Category: B*

## HOW SUPPLIED
*Ointment:* 2%

## ACTION
Unknown. Thought to inhibit bacterial protein and RNA synthesis.

## ONSET, PEAK, DURATION
Not applicable.

## INDICATIONS & DOSAGE
*Impetigo –*

**Adults and children:** apply to affected areas t.i.d. for 1 to 2 weeks.

## ADVERSE REACTIONS
**Skin:** burning, pruritus, stinging, rash, pain, erythema.

## INTERACTIONS
None significant.

## CONTRAINDICATIONS
Contraindicated in patients hypersensitive to the drug.

## NURSING CONSIDERATIONS
• Use cautiously in patients with burns or impaired renal function.

• Drug is not for ophthalmic use.

• Prolonged use may cause overgrowth of nonsusceptible bacteria and fungi.

• Local reactions appear to be caused by the polyethylene glycol vehicle.

---

Reactions may be *common,* uncommon, *life-threatening,* or **COMMON AND LIFE-THREATENING.**

☑ **PATIENT TEACHING**
- If no improvement occurs in 3 to 5 days or if condition worsens, tell patient to notify the doctor immediately.
- Warn patient about local adverse reactions associated with drug application.

---

## naftifine
Naftin

*Pregnancy Risk Category: B*

**HOW SUPPLIED**
*Cream:* 1%
*Gel:* 1%

**ACTION**
Unknown. A broad-spectrum fungicidal agent that is thought to inhibit sterol biosynthesis in susceptible fungi by blocking the enzyme squalene 2,3 epoxidase.

**ONSET, PEAK, DURATION**
Not applicable.

**INDICATIONS & DOSAGE**
*Tinea corporis, tinea cruris, and tinea pedis –*
**Adults:** apply to affected area once daily with the cream, or b.i.d. in the morning and evening with the gel.

**ADVERSE REACTIONS**
**Skin:** *burning, stinging,* dryness, pruritus, local irritation, erythema.

**INTERACTIONS**
None significant.

**CONTRAINDICATIONS**
Contraindicated in patients hypersensitive to the drug.

**NURSING CONSIDERATIONS**
- Therapy should be reevaluated if no improvement occurs after 4 weeks.
- Keep cream away from mucous membranes. Not for ophthalmic use.

☑ **PATIENT TEACHING**
- Tell the patient not to use occlusive dressings unless directed otherwise by the doctor.
- Instruct the patient to wash hands after application.
- Instruct the patient to discontinue therapy and notify the doctor if irritation or sensitivity develops.

---

## neomycin sulfate
Mycifradin†, Myciguent◇, Neo-Rx

*Pregnancy Risk Category: NR*

**HOW SUPPLIED**
*Cream:* 0.5%◇
*Ointment:* 0.5%◇

**ACTION**
Unknown. Thought to disrupt bacterial protein synthesis by binding to bacterial ribosomes.

**ONSET, PEAK, DURATION**
Not applicable.

**INDICATIONS & DOSAGE**
*Prevention or treatment of superficial bacterial infections –*
**Adults and children:** rub into affected area one to three times daily.

**ADVERSE REACTIONS**
**Skin:** *rashes, contact dermatitis,* urticaria.
**Systemic:** *possible nephrotoxicity, ototoxicity, and* **neuromuscular blockade***.*

**INTERACTIONS**
None significant.

**CONTRAINDICATIONS**
Contraindicated in patients hypersensitive to the drug.

**NURSING CONSIDERATIONS**
- Use cautiously in patients with extensive dermatologic conditions.

---

*Liquid form contains alcohol. **May contain tartrazine. †Canada only. ‡Australia only. ◇OTC.

Don't use on more than 20% of the body surface.
• Prolonged use may result in overgrowth of nonsusceptible organisms.
• In combination products containing corticosteroids, be aware that use of occlusive dressings increases corticosteroid absorption and the likelihood of systemic effects.
• Keep in mind that enhanced systemic absorption occurs on denuded or abraded areas.
• Watch for signs of hypersensitivity and contact dermatitis.
• *Alert:* Watch for signs of ototoxicity with prolonged or extended use.

☑ **PATIENT TEACHING**
• If no improvement occurs or if condition worsens, tell patient to stop using and notify the doctor.
• Tell patient to report adverse reactions, especially systemic reactions.

### nitrofurazone
Furacin

*Pregnancy Risk Category: C*

**HOW SUPPLIED**
*Cream:* 0.2%
*Ointment:* 0.2% (soluble dressing)
*Topical solution:* 0.2%

**ACTION**
Unknown. A broad-spectrum antibiotic that probably inhibits bacterial enzymes involved in carbohydrate metabolism.

**ONSET, PEAK, DURATION**
Not applicable.

**INDICATIONS & DOSAGE**
*Adjunctive treatment of second- and third-degree burns (especially when resistance to other antibiotics and sulfonamides occurs); prevention of skin allograft rejection –*
**Adults and children:** apply directly to lesion daily or every few days, de-

pending on severity of burn. May also be applied to dressings used to cover affected area.

**ADVERSE REACTIONS**
**Skin:** *erythema, pruritus,* burning, edema, severe reactions (vesiculation, denudation, ulceration), *allergic contact dermatitis.*

**INTERACTIONS**
None significant.

**CONTRAINDICATIONS**
Contraindicated in patients hypersensitive to the drug.

**NURSING CONSIDERATIONS**
• Use cautiously in patients with known or suspected renal impairment. Monitor serum creatinine levels regularly, as ordered.
• Clean wound, as indicated by the doctor, before reapplying dressings.
• Use sterile application technique to prevent further wound contamination.
• When using wet dressing, protect skin around wound with zinc oxide ointment.
• Be aware that drug may discolor in light but still retains its potency.
• Discard cloudy solutions if warming to 55° to 60° C (131° to 140° F) does not restore clarity.
• Store solution in tight, light-resistant containers (brown bottles). Avoid exposure to direct light, prolonged heat, and alkaline materials.

☑ **PATIENT TEACHING**
• Tell patient to report irritation, sensitization, or infection.
• Explain all procedures to patient.

Reactions may be *common,* uncommon, *life-threatening,* or COMMON AND LIFE-THREATENING.

# nystatin
Mycostatin, Nadostine†, Nilstat

*Pregnancy Risk Category: NR*

## HOW SUPPLIED
*Cream:* 100,000 units/g
*Ointment:* 100,000 units/g
*Powder:* 100,000 units/g
*Vaginal tablets:* 100,000 units

## ACTION
Disrupts integrity of fungal cell wall, promoting osmotic instability.

## ONSET, PEAK, DURATION
Not applicable for cream, ointment, or powder. Unknown for tablets.

## INDICATIONS & DOSAGE
*Cutaneous and mucocutaneous infections caused by* Candida albicans —
**Adults and children:** apply to affected area up to several times a day.
*Vulvovaginal candidiasis* —
**Adults:** 1 vaginal tablet daily or b.i.d. for 14 days.

## ADVERSE REACTIONS
**Skin:** occasional contact dermatitis from preservatives in some forms.

## INTERACTIONS
None significant.

## CONTRAINDICATIONS
Contraindicated in patients hypersensitive to the drug.

## NURSING CONSIDERATIONS
• Do not use occlusive dressings.
• Keep in mind that preparation does not stain skin or mucous membranes.
• Cream is recommended for intertriginous areas; powder, for moist areas; ointment, for dry areas.

## ☑ PATIENT TEACHING
• Instruct female patient how to administer vaginal tablets, and tell her to continue using the vaginal tablets during her menstrual period. Instruct her to refrigerate the tablets.
• Tell patient to use drug for full prescribed period, even if condition improves. Immunosuppressed patients may use the drug chronically.
• Instruct patient not to use occlusive dressings with skin application.

# oxiconazole nitrate
Oxistat

*Pregnancy Risk Category: B*

## HOW SUPPLIED
*Cream:* 1%
*Lotion:* 1%

## ACTION
Unknown. May inhibit ergosterol synthesis in fungal cell walls, causing osmotic instability and cell lysis.

## ONSET, PEAK, DURATION
Not applicable.

## INDICATIONS & DOSAGE
*Tinea pedis, cruris, and tinea corporis caused by* Trichophyton rubrum *or* T. mentagrophytes —
**Adults:** apply to affected area once or twice daily. Treat tinea cruris and tinea corporis for 2 weeks and tinea pedis for 1 month to minimize risk of recurrence.

## ADVERSE REACTIONS
**Skin:** pruritus, burning, stinging, contact dermatitis, irritation, scaling, tingling, pain, eczema.

## INTERACTIONS
None significant.

## CONTRAINDICATIONS
Contraindicated in patients hypersensitive to the drug.

## NURSING CONSIDERATIONS
• Know that drug is not for ophthalmic or vaginal administration.

---

*Liquid form contains alcohol.   **May contain tartrazine.   †Canada only.   ‡Australia only.   ◇OTC.

• Know that drug is for external use only.

☑ **PATIENT TEACHING**
• Inform patient that drug shouldn't touch the eyes or vagina.
• Tell patient to stop drug and call doctor if local irritation occurs.

## podofilox
Condylox*
*Pregnancy Risk Category: C*

**HOW SUPPLIED**
*Topical solution: 0.5%**

**ACTION**
Unknown; a keratolytic agent that probably causes local necrosis of wart tissue.

**ONSET, PEAK, DURATION**
Not applicable.

**INDICATIONS & DOSAGE**
*External genital warts (condylomata acuminata)* –
**Adults:** apply to affected areas q 12 hours for 3 consecutive days; then withhold for 4 consecutive days. Repeated as needed up to 4 weeks until warts disappear.

**ADVERSE REACTIONS**
**CNS:** insomnia, dizziness.
**GI:** vomiting.
**GU:** foreskin retraction, dyspareunia, hematuria.
**Skin:** *burning, pain, inflammation, erosion, pruritus,* tingling, *tenderness,* chafing, scarring, vesicle formation, crusting edema, dryness and peeling, ulceration.

**INTERACTIONS**
None significant.

**CONTRAINDICATIONS**
Contraindicated in patients with hypersensitivity to or intolerance of any component of the medication (contains 95% alcohol).

**NURSING CONSIDERATIONS**
• Know that drug should not be used to treat genital warts in the perianal area or on mucous membranes of the genital area, including the urethra, rectum, and vagina.
• *Alert:* Systemic use has caused hematologic toxicity, hematuria, seizures, and GI disturbances.
• If no response occurs after 4 weeks of therapy, anticipate using alternative therapy.

☑ **PATIENT TEACHING**
• Tell the patient that the drug is for external use only.
• Teach the patient how to apply the drug:
  – Dampen the supplied cotton-tipped applicator with drug and touch it to the wart.
  – Apply least amount needed to cover the lesion; 0.5 ml or less, and covering less than 10 cm$^2$ (4″) of wart tissue.
  – Let the area dry before allowing skin to retract.
  – Dispose of used applicator properly and wash hands thoroughly afterward.
• Tell the patient to avoid contact with eyes. If this occurs, he should flush the area with plenty of water and call the doctor at once.
• Tell the patient that additional applications will not improve efficacy but can increase adverse reactions and the risk of systemic absorption.

## silver sulfadiazine
Flamazine†, Flint SSD, Silvadene, SSD-AF, Thermazene
*Pregnancy Risk Category: B*

**HOW SUPPLIED**
*Cream: 1%*

## ACTION
Broad-spectrum sulfonamide that acts on cell membrane and cell wall; bactericidal for many gram-positive and gram-negative organisms.

## ONSET, PEAK, DURATION
Not applicable.

## INDICATIONS & DOSAGE
*Prevention and treatment of wound infection in second- and third-degree burns—*
**Adults and children:** apply 1/16" thickness to clean debrided burn wound daily or b.i.d.

## ADVERSE REACTIONS
**Hematologic:** *neutropenia.*
**Skin:** pain, burning, rashes, pruritus, skin necrosis, erythema multiforme, skin discoloration.

## INTERACTIONS
*Topical proteolytic enzymes:* inactivation of enzymes. Do not use together.

## CONTRAINDICATIONS
Contraindicated in premature and full-term neonates during first 2 months of life. Drug may increase possibility of kernicterus. Also contraindicated in patients with hypersensitivity to the drug or in pregnant women at or near term.

## NURSING CONSIDERATIONS
● Use with caution in patients hypersensitive to sulfonamides.
● Use sterile application technique to prevent wound contamination.
● Use only on affected areas. Keep these areas medicated at all times.
● Bathe the patient daily, if possible.
● Inspect the patient's skin daily, and note any changes. Notify the doctor if burning or excessive pain develops.
● Monitor serum sulfadiazine concentrations and renal function, as ordered, and check urine for sulfa crystals in patients with extensive burns.

● Tell doctor if hepatic or renal dysfunction occurs; drug may need to be stopped.
● Discard darkened cream, which indicates drug is ineffective.

☑ **PATIENT TEACHING**
● Instruct patient to report adverse reactions promptly, especially burning or excessive pain with application.
● Inform patient of need for frequent blood and urine tests to monitor for adverse effects.

# sulconazole nitrate
Exelderm
*Pregnancy Risk Category: C*

## HOW SUPPLIED
*Topical solution:* 1%
*Cream:* 1%

## ACTION
Unknown. A broad-spectrum antifungal imidazole derivative that inhibits the growth of both fungi and yeast.

## ONSET, PEAK, DURATION
Not applicable.

## INDICATIONS & DOSAGE
*Tinea cruris, tinea corporis, tinea pedis, or tinea versicolor—*
**Adults:** massage a small amount of drug into affected area daily to b.i.d. for 3 weeks. Treat tinea pedis with cream b.i.d. for 4 weeks.

## ADVERSE REACTIONS
**Skin:** pruritus, burning, stinging, redness.

## INTERACTIONS
None significant.

## CONTRAINDICATIONS
Contraindicated in patients hypersensitive to any component of the drug.

---

*Liquid form contains alcohol.   **May contain tartrazine.   †Canada only.   ‡Australia only.   ◇OTC.

## NURSING CONSIDERATIONS
• Use only cream for tinea pedia. Efficacy against tinea pedis (athlete's foot) has not been proven with the topical solution.
• Know that if no improvement occurs after 4 weeks, diagnosis should be reconsidered.

### ☑ PATIENT TEACHING
• Tell the patient to avoid touching the eyes with the drug and to wash hands thoroughly after applying.
• Explain to the patient the necessity of completing the full course of therapy to prevent recurrence. Clinical improvement is usually apparent within 1 week, with symptomatic relief in just a few days.
• If irritation develops during treatment, tell the patient to discontinue drug and contact the doctor.

---

## terbinafine hydrochloride
Lamisil
*Pregnancy Risk Category: B*

### HOW SUPPLIED
*Cream:* 1%

### ACTION
Fungicidal; selectively inhibits an early step in synthesis of sterols used by fungi for cell wall synthesis.

### ONSET, PEAK, DURATION
Not applicable.

### INDICATIONS & DOSAGE
*Interdigital tinea pedis, tinea cruris, and tinea corporis –*
**Adults:** cover affected area and immediate surrounding area daily or b.i.d. for at least 1 week.

### ADVERSE REACTIONS
**Skin:** irritation, burning, pruritus, dryness.

## INTERACTIONS
None significant.

### CONTRAINDICATIONS
Contraindicated in patients hypersensitive to the drug.

### NURSING CONSIDERATIONS
• Observe patients for 2 to 4 weeks after therapy is complete to determine if treatment was successful; review the diagnosis if the condition persists beyond this observation period.
• Be aware that therapy shouldn't exceed 4 weeks.

### ☑ PATIENT TEACHING
• Teach the patient proper use of drug. Tell the patient to use only as directed for the full recommended course, even if symptoms disappear and not to apply near the eyes, mouth, or mucous membranes or use occlusive dressings unless so directed.
• Tell the patient to discontinue drug and contact the doctor if irritation or sensitivity develops.

---

## terconazole
Terazol 3 Vaginal Suppositories, Terazol 7 Vaginal Cream
*Pregnancy Risk Category: C*

### HOW SUPPLIED
*Vaginal cream:* 0.4%, 0.8%
*Vaginal suppositories:* 80 mg

### ACTION
Unknown; may increase fungal cell membrane permeability (*Candida* species only).

### ONSET, PEAK, DURATION
Unknown.

### INDICATIONS & DOSAGE
*Vulvovaginal candidiasis –*
**Adults:** 1 applicatorful of cream or 1 suppository inserted into vagina h.s. 0.4% cream used for 7 consecutive

days; 0.8% cream or 80-mg suppository for 3 consecutive days. Course repeated, if necessary, after reconfirmation by smear or culture.

## ADVERSE REACTIONS
**CNS:** *headache.*
**GU:** dysmenorrhea, pain of the female genitalia, vulvovaginal burning.
**Skin:** irritation, *pruritus,* photosensitivity.
**Other:** fever, chills, body aches.

## INTERACTIONS
None significant.

## CONTRAINDICATIONS
Contraindicated in patients with known sensitivity to terconazole or any inactive ingredients in drug.

## NURSING CONSIDERATIONS
• Discontinue if the patient develops fever, chills, other flulike symptoms, or sensitivity and notify doctor
• Keep in mind that therapeutic effect of drug is unaffected by menstruation.

## ☑ PATIENT TEACHING
• Advise patient to continue treatment during the menstrual period. However, tell her not to use tampons.
• Tell patient to use for full treatment period prescribed. Explain how to prevent reinfection.

---

# tetracycline hydrochloride
Achromycin, Topicycline

*Pregnancy Risk Category: B*

## HOW SUPPLIED
*Ointment:* 3%
*Topical solution:* 2.2 mg/ml

## ACTION
Unknown. A broad-spectrum antibiotic that probably disrupts bacterial protein synthesis; usually bacteriostatic.

## ONSET, PEAK, DURATION
Unknown.

## INDICATIONS & DOSAGE
*Acne vulgaris –*
**Adults and children over 12 years:** rub solution generously into affected areas b.i.d. until skin is thoroughly covered.
*Prevention or treatment of superficial skin infections caused by susceptible bacteria –*
**Adults:** apply to affected area b.i.d. in morning and evening or t.i.d.

## ADVERSE REACTIONS
**Skin:** temporary stinging or burning on application; slight yellowing of treated skin, especially in patients with light complexions; severe dermatitis.

## INTERACTIONS
*Abrasive or medicated soaps or cleansers; acne preparations or other preparations containing peeling agents (benzoyl peroxide, resorcinol, salicylic acid, sulfur, tretinoin); alcohol-containing products (after-shave, cosmetics, perfumed toiletries, shaving creams or lotions); astringent soaps or cosmetics; isotretinoin; medicated cosmetics or cover-ups:* may cause cumulative dryness, resulting in excessive skin irritation. Use cautiously.

## CONTRAINDICATIONS
Contraindicated in patients hypersensitive to the drug.

## NURSING CONSIDERATIONS
• Use cautiously in patients with hepatic or renal impairment.
• Prolonged use may result in overgrowth of nonsusceptible organisms.
• Store at room temperature, away from excessive heat.
• Be aware that ointment form should not be used to treat acne vulgaris.

---

*Liquid form contains alcohol. **May contain tartrazine. †Canada only. ‡Australia only. ◊OTC.

## ☑ PATIENT TEACHING
● Tell the patient to wash area before applying.
● Explain that floating plug in bottle of Topicycline — an inert and harmless result of proper reconstitution of the preparation — shouldn't be removed.
● Tell the patient how to increase or decrease applicator pressure against skin to control flow rate of solution.
● Tell the patient that she may continue normal use of cosmetics.
● Tell the patient not to share medication with family members.
● Advise the patient to use or discard the drug within 2 months.
● If no improvement occurs or if condition worsens, advise the patient to stop using and notify the doctor.

---

## tioconazole
Vagistat

*Pregnancy Risk Category: C*

**HOW SUPPLIED**
*Vaginal ointment:* 6.5%

**ACTION**
A fungicidal imidazole that alters cell wall permeability.

**ONSET, PEAK, DURATION**
Unknown.

**INDICATIONS & DOSAGE**
*Vulvovaginal candidiasis —*
**Adults:** 1 applicatorful (about 4.6 g) inserted intravaginally h.s. one time only.

**ADVERSE REACTIONS**
**GU:** *burning, pruritus,* discharge, vaginal pain, dysuria, dyspareunia, vulvar edema, irritation.

**INTERACTIONS**
None significant.

**CONTRAINDICATIONS**
Contraindicated in patients hypersensitive to the drug or other imidazole antifungal agents (miconazole, ketoconazole).

**NURSING CONSIDERATIONS**
● Know that if patient is breast-feeding, she should temporarily stop doing so because drug it is not known if drug is excreted in breast milk.
● Notify the doctor if patient reports irritation or sensitivity.

## ☑ PATIENT TEACHING
● Review proper use of the drug with the patient. Written instructions for the patient are available with the product. Tell the patient to insert drug high into the vagina.
● To avoid contamination of the ointment, tell the patient to open the applicator just before using it.
● Tell the patient to use a sanitary napkin to avoid staining her clothing.
● Advise the patient to avoid sexual intercourse on the night after insertion, or advise her partner to use a condom to prevent reinfection.
● Emphasize the need to complete the full course of therapy, even after symptoms have improved. The patient should continue using the drug during her menstrual period.

---

## tolnaftate
Aftate for Athlete's Foot◊, Aftate for Jock Itch◊, Dr. Scholl's Athlete's Foot Powder◊, Dr. Scholl's Athlete's Foot Spray◊, Footwork◊, Fungatin◊, Genaspor◊, NP-27◊, Tinactin◊, Ting◊, Zeasorb-AF◊

*Pregnancy Risk Category: NR*

**HOW SUPPLIED**
*Aerosol liquid:* 1% (36% alcohol)◊
*Aerosol powder:* 1% (14% alcohol)◊
*Cream:* 1%◊
*Gel:* 1%◊

---

Reactions may be *common,* uncommon, *life-threatening,* or COMMON AND LIFE-THREATENING.

*Powder:* 1%◇
*Pump spray liquid:* 1% (36% alcohol)◇
*Topical solution:* 1%◇

## ACTION
Unknown, although drug has been demonstrated to distort the hyphae and stunt mycelial growth in susceptible fungi.

## ONSET, PEAK, DURATION
Not applicable.

## INDICATIONS & DOSAGE
*Superficial fungal infections of the skin; infections due to common pathogenic fungi; tinea pedis, tinea cruris, tinea corporis, and tinea versicolor* –
**Adults and children:** apply ¼″ to ½″ ribbon of cream or 2 to 3 drops of solution to cover area about the size of one hand; same amount of cream or 2 to 3 drops of solution to cover toes and interdigital webs of one foot; or gel, powder, or spray to cover affected area. Apply and massage gently into skin b.i.d. for 2 to 6 weeks.

## ADVERSE REACTIONS
**Skin:** possible irritation.

## INTERACTIONS
None significant.

## CONTRAINDICATIONS
Contraindicated in patients hypersensitive to the drug.

## NURSING CONSIDERATIONS
• Be aware that drug is not used to treat fungal infections of the hair or nails; tolnaftate is ineffective against these fungi.
• Know that drug is odorless and greaseless; it won't stain or discolor skin, hair, nails, or clothing.
• Know that powder or aerosol may be used inside socks and shoes of persons susceptible to tinea infections.

☑ **PATIENT TEACHING**
• Tell patient to continue using for full treatment period prescribed, even if condition has improved. Treatment should continue for at least 2 weeks after symptoms have resolved.
• Advise patient to use only a small quantity of cream or lotion; treated area should not be wet with solution.
• If no improvement occurs after 10 days, tell patient to call doctor.
• Tell patient to discontinue if condition worsens and to check with the doctor.

# 88

## Scabicides and pediculicides

**benzyl benzoate lotion**
**crotamiton**
**lindane**
**permethrin**
**pyrethrins**

**COMBINATION PRODUCTS**
None.

## benzyl benzoate lotion
Ascabiol‡

*Pregnancy Risk Category: C*

**HOW SUPPLIED**
*Lotion:* 14% (with benzocaine 2%)‡
*Emulsion:* 50%‡

**ACTION**
Unknown.

**ONSET, PEAK, DURATION**
Unknown.

**INDICATIONS & DOSAGE**
*Parasitic infestation (scabies,* Phthirus pubis, Pediculus humanus capitis) —
**Adults and children:** scrub entire body with soap and water. Remove scales or crusts. Then apply the lotion undiluted over affected area (include whole body for scabies), except the face and scalp, while still damp. Be sure to apply around nails. Let dry. Apply second coat on the most involved areas. Bathe after 24 hours.

Treatment may be repeated in 7 to 10 days if mites appear or new lesions develop.

**ADVERSE REACTIONS**
**Skin:** *irritation, pruritus; contact dermatitis* (with repeated applications).

**INTERACTIONS**
None significant.

**CONTRAINDICATIONS**
Contraindicated when skin is raw or inflamed or in patients hypersensitive to drug.

**NURSING CONSIDERATIONS**
● Do not apply to face, eyes, mucous membranes, or urethral meatus. If accidental contact with eyes occurs, flush with water and notify the doctor.
● Apply topical corticosteroids as prescribed if dermatitis develops from scratching.
● Do not apply to infants' or small children's hands because they put their hands into their mouths.
● Make sure hospitalized patients are placed in isolation, with linen-handling precautions, until treatment is completed.
● Store drug in light-resistant container; avoid exposure to excessive heat.

☑ **PATIENT TEACHING**
● Teach the patient how to administer drug.
● Tell the patient to discontinue drug and to wash it off skin and notify the doctor immediately if skin irritation or hypersensitivity develops.
● Instruct the patient to change and sterilize (boil, launder, dry clean, or apply very hot iron) all clothing and bed linen after drug is washed off.
● Instruct the patient to reapply drug if it is washed off during treatment time.
● After application for lice infestation, tell the patient to use a fine-tooth comb dipped in white vinegar to remove nits from hairy areas.

- Tell the patient to warn other family members and sexual contacts about infestation. Sexual contacts should be treated simultaneously.
- Reassure the patient that although itching may continue for several weeks, it will stop; continued itching does not indicate that therapy is ineffective.

---

## crotamiton
Eurax

*Pregnancy Risk Category: C*

### HOW SUPPLIED
*Cream:* 10%
*Lotion:* 10%

### ACTION
Unknown.

### ONSET, PEAK, DURATION
Unknown.

### INDICATIONS & DOSAGE
*Parasitic infestation (scabies) –*
**Adults and children:** scrub entire body with soap and water. Remove scales or crusts. Then apply a thin layer of cream over entire body, from chin down (with special attention to folds, creases, interdigital spaces, and genital area). Apply second coat in 24 hours. Wait additional 48 hours, then wash off. Treatment is repeated in 7 to 10 days if mites reappear or new lesions develop.
*Itching –*
**Adults and children:** applied locally and repeated p.r.n.

### ADVERSE REACTIONS
**Skin:** *irritation.*

### INTERACTIONS
None significant.

### CONTRAINDICATIONS
Contraindicated when skin is raw or inflamed and in patients hypersensitive to drug.

### NURSING CONSIDERATIONS
- Estimate amount of cream needed per application; most patients have a tendency to overuse scabicides. For most adults, a single tube of cream provides a sufficient amount for two applications.
- Apply topical corticosteroids, as prescribed, if dermatitis develops from scratching.
- Make sure hospitalized patients are placed in isolation, with special linen-handling precautions, until treatment is completed.
- Be aware that monthly maintenance treatments may be necessary in long-term care facilities, where infestation is a problem.

### ☑ PATIENT TEACHING
- Teach the patient how to apply drug. Tell the patient not to apply to face, eyes, mucous membranes, or urethral meatus. If accidental contact with eyes occurs, flush with water and notify the doctor.
- Tell the patient to discontinue drug and to wash it off skin and to notify the doctor immediately if skin irritation or hypersensitivity develops.
- Instruct the patient to change and sterilize (boil, launder, dry clean, or apply very hot iron) all clothing and bed linen after drug is washed off.
- After application for lice infestation, tell the patient to use a fine-tooth comb dipped in white vinegar to remove nits from hairy areas.
- Instruct the patient to reapply drug if it is washed off during treatment time.
- Tell the patient to warn other family members and sexual contacts about infestation. Sexual contacts should be treated simultaneously.

---

*Liquid form contains alcohol. **May contain tartrazine. †Canada only. ‡Australia only. ◇OTC.

# lindane

Gamma Benzene, gBh†, Kildane, Kwell, Kwellada†, Scabene

*Pregnancy Risk Category: B*

## HOW SUPPLIED
*Cream:* 1%
*Lotion:* 1%
*Shampoo:* 1%

## ACTION
Unknown. Appears to inhibit neuronal membrane function in arthropods, causing neuronal hyperactivity, seizures, and death after penetrating the parasites' exoskeleton.

## ONSET, PEAK, DURATION
Unknown.

## INDICATIONS & DOSAGE
*Parasitic infestation (scabies, pediculosis)* —

**Adults and children:** scrub entire body with soap and water; let skin dry thoroughly before using. Apply thin layer of cream or lotion over entire skin surface (with special attention to folds, creases, interdigital spaces, and genital area) for scabies, or to hairy areas for pediculosis. After 8 to 12 hours, wash off drug. Repeat process in 1 week if mites appear or new lesions develop.

Apply shampoo undiluted to affected area and work into lather for 4 to 5 minutes; small amounts of water may enhance formation of lather. Apply 30 ml of shampoo for short hair, 45 ml for medium-length hair, or 60 ml for long hair. Rinse thoroughly and rub dry with towel.

## ADVERSE REACTIONS
**CNS:** *dizziness, seizures.*
**Skin:** *irritation* (with repeated use).

## INTERACTIONS
None significant.

## CONTRAINDICATIONS
Contraindicated in patients hypersensitive to the drug, when skin is raw or inflamed, or in patients with seizure disorders. The lotion form is contraindicated in premature infants.

## NURSING CONSIDERATIONS
● Use cautiously in infants and young children, who are at greater risk for CNS toxicity.
● Apply topical corticosteroids or administer oral antihistamines, as prescribed, for pruritus.
● Make sure that hospitalized patients are placed in isolation, with special linen-handling precautions, until treatment is completed.
● Know that modest amounts (6% to 13%) are absorbed through intact skin. Absorption is increased if used with creams, oils, or lotions or if applied to face, scalp, axillae, neck, scrotum, or irritated or broken skin.

## ☑ PATIENT TEACHING
● Teach patient how to administer drug. Warn patient not to apply to open areas, acutely inflamed skin, or to face, eyes, mucous membranes, or urethral meatus. If accidental contact with eyes occurs, flush with water and notify the doctor. Avoid inhaling vapors.
● Tell patient to wash it off skin and to notify the doctor immediately if skin irritation or hypersensitivity develops.
● Discourage repeated use, which can lead to skin irritation, systemic toxicity, or seizures. Repeat use only if live lice or nits are found after 1 week.
● Instruct patient to change and sterilize (boil, launder, dry clean, or apply very hot iron) all clothing and bed linen after drug is washed off.
● After application for lice infestation, tell patient to use a fine-tooth comb dipped in white vinegar to remove nits from hairy areas.
● Advise patient to use shampoo to clean combs or brushes; wash them

---

Reactions may be *common,* uncommon, *life-threatening,* or **COMMON AND LIFE-THREATENING.**

thoroughly afterward. Warn the patient not to use routinely.
• Warn patient that itching may continue for several weeks after effective treatment, especially in scabies.
• Instruct patient to reapply drug if it is washed off during treatment time.
• Tell patient to warn other family members and sexual contacts about infestation. Sexual contacts should be treated simultaneously.

---

## permethrin
Elimite, Nix
*Pregnancy Risk Category: B*

### HOW SUPPLIED
*Topical liquid (cream-rinse):* 1%
*Cream:* 5%

### ACTION
Acts on the parasites' nerve cells to disrupt the sodium channel current, causing paralysis of the parasite.

### ONSET, PEAK, DURATION
Onset and peak unknown. Residual activity persists for about 10 days.

### INDICATIONS & DOSAGE
*Infestation with* Pediculus humanus capitis *(head lice) and its nits* –
**Adults and children:** use after hair has been washed with shampoo, rinsed with water, and towel-dried. Apply 25 to 50 ml of liquid to saturate the hair and scalp. Allow to remain on hair for 10 minutes before rinsing off with water.
*Treatment of* Sarcoptes scabiei –
**Adults and children:** thoroughly massage into the skin from the head to the soles. Infants should be treated on the hairline, neck, scalp, temple and forehead. Cream should be removed after 8 to 14 hours by washing.

### ADVERSE REACTIONS
**Skin:** pruritus, *burning, stinging,* edema, tingling, numbness or scalp discomfort, mild erythema, scalp rash.

### INTERACTIONS
None significant.

### CONTRAINDICATIONS
Contraindicated in patients hypersensitive to pyrethrins or chrysanthemums.

### NURSING CONSIDERATIONS
• Be aware that a single treatment is usually all that is necessary. Combing of nits is not required for effectiveness, but drug package supplies a fine-tooth comb for cosmetic use as desired.
• Retreat for lice, as prescribed, if lice are observed 7 days after the initial application.

### ☑ PATIENT TEACHING
• Explain to the patient that treatment with permethrin may temporarily worsen the symptoms of head lice infestation, such as pruritus, erythema, and edema.
• Tell the patient that headgear, scarves, coats, and bed linens should be disinfected by machine washing with hot water and machine drying for at least 20 minutes, using the hot cycle. Nonwashable items should be sealed in a plastic bag for 2 weeks, or sprayed with a product designed to eliminate lice and their nits.
• Tell the patient to warn other family members and sexual contacts about infestation. Sexual contacts should be treated simultaneously.

---

*Liquid form contains alcohol.  **May contain tartrazine.  †Canada only.  ‡Australia only.  ◇OTC.

## pyrethrins

A-200 Pyrinate◇, Barc◇, Blue Gel,
Pronto, Pyrinyl◇, R&C, RID◇,
TISIT◇, Triple X◇

*Pregnancy Risk Category: NR*

### HOW SUPPLIED

*Shampoo:* pyrethrins 0.17% and piperonyl butoxide 2%; pyrethrins 0.3%
and piperonyl butoxide 3%
*Topical gel:* pyrethrins 0.18% and piperonyl butoxide 2.2%; pyrethrins
0.33% and piperonyl butoxide 3%;
pyrethrins 0.3% and piperonyl butoxide 4%
*Topical solution:* pyrethrins 0.18%
and piperonyl butoxide 2%; pyrethrins 0.2%, piperonyl butoxide 2%,
and deodorized kerosene 0.8%; pyrethrins 0.3% and piperonyl butoxide
3%

### ACTION

Acts as contact poison that disrupts
parasite's nervous system, causing
parasite paralysis and death.

### ONSET, PEAK, DURATION

Not applicable.

### INDICATIONS & DOSAGE

*Infestations of head, body, and pubic
(crab) lice and their eggs –*
**Adults and children:** apply to hair,
scalp, or other infested areas until en-
tirely wet. Allow to remain for 10
minutes but no longer. Wash thoroughly with warm water and soap or
shampoo. Remove dead lice and eggs
with fine-tooth comb. Treatment repeated, if necessary, in 7 to 10 days to
kill newly hatched lice. Not to exceed
two applications within 24 hours.

### ADVERSE REACTIONS

**Skin:** *irritation* (with repeated use).

### INTERACTIONS

None significant.

### CONTRAINDICATIONS

Contraindicated in patients hypersensitive to the drug or to ragweed.

### NURSING CONSIDERATIONS

• Use cautiously in infants and small
children.
• Apply topical corticosteroids or oral
antihistamines as prescribed if dermatitis develops from scratching.
• Be aware that drug is not effective
against scabies.

### ☑ PATIENT TEACHING

• Instruct the patient not to apply to
open areas or acutely inflamed skin or
to face, eyes, mucous membranes, or
urethral meatus. If accidental contact
with eyes occurs, flush with water and
notify the doctor.
• Discourage repeated use, which can
lead to skin irritation and possible systemic toxicity.
• Tell the patient to discontinue drug
and to wash it off skin and to notify
the doctor immediately if skin irritation develops. All preparations contain petroleum distillates.
• Instruct the patient to change and
sterilize (boil, launder, dry clean, or
apply very hot iron) all clothing and
bed linen after drug is washed off.
• Teach the patient to remove dead
parasites with a fine-tooth comb.
• Tell the patient to warn other family
members and sexual contacts about
infestation. Sexual contacts should be
treated simultaneously.

---

# 89

# Topical corticosteroids

alclometasone dipropionate
amcinonide
betamethasone benzoate
betamethasone dipropionate
betamethasone valerate
clobetasol propionate
clocortolone pivalate
desonide
desoximetasone
dexamethasone
dexamethasone sodium
  phosphate
diflorasone diacetate
fluocinolone acetonide
fluocinonide
flurandrenolide
fluticasone propionate
halcinonide
halobetasol propionate
hydrocortisone
hydrocortisone acetate
hydrocortisone butyrate
hydrocortisone valerate
mometasone furoate
triamcinolone acetonide

## COMBINATION PRODUCTS
Corticosteroids for topical use are commonly combined with antibiotics and antifungals. (See Chapter 87, LOCAL ANTI-INFECTIVES.)

---

# alclometasone dipropionate
Alclovate, Logoderm‡

*Pregnancy Risk Category: C*

## HOW SUPPLIED
*Cream:* 0.05%
*Ointment:* 0.05%

## ACTION
Unknown. Diffuses across cell membranes to form complexes with specific cytoplasmic receptors. Exhibits anti-inflammatory, antipruritic, vasoconstrictive, and antiproliferative activity. Considered a group IV (low-potency) agent according to vasoconstrictive properties.

## ONSET, PEAK, DURATION
Onset and duration unknown. Plasma levels are highest when applied to inflamed or damaged skin, eyelids, or scrotal area; lowest when applied to intact normal skin, palms of hands, or soles of feet.

## INDICATIONS & DOSAGE
*Inflammation associated with corticosteroid-responsive dermatoses –*
**Adults:** apply a thin film to affected areas b.i.d. or t.i.d. Gently massage until the medication disappears.

## ADVERSE REACTIONS
**Skin:** burning, pruritus, irritation, dryness, erythema, folliculitis, striae, acneiform eruptions, perioral dermatitis, hypopigmentation, hypertrichosis, allergic contact dermatitis; *secondary infection, maceration, atrophy, striae, miliaria* (with occlusive dressings).
**Systemic:** *hypothalamic-pituitary-adrenal (HPA) axis suppression,* Cushing's syndrome, hyperglycemia, glucosuria.

## INTERACTIONS
None significant.

## CONTRAINDICATIONS
Contraindicated in patients hypersensitive to corticosteroids.

## NURSING CONSIDERATIONS
● Gently wash skin before applying. To prevent skin damage, rub medication in gently, leaving a thin coat.

---

When treating hairy sites, part hair and apply directly to lesions.
• Don't apply near eyes or mucous membranes or to face, armpits, groin, or under breasts, unless ordered.
• Change dressings as ordered. Stop drug and notify the doctor if skin infection, striae, or atrophy occurs.
• Notify the doctor and remove occlusive dressing if fever develops.
• If antifungal agents or antibiotics are used concomitantly, stop drug until infection is controlled, as ordered.
• Monitor the patient for systemic adverse reactions. Systemic absorption likely with use of occlusive dressings, prolonged treatment, or application to extensive body surface.
• Continue treatment for a few days after lesions clear, as ordered.
• Know that children may absorb larger amounts of drug and be more prone to systemic toxicity.
• Know that repeated application can result in diminished effectiveness.

☑ **PATIENT TEACHING**
• Teach patient how to apply drug.
• If an occlusive dressing is ordered, advise patient not to leave it in place longer than 16 hours each day or use it on infected or exudative lesions.
• Tell patient to stop drug and report signs of systemic absorption, skin irritation or ulceration, hypersensitivity, or infection.
• Warn patient not to use for more than 14 consecutive days.

## amcinonide
Cyclocort
*Pregnancy Risk Category: C*

**HOW SUPPLIED**
*Cream:* 0.1%
*Lotion:* 0.1%
*Ointment:* 0.1%

**ACTION**
Unknown. Diffuses across cell membranes to form complexes with specific cytoplasmic receptors. Exhibits anti-inflammatory, antipruritic, vasoconstrictive, and antiproliferative activity. Considered a group II (high-potency) agent according to vasoconstrictive properties.

**ONSET, PEAK, DURATION**
Onset and duration unknown. Plasma levels are highest when applied to inflamed or damaged skin, eyelids, or scrotal area; lowest when applied to intact normal skin, palms of hands, or soles of feet.

**INDICATIONS & DOSAGE**
*Inflammation associated with corticosteroid-responsive dermatoses —*
**Adults and children:** apply a light film to affected areas b.i.d. or t.i.d. Rub in gently until it disappears.

**ADVERSE REACTIONS**
**Skin:** burning, pruritus, irritation, dryness, erythema, folliculitis, striae, acneiform eruptions, perioral dermatitis, hypopigmentation, hypertrichosis, allergic contact dermatitis; *secondary infection, maceration, atrophy, striae, miliaria* (with occlusive dressings).
**Systemic:** *hypothalamic-pituitary-adrenal axis suppression,* Cushing's syndrome, hyperglycemia, glucosuria.

**INTERACTIONS**
None significant.

**CONTRAINDICATIONS**
Contraindicated in patients hypersensitive to the drug.

**NURSING CONSIDERATIONS**
• Gently wash skin before applying. To prevent skin damage, rub medication in gently, leaving a thin coat. Part

hair and apply directly to lesion when treating hairy sites.

• Avoid application near eyes or mucous membranes. Do not use on face, armpits, groin, in ear canal, or under breasts unless specifically ordered.

• For patients with eczematous dermatitis whose skin may be irritated by adhesive material, hold dressing in place with gauze, elastic bandages, stockings, or stockinette.

• Change dressings as ordered. Discontinue drug and notify the doctor if skin infection, striae, or atrophy occurs.

• Notify the doctor and remove occlusive dressing if fever develops.

• If antifungal agents or antibiotics are used concomitantly, stop drug until infection is controlled, as ordered.

• Avoid using plastic pants or tight-fitting diapers on treated areas in young children. Children may absorb larger amounts of drug and be more prone to systemic toxicity.

• Systemic absorption likely with use of occlusive dressings, prolonged treatment, or extensive body-surface treatment. Watch for symptoms.

• Continue treatment for a few days after lesions clear, as ordered.

### ☑ PATIENT TEACHING
• Teach patient how to apply drug.

• If an occlusive dressing is ordered, advise patient not to leave it in place longer than 16 hours each day or use it on infected or exudative lesions.

• Tell patient to stop drug and report signs of systemic absorption, skin irritation or ulceration, hypersensitivity, or infection.

---

# betamethasone benzoate
Benisone, Uticort

# betamethasone dipropionate
Alphatrex, Diprolene, Diprolene AF, Diprosone, Maxivate, Psorion

# betamethasone valerate
Betatrex, Beta-Val, Betnovate†‡, Valisone

*Pregnancy Risk Category: C*

## HOW SUPPLIED
**betamethasone benzoate**
*Cream:* 0.025%
*Gel:* 0.025%
*Lotion:* 0.025%
**betamethasone dipropionate**
*Aerosol:* 0.1%
*Cream:* 0.05%
*Lotion:* 0.05%
*Ointment:* 0.05%
**betamethasone valerate**
*Cream:* 0.01%, 0.1%
*Lotion:* 0.1%
*Ointment:* 0.1%

## ACTION
Unknown. Diffuses across cell membranes to form complexes with specific cytoplasmic receptors. Exhibits anti-inflammatory, antipruritic, vasoconstrictive, and antiproliferative activity. Considered a group III (medium-potency) agent according to vasoconstrictive properties.

## ONSET, PEAK, DURATION
Onset and duration unknown. Plasma levels are highest when applied to inflamed or damaged skin, eyelids, or scrotal area; lowest when applied to intact normal skin, palms of hands, or soles of feet.

## INDICATIONS & DOSAGE
*Inflammation associated with corticosteroid-responsive dermatoses –*
**Adults and children:** clean area; apply cream, ointment, lotion, aerosol spray, or gel sparingly daily to b.i.d.

## ADVERSE REACTIONS
**Skin:** burning, pruritus, irritation, dryness, erythema, folliculitis, striae, acneiform eruptions, perioral dermatitis, hypopigmentation, hypertrichosis, allergic contact dermatitis;

---

*secondary infection, maceration, atrophy, striae, miliaria* (with occlusive dressings).
**Systemic:** *hypothalamic-pituitary-adrenal axis suppression,* Cushing's syndrome, hyperglycemia, and glucosuria (with betamethasone dipropionate).

**INTERACTIONS**
None significant.

**CONTRAINDICATIONS**
Contraindicated in patients hypersensitive to corticosteroids.

**NURSING CONSIDERATIONS**
• Gently wash skin before applying. To prevent skin damage, rub medication in gently, leaving a thin coat. When treating hairy sites, part hair and apply directly to lesions.
• Avoid application near eyes, mucous membranes, or in ear canal.
• Because of alcohol content of vehicle, gel preparations may cause mild, transient stinging, especially when used on or near excoriated skin.
• For patients with eczematous dermatitis whose skin may be irritated by adhesive material, hold dressing in place with gauze, elastic bandages, stockings, or stockinette.
• Change dressings as ordered. Discontinue drug and notify the doctor if infection, striae, or atrophy occurs.
• Notify the doctor and remove occlusive dressing if fever develops.
• If antifungal agents or antibiotics are used concomitantly, stop drug until infection is controlled, as ordered.
• Systemic absorption likely with use of occlusive dressings, prolonged treatment, or extensive body-surface treatment. Watch for symptoms.
• Avoid using plastic pants or tight-fitting diapers on treated areas in young children. Children may absorb larger amounts of drug and be more prone to systemic toxicity.

• Continue drug for a few days after lesions clear.
• Diprolene and Diprolene AF may not be substituted generically because other products have different potencies.

☑ **PATIENT TEACHING**
• Teach patient how to apply drug.
• If an occlusive dressing is ordered, advise patient not to leave it in place longer than 16 hours each day and not to use occlusive dressings on infected or exudative lesions.
• Tell patient to stop drug and report signs of systemic absorption, skin irritation or ulceration, hypersensitivity, or infection.

---

## clobetasol propionate
Dermovate†, Temovate

*Pregnancy Risk Category: C*

**HOW SUPPLIED**
*Cream:* 0.05%
*Lotion:* 0.05%
*Ointment:* 0.05%

**ACTION**
Unknown. Diffuses across cell membranes to form complexes with specific cytoplasmic receptors. Exhibits anti-inflammatory, antipruritic, vasoconstrictive, and antiproliferative activity. Considered a group I (very high-potency) agent according to vasoconstrictive properties.

**ONSET, PEAK, DURATION**
Onset and duration unknown. Plasma levels are highest when applied to inflamed or damaged skin, eyelids, or scrotal area; lowest when applied to intact normal skin, palms of hands, or soles of feet.

**INDICATIONS & DOSAGE**
*Inflammation associated with corticosteroid-responsive dermatoses* –
**Adults:** apply a thin layer to affected skin areas b.i.d., in the morning and

---

evening for a maximum of 14 days. Total dosage should not exceed 50 g weekly.

**ADVERSE REACTIONS**
**Skin:** burning, pruritus, irritation, dryness, erythema, folliculitis, perioral dermatitis, allergic contact dermatitis, hypopigmentation, hypertrichosis, acneiform eruptions.
**Systemic:** *hypothalamic-pituitary-adrenal (HPA) axis suppression,* Cushing's syndrome, hyperglycemia, glucosuria.

**INTERACTIONS**
None significant.

**CONTRAINDICATIONS**
Contraindicated in patients hypersensitive to corticosteroids.

**NURSING CONSIDERATIONS**
• Gently wash skin before applying. To prevent skin damage, rub medication in gently, leaving a thin coat. When treating hairy sites, part hair and apply directly to lesions.
• Avoid application near eyes, mucous membranes, or in ear canal.
• *Alert:* Don't use occlusive dressings or bandage, cover, or wrap treated areas.
• If antifungal agents or antibiotics are used concomitantly, stop drug until infection is controlled, as ordered.
• Know that repeated application can result in diminished effectiveness.
• Discontinue drug and notify the doctor if skin infection, striae, or atrophy occurs.
• Do not refrigerate.

☑ **PATIENT TEACHING**
• Teach patient how to apply drug.
• Tell patient to stop drug and report signs of systemic absorption, skin irritation or ulceration, hypersensitivity, or infection.
• Warn patient not to use for longer than 14 consecutive days.

# clocortolone pivalate
Cloderm

*Pregnancy Risk Category: C*

**HOW SUPPLIED**
*Cream:* 0.1%

**ACTION**
Unknown. Diffuses across cell membranes to form complexes with specific cytoplasmic receptors. Exhibits anti-inflammatory, antipruritic, vasoconstrictive, and antiproliferative activity. Considered a group III (medium-potency) agent according to vasoconstrictive properties.

**ONSET, PEAK, DURATION**
Onset and duration unknown. Plasma levels are highest when applied to inflamed or damaged skin, eyelids, or scrotal area; lowest when applied to intact normal skin, palms of hands, or soles of feet.

**INDICATIONS & DOSAGE**
*Inflammation associated with corticosteroid-responsive dermatoses –*
**Adults and children:** apply cream sparingly to affected areas one to four times daily and rub in gently.

**ADVERSE REACTIONS**
**Skin:** burning, pruritus, irritation, dryness, erythema, folliculitis, striae, acneiform eruptions, perioral dermatitis, hypertrichosis, hypopigmentation, allergic contact dermatitis; *secondary infection, maceration, atrophy, striae, miliaria* (with occlusive dressings).
**Systemic:** *hypothalamic-pituitary-adrenal axis suppression,* Cushing's syndrome, hyperglycemia, glucosuria.

**INTERACTIONS**
None significant.

---

*Liquid form contains alcohol.    **May contain tartrazine.    †Canada only.    ‡Australia only.    ◊OTC.

## CONTRAINDICATIONS

Contraindicated in patients hypersensitive to the drug.

## NURSING CONSIDERATIONS

• Gently wash skin before applying. To prevent skin damage, rub medication in gently, leaving a thin coat. When treating hairy sites, part hair and apply directly to lesions.

• Avoid application near eyes or mucous membranes.

• For patients with eczematous dermatitis whose skin may be irritated by adhesive material, hold dressing in place with gauze, elastic bandages, or stockinette.

• Change dressings as ordered. Stop drug and tell the doctor if skin infection, striae, or atrophy occurs.

• Notify the doctor and remove occlusive dressing if fever develops.

• If antifungal agents or antibiotics are used concomitantly, stop drug until infection is controlled, as ordered.

• Systemic adverse reactions. Systemic absorption likely with use of occlusive dressings, prolonged treatment, or extensive body-surface treatment. Watch for symptoms.

• Avoid using plastic pants or tight-fitting diapers on treated areas in young children. Children may absorb larger amounts of drug and be more prone to systemic toxicity.

• Continue drug for a few days after lesions clear, as ordered.

☑ **PATIENT TEACHING**

• Teach patient how to apply drug.

• If an occlusive dressing is ordered, advise patient not to leave it in place longer than 16 hours each day and not to use occlusive dressings on infected or exudative lesions.

• Tell patient to stop drug and report signs of systemic absorption, skin irritation or ulceration, hypersensitivity, or infection.

# desonide

DesOwen, Tridesilon

*Pregnancy Risk Category: C*

## HOW SUPPLIED

*Cream:* 0.05%
*Ointment:* 0.05%
*Lotion:* 0.05%

## ACTION

Unknown. Diffuses across cell membranes to form complexes with specific cytoplasmic receptors. Exhibits anti-inflammatory, antipruritic, vasoconstrictive, and antiproliferative activity. Considered a group IV (low-potency) agent according to vasoconstrictive properties.

## ONSET, PEAK, DURATION

Onset and duration unknown. Plasma levels are highest when applied to inflamed or damaged skin, eyelids, or scrotal area; lowest when applied to intact normal skin, palms of hands, or soles of feet.

## INDICATIONS & DOSAGE

*Inflammation associated with corticosteroid-responsive dermatoses –*
**Adults and children:** clean area; apply sparingly b.i.d. to t.i.d.

## ADVERSE REACTIONS

**Skin:** burning, pruritus, irritation, dryness, erythema, folliculitis, perioral dermatitis, allergic contact dermatitis, hypertrichosis, hypopigmentation, acneiform eruptions; *maceration of skin, secondary infection, atrophy, striae, miliaria* (with occlusive dressings).
**Systemic:** *hypothalamic-pituitary-adrenal axis suppression,* Cushing's syndrome, hyperglycemia, glucosuria.

## INTERACTIONS

None significant.

---

Reactions may be *common,* uncommon, *life-threatening*, or **COMMON AND LIFE-THREATENING**.

## CONTRAINDICATIONS
Contraindicated in patients hypersensitive to the drug.

## NURSING CONSIDERATIONS
• Gently wash skin before applying. To prevent skin damage, rub medication in gently, leaving a thin coat. When treating hairy sites, part hair and apply directly to lesions.
• Avoid application near eyes, mucous membranes, or in ear canal.
• For patients with eczematous dermatitis whose skin may be irritated by adhesive material, hold dressing in place with gauze, elastic bandages, stockings, or stockinette.
• Change dressing as ordered. Stop drug and tell doctor if skin infection, striae, or atrophy occurs.
• Notify the doctor and remove occlusive dressing if fever develops.
• If antifungal agents or antibiotics are used concomitantly, stop drug until infection is controlled, as ordered.
• Systemic absorption likely with use of occlusive dressings, prolonged treatment, or extensive body-surface treatment. Watch for symptoms.
• Avoid using plastic pants or tight-fitting diapers on treated areas in young children. Children may absorb larger amounts of drug and be more prone to systemic toxicity.
• Continue treatment for a few days after lesions clear, as ordered.

## ☑ PATIENT TEACHING
• Teach patient how to apply drug.
• If an occlusive dressing is ordered, advise patient not to leave dressing in place longer than 16 hours each day and not to use occlusive dressings on infected or exudative lesions.
• Tell patient to stop drug and report signs of systemic absorption, skin irritation or ulceration, hypersensitivity, or infection.

# desoximetasone
Topicort

*Pregnancy Risk Category: C*

## HOW SUPPLIED
*Cream:* 0.05%, 0.25%
*Gel:* 0.05%
*Ointment:* 0.25%

## ACTION
Unknown. Diffuses across cell membranes to form complexes with specific cytoplasmic receptors. Exhibits anti-inflammatory, antipruritic, vasoconstrictive, and antiproliferative activity. Considered a group III (medium-potency) agent according to vasoconstrictive properties.

## ONSET, PEAK, DURATION
Onset and duration unknown. Plasma levels are highest when applied to inflamed or damaged skin, eyelids, or scrotal area; lowest when applied to intact, normal skin, palms of hands, or soles of feet.

## INDICATIONS & DOSAGE
*Inflammation associated with corticosteroid-responsive dermatoses –*
**Adults and children:** clean area; apply sparingly b.i.d.

## ADVERSE REACTIONS
**Skin:** burning, pruritus, irritation, dryness, erythema, folliculitis, hypertrichosis, acneiform eruptions, perioral dermatitis, hypopigmentation, allergic contact dermatitis; *maceration, secondary infection, atrophy, striae, miliaria* (with occlusive dressings).
**Systemic:** *hypothalamic-pituitary-adrenal axis suppression,* Cushing's syndrome, hyperglycemia, glucosuria.

## INTERACTIONS
None significant.

---

*Liquid form contains alcohol. **May contain tartrazine. †Canada only. ‡Australia only. ◇OTC.

## CONTRAINDICATIONS

Contraindicated in patients hypersensitive to the drug.

## NURSING CONSIDERATIONS

• Gently wash skin before applying. To prevent skin damage, rub medication in gently, leaving a thin coat. When treating hairy sites, part hair and apply directly to lesions.

• Avoid application near eyes, mucous membranes, or in ear canal.

• For patients with eczematous dermatitis whose skin may be irritated by adhesive material, hold dressing in place with gauze, elastic bandages, stockings, or stockinette.

• Change dressing as ordered. Stop drug and tell doctor if skin infection, striae, or atrophy occurs.

• Notify the doctor and remove occlusive dressing if fever develops.

• If antifungal agents or antibiotics are used concomitantly, stop drug until infection is controlled, as ordered.

• Systemic absorption likely with use of occlusive dressings, prolonged treatment, or extensive body-surface treatment. Watch for symptoms.

• Avoid using plastic pants or tight-fitting diapers on treated areas in young children. Children may absorb larger amounts of drug and be more prone to systemic toxicity.

• Continue drug for a few days after lesions clear, as ordered.

• Gel contains alcohol and may cause burning or irritation in open lesions.

• Store in tightly sealed containers.

## ☑ PATIENT TEACHING

• Teach patient how to apply drug.

• If an occlusive dressing is ordered, advise patient not to leave dressing in place longer than 16 hours each day and not to use occlusive dressings on infected or exudative lesions.

• Tell patient to stop drug and report signs of systemic absorption, skin irritation or ulceration, hypersensitivity, or infection.

# dexamethasone
Aeroseb-Dex, Decaderm, Decaspray

# dexamethasone sodium phosphate
Decadron Phosphate

*Pregnancy Risk Category: C*

## HOW SUPPLIED
**dexamethasone**
*Aerosol:* 0.01%, 0.04%
*Gel:* 0.1%
**dexamethasone sodium phosphate**
*Cream:* 0.1%

## ACTION
Unknown. Diffuses across cell membranes to form complexes with specific cytoplasmic receptors. Exhibits anti-inflammatory, antipruritic, vasoconstrictive, and antiproliferative activity. Considered a group IV (low-potency) agent according to vasoconstrictive properties.

## ONSET, PEAK, DURATION
Onset and duration unknown. Plasma levels are highest when applied to inflamed or damaged skin, eyelids, or scrotal area; lowest when applied to intact normal skin, palms of hands, or soles of feet.

## INDICATIONS & DOSAGE
*Inflammation associated with corticosteroid-responsive dermatoses –*
**Adults and children:** clean area; apply cream, gel, or aerosol sparingly t.i.d. to q.i.d.

For aerosol use on scalp, shake can well but gently, and apply to dry scalp after shampooing. Hold can upright. Slide applicator tube under hair so that it touches scalp. Spray while moving tube to all affected areas, keeping tube under hair and in contact with scalp throughout spraying, which should take about 2 seconds. Spot spray inadequately covered areas by sliding applicator tube through hair to touch scalp, then pressing and immediately releasing spray button. Don't massage medication into scalp or spray forehead or near eyes.

**ADVERSE REACTIONS**
**Skin:** burning, pruritus, irritation, dryness, erythema, folliculitis, hypertrichosis, acneiform eruptions, perioral dermatitis, hypopigmentation, allergic contact dermatitis; *maceration, secondary infection, atrophy, striae, miliaria* (with occlusive dressings).
**Systemic:** *hypothalamic-pituitary-adrenal axis suppression,* Cushing's syndrome, hyperglycemia, glucosuria.

**INTERACTIONS**
None significant.

**CONTRAINDICATIONS**
Contraindicated in patients hypersensitive to the drug.

**NURSING CONSIDERATIONS**
• Gently wash skin before applying. To prevent skin damage, rub medication in gently, leaving a thin coat. When treating hairy sites, part hair and apply directly to lesions.
• Avoid application near eyes, mucous membranes, or in ear canal.
• For patients with eczematous dermatitis whose skin may be irritated by adhesive material, hold dressing in place with gauze, elastic bandages, stockings, or stockinette.
• Change dressing as ordered. Stop drug and tell doctor if skin infection, striae, or atrophy occurs.
• Notify the doctor and remove occlusive dressing if fever develops.
• When using aerosol around the face, cover the patient's eyes and warn against inhalation of the spray. Aerosol preparation contains alcohol and may produce irritation or burning in open lesions. To avoid freezing tissues, do not spray longer than 3 seconds or closer than 6″ (15 cm).
• If antifungal agents or antibiotics are used concomitantly, stop drug until infection is controlled, as ordered.
• Systemic absorption likely with use of occlusive dressings, prolonged treatment, or extensive body-surface treatment. Watch for symptoms.
• Avoid using plastic pants or tight-fitting diapers on treated areas in young children. Children may absorb larger amounts of drug and be more prone to systemic toxicity.
• Continue treatment for a few days after lesions clear, as ordered.

☑ **PATIENT TEACHING**
• Teach patient how to apply drug.
• If an occlusive dressing is ordered, advise patient not to leave it in place longer than 16 hours each day and not to use occlusive dressings on infected or exudative lesions.
• Tell patient to stop drug and report signs of systemic absorption, skin irritation or ulceration, hypersensitivity, or infection.

---

## diflorasone diacetate
Florone, Flutone, Maxiflor, Psorcon
*Pregnancy Risk Category: C*

**HOW SUPPLIED**
*Cream:* 0.05%
*Ointment:* 0.05%

**ACTION**
Unknown. Diffuses across cell membranes to form complexes with specific cytoplasmic receptors. Exhibits anti-inflammatory, antipruritic, vasoconstrictive, and antiproliferative activity. Considered a group II (high-potency) agent according to vasoconstrictive properties.

**ONSET, PEAK, DURATION**
Onset and duration unknown. Plasma levels are highest when applied to in-

flamed or damaged skin, eyelids, or scrotal area; lowest when applied to intact normal skin, palms of hands, or soles of feet.

## INDICATIONS & DOSAGE
*Inflammation associated with corticosteroid-responsive dermatoses –*
**Adults and children:** clean area; apply sparingly in a thin film. Apply daily to q.i.d. as determined by severity of condition.

## ADVERSE REACTIONS
**Skin:** burning, pruritus, irritation, dryness, erythema, folliculitis, perioral dermatitis, hypertrichosis, hypopigmentation, acneiform eruptions; *maceration, secondary infection, atrophy, striae, miliaria* (with occlusive dressings).
**Systemic:** *hypothalamic-pituitary-adrenal axis suppression*, Cushing's syndrome, hyperglycemia, glucosuria.

## INTERACTIONS
None significant.

## CONTRAINDICATIONS
Contraindicated in patients hypersensitive to the drug.

## NURSING CONSIDERATIONS
• Before applying, gently wash skin. To prevent skin damage, rub medication in gently, leaving a thin coat. When treating hairy sites, part hair and apply directly to lesions.
• Avoid application near eyes, mucous membranes, or in ear canal.
• For patients with eczematous dermatitis whose skin may be irritated by adhesive material, hold dressing in place with gauze, elastic bandages, stockings, or stockinette.
• Change dressing as ordered. Stop drug and tell doctor if skin infection, striae, or atrophy occurs.
• Notify the doctor and remove occlusive dressing if fever develops.

• If antifungal agents or antibiotics are used concomitantly, stop drug until infection is controlled, as ordered.
• Systemic absorption likely with use of occlusive dressings, prolonged treatment, or extensive body-surface treatment. Watch for symptoms.
• Avoid using plastic pants or tight-fitting diapers on treated areas in young children. Children may absorb larger amounts of drug and be more prone to systemic toxicity.

## ☑ PATIENT TEACHING
• Teach patient how to apply drug.
• If an occlusive dressing is ordered, advise patient not to leave it in place longer than 16 hours each day and not to use occlusive dressings on infected or exudative lesions on in combination with Psorcon.
• Tell patient to stop drug and report signs of systemic absorption, skin irritation or ulceration, hypersensitivity, or infection.

---

# fluocinolone acetonide
Fluocet, Fluonid, Flurosyn, Synalar, Synemol

*Pregnancy Risk Category: C*

## HOW SUPPLIED
*Cream:* 0.01%, 0.025%, 0.2%
*Ointment:* 0.025%
*Topical solution:* 0.01%

## ACTION
Unknown. Diffuses across cell membranes to form complexes with specific cytoplasmic receptors. Exhibits anti-inflammatory, antipruritic, vasoconstrictive, and antiproliferative activity. Considered a group III (medium-potency) agent according to vasoconstrictive properties.

## ONSET, PEAK, DURATION
Onset and duration unknown. Plasma levels are highest when applied to inflamed or damaged skin, eyelids, or

---

scrotal area; lowest when applied to intact normal skin, palms of hands, or soles of feet.

## INDICATIONS & DOSAGE
*Inflammation associated with corticosteroid-responsive dermatoses –*
**Adults and children:** clean area; apply cream, ointment, or topical solution sparingly b.i.d. to q.i.d.

## ADVERSE REACTIONS
**Skin:** burning, pruritus, irritation, dryness, erythema, folliculitis, hypertrichosis, hypopigmentation, acneiform eruptions, perioral dermatitis, allergic contact dermatitis; *maceration, secondary infection, atrophy, striae, miliaria* (with occlusive dressings).
**Systemic:** *hypothalamic-pituitary-adrenal axis suppression,* Cushing's syndrome, hyperglycemia, glucosuria.

## INTERACTIONS
None significant.

## CONTRAINDICATIONS
Contraindicated in patients hypersensitive to the drug.

## NURSING CONSIDERATIONS
• Gently wash skin before applying. To prevent skin damage, rub medication in gently, leaving a thin coat. When treating hairy sites, part hair and apply directly to lesions.
• Avoid application near eyes, mucous membranes, or in ear canal.
• For patients with eczematous dermatitis whose skin may be irritated by adhesive material, hold dressing in place with gauze, elastic bandages, stockings, or stockinette.
• Change dressing as ordered. Stop drug and tell doctor if skin infection, striae, or atrophy occurs.
• Notify the doctor and remove occlusive dressing if fever develops.
• If antifungal agents or antibiotics

are used concomitantly, stop drug until infection is controlled, as ordered.
• Systemic absorption likely with use of occlusive dressings, prolonged treatment, or extensive body-surface treatment. Watch for symptoms.
• In young children, avoid using plastic pants or tight-fitting diapers on treated areas. Children may absorb larger amounts of drug and be more prone to systemic toxicity.
• Fluonid solution on dry lesions may increase dryness, scaling, or pruritus; on denuded or fissured areas, may produce burning or stinging. If either of these persists and dermatitis has not improved, discontinue use of solution and notify doctor.

### ☑ PATIENT TEACHING
• Teach patient how to apply drug.
• If an occlusive dressing is ordered, advise pateint not to leave it in place longer than 16 hours each day and not to use occlusive dressings on infected or exudative lesions.
• Tell patient to stop drug and report signs of systemic absorption, skin irritation or ulceration, hypersensitivity, or infection.

---

## fluocinonide
Lidemol†, Lidex, Lidex-E, Topsyn
*Pregnancy Risk Category: C*

## HOW SUPPLIED
*Cream:* 0.05%
*Gel:* 0.05%
*Ointment:* 0.05%
*Topical solution:* 0.05%

## ACTION
Unknown. Diffuses across cell membranes to form complexes with specific cytoplasmic receptors. Exhibits anti-inflammatory, antipruritic, vasoconstrictive, and antiproliferative activity. Considered a group II (high-potency) agent according to vasoconstrictive properties.

---

*Liquid form contains alcohol.   **May contain tartrazine.   †Canada only.   ‡Australia only.   ◊OTC.

## ONSET, PEAK, DURATION
Onset and duration unknown. Plasma levels are highest when applied to inflamed or damaged skin, eyelids, or scrotal area; lowest when applied to intact, normal skin, palms of hands, or soles of feet.

## INDICATIONS & DOSAGE
*Inflammation associated with corticosteroid-responsive dermatoses* –
**Adults and children:** clean area; apply cream, gel, ointment, or topical solution sparingly b.i.d. or q.i.d.

## ADVERSE REACTIONS
**Skin:** burning, pruritus, irritation, dryness, erythema, folliculitis, hypertrichosis, hypopigmentation, acneiform eruptions, perioral dermatitis, allergic contact dermatitis; *maceration, secondary infection, atrophy, striae, miliaria* (with occlusive dressings).
**Systemic:** *hypothalamic-pituitary-adrenal axis suppression,* Cushing's syndrome, hyperglycemia, glucosuria.

## INTERACTIONS
None significant.

## CONTRAINDICATIONS
Contraindicated in patients hypersensitive to the drug.

## NURSING CONSIDERATIONS
● Gently wash skin before applying. To prevent skin damage, rub medication in gently, leaving a thin coat. When treating hairy sites, part hair and apply directly to lesion.
● Avoid application near eyes, mucous membranes, or in ear canal.
● For patients with eczematous dermatitis whose skin may be irritated by adhesive material, hold dressing in place with gauze, elastic bandages, stockings, or stockinette.
● Change dressing as ordered. Stop drug and call doctor if skin infection, striae, or atrophy occurs.
● Notify the doctor and remove occlusive dressing if fever develops.
● If antifungal agents or antibiotics are used concomitantly, stop drug until infection is controlled, as ordered.
● Systemic absorption likely with use of occlusive dressings, prolonged treatment, or extensive body-surface treatment. Watch for symptoms.
● In young children, avoid using plastic pants or tight-fitting diapers on treated areas. Children may absorb larger amounts of drug and be more prone to systemic toxicity.
● Continue treatment for a few days after lesions clear, as ordered.

## ☑ PATIENT TEACHING
● Teach patient how to apply drug.
● If an occlusive dressing is ordered, advise patient not to leave it in place longer than 16 hours each day; don't use occlusive dressings on infected or exudative lesions.
● Tell patient to stop drug and report signs of systemic absorption, skin irritation or ulceration, hypersensitivity, or infection.

---

# flurandrenolide
Cordran, Cordran SP, Cordran Tape, Drenison†, Drenison ¼†, Drenison Tape†

*Pregnancy Risk Category: C*

## HOW SUPPLIED
*Cream:* 0.025%, 0.05%
*Lotion:* 0.05%
*Ointment:* 0.025%, 0.05%
*Tape:* 4 mcg/cm²

## ACTION
Unknown. Diffuses across cell membranes to form complexes with specific cytoplasmic receptors. Exhibits anti-inflammatory, antipruritic, vasoconstrictive, and antiproliferative activity. Considered a group III (me-

---

Reactions may be *common,* uncommon, *life-threatening,* or COMMON AND LIFE-THREATENING.

dium-potency) agent according to vasoconstrictive properties.

## ONSET, PEAK, DURATION
Onset and duration unknown. Plasma levels are highest when applied to inflamed or damaged skin, eyelids, or scrotal area; lowest when applied to intact normal skin, palms of hands, or soles of feet.

## INDICATIONS & DOSAGE
*Inflammation associated with corticosteroid-responsive dermatoses –*
**Adults and children:** clean area; apply cream, lotion, or ointment sparingly b.i.d. or t.i.d.

Apply Cordran tape q 12 to 24 hours. Before applying tape, clean skin carefully, removing scales, crust, and dried exudate. Let skin dry for 1 hour before applying new tape. Shave or clip hair to allow good contact with skin and comfortable removal. If tape ends loosen prematurely, trim off and replace with fresh tape.

## ADVERSE REACTIONS
**Skin:** burning, pruritus, irritation, dryness, erythema, folliculitis, hypertrichosis, hypopigmentation, acneiform eruptions, allergic contact dermatitis; *maceration, secondary infection, atrophy, striae, miliaria* (with occlusive dressings); purpura, stripping of epidermis, furunculosis (with tape).
**Systemic:** *hypothalamic-pituitary-adrenal axis suppression,* Cushing's syndrome, hyperglycemia, glucosuria.

## INTERACTIONS
None significant.

## CONTRAINDICATIONS
Contraindicated in patients hypersensitive to the drug.

## NURSING CONSIDERATIONS
• Gently wash skin before applying. To prevent skin damage, rub medication in gently, leaving a thin coat. When treating hairy sites, part hair and apply directly to lesions.
• Avoid application near eyes, mucous membranes, or in ear canal.
• *Alert:* Know that tape not advised for exudative lesions or lesions in intertriginous areas. Replace tape every 12 hours or, if well tolerated and adherence is satisfactory, every 24 hours. Do not tear Cordran tape; cut it with scissors.
• For patients with eczematous dermatitis whose skin may be irritated by adhesive material, hold dressing in place with gauze, elastic bandages, stockings, or stockinette.
• Stop drug and tell doctor if skin infection, striae, or atrophy occurs.
• Notify the doctor and remove occlusive dressing if fever develops.
• If antifungal agents or antibiotics are used concomitantly, stop drug until infection is controlled, as ordered.
• Systemic absorption likely with use of occlusive dressings, prolonged treatment, or extensive body-surface treatment. Watch for symptoms.
• Avoid using plastic pants or tight-fitting diapers on treated areas in young children. Children may absorb larger amounts of drug and be more prone to systemic toxicity.
• Continue treatment for a few days after lesions clear, as ordered.

## ☑ PATIENT TEACHING
• Teach patient how to apply drug.
• If an occlusive dressing is ordered, advise patient not to leave it in place longer than 16 hours each day and not to use occlusive dressings on infected or exudative lesions.
• Tell patient to stop drug and report signs of systemic absorption, skin irritation or ulceration, hypersensitivity, or infection.

# fluticasone propionate
Cutivate

*Pregnancy Risk Category: C*

## HOW SUPPLIED
*Cream:* 0.05%
*Ointment:* 0.005%

## ACTION
Unknown. Diffuses across cell membranes to form complexes with specific cytoplasmic receptors. Exhibits anti-inflammatory, antipruritic, vasoconstrictive, and antiproliferative activity. Considered a group III (medium-potency) agent according to vasoconstrictive properties.

## ONSET, PEAK, DURATION
Onset and duration unknown. Plasma levels are highest when applied to inflamed or damaged skin, eyelids, or scrotal area; lowest when applied to intact normal skin, palms of hands, or soles of feet.

## INDICATIONS & DOSAGE
*Inflammation associated with corticosteroid-responsive dermatoses* –
**Adults and children:** apply cream or ointment sparingly to affected area b.i.d., and rub in gently and completely.

## ADVERSE REACTIONS
**Skin:** stinging, burning, pruritus, irritation, dryness, erythema, folliculitis, skin atrophy, leukoderma, vesicles, numbness of fingers, rash, hypertrichosis, acneiform eruptions, hypopigmentation, perioral dermatitis, allergic contact dermatitis, secondary infection, striae, miliaria.
**Systemic:** *hypothalamic-pituitary-adrenal axis suppression,* Cushing's syndrome, hyperglycemia, glucosuria.

## INTERACTIONS
None significant.

## CONTRAINDICATIONS
Contraindicated in patients hypersensitive to the drug or its components and in patients with viral, fungal, herpetic, or tubercular skin lesions.

## NURSING CONSIDERATIONS
● Do not mix drug with other bases or vehicles; this may affect potency.
● If adverse reactions occur, the doctor may order a less potent agent.
● One-time coverage of the adult body requires 12 to 26 g. Use of more than 50 g weekly is not recommended.
● Discontinue drug if local irritation or systemic infection, absorption, or hypersensitivity occurs, as ordered.

## ☑ PATIENT TEACHING
● Teach the patient how to apply drug.
● Tell the patient to avoid prolonged use and contact with eyes. Warn him not to apply around eyes, genitals, or rectum; on face; and in skin creases.
● Tell the patient to notify the doctor if the condition persists or worsens or if burning or irritation develops.

# halcinonide
Halciderm, Halog

*Pregnancy Risk Category: C*

## HOW SUPPLIED
*Cream:* 0.025%, 0.1%
*Ointment:* 0.1%
*Topical solution:* 0.1%

## ACTION
Unknown. Diffuses across cell membranes to form complexes with specific cytoplasmic receptors. Exhibits anti-inflammatory, antipruritic, vasoconstrictive, and antiproliferative activity. Considered a group II (high-potency) agent according to vasoconstrictive properties.

---

Reactions may be *common,* uncommon, *life-threatening,* or **COMMON AND LIFE-THREATENING.**

## ONSET, PEAK, DURATION
Onset and duration unknown. Plasma levels are highest when applied to inflamed or damaged skin, eyelids, or scrotal area; lowest when applied to intact normal skin, palms of hands, or soles of feet.

## INDICATIONS & DOSAGE
*Inflammation associated with corticosteroid-responsive dermatoses –*
**Adults and children:** clean area; apply cream, ointment, or topical solution sparingly b.i.d. or t.i.d.

## ADVERSE REACTIONS
**Skin:** burning, pruritus, irritation, dryness, erythema, folliculitis, hypertrichosis, hypopigmentation, acneiform eruptions, allergic contact dermatitis; *maceration, secondary infection, atrophy, striae, miliaria* (with occlusive dressings).
**Systemic:** *hypothalamic-pituitary-adrenal axis suppression,* Cushing's syndrome, hyperglycemia, glucosuria.

## INTERACTIONS
None significant.

## CONTRAINDICATIONS
Contraindicated in patients hypersensitive to the drug.

## NURSING CONSIDERATIONS
• Gently wash skin before applying. To prevent skin damage, rub medication in gently, leaving a thin coat. When treating hairy sites, part hair and apply directly to lesions.
• Avoid application near eyes, mucous membranes, or in ear canal.
• Gently rub small amount of cream into lesion until it disappears. Reapply, leaving a thin coating on lesion, and cover with occlusive dressing, if ordered. Apply ointment to lesion and cover with occlusive dressing, if ordered. Do not leave dressing in place longer than 16 hours each day.

• Don't use occlusive dressings on infected or exudative lesions.
• For patients with eczematous dermatitis whose skin may be irritated by adhesive material, hold dressing in place with gauze, elastic bandages, stockings, or stockinette.
• Change dressing as ordered. Stop drug and tell doctor if skin infection, striae, or atrophy occurs.
• Be aware that good results have been obtained by applying occlusive dressings in the evening and removing them in the morning, providing 12-hour occlusion. Drug should then be reapplied and no occlusive dressings applied during the day.
• Notify the doctor and remove occlusive dressing if fever develops.
• If antifungal agents or antibiotics are used concomitantly, stop drug until infection is controlled, as ordered.
• Systemic absorption especially likely with use of occlusive dressings, prolonged treatment, or extensive body-surface treatment. Watch for symptoms.
• Avoid using plastic pants or tight-fitting diapers on treated areas in young children. Children may absorb larger amounts of drug and be more prone to systemic toxicity.
• Continue treatment for a few days after lesions clear, as ordered.

## ☑ PATIENT TEACHING
• Teach patient how to apply drug.
• If an occlusive dressing is ordered, advise patient not to leave it in place longer than 16 hours each day and not to use occlusive dressings on infected or exudative lesions.
• Tell patient to stop drug and report signs of systemic absorption, skin irritation or ulceration, hypersensitivity, or infection.

---

*Liquid form contains alcohol.   **May contain tartrazine.   †Canada only.   ‡Australia only.   ◇OTC.

## halobetasol propionate
Ultravate

*Pregnancy Risk Category: C*

### HOW SUPPLIED
*Cream:* 0.05%
*Ointment:* 0.05%

### ACTION
Unknown. Diffuses across cell membranes to form complexes with specific cytoplasmic receptors. Exhibits anti-inflammatory, antipruritic, vasoconstrictive, and antiproliferative activity. Considered a group I (very high-potency) agent according to vasoconstrictive properties.

### ONSET, PEAK, DURATION
Onset and duration unknown. Plasma levels are highest when applied to inflamed or damaged skin, eyelids, or scrotal area; lowest when applied to intact normal skin, palms of hands, or soles of feet.

### INDICATIONS & DOSAGE
*Inflammation associated with corticosteroid-responsive dermatoses –*
**Adults:** apply cream or ointment sparingly to affected area once daily or b.i.d., and rub in gently and completely. Treatment beyond 2 consecutive weeks is not recommended. Total dosage should not exceed 50 g weekly.

### ADVERSE REACTIONS
**Skin:** stinging, burning, pruritus, irritation, dryness, erythema, folliculitis, skin atrophy, leukoderma, vesicles, rash, hypertrichosis, acneiform eruptions, hypopigmentation, perioral dermatitis, allergic contact dermatitis, secondary infection, striae, miliaria.
**Systemic:** *hypothalamic-pituitary-adrenal (HPA) axis suppression,* Cushing's syndrome, hyperglycemia, glucosuria, fluid retention.

### INTERACTIONS
None significant.

### CONTRAINDICATIONS
Contraindicated in patients hypersensitive to the drug or any of its components.

### NURSING CONSIDERATIONS
- *Alert:* Do not use occlusive dressings with this drug.
- Avoid use on face, groin, or axilla.
- Be alert that some systemic absorption usually occurs and may cause HPA axis suppression, Cushing's syndrome, hyperglycemia, and glucosuria, which are reversible after discontinuation of therapy.
- Corticotropin stimulation, morning plasma cortisol, and urinary cortisol tests are useful in determining the extent of HPA axis suppression.
- If HPA axis suppression occurs, discontinue drug, reduce frequency of application, or substitute a less potent corticosteroid, as prescribed.
- Discontinue if infection occurs and notify the doctor.

### ☑ PATIENT TEACHING
- Teach the patient how to apply drug.
- Tell the patient that drug is for external use only, as directed by the doctor. Tell him to avoid contact with eyes and not to cover, bandage, or wrap treated area unless directed by the doctor. Tell the patient not to use more often or for any condition other than prescribed.
- Tell the patient to report any signs of stinging, burning, or irritation.

---

Reactions may be *common,* uncommon, *life-threatening,* or **COMMON AND LIFE-THREATENING.**

# hydrocortisone
Acticort, Aeroseb-HC, Bactine HC◇, CaldeCort, Carmol HC, Cetacort, Cort-Dome, Cortef◇, Cortenema, Cortinal, Cortizone 5◇, Cortril, Cremesone, Delacort, DermaCort◇, Dermolate◇, Dermtex HC, Durel-Cort, Ecosone, HC Cream, HI-Cor-2.5, Hycortole, Hydrocortex, HydroTex, Hytone, Ivocort, Maso-Cort, Microcort, Nutracort, Orabase HCA, Penecort, Proctocort, Rhus Tox HC, Rocort, Squibb-HC‡, Synacort, T/Scalp, Unicort

## hydrocortisone acetate
CortaGel, Cortaid◇, Cortamed†, Cortef, Corticaine, Corticreme†, Cortifoam, Dermacort‡, Dermacort Ointment‡, Epifoam, Gynecort, Hydrocortisone Acetate, Lanacort, MyCort Lotion, Proctofoam-HC

## hydrocortisone butyrate
Locoid

## hydrocortisone valerate
Westcort Cream

*Pregnancy Risk Category: C*

## HOW SUPPLIED
**hydrocortisone**
*Aerosol:* 0.5%
*Cream:* 0.25%◇, 0.5%◇, 1%◇, 2.5%
*Gel:* 0.5%, 1%
*Lotion:* 0.125%, 0.25%, 0.5%◇, 1%, 2%, 2.5%
*Ointment:* 0.5%◇, 1%◇, 2.5%
*Pledgets:* 0.5%, 1%
*Rectal cream:* 1%◇
*Topical solution:* 0.5%, 1%, 2.5%
**hydrocortisone acetate**
*Cream:* 0.5%◇
*Lotion:* 0.5%◇
*Ointment:* 0.5%◇, 1%
*Paste:* 0.5%
*Solution:* 1%
*Rectal foam:* 90 mg per application
**hydrocortisone butyrate**
*Cream:* 0.1%
*Ointment:* 0.1%
*Solution:* 0.1%
**hydrocortisone valerate**
*Cream:* 0.2%
*Ointment:* 0.2%

## ACTION
Unknown. Diffuses across cell membranes to form complexes with specific cytoplasmic receptors. Exhibits anti-inflammatory, antipruritic, vasoconstrictive, and antiproliferative activity. Considered a group IV (low-potency) agent according to vasoconstrictive properties.

## ONSET, PEAK, DURATION
Onset and duration unknown. Plasma levels are highest when applied to inflamed or damaged skin, eyelids, or scrotal area; lowest when applied to intact normal skin, palms of hands, or soles of feet.

## INDICATIONS & DOSAGE
*Inflammation associated with corticosteroid-responsive dermatoses; adjunctive topical management of seborrheic dermatitis of scalp—*
**Adults and children:** clean area; apply cream, gel, lotion, ointment, or topical solution sparingly daily to q.i.d. Spray aerosol onto affected area daily to q.i.d. until acute phase is controlled; then reduce dosage to one to three times weekly as needed.
*Inflammation associated with proctitis—*
**Adults:** 1 applicatorful of rectal foam P.R. daily or b.i.d. for 2 to 3 weeks, then every other day as necessary.

## ADVERSE REACTIONS
**Skin:** burning, pruritus, irritation, dryness, erythema, folliculitis, hypertrichosis, hypopigmentation, acneiform eruptions, allergic contact dermatitis; *maceration, secondary infection, atrophy, striae, miliaria* (with occlusive dressings).

---

*Liquid form contains alcohol. **May contain tartrazine. †Canada only. ‡Australia only. ◇OTC.

**Systemic:** *hypothalamic-pituitary-adrenal axis suppression,* Cushing's syndrome, hyperglycemia, glucosuria.

**INTERACTIONS**
None significant.

**CONTRAINDICATIONS**
Contraindicated in patients hypersensitive to the drug.

**NURSING CONSIDERATIONS**
• Gently wash skin before applying. To prevent skin damage, rub medication in gently, leaving a thin coat. When treating hairy sites, part hair and apply directly to lesions.
• Avoid application near eyes, mucous membranes, or in ear canal; may be safely used on face, groin, armpits, and under breasts.
• For patients with eczematous dermatitis whose skin may be irritated by adhesive material, hold dressing in place with gauze, elastic bandages, stockings, or stockinette.
• Notify the doctor, and remove occlusive dressing if fever develops.
• Change dressing as ordered. Stop drug and tell doctor if skin infection, striae, or atrophy occurs.
• When using aerosol around the face, cover the patient's eyes and warn against inhalation of the spray. Aerosol preparation contains alcohol and may produce irritation or burning in open lesions. Do not spray longer than 3 seconds or closer than 6″ (15 cm) to avoid freezing tissues. Apply to dry scalp after shampooing; no need to massage medication into scalp after spraying.
• If antifungal agents or antibiotics are used concomitantly, stop drug until infection is controlled, as ordered.
• Systemic absorption likely with use of occlusive dressings, prolonged treatment, or extensive body-surface treatment. Watch for symptoms.
• Avoid using plastic pants or tight-fitting diapers on treated areas in young children. Children may absorb larger amounts of drug and be more prone to systemic toxicity.
• Continue treatment for a few days after lesions clear, as ordered.

☑ **PATIENT TEACHING**
• Teach patient how to apply drug.
• If an occlusive dressing is ordered, advise patient not to leave it in place longer than 16 hours each day and not to use occlusive dressings on infected or exudative lesions.
• Tell patient to stop drug and report signs of systemic absorption, skin irritation or ulceration, hypersensitivity, or infection.

---

**mometasone furoate**
Elocon
*Pregnancy Risk Category: C*

**HOW SUPPLIED**
*Cream:* 0.1%
*Ointment:* 0.1%
*Lotion:* 0.1%

**ACTION**
Unknown. Diffuses across cell membranes to form complexes with specific cytoplasmic receptors. Exhibits anti-inflammatory, antipruritic, vasoconstrictive, and antiproliferative activity. Considered a group III (medium-potency) agent according to vasoconstrictive properties.

**ONSET, PEAK, DURATION**
Onset and duration unknown. Plasma levels are highest when applied to inflamed or damaged skin, eyelids, or scrotal area; lowest when applied to intact normal skin, palms of hands, or soles of feet.

**INDICATIONS & DOSAGE**
*Inflammation associated with corticosteroid-responsive dermatoses –*

---

Reactions may be *common,* uncommon, *life-threatening,* or **COMMON AND LIFE-THREATENING.**

**Adults:** apply to affected areas once daily.

## ADVERSE REACTIONS
**Skin:** burning, erythema, pruritus, atrophy, irritation, acneiform eruptions, hypopigmentation, allergic contact dermatitis.
**Systemic:** *hypothalamic-pituitary-adrenal axis suppression,* Cushing's syndrome, hyperglycemia, glucosuria.

## INTERACTIONS
None significant.

## CONTRAINDICATIONS
Contraindicated in patients hypersensitive to the drug or to other corticosteroids.

## NURSING CONSIDERATIONS
• Use cautiously in young children.
• Gently wash skin before applying. To prevent skin damage, rub medication in gently, leaving a thin coat. When treating hairy sites, part hair and apply directly to lesions.
• Don't apply near eyes, mucous membranes, or in ear canal.
• **Alert:** Do not use occlusive dressings with this drug.
• If antimicrobial agents are used concomitantly, stop drug until infection is controlled, as ordered.
• Systemic absorption likely with use of occlusive dressings, prolonged treatment, or extensive body-surface treatment. Watch for symptoms.
• Children may absorb larger amounts of drug and be more prone to systemic toxicity. Avoid using plastic pants or tight-fitting diapers on treated areas in young children.

## ☑ PATIENT TEACHING
• Teach patient how to apply drug.
• Tell patient to stop drug and report signs of systemic absorption, skin irritation or ulceration, hypersensitivity, or infection.

# triamcinolone acetonide
Aristocort, Flutex, Kenalog, Kenalone‡, Triacet

*Pregnancy Risk Category: C*

## HOW SUPPLIED
*Aerosol:* 0.2 mg/2-second spray
*Cream:* 0.02%‡, 0.025%, 0.1%, 0.5%
*Lotion:* 0.025%, 0.1%
*Ointment:* 0.02%‡, 0.025%, 0.1%, 0.5%
*Paste:* 0.1%
*Solution:* 0.1%

## ACTION
Unknown. Diffuses across cell membranes to form complexes with specific cytoplasmic receptors. Exhibits anti-inflammatory, antipruritic, vasoconstrictive, and antiproliferative activity. Considered a group III (medium-potency) agent according to vasoconstrictive properties.

## ONSET, PEAK, DURATION
Onset and duration unknown. Plasma levels are highest when applied to inflamed or damaged skin, eyelids, or scrotal area; low levels result when applied to intact, normal skin, palms of hands, or soles of feet.

## INDICATIONS & DOSAGE
*Inflammation associated with corticosteroid-responsive dermatoses –*
**Adults and children:** clean area; apply aerosol, cream, lotion, or ointment sparingly t.i.d. to q.i.d.
*Inflammation associated with oral lesions –*
**Adults and children:** apply paste h.s. and, if needed, two or three times daily, preferably after meals. Apply a small amount without rubbing, and press to lesion in mouth until a thin film develops.

## ADVERSE REACTIONS

**Skin:** burning, pruritus, irritation, dryness, erythema, folliculitis, hypertrichosis, hypopigmentation, acneiform eruptions, perioral dermatitis, allergic contact dermatitis; *maceration, secondary infection, atrophy, striae, miliaria* (with occlusive dressings).

**Systemic:** *hypothalamic-pituitary-adrenal axis suppression,* Cushing's syndrome, hyperglycemia, glucosuria.

## INTERACTIONS

None significant.

## CONTRAINDICATIONS

Contraindicated in patients hypersensitive to the drug.

## NURSING CONSIDERATIONS

• Gently wash skin before applying. To avoid skin damage, rub medication in gently, leaving a thin coat. When treating hairy sites, part hair and apply directly to lesions.
• Don't apply near eyes or in ear canal.
• Change dressing as ordered. Stop drug and tell doctor if skin infection, striae, or atrophy occurs.
• When using aerosol about the face, cover the patient's eyes and warn against inhalation of the spray. Aerosol preparation contains alcohol and may produce irritation or burning in open lesions. Do not spray longer than 3 seconds or closer than 6″ (15 cm) to avoid freezing tissues.
• If antifungal agents or antibiotics are used concomitantly, stop corticosteroids until infection is controlled, as ordered.
• Systemic absorption likely with use of occlusive dressings, prolonged treatment, or extensive body-surface treatment. Watch for symptoms.
• Avoid using plastic pants or tight-fitting diapers on treated areas in young children. Children may absorb larger amounts of drug and be more prone to systemic toxicity.

## ☑ PATIENT TEACHING

• Instruct patient how to apply drug.
• If an occlusive dressing is ordered, advise patient not to leave it in place longer than 16 hours each day; and not to use occlusive dressings on infected or exudative lesions.
• Tell patient to stop drug and report signs of systemic absorption, skin irritation or ulceration, hypersensitivity, or infection.

---

Reactions may be *common,* uncommon, *life-threatening,* or COMMON AND LIFE-THREATENING.

**vitamin A**

*vitamin B complex*
cyanocobalamin
hydroxocobalamin
folic acid
leucovorin calcium
niacin
niacinamide
pyridoxine hydrochloride
riboflavin
thiamine hydrochloride

**vitamin C**

**vitamin D**
cholecalciferol
ergocalciferol

**vitamin E**

*vitamin K analogue*
phytonadione

**sodium fluoride**
**sodium fluoride, topical**

*trace elements*
chromium
copper
iodine
manganese
selenium
zinc

## TRACE ELEMENT COMBINATION PRODUCTS

M.T.E.-4: zinc sulfate 1 mg, copper sulfate 0.4 mg, manganese sulfate 0.1 mg, and chromium chloride 4 mcg per ml.

M.T.E.-4 CONCENTRATED: zinc sulfate 5 mg, copper sulfate 1 mg, manganese sulfate 0.5 mg, and chromium chloride 10 mcg per ml.

M.T.E.-5: zinc sulfate 1 mg, copper sulfate 0.4 mg, manganese sulfate 0.1 mg, chromium chloride 4 mcg, and selenium (as selenious acid) 20 mcg per ml.

M.T.E.-5 CONCENTRATED: zinc sulfate 5 mg, copper sulfate 1 mg, manganese sulfate 0.5 mg, chromium chloride 10 mcg, and selenium (as selenious acid) 60 mcg per ml.

M.T.E.-6: zinc sulfate 1 mg, copper sulfate 0.4 mg, manganese sulfate 0.1 mg, chromium chloride 4 mcg, selenium (as selenious acid) 20 mcg, and sodium iodide 25 mcg per ml.

M.T.E.-6 CONCENTRATED: zinc sulfate 5 mg, copper sulfate 1 mg, manganese sulfate 0.5 mg, chromium chloride 10 mcg, selenium (as selenious acid) 60 mcg, and sodium iodide 75 mcg per ml.

M.T.E.-7: zinc sulfate 1 mg, copper sulfate 0.4 mg, manganese sulfate 0.1 mg, chromium chloride 4 mcg, selenium (as selenious acid) 20 mcg, and sodium iodide 25 mcg per ml.

MULTIPLE TRACE ELEMENT CONCENTRATED: zinc sulfate 5 mg, copper sulfate 1 mg, manganese sulfate 0.5 mg, and chromium chloride 10 mcg per ml.

MULTIPLE TRACE ELEMENT NEONATAL: zinc sulfate 0.5 mg, copper sulfate 0.1 mg, manganese sulfate 0.025 mg, chromium chloride 0.85 mcg.

MULTIPLE TRACE ELEMENT WITH SELENIUM: zinc sulfate 1 mg, copper sulfate 0.4 mg, manganese sulfate 0.1 mg, chromium chloride 4 mcg, and selenious acid 20 mcg.

MULTITRACE 5 CONCENTRATE: zinc chloride 5 mg, copper chloride 1 mg, manganese chloride 0.5 mg, chromium chloride 10 mcg per ml, and selenious acid 60 mcg.

NEOTRACE-4: zinc sulfate 1.5 mg,

---

*Liquid form contains alcohol. **May contain tartrazine. †Canada only. ‡Australia only. ◇OTC.

copper sulfate 0.1 mg, manganese sulfate 0.025 mg, and chromium chloride 0.85 mcg per ml.
PEDIATRIC MULTIPLE TRACE ELEMENT: zinc sulfate 0.5 mg, copper sulfate 0.1 mg, manganese sulfate 0.03 mg, and chromium chloride 1 mcg per ml.
PEDTRACE-4: zinc sulfate 0.5 mg, copper sulfate 0.1 mg, manganese sulfate 0.025 mg, and chromium chloride 0.85 mcg per ml.
P.T.E.-4: zinc sulfate 1 mg, copper sulfate 0.1 mg, manganese sulfate 0.025 mg, and chromium chloride 1 mcg per ml.
P.T.E.-5: zinc sulfate 1 mg, copper sulfate 0.1 mg, manganese sulfate 0.025 mg, chromium chloride 1 mcg, and selenium (as selenious acid) 15 mcg per ml.
TRACE METALS ADDITIVE: zinc chloride 0.8 mg, copper chloride 0.2 mg, manganese chloride 0.16 mg, and chromium chloride 2 mcg per ml.

## VITAMIN COMBINATION PRODUCTS
B complex vitamins◇
B complex vitamins with iron◇
B complex with vitamin C◇
B vitamin combinations◇
Calcium and vitamin products◇
Fluoride with vitamins◇
Geriatric supplements with multivitamins and minerals◇
Miscellaneous vitamins and minerals◇
Multivitamins◇
Multivitamins and minerals with hormones◇
Multivitamins with B₁₂◇
Vitamin A and D combinations◇

---

## vitamin A (retinol)
Acon, Aquasol A, Del-Vi-A
*Pregnancy Risk Category: NR*

## HOW SUPPLIED
*Tablets:* 10,000 IU
*Capsules:* 10,000 IU◇, 25,000 IU, 50,000 IU
*Drops:* 30 ml with dropper (50,000 IU/0.1 ml)
*Injection:* 2-ml vials (50,000 IU/ml with 0.5% chlorobutanol, polysorbate 80, butylated hydroxyanisol, and butylated hydroxytoluene)

## ACTION
Coenzyme that stimulates retinal function, bone growth, reproduction, and integrity of epithelial and mucosal tissues.

## ONSET, PEAK, DURATION
Onset and duration unknown. Peak levels occur in 3 to 5 hours.

## INDICATIONS & DOSAGE
*Recommended daily allowance (RDA)—*
*Note:* RDAs have been converted to retinol equivalents (RE). One RE has the activity of 1mcg all-*trans* retinol, 6 mcg beta carotene, or 12 mcg carotenoid provitamins.
**Neonates and infants to 1 year:** 375 mcg RE or 1,250 IU.
**Children 1 to 3 years:** 400 mcg RE or 1,330 IU.
**Children 4 to 6 years:** 500 mcg RE or 1,665 IU.
**Children 7 to 10 years:** 700 mcg RE or 2,330 IU.
**Males over 11 years:** 1,000 mcg RE or 3,330 IU.
**Females over 11 years:** 800 mcg RE or 2,665 IU.
**Pregnant women:** 800 mcg RE or 2,665 IU.
**Breast-feeding women (first 6 months):** 1,300 mcg RE or 4,330 IU.
**Breast-feeding women (second 6 months):** 1,200 mcg RE or 4,000 IU.
*Severe vitamin A deficiency—*
**Adults and children over 8 years:** 50,000 to 100,000 IU I.M. or 100,000 to 500,000 IU P.O. for 3

---

Reactions may be *common,* uncommon, *life-threatening,* or COMMON AND LIFE-THREATENING.

days, followed by 50,000 IU I.M. or P.O. for 2 weeks; then 10,000 to 20,000 IU P.O. for 2 months. Follow with adequate dietary nutrition and RDA vitamin A supplements.
**Infants under 1 year:** 7,500 to 15,000 IU I.M. daily for 10 days.
**Children 1 to 8 years:** 17,500 to 35,000 IU I.M. daily for 10 days.
*Maintenance dosage to prevent recurrence of vitamin A deficiency* –
**Children 1 to 8 years:** 5,000 to 10,000 IU P.O. daily for 2 months, then adequate dietary nutrition and RDA vitamin A supplements.

## ADVERSE REACTIONS
Adverse reactions usually occur only with toxicity.
**CNS:** irritability, headache, *increased intracranial pressure,* fatigue, lethargy, malaise.
**EENT:** papilledema, exophthalmos.
**GI:** anorexia, epigastric pain, vomiting, polydipsia.
**GU:** hypomenorrhea, polyuria.
**Hepatic:** jaundice, hepatomegaly, *cirrhosis,* elevated liver enzymes.
**Skeletal:** slow growth, decalcification, hypercalcemia, periostitis, premature closure of epiphyses, migratory arthralgia, cortical thickening over the radius and tibia.
**Skin:** alopecia; dry, cracked, scaly skin; pruritus; lip fissures; erythema; inflamed tongue, lips, and gums; massive desquamation; increased pigmentation; night sweats.
**Other:** splenomegaly, *anaphylactic shock.*

## INTERACTIONS
*Cholestyramine resin, mineral oil:* reduced GI absorption of fat-soluble vitamins. If needed, give mineral oil at bedtime.
*Isotretinoin, multivitamins containing vitamin A:* increased risk of toxicity. Avoid concomitant use.
*Warfarin:* increased risk of bleeding. Monitor PT closely.

## CONTRAINDICATIONS
Contraindicated orally in patients with malabsorption syndrome; if malabsorption is from inadequate bile secretion, oral route may be used with concurrent administration of bile salts (dehydrocholic acid). Also contraindicated in hypervitaminosis A and hypersensitivity to any ingredient in product. I.V. route contraindicated except for special water-miscible forms intended for infusion with large parenteral volumes. I.V. push of vitamin A of any type also contraindicated (anaphylaxis or anaphylactoid reactions and death have resulted).

## NURSING CONSIDERATIONS
• Use cautiously in pregnant patients, avoiding doses exceeding RDA.
• Assess the patient's vitamin A intake from all sources.
• Liquid preparations available for nasogastric route. Preparation may be mixed with cereal or fruit juice.
• Know that adequate vitamin A absorption requires suitable protein, vitamin E, and zinc intake and bile secretion; give supplemental salts as ordered. Zinc supplements may be needed in patients receiving long-term total parenteral nutrition.
• Monitor for adverse reactions if dosage is high.
• Acute toxicity has resulted from single doses of 25,000 IU/kg of body weight; 350,000 IU in infants and over 2 million IU in adults have also proved acutely toxic. Doses that do not exceed the RDA are usually nontoxic.
• Chronic toxicity in infants (3 to 6 months) has resulted from doses of 18,500 IU daily for 1 to 3 months. In adults, chronic toxicity has resulted from doses of 50,000 IU daily for over 18 months, 500,000 IU daily for 2 months, and 1 million IU daily for 3 days.
• Watch for skin disorders; high dosages may induce chronic toxicity.

---

*Liquid form contains alcohol. **May contain tartrazine. †Canada only. ‡Australia only. ◇OTC.

☑ **PATIENT TEACHING**
• To avoid toxicity, tell patient not to take megadoses of vitamins without specific indications.
• Stress that patient should not share prescribed vitamins with others.
• Tell patient to protect drug from light.

---

## cyanocobalamin (vitamin B₁₂)
Anacobin†, Bedoz†, Bioglan B₁₂Plus‡, Crystamine, Crysti-12, Cyanabin†, Cyanocobalamin, Cyanoject, Cyomin, Rubesol-1000, Rubion†, Rubramin

## hydroxocobalamin (vitamin B₁ₐ₂)
Codroxomin, Hydrobexan, Hydro-Cobex, Hydro-Crysti-12, LA-12

*Pregnancy Risk Category: NR*

**HOW SUPPLIED**
**cyanocobalamin**
*Tablets:* 25 mcg◊, 50 mcg◊, 100 mcg◊, 250 mcg◊, 500 mcg◊, 1,000 mcg◊
*Injection:* 1,000 mcg/ml
**hydroxocobalamin**
*Injection:* 1,000 mcg/ml

**ACTION**
Coenzyme that stimulates metabolic functions. Necessary for cell replication, hematopoiesis, and nucleoprotein and myelin synthesis.

**ONSET, PEAK, DURATION**
Onset and duration unknown. Time to peak plasma levels after oral administration is 8 to 12 hours; after I.M. administration, 1 hour.

**INDICATIONS & DOSAGE**
*Recommended daily allowance (RDA) for cyanocobalamin –*
**Neonates and infants to 6 months:** 0.3 mcg.
**Infants 6 months to 1 year:** 0.5 mcg.

**Children 1 to 3 years:** 0.7 mcg.
**Children 4 to 6 years:** 1 mcg.
**Children 7 to 10 years:** 1.4 mcg.
**Adults and children 11 years and over:** 2 mcg.
**Pregnant women:** 2.2 mcg.
**Breast-feeding women:** 2.6 mcg.
*Vitamin B₁₂ deficiency caused by inadequate diet, subtotal gastrectomy, or any other condition, disorder, or disease except malabsorption related to pernicious anemia or other GI disease –*
**Adults:** 30 mcg hydroxocobalamin I.M. daily for 5 to 10 days, depending on severity of deficiency. Maintenance dosage is 100 to 200 mcg I.M. once monthly. For subsequent prophylaxis, advise adequate nutrition and daily RDA vitamin B₁₂ supplements.
**Children:** 1 to 5 mg hydroxocobalamin spread over 2 or more weeks in doses of 100 mcg I.M., depending on severity of deficiency. Maintenance dosage is 30 to 50 mcg/month I.M. For subsequent prophylaxis, advise adequate nutrition and daily RDA vitamin B₁₂ supplements.
*Pernicious anemia or vitamin B₁₂ malabsorption –*
**Adults:** initially, 100 mcg cyanocobalamin I.M. or S.C. daily for 6 to 7 days, then 100 mcg I.M. or S.C. once monthly.
**Children:** 30 to 50 mcg I.M. or S.C. daily over 2 or more weeks; then 100 mcg I.M. or S.C. monthly for life.
*Methylmalonic aciduria –*
**Neonates:** 1,000 mcg cyanocobalamin I.M. daily.
*Schilling test flushing dose –*
**Adults and children:** 1,000 mcg hydroxocobalamin I.M. in a single dose.

**ADVERSE REACTIONS**
**CV:** peripheral vascular thrombosis, pulmonary edema, CHF.
**GI:** transient diarrhea.
**Skin:** itching, transitory exanthema, urticaria.
**Other:** *anaphylaxis, anaphylactoid reactions* (with parenteral administra-

---

Reactions may be *common,* uncommon, *life-threatening,* or COMMON AND LIFE-THREATENING.

tion), pain or burning at S.C. or I.M. injection sites.

## INTERACTIONS
*Aminoglycosides, chloramphenicol, colchicine, para-aminosalicylic acid and salts:* malabsorption of vitamin $B_{12}$. Don't use concomitantly.

## CONTRAINDICATIONS
Contraindicated in patients hypersensitive to vitamin $B_{12}$ or cobalt and in patients with early Leber's disease.

## NURSING CONSIDERATIONS
• Use cautiously in anemic patients with coexisting cardiac, pulmonary, or hypertensive disease; and in patients with severe vitamin $B_{12}$-dependent deficiencies.
• Use cautiously in premature infants. May contain benzyl alcohol, which may cause a "gasping syndrome."
• Determine reticulocyte count, hematocrit, $B_{12}$, iron, and folate levels before beginning therapy, as ordered.
• Don't mix parenteral liquids in same syringe with other medications.
• Drug is physically incompatible with dextrose solutions, alkaline or strongly acidic solutions, oxidizing or reducing agents, heavy metals, chlorpromazine, phytonadione, prochlorperazine, and many other drugs.
• Hydroxocobalamin is approved for I.M. use only. Its only advantage over cyanocobalamin is its longer duration.
• Don't give large oral doses of $B_{12}$ routinely; drug is lost through excretion.
• Monitor reticulocyte count, hematocrit, $B_{12}$, iron, and folate levels between the 5th and 7th day of therapy and periodically thereafter.
• Closely monitor serum potassium levels for first 48 hours. Give potassium supplement if ordered.
• Be aware that drug may cause false-positive intrinsic factor antibody test.
• Infection, tumors, or renal, hepatic,

and other debilitating diseases may reduce therapeutic response.
• Keep in mind that deficiencies are more common in strict vegetarians and their breast-fed infants.
• Be aware $B_{12}$ deficiency may suppress symptoms of polycythemia vera.
• Protect vitamin $B_{12}$ from light. Do not refrigerate or freeze.

## ☑ PATIENT TEACHING
• Stress need for patient with pernicious anemia to return for monthly injections. Although total body stores may last 3 to 6 years, anemia will recur if not treated monthly.
• Stress importance of follow-up visits and laboratory studies.

# folic acid (vitamin B₉)
Folvite, Novofolacid†

*Pregnancy Risk Category: NR*

## HOW SUPPLIED
*Tablets:* 0.4 mg, 0.8 mg, 1 mg
*Injection:* 10-ml vials (5 mg/ml with 1.5% benzyl alcohol or 10 mg/ml with 1.5% benzyl alcohol and 0.2% EDTA)

## ACTION
Stimulates normal erythropoiesis and nucleoprotein synthesis.

## ONSET, PEAK, DURATION
Onset and duration unknown. Serum levels peak in 30 to 60 minutes.

## INDICATIONS & DOSAGE
*Recommended daily allowance (RDA)* –
**Neonates and infants to 6 months:** 25 mcg.
**Infants 6 months to 1 year:** 35 mcg.
**Children 1 to 3 years:** 50 mcg.
**Children 4 to 6 years:** 75 mcg.
**Children 7 to 11 years:** 100 mcg.
**Children 11 to 14 years:** 150 mcg.
**Males 15 years and over:** 200 mcg.
**Females 15 years and over:** 180 mcg.
**Pregnant women:** 400 mcg.

**Breast-feeding women (first 6 months):** 280 mcg.

**Breast-feeding women (second 6 months):** 260 mcg.

*Megaloblastic or macrocytic anemia secondary to folic acid or other nutritional deficiency, hepatic disease, alcoholism, intestinal obstruction, excessive hemolysis –*

**Adults and children over 4 years:** 0.4 mg to 1 mg P.O., S.C., or I.M. daily. After anemia secondary to folic acid deficiency is corrected, proper diet and RDA supplements are necessary to prevent recurrence.

**Children under 4 years:** up to 0.3 mg P.O., S.C., or I.M. daily.

**Pregnant and breast-feeding women:** 0.8 mg P.O., S.C., or I.M. daily.

*Prevention of megaloblastic anemia during pregnancy to prevent fetal damage –*

**Adults:** up to 1 mg P.O., S.C., or I.M. daily throughout pregnancy.

*Nutritional supplement –*

**Adults:** 0.1 mg P.O., S.C., or I.M. daily.

**Children:** 0.05 mg P.O. daily.

*To test for folic acid deficiency in patients with megaloblastic anemia without masking pernicious anemia –*

**Adults and children:** 0.1 to 0.2 mg P.O. or I.M. for 10 days while maintaining a diet low in folate and vitamin $B_{12}$.

*Tropical sprue –*

**Adults:** 3 to 15 mg P.O. daily.

## ADVERSE REACTIONS
**Respiratory:** *bronchospasm.*
**Skin:** allergic reactions (rash, pruritus, erythema).
**Other:** general malaise.

## INTERACTIONS
*Aminosalicylic acid, chloramphenicol, methotrexate, sulfasalazine, trimethoprim:* antagonism of folic acid. Monitor for decreased folic acid effect. Use together cautiously.
*Anticonvulsants, such as phenobarbital and phenytoin:* increased anticonvulsant metabolism and decreased blood levels of the anticonvulsants. Monitor closely.

## CONTRAINDICATIONS
Contraindicated in patients with undiagnosed anemia because it may mask pernicious anemia. Also contraindicated in those with $B_{12}$ deficiency.

## NURSING CONSIDERATIONS
● Safety in pregnancy has not been established but pregnant women are more prone to develop folate deficiency. Folate-deficient mothers may be more prone to pregnancy-related complications and fetal abnormalities.
● Don't mix with other medications in same syringe for I.M. injections.
● Patients with small-bowel resections and intestinal malabsorption may require parenteral administration.
● Protect from light and heat; store at room temperature.

## ☑ PATIENT TEACHING
● Teach patient about proper nutrition to prevent recurrence of anemia.
● Stress importance of follow-up visits and laboratory studies.

# leucovorin calcium (citrovorum factor, folinic acid)
Wellcovorin

*Pregnancy Risk Category: C*

## HOW SUPPLIED
*Tablets:* 5 mg, 10 mg, 15 mg, 25 mg
*Injection:* 1-ml ampule (3 mg/ml with 0.9% benzyl alcohol)
*Powder for injection:* 50-mg vial, 100-mg vial, 350-mg vial

## ACTION
A reduced form of folic acid that is readily converted to other folic acid derivatives.

---

Reactions may be *common,* uncommon, *life-threatening,* or COMMON AND LIFE-THREATENING.

## ONSET, PEAK, DURATION

Onset occurs in 5 minutes after I.V. administration, 10 to 20 minutes after I.M. administration, 20 to 30 minutes after oral administration. Levels peak within 10 minutes after I.V. administration, less than 1 hour after I.M. administration, or 2 to 3 hours after oral administration. Effects persist for 3 to 6 hours for all routes.

## INDICATIONS & DOSAGE

*Overdose of folic acid antagonist –*
**Adults and children:** P.O., I.M., or I.V. dose equivalent to weight of antagonist given.
*Leucovorin rescue after high methotrexate dose in treatment of malignant disease –*
**Adults and children:** 10 mg/m² P.O., I.M., or I.V. q 6 hours until methotrexate levels fall below $5 \times 10^{-8}$ M.
*Megaloblastic anemia caused by congenital enzyme deficiency –*
**Adults and children:** 3 to 6 mg I.M., then 1 mg P.O. or I.M. daily for life.
*Folate-deficient megaloblastic anemia –*
**Adults and children:** up to 1 mg of leucovorin I.M daily. Duration of treatment depends on hematologic response.
*Prevention of hematologic toxicity caused by pyrimethamine or trimethoprim therapy –*
**Adults and children:** 400 mcg to 5 mg I.M. with each dose of the folic acid antagonist.
*Treatment of hematologic toxicity caused by pyrimethamine or trimethoprim therapy –*
**Adults and children:** 5 to 15 mg I.M. daily.
*Palliative treatment of advanced colorectal cancer –*
**Adults:** 20 mg/m² I.V., followed by fluorouracil 425 mg/m² I.V. daily for 5 consecutive days. Repeated at 4-week intervals for two additional courses; then at intervals of 4 to 5 weeks if tolerated.

## ADVERSE REACTIONS

**Skin:** hypersensitivity reactions (urticaria and anaphylactoid reactions).

## INTERACTIONS

*Fluorouracil:* may enhance fluorouracil toxicity. Avoid concomitant use.

## CONTRAINDICATIONS

Contraindicated in patients with pernicious anemia and other megaloblastic anemias secondary to the lack of vitamin $B_{12}$.

## NURSING CONSIDERATIONS

• **I.V. use:** When using powder for injection, reconstitute 50-mg vial with 5 ml, 100-mg vial with 10 ml, or 350-mg vial with 17 ml of sterile or bacteriostatic water for injection. When doses are more than 10 mg/m², don't use diluents containing benzyl alcohol.
• *Alert:* Don't exceed 160 mg/minute when giving by direct injection.
• Do not confuse leucovorin (folinic acid) with folic acid.
• Follow leucovorin rescue schedule and protocol closely.
• Do not administer leucovorin simultaneously with systemic methotrexate.
• Protect from light and heat, especially reconstituted parenteral drug.

## ☑ PATIENT TEACHING

• Explain need for drug use to patient and family, and answer any questions or concerns.
• Tell patient to report symptoms of hypersensitivity promptly.

---

# niacin (vitamin B₃, nicotinic acid)

Niac, Niacor, Nico-400, Nicobid◇, Nicolar**, Nicotinex

## niacinamide (nicotinamide)◇

*Pregnancy Risk Category: C*

## HOW SUPPLIED
**niacin**
*Tablets:* 25 mg◇, 50 mg◇, 100 mg◇, 250 mg◇, 500 mg
*Tablets (timed-release):* 150 mg◇, 250 mg◇, 500 mg◇, 750 mg◇
*Capsules (timed-release):* 125 mg◇, 250 mg◇, 300 mg◇, 400 mg◇, 500 mg
*Elixir:* 50 mg/5 ml◇
*Injection:* 100 mg/ml in 30-ml vials
**niacinamide**
*Tablets:* 50 mg◇, 100 mg◇, 125 mg◇, 250 mg◇, 500 mg◇

## ACTION
Niacin and niacinamide stimulate lipid metabolism, tissue respiration, and glycogenolysis; niacin decreases synthesis of low-density lipoproteins and inhibits lipolysis in adipose tissue.

## ONSET, PEAK, DURATION
Onset unknown. Triglyceride levels decrease within hours; cholesterol levels, within days. Serum levels peak 45 minutes after oral use. Duration unknown.

## INDICATIONS & DOSAGE
*Recommended daily allowance (RDA) –*
**Neonates and infants to 6 months:** 5 mg.
**Infants 6 months to 1 year:** 6 mg.
**Children 1 to 3 years:** 9 mg.
**Children 4 to 6 years:** 12 mg.
**Children 7 to 10 years:** 13 mg.
**Males 11 to 14 years:** 17 mg.
**Males 15 to 18 years:** 20 mg.
**Males 19 to 50 years:** 19 mg.
**Males 51 years and over:** 15 mg.
**Females 11 to 50 years:** 15 mg.
**Females 51 years and over:** 13 mg.
**Pregnant women:** 17 mg.
**Breast-feeding women:** 20 mg.
*Pellagra –*
**Adults:** 300 to 500 mg P.O., S.C., I.M., or I.V. daily in divided doses, depending on severity of deficiency.
**Children:** up to 300 mg P.O. or 100 mg I.V. daily, depending on severity of niacin deficiency.
  After symptoms subside, advise adequate nutrition and RDA supplements to prevent recurrence.
*Hartnup disease –*
**Adults:** 50 to 200 mg P.O. daily
*Niacin deficiency –*
**Adults:** up to 100 mg P.O. daily.
*Hyperlipidemias, especially with hypercholesterolemia –*
**Adults:** 1 to 2 g P.O. three times a day with or after meals, increased at intervals to 6 g daily.

## ADVERSE REACTIONS
Most reactions are dose-dependent.
**CV:** *excessive peripheral vasodilation (especially niacin),* hypotension, atrial fibrillation, cardiac arrhythmias.
**GI:** *nausea, vomiting, diarrhea,* possible activation of peptic ulceration, epigastric or substernal pain.
**Hepatic:** *hepatic dysfunction.*
**Skin:** *flushing,* pruritus, dryness, tingling.
**Other:** hyperglycemia, hyperuricemia, toxic amblyopia.

## INTERACTIONS
*Antihypertensive drugs (sympathetic or ganglionic blockers):* potential additive vasodilating effect, causing postural hypotension. Use together cautiously; also warn the patient about postural hypotension.

## CONTRAINDICATIONS
Contraindicated in patients with hepatic dysfunction, active peptic ulcers, severe hypotension, arterial hemorrhage, or drug hypersensitivity.

---

Reactions may be *common,* uncommon, *life-threatening,* or COMMON AND LIFE-THREATENING.

## NURSING CONSIDERATIONS
• Use cautiously in patients with gall-bladder disease, diabetes mellitus, or coronary artery disease and in patients with a history of liver disease, peptic ulcer, allergy, or gout.
• **I.V. use:** Give slow I.V. (no faster than 2 mg/minute). Explain harmlessness of flushing syndrome.
• To minimize adverse GI effects, give niacin with meals.
• Administer aspirin (325 mg P.O. 30 minutes before niacin dose), as ordered, to possibly reduce the flushing response to niacin.
• Timed-release niacin or niacinamide may prevent excessive flushing that occurs with large doses. However, timed-release niacin is linked with hepatic dysfunction, even at very low doses.
• Monitor hepatic function and blood glucose early in therapy, as ordered.

## ☑ PATIENT TEACHING
• Stress that this substance is a potent medication, not just a vitamin, and may cause serious adverse effects. Explain importance of adhering to therapeutic regimen.
• Advise patient against self-medicating for hyperlipidemia.

## pyridoxine hydrochloride (vitamin B₆)
Beesix, Hexa-Betalin, Nestrex◇, Rodex

*Pregnancy Risk Category: A*

## HOW SUPPLIED
*Tablets:* 10 mg◇, 25 mg◇, 50 mg◇, 100 mg◇, 200 mg◇, 250 mg◇, 500 mg◇
*Capsules (timed-release):* 100 mg
*Capsules:* 500 mg
*Tablets (timed-release):* 100 mg
*Injection:* 100 mg/ml

## ACTION
Acts as a coenzyme that stimulates various metabolic functions, including amino acid metabolism.

## ONSET, PEAK, DURATION
Unknown.

## INDICATIONS & DOSAGE
*Recommended daily allowance (RDA) –*
**Neonates and infants to 6 months:** 0.3 mg.
**Infants 6 months to 1 year:** 0.6 mg.
**Children 1 to 3 years:** 1 mg.
**Children 4 to 6 years:** 1.1 mg.
**Children 7 to 10 years:** 1.4 mg.
**Males 11 to 14 years:** 1.7 mg.
**Males 15 years and over:** 2 mg.
**Females 11 to 14 years:** 1.4 mg.
**Females 15 to 18 years:** 1.5 mg.
**Females 19 years and over:** 1.6 mg.
**Pregnant women:** 2.2 mg.
**Breast-feeding women:** 2.1 mg.
*Dietary vitamin B₆ deficiency –*
**Adults:** 10 to 20 mg P.O., I.M., or I.V. daily for 3 weeks, then 2 to 5 mg daily as a supplement to a proper diet.
*Seizures related to vitamin B₆ deficiency or dependency –*
**Adults and children:** 100 mg I.M. or I.V. in single dose.
*Vitamin B₆-responsive anemias or dependency syndrome (inborn errors of metabolism) –*
**Adults:** up to 600 mg P.O., I.M., or I.V. daily until symptoms subside, then 30 mg daily for life.
*Prevention of vitamin B₆ deficiency during drug therapy –*
**Adults:** 6 to 100 mg P.O. daily for isoniazid therapy.
*Drug-induced vitamin B₆ deficiency –*
**Adults and children:** 50 to 200 mg P.O., I.M., or I.V. daily for 3 weeks, followed by 25 to 100 mg P.O., I.M., or I.V. daily to prevent relapse.
*Antidote for isoniazid poisoning –*
**Adults:** 4 g I.V., followed by 1 g I.M. q 30 minutes until the amount of pyri-

doxine administered equals the amount of isoniazid ingested.

## ADVERSE REACTIONS
**CNS:** paresthesia, unsteady gait, numbness, somnolence.

## INTERACTIONS
*Levodopa:* decreased levodopa effect. Avoid concomitant use.
*Phenobarbital, phenytoin:* decreased anticonvulsant serum levels, increasing risk of seizures. Avoid concomitant use.

## CONTRAINDICATIONS
Contraindicated in patients hypersensitive to pyridoxine.

## NURSING CONSIDERATIONS
• **I.V. use:** Inject undiluted drug into I.V. line of a free-flowing compatible solution. Or, infuse diluted drug over prescribed duration for intermittent infusion. Don't use for continuous infusion.
• Protect from light. Do not use solution if it contains a precipitate, although slight darkening is acceptable.
• When used to treat isoniazid toxicity, expect to also give anticonvulsants.
• If sodium bicarbonate is needed to control acidosis in isoniazid toxicity, don't mix in same syringe with pyridoxine.
• Patients taking high doses (2 to 6 g/ day) may experience difficulty walking because of diminished proprioceptive and sensory function.
• Carefully monitor the patient's diet. Excessive protein intake increases daily pyridoxine requirements.

## ☑ PATIENT TEACHING
• Stress importance of compliance and of good nutrition if prescribed for maintenance therapy to prevent recurrence of deficiency. Explain that pyridoxine, in combination therapy with isoniazid, has a specific therapeutic purpose and is not just a vitamin.
• Advise patient taking levodopa alone to avoid multivitamins containing pyridoxine because of decreased levodopa effect.

---

# riboflavin (vitamin B₂)◊
*Pregnancy Risk Category: NR*

## HOW SUPPLIED
*Tablets:* 10 mg◊, 25 mg◊, 50 mg◊, 100 mg◊
*Tablets (sugar-free):* 50 mg◊, 100 mg◊

## ACTION
Converts to two other coenzymes necessary for normal tissue respiration.

## ONSET, PEAK, DURATION
Unknown.

## INDICATIONS & DOSAGE
*Recommended daily allowance (RDA) –*
**Neonates and infants to 6 months:** 0.4 mg.
**Infants 6 months to 1 year:** 0.5 mg.
**Children 1 to 3 years:** 0.8 mg.
**Children 4 to 6 years:** 1.1 mg.
**Children 7 to 10 years:** 1.2 mg.
**Males 11 to 14 years:** 1.5 mg.
**Males 15 to 18 years:** 1.8 mg.
**Males 19 to 50 years:** 1.7 mg.
**Males 51 years and over:** 1.4 mg.
**Females 11 to 50 years:** 1.3 mg.
**Females 51 years and over:** 1.2 mg.
**Pregnant women:** 1.6 mg.
**Breast-feeding women (first 6 months):** 1.8 mg.
**Breast-feeding women (second 6 months):** 1.7 mg.
*Riboflavin deficiency or adjunct to thiamine treatment for polyneuritis or cheilosis secondary to pellagra –*
**Adults and children over 12 years:** 5 to 30 mg P.O. daily, depending on severity.
**Children under 12 years:** 3 to 10 mg P.O. daily, depending on severity.
 For maintenance, increase nutri-

---

tional intake and supplement with vitamin B complex.

**ADVERSE REACTIONS**
**GU:** bright yellow urine (with high doses).

**INTERACTIONS**
*Propantheline, other anticholinergics:* decreased rate and extent of absorption. Avoid concomitant use.

**CONTRAINDICATIONS**
None known.

**NURSING CONSIDERATIONS**
• Drug may be given I.M. or I.V. as a component of multiple vitamins.
• Know that riboflavin deficiency usually accompanies other vitamin B complex deficiencies and may require multivitamin therapy.
• Protect from air and light.

☑ **PATIENT TEACHING**
• Tell patient to take riboflavin with meals; food increases its absorption.
• Stress proper nutritional habits to prevent recurrence of deficiency.

---

## thiamine hydrochloride (vitamin B₁)

Betamin‡, Beta-Sol‡, Biamine, Thiamilate

*Pregnancy Risk Category: A*

**HOW SUPPLIED**
*Tablets:* 5 mg◇, 10 mg◇, 25 mg◇, 50 mg◇, 100 mg◇, 250 mg◇, 500 mg◇
*Tablet (enteric-coated):* 20 mg
*Elixir†:* 250 mcg/5 ml
*Injection:* 100 mg/ml, 200 mg/ml

**ACTION**
Combines with adenosine triphosphate to form a coenzyme necessary for carbohydrate metabolism.

**ONSET, PEAK, DURATION**
Unknown.

**INDICATIONS & DOSAGE**
*Recommended daily allowance (RDA) –*
**Neonates and infants to 6 months:** 0.3 mg.
**Infants 6 months to 1 year:** 0.4 mg.
**Children 1 to 3 years:** 0.7 mg.
**Children 4 to 6 years:** 0.9 mg.
**Children 7 to 10 years:** 1 mg.
**Males 11 to 14 years:** 1.3 mg.
**Males 15 to 50 years:** 1.5 mg.
**Males 51 years and over:** 1.2 mg.
**Females 11 to 50 years:** 1.1 mg.
**Females 51 years and over:** 1 mg.
**Pregnant women:** 1.5 mg.
**Breast-feeding women:** 1.6 mg.
*Beriberi –*
**Adults:** depending on severity, 10 to 20 mg I.M. t.i.d. for 2 weeks, followed by dietary correction and multivitamin supplement containing 5 to 10 mg thiamine daily for 1 month.
**Children:** depending on severity, 10 to 50 mg I.M. daily for several weeks with adequate diet.
*Wet beriberi with myocardial failure –*
**Adults and children:** 10 to 30 mg I.V. t.i.d.
*Wernicke's encephalopathy –*
**Adults:** initially, 100 mg I.V., followed by 50 to 100 mg I.V. or I.M. daily until patient is consuming a regular balanced diet.

**ADVERSE REACTIONS**
**CNS:** restlessness.
**CV:** *angioedema,* cyanosis, *CV collapse.*
**EENT:** tightness of throat (allergic reaction).
**GI:** nausea, hemorrhage.
**Respiratory:** pulmonary edema.
**Skin:** feeling of warmth, pruritus, urticaria, diaphoresis.
**Other:** weakness; tenderness and induration following I.M. administration.

**INTERACTIONS**
None significant.

---

*Liquid form contains alcohol.   **May contain tartrazine.   †Canada only.   ‡Australia only.   ◇OTC.

## CONTRAINDICATIONS

Contraindicated in patients hypersensitive to thiamine products.

## NURSING CONSIDERATIONS

• Know that parenteral administration should be used only when P.O. route is not feasible.

• **I.V. use:** Dilute before giving.

• **Alert:** Administer large I.V. doses cautiously; give the patient a skin test before therapy if he has a history of hypersensitivity reactions. Have epinephrine on hand to treat anaphylaxis.

• Do not use with materials that yield alkaline solutions. Thiamine is unstable in alkaline solutions.

• Know that thiamine malabsorption is most likely in alcoholism, cirrhosis, or GI disease.

• Clinically significant deficiency can occur in approximately 3 weeks of totally thiamine-free diet. Thiamine deficiency usually requires concurrent treatment for multiple deficiencies.

• Keep in mind that doses larger than 30 mg t.i.d. may not be fully utilized. After tissue saturation with thiamine, it is excreted in urine as pyrimidine.

### ☑ PATIENT TEACHING

• Inform breast-feeding patient that if beriberi occurs in infant, both she and her child should be treated with thiamine.

• Stress proper nutritional habits to prevent recurrence of deficiency.

---

## vitamin C (ascorbic acid)

Ascorbicap◇, Cebid Timecelles◇, Cecon◇, Cee-1000 T.D.◇, Cenolate◇, Cetane◇, Cevalin◇, Cevi-Bid, Ce-Vi-Sol*, Cevita◇, C-Span◇, Dull-C◇, Flavettes‡, Flavorcee◇, N'ice Vitamin C Drops◇, Redoxon†, Vita C Crystals◇

*Pregnancy Risk Category: C*

## HOW SUPPLIED

*Tablets:* 25 mg◇, 50 mg◇, 100 mg◇, 250 mg◇, 500 mg◇, 1,000 mg◇
*Tablets (chewable):* 50 mg, 100 mg◇, 250 mg◇, 500 mg◇, 1,000 mg◇
*Tablets (effervescent):* 1,000 mg sugar-free◇
*Tablets (timed-release):* 500 mg◇, 1,000 mg◇, 1,500 mg
*Capsules (timed-release):* 500 mg◇
*Crystals:* 100 g (4 g/tsp)◇, 500 g (4 g/tsp)◇
*Lozenges:* 60 mg◇
*Oral liquid:* 50 ml (35 mg/0.6 ml)*◇
*Oral solution:* 60 mg/ml◇, 100 mg/ml◇
*Powder:* 100 g (4 g/tsp)◇, 500 g (4 g/tsp)◇
*Syrup:* 20 mg/ml in 120 ml, 480 ml◇; 500 mg/5 ml in 5 ml◇, 120 ml◇, 480 ml◇
*Injection:* 100 mg/ml; 250 mg/ml; 500 mg/ml

## ACTION

Stimulates collagen formation and tissue repair; involved in oxidation-reduction reactions.

## ONSET, PEAK, DURATION

Unknown.

## INDICATIONS & DOSAGE

*Recommended daily allowance (RDA) –*
**Neonates and infants to 6 months:** 30 mg.
**Infants 6 months to 1 year:** 35 mg.
**Children 1 to 3 years:** 40 mg.
**Children 4 to 10 years:** 45 mg.
**Children 11 to 14 years:** 50 mg.
**Adults and children 15 years and over:** 60 mg.
**Pregnant women:** 70 mg.
**Breast-feeding women (first 6 months):** 95 mg.
**Breast-feeding women (second 6 months):** 90 mg.
*Frank and subclinical scurvy –*
**Adults:** depending on severity, 300 mg to 1 g P.O., S.C., I.M., or I.V.

---

daily, then at least 50 mg daily for maintenance.

**Children:** depending on severity, 100 to 300 mg P.O., S.C., I.M., or I.V. daily, then at least 30 mg daily for maintenance.

**Premature infants:** 75 to 100 mg P.O., I.M., I.V., or S.C. daily.

*Extensive burns, delayed fracture or wound healing, postoperative wound healing, severe febrile or chronic disease states—*

**Adults:** 300 to 500 mg S.C., I.M., or I.V. daily for 7 to 10 days. 1 to 2 g daily for extensive burns.

**Children:** 100 to 200 mg P.O., S.C., I.M., or I.V. daily.

*Prevention of vitamin C deficiency in patients with poor nutritional habits or increased requirements—*

**Adults:** 70 to 150 mg P.O., S.C., I.M., or I.V. daily.

**Pregnant and breast-feeding women:** at least 70 to 150 mg P.O., S.C., I.M., or I.V. daily.

**Children:** at least 40 mg P.O., S.C., I.M., or I.V. daily.

**Infants:** at least 35 mg P.O., S.C., I.M., or I.V. daily.

*Potentiation of methenamine in urine acidification—*

**Adults:** 4 to 12 g P.O. daily in divided doses.

## ADVERSE REACTIONS

**CNS:** faintness or dizziness with too-rapid I.V. administration.
**GI:** diarrhea.
**GU:** acid urine, oxaluria, renal calculi.
**Other:** discomfort at injection site.

## INTERACTIONS

*Aspirin (high doses):* increased risk of ascorbic acid deficiency. Monitor the patient closely.
*Oral iron supplements:* increased iron absorption (a beneficial interaction).
*Warfarin:* decreased anticoagulant effect. Monitor closely.

## CONTRAINDICATIONS
None known.

## NURSING CONSIDERATIONS
● **I.V. use:** Infuse cautiously in patients with renal insufficiency.
● *Alert:* Avoid too-rapid I.V. administration.
● When giving for urine acidification, check urine pH to ensure efficacy.
● Protect solution from light, and refrigerate ampules.

## ☑ PATIENT TEACHING
● For patient receiving vitamin C I.M., explain that I.M. route may promote better utilization.
● Stress proper nutritional habits to prevent recurrence of deficiency.

# vitamin D

## cholecalciferol (vitamin D₃)
Delta-D◇, Vitamin D₃◇

## ergocalciferol (vitamin D₂)
Calciferol, Deltalin Gelseals, Drisdol, Radiostol†, Radiostol Forte†, Vitamin D

*Pregnancy Risk Category: C*

## HOW SUPPLIED
*Tablets:* 1.25 mg (50,000 IU)
*Capsules:* 1.25 mg (50,000 IU)
*Oral liquid:* 8,000 IU/ml in 60-ml dropper bottle◇
*Injection:* 12.5 mg (500,000 IU)/ml

## ACTION
Promotes absorption and utilization of calcium and phosphate, helping to regulate calcium homeostasis.

## ONSET, PEAK, DURATION
According to metabolites formed or derivative, onset is as follows: oral calcitriol, 2 to 6 hours; dihydrotachysterol, several hours to 1 day; ergocalciferol, 12 to 24 hours although therapeutic onset may take 10 to 14 days.

Time to peak as follows: alfacalcidol, about 12 hours; calcifediol, about 4 hours; calcitriol, about 3 to 6 hours. Duration as follows: alfacalcidol, up to 48 hours; calcifediol, 15 to 20 days; calcitriol, 3 to 5 days; dihydrotachysterol, up to 9 weeks; ergocalciferol, up to 6 months.

## INDICATIONS & DOSAGE
*Recommended daily allowance (RDA) for cholecalciferol –*
**Neonates and infants to 6 months:** 300 IU.
**Infants 6 months to adults 24 years:** 400 IU.
**Adults 25 years and over:** 200 IU.
**Pregnant or lactating women:** 400 IU.
*Rickets and other vitamin D deficiency diseases; renal osteodystrophy –*
**Adults:** initially, 12,000 IU P.O. or I.M. daily, usually increased based on response up to 500,000 IU daily.
**Children:** 1,500 to 5,000 IU P.O. or I.M. daily for 2 to 4 weeks, repeated after 2 weeks, if necessary. Alternatively, give single dose of 600,000 IU.

After correction of deficiency, maintenance includes adequate diet and RDA supplements.
*Hypoparathyroidism –*
**Adults and children:** 50,000 to 200,000 IU P.O. or I.M. daily, with calcium supplement.
*Familial hypophosphatemia –*
**Adults:** 50,000 to 200,000 IU daily with phosphorus supplement.

## ADVERSE REACTIONS
Adverse reactions listed usually occur only in vitamin D toxicity.
**CNS:** headache, weakness, somnolence, decreased libido, overt psychosis, irritability.
**CV:** *calcifications of soft tissues, including the heart,* hypertension, cardiac arrhythmias.
**EENT:** rhinorrhea, conjunctivitis (calcific), photophobia.
**GI:** anorexia, nausea, vomiting, con-

stipation, dry mouth, metallic taste, polydipsia.
**GU:** polyuria, albuminuria, hypercalciuria, nocturia, *impaired renal function,* reversible azotemia.
**Skin:** pruritus.
**Other:** bone and muscle pain, bone demineralization, weight loss, *hypercalcemia,* hyperthermia.

## INTERACTIONS
*Cholestyramine resin, mineral oil:* inhibited GI absorption of oral vitamin D. Space doses. Use together cautiously.
*Corticosteroids:* antagonized effect of vitamin D. Monitor vitamin D levels closely.
*Digitalis glycosides:* increased risk of arrhythmias. Monitor serum calcium levels.
*Magnesium-containing antacids:* possible hypermagnesemia, especially in patients with chronic renal failure. Monitor serum magnesium levels.
*Phenobarbital, phenytoin:* increased vitamin D metabolism and decreased effectiveness. Monitor closely.
*Thiazide diuretics:* may cause hypercalcemia in patients with hypoparathyroidism. Monitor closely.

## CONTRAINDICATIONS
Contraindicated in patients with hypercalcemia, hypervitaminosis A, or renal osteodystrophy with hyperphosphatemia.

## NURSING CONSIDERATIONS
● Ergocalciferol should be given with extreme caution, if at all, to patients with impaired renal function, heart disease, renal stones, or arteriosclerosis.
● Use cautiously in cardiac patients, especially those taking digitalis glycosides, as well as in patients with increased sensitivity to these drugs.
● Use I.M. injection of vitamin D dispersed in oil for patients unable to absorb the oral form, as ordered.

---

- *Alert:* Monitor the patient's eating and bowel habits; dry mouth, nausea, vomiting, metallic taste, and constipation may be early signs of toxicity.
- Monitor serum and urine calcium, potassium, and urea levels when high therapeutic dosages are used.
- Dosages of 60,000 IU/day can cause hypercalcemia.
- Be aware that malabsorption from inadequate bile or hepatic dysfunction may require addition of exogenous bile salts to oral form.
- Patients with hyperphosphatemia require dietary phosphate restrictions and binding agents to avoid metastatic calcifications and renal calculi.

☑ **PATIENT TEACHING**
- Warn patient of the dangers of increasing dosage without asking the doctor. This vitamin is fat-soluble.
- Tell the patient taking vitamin D to restrict intake of magnesium-containing antacids.

## vitamin E (tocopherol)
Amino-Opti-E◊, Aquasol E◊, E-Complex-600◊, E-200 I.U. Softgels◊, E-400 I.U. Softgels◊, E Vitamin Succinate◊, Vita-Plus E Softgels◊

*Pregnancy Risk Category: NR*

**HOW SUPPLIED**
*Tablets (chewable):* 200 IU◊, 400 IU◊
*Capsules:* 200 IU◊, 400 IU◊, 500 IU◊, 600 IU◊, 1,000 IU◊, 330 mg, 147 mg, 73.5 mg
*Oral solution:* 50 mg/ml◊

**ACTION**
Unknown. Thought to act as an antioxidant and protect RBC membranes against hemolysis.

**ONSET, PEAK, DURATION**
Unknown.

**INDICATIONS & DOSAGE**
*Recommended daily allowance (RDA) –*
*Note:* RDAs for vitamin E have been converted to alpha-tocopherol equivalents (α-TE). One α-TE equals 1 mg of D-alpha tocopherol or 1.49 IU.
**Neonates and infants to 6 months:** 3 α-TE or 4 IU.
**Infants 6 months to 1 year:** 4 α-TE or 6 IU.
**Children 1 to 3 years:** 6 α-TE or 9 IU.
**Children 4 to 10 years:** 7 α-TE or 10 IU.
**Males 11 years and over:** 10 α-TE or 15 IU.
**Females 11 years and over:** 8 α-TE or 12 IU.
**Pregnant women:** 10 α-TE or 15 IU.
**Breast-feeding women (first 6 months):** 12 α-TE or 18 IU.
**Breast-feeding women (second 6 months):** 11 α-TE or 16 IU.
*Vitamin E deficiency in premature neonates and in patients with impaired fat absorption –*
**Adults:** depending on severity, 60 to 75 IU P.O. daily.
**Children:** 1 IU/kg daily.

**ADVERSE REACTIONS**
None reported with recommended dosages. Hypervitaminosis E symptoms include fatigue, weakness, nausea, headache, blurred vision, flatulence, diarrhea.

**INTERACTIONS**
*Anticoagulants (oral):* hypoprothrombinemic effects may be increased, possibly causing bleeding. Monitor closely.
*Cholestyramine resin, mineral oil:* inhibited GI absorption of oral vitamin E. Space doses. Use together cautiously.
*Vitamin K:* antagonized effects of vitamin K possible with large doses of vitamin E. Avoid concurrent use.

**CONTRAINDICATIONS**
None known.

---

*Liquid form contains alcohol. **May contain tartrazine. †Canada only. ‡Australia only. ◊OTC.

## NURSING CONSIDERATIONS
• Monitor the patient with liver or gallbladder disease for response to therapy. Adequate bile is essential for vitamin E absorption.
• Be aware that water-miscible forms more completely absorbed in GI tract.
• Requirements increase with rise in dietary polyunsaturated acids.

### ☑ PATIENT TEACHING
• Tell patient that he shouldn't crush tablets or open capsules. An oral solution and chewable tablets are commercially available.
• Discourage the patient from self-medication with megadoses, which can cause thrombophlebitis. This vitamin is fat-soluble.

---

## phytonadione (vitamin K₁)
AquaMEPHYTON, Konakion, Mephyton

*Pregnancy Risk Category: C*

### HOW SUPPLIED
*Tablets:* 5 mg
*Injection (aqueous colloidal solution):* 2 mg/ml, 10 mg/ml
*Injection (aqueous dispersion):* 2 mg/ml, 10 mg/ml

### ACTION
An antihemorrhagic factor that promotes hepatic formation of active prothrombin.

### ONSET, PEAK, DURATION
Onset occurs in 6 to 12 hours after oral administration, 1 to 2 hours (with hemorrhage controlled in 3 to 6 hours) after parenteral administration. Peak unknown. Normal prothrombin concentrations are often obtained in 12 to 14 hours.

### INDICATIONS & DOSAGE
*Recommended daily allowance (RDA) –*

**Neonates and infants to 6 months:** 5 mcg.
**Infants 6 months to 1 year:** 10 mcg.
**Children 1 to 3 years:** 15 mcg.
**Children 4 to 6 years:** 20 mcg.
**Children 7 to 10 years:** 30 mcg.
**Children 11 to 14 years:** 45 mcg.
**Males 15 to 18 years:** 65 mcg.
**Males 19 to 24 years:** 70 mcg.
**Males 25 years and over:** 80 mcg.
**Females 15 to 18 years:** 55 mcg.
**Females 19 to 24 years:** 60 mcg.
**Females 25 years and over and pregnant or breast-feeding women:** 65 mcg.
*Hypoprothrombinemia secondary to vitamin K malabsorption, drug therapy, or excessive vitamin A dosage –*
**Adults:** depending on severity – 2.5 to 10 mg P.O., S.C., or I.M. repeated and increased up to 50 mg if necessary.
**Infants:** 2 mg P.O. or parenterally.
**Children:** 5 to 10 mg P.O. or parenterally.
  I.V. injection rate for infants and children should not exceed 3 mg/m²/minute or a total of 5 mg.
*Hypoprothrombinemia secondary to effect of oral anticoagulants –*
**Adults:** 2.5 to 10 mg P.O., S.C., or I.M. based on PT, repeated if necessary within 12 to 48 hours after oral dose or within 6 to 8 hours after parenteral dose. In emergency, 10 to 50 mg slow I.V., rate not to exceed 1 mg/minute, repeated q 4 hours, p.r.n.
*Prevention of hemorrhagic disease of newborn –*
**Neonates:** 0.5 to 1 mg I.M. within 1 hour after birth.
*Treatment of hemorrhagic disease of newborn –*
**Neonates:** 1 mg S.C. or I.M. Higher doses may be necessary if mother has been receiving oral anticoagulants.
*To differentiate between hepatocellular disease or biliary obstruction as source of hypoprothrombinemia –*
**Adults and children:** 10 mg I.M. or S.C.
*Prevention of hypoprothrombinemia*

---

Reactions may be *common,* uncommon, *life-threatening,* or COMMON AND LIFE-THREATENING.

*related to vitamin K deficiency in long-term parenteral nutrition –*
**Adults:** 5 to 10 mg I.M. weekly.
**Children:** 2 to 5 mg I.M. weekly.
*Prevention of hypoprothrombinemia in infants receiving less than 0.1 mg/liter vitamin K in breast milk or milk substitutes –*
**Infants:** 1 mg I.M. monthly.

### ADVERSE REACTIONS
**CNS:** dizziness.
**CV:** transient hypotension after I.V. administration, rapid and weak pulse.
**Skin:** diaphoresis, flushing, erythema.
**Other:** *anaphylaxis and anaphylactoid reactions* (usually after too-rapid I.V. administration); pain, swelling, and hematoma at injection site.

### INTERACTIONS
*Anticoagulants:* temporary resistance to prothrombin-depressing anticoagulants may result, especially when larger doses of phytonadione are used. Monitor closely.
*Cholestyramine resin, mineral oil:* inhibited GI absorption of oral vitamin K. Space doses. Use together cautiously.

### CONTRAINDICATIONS
Contraindicated in patients with hypersensitivity to drug.

### NURSING CONSIDERATIONS
• Check brand name labels for administration route restrictions.
• Effects of I.V. injection are more rapid but shorter-lived than S.C. or I.M. injections.
• **I.V. use:** Dilute with 0.9% sodium chloride for injection, $D_5W$, or $D_5W$ in 0.9% sodium chloride for injection. Give I.V. by slow infusion over 2 to 3 hours. Rate shouldn't exceed 1 mg/minute in adults or 3 mg/m$^2$/minute in children.
• Protect parenteral products from light. Wrap infusion container with aluminum foil.

• For I.M. administration in adults and older children, administer in upper outer quadrant of buttocks; for infants, administer in the anterolateral aspect of the thigh or deltoid region.
• Anticipate order of weekly addition of 5 to 10 mg of phytonadione to total parenteral nutrition solutions.
• Monitor PT to determine dosage effectiveness, as ordered.
• If severe bleeding occurs, don't delay other measures, such as fresh frozen plasma or whole blood.
• **Alert:** Watch for signs of flushing, weakness, tachycardia, and hypotension; may progress to shock.
• Be aware that phytonadione therapy for hemorrhagic disease in infants causes fewer adverse reactions than do other vitamin K analogues.
• Failure to respond to vitamin K may indicate coagulation defects.

### ☑ PATIENT TEACHING
• Explain the drug's purpose.
• Tell patient to avoid hazardous activities if dizziness occurs.

## sodium fluoride
Fluor-A-Day†, Fluoritab, Fluorodex, Fluotic†, Flura, Flura-Drops, Flura-Loz, Karidium, Luride, Luride Lozi-Tabs, Luride-SF, Luride-SF Lozi-Tabs, Pediaflor, Pedi-Dent†, Pharmaflur, Pharmaflur df, Pharmaflur 1.1, Phos-Flur, Solu-Flur†

## sodium fluoride, topical
ACT◊, Fluorigard◊, Fluorinse, Gel Kam, Gel-Tin◊, Karigel, Karigel-N, Listermint with Fluoride, Minute Gel, Point-Two, PreviDent, Stop◊, Thera-Flur, Thera-Flur-N

*Pregnancy Risk Category: NR*

### HOW SUPPLIED
**sodium fluoride**
*Tablets:* 1 mg
*Tablets (chewable):* 0.5 mg, 1 mg

---

*Liquid form contains alcohol. **May contain tartrazine. †Canada only. ‡Australia only. ◊OTC.

*Drops:* 0.125 mg/drop, 0.25 mg/drop, 0.2 mg/ml, 0.5 mg/ml
*Lozenges:* 1 mg
**sodium fluoride, topical**
*Gel:* 0.1%, 0.5%, 1.23%
*Gel drops:* 0.5%
*Rinse:* 0.01%◇, 0.02%◇, 0.09%

## ACTION
Stabilizes the apatite crystal of bone and teeth.

## ONSET, PEAK, DURATION
Onset and duration unknown. Peaks in 30 to 60 minutes.

## INDICATIONS & DOSAGE
*Prevention of dental caries –*
**Adults and children over 6 years:** 5 to 10 ml of rinse or thin ribbon of gel applied to teeth with toothbrush or mouth trays for at least 1 minute h.s.
**Children under 2 years:** 0.25 mg P.O. (tablet or drops) daily.
**Children 2 to 3 years:** 0.5 mg P.O. (tablet or drops) daily.
**Children 3 to 6 years:** 1 mg P.O. (tablet or lozenge) daily.

## ADVERSE REACTIONS
**CNS:** headache, weakness.
**GI:** gastric distress.
**Skin:** hypersensitivity reactions, such as atopic dermatitis, eczema, and urticaria.
**Other:** staining of teeth.

## INTERACTIONS
*Dairy products:* incompatibility may occur due to formation of calcium fluoride, which is poorly absorbed.

## CONTRAINDICATIONS
Contraindicated in patients hypersensitive to fluoride or when intake from drinking water exceeds 0.7 ppm.

## NURSING CONSIDERATIONS
• Administer oral drops undiluted or mixed with fluids or food.
• Know that chronic toxicity (fluo-

rosis) may result from prolonged use of higher-than-recommended doses.

## ☑ PATIENT TEACHING
• Tell patient that tablets may be dissolved in mouth, chewed, or swallowed whole.
• Advise patient that topical rinses and gels should not be swallowed by children under 3 years or used if water supply is fluorinated. Most effective when used right after brushing teeth. Tell patient to rinse around and between teeth for 1 minute, then spit out.
• Tell patient to dilute drops or rinses in plastic, not glass, containers.
• Advise patient to notify the dentist if tooth mottling occurs.

# trace elements

## chromium (chromic chloride)
Chroma-Pak, Chromic Chloride, Chromium Chloride

## copper (cupric chloride, cupric sulfate)
Cupric Sulfate

## iodine (sodium iodide)
Iodopen

## manganese (manganese chloride, manganese sulfate)

## selenium (selenious acid)
Sele-Pak, Selepen

## zinc (zinc chloride, zinc sulfate)
Zinca-Pak

*Pregnancy Risk Category: C*

## HOW SUPPLIED
**chromium**
*Injection:* 4 mcg/ml, 20 mcg/ml
**copper**
*Injection:* 0.4 mg/ml, 2 mg/ml

**iodine**
*Injection:* 100 mcg/ml
**manganese**
*Injection:* 0.1 mg/ml
**selenium**
*Injection:* 40 mcg/ml
**zinc**
*Injection:* 1 mg/ml, 5 mg/ml

## ACTION
Participates in synthesis and stabilization of proteins and nucleic acids in subcellular and membrane transport systems.

## ONSET, PEAK, DURATION
Onset and peak occur right after an I.V. infusion. Duration unknown.

## INDICATIONS & DOSAGE
*Prevention of individual trace element deficiencies in patients receiving long-term total parenteral nutrition (TPN)* –
*Chromium* –
**Adults:** 10 to 15 mcg I.V. daily.
**Children:** 0.14 to 0.20 mcg/kg I.V. daily.
*Copper* –
**Adults:** 0.5 to 1.5 mg I.V. daily.
**Children:** 20 mcg/kg I.V. daily.
*Iodine* –
**Adults:** 1 to 2 mcg/kg I.V. daily.
*Manganese* –
**Adults:** 0.15 to 0.8 mg I.V. daily.
**Children:** 2 to 10 mcg/kg I.V. daily.
*Selenium* –
**Adults:** 20 to 40 mcg I.V. daily.
**Children:** 3 mcg/kg I.V. daily.
*Zinc* –
**Adults:** 2.5 to 4 mg I.V. daily.
**Children:** 0.05 to 0.1 mg/kg I.V. daily.

## ADVERSE REACTIONS
None reported when used at recommended dosages except for hypersensitivity to iodides.

## INTERACTIONS
None significant at recommended dosages.

## CONTRAINDICATIONS
None known.

## NURSING CONSIDERATIONS
• **I.V. use:** Cautiously infuse diluted solution through a patent I.V. line over the ordered duration.
• Do not administer undiluted due to potential for phlebitis.
• Check serum levels of trace elements in patients who have received TPN for 2 months or longer, as ordered. Give supplement, if ordered. Report low serum levels of these elements.
• Normal serum levels are 0.85 ng/ml chromium; 0.07 to 0.15 mg/ml copper; 4 to 20 mcg/100 ml manganese; 0.1 to 0.19 mcg/ml selenium; and 0.05 to 0.15 mg/100 ml zinc.
• Be aware that solutions of trace elements are compounded by the pharmacist for addition to TPN solutions according to various formulas. One common trace element solution is Shil's solution, which contains copper 1 mg/ml, iodide 0.06 mg/ml, manganese 0.4 mg/ml, and zinc 2 mg/ml.

☑ **PATIENT TEACHING**
• Explain need for zinc administration to patient and family.
• Tell patient to report signs of hypersensitivity promptly.

---

amino acid infusions, crystalline
amino acid infusions in dextrose
amino acid infusions with electrolytes
amino acid infusions with electrolytes in dextrose
amino acid infusions for hepatic failure
amino acid infusions for high metabolic stress
amino acid infusions for renal failure
dextrose
fat emulsions
medium-chain triglycerides

### COMBINATION PRODUCTS
Various products contain dextrose or invert sugar in combination with electrolytes.

## amino acid infusions, crystalline
Aminosyn, Aminosyn II, Aminosyn-PF, FreAmine III, Novamine, Travasol, TrophAmine

## amino acid infusions in dextrose
Aminosyn II with dextrose

## amino acid infusions with electrolytes
Aminosyn with electrolytes, Aminosyn II with electrolytes, FreAmine III with electrolytes, ProcalAmine with electrolytes, Travasol with electrolytes

## amino acid infusions with electrolytes in dextrose
Aminosyn II with electrolytes in dextrose

## amino acid infusions for hepatic failure
HepatAmine

## amino acid infusions for high metabolic stress
Aminosyn-HBC, BranchAmin, FreAmine HBC

## amino acid infusions for renal failure
Aminess, Aminosyn-RF, NephrAmine, RenAmin

*Pregnancy Risk Category: C*

### HOW SUPPLIED
*Injection:* 250 ml, 500 ml, 1,000 ml, 2,000 ml containing amino acids in various concentrations
**amino acid infusions, crystalline**
Aminosyn: 3.5%, 5%, 7%, 8.5%, 10%
Aminosyn II: 3.5%, 5%, 7%, 8.5%, 10%
Aminosyn-PF: 7%, 10%
FreAmine III: 8.5%, 10%
Novamine: 11.4%, 15%
Travasol: 5.5%, 8.5%, 10%
TrophAmine: 6%, 10%
**amino acid infusions in dextrose**
Aminosyn II: 3.5% in 5% dextrose, 3.5% in 25% dextrose, 4.25% in 10% dextrose, 4.25% in 20% dextrose, 4.25% in 25% dextrose, 5% in 25% dextrose
**amino acid infusions with electrolytes**
Aminosyn: 3.5%, 7%, 8.5%
Aminosyn II: 3.5%, 7%, 8.5%, 10%
FreAmine III: 3%, 8.5%
ProcalAmine: 3%
Travasol: 3.5%, 5.5%, 8.5%
**amino acid infusions with electrolytes in dextrose**
Aminosyn II: 3.5% with electrolytes

---

Reactions may be *common,* uncommon, *life-threatening,* or COMMON AND LIFE-THREATENING.

in 5% dextrose, 4.25% with electrolytes in 10% dextrose
**amino acid infusions for hepatic failure**
HepatAmine: 8%
**amino acid infusions for high metabolic stress**
Aminosyn-HBC: 7%
BranchAmin: 4%
FreAmine HBC: 6.9%
**amino acid infusions for renal failure**
Aminess: 5.2%
Aminosyn-RF: 5.2%
NephrAmine: 5.4%
RenAmin: 6.5%

## ACTION
Provides a substrate for protein synthesis or enhances conservation of existing body protein. Formulations for hepatic failure and high metabolic stress contain essential and nonessential amino acids, with high concentrations of the branched chain amino acids isoleucine, leucine, and valine. Formulations for patients with renal failure contain histidine and minimal amounts of essential amino acids; nonessential amino acids are synthesized from excess ammonia in the blood of the uremic patient, thus lowering azotemia.

## ONSET, PEAK, DURATION
Onset and peak occur immediately after an I.V. infusion. Duration unknown.

## INDICATIONS & DOSAGE
*Total parenteral nutrition in patients who cannot or will not eat –*
**Adults:** 1 to 1.5 g/kg I.V. daily.
**Children under 10 kg:** 2 to 4 g/kg I.V. daily.
**Children over 10 kg:** 20 to 25 g/kg I.V. daily for the first 10 kg, then 1 to 1.25 g/kg I.V. daily for each kg over 10 kg.

*Nutritional support in patients with cirrhosis, hepatitis, and hepatic encephalopathy –*
**Adults:** 80 to 120 g of amino acids (12 to 18 g of nitrogen) I.V. daily of the formulation for hepatic failure.
*Nutritional support in patients with high metabolic stress –*
**Adults:** 1.5 g/kg I.V. daily of the formulation for high metabolic stress.
*Nutritional support in patients with renal failure –*
**Adults:** 0.3 to 0.5 g/kg I.V. daily (up to total of 26 g daily). Patients on dialysis may require 1 to 1.2 g/kg daily.

## ADVERSE REACTIONS
**CV:** thrombophlebitis, edema, thrombosis.
**GI:** nausea.
**GU:** glycosuria, osmotic diuresis.
**Hepatic:** elevated liver enzyme levels.
**Skin:** flushing.
**Other:** hypersensitivity reactions, tissue sloughing at infusion site caused by extravasation, *catheter sepsis, rebound hypoglycemia* (when long-term infusions are abruptly stopped), hyperglycemia, osteoporosis, metabolic acidosis, alkalosis, hypophosphatemia, *hyperosmolar nonketotic syndrome,* hyperammonemia, *electrolyte imbalances,* fever, weight gain.

## INTERACTIONS
*Tetracycline:* may reduce the protein-sparing effects of infused amino acids because of its antianabolic activity.

## CONTRAINDICATIONS
Contraindicated in patients with anuria and in patients with inborn errors of amino acid metabolism, such as maple syrup urine disease and isovaleric acidemia. Also contraindicated in patients with severe uncorrected electrolyte or acid-base imbalances, hyperammonemia, and decreased circulating blood volume.

---

*Liquid form contains alcohol.  **May contain tartrazine.  †Canada only.  ‡Australia only.  ◇OTC.

## NURSING CONSIDERATIONS

• Use with extreme caution in pediatric patients and in neonates, especially those with low birth weight.

• Use cautiously in patients with renal insufficiency or failure, cardiac disease, or hepatic impairment.

• Administer cautiously to diabetic patients; insulin may be required to prevent hyperglycemia. Administer cautiously in cardiac insufficiency; may cause circulatory overload. Patients with fluid restriction may tolerate only 1 to 2 liters.

• Obtain baseline serum electrolytes, glucose, BUN, calcium and phosphorus levels before therapy, as ordered, and then monitor these levels periodically throughout therapy.

• Know that safe and effective use of parenteral nutrition requires a knowledge of nutrition as well as clinical expertise in the recognition and treatment of potential complications. Frequent evaluation of the patient and laboratory studies are necessary.

• **I.V. use:** Control infusion rate carefully with infusion pump. If infusion rate falls behind, notify the doctor; do not increase the rate to catch up.

• Know that peripheral infusions should be limited to 2.5% amino acids and dextrose 10%. Check infusion site frequently for erythema, inflammation, irritation, tissue sloughing, necrosis, and phlebitis. Change peripheral I.V. sites routinely to prevent irritation and infection. If a subclavian catheter is used, administer solution into the midsuperior vena cava.

• Add vitamins, electrolytes, and trace elements, as ordered.

• Check fractional urine every 6 hours for glycosuria initially, then every 12 to 24 hours in stable patients. Abrupt onset of glycosuria may be an early sign of impending sepsis.

• Assess body temperature every 4 hours; elevation may indicate sepsis or infection.

• Monitor for extraordinary electrolyte losses that may occur during nasogastric suction, vomiting, diarrhea, or drainage from GI fistula.

• Be prepared to individualize dosage to metabolic and clinical response as determined by nitrogen balance and body weight corrected for fluid balance.

• If the patient has chills, fever, or other signs of sepsis, replace I.V. tubing and bottle and send them to the laboratory to be cultured.

### ☑ PATIENT TEACHING

• Explain need for use to patient and family, and answer any questions.

• Tell patient to report adverse reactions promptly.

# dextrose (D-glucose)

*Pregnancy Risk Category: C*

## HOW SUPPLIED

*Injection:* 3-ml ampule (10%); 5-ml ampule (10%); 10 ml (25%); 50 ml (5% and 50% available in vial, ampule, and Bristoject); 70-ml pin-top vial (70% for additive use only); 100 ml (5%); 250 ml (5%, 10%); 400 ml (5%); 500 ml (5%, 10%, 20%, 30%, 40%, 50%, 60%, 70%); 650 ml (38.5%); 1,000 ml (2.5%, 5%, 10%, 20%, 30%, 40%, 50%, 60%, 70%)

## ACTION

A simple water-soluble sugar that minimizes glyconeogenesis and promotes anabolism in patients whose oral caloric intake is limited.

## ONSET, PEAK, DURATION

Onset and serum levels peak immediately after I.V. infusion. Duration unknown.

## INDICATIONS & DOSAGE

*Fluid replacement and caloric supplementation in patients who can't maintain adequate oral intake or who are restricted from doing so –*

---

**Adults and children:** dosage depends on fluid and caloric requirements. Peripheral I.V. infusion of 2.5%, 5%, or 10% solution or central I.V. infusion of 20% solution is used for minimal fluid needs. A 25% solution is used to treat acute hypoglycemia in neonate or older infant. A 50% solution is used to treat insulin-induced hypoglycemia. Solutions of 10%, 20%, 30%, 40%, 50%, 60%, and 70% are diluted in admixtures, usually amino acid solutions, for total parenteral nutrition (TPN) given through a central vein.

## ADVERSE REACTIONS
**CNS:** confusion, *unconsciousness in hyperosmolar nonketotic syndrome.*
**CV:** with fluid overload — *pulmonary edema, exacerbated hypertension, and CHF* in susceptible patients. Prolonged or concentrated infusions may cause *phlebitis, venous sclerosis,* and tissue necrosis, especially when administered peripherally.
**GU:** glycosuria, osmotic diuresis.
**Skin:** sloughing and tissue necrosis, if extravasation occurs with concentrated solutions.
**Other:** with rapid infusion of concentrated solution or prolonged infusion — hyperglycemia, hypervolemia, hypovolemia, dehydration, fever, hyperosmolarity. Rapid termination of long-term infusions may cause hypoglycemia from rebound hyperinsulinemia.

## INTERACTIONS
None significant.

## CONTRAINDICATIONS
Contraindicated in patients in diabetic coma while blood glucose remains excessively high. Use of concentrated solutions contraindicated in patients with intracranial or intraspinal hemorrhage, or in dehydrated patients with delirium tremens or in patients with severe dehydration, anuria, hepatic coma, or glucose-galactose malabsorption syndrome.

## NURSING CONSIDERATIONS
● Use cautiously in patients with cardiac or pulmonary disease, hypertension, renal insufficiency, urinary obstruction, or hypovolemia.
● **I.V. use:** Control infusion rate carefully; maximum rate is 0.5 g/kg/hour. Use infusion pump when infusing with amino acids for TPN. Never infuse concentrated solutions rapidly, which may cause hyperglycemia and fluid shift.
● Monitor serum glucose levels carefully. Prolonged therapy with $D_5W$ can cause depletion of pancreatic insulin production and secretion.
● *Alert:* Never stop hypertonic solutions abruptly. If necessary, have dextrose 10% in water solution available to treat hypoglycemia if rebound hyperinsulinemia occurs.
● Don't give dextrose solutions without sodium chloride solution in blood transfusions; may cause clumping of RBCs. Use central veins to infuse dextrose solutions with concentrations greater than 10%.
● Take care to prevent extravasation. Check injection site frequently to prevent irritation, tissue sloughing, necrosis, and phlebitis.
● Check vital signs frequently. Report adverse effects promptly.
● Monitor fluid intake and output and weight carefully, especially patients with renal function impairment.
● Watch closely for signs of fluid overload, especially if fluid intake is restricted.

## ☑ PATIENT TEACHING
● Explain need for drug to patient and family, and answer any questions.
● Tell patient to report adverse reactions promptly.

---

*Liquid form contains alcohol.  **May contain tartrazine.  †Canada only.  ‡Australia only.  ◇OTC.

# fat emulsions
Intralipid 10%, Intralipid 20%,
Liposyn II 10%, Liposyn II 20%,
Liposyn III 10%, Liposyn III 20%

*Pregnancy Risk Category: C*

## HOW SUPPLIED
*Injection:* 50 ml (10%, 20%), 100 ml
(10%, 20%), 200 ml (10%, 20%),
250 ml (10%, 20%), 500 ml (10%,
20%)

## ACTION
Provides neutral triglycerides, predominantly unsaturated fatty acids;
acts as a source of calories; and prevents fatty acid deficiency. When substituted for dextrose as a source of
calories, fat emulsions decrease carbon dioxide production.

## ONSET, PEAK, DURATION
Onset and serum levels peak immediately after I.V. infusion. Duration unknown.

## INDICATIONS & DOSAGE
Intralipid:
*Source of calories as adjunct to total
parenteral nutrition (TPN) –*
**Adults:** 1 ml/minute I.V. for 15 to 30
minutes (10% emulsion); 0.5 ml/min-
ute I.V. for 15 to 30 minutes (20%
emulsion). If no adverse reactions occur, rate increased to deliver 500 ml
over 4 to 8 hours; total daily dosage
should not exceed 2.5 g/kg.
**Children:** 0.1 ml/minute for 10 to 15
minutes (10% emulsion), 0.05 ml/
minute I.V. for 10 to 15 minutes (20%
emulsion). If no adverse reactions occur, rate increased to deliver 1 g/kg
over 4 hours; daily dosage should not
exceed 4 g/kg. Equals 60% of daily
caloric intake; protein-carbohydrate
TPN should supply remaining 40%.
*Fatty acid deficiency –*
**Adults and children:** 8% to 10% of
total caloric intake I.V.
Liposyn:

*Prevention of fatty acid deficiency –*
**Adults:** 500 ml (10% emulsion) I.V.
twice weekly. Infused initially at a
rate of 1 ml/minute for 30 minutes.
Rate may be increased to, but should
not exceed, 500 ml over 4 to 6 hours.
**Children:** 5 to 10 ml/kg (10% emulsion) I.V. daily. Initially infused at a
rate of 0.1 ml/minute for 30 minutes.
Rate may be increased to, but should
not exceed, 100 ml/hour.

## ADVERSE REACTIONS
*Early reactions to fat overload:*
**CNS:** headache, sleepiness, dizzi-
ness.
**EENT:** pressure over eyes.
**GI:** nausea, vomiting.
**Hematologic:** *hypercoagulability,
thrombocytopenia in neonates* (rare).
**Respiratory:** dyspnea, cyanosis.
**Skin:** flushing, diaphoresis.
**Other:** hyperlipidemia, fever, chest
and back pains, hypersensitivity reac-
tions, irritation at infusion site.
*Delayed reactions:*
**CNS:** *focal seizures*.
**Hematologic:** *thrombocytopenia,*
leukopenia, leukocytosis.
**Hepatic:** transient increases in liver
function test values, hepatomegaly.
**Other:** fever, splenomegaly.

## INTERACTIONS
None significant.

## CONTRAINDICATIONS
Contraindicated in hyperlipidemia,
lipid nephrosis, or acute pancreatitis
accompanied by hyperlipidemia; and
in patients with severe egg allergies.

## NURSING CONSIDERATIONS
● Use cautiously in patients with severe hepatic disease; pulmonary disease; anemia; or blood coagulation
disorders, including thrombocytopenia; and in patients at risk for fat
embolism.
● Also use cautiously in jaundiced or
premature infants.

---

Reactions may be *common*, uncommon, *life-threatening*, or **COMMON AND LIFE-THREATENING**.

- **I.V. use:** Avoid rapid infusion, and use an infusion pump to regulate rate.
- Be aware that drug may be mixed with amino acid solution, dextrose, electrolytes, and vitamins in the same I.V. container. Check with the pharmacist for acceptable proportions and compatibility information.
- Know that an in-line filter with pores of 1.2 micron or larger is sometimes used to remove particulate matter.
- Do not use fat emulsion if it separates or becomes oily.
- Lipids support bacterial growth, so change all I.V. tubing before each infusion. Check injection site daily. Report signs of inflammation or infection promptly.
- Watch for adverse reactions, especially during first half of infusion.
- Monitor serum lipid levels closely when the patient is receiving fat emulsion therapy. Lipemia must clear between dosing.
- Monitor hepatic function carefully in long-term therapy.
- Check platelet count frequently in neonates receiving fat emulsions I.V.
- Carefully monitor serum triglycerides and free fatty acids in infants.
- Refrigeration is not necessary.
- Intralipid and Liposyn differ mainly by their fatty acid components.

**PATIENT TEACHING**
- Explain need for fat emulsion therapy, and answer any questions.
- Tell patient to report adverse reactions promptly.

---

## medium-chain triglycerides
M.C.T.◇

*Pregnancy Risk Category: NR*

**HOW SUPPLIED**
*Oil:* 960 ml (115 calories/15 ml)◇

**ACTION**
Source of rapidly hydrolyzable lipid.

**ONSET, PEAK, DURATION**
Unknown.

**INDICATIONS & DOSAGE**
*Inadequate digestion or absorption of food fats –*
**Adults:** 15 ml P.O. t.i.d. or q.i.d.

**ADVERSE REACTIONS**
**CNS:** reversible *coma* in susceptible patients (such as those with advanced hepatic cirrhosis).
**GI:** *nausea, vomiting, diarrhea, abdominal distention, cramps.*

**INTERACTIONS**
None significant.

**CONTRAINDICATIONS**
None known.

**NURSING CONSIDERATIONS**
- Use cautiously in patients with hepatic cirrhosis and complications such as portacaval shunts or tendency to encephalopathy.
- To minimize GI adverse reactions, give smaller, more frequent doses with meals, mixed with salad dressing, or in chilled fruit juice.
- Know that drug is more easily absorbed than long-chain fats; not dependent on bile salts for emulsification.
- Know that drug's rapid metabolism provides quick energy.
- Drug provides 7.7 calories/ml. No essential fatty acids are provided.

**☑ PATIENT TEACHING**
- Instruct patient when and how to take drug to minimize GI adverse reactions.
- Tell patient to report persistent or severe adverse reactions promptly.
- Tell patient not to use plastic containers or utensils to give the drug.

---

# Antigout drugs

allopurinol
colchicine
probenecid
sulfinpyrazone

**COMBINATION PRODUCTS**
COLBENEMID, PROBEN-C, PROBEN-
ECID WITH COLCHICINE: probenecid
500 mg and colchicine 0.5 mg.

---

# allopurinol

Alloremed‡, Apo-Allopurinol†,
Capurate‡, Lopurin, Purinol†,
Zyloprim

*Pregnancy Risk Category: C*

**HOW SUPPLIED**
*Tablets (scored):* 100 mg, 300 mg
*Capsules:* 100 mg‡, 300 mg‡

**ACTION**
Reduces uric acid production by inhibiting the biochemical reactions
preceding its formation.

**ONSET, PEAK, DURATION**
Onset occurs within 2 or 3 days. Allopurinol levels peak in 0.5 to 2 hours;
oxypurinol (active metabolite) levels
in 4.5 to 5 hours. Effects persist for 1
to 2 weeks.

**INDICATIONS & DOSAGE**
*Gout, primary or secondary to hyper-
uricemia; secondary to diseases such
as acute or chronic leukemia, polycythemia vera, multiple myeloma, and
psoriasis –*
Dosage varies with severity of disease; can be given as single dose or
divided, but doses larger than 300 mg
should be divided.
**Adults:** mild gout, 200 to 300 mg
P.O. daily; severe gout with large to-
phi, 400 to 600 mg P.O. daily. Same

dosage for maintenance in secondary
hyperuricemia.
*Hyperuricemia secondary to malig-
nancies –*
**Children under 6 years:** 50 mg P.O.
t.i.d.
**Children 6 to 10 years:** 300 mg P.O.
daily or divided t.i.d.
*Prevention of acute gouty attacks –*
**Adults:** 100 mg P.O. daily; increase
at weekly intervals by 100 mg without
exceeding maximum dose (800 mg),
until serum uric acid falls to 6 mg/100
ml or less.
*Prevention of uric acid nephropathy
during cancer chemotherapy –*
**Adults:** 600 to 800 mg P.O. daily for
2 to 3 days, with high fluid intake.
*Recurrent calcium oxalate calculi –*
**Adults:** 200 to 300 mg P.O. daily in
single or divided doses.
  In impaired renal function in
adults: 200 mg P.O. daily if creatinine
clearance is 10 to 20 ml/minute; 100
mg P.O. daily if less than 10 ml/min-
ute; 100 mg P.O. more than 24 hours
apart if less than 3 ml/minute.

**ADVERSE REACTIONS**
**CNS:** drowsiness, headache, paresthesia, peripheral neuropathy, neuritis.
**CV:** hypersensitivity vasculitis, necrotizing angiitis.
**EENT:** epistaxis.
**GI:** nausea, vomiting, diarrhea, abdominal pain, gastritis, dyspepsia.
**GU:** *renal failure,* uremia.
**Hematologic:** *agranulocytosis,* anemia, *aplastic anemia, thrombocytopenia,* leukopenia, leukocytosis, eosinophilia.
**Hepatic:** altered liver function studies, *hepatitis, hepatic necrosis,* hepatomegaly, cholestatic jaundice.
**Skin:** *rash,* (usually maculopapular);

---

Reactions may be *common,* uncommon, *life-threatening,* or COMMON AND LIFE-THREATENING.

*exfoliative, urticarial, and purpuric lesions; erythema multiforme;* severe furunculosis of nose; ichthyosis, *toxic epidermal necrolysis.*
**Other:** arthralgia, ecchymoses, fever, myopathy, taste loss or perversion, alopecia, chills.

## INTERACTIONS
*Amoxicillin, ampicillin, bacampicillin:* increased possibility of rash. Avoid concomitant use.
*Anticoagulants:* potentiation of anticoagulant effect. Dosage adjustments may be necessary.
*Antineoplastic agents:* increased potential for bone marrow suppression. Monitor the patient carefully.
*Chlorpropamide:* possible increased hypoglycemic effect. Avoid concomitant use.
*Diazoxide, diuretics, ethanol, mecamylamine, pyrazinamide:* increased serum acid concentration. Adjust dosage of allopurinol.
*Ethacrynic acid, thiazide diuretics:* increased risk of allopurinol toxicity. Reduce dosage of allopurinol, and closely monitor renal function.
*Uricosuric agents:* additive effect. May enhance therapy.
*Urine-acidifying agents (ammonium chloride, ascorbic acid, potassium or sodium phosphate):* may increase the possibility of kidney stone formation. Monitor the patient carefully.
*Xanthines:* increased serum theophylline levels. Adjust dosage of theophyllines.

## CONTRAINDICATIONS
Contraindicated in patients with hypersensitivity to the drug and in those with idiopathic hemochromatosis.

## NURSING CONSIDERATIONS
● Monitor serum uric acid levels to evaluate drug's effectiveness.
● Monitor fluid intake and output; daily urine output of at least 2 liters

and maintenance of neutral or slightly alkaline urine are desirable.
● Periodically monitor CBC and hepatic and renal function, especially at start of therapy, as ordered.
● If renal insufficiency occurs at any time during treatment, be prepared to reduce dosage, as ordered.
● Optimal benefits may require 2 to 6 weeks of therapy. Because acute gouty attacks may occur during this time, concurrent use of colchicine may be prescribed prophylactically.

## ☑ PATIENT TEACHING
● To minimize GI adverse reactions, tell patient to take with or immediately after meals.
● Encourage the patient to drink plenty of fluids while taking this drug unless otherwise contraindicated.
● Drug may cause drowsiness; tell patient not to drive or perform hazardous tasks requiring mental alertness until CNS effects of the drug are known.
● If the patient is taking allopurinol for treatment of recurrent calcium oxalate stones, advise him to also reduce his dietary intake of animal protein, sodium, refined sugars, oxalate-rich foods, and calcium.
● Tell patient to discontinue at first sign of rash, which may precede severe hypersensitivity or other adverse reaction. Rash is more common in patient taking diuretics and in those with renal disorders. Tell the patient to report all adverse reactions.

## colchicine
Colchicine MR‡, Colgout‡, Colsalide, Novocolchicine†
*Pregnancy Risk Category: D*

### HOW SUPPLIED
*Tablets:* 0.5 mg ( 1/120 grain), 0.6 mg (1/100 grain) as sugar-coated granules
*Injection:* 1 mg (1/60 grain)/2 ml

---

## ACTION
Unknown. As antigout agent, apparently decreases WBC motility, phagocytosis, and lactic acid production, decreasing urate crystal deposits and reducing inflammation. As antiosteolytic agent, apparently inhibits mitosis of osteoprogenitor cells and decreases osteoclast activity.

## ONSET, PEAK, DURATION
Onset is 6 to 12 hours after I.V. administration; within 12 hours after oral administration. Levels peak in 0.5 to 2 hours after oral administration; unknown after I.V. administration. Duration unknown.

## INDICATIONS & DOSAGE
*Prevention of acute gout attacks as prophylactic or maintenance therapy –*
**Adults:** 0.5 or 0.6 mg P.O. daily. Patients who normally have one attack per year or less should receive drug only 1 to 4 days per week; patients who have more than one attack per year should receive drug daily. In severe cases, 1.5 to 1.95 mg P.O. daily.
*Prevention of gout attacks in patients undergoing surgery –*
**Adults:** 0.5 to 0.6 mg P.O. t.i.d. 3 days before and 3 days after surgery.
*Acute gout, acute gouty arthritis –*
**Adults:** initially, 0.5 to 1.2 mg P.O., then 0.5 or 0.6 mg q 1 to 2 hours until pain is relieved; nausea, vomiting, or diarrhea ensues; or the maximum dosage of 8 mg is reached. Alternatively, 2 mg I.V., followed by 0.5 mg I.V. q 6 hours if necessary. (Note that some clinicians prefer to give a single I.V. injection of 3 mg.) Total I.V. dosage over 24 hours (one course of treatment) should not exceed 4 mg.

## ADVERSE REACTIONS
**CNS:** peripheral neuritis.
**GI:** *nausea, vomiting, abdominal pain, diarrhea.*
**Hematologic:** *aplastic anemia, thrombocytopenia, and agranulocytosis* (with long-term use); nonthrombocytopenic purpura.
**Skin:** urticaria, dermatitis, hypersensitivity reactions.
**Other:** alopecia, severe local irritation if extravasation occurs, myopathy, reversible azoospermia.

## INTERACTIONS
*Ethanol:* may impair efficacy of colchicine prophylaxis. Don't use together.
*Loop diuretics:* may decrease efficacy of colchicine prophylaxis. Avoid concomitant use.
*Phenylbutazone:* may increase risk of leukopenia or thrombocytopenia. Avoid concomitant use.
*Vitamin B$_{12}$:* impaired absorption of vitamin B$_{12}$. Avoid concomitant use.

## CONTRAINDICATIONS
Contraindicated in patients with hypersensitivity to drug, blood dyscrasias, or serious CV disease, renal disease, or GI disorders.

## NURSING CONSIDERATIONS
• Use cautiously in elderly or debilitated patients or in those with early signs of CV, renal, or GI disease.
• Obtain baseline laboratory studies, including CBC, prior to therapy, as ordered, and then periodically throughout therapy.
• **I.V. use:** Give by slow I.V. push over 2 to 5 minutes. Avoid extravasation because colchicine irritates tissues. Don't dilute colchicine injection with dextrose 5% injection or any other fluid that might change pH of colchicine solution. If lower concentration of colchicine injection is needed, dilute with 0.9% sodium chloride solution or sterile water for injection and give over 2 to 5 minutes by direct injection. Preferably, inject into the tubing of a free-flowing I.V. solution. Don't inject if diluted solution becomes turbid.

---

Reactions may be *common,* uncommon, *life-threatening,* or **COMMON AND LIFE-THREATENING.**

• Do not administer I.M. or S.C.; severe local irritation occurs.

• Give with meals to reduce GI effects as maintenance therapy. May be used with uricosuric agents, as ordered.

• Monitor fluid intake and output, and keep output at 2,000 ml daily.

• **Alert:** Know that after a full course of I.V. colchicine (4 mg), no more colchicine should be given by any route for at least 7 days. Colchicine is a toxic drug and fatalities have resulted from overdose.

• The first sign of acute overdose may be GI symptoms, followed by vascular damage, muscle weakness, and ascending paralysis. Delirium and seizures may occur without the patient losing consciousness.

• Discontinue drug as soon as gout pain is relieved or at the first sign of GI symptoms, as ordered.

• Be aware that colchicine has no effect on non-gouty arthritis.

• Store in tightly closed, light-resistant container.

☑ **PATIENT TEACHING**
• Teach the patient how to take the drug and tell him to drink extra fluids.
• Tell the patient to report adverse reactions, especially signs of acute overdose.

## probenecid
Benemid, Benn, Benuryl†,
Probalan, Robenecid

*Pregnancy Risk Category: NR*

**HOW SUPPLIED**
*Tablets:* 500 mg

**ACTION**
Blocks renal tubular reabsorption of uric acid, increasing excretion, and inhibits active renal tubular secretion of many weak organic acids, such as penicillins and cephalosporins.

**ONSET, PEAK, DURATION**
Onset unknown. Serum levels peak in 2 to 4 hours; peak effects occur in 30 minutes for uricosuric effects and 2 hours for suppression of penicillin excretion. Duration unknown for uricosuric effects; effects persist for about 8 hours for suppression of penicillin excretion.

**INDICATIONS & DOSAGE**
*Adjunct to penicillin therapy –*
**Adults and children over 50 kg:** 500 mg P.O. q.i.d.
**Children 2 to 14 years or 50 kg or under:** initially, 25 mg/kg P.O., then 40 mg/kg/day in divided doses q.i.d.
*Gonorrhea –*
**Adults:** 3.5 g ampicillin P.O. with 1 g probenecid P.O. given together; or 1 g probenecid P.O. 30 minutes before dose of 4.8 million units of aqueous penicillin G procaine I.M., injected at two different sites.
*Hyperuricemia of gout, gouty arthritis –*
**Adults:** 250 mg P.O. b.i.d. for 1st week, then 500 mg b.i.d., to maximum of 2 g daily. Maintenance dosage should be reviewed every 6 months and reduced by increments of 500 mg if indicated.

**ADVERSE REACTIONS**
**CNS:** *headache,* dizziness.
**GI:** anorexia, nausea, vomiting, sore gums.
**GU:** urinary frequency, renal colic, nephrotic syndrome.
**Hematologic:** *hemolytic anemia,* anemia, *aplastic anemia.*
**Skin:** dermatitis, pruritus.
**Other:** flushing, fever, exacerbation of gout, *hepatic necrosis,* hypersensitivity reactions (including *anaphylaxis,* fever).

**INTERACTIONS**
*Ethanol:* increased urate levels. Avoid use.
*Indomethacin:* decreased indometha-

cin excretion. Lower indomethacin dosages may be required.
*Methotrexate:* decreased methotrexate excretion. Lower methotrexate dosage may be required. Serum levels should be determined.
*Oral antidiabetic agents:* enhanced hypoglycemic effect. Monitor blood glucose levels closely. Dosage adjustment may be required.
*Salicylates:* inhibited uricosuric effect of probenecid, causing urate retention. Do not use together.

## CONTRAINDICATIONS
Contraindicated in patients with hypersensitivity to drug, uric acid kidney stones, or blood dyscrasias; in acute gout attack; and in children under 2 years.

## NURSING CONSIDERATIONS
• Use cautiously in patients with peptic ulcer or renal impairment.
• To minimize GI distress, give with milk, food, or antacids. Continued disturbances might indicate need to lower dosage.
• Monitor periodic BUN and renal function tests in long-term therapy.
• Force fluids to maintain minimum daily output of 2 to 3 liters. Alkalinize urine with sodium bicarbonate or potassium citrate, as ordered. These measures will prevent hematuria, renal colic, urate stone development, and costovertebral pain.
• Keep in mind that therapy is not initiated until acute attack subsides. Contains no analgesic or anti-inflammatory agent, and is of no value during acute gout attacks.
• Be aware that drug is suitable for long-term use; no cumulative effects or tolerance reported.
• Drug is ineffective in patients with chronic renal insufficiency (glomerular filtration rate less than 30 ml/minute).
• Drug may increase frequency, severity, and length of acute gout attacks during first 6 to 12 months of therapy. Prophylactic colchicine or another anti-inflammatory agent is given during first 3 to 6 months.
• Be aware that drug may produce false-positive glucose tests with Benedict's solution or Clinitest, but not with glucose oxidase method (Clinistix, Diastix, Tes-Tape).
• Drug decreases urinary excretion of 17-ketosteroids, Bromsulphalein (BSP), aminohippuric acid, and iodine-related organic acids, interfering with laboratory procedures.

## ☑ PATIENT TEACHING
• Instruct patient and family that drug must be taken regularly as ordered or gout attacks may result.
• Tell him to visit the doctor regularly so that uric acid can be monitored and dosage adjusted, if necessary. Lifelong therapy may be required in patients with hyperuricemia.
• Advise patient with gout to avoid all medications that contain aspirin, which may precipitate gout. Acetaminophen may be used for pain.
• Tell patient with gout to avoid alcohol; it increases urate level.
• Tell patient with gout to limit intake of foods high in purine: anchovies, liver, sardines, kidneys, sweetbreads, peas, and lentils. Also tell patient to force fluids.

## sulfinpyrazone
Anturant†, Anturane
*Pregnancy Risk Category: NR*

### HOW SUPPLIED
*Tablets:* 100 mg
*Capsules:* 200 mg

### ACTION
Blocks renal tubular reabsorption of uric acid, increasing excretion, and inhibits platelet aggregation.

## ONSET, PEAK, DURATION
Onset unknown. Serum levels peak 1 to 2 hours after administration. Effects persist for 4 to 6 hours.

## INDICATIONS & DOSAGE
*Intermittent or chronic gouty arthritis* —
**Adults:** 200 to 400 mg P.O. b.i.d. 1st week, then 400 mg P.O. b.i.d. Maximum dosage is 800 mg daily.

## ADVERSE REACTIONS
**GI:** *nausea, dyspepsia,* epigastric pain, reactivation of peptic ulcerations.
**Hematologic:** *blood dyscrasias* (for example, anemia, leukopenia, *agranulocytosis, thrombocytopenia, aplastic anemia*).
**Respiratory:** bronchoconstriction in patients with aspirin-induced asthma.
**Skin:** rash.

## INTERACTIONS
*Oral anticoagulants:* increased anticoagulant effect and risk of bleeding. Use together cautiously.
*Oral antidiabetic agents:* increased effects. Monitor closely.
*Probenecid:* inhibited renal excretion of sulfinpyrazone. Use together cautiously.
*Salicylates, aspirin:* inhibited uricosuric effect of sulfinpyrazone. Do not use together.

## CONTRAINDICATIONS
Contraindicated in patients with hypersensitivity to pyrazole derivatives (including oxyphenbutazone and phenylbutazone), blood dyscrasias, active peptic ulcer, or symptoms of GI inflammation or ulceration.

## NURSING CONSIDERATIONS
• Use cautiously in patients with healed peptic ulcer and in pregnant patients.
• To minimize GI disturbances, give with milk, food, or antacids.

• Monitor periodic BUN, CBC, and renal function studies advised during long-term use, as ordered.
• Monitor fluid intake and output closely. Therapy, especially at start, may lead to renal colic and formation of uric acid stones until acid levels are normal (about 6 mg/dl).
• Force fluids to maintain minimum daily output of 2 to 3 liters. Alkalinize urine with sodium bicarbonate or other agent, as ordered.
• Drug contains no analgesic or anti-inflammatory agent and is of no value during acute gout attacks.
• Drug may increase frequency, severity, and length of acute gout attacks during first 6 to 12 months of therapy. Prophylactic colchicine or another anti-inflammatory agent is given during first 3 to 6 months.
• Lifelong therapy may be required in patients with hyperuricemia.
• Drug decreases urinary excretion of aminohippuric acid, interfering with laboratory test results.
• Keep in mind that alkalinizing agents are used therapeutically to increase sulfinpyrazone activity, preventing urolithiasis.

## ☑ PATIENT TEACHING
• Instruct patient and family that drug must be taken regularly as ordered or gout attacks may result.
• Tell patient to visit the doctor regularly so blood levels can be monitored and dosage adjusted if necessary.
• Warn patient with gout not to take any aspirin-containing medications because these may precipitate gout. Acetaminophen may be used for pain.
• Tell patient with gout to avoid foods high in purine: anchovies, liver, sardines, kidneys, sweetbreads, peas, and lentils. Tell him to force fluids.

---

*Liquid form contains alcohol.    **May contain tartrazine.    †Canada only.    ‡Australia only.    ◇OTC.

chymopapain
fibrinolysin and
   desoxyribonuclease
hyaluronidase

## COMBINATION PRODUCTS
None.

---

## chymopapain
Chymodiactin

*Pregnancy Risk Category: C*

### HOW SUPPLIED
*Powder for injection:* 4,000 units/vial,
10,000 units/vial; each unit of chymopapain also known as 1 picoKatal
(pKat)

### ACTION
Hydrolyzes noncollagenous proteins
in the chondromucoprotein of the nucleus pulposus.

### ONSET, PEAK, DURATION
Onset and peak unknown. Effects persist for at least 1 week.

### INDICATIONS & DOSAGE
*Herniated lumbar intervertebral disk—*
**Adults:** 2,000 to 4,000 pKat units/
disk injected intradiskally. Maximum
dosage in patients with multiple disk
herniation is 8,000 units.

### ADVERSE REACTIONS
**Systemic:** *anaphylaxis, anaphylactoid
reaction; paraplegia, subarachnoid
and intracerebral hemorrhage, seizures, acute transverse myelitis,* nausea, headache, dizziness, leg weakness,
paresthesia, numbness of legs and toes,
various GI disturbances.
**Other:** *back pain, stiffness, back
spasm, soreness,* erythema, rash, pru-

ritic urticaria, conjunctivitis, vasomotor rhinitis, angioedema.

### INTERACTIONS
*Radiographic contrast media:* potential adverse reactions when injected
concomitantly with chymopapain.
Avoid concurrent use.

### CONTRAINDICATIONS
Contraindicated in patients with history of allergy to the drug, papaya, or
papaya derivatives (such as meat tenderizers); in patients who have previously received an injection of chymopapain; and in those with severe spon-
dylolisthesis in addition to spinal stenosis, severe progressing paralysis, or
evidence of spinal cord tumor or a
cauda equina lesion.

### NURSING CONSIDERATIONS
• A ChymoFAST test can detect hypersensitivity to this drug. Giving histamine receptor antagonists prior to
drug may lessen the severity of anaphylactoid reactions.
• Drug should be used only by doctors qualified and experienced to perform laminectomy, diskectomy, or
other spinal procedures, and who
have received specialized training in
chemonucleolysis. It shouldn't be injected in any region other than the
lumbar spine; extremely toxic if injected into the subarachnoid space.
• Use within 1 hour after reconstitution. Discard unused drug.
• Watch very closely for anaphylactoid
reaction (0.5% of patients). Reaction
may be immediate or delayed up to 1
hour after injection and last for minutes
to several hours. Watch for hypotension
and bronchospasm, possibly leading to
laryngeal edema, arrhythmias, cardiac
arrest, coma, and death. Other signs of

---

Reactions may be *common,* uncommon, *life-threatening,* or COMMON AND LIFE-THREATENING.

allergic response include erythema, pilomotor erection, rash, pruritic urticaria, conjunctivitis, vasomotor rhinitis, angioedema, or various GI disturbances.
• Keep an I.V. line open to manage anaphylaxis quickly, if needed. Keep epinephrine and steroids also available.

☑ **PATIENT TEACHING**
• Instruct the patient to anticipate delayed allergic reactions, such as rash, urticaria, or pruritus, which may occur up to 15 days after injection. He should report these at once.
• Warn the patient that he may experience back pain or involuntary muscle spasm in the lower back for several days after injection. Reassure him that this is common and not chronic.

---

## fibrinolysin and desoxyribonuclease
Elase

*Pregnancy Risk Category: NR*

**HOW SUPPLIED**
*Powder for solution:* 25 units fibrinolysin and 15,000 units desoxyribonuclease in 30-ml vial
*Ointment:* 30 units fibrinolysin and 20,000 units desoxyribonuclease in 30-g tube (with applicator)

**ACTION**
Fibrinolysin attacks fibrin of blood clots and fibrinous exudates; desoxyribonuclease attacks DNA. Combined enzymatic action debrides wound surfaces and promotes healing.

**ONSET, PEAK, DURATION**
Unknown.

**INDICATIONS & DOSAGE**
*Debridement of inflammatory and infected lesions, including surgical wounds, ulcerative lesions, second- and third-degree burns, circumcision,* *episiotomy, abscesses, fistulas, and sinus tracts –*
**Adults and children:** ointment applied to lesions daily to t.i.d. for as long as enzyme action is desired. Alternatively, solution prepared from powder applied topically as a liquid, spray, or wet dressing.
For wet-to-dry dressing, mix 1 vial of Elase powder with 10 to 50 ml of 0.9% sodium chloride solution; saturate strips of fine gauze with solution. Pack ulcerated area with Elase gauze. Let gauze dry in contact with ulcerated lesion for 6 to 8 hours. Remove dried gauze and repeat t.i.d. or q.i.d.
*Mild-to-moderate cervicitis or vaginitis –*
**Adults:** 5 ml of ointment inserted intravaginally using applicator supplied, once daily h.s. for 5 days or until tube is empty.
*Irrigation of infected wounds, empyema cavities, abscesses, otorhinolaryngologic wounds, subcutaneous hematomas –*
**Adults and children:** dilute prepared solution and irrigate wound p.r.n., depending on extent and severity.
For solution as irrigating agent, drain cavity and replace Elase every 6 to 10 hours to reduce amount of byproduct accumulation and to minimize loss of enzyme activity.

**ADVERSE REACTIONS**
**Systemic:** hyperemia with high doses, hypersensitivity reactions.

**INTERACTIONS**
None significant.

**CONTRAINDICATIONS**
Contraindicated in patients with hypersensitivity to the drug or to bovine products; not for parenteral use (fibrinolysin may be antigenic).

**NURSING CONSIDERATIONS**
• Dense, dry eschar is surgically removed before enzymatic debridement.

---

Enzyme must be in constant contact with substrate. Necrotic debris is removed periodically; the enzyme is replenished at least once daily.

● Prepare solution just before use and discard after 24 hours.

● Clean wound with water, 0.9% sodium chloride solution, or hydrogen peroxide and dry; cover with thin layer of Elase and nonadherent dressing.

● Ensure that wound-dressing techniques are performed carefully under aseptic conditions and that antibiotic therapy is instituted, as ordered.

● Change dressing up to three times daily. Flush away necrotic debris and reapply ointment. Frequency of application may be more important than the amount of drug used.

☑ **PATIENT TEACHING**

● Explain drug use and administration to patient and family.

● Tell patient to report hypersensitivity reactions promptly.

## hyaluronidase
Wydase

*Pregnancy Risk Category: C*

**HOW SUPPLIED**
*Injection:* 150 units/ml in 1-ml, 10-ml vials

**ACTION**
Hydrolyzes hyaluronic acid, promoting diffusion of fluids in tissues.

**ONSET, PEAK, DURATION**
Unknown.

**INDICATIONS & DOSAGE**
*Adjunct to increase absorption and dispersion of other injected drugs –*
**Adults and children:** 150 units added to solution containing other drug.
*Hypodermoclysis –*
**Adults and children over 3 years:** 150 units injected S.C. before clysis

or injected into clysis tubing near needle for each 1,000 ml clysis solution.
*Excretory urography when contrast medium is given S.C. –*
**Adults and children:** with the patient in a prone position, 75 units S.C. over each scapula, followed by injection of contrast medium at same sites.

**ADVERSE REACTIONS**
**Skin:** allergic reactions (rare).

**INTERACTIONS**
*Local anesthetics:* increased potential for toxic local reaction. Use together cautiously.

**CONTRAINDICATIONS**
Contraindicated in patients with hypersensitivity to drug.

**NURSING CONSIDERATIONS**
● Perform a skin test for sensitivity. Don't inject into diseased areas. Watch for local reactions.

● Do not inject into acutely inflamed or cancerous areas.

● Drug not recommended for I.V. use.

● For children, add 15 units to each 100 ml of solution. The drip rate should not exceed 2 ml/minute.

● Don't add to any solutions containing epinephrine and heparin. Drug is incompatible with these drugs.

● In patients with hypodermoclysis, adjust dosage, rate of injection, and type of solution according to the patient's response, as ordered.

● Don't get solution in eyes; if solution does get in eyes, flush with water.

● Protect from heat. Don't use cloudy or discolored solution. Store reconstituted solution below 30° C (86° F), and use within 14 days.

☑ **PATIENT TEACHING**

● Explain need for drug to patient and family, and describe how drug is given.

● Inform patient about possible adverse skin reactions.

---

Reactions may be *common*, uncommon, *life-threatening*, or **COMMON AND LIFE-THREATENING**.

carboprost tromethamine
dinoprostone
methylergonovine maleate
oxytocin, synthetic injection
oxytocin, synthetic nasal
solution

**COMBINATION PRODUCTS**
None.

## carboprost tromethamine
Hemabate

*Pregnancy Risk Category: C*

**HOW SUPPLIED**
*Injection:* 250 mcg/ml

**ACTION**
A prostaglandin that produces strong, prompt contractions of uterine smooth muscle, possibly mediated by calcium and cAMP.

**ONSET, PEAK, DURATION**
Onset unknown. Serum levels peak in 15 to 60 minutes. Average time to abortion, 16 hours; elimination complete in 24 hours.

**INDICATIONS & DOSAGE**
*To abort pregnancy between 13th and 20th weeks of gestation* –
**Adults:** initially, 250 mcg deep I.M. Subsequent doses of 250 mcg administered at intervals of 1½ to 3½ hours, depending on uterine response. Dosage may be increased in increments to 500 mcg if contractility is inadequate after several 250-mcg doses. Total dosage should not exceed 12 mg.
*Postpartum hemorrhage caused by uterine atony not managed by conventional methods* –
**Adults:** 250 mcg by deep I.M. injec-

tion. Repeat doses administered at 15- to 90-minute intervals, as necessary. Maximum total dosage is 2 mg.

**ADVERSE REACTIONS**
**CNS:** headache, anxiety, hot flashes, paresthesia, syncope, weakness.
**CV:** chest pain, arrhythmias.
**EENT:** blurred vision, eye pain.
**GI:** *vomiting, diarrhea, nausea.*
**GU:** endometritis, uterine rupture, uterine or vaginal pain.
**Respiratory:** coughing, wheezing.
**Skin:** flushing, rash.
**Other:** *fever,* chills, backache, breast tenderness, diaphoresis, leg cramps.

**INTERACTIONS**
None significant.

**CONTRAINDICATIONS**
Contraindicated in patients with hypersensitivity to drug, acute pelvic inflammatory disease, or active cardiac, pulmonary, renal, or hepatic disease.

**NURSING CONSIDERATIONS**
• Use cautiously in patients with history of asthma; hypotension; hypertension; CV, adrenal, renal, or hepatic disease; anemia; jaundice; diabetes; seizure disorders; or previous uterine surgery.
• Unlike other prostaglandin abortifacients, carboprost is administered by I.M. injection. Injectable form avoids risk of expelling vaginal suppositories, which may occur in the presence of profuse vaginal bleeding.
• Know that carboprost should be used only by trained personnel in a hospital setting.

---

*Liquid form contains alcohol.  **May contain tartrazine.  †Canada only.  ‡Australia only.  ◇OTC.

☑ **PATIENT TEACHING**
- Explain to patient and family how drug works and how it is administered.
- Instruct patient to report adverse reactions promptly.

---

# dinoprostone
Prepidil, Prostin E₂

*Pregnancy Risk Category: C*

## HOW SUPPLIED
*Vaginal suppositories:* 20 mg
*Endocervical gel:* 0.5 mg per application (2.5-ml syringe)

## ACTION
A prostaglandin that produces strong, prompt contractions of uterine smooth muscle, possibly mediated by calcium and cAMP.

## ONSET, PEAK, DURATION
Onset occurs within 10 minutes for suppositories, 15 to 30 minutes for gel. Peak unknown. Contractions persist for 2 to 6 hours following insertion of suppository. Average time to abortion is 17 hours for suppositories; unknown for gel.

## INDICATIONS & DOSAGE
*To abort second-trimester pregnancy; to evacuate uterus in missed abortion, intrauterine fetal deaths up to 28 weeks of gestation, or benign hydatidiform mole (suppository only) –*
**Adults:** 20-mg suppository inserted high into posterior vaginal fornix. Repeated q 3 to 5 hours until abortion is complete.
*Ripening of an unfavorable cervix in pregnant patients at or near term (gel only) –*
**Adults:** contents of one syringe administered intravaginally; if cervix remains unfavorable after 6 hours, dosage repeated. No more than 1.5 mg (three applications) should be given within 24-hour period.

## ADVERSE REACTIONS
**CNS:** *headache, dizziness,* anxiety, hot flashes, paresthesia, weakness, syncope.
**CV:** chest pain, arrhythmias.
**EENT:** blurred vision, eye pain.
**GI:** *nausea, vomiting, diarrhea.*
**GU:** vaginal pain, vaginitis, endometritis.
**Respiratory:** coughing, dyspnea.
**Skin:** rash.
**Other:** *nocturnal leg cramps, fever, shivering, chills,* backache, breast tenderness, diaphoresis, muscle cramps.

## INTERACTIONS
*Ethanol:* inhibited effectiveness of dinoprostone with high doses. Avoid concomitant use.
*Other oxytocics:* may potentiate action. Avoid concomitant use.

## CONTRAINDICATIONS
The gel form is contraindicated where prolonged contractions of the uterus are considered inappropriate and in patients with hypersensitivity to prostaglandins or constituents of the gel. Also contraindicated in patients with placenta previa or unexplained vaginal bleeding during this pregnancy and in whom vaginal delivery is not indicated (that is, because of vasa previa or active herpes genitalia). The suppository form is contraindicated in patients with hypersensitivity to the drug, acute pelvic inflammatory disease, and active cardiac, pulmonary, renal, or hepatic disease.

## NURSING CONSIDERATIONS
- Use suppository form cautiously in patients with asthma; seizure disorders; anemia; diabetes; hypertension or hypotension; jaundice; CV , renal, or hepatic disease; scarred uterus; cervicitis; or acute vaginitis.
- Use gel form cautiously in patients with asthma or history of asthma, glaucoma or raised intraocular pres-

---

# OXYTOCICS 1179

sure, renal or hepatic dysfunction, and in patients with ruptured membranes.
- Administer only when critical care facilities are available.
- Just before use, warm dinoprostone suppositories in their wrapping to room temperature. After administration, patient should remain supine for 10 minutes.
- When used as an abortifacient, be prepared to pretreat the patient with an antiemetic and an antidiarrheal agent.
- When used for cervical ripening, have the patient lying on her back, with the cervix visualized using a speculum. Assist with insertion: using aseptic technique, catheter provided with the drug is used to administer the gel into the cervical canal just below the level of the internal os.
- Be aware that when gel form is used, contents of the syringe are used for one patient only. Discard the syringe, catheter, and any unused drug after administration; do not attempt to administer the small amount of drug remaining in the catheter.
- Treat dinoprostone-induced fever (self-limiting and transient and occurs in approximately 50% of all patients) with water or alcohol sponging and increased fluid intake, not with aspirin.
- Check vaginal discharge regularly.
- Keep in mind that abortion should be complete within 30 hours when suppository form is used.
- Freeze suppositories at −20° C (−4° F).

☑ **PATIENT TEACHING**
- Explain to patient and family how drug works and how it is administered.
- Instruct patient to report adverse reactions promptly.

---

**methylergonovine maleate**
Methergine

*Pregnancy Risk Category: C*

**HOW SUPPLIED**
*Tablets:* 0.2 mg
*Injection:* 0.2 mg/ml

**ACTION**
Increases motor activity of the uterus by direct stimulation.

**ONSET, PEAK, DURATION**
Onset occurs in 2 to 5 minutes after I.M. use, 5 to 10 minutes after oral use, immediately after I.V. use. Serum levels peak 30 minutes after oral use; unknown for other forms of administration. Effects persist for 3 hours or more after oral or I.M. use; 45 minutes after I.V. administration.

**INDICATIONS & DOSAGE**
*Prevention and treatment of postpartum hemorrhage caused by uterine atony or subinvolution* –
**Adults:** 0.2 mg I.M. q 2 to 4 hours; for excessive uterine bleeding or other emergencies, 0.2 mg I.V. over 1 minute while blood pressure and uterine contractions are monitored. After initial I.M. or I.V. dose, 0.2 mg P.O. q 6 to 8 hours for 2 to 7 days. Dosage decreased if severe cramping occurs.

**ADVERSE REACTIONS**
**CNS:** dizziness, headache, *seizures, CVA* (with I.V. use), hallucinations.
**CV:** hypertension, transient chest pain, palpitations, hypotension.
**EENT:** tinnitus, nasal congestion, foul taste.
**GI:** *nausea, vomiting,* diarrhea.
**GU:** hematuria.
**Respiratory:** dyspnea.
**Other:** diaphoresis, thrombophlebitis, leg cramps.

**INTERACTIONS**
*Dopamine, I.V. oxytocin, regional anesthetics, vasoconstrictors:* excessive vasoconstriction. Use together cautiously.

## CONTRAINDICATIONS
Contraindicated in patients with hypertension, toxemia, or sensitivity to ergot preparations and in pregnant patients.

## NURSING CONSIDERATIONS
• Use cautiously in patients with sepsis, obliterative vascular disease, or hepatic or renal disease and during last stage of labor.
• **Alert: I.V. use:** Keep in mind that drug should not be routinely administered I.V. because of the risk of severe hypertension and CVA. If it must be given by this route, administer slowly over 1 minute with careful blood pressure monitoring. I.V. dose may be diluted to 5 ml with 0.9% sodium chloride solution prior to administration. Contractions begin immediately after I.V. use and continue for up to 45 minutes.
• Monitor and record blood pressure, pulse rate, and uterine response; report any sudden change in vital signs, frequent periods of uterine relaxation, and character and amount of vaginal bleeding.
• Monitor contractions which may continue 3 hours or more after P.O. or I.M. administration.
• Store tablets in tightly closed, light-resistant containers. Discard if discolored.
• Store I.V. solutions below 8° C (46.4° F). Daily stock may be kept at room temperature for 60 to 90 days.

## ☑ PATIENT TEACHING
• Explain to patient and family how drug works and how it is administered.
• Instruct patient to report adverse reactions promptly.

# oxytocin, synthetic injection
Oxytocin, Pitocin, Syntocinon

*Pregnancy Risk Category: NR*

## HOW SUPPLIED
*Injection:* 10 units/ml ampule, vial, or tubex

## ACTION
Causes potent and selective stimulation of uterine and mammary gland smooth muscle.

## ONSET, PEAK, DURATION
Onset occurs 3 to 5 minutes after I.M. use, immediately after I.V. use. Peak unknown. Effects persist 1 hour after I.V. use, 2 to 3 hours after I.M. use.

## INDICATIONS & DOSAGE
*Induction or stimulation of labor –*
**Adults:** initially, 1-ml (10 units) ampule in 1,000 ml of dextrose 5% injection or 0.9% sodium chloride solution I.V. infused at 1 to 2 milliunits/minute. Rate increased in increments of no more than 1 to 2 milliunits/minute at 15- to 30-minute intervals until normal contraction pattern is established. Rate decreased when labor is firmly established.
*Reduction of postpartum bleeding after expulsion of placenta –*
**Adults:** 10 to 40 units added to 1,000 ml of $D_5W$ or 0.9% sodium chloride solution infused at rate necessary to control bleeding, usually 20 to 40 milliunits/minute. Also, 1 ml (10 units) can be given I.M. after delivery of the placenta.
*Incomplete or inevitable abortion –*
**Adults:** 10 units of oxytocin I.V. in 500 ml of 0.9% sodium chloride solution or dextrose 5% in 0.9% sodium chloride solution. Infuse at rate of 20 to 40 drops/minute.

---

Reactions may be *common*, uncommon, *life-threatening*, or COMMON AND LIFE-THREATENING.

## ADVERSE REACTIONS
*Maternal* –
**CNS: *subarachnoid hemorrhage***
(from hypertension); ***seizures or coma***
(from water intoxication).
**CV: *hypertension;*** increased heart
rate, systemic venous return, and cardiac output; ***arrhythmias.***
**GI:** nausea, vomiting.
**Hematologic: *afibrinogenemia*** (may
be related to postpartum bleeding).
**Other:** hypersensitivity reactions
*(anaphylaxis),* tetanic uterine contractions, ***abruptio placentae, im-***
***paired uterine blood flow,*** pelvic hematoma, ***increased uterine motility,***
***uterine rupture, postpartum hemor-***
***rhage.***
*Fetal* –
**CV:** bradycardia, ***PVCs,*** arrhythmias.
**Respiratory: *anoxia, asphyxia.***
**Other: *infant brain damage.***

## INTERACTIONS
*Cyclopropane anesthetics:* less pronounced bradycardia and hypotension. Use together cautiously.
*Thiopental anesthetics:* possible delayed induction. Use together cautiously.
*Vasoconstrictors:* severe hypertension
if oxytocin is given within 3 to 4
hours of vasoconstrictor in patients
receiving caudal block anesthetic.
Avoid concomitant use.

## CONTRAINDICATIONS
Contraindicated when cephalopelvic
disproportion is present or when delivery requires conversion, as in
transverse lie; in fetal distress when
delivery isn't imminent, prematurity,
and other obstetric emergencies; and
in patients with severe toxemia, hypertonic uterine patterns, hypersensitivity to drug, total placenta previa,
and vasoprevia.

## NURSING CONSIDERATIONS
● Use with extreme caution during
first and second stages of labor because cervical laceration, uterine rupture, and maternal and fetal death
have been reported.
● Use with extreme caution, if at all,
in patients with history of cervical or
uterine surgery (including cesarean
section), grand multiparity, uterine
sepsis, traumatic delivery, or overdis-
tended uterus and in invasive cervical
cancer.
● **I.V. use:** Don't give by I.V. bolus injection. Administer by infusion only;
give by piggyback infusion so the
drug may be discontinued without interrupting the I.V. line. Use an infusion pump.
● Know that drug is not recommended
for routine I.M. use. However, 10
units may be given I.M. after delivery
of placenta to control postpartum
uterine bleeding.
● Never give oxytocin simultaneously
by more than one route.
● Be aware that drug is used to induce
or reinforce labor only when pelvis is
known to be adequate, when vaginal
delivery is indicated, when fetal ma-
turity is assured, and when fetal position is favorable. Should be used only
in hospital where critical care facilities and doctor are immediately available.
● Monitor fluid intake and output.
Antidiuretic effect may lead to fluid
overload, seizures, and coma.
● Monitor and record uterine contractions, heart rate, blood pressure, intrauterine pressure, fetal heart rate,
and character of blood loss every 15
minutes.
● Have magnesium sulfate (20% solution) available for relaxation of the
myometrium.
● If contractions occur less than 2
minutes apart and if contractions
above 50 mm Hg are recorded, or if
contractions last 90 seconds or longer,

---

*Liquid form contains alcohol.    **May contain tartrazine.    †Canada only.    ‡Australia only.    ◊OTC.

stop infusion, turn the patient on her side, and notify the doctor.
● Oxytocin is not known to present a risk of fetal abnormalities when used as indicated.

☑ **PATIENT TEACHING**
● Explain to patient and family how drug works and how it is administered.
● Instruct patient to report adverse reactions promptly.

---

# oxytocin, synthetic nasal solution
Syntocinon

*Pregnancy Risk Category: X*

**HOW SUPPLIED**
*Nasal solution:* 40 units/ml

**ACTION**
Stimulates smooth muscle to facilitate ejection of milk from breasts.

**ONSET, PEAK, DURATION**
Onset occurs within a few minutes. Peak unknown. Effects persist for 20 minutes.

**INDICATIONS & DOSAGE**
*Promotion of initial milk ejection –*
**Adults:** 1 spray into one or both nostrils 2 or 3 minutes before breast-feeding or pumping breasts.

**ADVERSE REACTIONS**
**EENT:** nasal irritation, rhinorrhea, lacrimation.
**Other:** uterine bleeding, uterine contractions.

**INTERACTIONS**
None significant.

**CONTRAINDICATIONS**
Contraindicated in patients with hypersensitivity to the drug and during pregnancy.

**NURSING CONSIDERATIONS**
● Inspect nasal cavity for signs of irritation.

☑ **PATIENT TEACHING**
● Teach patient how to administer drug. Instruct her to clear nasal passages first, then hold her head in a vertical position and, holding squeeze bottle upright, eject solution into nostril.
● Inform patient of adverse reactions associated with drug and to notify doctor if severe.

---

# 95

## Spasmolytics

**flavoxate hydrochloride**
**oxybutynin chloride**
**phenazopyridine hydrochloride**

**COMBINATION PRODUCTS**
None.

---

## flavoxate hydrochloride
Urispas

*Pregnancy Risk Category: B*

**HOW SUPPLIED**
*Tablets:* 100 mg

**ACTION**
Produces direct spasmolytic effect on smooth muscles of the urinary tract and provides some local anesthesia and analgesia.

**ONSET, PEAK, DURATION**
Onset and duration unknown. Levels peak within 2 hours.

**INDICATIONS & DOSAGE**
*Symptomatic relief of dysuria, urinary frequency and urgency, nocturia, incontinence, and suprapubic pain associated with urologic disorders –*
**Adults and children over 12 years:**
100 to 200 mg P.O. t.i.d. to q.i.d. Dosage may be reduced with improvement of symptoms.

**ADVERSE REACTIONS**
**CNS:** *confusion* (especially in elderly patients), nervousness, dizziness, headache, drowsiness.
**CV:** tachycardia, palpitations.
**EENT:** *blurred vision,* disturbed eye accommodation, increased ocular tension.
**GI:** dry mouth, nausea, vomiting.
**GU:** dysuria.

**Hematologic:** eosinophila, leukopenia.
**Skin:** urticaria, dermatoses.
**Other:** fever.

**INTERACTIONS**
None significant.

**CONTRAINDICATIONS**
Contraindicated in patients with pyloric or duodenal obstruction, obstructive intestinal lesions or ileus, achalasia, GI hemorrhage, or obstructive uropathies of lower urinary tract.

**NURSING CONSIDERATIONS**
• Use cautiously in patients suspected of having glaucoma.
• Know that safety and effectiveness in children 12 years and under is unknown.
• Check history for other drug use before giving drugs with anticholinergic adverse reactions. Such reactions may be intensified by flavoxate.

☑ **PATIENT TEACHING**
• Warn patient to avoid hazardous activities, such as operating machinery or driving, until CNS effects of the drug are known.
• Tell patient to contact the doctor if he experiences adverse reactions to the drug or if symptoms don't diminish.

---

## oxybutynin chloride
Ditropan

*Pregnancy Risk Category: B*

**HOW SUPPLIED**
*Tablets:* 5 mg
*Syrup:* 5 mg/5 ml

---

## ACTION
Produces a direct spasmolytic effect and an antimuscarinic (atropine-like) effect on urinary tract smooth muscles, increasing urinary bladder capacity and providing some local anesthesia and mild analgesia.

## ONSET, PEAK, DURATION
Onset occurs in 30 to 60 minutes. Levels peak within 3 to 4 hours. Effects persist for 6 to 10 hours.

## INDICATIONS & DOSAGE
*Antispasmodic for uninhibited or reflex neurogenic bladder–*
**Adults:** 5 mg P.O. b.i.d. to t.i.d., to maximum of 5 mg q.i.d.
**Children over 5 years:** 5 mg P.O. b.i.d., to maximum of 5 mg t.i.d.

## ADVERSE REACTIONS
**CNS:** dizziness, insomnia. restlessness, hallucinations, asthenia.
**CV:** *palpitations, tachycardia,* vasodilation.
**EENT:** mydriasis, cycloplegia, decreased lacrimation, amblyopia.
**GI:** nausea, vomiting, *constipation, dry mouth,* decreased GI motility.
**GU:** *urinary hesitancy or urine retention.*
**Skin:** rash.
**Other:** decreased diaphoresis, fever, suppression of lactation.

## INTERACTIONS
None significant.

## CONTRAINDICATIONS
Contraindicated in patients with hypersensitivity to drug, myasthenia gravis, GI obstruction, glaucoma, adynamic ileus, megacolon, severe colitis, ulcerative colitis when megacolon is present, or obstructive uropathy; in elderly or debilitated patients with intestinal atony; and in hemorrhaging patients with unstable CV status.

## NURSING CONSIDERATIONS
• Use cautiously in elderly patients and in patients with autonomic neuropathy, reflux esophagitis, and hepatic or renal disease.
• Before giving oxybutynin, anticipate confirmation of neurogenic bladder by cystometry and rule out partial intestinal obstruction in patients with diarrhea, especially those with colostomy or ileostomy.
• If urinary tract infection is present, administer antibiotics, as ordered.
• Be aware that drug may aggravate symptoms of hyperthyroidism, coronary artery disease, CHF, arrhythmias, tachycardia, hypertension, or prostatic hyperplasia.
• Periodically prepare patient for cystometry to evaluate response to therapy.
• To minimize tendency toward tolerance, be prepared to stop therapy periodically to determine tolerance.

## ☑ PATIENT TEACHING
• Warn patient to avoid hazardous activities, such as operating machinery or driving, until CNS effects of the drug are known.
• Caution patient that using oxybutynin during very hot weather may precipitate fever or heatstroke because it suppresses diaphoresis.
• Advise patient to store the drug in tightly closed containers at 59° to 86° F (15° to 30° C).

---

Reactions may be *common,* uncommon, *life-threatening,* or COMMON AND LIFE-THREATENING.

# phenazopyridine hydrochloride (phenylazo diamino pyridine hydrochloride)

Azo-Standard◇, Baridium◇, Di-Azo◇, Eridium◇, Geridium◇, Phenazo†, Phenazodine◇, Prodium◇, Pyrazodine◇, Pyridiate◇, Pyridin◇, Pyridium, Pyronium†, Urodine◇, Urogesic◇, Viridium◇

*Pregnancy Risk Category: B*

## HOW SUPPLIED
*Tablets:* 100 mg◇, 200 mg

## ACTION
Unknown. Exerts local anesthetic action on urinary mucosa through unknown mechanism.

## ONSET, PEAK, DURATION
Unknown.

## INDICATIONS & DOSAGE
*Pain with urinary tract irritation or infection –*
**Adults:** 200 mg P.O. t.i.d. after meals
**Children:** 12 mg/kg P.O. daily in 3 equally divided doses after meals.

## ADVERSE REACTIONS
**CNS:** headache.
**GI:** nausea, GI disturbances.
**Hematologic:** hemolytic anemia.
**Skin:** rash, pruritus.
**Other:** anaphylactoid reactions, methemoglobinemia.

## INTERACTIONS
None significant.

## CONTRAINDICATIONS
Contraindicated in patients with hypersenstivity to drug, glomerulonephritis, severe hepatitis, uremia, pyelonephritis during pregnancy, or renal insufficiency.

## NURSING CONSIDERATIONS
• Know that when drug is used with an antibacterial agent, therapy should not extend beyond 2 days.

## ☑ PATIENT TEACHING
• Advise patient that taking the drug with meals may minimize GI distress.
• Caution patient to stop taking drug and to notify the doctor immediately if skin or sclera becomes yellow-tinged. These signs may indicate drug accumulation caused by impaired renal excretion.
• Alert patient that drug colors urine red or orange. May stain fabrics or contact lenses.
• Tell diabetic patient that drug may alter Clinistix or Tes-Tape results. He should use Clinitest for accurate urine glucose test results. Also tell patient drug may interfere with urinary ketone tests (Acetest or Ketostix).

---

*Liquid form contains alcohol. **May contain tartrazine. †Canada only. ‡Australia only. ◇OTC.

auranofin
aurothioglucose
gold sodium thiomalate

## COMBINATION PRODUCTS
None.

## auranofin
Ridaura

*Pregnancy Risk Category: C*

## HOW SUPPLIED
*Capsules:* 3 mg

## ACTION
Unknown. Anti-inflammatory effects in rheumatoid arthritis are probably caused by inhibition of sulfhydryl systems, which alters cellular metabolism. Auranofin may also alter enzyme function and immune response and suppress phagocytic activity.

## ONSET, PEAK, DURATION
Onset occurs in 1 to 3 months, possibly 6 months. Serum levels peak within 2 hours. Effects may last for months after drug is discontinued.

## INDICATIONS & DOSAGE
*Rheumatoid arthritis –*
**Adults:** 6 mg P.O. daily, either as 3 mg b.i.d. or 6 mg once daily. After 6 months, may be increased to 9 mg daily.

## ADVERSE REACTIONS
**CNS:** confusion, hallucinations, *seizures.*
**EENT:** conjunctivitis.
**GI:** *diarrhea, abdominal pain, nausea, stomatitis,* glossitis, anorexia, metallic taste, dyspepsia, flatulence, constipation, dysgeusia, *ulcerative colitis.*
**GU:** proteinuria, hematuria, nephrotic syndrome, glomerulonephritis, *acute renal failure.*
**Hematologic:** *thrombocytopenia* (with or without purpura), *aplastic anemia, agranulocytosis,* leukopenia, eosinophilia, anemia.
**Hepatic:** jaundice, elevated liver enzymes.
**Respiratory:** interstitial pneumonitis.
**Skin:** *rash, pruritus, dermatitis, exfoliative dermatitis,* urticaria, erythema, alopecia.

## INTERACTIONS
*Phenytoin:* may increase phenytoin blood levels. Monitor for toxicity.

## CONTRAINDICATIONS
Contraindicated in patients with history of severe gold toxicity, necrotizing enterocolitis, pulmonary fibrosis, exfoliative dermatitis, bone marrow aplasia, severe hematologic disorders or history of severe toxicity caused by previous exposure to other heavy metals. Also contraindicated in patients with urticaria, eczema, colitis, severe debilitation, hemorrhagic conditions, or systemic lupus erythematosus and in patients who have recently received radiation therapy.

## NURSING CONSIDERATIONS
● Use cautiously with other drugs that cause blood dyscrasias. Also use cautiously in patients who have preexisting renal, hepatic, or inflammatory bowel disease; skin rash; or a history of bone marrow depression.
● Monitor patient's platelet count monthly. Auranofin should be stopped if platelet count falls below 100,000/mm$^3$, if hemoglobin drops suddenly, if granulocytes are below 1,500/mm$^3$, or if leukopenia (WBC count below 4,000/mm$^3$) or eosinophilia (eosinophils greater than 75%) is present.

---

Reactions may be *common,* uncommon, *life-threatening,* or COMMON AND LIFE-THREATENING.

• Monitor patient's urinalysis results. If proteinuria or hematuria is detected, stop drug because it can cause nephrotic syndrome or glomerulonephritis, and notify doctor.

### ☑ PATIENT TEACHING
• Encourage patient to take drug as prescribed.
• Tell patient to continue concomitant drug therapy if prescribed.
• Remind patient to see the doctor for monthly platelet counts.
• Suggest patient have regular urinalysis.
• Tell patient to keep taking drug if mild diarrhea occurs but to immediately report blood in stool. Diarrhea is the most common adverse reaction.
• Advise patient to report rashes or other skin problems and stop drug until reaction subsides. Pruritus may precede dermatitis; any pruritic skin eruption while patient is receiving auranofin should be considered a reaction until proven otherwise.
• Advise patient that stomatitis may be preceded by a metallic taste, which he should report. Promote careful oral hygiene during therapy.
• Inform patient that beneficial effect may be delayed as long as 3 months. If response is inadequate and maximum dose has been reached, expect the doctor to discontinue drug.
• Warn patient not to give the drug to others. Auranofin should be prescribed only for selected rheumatoid arthritis patients.

---

## aurothioglucose
Gold-50‡, Solganal

## gold sodium thiomalate
Myochrysine

*Pregnancy Risk Category: C*

### HOW SUPPLIED
**aurothioglucose**
*Injection (suspension):* 50 mg/ml in sesame oil in 10-ml vial

**gold sodium thiomalate**
*Injection:* 25 mg/ml, 50 mg/ml with benzyl alcohol

### ACTION
Unknown. Anti-inflammatory effects in rheumatoid arthritis are probably caused by inhibition of sulfhydryl systems, which alters cellular metabolism. Gold salts may also alter enzyme function and immune response and suppress phagocytic activity.

### ONSET, PEAK, DURATION
Onset and duration unknown. Serum levels peak within 3 to 6 hours.

### INDICATIONS & DOSAGE
*Rheumatoid arthritis –*
**aurothioglucose**
**Adults:** initially, 10 mg I.M., followed by 25 mg for second and third doses at weekly intervals. Then, 50 mg weekly until 1 g has been given. If improvement occurs without toxicity, 25 to 50 mg is continued at 3- to 4-week intervals indefinitely.
**Children 6 to 12 years:** one-fourth the usual adult dosage. Or 1 mg/kg I.M. once weekly for 20 weeks.
**gold sodium thiomalate**
**Adults:** initially, 10 mg I.M., followed by 25 mg in 1 week. Then, 25 to 50 mg weekly until 14 to 20 doses have been given. If improvement occurs without toxicity, 25 to 50 mg q 2 weeks for four doses; then, 25 to 50 mg q 3 weeks for four doses; then, 25 to 50 mg every month indefinitely as maintenance therapy. If relapse occurs during maintenance therapy, injections are resumed at weekly intervals.
**Children:** initially, 10 mg I.M., followed by 1 mg/kg I.M. weekly for 20 weeks. If response is good, may be given q 3 to 4 weeks indefinitely.

### ADVERSE REACTIONS
**CNS:** confusion, hallucinations, *seizures.*
**CV:** bradycardia, hypotension.

---

**EENT:** corneal gold deposition, corneal ulcers.

**GI:** *metallic taste, stomatitis, diarrhea,* anorexia, abdominal cramp, nausea, vomiting, ulcerative enterocolitis.

**GU:** albuminuria, proteinuria, ***nephrotic syndrome,*** nephritis, acute tubular necrosis, hematuria, ***acute renal failure.***

**Hematologic:** *thrombocytopenia* (with or without purpura), *aplastic anemia, agranulocytosis,* leukopenia, eosinophilia, anemia.

**Hepatic:** hepatitis, jaundice, elevated liver function tests.

**Skin:** photosensitivity, *rash, dermatitis,* erythema, exfoliative dermatitis.

**Other:** *anaphylaxis, angioedema,* diaphoresis.

**INTERACTIONS**
None significant.

**CONTRAINDICATIONS**
Contraindicated in patients with hypersensitivity to the drug; in those with a history of severe toxicity from previous exposure to gold or other heavy metals, hepatitis, or exfoliative dermatitis; and in patients with severe uncontrollable diabetes, renal disease, hepatic dysfunction, uncontrolled heart failure, systemic lupus erythematosus, colitis, or Sjögren's syndrome. Also contraindicated in patients with urticaria, eczema, hemorrhagic conditions, or severe hematologic disorders and in those who have recently received radiation therapy.

**NURSING CONSIDERATIONS**
● Use with extreme caution, if at all, in patients with rash, marked hypertension, compromised cerebral or CV circulation, or history of renal or hepatic disease, drug allergies, or blood dyscrasias.
● Give only under constant supervision of doctor thoroughly familiar with drug's toxicities and benefits.
● Give all gold salts I.M., as ordered, preferably intragluteally. Drug is pale yellow; don't use if it darkens.
● Immerse aurothioglucose (a suspen-

sion) vial in warm water, and shake vigorously before injecting.
● When giving gold sodium thiomalate, have patients lie down and stay down for 10 to 20 minutes after injection to minimize hypotension.
● Watch for anaphylactoid reaction for 30 minutes after administration.
● *Alert:* Keep dimercaprol on hand to treat acute toxicity.
● Analyze urine for protein and sediment changes before each injection.
● Monitor CBC, including platelet count, before every second injection.
● Monitor platelet counts if patients develop purpura or ecchymoses.
● Know that gold therapy may alter liver function studies.
● Most adverse reactions are readily reversible if drug is stopped at once.
● If adverse reactions are mild, some rheumatologists resume gold therapy after 2 to 3 weeks' rest.

☑ **PATIENT TEACHING**
● Advise patient that increased joint pain may occur for 1 to 2 days after injection but usually subsides.
● Advise patient to report rashes or skin problems and stop drug until reaction subsides. Pruritus may precede dermatitis; any pruritic skin eruption while patient is receiving gold therapy should be considered a reaction until proven otherwise.
● Advise patient that stomatitis may be preceded by a metallic taste, which he should report. Promote careful oral hygiene during therapy.
● Tell patient to avoid sunlight and artificial ultraviolet light to minimize the risk of photosensitivity.
● Tell patient that benefits may not appear for 3 to 4 months.
● Stress need for close medical follow-up and blood and urine tests.

---

Reactions may be *common,* uncommon, *life-threatening,* or COMMON AND LIFE-THREATENING.

activated charcoal
aminocaproic acid
ammonia, aromatic spirits
deferoxamine mesylate
digoxin immune FAB
dimercaprol
disulfiram
D-penicillamine
edetate calcium disodium
edetate disodium
flumazenil
ipecac syrup
nalmefene hydrochloride
naloxone hydrochloride
naltrexone hydrochloride
pralidoxime chloride
protamine sulfate
sodium polystyrene sulfonate
succimer
trientine hydrochloride

(See also Chapter 38, ANTICHOLINERGICS.)
(See also Chapter 40, ADRENERGIC
   BLOCKERS [SYMPATHOLYTICS].)

**COMBINATION PRODUCTS**
None.

## activated charcoal
Actidose◇, Actidose-Aqua◇,
Charcoaide◇, Charcocaps◇, Liqui-
Char◇, Superchar◇

*Pregnancy Risk Category: NR*

### HOW SUPPLIED
*Tablets:* 200 mg‡◇, 300 mg‡◇, 325
mg◇, 650 mg◇
*Capsules:* 260 mg◇
*Powder:* 30 g◇, 50 g◇
*Oral suspension:* 0.625 g/5 ml◇, 0.83
g/5 ml◇, 1 g/5 ml◇, 1.25 g/5 ml◇

### ACTION
An adsorbent that adheres to many
drugs and chemicals, inhibiting their
absorption from the GI tract.

### ONSET, PEAK, DURATION
Onset immediate upon contact. Peak
and duration not applicable because
drug is not absorbed.

### INDICATIONS & DOSAGE
*Flatulence or dyspepsia –*
**Adults:** 600 mg to 5 g P.O. as a single
dose or 0.975 mg to 3.9 g P.O. t.i.d.
after meals.
*Poisoning –*
**Adults:** initially, 1 g/kg (30 to 100 g)
P.O. or 5 to 10 times the amount of
poison ingested as a suspension in 180
to 240 ml (6 to 8 oz) of water.
**Children:** 5 to 10 times estimated
weight of drug or chemical ingested.
Minimum dose is 30 g P.O. in 240 ml
of water to make a slurry. Given preferably within 30 minutes of poisoning. Larger dose is necessary if food
is in the stomach.

   Commonly used for treating poisoning or overdosage with acetaminophen, aspirin, atropine, barbiturates,
dextropropoxyphene, digitalis glycosides, poisonous mushrooms, oxalic
acid, parathion, phenol, phenylpropanolamine, phenytoin, propantheline,
propoxyphene, strychnine, or tricyclic antidepressants.

   Check with poison control center
for use in other types of poisonings or
overdoses.

### ADVERSE REACTIONS
**GI:** black stools, nausea, constipation.

---

*Liquid form contains alcohol.   **May contain tartrazine.   †Canada only.   ‡Australia only.   ◇OTC.

## INTERACTIONS

*Acetylcysteine, ipecac:* render charcoal ineffective. Don't administer together, or lavage stomach until all charcoal is removed.

## CONTRAINDICATIONS

None known.

## NURSING CONSIDERATIONS

• Know that although there are no contraindications for the drug, it is not effective in the treatment of all acute poisonings.
• Give after emesis is complete because activated charcoal absorbs and inactivates syrup of ipecac.
• Mix powder form (most effective) with tap water to form consistency of thick syrup. Adding a small amount of fruit juice or flavoring will make mix more palatable. Do not mix with ice cream, milk, or sherbet because these will decrease the absorptive capacity of activated charcoal.
• Give by large bore nasogastric tube after lavage if necessary.
• If patient vomits shortly after administration, be prepared to repeat dose.
• Space doses at least 1 hour apart from other drugs if treatment is for any indication other than poisoning.
• Follow treatment with stool softener or laxative, as ordered, to prevent constipation unless sorbitol is part of product ingredients.
• Be aware that preparations made with sorbitol have a laxative effect that lessens the risk of severe constipation or fecal impaction.

## ☑ PATIENT TEACHING

• Explain to patient (if awake) and family purpose of drug and how it will be administered.
• Warn patient that stools will be black.

# aminocaproic acid
Amicar
*Pregnancy Risk Category: C*

## HOW SUPPLIED

*Tablets:* 500 mg
*Syrup:* 250 mg/ml
*Injection:* 250 mg/ml

## ACTION

Inhibits plasminogen activator substances and, to a lesser degree, blocks antiplasmin activity by inhibiting fibrinolysis.

## ONSET, PEAK, DURATION

Onset occurs within 1 hour. Levels peak within 2 hours after oral administration; unknown after I.V. administration. Effects persist for less than 3 hours after I.V. administration, unknown for oral administration.

## INDICATIONS & DOSAGE

*Excessive bleeding resulting from hyperfibrinolysis –*
**Adults:** initially, 5 g P.O. or slow I.V. infusion, followed by 1 to 1.25 g hourly until bleeding is controlled. Maximum dosage is 30 g daily.

## ADVERSE REACTIONS

**CNS:** dizziness, malaise, headache, delirium, *seizures,* hallucinations, weakness.
**CV:** hypotension, bradycardia, *arrhythmias* (with rapid I.V. infusion).
**EENT:** tinnitus, nasal congestion, conjunctival suffusion.
**GI:** nausea, cramps, diarrhea.
**Hematologic:** generalized thrombosis.
**Skin:** rash.
**Other:** malaise, myopathy, *acute renal failure.*

## INTERACTIONS

*Estrogens, oral contraceptives:* increased probability of hypercoagulability. Use together cautiously.

---

Reactions may be *common,* uncommon, *life-threatening,* or COMMON AND LIFE-THREATENING.

## CONTRAINDICATIONS

Contraindicated in patients with active intravascular clotting or presence of disseminated intravascular coagulation unless heparin is used concomitantly. Injectable form is contraindicated in newborns.

## NURSING CONSIDERATIONS

• Use cautiously in patients with cardiac, hepatic, or renal disease.
• **I.V. use:** Dilute solution with sterile water for injection, 0.9% sodium chloride for injection, $D_5W$, or Ringer's injection. Infuse slowly. Don't give by direct or intermittent injection.
• **Alert:** Monitor coagulation studies as ordered and heart rhythm and blood pressure. Notify the doctor of any change immediately.

☑ **PATIENT TEACHING**
• Explain drug use and how it will be administered to patient and family.
• Instruct patient to report adverse reactions promptly.

## ammonia, aromatic spirits◊

Pregnancy Risk Category: NR

**HOW SUPPLIED**
*Solution:* 30 ml◊, 60 ml◊, 120 ml◊; pints◊; gallons◊
*Inhalant:* 0.33 ml◊, 0.4 ml◊

**ACTION**
Irritates the sensory receptors in the nasal membranes, producing reflex stimulation of the respiratory centers.

**ONSET, PEAK, DURATION**
Onset immediate. Peak and duration unknown.

**INDICATIONS & DOSAGE**
*Treatment or prevention of fainting –*
**Adults and children:** inhaled as 2 to 4 ml P.O., diluted in at least 30 ml of water, p.r.n.

## ADVERSE REACTIONS
**EENT:** irritation.

## INTERACTIONS
None significant.

## CONTRAINDICATIONS
None known.

## NURSING CONSIDERATIONS
• Avoid inhaling vapors when administering drug.
• Monitor patient closely for response.

☑ **PATIENT TEACHING**
• Instruct patient how to use drug.
• Tell patient to store in refrigerator.

---

## deferoxamine mesylate
Desferal

Pregnancy Risk Category: C

**HOW SUPPLIED**
*Powder for injection:* 500 mg

**ACTION**
Chelates iron by binding ferric ions.

**ONSET, PEAK, DURATION**
Unknown.

**INDICATIONS & DOSAGE**
*Adjunctive treatment of acute iron intoxication –*
**Adults and children:** 1 g I.M. or I.V., followed by 500 mg I.M. or I.V. for two doses q 4 hours; then 500 mg I.M. or I.V. q 4 to 12 hours. Maximum dosage is 6 g in 24 hours.
*Chronic iron overload from multiple transfusions –*
**Adults and children:** 500 mg to 1 g I.M. daily and 2 g by slow I.V. infusion in separate solution along with each unit of blood transfused. Maximum dosage is 6 g daily. Alternatively, 20 to 40 mg/kg via S.C. infusion pump daily.

---

## ADVERSE REACTIONS
**CV:** tachycardia with long-term use.
**EENT:** blurred vision, cataracts, hearing loss.
**GI:** diarrhea and abdominal discomfort with long-term use.
**GU:** dysuria with long-term use.
**Other:** hypersensitivity reactions (cutaneous wheal formation, pruritus, rash, *anaphylaxis*); pain and induration at injection site; leg cramps, fever; after too-rapid I.V. administration—*erythema, urticaria, hypotension, shock*.

## INTERACTIONS
*Ascorbic acid:* may enhance the effects of deferoxamine and increase tissue toxicity of iron. Use together with extreme caution and close monitoring.

## CONTRAINDICATIONS
Contraindicated in patients with severe renal disease or anuria.

## NURSING CONSIDERATIONS
• Use cautiously in patients with impaired renal function.
• To reconstitute, add 2 ml of sterile water for injection to each ampule. Make sure drug is completely dissolved. Reconstituted solution is good for 1 week at room temperature. Protect from light.
• After reconstitution, administer I.M. or add to 0.9% sodium chloride solution, D$_5$W, or lactated Ringer's solution and infuse at a rate not exceeding 15 mg/kg hourly.
• Have epinephrine 1:1,000 available to treat hypersensitivity reaction.
• Monitor fluid intake and output carefully.

## ☑ PATIENT TEACHING
• Warn patient that urine may be red. Tell patient to report persistent or serious adverse reactions promptly.
• Advise patient to have regular eye examinations during long-term therapy because cataract formation has been reported.

---

# digoxin immune FAB (ovine)
Digibind
*Pregnancy Risk Category: C*

## HOW SUPPLIED
*Injection:* 40-mg vial

## ACTION
Binds molecules of unbound digoxin and digitoxin, making them unavailable for binding at site of action on cells.

## ONSET, PEAK, DURATION
Onset variable but thought to occur within 30 minutes. Peak occurs at completion of I.V. infusion. Effects persist for 2 to 6 hours.

## INDICATIONS & DOSAGE
*Potentially life-threatening digoxin or digitoxin intoxication—*
**Adults and children:** I.V. dosage varies according to the amount of digoxin or digitoxin to be neutralized. Each vial binds about 0.6 mg of digoxin or digitoxin. Average dosage is 6 vials (240 mg). However, if the toxicity resulted from acute digoxin ingestion and neither a serum digoxin level nor an estimated ingestion amount is known, 20 vials (800 mg) may be required. See package insert for complete, specific dosage instructions.

## ADVERSE REACTIONS
**CV:** *CHF* and rapid ventricular rate (both caused by reversal of the digitalis glycoside's therapeutic effects).
**Other:** hypersensitivity reactions, hypokalemia, *anaphylaxis*.

## INTERACTIONS
None significant.

---

Reactions may be *common*, uncommon, *life-threatening*, or COMMON AND LIFE-THREATENING.

## CONTRAINDICATIONS
None known.

## NURSING CONSIDERATIONS
• Use cautiously in patients known to be allergic to ovine proteins. In these high-risk patients, skin testing is recommended because the drug is derived from digoxin-specific antibody fragments obtained from immunized sheep.

• Know that drug is used only for life-threatening overdose in patients in shock or cardiac arrest; with ventricular arrhythmias, such as ventricular tachycardia or fibrillation; with progressive bradycardia, such as severe sinus bradycardia; or with second- or third-degree AV block not responsive to atropine.

• **I.V. use:** Reconstitute 40-mg vial with 4 ml of sterile water for injection. Gently roll vial to dissolve the powder. Reconstituted solution contains 10 mg/ml. Drug may be given by direct injection if cardiac arrest seems imminent. Alternatively, dilute with 0.9% sodium chloride for injection to an appropriate volume and give by intermittent infusion over 30 minutes.

• Infuse the drug through a 0.22-micron membrane filter.

• Refrigerate powder for injection. Reconstitute drug immediately before use. Reconstituted solutions may be refrigerated for 4 hours.

• Monitor potassium level closely, as ordered.

• Know that in most patients, signs of digitalis toxicity disappear within a few hours.

• Be aware that because drug will interfere with digitalis immunoassay measurements, standard serum digoxin levels will be misleading until drug is cleared from body (about 2 days).

## ☑ PATIENT TEACHING
• Explain need for drug and how drug is administered to patient and family.

• Instruct patient to report adverse reactions promptly.

---

# dimercaprol
BAL in Oil
*Pregnancy Risk Category: NR*

## HOW SUPPLIED
*Injection:* 100 mg/ml

## ACTION
Forms complexes with heavy metals.

## ONSET, PEAK, DURATION
Onset unknown. Levels peak within 30 to 60 minutes. Effects persist for 4 hours.

## INDICATIONS & DOSAGE
*Severe arsenic or gold poisoning –*
**Adults and children:** 3 mg/kg deep I.M. q 4 hours for 2 days, then q.i.d. on 3rd day, then b.i.d. for 10 days.
*Mild arsenic or gold poisoning –*
**Adults and children:** 2.5 mg/kg deep I.M. q.i.d. for 2 days, then b.i.d. on 3rd day, then once daily for 10 days.
*Mercury poisoning –*
**Adults and children:** initially, 5 mg/kg deep I.M., then 2.5 mg/kg daily or b.i.d. for 10 days.
*Acute lead encephalopathy or lead level greater than 100 mcg/ml –*
**Adults and children:** 4 mg/kg deep I.M., then q 4 hours with edetate calcium disodium (250 mg/m² I.M.) for 2 to 7 days. Use separate sites. Maximum dosage is 5 mg/kg per dose.

## ADVERSE REACTIONS
**CNS:** pain or tightness in throat, chest, or hands; headache; paresthesia; muscle pain or weakness, anxiety.
**CV:** *transient increase in blood pressure* (returns to normal in 2 hours), *tachycardia.*
**EENT:** blepharospasm, conjunctivitis, lacrimation, rhinorrhea, excessive salivation.
**GI:** *nausea; vomiting; burning sensa-*

---

*Liquid form contains alcohol.   **May contain tartrazine.   †Canada only.   ‡Australia only.   ◇OTC.

*tion in lips, mouth, and throat; abdominal pain.*
**Other:** *fever* (especially in children).

## INTERACTIONS
*Iron:* toxic metal complex formed; concurrent therapy contraindicated. Wait 24 hours after last dimercaprol dose.
*Iodine 131 uptake thyroid tests:* decreased. Don't schedule patient for this test during course of dimercaprol therapy.

## CONTRAINDICATIONS
Contraindicated in patients with hepatic dysfunction (except postarsenical jaundice).

## NURSING CONSIDERATIONS
• Use cautiously in patients with hypertension or oliguria.
• Know that safe use in pregnancy has not been established and drug should not be used unless judged by doctor to be necessary to treat a life-threatening acute poisoning.
• Don't give I.V.; give by deep I.M. route only.
• Be careful not to let drug come in contact with skin because it may cause a skin reaction.
• Be aware that drug has an unpleasant, garlic-like odor.
• Know that solution with slight sediment is usable.
• Use ephedrine or antihistamine, as ordered, to prevent or relieve mild adverse reactions.
• Keep urine alkaline to prevent renal damage. Oral sodium bicarbonate may be ordered.

## ☑ PATIENT TEACHING
• Explain need for drug and how drug is administered to patient and family.
• Instruct patient to report adverse reactions promptly.

# disulfiram
Antabuse

*Pregnancy Risk Category: NR*

## HOW SUPPLIED
*Tablets:* 250 mg, 500 mg

## ACTION
Blocks oxidation of ethanol at the acetaldehyde stage. Excess acetaldehyde produces a highly unpleasant reaction in the presence of even small amounts of ethanol.

## ONSET, PEAK, DURATION
Onset occurs in 1 to 2 hours. Peak unknown. Effects persist for 14 days after drug discontinuation.

## INDICATIONS & DOSAGE
*Adjunct in management of chronic alcoholism –*
**Adults:** 250 to 500 mg P.O. as a single dose in the morning for 1 to 2 weeks or in evening if drowsiness occurs. Maintenance dosage is 125 to 500 mg P.O. daily (average dosage 250 mg) until permanent self-control is established. Treatment may continue for months or years.

## ADVERSE REACTIONS
**CNS:** drowsiness, headache, fatigue, delirium, depression, neuritis, peripheral neuritis, polyneuritis, restlessness, psychotic reactions.
**EENT:** optic neuritis.
**GI:** metallic or garlic aftertaste.
**GU:** impotence.
**Skin:** acneiform or allergic dermatitis, occasional eruptions.
**Other:** disulfiram reaction (precipitated by ethanol use), which may include flushing, throbbing headache, dyspnea, nausea, copious vomiting, diaphoresis, thirst, chest pain, palpitations, hyperventilation, hypotension, syncope, anxiety, weakness, blurred vision, confusion, arthropathy. *In severe reactions – respiratory*

---

Reactions may be *common,* uncommon, *life-threatening,* or COMMON AND LIFE-THREATENING.

*depression, CV collapse, arrhyth-*
*mias, MI, acute CHF, seizures, un-*
*consciousness, or death.*

## INTERACTIONS
*Alfentanil:* prolonged duration of effect. Closely monitor patient.
*Anticoagulants:* increased anticoagulant effect. Adjust dosage of anticoagulant.
*Bacampicillin:* lowered concentrations of ethanol and acetaldehyde.
*CNS depressants:* increased CNS depression. Use together cautiously.
*Ethanol:* precipitated disulfiram reaction. Do not use concomitantly.
*Isoniazid:* ataxia or marked change in behavior. Do not use concomitantly.
*Metronidazole:* psychotic reaction. Do not use concomitantly.
*Midazolam:* increased plasma levels of midazolam. Use together cautiously.
*Paraldehyde:* toxic levels of acetaldehyde. Do not use concomitantly.
*Phenytoin:* increased blood levels of phenytoin. Monitor phenytoin blood levels, and expect the doctor to adjust phenytoin dosages.
*Tricyclic antidepressants, especially amitriptyline:* transient delirium. Closely monitor the patient.

## CONTRAINDICATIONS
Contraindicated during alcohol intoxication and within 12 hours of alcohol ingestion; in patients with hypersensitivity to disulfiram or to other thiuram derivatives used in pesticides and rubber vulcanization; and in patients with psychoses, myocardial disease, or coronary occlusion; and in patients receiving metronidazole, paraldehyde, alcohol, or alcohol-containing preparations.

## NURSING CONSIDERATIONS
• Know that drug should not be administered during pregnancy.
• Use with extreme caution in patients with diabetes mellitus, hypo-

thyroidism, seizure disorder, cerebral damage, nephritis or hepatic cirrhosis or insufficiency and with concurrent phenytoin therapy.
• Use only under close medical and nursing supervision. Never administer until the patient has abstained from alcohol for at least 12 hours. Patients should clearly understand consequences of disulfiram therapy and give permission for its use. Use drug only in patients who are cooperative, well motivated, and receiving supportive psychiatric therapy.
• Know that complete physical examination and laboratory studies, including CBC, SMA-12, and transaminase level, should precede therapy and be repeated regularly, as ordered.

☑ **PATIENT TEACHING**
• *Alert:* Caution patient's family that disulfiram should never be given to the patient without his knowledge; severe reaction or death could result if patient ingests alcohol.
• Warn patient to avoid all sources of alcohol (for example, sauces and cough syrups). Even external application of liniments, shaving lotion, and back-rub preparations may precipitate disulfiram reaction. Tell patient that alcohol reaction may occur as long as 2 weeks after single dose of disulfiram; the longer patient remains on drug, the more sensitive he becomes to alcohol.
• Tell patient to wear a bracelet or carry a card supplied by drug manufacturer identifying him as disulfiram user. *Note:* Mild reactions may occur in sensitive patient with blood alcohol levels of 5 to 10 mg/100 ml; symptoms are fully developed at 50 mg/100 ml; unconsciousness typically occurs at 125 to 150 mg/100 ml level. Reaction may last from 30 minutes to several hours or as long as alcohol remains in blood.
• Reassure patient that disulfiram-induced adverse reactions (unrelated to

concomitant alcohol use), such as drowsiness, fatigue, impotence, headache, peripheral neuritis, and metallic or garlic taste, subside after about 2 weeks of therapy.

---

# D-penicillamine
Cuprimine, Depen, D-Penamine‡

*Pregnancy Risk Category: NR*

## HOW SUPPLIED
*Tablets:* 125 mg‡, 250 mg
*Capsules:* 125 mg, 250 mg

## ACTION
Chelates heavy metals and may inhibit collagen formation. Unknown for rheumatoid arthritis.

## ONSET, PEAK, DURATION
Onset and duration unknown. Peak levels occur in 1 hour.

## INDICATIONS & DOSAGE
*Wilson's disease –*
**Adults and children:** 250 mg P.O. q.i.d. 30 to 60 minutes before meals. Dosage adjusted to achieve urinary copper excretion of 0.5 to 1 mg daily.
*Cystinuria –*
**Adults:** 250 mg to 1 g P.O. q.i.d. before meals. Dosage adjusted to achieve urinary cystine excretion of less than 100 mg daily when renal calculi are present, or 100 to 200 mg daily when no calculi are present. Maximum dosage is 4 g daily.
**Children:** 30 mg/kg P.O. daily, divided q.i.d. before meals. Dosage adjusted to achieve urinary cystine excretion of less than 100 mg daily when renal calculi are present, or 100 to 200 mg daily when no calculi are present.
*Rheumatoid arthritis –*
**Adults:** initially, 125 to 250 mg P.O. daily, with increases of 125 to 250 mg q 1 to 3 months, if necessary. Maximum dosage is 1.5 g daily.

## ADVERSE REACTIONS
**EENT:** tinnitus, *optic neuritis.*
**GI:** *anorexia, epigastric pain, nausea, vomiting, diarrhea, loss of or altered taste perception, stomatitis.*
**GU: nephrotic syndrome, glomerulonephritis,** proteinuria, hematuria.
**Hematologic:** *leukopenia, eosinophilia,* **thrombocytopenia,** *monocytosis,* **agranulocytosis, aplastic anemia,** lupuslike syndrome.
**Hepatic:** hepatotoxicity.
**Skin:** friability, especially at pressure spots; wrinkling; erythema; urticaria; ecchymoses.
**Other:** hair loss, myasthenia gravis syndrome with long-term use, allergic reactions *(rash, pruritus, fever),* arthralgia, lymphadenopathy, or pneumonitis.

## INTERACTIONS
*Antacids, oral iron:* decreased effectiveness of D-penicillamine. Give at least 2 hours apart.

## CONTRAINDICATIONS
Contraindicated in pregnant patients with cystinuria, in patients with previous penicillamine-related aplastic anemia or granulocytosis, and in rheumatoid arthritis patients with renal insufficiency.

## NURSING CONSIDERATIONS
• Use with extreme caution, if at all, in patients with hypersensitivity to penicillin.
• Give dose on empty stomach to facilitate absorption, preferably 1 hour before or 3 hours after meals.
• Keep in mind patients should receive supplemental pyridoxine daily.
• If patients have a skin reaction, give antihistamines as prescribed. Handle patients carefully to avoid skin damage.
• Monitor CBC and renal and hepatic function every 2 weeks for the first 6 months, then monthly, as ordered.
• Monitor urinalysis regularly for protein loss.

---

Reactions may be *common,* uncommon, *life-threatening,* or COMMON AND LIFE-THREATENING.

- ***Alert:*** Report rash and fever (important signs of toxicity) to the doctor immediately.
- Withhold drug and notify the doctor if WBC count falls below 3,500/mm³ or platelet count falls below 100,000/mm³. A progressive decline in platelet or WBC count in three successive blood tests may necessitate temporary cessation of therapy, even if such counts are within normal limits.

☑ **PATIENT TEACHING**
- Tell patient that therapeutic effect may be delayed up to 3 months in treatment of rheumatoid arthritis.
- Tell patient to take drug on an empty stomach and to maintain adequate fluid intake, especially at night.
- Advise patient to report early signs of granulocytopenia: fever, sore throat, chills, bruising, and prolonged bleeding time.
- Reassure patient that taste impairment usually resolves in 6 weeks without changes in dosage.

---

## edetate calcium disodium
Calcium Disodium Versenate,
Calcium EDTA

*Pregnancy Risk Category: NR*

**HOW SUPPLIED**
*Injection:* 200 mg/ml

**ACTION**
Forms stable, soluble complexes with metals, particularly lead.

**ONSET, PEAK, DURATION**
Onset occurs in 1 hour. Effects peak after 24 to 48 hours. Duration unknown.

**INDICATIONS & DOSAGE**
*Acute lead encephalopathy or blood lead levels above 70 mcg/dl –*
**Adults and children:** 1.5 g/m² I.V. or I.M. daily in divided doses at 12-hour intervals for 3 to 5 days, usually in

conjunction with dimercaprol. A second course may be administered in 5 to 7 days.
*Lead poisoning without encephalopathy or asymptomatic with blood levels greater than 70 mcg/dl –*
**Children:** 1 g/m² I.V. or I.M. daily in divided doses.

**ADVERSE REACTIONS**
**GU:** proteinuria, hematuria; ***nephrotoxicity with renal tubular necrosis leading to fatal nephrosis.***

**INTERACTIONS**
None significant.

**CONTRAINDICATIONS**
Contraindicated in patients with anuria, hepatitis, and acute renal disease.

**NURSING CONSIDERATIONS**
- Use with extreme caution in patients with mild renal disease. Expect dosages to be reduced.
- **I.V. use:** Dilute with D₅W or 0.9% sodium chloride for injection to a concentration of 2 to 4 mg/ml. Infuse one-half of the daily dose over 1 hour in asymptomatic patients or 2 hours in symptomatic patients. Give the rest of the infusion at least 6 hours later. Alternatively, give by slow infusion over at least 8 hours.
- Add procaine hydrochloride, as ordered, to I.M. solution to minimize pain. Watch for local reactions.
- Because I.V. use may increase intracranial pressure, do not administer by that route to treat lead encephalopathy. Give by I.M. route instead.
- Know that I.M. route preferred, especially for children and patients with lead encephalopathy.
- Monitor fluid intake and output, urinalysis, BUN level, and ECGs daily, as ordered.
- To avoid toxicity, use with dimercaprol, as ordered.
- Do not confuse with edetate diso-

dium, which is used to treat hypercalcemia.

☑ **PATIENT TEACHING**
• Explain need for drug and how drug is administered to patient and family.
• Instruct patient to force fluids to facilitate lead excretion (except in patients with lead encephalopathy).

---

## edetate disodium
Disodium EDTA, Disotate, Endrate

*Pregnancy Risk Category: NR*

**HOW SUPPLIED**
*Injection:* 150 mg/ml

**ACTION**
Chelates with metals, such as calcium, to form a stable, soluble complex.

**ONSET, PEAK, DURATION**
Unknown.

**INDICATIONS & DOSAGE**
*Hypercalcemic crisis –*
**Adults:** 50 mg/kg by slow I.V. infusion added to 500 ml of $D_5W$ or 0.9% sodium chloride solution administered over 3 or more hours. Maximum dosage is 3 g/day.
**Children:** 40 to 70 mg/kg by slow I.V. infusion, diluted to a maximum concentration of 30 mg/ml in $D_5W$ or 0.9% sodium chloride solution administered over 3 or more hours. Maximum dosage is 70 mg/kg/day.
*Digitalis-induced cardiac arrhythmias –*
**Adults and children:** 15 mg/kg/hour I.V. with maximum daily dosage 60 mg/kg daily.

**ADVERSE REACTIONS**
**CNS:** circumoral paresthesia, numbness, headache.
**CV:** hypotension.
**EENT:** erythema.
**GI:** nausea, vomiting, diarrhea.

**GU:** in excessive doses – nephrotoxicity with urinary urgency, nocturia, dysuria, polyuria, proteinuria, renal insufficiency, *renal failure, tubular necrosis.*
**Skin:** exfoliative dermatitis.
**Other:** *severe hypocalcemia,* decreased magnesium, pain at site of infusion, thrombophlebitis.

**INTERACTIONS**
None significant.

**CONTRAINDICATIONS**
Contraindicated in patients with hypersensitivity to drug, anuria, known or suspected hypocalcemia, significant renal disease, active or healed tubercular lesions, or history of seizures or intracranial lesions.

**NURSING CONSIDERATIONS**
• Use cautiously in patients with limited cardiac reserve, CHF, or hypokalemia.
• **I.V. use:** Dilute before use. Avoid rapid I.V. infusion; profound hypocalcemia may occur, leading to tetany, seizures, arrhythmias, and respiratory arrest. Not recommended for direct or intermittent injection. Avoid extravasation.
• Record I.V. site used, and avoid repeated use of the same site, which increases likelihood of thrombophlebitis.
• Keep I.V. calcium available to treat hypocalcemia.
• Keep patients in bed for 15 minutes after infusion to avoid orthostatic hypotension. Monitor blood pressure closely.
• Monitor ECG and renal function tests frequently, as ordered.
• Obtain serum calcium after each dose, as ordered.
• If generalized systemic reactions – fever, chills, back pain, emesis, muscle cramps, urinary urgency – occur 4 to 8 hours after infusion, report them to the doctor. Treatment is usually

---

Reactions may be *common,* uncommon, *life-threatening,* or **COMMON AND LIFE-THREATENING.**

supportive. Symptoms generally subside within 12 hours.
• Don't use to treat lead toxicity; know that edetate calcium disodium should be used instead.

### ☑ PATIENT TEACHING
• Explain need for drug and how drug is administered to patient and family.
• Instruct patient to report adverse reactions promptly.

---

## flumazenil
Romazicon

*Pregnancy Risk Category: C*

### HOW SUPPLIED
*Injection:* 0.1 mg/ml in 5- and 10-ml multiple-dose vials

### ACTION
Benzodiazepine antagonist that competitively inhibits the actions of benzodiazepines on the gamma-aminobutyric acid-benzodiazepine receptor complex.

### ONSET, PEAK, DURATION
Onset occurs in 1 to 2 minutes after completion of injection. Peak levels are obtained in 6 to 10 minutes. Duration of drug is related to plasma concentration of the sedating benzodiazepin as well as the dose of flumazenil given.

### INDICATIONS & DOSAGE
*Complete or partial reversal of sedative effects of benzodiazepines after anesthesia or short diagnostic procedures (conscious sedation)* –
**Adults:** initially, 0.2 mg I.V. over 15 seconds. If patient does not reach the desired level of consciousness after 45 seconds, dose is repeated. Repeated at 1-minute intervals until a cumulative dose of 1 mg has been given (initial dose plus four additional doses), if needed. Most patients respond after 0.6 to 1 mg of drug. In case of reseda-

tion, dosage may be repeated after 20 minutes; however, no more than 1 mg should be given at any one time and no more than 3 mg/hour.
*Suspected benzodiazepine overdose* –
**Adults:** initially, 0.2 mg I.V. over 15 seconds. If patient does not reach the desired level of consciousness after 30 seconds, 0.3 mg is administered over 30 seconds. If patient still does not respond adequately, 0.5 mg is administered over 30 seconds; 0.5-mg doses are repeated as needed at 1-minute intervals until a cumulative dose of 3 mg has been given. Most patients suffering from benzodiazepine overdose respond to cumulative doses between 1 and 3 mg; rarely, patients who respond partially after 3 mg may require additional doses. No more than 5 mg over 5 minutes should be given initially. Sedation that persists after this dosage is unlikely to be caused by benzodiazepines. In case of resedation, dosage may be repeated after 20 minutes; however, no more than 1 mg should be given at any one time and no more than 3 mg/hour.

### ADVERSE REACTIONS
**CNS:** *dizziness, abnormal or blurred vision, headache, seizures,* agitation, emotional lability, tremor, insomnia.
**CV:** *arrhythmias,* cutaneous vasodilation, palpitations.
**GI:** *nausea, vomiting.*
**Respiratory:** dyspnea, hyperventilation.
**Other:** *diaphoresis, pain at injection site.*

### INTERACTIONS
*Antidepressants; drugs that can cause seizures or arrhythmias:* seizures or arrhythmias can develop after effect of benzodiazepine overdose is removed. Use flumazenil with caution in cases of mixed overdose.

---

## CONTRAINDICATIONS

Contraindicated in patients hypersensitive to flumazenil or benzodiazepines; in patients who show evidence of serious tricyclic antidepressant overdose; and in those who received benzodiazepine to treat a potentially life-threatening condition (such as status epilepticus).

## NURSING CONSIDERATIONS

● Use cautiously in patients at high risk for developing seizures; patients who have recently received multiple doses of a parenteral benzodiazepine; patients displaying some signs of seizure activity; patients who may be at risk for unrecognized benzodiazepine dependence, such as intensive care unit patients; patients with head injury; psychiatric patients; and alcohol-dependent patients.

● Be aware that safety and efficacy in children have not been established.

● **I.V. use:** Administer by direct injection or dilute with a compatible solution. Discard unused drug that has been drawn into a syringe or diluted within 24 hours.

● Administer drug into an I.V. line in a large vein with a free-flowing I.V. solution to minimize pain at the injection site. Compatible solutions include $D_5W$, lactated Ringer's injection, and 0.9% sodium chloride.

● Monitor patients closely for resedation that may occur after reversal of benzodiazepine effects because flumazenil's duration of action is shorter than that of all benzodiazepines. Duration of monitoring period depends on specific drug being reversed. Monitor closely after long-acting benzodiazepines, such as diazepam, or after high doses of short-acting benzodiazepines, such as 10 mg of midazolam. In most cases, severe resedation is unlikely in patients who fail to show signs of resedation 2 hours after a 1-mg dose of flumazenil.

## ☑ PATIENT TEACHING

● Warn patient not to perform hazardous activities, such as operating heavy equipment or driving, within 24 hours of procedure because of resedation risk.

● Tell patient to avoid alcohol, CNS depressants, and OTC drugs for 24 hours.

● Give family members necessary instructions or provide patient with written instructions. The patient will not recall information given in the postprocedure period because drug does not reverse the amnesic effects of benzodiazepines.

## ipecac syrup

*Pregnancy Risk Category: C*

### HOW SUPPLIED

*Syrup\*:* 70 mg powdered ipecac/ml (contains glycerin 10% and alcohol 1% to 2.5%)

### ACTION

Induces vomiting by acting locally on the gastric mucosa and centrally on the chemoreceptor trigger zone.

### ONSET, PEAK, DURATION

Onset occurs in 20 to 30 minutes. Peak unknown. Effects persist for 20 to 25 minutes.

### INDICATIONS & DOSAGE

*To induce vomiting in poisoning –*
**Adults and children over 12 years:** 30 ml P.O., followed by 200 to 300 ml of water.
**Children 6 months to 1 year:** 5 ml P.O., followed by 100 to 200 ml of water or milk. If necessary, repeat dose once after 20 minutes.
**Children 1 to 12 years:** 15 ml P.O., followed by about 200 ml of water or milk.

---

Reactions may be *common,* uncommon, *life-threatening,* or **COMMON AND LIFE-THREATENING.**

## ADVERSE REACTIONS
**CNS:** depression, *drowsiness.*
**CV:** *arrhythmias,* bradycardia, hypotension, atrial fibrillation or *fatal myocarditis* after ingestion of excessive dose.
**GI:** *diarrhea.*

## INTERACTIONS
*Activated charcoal:* neutralized emetic effect. Don't give together; may give activated charcoal after vomiting.

## CONTRAINDICATIONS
Contraindicated in semicomatose or unconscious patients, or those with severe inebriation, seizures, shock, or loss of gag reflex.

## NURSING CONSIDERATIONS
• Unless advised otherwise by a poison control center, don't give after ingestion of petroleum distillates (for example, kerosene, gasoline) or volatile oils; retching and vomiting may cause aspiration and lead to bronchospasm, pulmonary edema, or aspiration pneumonitis. Vegetable oil will delay absorption of these substances. Don't give after ingestion of caustic substances, such as lye; additional injury to the esophagus and mediastinum can occur.
• Keep in mind that stomach is usually emptied completely; vomitus also may contain some intestinal material.
• If two doses do not induce vomiting, be prepared for gastric lavage.
• Know that ipecac syrup usually induces vomiting within 20 to 30 minutes.
• In antiemetic toxicity, know that ipecac syrup is usually effective if less than 1 hour has passed since ingestion of antiemetic.
• Be aware that no systemic toxicity occurs with doses of 30 ml (1 oz) or less.
• Clearly indicate ipecac *syrup,* not single word "ipecac," to avoid confusion with fluidextract, which is 14 times more concentrated and, if inadvertently used instead of syrup, may cause death. Fluidextract is no longer commercially available in the United States.
• Be aware that ipecac syrup is now commonly abused by bulimics who binge and then purge.

## ☑ PATIENT TEACHING
• Recommend to parents that 1 oz (30 ml) of syrup be available in the home when child becomes 1 year old for immediate use in case of emergency.
• Instruct parents how to administer the drug and what to do in case of accidental poisoning.

---

# nalmefene hydrochloride
Revex
*Pregnancy Risk Category: B*

## HOW SUPPLIED
*Injection:* 100 mcg/ml, 1 mg/ml

## ACTION
Blocks opioid receptors and thereby prevents or reverses the effects of opioids, including respiratory depression, sedation, and hypotension.

## ONSET, PEAK, DURATION
Onset and peak occur almost immediately after I.V. administration. Duration varies, but usually is as long as most opioid analgesics. Low doses (1 mcg/kg) may last for 30 to 60 minutes; fully reversing doses (1 mg/70 kg) may last for many hours.

## INDICATIONS & DOSAGE
*Reversal of postoperative opioid effects* –
**Adults:** use 100 mcg/ml dosage strength as follows: initially, 0.25 mcg/kg I.V., followed by 0.25-mcg/kg incremental doses at 2- to 5-minute intervals, p.r.n. A cumulative total

---

*Liquid form contains alcohol.   **May contain tartrazine.   †Canada only.   ‡Australia only.   ◇OTC.

dose above 1 mcg/kg does not provide additional therapeutic effect.

*Management of opioid overdose* –

**Adults:** use 1-mg/ml dosage strength as follows: initially, 0.5 mg/70 kg I.V., followed by 1 mg/70 kg in 2 to 5 minutes, p.r.n.

## ADVERSE REACTIONS

**CNS:** *dizziness, headache,* somnolence, depression, agitation, nervousness, tremor, confusion, withdrawal syndrome, myoclonus.

**CV:** *tachycardia, hypertension or hypotension, vasodilation,* bradycardia, arrhythmias.

**GI:** *nausea, vomiting,* diarrhea, dry mouth.

**GU:** urine retention.

**Other:** *postoperative pain, fever, chills.*

## INTERACTIONS

None significant.

## CONTRAINDICATIONS

Contraindicated in patients with hypersensitivity to the drug.

## NURSING CONSIDERATIONS

• Use with extreme caution in patients with known physical dependence on opioids or following surgery involving high doses of opioids. Know that excessive doses of opioid antagonists in the postoperative setting has been associated with hypertension, tachycardia, and excessive mortality in patients at high risk for CV complications.

• Use with caution in patients with CV disease and in those who are receiving potentially cardiotoxic drugs or who are breast-feeding.

• Be aware that nalmefene may not completely reverse buprenorphine-induced respiratory depression.

• *Alert:* For I.V. use, drug is supplied in two concentrations: an ampule with a blue label contains 1 ml at a concentration suitable for postoperative use (100 mcg/ml), and an ampule with a green label contains 2 ml at a concentration suitable for management of overdose (1 mg/ml). Check concentration carefully before administering drug.

• In postoperative cases where the patient is known to be at increased risk for CV complications, be aware that doctor may order drug to be diluted 1:1 with saline solution or sterile water and smaller initial and incremental doses of 0.1 mcg/kg.

• Be aware that patients with renal failure may require incremental doses given slowly (over 60 seconds) to minimize the hypertension and dizziness that has been reported following the abrupt administration of the drug to such patients.

• Know that a cumulative total dose above 1.5 mg/70 kg is unlikely to have an effect.

• Know that if drug cannot be administered I.V., a single 1-mg dose may produce therapeutic results within 5 to 15 minutes if administered I.M. or S.C.

• Monitor patient's respiratory depth and rate closely. Duration of action of the opioid may exceed that of nalmefene, causing the patient to relapse into respiratory depression. Keep patient under close observation until there is no reasonable risk of recurring respiratory depression.

• Know that nalmefene may produce acute withdrawal symptoms in patients with known physical dependence on opioids. If suspicion of opioid dependency is present, administer a test dose of 0.1 mg/70 kg I.V., as ordered. If no evidence of withdrawal occurs in 2 minutes, the recommended dose may be administered, as ordered.

☑ **PATIENT TEACHING**

• Inform family of need for drug and explain how it will be administered.

• Reassure family that patient will be

---

monitored closely until narcotic effects are alleviated.

---

# naloxone hydrochloride
Narcan

*Pregnancy Risk Category: B*

## HOW SUPPLIED
*Injection:* 0.02mg/ml, 0.4 mg/ml, 1 mg/ml

## ACTION
Unknown. Thought to displace previously administered narcotic analgesics from their receptors (competitive antagonism). Has no pharmacologic activity of its own.

## ONSET, PEAK, DURATION
Onset occurs in 1 to 2 minutes after I.V. use, 2 to 5 minutes after S.C. or I.M. use. Peak unknown. Duration depends on dose and route of administration. I.M. administration provides a more prolonged duration.

## INDICATIONS & DOSAGE
*Known or suspected narcotic-induced respiratory depression, including that caused by pentazocine and propoxyphene –*
**Adults:** 0.4 to 2 mg I.V., S.C., or I.M. Repeated q 2 to 3 minutes, p.r.n. If no response is observed after 10 mg has been administered, the diagnosis of narcotic-induced toxicity should be questioned.
**Children:** 0.01 mg/kg I.V., followed by a second dose of 0.1 mg/kg I.V., if needed. If I.V. route is not available, drug may be administered I.M. or S.C. in divided doses.
**Neonates:** 0.01 mg/kg I.V., I.M., or S.C. Dose may be repeated q 2 to 3 minutes p.r.n.
*Postoperative narcotic depression –*
**Adults:** 0.1 to 0.2 mg I.V. q 2 to 3 minutes p.r.n. Dosage may be repeated within 1 to 2 hours, if needed.

**Children:** 0.005 to 0.01 mg/kg dose I.V. Repeated q 2 to 3 minutes p.r.n.
**Neonates (asphyxia neonatorum):** 0.01 mg/kg I.V. into umbilical vein. May be repeated q 2 to 3 minutes.

## ADVERSE REACTIONS
**CV:** tachycardia and hypertension with higher-than-recommended doses, hypotension, *ventricular fibrillation.*
**GI:** nausea and vomiting with higher-than-recommended doses.
**Other:** tremors and withdrawal symptoms in narcotic-dependent patients with higher-than-recommended doses, diaphoresis, *seizures,* pulmonary edema.

## INTERACTIONS
None significant.

## CONTRAINDICATIONS
Contraindicated in patients with hypersensitivity to the drug.

## NURSING CONSIDERATIONS
• Use cautiously in patients with cardiac irritability and opiate addiction. Abrupt reversal of opiate-induced CNS depression may result in nausea, vomiting, diaphoresis, tachycardia, CNS excitement, and increased blood pressure.
• **I.V. use:** Be prepared to administer continuous I.V. infusion (necessary in many instances to control adverse effects of epidurally administered morphine). If 0.02 mg/ml is not available know that the adult concentration (0.4 mg) may be diluted by mixing 0.5 ml with 9.5 ml of sterile water or sodium chloride for injection to make neonatal concentration (0.02 mg/ml).
• Keep in mind that duration of action of the narcotic may exceed that of naloxone and patients may relapse into respiratory depression.
• Know that respiratory rate increases within 1 to 2 minutes.
• Be aware that drug is effective only

---

in reversing respiratory depression caused by opiates, not against other drug-induced respiratory depression.
• Be aware that patients who receive naloxone to reverse opioid-induced respiratory depression may exhibit tachypnea.
• Monitor respiratory depth and rate. Be prepared to provide oxygen, ventilation, and other resuscitation measures.

### ☑ PATIENT TEACHING
• Inform family of need for drug and explain how it is administered.
• Reassure family that patient will be monitored closely until effects of narcotic are alleviated.

---

## naltrexone hydrochloride
Re Via

*Pregnancy Risk Category: C*

### HOW SUPPLIED
*Tablets:* 50 mg

### ACTION
Unknown. Probably reversibly blocks the subjective effects of opioids administered I.V. by occupying opiate receptors in the brain.

### ONSET, PEAK, DURATION
Onset occurs in 15 to 30 minutes. Effects peak after 12 hours. Effects persist about 24 hours.

### INDICATIONS & DOSAGE
*Adjunct for maintenance of opioid-free state in detoxified individuals –*
**Adults:** initially, 25 mg P.O. If no withdrawal signs occur within 1 hour, an additional 25 mg is given. Once patient has been started on 50 mg q 24 hours, flexible maintenance schedule may be used. From 50 to 150 mg may be given daily, depending on the schedule prescribed.
*Treatment of alcohol dependence –*
**Adults:** 50 mg P.O. once daily.

### ADVERSE REACTIONS
**CNS:** *insomnia, anxiety, nervousness, headache,* depression, dizziness, fatigue, somnolence, ***suicide ideation.***
**GI:** *nausea, vomiting,* anorexia, *abdominal pain,* constipation, increased thirst.
**GU:** delayed ejaculation, decreased potency.
**Hepatic:** hepatotoxicity.
**Skin:** rash.
**Other:** *muscle and joint pain,* chills.

### INTERACTIONS
*Thioridazine:* causes increased somnolence and lethargy.

### CONTRAINDICATIONS
Contraindicated in patients receiving opioid analgesics, in opioid-dependent patients, in patients in acute opioid withdrawal, and in those with positive urine screen for opioids or in acute hepatitis or liver failure. Also contraindicated in patients with hypersensitivity to drug.

### NURSING CONSIDERATIONS
• Use cautiously in patients with mild hepatic disease or history of recent hepatic disease.
• Be aware that treatment for opioid dependency shouldn't begin until patients receive naloxone challenge, a provocative test of opioid dependency. If signs of opioid withdrawal persist after naloxone challenge, don't administer naltrexone.
• Keep in mind that patients must be completely free of opioids before taking naltrexone or severe withdrawal symptoms may occur. Patients who have been addicted to short-acting opioids, such as heroin and meperidine, must wait at least 7 days after the last opioid dose before starting naltrexone. Patients who have been addicted to longer-acting opioids, such as methadone, should wait at least 10 days.

---

Reactions may be *common,* uncommon, *life-threatening,* or COMMON AND LIFE-THREATENING.

• In an emergency, anticipate that patients receiving naltrexone may be given an opioid analgesic, but the dose must be higher than usual to surmount naltrexone's effect. Monitor for respiratory depression from the opioid; it may be longer and deeper.
• For patients being treated because of a history of opioid dependency and who are expected to be noncompliant, be prepared to try a flexible maintenance dosage regimen of 100 mg on Monday and Wednesday and 150 mg on Friday, as ordered.
• Know that naltrexone should be used only as part of a comprehensive rehabilitation program.

☑ **PATIENT TEACHING**
• Advise patient to carry a medical identification card. Warn him about telling medical personnel that he takes naltrexone.
• Give patient names of nonopioid drugs that they can continue to take for pain, diarrhea, or cough.

---

## pralidoxime chloride (pyridine-2-aldoxime methochloride; 2-PAM)
Protopam Chloride
*Pregnancy Risk Category: C*

**HOW SUPPLIED**
*Injection:* 1 g/20 ml in 20-ml vial without diluent or syringe; 1 g/20 ml in 20-ml vial with diluent, syringe, needle, and alcohol swab (emergency kit); 600 mg/2 ml auto-injector, parenteral

**ACTION**
Reactivates cholinesterase that has been inactivated by organophosphorus pesticides and related compounds, permitting degradation of accumulated acetylcholine and facilitating normal functioning of neuromuscular junctions.

**ONSET, PEAK, DURATION**
Onset and duration unknown. Levels peak within 5 to 15 minutes after I.V. administration; 10 to 20 minutes after I.M. administration; unknown after S.C. administration.

**INDICATIONS & DOSAGE**
*Antidote for organophosphate poisoning* –
**Adults:** 1 to 2 g in 100 ml of sodium chloride solution by I.V. infusion over 15 to 30 minutes. If pulmonary edema is present, give by slow I.V. push over 5 minutes. Repeated in 1 hour if muscle weakness persists. Additional doses may be given cautiously. I.M. or S.C. injection may be used if I.V. is not feasible.
**Children:** 20 to 40 mg/kg I.V., administered as for adults.
*Cholinergic crisis in myasthenia gravis* –
**Adults:** 1 to 2 g I.V., followed by 250 mg I.V. q 5 minutes as needed.

**ADVERSE REACTIONS**
**CNS:** dizziness, headache, drowsiness.
**CV:** tachycardia.
**EENT:** blurred vision, diplopia, impaired accommodation.
**GI:** nausea.
**Other:** muscular weakness, hyperventilation, mild to moderate pain at injection site, transient elevation of liver enzymes.

**INTERACTIONS**
None significant.

**CONTRAINDICATIONS**
None known.

**NURSING CONSIDERATIONS**
• Use with extreme caution in patients with myasthenia gravis (overdose may trigger myasthenic crisis).
• Initially, remove secretions, maintain patent airway, and institute mechnical ventilation if needed. After

---

dermal exposure to organophosphate, remove the patient's clothing and wash his skin and hair with sodium bicarbonate, soap, water, and alcohol as soon as possible. A second washing may be necessary. When washing the patient, wear protective gloves and clothes to avoid exposure.
• Draw blood for cholinesterase levels before giving pralidoxime.
• Drug should be used in hospitalized patients only; have respiratory and other supportive measures available. If possible, obtain accurate medical history and chronology of poisoning. Drug should be given as soon as possible after poisoning; treatment is most effective if initiated within 24 hours after exposure.
• **I.V. use:** Give I.V. preparation slowly as diluted solution. Dilute with sterile water without preservatives.
• To ameliorate muscarinic effects and block accumulation of acetylcholine associated with organophosphate poisoning, give atropine 2 to 4 mg I.V. with pralidoxine if cyanosis is not present, as ordered. (If cyanosis is present, give atropine I.M.) Give atropine every 5 to 6 minutes, as ordered, until signs of atropine toxicity (flushing, tachycardia, dry mouth, blurred vision, excitement, delirium, and hallucinations) appear; atropinization should be maintained for at least 48 hours.
• Observe patient for 48 to 72 hours if poison was ingested. Delayed absorption may occur from lower bowel. It is difficult to distinguish between toxic effects produced by atropine or by organophosphate compounds and those resulting from pralidoxime.
• Watch the patient with myasthenia gravis treated for overdose of cholinergic drugs for signs of rapid weakening. He can pass quickly from cholinergic crisis to myasthenic crisis and requires more cholinergic drugs to treat myasthenia. Keep edrophonium

(Tensilon) available for establishing differential diagnosis.
• Drug is not effective against poisoning due to phosphorus, inorganic phosphates, or organophosphates with no anticholinesterase activity.

### ☑ PATIENT TEACHING
• Explain need for drug and how it is administered to patient and family.
• Tell patient to report adverse effects.
• Caution patient treated for organophosphate poisoning to avoid contact with insecticides for several weeks.

## protamine sulfate
*Pregnancy Risk Category: C*

**HOW SUPPLIED**
*Injection:* 10 mg/ml

**ACTION**
A heparin antagonist that forms a physiologically inert complex with heparin sodium.

**ONSET, PEAK, DURATION**
Onset within 30 seconds to 1 minute. Peak unknown. Effects last 2 hours.

**INDICATIONS & DOSAGE**
*Heparin overdose –*
**Adults:** dosage based on venous blood coagulation studies, usually 1 mg for each 90 to 115 units of heparin. Give by slow I.V. injection over 10 minutes in doses not to exceed 50 mg.

**ADVERSE REACTIONS**
**CV:** fall in blood pressure, bradycardia, *circulatory collapse.*
**GI:** nausea, vomiting.
**Respiratory:** dyspnea, *pulmonary edema, acute pulmonary hypertension.*
**Other:** transitory flushing, feeling of warmth, *anaphylaxis, anaphylactoid reactions,* lassitude.

---

## INTERACTIONS
None significant.

## CONTRAINDICATIONS
Contraindicated in patients with hypersensitivity to drug.

## NURSING CONSIDERATIONS
• Use cautiously after cardiac surgery.
• Calculate dosage carefully. One mg of protamine neutralizes 90 to 115 units of heparin depending on salt (heparin calcium or heparin sodium) and source of heparin (beef or pork).
• **I.V. use:** Administer slowly by direct I.V. injection. Have emergency equipment available to treat shock.
• Know that risk of a hypersensitivity reaction is increased in patients with known hypersensitivity to fish, vasectomized or infertile males, or patients taking protamine-insulin products.
• Monitor patient continually.
• Watch for spontaneous bleeding (heparin "rebound"), especially in dialysis patients and in those who have undergone cardiac surgery.
• Protamine sulfate may act as anticoagulant in very high doses.

### ☑ PATIENT TEACHING
• Explain need for drug and how it is administered to patient and family.
• Tell patient to report adverse effects.

---

## sodium polystyrene sulfonate
Kayexalate, Resonium A, SPS
*Pregnancy Risk Category: C*

## HOW SUPPLIED
*Powder:* 1-lb jar (3.5 g/tsp)
*Suspension:* 15 g/60 ml\*

## ACTION
Potassium-removing resin exchanges sodium ions for potassium ions in the intestine: 1 g of sodium polystyrene sulfonate is exchanged for 0.5 to 1 mEq of potassium. The resin is then eliminated. Much of the exchange capacity is used for cations other than potassium (calcium and magnesium) and possibly for fats and proteins.

## ONSET, PEAK, DURATION
Unknown.

## INDICATIONS & DOSAGE
*Hyperkalemia* –
**Adults:** 15 g P.O. daily to q.i.d. in water or sorbitol (3 to 4 ml/g of resin). Alternatively, mix powder with appropriate medium – aqueous suspension or diet appropriate for renal failure – and instill through a nasogastric (NG) tube.

Or 30 to 50 g/100 ml of sorbitol q 6 hours as warm emulsion deep into sigmoid colon (20 cm). In persistent vomiting or paralytic ileus, high-retention enema of sodium polystyrene sulfonate (30 g) suspended in 200 ml of 10% methylcellulose, 10% dextrose, or 25% sorbitol solution may be given.
**Children:** 1 g of resin P.O. or P.R. for each mEq of potassium to be removed.

Oral administration preferred because drug should remain in intestine for at least 6 hours.

## ADVERSE REACTIONS
**GI:** *constipation,* fecal impaction (in elderly patients), anorexia, gastric irritation, nausea, vomiting, *diarrhea* (with sorbitol emulsions).
**Other:** *hypokalemia,* hypocalcemia, sodium retention.

## INTERACTIONS
*Antacids and laxatives (nonabsorbable cation-donating types, including magnesium hydroxide):* systemic alkalosis and reduced potassium exchange capability. Don't use together.

---

## CONTRAINDICATIONS

Contraindicated in patients with hypokalemia or hypersensitivity to drug.

## NURSING CONSIDERATIONS

• Use cautiously in patients with severe CHF, severe hypertension, or marked edema.

• Don't heat resin; this impairs drug's effect. Mix resin only with water or sorbitol for P.O. administration. *Never* mix with orange juice (high potassium content) to disguise taste.

• Chill oral suspension for greater palatability.

• If sorbitol is given, mix with resin suspension.

• Consider solid form. Resin cookie and candy recipes are available; ask pharmacist or dietitian to supply.

• Know that premixed forms are available (SPS and others). If preparing manually, mix polystyrene resin only with water and sorbitol for rectal use. Do not use mineral oil for rectal administration to prevent impaction; ion exchange requires aqueous medium. Sorbitol content prevents impaction.

• Prepare rectal dose at room temperature. Stir emulsion gently during administration.

• Use #28 French rubber tube for rectal dose; insert 20 cm into sigmoid colon. Tape tube in place. Or, consider an indwelling urianry (Foley) catheter with a 30-ml balloon inflated distal to anal sphincter to aid in retention. This is especially helpful for patients with poor sphincter control. Use gravity flow. Drain returns constantly through Y-tube connection. Place patient in knee-chest position or with hips on pillow for a while if back-leakage occurs.

• After rectal administration, flush tubing with 50 to 100 ml of nonsodium fluid to ensure delivery of all drug. Flush rectum to remove the resin.

• Prevent fecal impaction in elderly patients by administering resin rectally, as ordered. Give cleansing enema before rectal administration. Have patients retain enema — for 6 to 10 hours if possible, but 30 to 60 minutes is acceptable.

• Watch for constipation in oral or NG administration. Use sorbitol (10 to 20 ml of 70% syrup every 2 hours as needed) to produce one or two watery stools daily.

• Monitor serum potassium levels at least once daily. Treatment may result in potassium deficiency and is usually stopped when potassium is reduced to 4 or 5 mEq/L.

• Watch for signs of hypokalemia: irritability, confusion, arrhythmias, ECG changes, severe muscle weakness and sometimes paralysis, and digitalis toxicity in digitalized patients.

• If hyperkalemia is severe, know that doctor does not depend solely on polystyrene resin to lower serum potassium. Dextrose 50% with regular insulin I.V. push may be given.

• Monitor for symptoms of other electrolyte deficiencies (magnesium, calcium) because drug is nonselective. Monitor serum calcium in patients receiving sodium polystyrene therapy for more than 3 days. Supplementary calcium may be needed.

• Watch for sodium overload. Drug contains about 100 mg sodium/g. About one-third of resin's sodium is retained.

☑ **PATIENT TEACHING**

• Explain need for drug and how it is to be administered to patient.

• Instruct patient to report adverse reactions promptly.

## succimer

Chemet

*Pregnancy Risk Category: C*

## HOW SUPPLIED

*Capsules:* 100 mg

---

Reactions may be *common,* uncommon, *life-threatening,* or **COMMON AND LIFE-THREATENING.**

## ACTION
A chelating agent that forms water-soluble complexes with lead and increases its excretion in urine.

## ONSET, PEAK, DURATION
Onset and duration unknown. Serum levels peak in 1 to 2 hours.

## INDICATIONS & DOSAGE
*Lead poisoning in children with blood lead levels above 45 mcg/dl* –
**Children:** initially, 10 mg/kg or 350 mg/m² q 8 hours for 5 days. Dosage rounded as appropriate to nearest 100 mg (see chart). Then, frequency of administration decreased to q 12 hours for an additional 2 weeks of therapy.

| Weight (kg) | Dose (mg) |
|-------------|-----------|
| 8 to 15     | 100       |
| 16 to 23    | 200       |
| 24 to 34    | 300       |
| 35 to 44    | 400       |
| >45         | 500       |

## ADVERSE REACTIONS
**CNS:** *drowsiness, dizziness, sensory motor neuropathy, sleepiness, paresthesia, headache.*
**CV:** arrhythmias.
**EENT:** plugged ears, cloudy film in eyes, otitis media, watery eyes, sore throat, rhinorrhea, nasal congestion.
**GI:** *nausea, vomiting, diarrhea, loss of appetite, abdominal cramps, hemorrhoidal symptoms, metallic taste in mouth, loose stools.*
**GU:** decreased urination, difficult urination, proteinuria.
**Hematologic:** increased platelet count, intermittent eosinophilia.
**Respiratory:** cough, head cold.
**Skin:** papular rash, herpetic rash, mucocutaneous eruptions, pruritus.
**Other:** *leg, kneecap, back, stomach, rib, or flank pain; flulike symptoms;* moniliasis; *elevated serum AST, ALT, alkaline phosphatase, or cholesterol levels.*

## INTERACTIONS
None significant.

## CONTRAINDICATIONS
Contraindicated in patients with hypersensitivity to the drug.

## NURSING CONSIDERATIONS
• Use cautiously in patients with compromised renal function.
• Measure severity by initial blood lead level and by rate and degree of rebound of blood lead level. Severity should be used as a guide for more frequent blood lead monitoring.
• Monitor serum transaminase before and at least weekly during therapy. Transient mild elevations of serum transaminases have been observed. Patients with history of hepatic disease need close monitoring.
• Monitor patients at least once weekly for rebound blood lead levels. Elevated levels and associated symptoms may return rapidly after drug is stopped because of redistribution of lead from bone to soft tissues and blood.
• Be aware that course of treatment lasts 19 days. Repeated courses may be necessary if indicated by weekly monitoring of blood lead levels.
• Know that a minimum of 2 weeks between courses is recommended unless high blood lead levels indicate need for immediate therapy.
• Know that false-positive results for ketones in urine using nitroprusside reagents (Ketostix) and falsely decreased levels of serum uric acid and CK have been reported.
• Know that concurrent administration of succimer with other chelating agents is not recommended. Patients who have received edetate calcium disodium with or without dimercaprol may use succimer as subsequent therapy after a 4-week interval.

---

*Liquid form contains alcohol.   **May contain tartrazine.   †Canada only.   ‡Australia only.   ◊OTC.

## ☑ PATIENT TEACHING
• Explain to parents and child need for drug and how it will be given. Stress importance of complying with frequently ordered blood tests.
• Tell parents of young child who cannot swallow capsules that capsule can be opened and its contents sprinkled on a small amount of soft food. Alternatively, medicated beads from capsule may be poured on a spoon; follow with flavored beverage.
• Assist parents with identifying and removing sources of lead in child's environment. Chelation therapy is not a substitute for preventing further exposure and should not be used to permit continued exposure.
• Tell patients to consult the doctor if rash occurs. Consider possibility of allergic or other mucocutaneous reactions each time drug is used.

## trientine hydrochloride
Syprine

*Pregnancy Risk Category: C*

## HOW SUPPLIED
*Capsules:* 250 mg

## ACTION
Chelates copper and increases its urinary excretion.

## ONSET, PEAK, DURATION
Unknown.

## INDICATIONS & DOSAGE
*Wilson's disease in patients who cannot tolerate penicillamine –*
**Adults:** 750 to 1,250 mg P.O. daily in two, three, or four divided doses. Dosage may then be increased up to 2,000 mg daily, p.r.n.
**Children age 12 and under:** 500 to 750 mg P.O. daily in two, three, or four divided doses. Dosage may then be increased up to 1,500 mg daily, p.r.n.
  Long-term maintenance dosage should be determined q 6 to 12 months, based on serum copper analysis.

## ADVERSE REACTIONS
**Hematologic:** iron-deficiency anemia.
**Other:** hypersensitivity reactions (rash), systemic lupus erythematosus.

## INTERACTIONS
*Mineral supplements, including iron:* may block trientine absorption. Administer at least 2 hours apart.

## CONTRAINDICATIONS
Contraindicated in patients with hypersensitivity to the drug.

## NURSING CONSIDERATIONS
• Monitor patients (especially women) closely for signs of iron-deficiency anemia throughout therapy.
• Watch for signs of hypersensitivity reactions, such as rash.

## ☑ PATIENT TEACHING
• Tell patient to take drug on an empty stomach at least 1 hour before or 2 hours after meals, and at least 1 hour apart from other drugs, food, or milk.
• Tell patient to swallow capsules whole with water.
• If capsule is accidentally opened and contents spilled on skin, tell patient to wash site thoroughly. Exposure to capsule contents may cause contact dermatitis.
• Tell patient to take his temperature every night and report any fevers or skin eruptions, especially during the first month of therapy.
• Urge patients to follow regimen and low-copper diet as prescribed.

abciximab
acetohydroxamic acid
alendronate sodium
alglucerase
alprostadil
aminoglutethimide
aprotinin
calcipotriene
capsaicin
cisapride
clomiphene citrate
cysteamine bitartrate
dexrazoxane
diazoxide, oral
etretinate
finasteride
gallium nitrate
imiglucerase
isotretinoin
levocarnitine
levomethadyl acetate
  hydrochloride
masoprocol
mesalamine
mesna
methoxsalen
minoxidil (topical)
nimodipine
olsalazine sodium
pamidronate disodium
pilocarpine hydrochloride
riluzole
ritodrine hydrochloride
sodium benzoate and sodium
  phenylacetate
strontium 89 ($^{89}$SR) chloride
sulfasalazine
tiopronin
tretinoin
trilostane

**COMBINATION PRODUCTS**
None.

## abciximab
ReoPro
*Pregnancy Risk Category: C*

**HOW SUPPLIED**
*Injection:* 2 mg/ml

**ACTION**
Binds to the glycoprotein 11b/111a
(GP11b/111a) receptor of human
platelets and inhibits platelet aggregation.

**ONSET, PEAK, DURATION**
Onset and peak occur almost immediately after I.V. infusion. Effects on
platelet aggregation persist for about
48 hours.

**INDICATIONS & DOSAGE**
*Adjunct to percutaneous transluminal
coronary angioplasty (PTCA) or atherectomy for the prevention of acute
cardiac ischemic complications in patients at high risk for abrupt closure of
the treated coronary vessel –*
**Adults:** 0.25 mg/kg as an I.V. bolus
administered 10 to 60 minutes before
start of PTCA or atherectomy, followed by a continuous I.V. infusion of
10 mcg/minute for 12 hours.

**ADVERSE REACTIONS**
**CNS:** hyperesthesia, hypoesthesia,
confusion.
**CV:** *hypotension,* bradycardia, pe-
ripheral edema.
**EENT:** abnormal vision.
**GI:** *nausea, vomiting.*
**Hematologic:** *bleeding, **thrombocy-
topenia,*** anemia, leukocytosis.
**Respiratory:** pleural effusion, pleu-
risy, pneumonia.
**Other:** pain.

---

*Liquid form contains alcohol.   **May contain tartrazine.   †Canada only.   ‡Australia only.   ◇OTC.

### INTERACTIONS

*Antiplatelet agents, heparin, NSAIDs, other anticoagulants, thrombolytics:* increased risk of bleeding. Monitor patient closely.

### CONTRAINDICATIONS

Contraindicated in patients with hypersensitivity to any component of the drug or to murine proteins; in those with active internal bleeding, recent (within 6 weeks) GI or GU bleeding of clinical significance, history of CVA within past 2 years or CVA with significant residual neurologic deficit, bleeding diathesis, thrombocytopenia (less than 100,000/mm$^2$), recent (within 6 weeks) major surgery or trauma, intracranial neoplasm, intracranial arteriovenous malformation, intracranial aneurysm, severe uncontrolled hypertension, or history of vasculitis; when oral anticoagulants have been administered within past 7 days unless PT is equal to or less than 1.2 times control; or with use of I.V. dextran before PTCA or intent to use it during PTCA.

### NURSING CONSIDERATIONS

• Use with caution in patients at increased risk for bleeding. Patients at risk include those who weigh less than 75 kg, are over age 65, have a history of GI disease, or are receiving thrombolytic agents. Conditions that also increase the patient's risk of bleeding include PTCA within 12 hours of onset of symptoms for acute MI, prolonged PTCA (lasting more than 70 minutes), or failed PTCA. Heparin used in conjunction with abciximab also may contribute to the risk of bleeding.

• Know that patients who are at risk for abrupt closure and thus would be candidates for abciximab therapy include those undergoing PTCA with at least one of the following conditions: unstable angina or a non-Q-wave MI, an acute Q-wave MI within 12 hours of onset of symptoms, the presence of two type B lesions in the artery to be dilated, the presence of one type B lesion in the artery to be dilated in a woman over age 65 or in a patient with diabetes, the presence of one type C lesion in the artery to be dilated, or angioplasty of an infarct-related lesion within 7 days of MI.

• Be aware that abciximab is intended for use with aspirin and heparin.

• Keep epinephrine, dopamine, theophylline, antihistamines, and corticosteroids readily available in case anaphylaxis occurs.

• **I.V. use:** Inspect solution for particulate matter before administration. If any visibly opaque particles are found, discard solution and obtain new vial. Withdraw the necessary amount of abciximab for I.V. bolus injection through a sterile, nonpyrogenic, low-protein-binding 0.2- or 0.22-micron filter into a syringe. The I.V. bolus should be administered 10 to 60 minutes before the procedure.

• Withdraw 4.5 ml of abciximab for continuous I.V. infusion through a sterile, nonpyrogenic, low-protein-binding 0.2-or 0.22-micron filter into a syringe. Inject into 250 ml of sterile 0.9% sodium chloride solution or 5% dextrose, and infuse at a rate of 17 ml/hour for 12 hours via a continuous infusion pump equipped with an in-line filter. Discard the unused portion at the end of the 12-hour infusion.

• Administer abciximab in a separate I.V. line; no other medication should be added to the infusion solution.

• Monitor the patient closely for bleeding. Bleeding associated with therapy falls into two broad categories: that observed at the arterial access site used for cardiac catheterization and internal bleeding involving the GI or GU tract, or retroperitoneal sites.

• Institute bleeding precautions. Maintain patient on bed rest for 6 to 8 hours following sheath removal or discontinuation of abciximab infusion, whichever is later. Minimize or avoid, if possible, arterial and venous punctures; I.M. injections; use of urinary catheters, nasogastric tubes, or automatic blood pressure cuffs; and nasotracheal intubation.

### ☑ PATIENT TEACHING
• Explain need for drug and how it is administered to patient and family
• Instruct patient to report adverse reactions immediately.

---

### acetohydroxamic acid
Lithostat

*Pregnancy Risk Category: X*

### HOW SUPPLIED
*Tablets (scored):* 250 mg

### ACTION
Prevents formation of renal stones by inhibiting bacterial urease activity.

### ONSET, PEAK, DURATION
Onset and duration unknown. Serum levels peak within 15 to 60 minutes.

### INDICATIONS & DOSAGE
*Urinary tract infection caused by kidney stones –*
**Adults:** 250 mg P.O. t.i.d. or q.i.d. at 6- to 8-hour intervals when the stomach is empty. Maximum daily dosage is 1.5 g.
**Children:** 10 mg/kg/day P.O. in two or three divided doses.

### ADVERSE REACTIONS
**CNS:** *mild headache, depression, anxiety, nervousness, malaise, tremulousness.*
**CV:** phlebitis, palpitations.
**GI:** *nausea, vomiting, diarrhea, constipation, anorexia.*
**Hematologic:** *hemolytic anemia*, reticulocytosis.
**Skin:** *nonpruritic, macular rash on arms and face.*

**Other:** alopecia, deep vein thrombosis.

### INTERACTIONS
*Methenamine:* may produce synergistic effects.
*Oral iron supplements:* reduced absorption of acetohydroxamic acid. Consult the doctor, who may prescribe I.M. administration of iron.

### CONTRAINDICATIONS
Contraindicated in patients whose physical state and disease are amenable to surgery and appropriate antibiotics, in patients whose urine is infected by nonurease-producing organisms, during pregnancy, and in patients with poor renal function.

### NURSING CONSIDERATIONS
• Monitor CBC, including reticulocyte count, after 2 weeks of therapy, then at 3-month intervals for duration of treatment, as ordered. If laboratory findings indicate hemolytic anemia, discontinue drug and notify doctor.
• Anticipate using a reduced dosage in renal impairment.
• Be aware that a negative Coombs' test for hemolytic anemia has occurred in patients receiving acetohydroxamic acid.
• Keep in mind that patients may also be given methenamine to enhance response to acetohydroxamic acid.
• Monitor for skin rash, more common during prolonged use and with concomitant use of alcoholic beverages. The rash appears 30 to 45 minutes after ingestion of alcoholic beverages and disappears spontaneously in 30 to 60 minutes.

### ☑ PATIENT TEACHING
• Instruct patient to take drug on an empty stomach.
• Although rash doesn't usually require treatment, advise patient to avoid drinking alcoholic beverages.

---

▼ *NEW DRUG*

# alendronate sodium
Fosamax

*Pregnancy Risk Category: C*

## HOW SUPPLIED
*Tablets:* 10 mg, 40 mg

## ACTION
Suppresses osteoclast activity on newly formed resorption surfaces, which reduces bone turnover. Bone formation exceeds resorption at remodeling sites, leading to progressive gains in bone mass.

## ONSET, PEAK, DURATION
Decreased rate of bone resorption is evident in 1 month; in 3 to 6 months, it reaches a plateau that is maintained for duration of therapy.

## INDICATIONS & DOSAGE
*Osteoporosis in postmenopausal women* –
**Adults:** 10 mg P.O. daily, taken with plain water only, at least 30 minutes before first food, beverage, or medication of day.
*Paget's disease of bone* –
**Adults:** 40 mg P.O. daily for 6 months, taken with plain water only, at least 30 minutes before first food, beverage, or medication of day.

## ADVERSE REACTIONS
**CNS:** headache.
**GI:** abdominal pain, nausea, dyspepsia, constipation, diarrhea, flatulence, acid regurgitation, esophageal ulcer, vomiting, dysphagia, abdominal distention, gastritis.
**Other:** musculoskeletal pain, taste perversion.

## INTERACTIONS
*Antacids, calcium supplements:* interferes with absorption of alendronate. Have patient wait at least 30 minutes after taking alendronate before taking any other drug.
*Aspirin, NSAIDs:* increased risk of upper GI adverse reactions with alendronate doses greater than 10 mg/day. Monitor patient closely.
*Hormone replacement therapy:* not recommended for use with alendronate in treating osteoporosis; evidence of effectiveness is lacking.

## CONTRAINDICATIONS
Contraindicated in patients with hypersensitivity to drug, hypocalcemia, or severe renal insufficiency.

## NURSING CONSIDERATIONS
● Use cautiously in patients with active upper GI problems (dysphagia, symptomatic esophageal diseases, gastritis, duodenitis, ulcers) or mild to moderate renal insufficiency.
● Hypocalcemia and other disturbances of mineral metabolism (such as vitamin D deficiency) should be corrected before therapy begins.
● When drug is used to treat osteoporosis in postmenopausal women, osteoporosis may be confirmed by findings of low bone mass on diagnostic studies or by history of osteoporotic fracture.
● When used to treat Paget's disease, drug is indicated for patients with alkaline phosphatase level at least two times the upper limit of normal, in those who are symptomatic, and in those at risk for future complications from the disease.
● Monitor patient's serum calcium and phosphate levels throughout therapy, as ordered.

## ☑ PATIENT TEACHING
● Stress importance of taking tablet with a glass of plain water at least 30 minutes before ingesting anything else, including food, beverages, and other medications. Tell the patient that waiting longer than 30 minutes will improve absorption.

---

Reactions may be *common,* uncommon, *life-threatening,* or COMMON AND LIFE-THREATENING.

- Warn the patient not to lie down for at least 30 minutes after taking drug to facilitate delivery to stomach and to reduce potential for esophageal irritation.
- Advise the patient to take supplemental calcium and vitamin D, if dietary intake is inadequate.
- Tell the patient about the benefits of weight-bearing exercises in increasing bone mass. If applicable, explain the importance of reducing or eliminating cigarette smoking and alcohol use.

---

## alglucerase (glucocerebrosidase, glucosylceramidase, glucocerebrosidase-beta-glucosidase)
Ceredase

*Pregnancy Risk Category: C*

### HOW SUPPLIED
*Injection:* 10 IU/ml in 5-ml bottles, 80 IU/ml in 5-ml bottles

### ACTION
Reduces glycolipid accumulation by acting as a catalyst for the hydrolysis of glucocerebroside to glucose and ceramide—part of the normal degradation pathway for lipids.

### ONSET, PEAK, DURATION
Onset and duration unknown. Serum levels peak in 1 hour following I.V. administration.

### INDICATIONS & DOSAGE
*Long-term endogenous enzyme (glucosylceramidase) replacement therapy in confirmed type I Gaucher's disease—*
**Adults and children:** individualized dosage; initially, 2.5 units/kg I.V. three times weekly up to as much as 60 units/kg once a week or as infrequently as q 4 weeks. Infusion should run over 1 to 2 hours. Once response is established, dosage reduced for maintenance at 3- to 6-month intervals.

### ADVERSE REACTIONS
**GI:** abdominal discomfort, nausea, vomiting.
**Other:** chills, slight fever, discomfort, burning, swelling at injection site.

### INTERACTIONS
None significant.

### CONTRAINDICATIONS
None known.

### NURSING CONSIDERATIONS
- Use cautiously in patients with symptoms of hypersensitivity to drug. Know that pretreatment with antihistamines may be required. Also use cautiously in patients with androgen-sensitive malignant disease such as prostate cancer and patients with known prior allergies to human chorionic gonadotropin.
- **I.V. use:** To prepare solution, dilute appropriate amount of alglucerase with 0.9% sodium chloride solution to a final volume not to exceed 100 ml. Use an in-line particulate filter during administration. Because alglucerase is preservative-free, use immediately.
- Do not shake bottle. Shaking may denature the glycoprotein and render it biologically inactive.
- Monitor response parameters to use lowest effective dose.
- Be aware that alglucerase is purified from a large pool of human placental tissue collected from selected donors. Although the risk of viral contamination from slow-acting or latent viruses is believed to be remote, the risks and benefits of therapy must be carefully assessed before administration.
- Keep in mind that hemoglobin levels may normalize after 6 months of

---

therapy. Improved mineralization may also occur after prolonged treatment.

● Store at 39° F (4° C). Do not use solution that is discolored or that contains particles.

☑ **PATIENT TEACHING**
● Explain to patient and family how drug works and is administered. Stress importance of compliance with administration schedule.
● Tell patient to report discomfort at I.V. site promptly.

# alprostadil
Caverject

*Pregnancy Risk Category: NR*

## HOW SUPPLIED
*Injections:* 11.9 mcg/vial, 23.2 mcg/vial

## ACTION
A prostaglandin derivative that induces erection by relaxing trabecular smooth muscle and dilating cavernosal arteries. This leads to expansion of lacunar spaces and entrapment of blood by compressing venules against the tunica albuginea, a process referred to as the corporal veno-occlusive mechanism.

## ONSET, PEAK, DURATION
Onset and peak occur in 5 to 20 minutes. Duration is preferably no longer than 1 hour but can last longer than 6 hours.

## INDICATIONS & DOSAGE
*Erectile dysfunction due to vasculogenic, psychogenic, or mixed etiology* –
**Adults:** dosages are highly individualized, with initial dose of 2.5 mcg intracavernously. If partial response occurs, second dose of 2.5 mcg is given, then increased further in increments of 5 to 10 mcg until patient achieves erection (one suitable for in-

tercourse and preferably not exceeding 1 hour's duration). If no response occurs to initial dose, second dose may be increased to 7.5 mcg within 1 hour, then increased further in increments of 5 to 10 mcg until patient achieves suitable erection. Patient must remain in doctor's office until complete detumescence occurs. Procedure should not be repeated for at least 24 hours.
*Erectile dysfunction of neurogenic etiology (spinal cord injury)* –
**Adults:** dosages are highly individualized, with initial dose of 1.25 mcg intracavernously. If partial response occurs, second dose of 1.25 mcg is given, followed by a third dose of 2.5 mcg, then increased further in increments of 5 mcg until patient achieves suitable erection. If no response occurs to initial dose, second dose may be increased to 2.5 mcg within 1 hour, then increased further in increments of 5 mcg until patient achieves suitable erection. Patient must remain in doctor's office until complete detumescence occurs. Procedure should not be repeated for at least 24 hours.

## ADVERSE REACTIONS
**CNS:** headache, dizziness.
**CV:** hypertension.
**GU:** *penile pain;* prolonged erection; penile fibrosis, rash, or edema; penis disorder; prostatic disorder.
**Respiratory:** upper respiratory infection, flu syndrome, sinusitis, nasal congestion, cough.
**Other:** injection site hematoma or ecchymosis, back pain, localized trauma or pain.

## INTERACTIONS
*Anticoagulants:* increased risk of bleeding from intracavernosal injection site. Monitor patient closely.
*Vasoactive agents:* safety and efficacy of concomitant use have not been studied. Avoid concomitant use.

---

Reactions may be *common,* uncommon, *life-threatening,* or COMMON AND LIFE-THREATENING.

## CONTRAINDICATIONS

Contraindicated in patients with hypersensitivity to drug, conditions associated with predisposition to priapism (sickle cell anemia or trait, multiple myeloma, leukemia), or penile deformation (angulation, cavernosal fibrosis, Peyronie's disease). Drug also should not be used in men who have penile implants or for whom sexual activity is inadvisable or contraindicated. Drug is not given to women or children.

## NURSING CONSIDERATIONS

● Ensure that the patient has had underlying medical causes of erectile dysfunction diagnosed and treated before therapy begins.
● Know that regular follow-up care, with thorough examination of the penis, is strongly recommended to detect signs of penile fibrosis. Drug should be discontinued in patients who develop penile angulation, cavernosal fibrosis, or Peyronie's disease.

## ☑ PATIENT TEACHING

● Teach the patient how to prepare and administer drug before he begins treatment at home. Stress importance of reading and following patient instructions in each package insert.
● Tell him not to shake contents of reconstituted vial, and remind him that vial is designed for single use only. Tell him to discard vial if solution is discolored or contains precipitate.
● Inform him that he can expect an erection 5 to 20 minutes after administration, with a preferable duration of no more than 1 hour. If his erection lasts significantly longer than 1 hour, tell him to seek medical attention immediately.
● Remind him to take drug as prescribed (generally, no more than 3 times weekly, with at least 24 hours between each use). Warn him not to change dosage without consulting the doctor.

● Review possible adverse reactions. Tell him to inspect his penis daily and to report redness, swelling, tenderness, curvature, priapism, unusual pain, nodules, or hard tissue.
● Urge him not to reuse or share needles, syringes, or medication.
● Warn him that drug does not protect against sexually transmitted diseases. Also caution him that bleeding at injection site can increase risk of transmitting blood-borne diseases to his partner.
● Remind him to keep regular follow-up appointments so the doctor can evaluate drug effectiveness and safety.

# aminoglutethimide
Cytadren

*Pregnancy Risk Category: D*

## HOW SUPPLIED
*Tablets:* 250 mg

## ACTION
Blocks conversion of cholesterol to delta-5-pregnenolone in the adrenal cortex, inhibiting the synthesis of adrenal steroids.

## ONSET, PEAK, DURATION
Suppression of adrenal function occurs in 3 to 5 days. Time to peak concentration occurs in 1½ hours. Adrenal function usually returns to normal 1½ to 3 days after discontinuing drug, although recovery may take a year or longer after prolonged therapy.

## INDICATIONS & DOSAGE
*Suppression of adrenal function in Cushing's syndrome and adrenal cancer –*
**Adults:** 250 mg q.i.d. at 6-hour intervals. Dosage may be increased in increments of 250 mg daily q 1 to 2 weeks to a maximum daily dosage of 2 g.

## ADVERSE REACTIONS
**CNS:** *drowsiness,* headache, dizziness.
**CV:** hypotension, tachycardia.
**GI:** *nausea, anorexia,* vomiting.
**Hematologic:** transient leukopenia, **agranulocytosis, thrombocytopenia.**
**Skin:** *morbilliform rash,* pruritus, urticaria.
**Other:** fever, myalgia, adrenal insufficiency, masculinization, hirsutism, hypothyroidism.

## INTERACTIONS
*Dexamethasone, medroxyprogesterone:* increased hepatic metabolism of these agents. Monitor patient closely.
*Ethanol:* may potentiate the effects of aminoglutethimide. Avoid concomitant use.
*Oral anticoagulants:* decreased anticoagulant effect. Monitor P.T.

## CONTRAINDICATIONS
Contraindicated in patients hypersensitive to the drug or to glutethimide.

## NURSING CONSIDERATIONS
● Perform baseline hematologic studies, as ordered.
● Monitor blood pressure frequently.
● Monitor CBC periodically, as ordered.
● Be aware that drug may cause adrenal hypofunction, especially under stressful conditions, such as surgery, trauma, or acute illness. Patients may need mineralocorticoid supplements to treat hyponatremia and orthostatic hypotension. Glucocorticoid replacement may also be necessary, especially in patients with breast cancer. Monitor such patients carefully.
● Know that drug may cause a decrease in thyroid hormone production. Monitor thyroid function studies.

## ☑ PATIENT TEACHING
● Warn patient to watch for signs of infection (fever, sore throat, fatigue) and bleeding (easy bruising, nosebleeds, bleeding gums, melena). He should take his temperature daily.
● Warn patient to avoid activities that require alertness and good motor coordination until CNS effects of the drug are known.
● Advise patient to stand up slowly to minimize orthostatic hypotension.
● Tell patient to report rash that persists for more than 8 days. Reassure patient that drowsiness, nausea, and loss of appetite usually diminish within 2 weeks after start of aminoglutethimide therapy, but advise him to notify the doctor if these symptoms persist.

---

# aprotinin
Trasylol
*Pregnancy Risk Category: B*

## HOW SUPPLIED
*Injection:* 10,000 KIU (kallikrein inactivator units)/ml (1.4 mg/ml) in 100-ml and 200-ml vials

## ACTION
A naturally occurring protease inhibitor that acts as a systemic hemostatic agent, decreasing bleeding and turnover of coagulation factors. It inhibits fibrinolysis by affecting kallikrein and plasmin, prevents triggering of the contact phase of the coagulation pathway, and increases the resistance of platelets to damage from mechanical injury and high plasmin levels that occur during cardiopulmonary bypass.

## ONSET, PEAK, DURATION
Unknown.

## INDICATIONS & DOSAGE
*To reduce blood loss or the need for transfusion in patients undergoing coronary artery bypass grafts –*
**Adults:** started with 10,000 units test dose at least 10 minutes before the loading dose. If no allergic reaction is

---

evident, anesthesia may be induced while the loading dose of 2 million units is given slowly over 20 to 30 minutes. When the loading dose is complete, sternotomy may be performed. Before bypass is initiated, the cardiopulmonary bypass circuit is primed with 2 million units of the drug by replacing an aliquot of the priming fluid with the drug. A continuous infusion at a rate of 500,000 units/hour is then given until the patient leaves the operating room. This is known as *regimen A.* Alternatively, a second regimen known as *regimen B* may be given which is half the dosage of *regimen A* (except for test dose).

## ADVERSE REACTIONS

**CV:** *cardiac arrest, CHF, heart failure, ventricular tachycardia,* MI, heart block, *atrial fibrillation,* atrial flutter, hypotension, supraventricular tachycardia.
**GU:** nephrotoxicity, *renal failure.*
**Respiratory:** pneumonia, respiratory disorder, apnea, asthma, dyspnea.
**Other:** hypersensitivity reactions, *anaphylaxis,* fever, *shock,* sepsis.

## INTERACTIONS
None significant.

## CONTRAINDICATIONS
Contraindicated in patients hypersensitive to beef because the drug is prepared from bovine lung.

## NURSING CONSIDERATIONS
• **Alert:** Use drug cautiously and monitor patients closely for hypersensitivity reaction. Patients may experience anaphylaxis after the full therapeutic dose even if they remained asymptomatic after the test dose. If symptoms of hypersensitivity occur (skin eruptions, itching, dyspnea, nausea, tachycardia), discontinue the infusion immediately, make doctor aware, and provide supportive treatment.
• Obtain history of possible allergies.

Patients with a history of allergies to drugs or other substances may be at higher risk of developing an allergic reaction to aprotinin.
• Be prepared to administer a test dose. Test dose is particularly important in patients who have previously received the drug because they have a higher risk of anaphylaxis. In such patients, pretreat with an antihistamine, as ordered.
• **I.V. use:** Keep in mind that aprotinin is incompatible with amino acids, corticosteroids, fat emulsions, heparin, and tetracyclines. Don't add any drugs to the I.V. container and use a separate I.V. line.
• Administer all doses through a central line.
• To avoid hypotension, make sure patients are supine when the loading dose is given.
• Monitor laboratory studies, as ordered. Aprotinin will prolong activated clotting time and PTT. It may increase CK and transaminase levels and may falsely prolong whole blood clotting times when determined by surface activation methods, such as the Hemachron method.
• Monitor patients for increased serum creatinine levels and other signs of nephrotoxicity. If nephrotoxicity occurs, it is usually mild and reversible.
• Store between 36° and 77° F (2° and 25° C). Protect from freezing.

☑ **PATIENT TEACHING**
• Explain need for drug and how drug is administered to patient and family.
• Reassure patient and family that patient will be monitored continuously throughout drug administration for adverse reactions.

---

*Liquid form contains alcohol.   **May contain tartrazine.   †Canada only.   ‡Australia only.   ◇OTC.

# calcipotriene
Dovonex

*Pregnancy Risk Category: C*

## HOW SUPPLIED
*Ointment:* 0.005%

## ACTION
A synthetic vitamin D$_3$ analogue that regulates the development and production of skin cells.

## ONSET, PEAK, DURATION
Unknown.

## INDICATIONS & DOSAGE
*Moderate plaque psoriasis* –
**Adults:** apply a thin layer to the affected area b.i.d. Rub in gently and completely.

## ADVERSE REACTIONS
**Skin:** *burning, pruritus, irritation,* atrophy, dermatitis, dry skin, erythema, folliculitis, hyperpigmentation, peeling, rash, worsening of psoriasis.
**Other:** hypercalcemia.

## INTERACTIONS
None significant.

## CONTRAINDICATIONS
Contraindicated in patients hypersensitive to the drug or any components in the preparation. Also contraindicated in patients with hypercalcemia or evidence of vitamin D toxicity.

## NURSING CONSIDERATIONS
● Use cautiously in breast-feeding patients.
● Use cautiously in elderly patients; they may experience more severe adverse skin reactions.

## ☑ PATIENT TEACHING
● Advise patients to apply only a thin layer of ointment. Transient eleva-tions of serum calcium can occur, especially when applied excessively.
● Advise patients not to use the drug on the face, in the eyes, orally, or vaginally. Tell them to wash their hands after applying the ointment.
● Tell patients discontinue drug and call doctor if drug irritates lesions or surrounding uninvolved skin.

# capsaicin
Axsain◇, Zostrix◇, Zostrix-HP
0.075%

*Pregnancy Risk Category: NR*

## HOW SUPPLIED
*Cream:* 0.025%◇ (Zostrix◇),
0.075%◇ (Axsain◇)

## ACTION
Unknown. May deplete substance P, the principal neurotransmitter for pain, in peripheral type C sensory fibers.

## ONSET, PEAK, DURATION
Unknown.

## INDICATIONS & DOSAGE
*Temporary relief of pain after herpes zoster infections, neuralgias, such as postoperative pain and painful diabetic neuropathy; pain associated with osteoarthritis or rheumatoid arthritis* –
**Adults and children over 2 years:** applied to affected areas not more than q.i.d.

## ADVERSE REACTIONS
**Respiratory:** cough, irritation.
**Skin:** redness, *stinging or burning on application.*

## INTERACTIONS
None significant.

## CONTRAINDICATIONS
Contraindicated in patients hypersensitive to the drug.

---

Reactions may be *common,* uncommon, *life-threatening,* or COMMON AND LIFE-THREATENING.

## NURSING CONSIDERATIONS
• Know that drug is for external use only.

☑ **PATIENT TEACHING**
• Warn patient to avoid getting drug in eyes or on broken skin.
• Advise patient not to bandage area tightly after applying drug.
• Tell patient to wash hands after applying drug.
• Inform patient that transient burning or stinging with application is usually evident at initial therapy but will decrease with cautious use. However, this effect will persist in patient who uses the drug less frequently than three times a day.
• Tell patient who is self-medicating with capsaicin to contact the doctor if symptoms persist beyond 2 to 4 weeks or resolve and shortly reappear.

---

# cisapride
Propulsid

*Pregnancy Risk Category: C*

## HOW SUPPLIED
*Tablets:* 10 mg, 20 mg

## ACTION
Stimulates serotonin-4 (5-HT$_4$) receptors, enhancing the release of acetylcholine at the myenteric plexus and increasing GI motility.

## ONSET, PEAK, DURATION
Onset occurs in 30 to 60 minutes. Plasma levels peak within 1 to 2 hours. Duration unknown.

## INDICATIONS & DOSAGE
*Symptoms of nocturnal heartburn caused by gastroesophageal reflux disease* –
**Adults:** initially, 10 mg P.O. q.i.d. 15 minutes before meals and h.s. If response is inadequate, increased to 20 mg q.i.d.

## ADVERSE REACTIONS
**CNS:** *headache,* insomnia, anxiety, nervousness.
**EENT:** abnormal vision.
**GI:** *diarrhea, abdominal pain,* nausea, constipation, flatulence, dyspepsia.
**GU:** frequency, urinary tract infection, vaginitis.
**Respiratory:** rhinitis, sinusitis, cough, upper respiratory tract infections.
**Skin:** rash, pruritus.
**Other:** pain, fever, viral infections, arthralgia.

## INTERACTIONS
*Anticholinergics:* decreased effectiveness of cisapride. Avoid concomitant use.
*Anticoagulants:* may increase clotting times. Monitor closely.
*Benzodiazepines, ethanol:* enhanced sedation. Avoid concomitant use.
*Cimetidine, ranitidine:* increased absorption of these agents; cimetidine increases cisapride levels. Use together cautiously.
*Itraconazole, ketoconazole, I.V. miconazole, troleandomycin:* increased cisapride levels which may cause ventricular arrhythmias. Avoid concomitant use.

## CONTRAINDICATIONS
Contraindicated in patients hypersensitive to the drug. Also contraindicated in patients in whom increased GI motility may be harmful, such as those with mechanical obstruction, hemorrhage, or perforation of the GI tract.

## NURSING CONSIDERATIONS
• Use cautiously in breast-feeding patients because small amounts of the drug are excreted in breast milk.

☑ **PATIENT TEACHING**
• Remind patient to avoid alcohol and sedatives while using this drug.

---

• Advise patient to immediately report any adverse effects to the doctor.

---

## clomiphene citrate
Clomid, Milophene, Serophene

*Pregnancy Risk Category: NR*

### HOW SUPPLIED
*Tablets:* 50 mg

### ACTION
Unknown. Appears to stimulate release of pituitary gonadotropins, follicle-stimulating hormone, and luteinizing hormone. This results in maturation of the ovarian follicle, ovulation, and development of the corpus luteum.

### ONSET, PEAK, DURATION
Not clearly defined although ovulation usually occurs 4 to 10 days after last day of treatment; this period of time may vary among patients and for each cycle.

### INDICATIONS & DOSAGE
*To induce ovulation –*
**Adults:** 50 to 100 mg P.O. daily for 5 days, starting any time; or 50 to 100 mg P.O. daily starting on day 5 of menstrual cycle (first day of menstrual flow is day 1). Repeated until conception occurs or until three courses of therapy are completed.

### ADVERSE REACTIONS
**CNS:** headache, restlessness, insomnia, dizziness, light-headedness, depression, fatigue.
**EENT:** blurred vision, diplopia, scotoma, photophobia.
**GI:** nausea, vomiting, bloating, distention, weight gain.
**GU:** urinary frequency and polyuria; abnormal uterine bleeding; *ovarian enlargement* and cyst formation, which regress spontaneously when drug is stopped.
**Skin:** urticaria, rash, dermatitis.

**Other:** *hot flashes,* reversible alopecia, *breast discomfort.*

### INTERACTIONS
None significant.

### CONTRAINDICATIONS
Contraindicated during pregnancy and in patients with undiagnosed abnormal genital bleeding, ovarian cyst not due to polycystic ovarian syndrome, hepatic disease or dysfunction, uncontrolled thyroid or adrenal dysfunction, or presence of organic intracranial lesion (such as a pituitary tumor).

### NURSING CONSIDERATIONS
• Know that patient must be monitored closely because of potentially serious adverse reactions.

### ☑ PATIENT TEACHING
• Tell patient there is a possibility of multiple births with this drug. Risk increases with higher doses.
• Teach patient to take and chart basal body temperature to ascertain whether ovulation has occurred.
• Reassure patient that ovulation generally occurs after the first course of therapy. If pregnancy does not occur, course of therapy may be repeated twice.
• Advise patient to stop drug and contact the doctor immediately if pregnancy is suspected because the drug may have teratogenic effect.
• *Alert:* Advise patient to stop drug and contact the doctor immediately if abdominal symptoms or pain occurs because these may indicate ovarian enlargement or ovarian cyst. Also tell patient to report signs of impending visual toxicity – blurred vision, diplopia, scotoma, or photophobia – to the doctor immediately.
• Warn patient to avoid hazardous activities, such as driving or operating machinery, until CNS effects are

---

Reactions may be *common,* uncommon, *life-threatening,* or COMMON AND LIFE-THREATENING.

known. Drug may cause dizziness or visual disturbances.

# cysteamine bitartrate
Cystagon

*Pregnancy Risk Category: C*

## HOW SUPPLIED
*Capsules:* 50 mg, 150 mg

## ACTION
Reacts with cystine, thereby decreasing the cystine level in cells.

## ONSET, PEAK, DURATION
Unknown.

## INDICATIONS & DOSAGE
*Management of nephropathic cystinosis –*

**Adults and children over age 12 and weighing more than 50 kg:** initially, one-fourth to one-sixth of the maintenance dosage, then increased gradually over 4 to 6 weeks to achieve maintenance dosage. Maintenance dosage is 2 g (free base) P.O. in four divided doses.

**Children 12 years and under:** initially, one-fourth to one-sixth of the maintenance dosage, then increased gradually over 4 to 6 weeks to achieve maintenance dosage. Maintenance dosage is 1.3 g/m$^2$ (free base) P.O. daily in four divided doses.

## ADVERSE REACTIONS
**CNS:** *lethargy,* somnolence, encephalopathy, headache, *seizures,* ataxia, confusion, tremor, hyperkinesis, decreasing hearing, dizziness, jitteriness, nervousness, abnormal thinking, depression, emotional lability, hallucinations, nightmares.
**CV:** hypertension.
**GI:** *vomiting, anorexia, diarrhea,* nausea, abdominal pain, dyspepsia, constipation, gastroenteritis, duodenitis, duodenal ulcer.
**Hepatic:** abnormal liver function.

**Hematologic:** anemia, leukopenia.
**Skin:** *rash,* urticaria.
**Other:** *fever,* dehydration, bad breath.

## INTERACTIONS
None significant.

## CONTRAINDICATIONS
Contraindicated in patients with hypersensitivity to the drug, cysteamine, or penicillamine.

## NURSING CONSIDERATIONS
• Know that drug therapy should begin as soon as the diagnosis of nephropathic cystinosis has been confirmed by increased level of cystine in increased WBCs.
• Monitor patient for a rash. If one develops, notify the doctor because the drug will need to be withheld until the rash clears. The doctor may then restart the drug at a lower dosage and slowly titrate dosage to achieve therapeutic effect. However, if a severe rash (such as erythema multiforme bullosa or toxic epidermal necrolysis) develops, know that the drug should not be restarted.
• Monitor patient closely for adverse CNS or GI reactions. If any develop, notify the doctor because the dosage will need to be adjusted or the drug temporarily withheld.
• Monitor patient's CBC and liver function studies, as ordered, to detect adverse hematologic reactions. Notify the doctor if any laboratory abnormalities are present.
• Be aware that measurements of cystine level in leukocytes may be ordered because they are useful in determining adequate dosage and compliance. When the drug is well tolerated, the goal of therapy is to keep leukocyte cystine levels below 1 mmol/½ cystine/mg protein 5 to 6 hours after administration of the drug. Measurements should be done at least every 3 months.

---

• Know that patients with cystinosis taking cysteamine hydrochloride or phosphocysteamine solutions may be transferred to equimolar doses of the drug.

☑ **PATIENT TEACHING**
• Inform the patient and parents that dosage of cysteamine is based on the patient's weight and that patient must follow doctor's directions exactly.
• Instruct the patient and parents that if a dose of the drug is missed, it should be taken as soon as possible. However, if within 2 hours of the next dose, patient should skip the missed dose and resume the regular dosing schedule. Tell patient not to double the dose.
• Tell parents of a child under age 6 not to give the child the capsule to swallow because the child may choke or aspirate it. Instead, the capsule may be opened and the contents sprinkled on food or mixed in formula.
• Inform the patient or parents that supplements also will be given to replace electrolytes lost through the kidneys and that periodic blood tests will need to be performed to help determine the correct dosage of the drug. Compliance with these measures is extremely important for maximal effectiveness of the drug.
• Instruct the patient not to engage in hazardous activities (such as driving) until the drug's CNS effects are known.
• Advise patient and parents to store the drug in a dry place, away from light.

▼ *NEW DRUG*

# dexrazoxane
Zinecard

*Pregnancy Risk Category: C*

**HOW SUPPLIED**
*Injection:* 250 mg, 500 mg

**ACTION**
Unknown. A cyclic derivative of EDTA that readily penetrates cell membranes, drug may be converted to ring-opened chelating agent that interferes with iron-mediated free radical generation thought to be partly responsible for anthracycline-induced cardiomyopathy.

**ONSET, PEAK, DURATION**
Onset and duration unknown. Peak plasma levels occur in 15 minutes.

**INDICATIONS & DOSAGE**
*Reduction of incidence and severity of doxorubicin-induced cardiomyopathy in women with metastatic breast cancer who have received a cumulative doxorubicin dose of 300 mg/m² but would benefit from continued doxorubicin therapy —*
**Adults:** Dosage ratio of dexrazoxane to doxorubicin must be 10:1 (such as 500 mg/m² of dexrazoxane:50 mg/m² of doxorubicin). After reconstitution, dexrazoxane should be administered by slow I.V. push or rapid drip I.V. infusion. After completion of dexrazoxane administration and before 30 minutes have elapsed from its start, the I.V. injection of doxorubicin should be given.

**ADVERSE REACTIONS**
*Note:* The following reactions (except for pain on injection) may be attributed to the FAC regimen (fluorouracil, anthracycline, cyclophosphamide) given shortly after dexrazoxane.
**CNS:** *fatigue, malaise, neurotoxicity.*
**GI:** *nausea, vomiting, anorexia, stomatitis, diarrhea,* esophagitis, dysphagia.
**Hematologic:** immunosuppression, hemorrhage.
**Skin:** urticaria.
**Other:** *alopecia, fever, infection, pain on injection, sepsis,* streaking at I.V. insertion site, erythema, phlebitis, extravasation.

---

Reactions may be *common,* uncommon, *life-threatening,* or **COMMON AND LIFE-THREATENING**.

## INTERACTIONS
None known.

## CONTRAINDICATIONS
Contraindicated in patients who are not receiving anthracycline as part of the chemotherapy regimen.

## NURSING CONSIDERATIONS
• Drug is not recommended for use in pregnant or breast-feeding women.
• Use cautiously in all patients because additive effects of immunosuppression may occur from concomitant administration of cytotoxic drugs.
• *Alert:* Dexrazoxane is not recommended for use until after patient has an accumulated doxorubicin dose of 300 mg/m$^2$ and continuation of doxorubicin is desired. With combination therapy, dexrazoxane should be administered before doxorubicin.
• **I.V. use:** Drug must be diluted with diluent supplied with drug (0.167 Molar Sodium Lactate Injection) to give concentration of 10 mg dexrazoxane per 1 ml of sodium lactate. Reconstituted drug should be given by slow I.V. push or rapid drip I.V. infusion from a bag.
• When transferred to empty infusion bag, reconstituted drug is stable for 6 hours when stored at 36° to 46° F (2° to 8° C). Discard unused solution.
• Reconstituted drug may be diluted with normal saline solution or 5% dextrose injection to concentration of 1.3 to 5.0 mg/ml in I.V. infusion bags. Resultant solution is stable for 6 hours under same storage conditions as those for diluted drug.
• When handling and preparing reconstituted solution, wear gloves and use same precautions as those for handling antineoplastic drugs. If drug powder or solution contacts skin or mucosa, immediately wash affected areas thoroughly with soap and water.
• Don't mix dexrazoxane with other drugs.
• Monitor CBC closely, as ordered, because drug may add to myelosuppressive effects of cytotoxic drugs. Institute infection control and bleeding precautions, as indicated by CBC results.

## ☑ PATIENT TEACHING
• Explain the drug's purpose to patient.
• Instruct her to watch for and report signs of infection (fever, sore throat, fatigue) and bleeding (easy bruising, nose bleeds, bleeding gums, melena). Tell her to take her temperature daily, and teach her infection control and bleeding precautions.
• Reassure her that alopecia is usually reversible.

---

# diazoxide, oral
Proglycem
*Pregnancy Risk Category: C*

## HOW SUPPLIED
*Capsules:* 50 mg
*Oral suspension:* 50 mg/ml in 30-ml bottle

## ACTION
Inhibits release of insulin from the pancreas and decreases peripheral utilization of glucose.

## ONSET, PEAK, DURATION
Onset occurs in 1 hour. Peak unknown. Effects persist for 8 hours.

## INDICATIONS & DOSAGE
*Hypoglycemia from a variety of conditions resulting in hyperinsulinism* —
**Adults and children:** 3 to 8 mg/kg P.O. daily, in two or three equally divided doses q 8 to 12 hours.
**Infants and neonates:** 8 to 15 mg/kg P.O. daily, in two or three equally divided doses q 8 to 12 hours.

---

## ADVERSE REACTIONS

**CNS:** headache, weakness, malaise, anxiety, dizziness, insomnia, paresthesia.

**CV:** arrhythmias, tachycardia, hypotension, hypertension.

**EENT:** diplopia, transient cataracts, blurred vision, lacrimation.

**GI:** nausea, vomiting, anorexia, taste alteration, abdominal pain, diarrhea.

**GU:** azotemia, reversible nephrotic syndrome, decreased urinary output, hematuria, albuminuria.

**Hematologic:** leukopenia, *thrombocytopenia,* anemia, eosinophilia, excessive bleeding.

**Skin:** rash, pruritus.

**Other:** *sodium and fluid retention, ketoacidosis and hyperosmolar nonketotic syndrome, hyperuricemia,* hirsutism, fever.

## INTERACTIONS

*Alpha-adrenergic blockers:* antagonism of diazoxide inhibition of insulin release. Avoid concomitant use.

*Anticoagulants:* increased anticoagulant effect. Adjust dosage of anticoagulant.

*Antigout agents:* increased serum uric acid. Adjust dosage of antigout agent.

*Antihypertensives, peripheral vasodilators:* additive hypotensive effects. Monitor blood pressure.

*Beta-adrenergic blockers:* increased hypotensive effect. Monitor blood pressure.

*Hydantoin anticonvulsants:* decreased anticonvulsant effects and decreased hyperglycemic effect of diazoxide. Don't use together.

*Thiazide diuretics:* may potentiate hyperglycemic, hyperuricemic, and hypotensive effects. Monitor appropriate laboratory values.

## CONTRAINDICATIONS

Contraindicated in patients hypersensitive to the drug or other thiazides and in patients with functional hypoglycemia.

## NURSING CONSIDERATIONS

• Monitor urine regularly for glucose and ketones; report any abnormalities to the doctor.

• If not effective after 2 or 3 weeks, be prepared to stop drug, as ordered.

• Be aware that oral diazoxide does not significantly lower blood pressure in the dosages used to treat hypoglycemia.

### ☑ PATIENT TEACHING

• Explain to patient and family importance of following dietary restrictions for successful therapy.

• Reassure patient that hair growth on arms and forehead is a common adverse reaction that subsides when drug treatment is completed.

• Advise patient to report to the doctor any adverse reactions, including excessive thirst, fruity breath odor, or urinary frequency.

---

## etretinate
Tegison

*Pregnancy Risk Category: X*

### HOW SUPPLIED
*Capsules:* 10 mg, 25 mg

### ACTION
Unknown. Thought to inhibit ornithine decarboxylase, an enzyme that regulates cell growth and differentiation. May also block neutrophil migration into the epidermis.

### ONSET, PEAK, DURATION
Onset and duration unknown. Peak concentration occurs in 2 to 6 hours.

### INDICATIONS & DOSAGE
*Severe recalcitrant psoriasis, including erythrodermia and generalized pustular types in patients unresponsive to standard therapy (topical tar plus UVB light, psoralens plus UVA light, systemic corticosteroids, and methotrexate) —*

---

Reactions may be *common,* uncommon, *life-threatening,* or **COMMON AND LIFE-THREATENING.**

**Adults:** initially, 0.75 to 1 mg/kg P.O. daily in divided doses. Maximum initial dosage is 1.5 mg/kg daily. After initial response, maintenance dosage is 0.5 to 0.75 mg/kg daily.

## ADVERSE REACTIONS
**CNS:** *benign intracranial hypertension (pseudotumor cerebri), fatigue,* headache, dizziness, lethargy, pain, rigors.
**CV:** thrombosis, edema.
**EENT:** *eye pain, blurred vision, dry eyes,* photosensitivity, decreased night vision, *conjunctivitis, diplopia, dry nose, sore mouth,* gingival bleeding.
**GI:** *appetite change, nausea, sore tongue, chapped lips, dry mouth, thirst, abdominal pain.*
**GU:** *WBCs in urine,* proteinuria, hematuria, glycosuria.
**Hematologic:** *blood dyscrasia,* anemia, altered PT, *thrombocytopenia.*
**Hepatic:** *hepatitis,* elevated liver enzymes.
**Respiratory:** dyspnea.
**Skin:** *peeling, pruritus, alopecia, dry skin, rash, red scaly face, bruising, sunburn, nail disorders.*
**Other:** *bone pain, hypokalemia or hyperkalemia, hyperlipidemia, hyperostosis, muscle cramps, myalgia, fever.*

## INTERACTIONS
*Ethanol:* increased risk of hypertriglyceridemia. Avoid concomitant use.
*Hepatotoxic medications (including methotrexate):* increased risk of hepatotoxicity. Monitor closely.
*Tetracyclines:* increased risk of pseudotumor cerebri. Avoid concomitant use.
*Vitamin A:* additive toxic effects. Avoid concomitant use.

## CONTRAINDICATIONS
Contraindicated in patients who are pregnant, who intend to become pregnant, or who may not use reliable contraception during and after treatment (drug causes severe birth defects).

## NURSING CONSIDERATIONS
● Be aware that women of childbearing age must not receive etretinate unless pregnancy is excluded by a pregnancy test within 2 weeks before initiating therapy. Therapy may begin on 2nd or 3rd day of next normal menstrual period.
● Monitor liver function tests every 1 to 2 weeks for the first 1 to 2 months of therapy, and every 1 to 3 months thereafter, as ordered. Suspected hepatotoxicity requires discontinuation of drug.
● Monitor blood lipids every 1 to 2 weeks during treatment, as ordered.
● **Alert:** Monitor patient for pseudotumor cerebri. If symptoms occur, immediately check for papilledema. If present, discontinue drug immediately and notify doctor.

## ☑ PATIENT TEACHING
● Warn patient to use effective contraception for 1 month before therapy begins, during treatment, and for an indefinite time after treatment is discontinued. Know that significant residual blood levels of etretinate have been reported as long as 3 years after discontinuation of treatment. Consequently, the period after treatment during which pregnancy must be avoided to prevent teratogenicity is unknown.
● Advise patient to take drug with milk or fatty food to enhance absorption.
● Advise patient never to double the dose but to take a missed dose as soon as possible. If it's nearly time for the next dose, the missed dose should be skipped and the schedule resumed.
● Warn patient not to take vitamin A supplements to avoid possible additive adverse reactions.
● Reassure patient that transient exacerbation of psoriasis is common during beginning of therapy.

---

*Liquid form contains alcohol.   **May contain tartrazine.   †Canada only.   ‡Australia only.   ◇OTC.

• Advise patient to expect dry skin and possible difficulty tolerating contact lenses during treatment.
• Tell patient to avoid bright sun and to use a sunblock to prevent photosensitivity reactions.
• Advise patient to use ice or sugarless hard candy or gum for dry mouth and to check with the dentist if this continues beyond 2 weeks.
• Advise patient to report visual difficulties.
• Advise diabetic patient to monitor blood glucose closely. Adjustments of hypoglycemic medications may be necessary.
• Tell patient to report possible early signs of pseudotumor cerebri—headache, nausea and vomiting, and visual disturbances—to the doctor promptly.

---

## finasteride
Proscar

*Pregnancy Risk Category: X*

### HOW SUPPLIED
*Tablets:* 5 mg

### ACTION
Competitively inhibits steroid 5 alpha-reductase, an enzyme responsible for formation of the potent androgen 5 alpha-dihydrotestosterone (DHT) from testosterone. Because DHT influences development of the prostate gland, decreasing levels of this hormone in adult males should relieve the symptoms associated with benign prostatic hyperplasia (BPH).

### ONSET, PEAK, DURATION
Onset unknown. Serum levels peak in 1 to 2 hours. Effects persist for 24 hours after single dose; about 2 weeks after withdrawal of therapy.

### INDICATIONS & DOSAGE
*Symptomatic BPH* –
**Adults:** 5 mg P.O. daily.

### ADVERSE REACTIONS
**GU:** impotence, decreased volume of ejaculate.
**Other:** decreased libido.

### INTERACTIONS
*Theophylline:* may increase theophylline clearance and decrease theophylline half-life. Monitor theophylline levels.

### CONTRAINDICATIONS
Contraindicated in patients hypersensitive to the drug. Know that although drug is not used in women, manufacturer indicates pregnancy as a contraindication.

### NURSING CONSIDERATIONS
• Before therapy, know that patient should be evaluated for conditions that might mimic BPH, including hypotonic bladder; prostate cancer, infection, or stricture; or relevant neurologic conditions.
• Anticipate baseline and periodic digital rectal examinations. Drug will decrease serum prostate-specific antigen (PSA) levels, even in prostate cancer. However, in clinical trials, drug didn't appear to decrease the rate of prostate cancer detection.
• Carefully monitor patients who have a large residual urine volume or severely diminished urine flow. Know that these patients may not be candidates for finasteride therapy.
• Carefully evaluate sustained increases in serum PSA levels, which could indicate noncompliance with therapy.
• Be aware that although drug's elimination rate is decreased in elderly patients, dosage adjustments aren't necessary.
• Because it's impossible to identify which patients will respond to finasteride, know that a minimum of 6 months of therapy may be necessary.
• Keep in mind that the long-term effects on the complications of BPH, in-

---

Reactions may be *common,* uncommon, *life-threatening,* or **COMMON AND LIFE-THREATENING.**

cluding acute urinary obstruction, and incidence of surgery are unknown.

### ☑ PATIENT TEACHING
• Warn woman who is or may become pregnant not to handle crushed tablets because of risk of adverse effects on a male fetus.
• Caution patient whose sexual partner is or may become pregnant to discontinue drug or take precautions to avoid exposing her to his semen.
• Reassure patient that finasteride may decrease volume of ejaculate but doesn't appear to impair normal sexual function. However, impotence and decreased libido have occurred in less than 4% of patients.

---

### gallium nitrate
Ganite

*Pregnancy Risk Category: C*

### HOW SUPPLIED
*Injection:* 25 mg/ml

### ACTION
Unknown. Appears to reduce hypercalcemia by inhibiting resorption of bone and reducing bone turnover in patients with increased bone turnover.

### ONSET, PEAK, DURATION
Onset and peak unknown. Effects persist for 6 days.

### INDICATIONS & DOSAGE
*Symptomatic, unresponsive hypercalcemia caused by cancer –*
**Adults:** 200 mg/m$^2$ as a continuous I.V. infusion daily for 5 consecutive days or until serum calcium is normal. Lower doses (100 mg/m$^2$) may be given to patients with mild hypercalcemia.

### ADVERSE REACTIONS
**CNS:** lethargy, confusion, paresthesia.
**CV:** tachycardia, lower extremity edema, decreased mean systolic and diastolic blood pressures.
**EENT:** visual or hearing impairment, acute optic neuritis.
**GI:** nausea and vomiting, diarrhea, constipation.
**GU:** *acute renal failure, increased BUN and creatinine levels.*
**Hematologic:** anemia, leukopenia.
**Respiratory:** dyspnea, rales and rhonchi, pulmonary infiltrates, pleural effusion.
**Skin:** rash.
**Other:** *hypophosphatemia, hypocalcemia, decreased serum bicarbonate,* fever, hypothermia.

### INTERACTIONS
*Nephrotoxic drugs, such as aminoglycosides or amphotericin B:* increased risk of nephrotoxicity. Avoid concomitant use.

### CONTRAINDICATIONS
Contraindicated in patients with severe renal impairment.

### NURSING CONSIDERATIONS
• Make sure that patients are adequately hydrated, either with oral fluids or I.V. sodium chloride solution, as ordered, before using drug. Establish adequate urine flow (2 liters/day) before treatment. Diuretic therapy is not recommended before correction of hypovolemia. Avoid overhydration, especially in patients with decreased CV function.
• **I.V. use:** Dilute daily dose in 1 liter of 0.9% sodium chloride for injection or D$_5$W. Discard unused portion (drug contains no preservatives).
• Know that rapid I.V. infusion or dosage over 200 mg/m$^2$ may increase risk of nephrotoxicity or cause nausea and vomiting.
• Monitor BUN and serum creatinine levels, as ordered, during therapy. Discontinue drug if serum creatinine rises above 2.5 mg/dl, and notify doctor.

---

*Liquid form contains alcohol.  **May contain tartrazine.  †Canada only.  ‡Australia only.  ◇OTC.

• Carefully monitor fluid intake and output and renal function, as ordered. Short-term therapy with I.V. calcium may also be needed. Overdosage is usually treated with vigorous hydration, sometimes with diuretics, for 2 to 3 days.

• In patients who require treatment with a potentially nephrotoxic drug, such as an aminoglycoside, be prepared to discontinue gallium nitrate therapy and continue hydration for several days after administration of the nephrotoxic drug, as ordered. Monitor renal function closely.

• Monitor serum calcium levels, as ordered, and assess patients for signs of hypocalcemia, including a positive Chvostek's sign. If hypocalcemia occurs, discontinue drug and notify doctor. Treatment of hypocalcemia may be required.

• Be aware that transient hypophosphatemia is common. Patients may require oral phosphorus supplements.

☑ **PATIENT TEACHING**

• Stress importance of forcing fluids as directed throughout therapy.

• Advise patient to report hearing or vision problems. In early clinical trials, a few patients experienced hearing loss and optic neuritis after high-dose gallium nitrate therapy when combined with investigational antineoplastic agents.

---

# imiglucerase
Cerezyme

*Pregnancy Risk Category: C*

## HOW SUPPLIED
*Injection:* 200 units/vial

## ACTION
Catalyzes the hydrolysis of glucocerebroside to glucose and ceramide (part of the normal degradation pathway for lipids) and thus prevents the sequelae of Gaucher's disease, which normally occur as a result of the accumulation of glucocerebroside.

## ONSET, PEAK, DURATION
Onset and duration unknown. Levels peak in 1 hour.

## INDICATIONS & DOSAGE
*Long-term endogenous enzyme (glucosylceramidase) replacement therapy in confirmed type I Gaucher's disease –*
**Adults and children:** dosage individualized; initially, up to 60 U/kg I.V. administered over 1 to 2 hours. Frequency of dosing typically is once q 2 weeks, but may range from three times weekly to once monthly, depending on severity of the disease. Dosage may be reduced for maintenance therapy, at intervals of 3 to 6 months, while response parameters are carefully monitored.

## ADVERSE REACTIONS
**CNS:** headache, dizziness.
**CV:** mild hypotension.
**GI:** nausea, abdominal discomfort.
**GU:** decreased urinary frequency.
**Skin:** pruritus, rash.
**Other:** hypersensitivity reactions.

## INTERACTIONS
None significant.

## CONTRAINDICATIONS
None known.

## NURSING CONSIDERATIONS
• Use with caution in patients who have exhibited symptoms of hypersensitivity to the product and in those who have previously been treated with alglucerase and who have developed antibody to alglucerase or exhibited symptoms of hypersensitivity to alglucerase.

• **I.V. use:** Reconstitute each vial with 5.1 ml of sterile water for injection USP. Inspect solution for particulate matter and discoloration before use; if either is present, do not use.

---

Reactions may be *common,* uncommon, *life-threatening,* or **COMMON AND LIFE-THREATENING.**

Dilute solution further with 0.9% sodium chloride solution to a final volume of 100 to 200 ml. Because imiglucerase is preservative-free, use immediately. Administer by I.V. infusion over 1 to 2 hours.

• Know that when diluted to 50 ml, imiglucerase has been shown to be stable for up to 24 hours when stored at 2° to 8° C (36° to 46° F).

• Monitor response parameters for doctor to determine lowest effective dosage.

### ☑ PATIENT TEACHING
• Explain to patient and family how drug works and how it is administered. Stress importance of compliance with administration schedule.

• Tell patient to report persistent or severe adverse reactions promptly.

---

## isotretinoin
Accutane, Roaccutane‡

*Pregnancy Risk Category: X*

### HOW SUPPLIED
*Capsules:* 10 mg, 20 mg, 40 mg

### ACTION
Unknown. Thought to normalize keratinization, reversibly decrease size of sebaceous glands, and alter composition of sebum to a less viscous form that is less likely to cause follicular plugging.

### ONSET, PEAK, DURATION
Onset and duration unknown. Plasma levels peak in about 3 hours.

### INDICATIONS & DOSAGE
*Severe recalcitrant nodular acne unresponsive to conventional therapy –*
**Adults and adolescents:** 0.5 to 2 mg/kg P.O. daily in two divided doses for 15 to 20 weeks.

### ADVERSE REACTIONS
**CNS:** headache, fatigue, *pseudotumor cerebri* (benign intracranial hypertension).
**EENT:** *conjunctivitis,* corneal deposits, dry eyes, visual disturbances, *epistaxis, dry nose.*
**GI:** nonspecific GI symptoms, gum bleeding and inflammation, *nausea, vomiting,* anorexia, *dry mouth, abdominal pain.*
**Hematologic:** anemia, elevated platelet count.
**Hepatic:** elevated AST, ALT, and alkaline phosphatase levels.
**Skin:** *cheilosis, rash, dry skin, facial skin desquamation,* peeling of palms and toes, skin infection, photosensitivity, *cheilitis, pruritus, fragility.*
**Other:** *hypertriglyceridemia, musculoskeletal pain (skeletal hyperostosis), drying of mucous membranes, petechiae, nail brittleness,* thinning of hair, hyperglycemia.

### INTERACTIONS
*Ethanol:* increased risk of hypertriglyceridemia. Avoid concomitant use.
*Tetracyclines:* increased risk of pseudotumor cerebri. Avoid concomitant use.
*Vitamin A, products containing vitamin A:* increased toxic effects of isotretinoin. Don't use together without the doctor's permission.

### CONTRAINDICATIONS
Contraindicated in women of childbearing age unless patient has had a negative serum pregnancy test within 2 weeks before beginning therapy; will begin drug therapy on 2nd or 3rd day of next menstrual period; and will comply with stringent contraceptive measures for 1 month before therapy, during therapy, and for at least 1 month after therapy. *Severe fetal abnormalities may occur if used during pregnancy.* Also contraindicated in patients hypersensitive to parabens, which are used as preservatives.

---

## NURSING CONSIDERATIONS

• Monitor baseline serum lipid studies and liver function tests prior to therapy, as ordered.

• Monitor serum lipid studies and liver function tests at regular intervals until response to drug is established, usually about 4 weeks.

• Monitor blood glucose level regularly.

• Monitor CK levels in patients who participate in vigorous physical activity, as ordered.

• Know that most adverse reactions appear to be dose-related, occurring at dosages greater than 1 mg/kg daily. They are generally reversible when therapy is discontinued or dosage is reduced.

• **Alert:** Be aware that patients who experience headache, nausea and vomiting, or visual disturbances should be screened for papilledema. Signs and symptoms of pseudotumor cerebri require immediate discontinuation of therapy and prompt neurologic intervention.

• Anticipate a second course of therapy, if needed, not to start for at least 8 weeks after completion of first course because improvement may continue after withdrawal of drug.

### ☑ PATIENT TEACHING

• Advise patient to take drug with or shortly after meals to ensure adequate absorption.

• Tell patient to immediately report any visual disturbances and bone, muscle, or joint pain.

• Warn patient that contact lenses may feel uncomfortable during isotretinoin therapy.

• Warn patient against using abrasives, medicated soaps and cleansers, acne preparations containing peeling agents, and topical alcohol preparations (including cosmetics, aftershave, cologne) because these agents cause cumulative irritation or excessive drying of skin.

• Tell patient to avoid prolonged exposure to the sun and to use sunblock. Drug may have additive effect if used with other agents that cause photosensitivity.

---

# levocarnitine (L-carnitine)
Carnitor, VitaCarn

*Pregnancy Risk Category: B*

## HOW SUPPLIED
*Tablets:* 330 mg
*Capsules:* 250 mg
*Oral liquid:* 100 mg/ml
*Injection:* 1 g/5 ml

## ACTION
Facilitates transport of fatty acids into cellular mitochondria. The fatty acids are then used to produce energy.

## ONSET, PEAK, DURATION
Unknown.

## INDICATIONS & DOSAGE
*Primary and secondary systemic carnitine deficiency –*
**Adults:** 990 mg P.O. b.i.d. or t.i.d. Alternately, 10 to 30 ml (1 to 3 g) of oral liquid daily.
**Children:** 50 to 100 mg/kg/day P.O. in divided doses.

All dosages depend on the clinical response. Higher dosages may be given. However, for children, maximum dosage is 3 g/day.
*Acute and chronic treatment of secondary carnitine deficiency –*
**Adults:** 50 mg/kg I.V. slowly over 2 to 3 minutes q 3 to 4 hours.

## ADVERSE REACTIONS
**GI:** *nausea, vomiting, cramps, diarrhea.*
**Other:** *body odor.*

## INTERACTIONS
*D,L-carnitine (sold as vitamin $B_T$):* inhibition of levocarnitine and possible deficiency. Avoid concomitant use.

---

Reactions may be *common,* uncommon, *life-threatening,* or **COMMON AND LIFE-THREATENING.**

*Valproic acid:* increased requirement for carnitine. Adjust dosage as ordered.

## CONTRAINDICATIONS
None known.

## NURSING CONSIDERATIONS
• Give enteral liquid alone or dissolved in drinks or liquid food.
• Space doses evenly every 3 to 4 hours and give drug with or after meals, if possible.
• Use entire or partial contents of containers of liquid immediately after opening; discard any unused contents.
• Do not refrigerate solution.
• Monitor patient's tolerance during 1st week of therapy and after increasing dosage, as ordered.
• Monitor blood chemistry results and plasma carnitine concentrations periodically, as ordered, as well as vital signs and patient's overall clinical condition.

## ☑ PATIENT TEACHING
• Tell patient to consume oral liquid slowly to minimize GI distress. If GI intolerance persists, dosage may have to be reduced.
• Warn patient to avoid "vitamin $B_T$" in health food stores. This will interact with the drug and render it ineffective.
• Caution patient not to share drug with others. Some people have used it to improve athletic performance.
• Warn patient about possible body odor.

---

# levomethadyl acetate hydrochloride
ORLAAM
Controlled Substance Schedule II
*Pregnancy Risk Category: C*

## HOW SUPPLIED
*Oral solution:* 10 mg/ml

## ACTION
A synthetic opiate agonist structurally similar to methadone that suppresses symptoms of withdrawal in opiate-tolerant persons by cross-substituting for opiate agonists. Long-term administration may produce sufficient tolerance to block the euphoric effects of opiate agonists.

## ONSET, PEAK, DURATION
Onset and peak unknown. Effects persist for 48 to 72 hours.

## INDICATIONS & DOSAGE
*Opiate addiction –*
**Adults:** dosage is highly individualized. Initially, 20 to 40 mg q 48 to 72 hours. Subsequent doses increased in increments of 5 to 10 mg at 48 to 72 hour intervals until steady state is reached, usually within 1 to 2 weeks. Most patients are stable on 60 to 90 mg three times a week.

## ADVERSE REACTIONS
**CNS:** drowsiness, sedation.
**CV:** bradycardia, edema, prolonged QT interval.
**EENT:** blurred vision, rhinitis.
**GI:** *abdominal pain, diarrhea, constipation, dry mouth, nausea, vomiting.*
**GU:** *impotence, difficulty with ejaculation.*
**Respiratory:** *cough.*
**Skin:** *rash, diaphoresis.*
**Other:** yawning, arthralgia, asthenia, back pain, chills, flulike syndrome, malaise, abstinence syndrome with sudden withdrawal.

## INTERACTIONS
*Carbamazepine, phenobarbital, phenytoin, rifampin:* increased hepatic enzyme activity; may increase levomethadyl's peak activity or shorten its duration of action. Monitor closely.
*Cimetidine, erythromycin, ketoconazole:* decreased hepatic enzyme activity; may decrease levomethadyl's peak

---

activity or prolong its duration of action. Monitor closely.
*Naloxone, pentazocine or other opioid agonist-antagonists:* may precipitate abstinence syndrome. Don't use together.

**CONTRAINDICATIONS**
Contraindicated in patients hypersensitive to the drug.

**NURSING CONSIDERATIONS**
• Use cautiously in patients with cardiac conduction defects or with hepatic or renal failure.
• Be aware that levomethadyl is to be used only by certain licensed and approved clinics. There are no recognized clinical uses for the drug outside of addiction treatment programs. Levomethadyl may only be dispensed by treatment programs approved by the FDA, DEA, and designated state authority. By law, take-home doses are forbidden.
• If administering to women of childbearing age, anticipate monthly pregnancy tests. Patients should be switched to methadone if pregnancy occurs.
• *Alert:* Know that this drug should never be administered on a daily basis because of the risk of fatal overdose.
• Know that most patients can tolerate the 72-hour interval between weekly regimens. If withdrawal is a problem during the 72-hour interval, be prepared to increase the preceding dose or switch to an alternate-day schedule as ordered. Never give levomethadyl on 2 consecutive days; instead, give small supplemental doses of methadone. Consider the risk of drug diversion before giving patients take-home methadone.
• When used to replace methadone, keep in mind that the suggested initial dose is 1.2 to 1.3 times the daily methadone dose three times a week, not to exceed 120 mg. Adjust dosage according to clinical response as or-

dered. The crossover to methadone should be done in a single dose rather than decreasing doses of methadone and increasing doses of levomethadyl.

☑ **PATIENT TEACHING**
• Explain how drug is administered, and review administration schedule with patient and family.
• Inform female patient of need for monthly pregnancy tests. Advise patient to avoid pregnancy but if pregnancy is suspected to call doctor immediately because drug will need to be discontinued.

# masoprocol
Actinex
*Pregnancy Risk Category: B*

**HOW SUPPLIED**
*Cream:* 10%

**ACTION**
Unknown. Has antiproliferative activity against keratinocytes in vitro.

**ONSET, PEAK, DURATION**
Unknown.

**INDICATIONS & DOSAGE**
*Actinic (solar) keratoses –*
**Adults:** a sufficient amount of cream to cover area b.i.d., in morning and evening, for 28 days.

**ADVERSE REACTIONS**
**EENT:** eye irritation.
**Skin:** *erythema, flaking, dryness, edema, pruritus, burning, soreness,* bleeding, crusting, blistering, oozing, rash, irritation, stinging, tightness, tingling.

**INTERACTIONS**
None significant.

## CONTRAINDICATIONS
Contraindicated in patients hypersensitive to the drug or any component of the formulation.

## NURSING CONSIDERATIONS
• Drug contains sulfites, which may cause allergic reactions in sensitive persons.
• Use cautiously near the eyes because drug may cause pain and burning if it comes into contact with them. If such contact occurs, rinse with plenty of water.

## ☑ PATIENT TEACHING
• Instruct patient to wash and dry the area, then gently massage in the cream (avoiding eyes and mucous membranes of nose and mouth) until evenly distributed; and to wash hands after applying drug with fingers.
• Occlusive dressings, makeup, and other skin products should not be used without the doctor's approval.
• Explain to patient that local skin reactions will clear within 2 weeks of discontinuing drug. Local skin reactions are common but don't interfere with drug's effectiveness. However, if severe reactions occur, such as oozing or blistering, tell patient to discontinue drug and contact the doctor immediately.
• Warn patient to avoid unnecessary exposure to sun to prevent actinic (solar) keratoses. Advise patient to wear protective clothing and to use sunblock.
• Tell patient that drug may stain clothing or fabrics.

---

# mesalamine
Asacol, Pentasa, Rowasa

*Pregnancy Risk Category: B*

## HOW SUPPLIED
*Tablets (delayed-release):* 400 mg.
*Capsules (controlled-release):* 250 mg
*Rectal suspension:* 4 g/60 ml

*Suppositories:* 500 mg

## ACTION
Unknown. An active metabolite of sulfasalazine; probably acts topically by inhibiting prostaglandin production in the colon. Exact mechanism unknown.

## ONSET, PEAK, DURATION
Onset and duration unknown. Peak levels occur within 3 to 6 hours.

## INDICATIONS & DOSAGE
*Active mild to moderate distal ulcerative colitis, proctitis, or proctosigmoiditis –*
**Adults:** 800 mg P.O. (tablets) t.i.d. for total dose of 2.4 g/day for 6 weeks; 1 g P.O. (capsules) 4 times daily for a total dose of 4 g up to 8 weeks; 500 mg P.R. (suppository) b.i.d., or 4 g as a retention enema once daily (preferably h.s.). Rectal dosage form should be retained overnight (for about 8 hours). Usual course of therapy for rectal form is 3 to 6 weeks.

## ADVERSE REACTIONS
**CNS:** headache, dizziness, fatigue, malaise, asthenia, chills.
**GI:** abdominal pain, cramps, discomfort, flatulence, diarrhea, rectal pain, bloating, nausea, *pancolitis,* vomiting, constipation, eructation.
**Respiratory:** wheezing.
**Skin:** itching, rash, urticaria, hair loss.
**Other:** *anaphylaxis* (rare), fever, arthralgia, chest pain, myalgia, back pain, hypertonia.

## INTERACTIONS
None significant.

## CONTRAINDICATIONS
Contraindicated in patients hypersensitive to the drug, its components, or salicylates.

---

*Liquid form contains alcohol.   **May contain tartrazine.   †Canada only.   ‡Australia only.   ◇OTC.

## NURSING CONSIDERATIONS
• Use cautiously in patients with renal impairment. Problems have not been documented, but nephrotoxic potential from absorbed mesalamine exists.
• Monitor periodic renal function studies in patients on long-term therapy, as ordered.
• Because it contains potassium metabisulfite, keep in mind that mesalamine may cause hypersensitivity reactions in patients sensitive to sulfites.

### ☑ PATIENT TEACHING
• Instruct patient to carefully follow instructions supplied with medication.
• Instruct patient to discontinue drug if he experiences a fever or rash. Patient intolerant of sulfasalazine may also be hypersensitive to mesalamine.

---

## mesna
Mesnex

*Pregnancy Risk Category: B*

### HOW SUPPLIED
*Injection:* 100 mg/ml

### ACTION
Prevents ifosfamide-induced hemorrhagic cystitis by reacting with urotoxic ifosfamide metabolites.

### ONSET, PEAK, DURATION
Unknown.

### INDICATIONS & DOSAGE
*Prophylaxis of hemorrhagic cystitis in patients receiving ifosfamide –*
**Adults:** dosage varies with amount of ifosfamide administered. Usual dosage is 240 mg/m$^2$ as an I.V. bolus with administration of ifosfamide. Dosage repeated at 4 hours and 8 hours after administration of ifosfamide.

## ADVERSE REACTIONS
**CNS:** *headache, fatigue.*
**GI:** *soft stools, nausea, vomiting, diarrhea, dysgeusia.*
**Other:** *limb pain, hypotension, allergy.*
   *Note:* Because mesna is used concomitantly with ifosfamide and other chemotherapeutic agents, it is difficult to determine adverse reactions attributable solely to mesna.

## INTERACTIONS
None significant.

## CONTRAINDICATIONS
Contraindicated in patients hypersensitive to mesna or thiol-containing compounds.

## NURSING CONSIDERATIONS
• **I.V. use:** Prepare I.V. solution by diluting commercially available ampules with D$_5$W solution, dextrose 5% and 0.9% sodium chloride for injection, 0.9% sodium chloride for injection, or lactated Ringer's solution to obtain a final solution of 20 mg mesna/ml.
• Do not mix mesna I.V. with cisplatin. Mesna I.V. is incompatible with cisplatin.
• Refrigerate diluted solutions after preparation and use within 6 hours. Diluted solutions are stable for 24 hours at room temperature. After opening ampule, discard any unused drug because it decomposes quickly into an inactive compound.
• Monitor urine samples daily in patients receiving mesna for hematuria.
• Know that mesna is not effective in preventing hematuria from other causes (such as thrombocytopenia).
• Although formulated to prevent hemorrhagic cystitis from ifosfamide, be aware that drug will not protect against other toxicities associated with ifosfamide therapy.
• Keep in mind that up to 6% of pa-

---

tients may not respond to drug's protective effects.
• Be aware that mesna may interfere with diagnostic tests for urine ketones.

☑ **PATIENT TEACHING**
• Explain need for drug and how it is administered to patient and family.
• Instruct patient to report persistent or severe adverse reactions.

---

## methoxsalen (topical)
Oxsoralen

*Pregnancy Risk Category: C*

**HOW SUPPLIED**
*Lotion:* 1%

**ACTION**
Unknown. May enhance melanogenesis, either directly or secondarily, to an inflammatory process.

**ONSET, PEAK, DURATION**
Unknown.

**INDICATIONS & DOSAGE**
*To induce repigmentation in vitiligo; psoriasis –*
**Adults and children over 12 years:** lotion applied to small, well-defined vitiliginous lesions. For optimum effect, the lotion should be applied about 1 to 2 hours before exposure to UV light. The treated area may be exposed to UV light for a limited time.
    After exposure, wash lesions with soap and water, and protect area with sunblock. Manufacturer recommends weekly treatment.

**ADVERSE REACTIONS**
**Skin:** edema, erythema, painful blistering, burning, peeling, pruritus.

**INTERACTIONS**
*Photosensitizing agents:* may increase methoxsalen toxicity. Don't use together.

**CONTRAINDICATIONS**
Contraindicated in patients sensitive to psoralen compounds and in patients with diseases associated with photosensitivity (such as porphyria, acute lupus erythematosus, xeroderma, or hydromorphic and polymorphic light eruptions). Also contraindicated in patients with melanoma, invasive squamous cell carcinoma, and aphakia.

**NURSING CONSIDERATIONS**
• Use cautiously in patients with familial history of sunlight allergy, GI diseases, or chronic infection.
• Be prepared to regulate therapy carefully. Overdosage or overexposure to light can cause serious burning or blistering.
• Protect patient's eyes and lips during light exposure treatments.
• Obtain monthly liver function tests for patients with vitiligo (especially at beginning of therapy), as ordered.

☑ **PATIENT TEACHING**
• Tell patient to avoid excessive sunlight during therapy.
• Inform patient of need for monthly blood tests, and stress importance of compliance to test schedule.

---

## minoxidil (topical)
Rogaine

*Pregnancy Risk Category: C*

**HOW SUPPLIED**
*Topical solution:* 2%

**ACTION**
Unknown. Stimulates hair growth, possibly by dilating arterial microcapillaries around hair follicles.

**ONSET, PEAK, DURATION**
Unknown.

---

*Liquid form contains alcohol. **May contain tartrazine. †Canada only. ‡Australia only. ◇OTC.

## INDICATIONS & DOSAGE
*Androgentic alopecia* –
**Adults:** 1 ml of 2% solution applied to affected area b.i.d. Maximum daily dosage is 2 ml.

## ADVERSE REACTIONS
**CNS:** headache, dizziness, faintness, light-headedness.
**CV:** edema, chest pain, hypertension, hypotension, palpitations, increased or decreased pulse rate.
**EENT:** sinusitis.
**GI:** diarrhea, nausea, vomiting.
**GU:** urinary tract infection, renal calculi, urethritis.
**Respiratory:** bronchitis, upper respiratory infection.
**Skin:** irritant dermatitis, allergic contact dermatitis, eczema, hypertrichosis, local erythema, pruritus, dry skin or scalp, flaking, alopecia, exacerbation of hair loss.
**Other:** back pain, tendinitis, edema, weight gain.

## INTERACTIONS
*Topical corticosteroids, petrolatum, topical retinoids, or other drugs that may enhance skin absorption:* increased risk of systemic effects of minoxidil. Do not apply minoxidil with other drugs.

## CONTRAINDICATIONS
Contraindicated in patients hypersensitive to the drug or any component of the solution.

## NURSING CONSIDERATIONS
• Use cautiously in individuals over 50 years, and in those with cardiac, renal, or hepatic disease.
• Know that patients need to have normal, healthy scalps before beginning therapy, because absorption of drug through irritated skin may cause adverse systemic effects.
• Be aware that treatment is most likely to succeed in patients with balding area smaller than 4″ (10 cm) that developed within the past 10 years.

☑ **PATIENT TEACHING**
• Teach patient how to apply topical minoxidil. Hair and scalp should be thoroughly dry before application, and drug should not be applied to any other body areas. Tell patient not to use drug on irritated or sunburned scalp or with any other medication on scalp. Tell him to thoroughly wash hands after application.
• Warn patient to avoid inhaling any spray or mist from drug. He should avoid spraying around eyes because solution contains alcohol and may be irritating.
• Teach patient to monitor pulse rate and body weight.
• Advise patient of need for medical follow-ups 1 month after therapy starts and every 6 months thereafter.
• Advise patient that therapy will be prolonged and will continue for at least 4 months before clinical effects appear. About 40% of patients will see moderate to dense hair growth.
• Tell patient that discontinuing drug may result in loss of new hair growth. New hair growth is usually fine and may be colorless, but will resemble existing hair after continued treatment.

## nimodipine
Nimotop

*Pregnancy Risk Category: C*

## HOW SUPPLIED
*Capsules:* 30 mg

## ACTION
Inhibits calcium ion influx across cardiac and smooth muscle cells, decreasing myocardial contractility and oxygen demand, and dilates coronary and cerebral arteries and arterioles.

**ONSET, PEAK, DURATION**
Onset and duration unknown. Peak effect occurs within 1 hour.

**INDICATIONS & DOSAGE**
*Improvement of neurologic deficits in patients after subarachnoid hemorrhage from ruptured congenital aneurysms –*
**Adults:** 60 mg P.O. q 4 hours for 21 days. Therapy begun within 96 hours after subarachnoid hemorrhage.
　In patients with hepatic failure, 30 mg P.O. q 4 hours for 21 days.

**ADVERSE REACTIONS**
**CNS:** headache, psychic disturbances.
**CV:** decreased blood pressure, flushing, edema, tachycardia.
**GI:** nausea, diarrhea, abdominal discomfort.
**Respiratory:** dyspnea.
**Skin:** dermatitis, rash.
**Other:** muscle cramps.

**INTERACTIONS**
*Antihypertensives:* possible enhanced hypotensive effect. Monitor patient closely.
*Calcium channel blockers:* possible enhanced CV effects. Monitor patient closely.

**CONTRAINDICATIONS**
None known.

**NURSING CONSIDERATIONS**
• Use cautiously in patients with hepatic failure.
• Know that nimodipine should be reserved for patients who are in good neurologic condition (for example, Hunt and Hess grades I to III).
• Monitor blood pressure and heart rate in all patients, especially at start of therapy.

**☑ PATIENT TEACHING**
• Explain need for drug, and review administration schedule with patient

and family. Stress importance of compliance for maximum drug effectiveness.
• Instruct patient to report persistent or severe adverse reactions promptly.

# olsalazine sodium
Dipentum

*Pregnancy Risk Category: C*

**HOW SUPPLIED**
*Capsules:* 250 mg

**ACTION**
Unknown. After oral administration, converts to 5-aminosalicylic acid (5-ASA or mesalamine) in the colon, where it has a local anti-inflammatory effect.

**ONSET, PEAK, DURATION**
Onset and duration unknown. Time to peak concentration is 1 hour.

**INDICATIONS & DOSAGE**
*Maintenance of remission of ulcerative colitis in patients intolerant of sulfasalazine –*
**Adults:** 500 mg P.O. b.i.d. with meals.

**ADVERSE REACTIONS**
**CNS:** headache, depression, vertigo, dizziness, fatigue.
**GI:** *diarrhea,* nausea, *abdominal pain,* dyspepsia, bloating, anorexia.
**Skin:** rash, itching.
**Other:** arthralgia.

**INTERACTIONS**
None significant.

**CONTRAINDICATIONS**
Contraindicated in patients hypersensitive to salicylates.

**NURSING CONSIDERATIONS**
• Use cautiously in patients with preexisting renal disease. Although problems have not been reported with this

---

*Liquid form contains alcohol.   **May contain tartrazine.   †Canada only.   ‡Australia only.   ◇OTC.

drug, the possibility of renal tubular damage from absorbed mesalamine or its metabolites must be considered.

• Regularly monitor BUN and creatinine levels and urinalysis in patients with preexisting renal disease, as ordered.

• Be aware that in clinical trials, 17% of all patients reported diarrhea during therapy. Although diarrhea appears dose-related, it is difficult to distinguish from worsening of disease symptoms. Exacerbation of disease has been noted with similar drugs.

☑ **PATIENT TEACHING**
• Teach patient to take drug in evenly divided doses and with food to minimize adverse GI reactions.

• Instruct patient to report persistent or severe adverse reactions promptly.

## pamidronate disodium
Aredia
*Pregnancy Risk Category: C*

**HOW SUPPLIED**
*Injection:* 30-mg vial

**ACTION**
An antihypercalcemic agent that inhibits resorption of bone. Adsorbs to hydroxyapatite crystals in bone and may directly block dissolution of calcium phosphate. Drug apparently doesn't inhibit bone formation or mineralization.

**ONSET, PEAK, DURATION**
Unknown.

**INDICATIONS & DOSAGE**
*Moderate to severe hypercalcemia associated with cancer (with or without bone metastases)* –
**Adults:** dosage depends on severity of hypercalcemia. Serum calcium levels should be corrected for serum albumin:

$$\text{Corrected serum} \atop \text{calcium (CCa)} \atop \text{(in mg/dl)} = \text{serum calcium} \atop \text{(in mg/dl)} + 0.8 \, (4 - \text{serum} \atop \text{albumin)} \atop \text{(in g/dl)}$$

Patients with moderate hypercalcemia (CCa levels of 12 to 13.5 mg/dl) may receive 60 to 90 mg by I.V. infusion over 4 hours for 60-mg dose and over 24 hours for 90-mg dose. Patients with severe hypercalcemia (CCa levels over 13.5 mg/dl) may receive 90 mg by I.V. infusion over 24 hours. A minimum of 7 days should elapse before retreatment to allow for full response to the initial dose.
*Moderate to severe Paget's disease* –
**Adults:** 30 mg I.V. as a 4-hour infusion on 3 consecutive days for total dose of 90 mg. Cycle repeated, as needed.

**ADVERSE REACTIONS**
**CNS:** *seizures, fatigue,* somnolence.
**CV:** atrial fibrillation, syncope, tachycardia, *hypertension.*
**GI:** *abdominal pain, anorexia, constipation, nausea, vomiting,* GI hemorrhage.
**Hematologic:** *leukopenia,* **thrombocytopenia,** *anemia.*
**Other:** *hypophosphatemia, hypokalemia, hypomagnesemia, hypocalcemia, fever, infusion-site reaction.*

**INTERACTIONS**
None significant.

**CONTRAINDICATIONS**
Contraindicated in patients hypersensitive to the drug or to other biphosphonates, such as etidronate.

**NURSING CONSIDERATIONS**
• Use with extreme caution, and consider the risks versus benefits in patients with renal impairment.

• Assess hydration status prior to treatment. Know that drug should be used only after patients have been vigorously hydrated with sodium chloride solution. In patients with mild to

---

Reactions may be *common,* uncommon, *life-threatening,* or **COMMON AND LIFE-THREATENING.**

moderate hypercalcemia, hydration alone may be sufficient.

• **I.V. use:** Reconstitute vial with 10 ml of sterile water for injection. After drug is completely dissolved, add to 1,000 ml of 0.45% or 0.9% sodium chloride for injection or D₅W. Do not mix with infusion solutions that contain calcium, such as Ringer's injection or lactated Ringer's injection. Visually inspect for precipitate before administering.

• Give only by I.V. infusion. Animal studies have shown evidence of nephropathy when drug is given as a bolus.

• Because drug can cause electrolyte disturbances, carefully monitor serum electrolytes, especially calcium, phosphate, and magnesium, as ordered. Short-term administration of calcium may be necessary in patients with severe hypocalcemia. Also monitor creatinine level, CBC and differential count, and hematocrit and hemoglobin levels, as ordered.

• Carefully monitor patients with preexisting anemia, leukopenia, or thrombocytopenia during first 2 weeks of therapy.

• Monitor patient's temperature. In clinical trials, 27% of patients experienced an elevation of 1° C (1.8° F) for 24 to 48 hours after therapy.

• Solution is stable for 24 hours at room temperature.

☑ **PATIENT TEACHING**
• Explain need for drug and how it is administered to patient and family.
• Instruct patient to report adverse reactions promptly.

---

**pilocarpine hydrochloride**
Salagen

*Pregnancy Risk Category: C*

**HOW SUPPLIED**
*Tablets:* 5 mg

**ACTION**
A cholinergic parasympathomimetic agent that increases secretion of salivary glands, eliminating dryness.

**ONSET, PEAK, DURATION**
Unknown.

**INDICATIONS & DOSAGE**
*Treatment of xerostomia from salivary gland hypofunction caused by radiotherapy for cancer of head and neck* –
**Adults:** 5 mg P.O. t.i.d.; may be increased to 10 mg P.O. t.i.d, as needed.

**ADVERSE REACTIONS**
**CNS:** *dizziness, headache,* tremor.
**CV:** hypertension, tachycardia.
**EENT:** *rhinitis, lacrimation, amblyopia, pharyngitis, voice alteration, conjunctivitis, epistaxis, sinusitis, abnormal vision.*
**GI:** *nausea,* dyspepsia, diarrhea, abdominal pain, vomiting, dysphagia.
**GU:** *urinary frequency.*
**Skin:** *flushing,* rash, pruritus.
**Other:** *sweating, chills, asthenia,* edema, taste perversion, myalgia.

**INTERACTIONS**
*Beta-adrenergic antagonists:* may increase risk of conduction disturbances. Use together cautiously.
*Drugs with parasympathomimetic effects:* may result in additive pharmacologic effects. Monitor patient closely.
*Drugs with anticholinergic effects:* may antagonize anticholinergic effects. Use together cautiously.

**CONTRAINDICATIONS**
Contraindicated in patients with uncontrolled asthma or hypersensitivity to pilocarpine and when miosis is undesirable, such as in acute iritis or narrow-angle glaucoma.

---

*Liquid form contains alcohol.   **May contain tartrazine.   †Canada only.   ‡Australia only.   ◇OTC.

## NURSING CONSIDERATIONS

• Use cautiously in patients with cardiovascular disease, controlled asthma, chronic bronchitis, chronic obstructive pulmonary disease, cholelithiasis, biliary tract disease, nephrolithiasis, or cognitive or psychiatric disturbances.
• Drug should not be used in breast-feeding women.
• Safety and efficacy in children have not been established.
• Because retinal detachment has been reported with pilocarpine use in patients with retinal disease, examine the patient's fundus carefully before therapy begins.
• Monitor the patient for signs of toxicity: headache, visual disturbance, lacrimation, sweating, respiratory distress, gastrointestinal spasm, nausea, vomiting, diarrhea, atrioventricular block, tachycardia, bradycardia, hypotension, hypertension, shock, mental confusion, arrhythmia, and tremors. Immediately notify the doctor of suspected toxicity.

## ☑ PATIENT TEACHING

• Warn the patient that driving ability may be impaired by drug-induced visual disturbances, especially at night.
• Advise the patient to drink plenty of fluids to prevent dehydration.

▼ NEW DRUG

# riluzole
Rilutek

*Pregnancy Risk Category: C*

## HOW SUPPLIED
*Tablets:* 50 mg

## ACTION
Unknown.

## ONSET, PEAK, DURATION
Unknown.

## INDICATIONS & DOSAGE
*Amyotrophic lateral sclerosis –*
**Adults:** 50 mg P.O. q 12 hours, taken on empty stomach.

## ADVERSE REACTIONS
**CNS:** headache, aggravation reaction, hypertonia, depression, dizziness, insomnia, somnolence, vertigo, circumoral paresthesia.
**CV:** hypertension, tachycardia, palpitation, postural hypotension.
**GI:** abdominal pain, *nausea,* vomiting, dyspepsia, anorexia, diarrhea, flatulence, stomatitis.
**GU:** urinary tract infection, dysuria.
**Respiratory:** *decreased lung function,* rhinitis, increased cough, sinusitis.
**Skin:** pruritus, eczema, alopecia, exfoliative dermatitis.
**Other:** *asthenia,* back pain, malaise, dry mouth, tooth disorder, oral moniliasis, phlebitis, weight loss, peripheral edema, arthralgia.

## INTERACTIONS
No clinical trials have studied riluzole's interaction with other drugs. Closely monitor patients receiving concomitant therapy, and use caution when giving potentially hepatotoxic drugs (allopurinol, methyldopa, sulfasalazine) concomitantly.

## CONTRAINDICATIONS
Contraindicated in patients with history of severe hypersensitivity to riluzole or any component of drug.

## NURSING CONSIDERATIONS
• Use cautiously in patients with hepatic or renal dysfunction, in elderly patients, and in females and Japanese patients (who may have a lower metabolic capacity to eliminate riluzole than do males and Caucasians, respectively).
• Be aware that elevations in baseline liver function studies (especially bilirubin) preclude use of riluzole. Liver

---

Reactions may be *common*, uncommon, *life-threatening*, or **COMMON AND LIFE-THREATENING**.

function studies should be done periodically during therapy, as ordered. In many patients, drug may increase serum aminotransferase; if level exceeds 10 times the upper limit of normal or if clinical jaundice develops, notify the doctor.
• Give drug at least 1 hour before or 2 hours after a meal to avoid decreased bioavailability.
• Institute safety precautions until adverse effects are known.

☑ **PATIENT TEACHING**
• Tell the patient to take drug at same time each day. If a dose is missed, tell him to take next tablet when planned.
• Instruct him to report fever to the doctor, who will want to order a WBC count.
• Warn him to avoid hazardous activities until CNS effects of drug are known and to limit alcohol use while taking drug.
• Tell him to store drug at room temperature, protected from bright light, and to keep it out of children's reach.

---

## ritodrine hydrochloride
Yutopar

*Pregnancy Risk Category: B*

**HOW SUPPLIED**
*Tablets:* 10 mg
*Injection:* 10 mg/ml, 15 mg/ml

**ACTION**
A beta-receptor agonist that stimulates the beta$_2$-adrenergic receptors in uterine smooth muscle, inhibiting contractility.

**ONSET, PEAK, DURATION**
Onset occurs in 30 to 60 minutes after oral administration, 5 minutes after I.V. administration. Serum levels peak 30 to 60 minutes after oral administration in nonpregnant women; 60 minutes after I.V. administration in nonpregnant women. Duration unknown.

**INDICATIONS & DOSAGE**
*Preterm labor* –
**Adults:** dilute 150 mg (three ampules) in 500 ml of fluid, yielding a final concentration of 0.3 mg/ml. Usual initial dose is 0.05 mg/minute I.V., gradually increased by 0.05 mg/minute q 10 minutes until desired result is obtained. Effective dosage usually ranges from 0.15 to 0.35 mg/minute.

*Note:* I.V. infusion should be continued for 12 hours after contractions have stopped. Oral maintenance: 10 mg approximately 30 minutes before termination of I.V. therapy. Usual dosage for first 24 hours of maintenance is 10 mg P.O. q 2 hours. Thereafter, usual dosage is 10 to 20 mg P.O. q 4 to 6 hours. Total daily dosage should not exceed 120 mg.

**ADVERSE REACTIONS**
*Intravenous:*
**CNS:** nervousness, anxiety, *headaches,* emotional upset, malaise.
**CV:** *dose-related alterations in blood pressure, palpitations,* **pulmonary edema,** *tachycardia.*
**GI:** *nausea, vomiting.*
**Hematologic:** leukopenia, *agranulocytosis.*
**Other:** *erythema, hyperglycemia,* hypokalemia, *anaphylactic shock.*
*Oral:*
**CNS:** *tremor,* nervousness.
**CV:** *palpitations.*
**GI:** *nausea, vomiting.*
**Skin:** rash.

**INTERACTIONS**
*Beta-adrenergic blockers:* may inhibit ritodrine's action. Avoid concurrent use.
*Corticosteroids:* may produce pulmonary edema in mother. Monitor patient closely.
*Inhalation anesthetics:* potentiated ad-

---

verse cardiac effects, arrhythmias, and hypotension. Monitor patient closely.
*Sympathomimetics:* additive sympathomimetic effects. Use together cautiously.

## CONTRAINDICATIONS

Contraindicated in pregnant women before 20th week of pregnancy and in women with antepartum hemorrhage, eclampsia, intrauterine fetal death, chorioamnionitis, maternal cardiac disease, pulmonary hypertension, maternal hyperthyroidism, or uncontrolled maternal diabetes mellitus. Also contraindicated in patients hypersensitive to the drug or with pre-existing maternal medical conditions that would seriously be affected by the known pharmacologic properties of this drug, such as hypovolemia, pheochromocytoma, or uncontrolled hypertension.

## NURSING CONSIDERATIONS

• Use cautiously in patients with a sulfite sensitivity.
• **I.V. use:** Don't use ritodrine I.V. if solution is discolored or contains a precipitate.
• *Alert:* Because CV responses are common and more pronounced during I.V. administration, closely monitor CV effects — including maternal pulse rate and blood pressure, and fetal heart rate. Maternal tachycardia of over 140 beats/minute or persistent respiratory rate of over 20 breaths/minute may be a sign of impending pulmonary edema. Discontinue drug if pulmonary edema develops and notify doctor.
• Monitor blood glucose concentrations during infusion, especially in diabetic mother.
• Monitor amount of fluids administered I.V. to prevent circulatory overload.

☑ **PATIENT TEACHING**
• Explain need for drug and how drug is administered to patient and family.
• Instruct patient to report adverse reactions promptly.

## sodium benzoate and sodium phenylacetate
Ucephan

*Pregnancy Risk Category: C*

### HOW SUPPLIED
*Oral solution:* 10 g sodium benzoate and 10 g sodium phenylacetate per 100 ml

### ACTION
Activates metabolic pathways that are ineffective in patients with urea cycle enzymopathies, resulting in decreased ammonia formation.

### ONSET, PEAK, DURATION
Onset and duration unknown. Serum levels peak within 1 hour.

### INDICATIONS & DOSAGE
*Prevention or treatment of hyperammonemia in patients with urea cycle enzymopathy –*
**Children:** 2.5 ml/kg P.O. daily in three to six equally divided doses. Maximum daily dosage is 100 ml.

### ADVERSE REACTIONS
**GI:** nausea, vomiting.

### INTERACTIONS
*Penicillin, probenecid:* may impair renal excretion of conjugated metabolites. Monitor the patient for toxicity.

### CONTRAINDICATIONS
Contraindicated in patients hypersensitive to sodium benzoate or sodium phenylacetate and in patients who have CHF or renal impairment.

---

Reactions may be *common,* uncommon, *life-threatening,* or COMMON AND LIFE-THREATENING.

## NURSING CONSIDERATIONS

• Use cautiously in neonates with hyperbilirubinemia.

• Carefully measure required dosage because stock solution is very concentrated.

• Dilute each dose in 120 to 240 ml (4 to 8 oz) of infant formula or milk and administer with meals. Inspect mixture for compatibility if other liquids are used. Drug may precipitate in some solutions, especially acidic solutions such as fruit juice, depending on concentration and pH.

• Avoid getting solution on skin or clothing; lingering odor of drug may be offensive.

• Watch for salicylate-associated adverse reactions, including mild respiratory alkalosis and exacerbation of peptic ulcerations. Drug is structurally similar to salicylates.

• Know that drug may compete with bilirubin for binding sites on serum albumin.

• Be aware that drug is not intended as sole therapy for patients with urea cycle enzymopathies. It is most effective when combined with a low-protein diet and amino acid supplementation.

## ☑ PATIENT TEACHING

• Explain need for drug and how it is administered to child (if appropriate) and parents.

• Instruct parents to report persistent or severe nausea and vomiting.

---

## strontium 89 ($^{89}$Sr) chloride
Metastron

*Pregnancy Risk Category: D*

## HOW SUPPLIED
*Injection:* 4 millicuries (mCi)/10 ml

## ACTION
Acts as a calcium analogue that is actively taken up by bone, particularly in areas of active osteogenesis such as metastatic bone tumors. The drug locally irradiates tissue with beta radiation.

## ONSET, PEAK, DURATION
Rapidly taken up by bone within hours of injection. Pain relief typically takes 7 to 20 days. Effects persist for 4 to 12 months.

## INDICATIONS & DOSAGE
*Relief of bone pain in patients with painful metastatic lesions –*
**Adults:** 4 mCi by slow I.V. injection over 1 to 2 minutes.

## ADVERSE REACTIONS
**CV:** cutaneous flushing with rapid injection.
**Hematologic:** *bone marrow suppression.*
**Other:** transient increase in pain ("flare" reaction).

## INTERACTIONS
*Calcium supplements:* decreased effectiveness of $^{89}$Sr Discontinue calcium supplements about 2 weeks before $^{89}$Sr administration.
*Cytotoxic agents:* additive bone marrow suppression. Monitor closely.

## CONTRAINDICATIONS
None known.

## NURSING CONSIDERATIONS
• Use cautiously in patients with platelet counts below 60,000/mm³ or WBC counts below 2,400/mm³.
• *Alert:* Follow institutional safety measures to minimize radiation exposure. Urinary excretion of radiation is greatest during the first 2 days after administration.
• Consider placing an indwelling urinary catheter in incontinent patients to minimize contamination of the environment with radiation.
• Frequently assess the degree of pain relief after administration of the drug. During the lst week, a transient in-

crease in pain may necessitate a dosage increase in concomitantly administered analgesics. Pain relief from [89]SR usually occurs after 2 to 3 weeks. In clinical trials, over 75% of patients received substantial pain relief, allowing a reduction or elimination of opioid analgesics.

• Because the drug is a potential carcinogen, know that use should be restricted to patients with documented metastatic bone cancer.

• Because of the delayed onset of pain relief, be aware that this drug should not be used in patients with a short life expectancy.

☑ **PATIENT TEACHING**
• Teach patient proper radiation precautions; during the first few days of treatment, patient should flush the toilet twice, wipe any spilled urine with a tissue that is subsequently flushed, and immediately launder any linens soiled with blood or urine. Make sure patient understands that the drug has a low level of radioactivity and that he will pose no risk to family members.
• Advise female patient of childbearing age to avoid becoming pregnant while taking this drug.

# sulfasalazine (salazosulfapyridine, sulphasalazine)

Azulfidine, Azulfidine EN-Tabs, PMS Sulfasalazine E.C.†, Salazopyrin†‡, Salazopyrin EN-Tabs†‡, S.A.S., S.A.S.-Enteric

*Pregnancy Risk Category: B*

## HOW SUPPLIED
*Tablets:* 500 mg with or without enteric coating
*Oral suspension:* 250 mg/5 ml

## ACTION
Unknown.

## ONSET, PEAK, DURATION
Onset and duration unknown. Peak serum levels of parent drug occur within 1½ to 6 hours; peak levels of metabolites, within 12 to 24 hours.

## INDICATIONS & DOSAGE
*Mild to moderate ulcerative colitis, adjunctive therapy in severe ulcerative colitis, Crohn's disease –*
**Adults:** initially, 3 to 4 g P.O. daily in evenly divided doses; usual maintenance dosage is 1.5 to 2 g P.O. daily in divided doses q 6 hours. Dosage may be started with 1 to 2 g, with a gradual increase in dosage to minimize adverse effects.
**Children over 2 years:** initially, 40 to 60 mg/kg P.O. daily, divided into three to six doses; then 30 mg/kg daily in four doses. Dosage may be started at lower dose if GI intolerance occurs.

## ADVERSE REACTIONS
**CNS:** headache, depression, *seizures,* hallucinations.
**GI:** *nausea, vomiting, diarrhea,* abdominal pain, anorexia, stomatitis.
**GU:** *toxic nephrosis with oliguria and anuria,* crystalluria, hematuria, oligospermia, infertility.
**Hematologic:** *agranulocytosis, aplastic anemia,* megaloblastic anemia, *thrombocytopenia,* leukopenia, *hemolytic anemia.*
**Hepatic:** jaundice, hepatotoxicity.
**Skin:** *erythema multiforme (Stevens-Johnson syndrome), generalized skin eruption, epidermal necrolysis, exfoliative dermatitis,* photosensitivity, urticaria, pruritus.
**Other:** hypersensitivity reactions (*serum sickness, drug fever, anaphylaxis* ).

## INTERACTIONS
*Antibiotics:* may alter action of sulfasalazine by altering internal flora. Monitor closely.

---

Reactions may be *common,* uncommon, *life-threatening,* or **COMMON AND LIFE-THREATENING.**

*Digoxin:* may reduce absorption of digoxin. Monitor closely.
*Folic acid:* absorption may be decreased. No intervention necessary.
*Iron:* lowered blood concentrations of sulfasalazine caused by iron chelation. Monitor closely.
*Oral anticoagulants:* increased anticoagulant effect. Monitor for bleeding.
*Oral antidiabetic agents:* increased hypoglycemic effect. Monitor blood glucose levels.
*Oral contraceptives:* decreased contraceptive effectiveness and increased risk of breakthrough bleeding. Suggest a nonhormonal form of contraception.

## CONTRAINDICATIONS
Contraindicated in patients with hypersensitivity to the drug or its metabolites, porphyria, or intestinal and urinary obstruction and in infants under age 2.

## NURSING CONSIDERATIONS
• Use cautiously and in reduced dosages in patients with impaired hepatic or renal function, severe allergy, bronchial asthma, and G6PD deficiency.
• Be aware that drug colors alkaline urine orange-yellow.
• *Alert:* Discontinue immediately if the patient shows signs and symptoms of hypersensitivity and notify doctor.

### ☑ PATIENT TEACHING
• Instruct patient to take drug after food intake and to space doses evenly.
• Warn the patient to avoid direct sunlight and ultraviolet light to prevent photosensitivity reaction.

---

## tiopronin
Thiola
*Pregnancy Risk Category: C*

## HOW SUPPLIED
*Tablets:* 100 mg

## ACTION
Forms a water-soluble chemical complex with cysteine in the urine, increasing cysteine solubility and preventing formation of urinary cysteine stones.

## ONSET, PEAK, DURATION
Onset rapid. Peak unknown. Effects persist less than 10 hours.

## INDICATIONS & DOSAGE
*Prevention of urinary cysteine stone formation in patients with severe homozygous cysteinuria (urinary cysteine excretion exceeding 500 mg/day) unresponsive to other therapies –*
**Adults:** 800 mg P.O. daily, divided t.i.d.
**Children:** 15 mg/kg P.O. daily, divided t.i.d.

## ADVERSE REACTIONS
**GI:** hypogeusia.
**Skin:** rash, pruritus, wrinkling, friability.
**Other:** drug fever, lupus erythematosus-like reaction.

## INTERACTIONS
None significant.

## CONTRAINDICATIONS
Contraindicated in patients with a history of agranulocytosis, aplastic anemia, or thrombocytopenia.

## NURSING CONSIDERATIONS
• Keep in mind that the following conservative measures to treat cysteinuria should be attempted before tiopronin is administered. Patients should drink at least 3 liters (or quarts) of fluid daily, including at least two 8-oz (480 ml) glasses of water at each meal and at bedtime. Urine output should be at least 3 liters daily, and urine pH should be 6.5 to

---

7. Excessive alkalization of urine may precipitate calcium stones. Urine pH should not exceed 7.

• Monitor CBC, platelet counts, hemoglobin, serum albumin, liver function tests, 24-hour urine protein, and routine urinalysis at 3- to 6-month intervals during treatment, as ordered.

• Frequently monitor urine cysteine during first 6 months of treatment to identify optimal dosage level and then at least every 6 months, as ordered.

• Inspect skin for rash. Generalized rash with mild pruritus that develops in first few months of therapy may be controlled with antihistamines and will disappear after discontinuing the drug. A rash accompanied by intense pruritus may appear on the trunk after 6 months of therapy. This rash disappears slowly after discontinuing drug.

• Drug fever may develop, especially during 1st month of therapy. Expect drug to be discontinued until fever subsides and to be reinstituted at lower dosages.

• Know that dosage is usually adjusted to keep urine cysteine levels below 250 mg/L.

• Be aware that studies indicate that about two-thirds of patients who cannot tolerate penicillamine will tolerate tiopronin.

☑ **PATIENT TEACHING**
• Whenever possible, tell patient to take tiopronin at least 1 hour before or 2 hours after meals.

• Advise patient to have annual abdominal X-ray to assess for presence of stones.

• Tell patient to report any signs or symptoms of hematologic abnormalities, including fever, sore throat, bleeding or bruising, and chills. Blood dyscrasias have been reported in patients receiving other drugs for cysteinuria.

# tretinoin (vitamin A acid, retinoic acid)
Renova, Retin-A, StieVAA†

*Pregnancy Risk Category: C*

## HOW SUPPLIED
*Cream:* 0.025%, 0.05%, 0.1%
*Gel:* 0.025%, 0.01%
*Solution:* 0.05%

## ACTION
Inhibits comedones by increasing epidermal cell mitosis and turnover.

## ONSET, PEAK, DURATION
Unknown.

## INDICATIONS & DOSAGE
*Acne vulgaris (especially grades I, II, and III) –*
**Adults and children:** clean affected area and lightly apply once daily h.s.
*Adjunct therapy to skin care and sun avoidance program –*
**Adults:** apply to affected area once daily h.s.

## ADVERSE REACTIONS
**Skin:** *feeling of warmth, slight stinging, local erythema, peeling,* chapping, swelling, blistering, crusting, temporary hyperpigmentation or hypopigmentation.

## INTERACTIONS
*Topical preparations containing sulfur, resorcinol, or salicylic acid:* increased risk of skin irritation. Don't use together.

## CONTRAINDICATIONS
Contraindicated in patients hypersensitive to any tretinoin component.

## NURSING CONSIDERATIONS
• Use cautiously in patients with eczema.

• Know that relapses generally occur within 3 to 6 weeks after therapy is stopped.

---

Reactions may be *common,* uncommon, *life-threatening,* or **COMMON AND LIFE-THREATENING.**

## ☑ PATIENT TEACHING

- Instruct patient to clean area thoroughly before application and to avoid getting drug in eyes, mouth, or mucous membranes.
- Tell patient to wash face with mild soap no more than two or three times a day. Warn against using strong or medicated cosmetics, soaps, or other skin cleansers. Also advise patient to avoid topical products containing alcohol, astringents, spices, and lime because they may interfere with drug.
- Advise patient not to discontinue the drug if it causes transient exacerbation of inflammatory lesions. If severe local irritation develops, advise patient to discontinue temporarily and notify doctor. Dosage will be readjusted when application is resumed. Some redness and scaling are normal reactions.
- Warn patient that he may experience increased sensitivity to wind or cold temperatures.
- Instruct patient to minimize exposure to sunlight or ultraviolet rays during treatment. If patient become sunburned, he should delay therapy until sunburn subsides. Tell patient who can't avoid exposure to sunlight to use SPF-15 sunblock and to wear protective clothing.

---

## trilostane
Modrastane

*Pregnancy Risk Category: X*

### HOW SUPPLIED
*Capsules:* 30 mg, 60 mg

### ACTION
Reversibly lowers elevated circulating levels of glucocorticoids by inhibiting the enzyme system essential for their production in the adrenal gland.

### ONSET, PEAK, DURATION
Unknown.

### INDICATIONS & DOSAGE
*Adrenocortical hyperfunction in Cushing's syndrome –*
**Adults:** 30 mg P.O. q.i.d. initially. May be increased at intervals of 3 to 4 days to maximum of 480 mg/day. Most patients respond to doses below 360 mg/day.

### ADVERSE REACTIONS
**CNS:** headache, dizziness, light-headedness.
**CV:** *orthostatic hypotension.*
**EENT:** burning of oral and nasal membranes.
**GI:** *diarrhea, upset stomach,* nausea, flatulence, cramps, bloating.
**Skin:** flushing, rash.
**Other:** fever, fatigue, hot flashes, muscle aches, hyperkalemia.

### INTERACTIONS
*Aminoglutethimide, mitotane:* may cause severe adrenocortical hypofunction.
*Loop diuretics, thiazides:* decreased potassium loss because trilostane inhibits aldosterone production.

### CONTRAINDICATIONS
Contraindicated in patients with severe renal or hepatic disease.

### NURSING CONSIDERATIONS
- Use cautiously in patients who are receiving other drugs that suppress adrenal function.
- Because the drug may cause orthostatic hypotension by suppressing aldosterone production, monitor blood pressure regularly in all patients.
- Be aware that trilostane may prevent normal response to physiologically stressful situation. Therefore, patients who develop a severe illness or need surgery may need to have this drug temporarily discontinued. Supplemental corticosteroids may be necessary.

---

*Liquid form contains alcohol.  **May contain tartrazine.  †Canada only.  ‡Australia only.  ◇OTC.

### ☑ PATIENT TEACHING
• Trilostane is prescribed when surgery or pituitary radiation therapy is inappropriate or must be delayed. Explain to patient that the drug does not cure the underlying disease.
• Tell patient to seek medical attention if stressful situation arises because drug therapy will need to be re-evaluated.

# Appendices
# and Index

# Selected local and topical anesthetics

| DRUG, INDICATIONS, DOSAGE | ADVERSE REACTIONS |
|---|---|

## Local

**bupivacaine hydrochloride**
(Marcain‡, Marcaine, Sensorcaine)
Dosages given are for the drug without epinephrine
and for adults. Volume listed below refers to the total
volume of anesthetic given, sometimes in incremental doses of 2 to 6 ml.
*Epidural block—*
0.25% solution: 10 to 20 ml (25 to 50 mg)
0.5% solution: 10 to 20 ml (50 to 100 mg)
0.75% solution: 10 to 20 ml (75 to 150 mg)
*Caudal block—*
0.25% solution: 15 to 30 ml (37.5 to 75 mg)
0.5% solution: 15 to 30 ml (75 to 150 mg)
*Spinal block—*
0.75% solution (in dextrose 8.25%): 1 to 1.6 ml (7.5
to 12 mg)
*Peripheral nerve block—*
0.25% solution: 5 ml (12.5 mg)
0.5% solution: 5 ml (25 mg)

**Skin:** dermatologic reactions.
**Other:** edema, *status asthmaticus, anaphylaxis, anaphylactoid reactions.*
Systemic effects from high
blood levels of the drug—
**CNS:** anxiety, nervousness,
*seizures* followed by drowsiness.
**CV:** bradycardia, hypotension,
myocardial depression, *arrhythmias, cardiac arrest.*
**EENT:** blurred vision, tinnitus.
**GI:** nausea, vomiting.
**Respiratory:** *respiratory
arrest.*

---

**chloroprocaine hydrochloride**
(Nesacaine, Nesacaine MPF)
Dosages given are for the drug without epinephrine
and for adults. Volume listed below refers to the total
volume of anesthetic given, sometimes in incremental doses of 2 to 6 ml.
*Infiltration and nerve block—*
1% solution: 3 to 20 ml (30 to 200 mg)
2% solution: 2 to 40 ml (40 to 800 mg)
*Caudal and epidural block—*
2% to 3% solution: 15 to 25 ml (300 to 750 mg).
    May be repeated with smaller doses q 40 to 50 min-
utes. Dose and interval may be increased when combined with epinephrine. Maximum adult dosage is 800
mg or 11 mg/kg; when combined with epinephrine, maximum dosage is 1 g.

**Skin:** dermatologic reactions.
**Other:** edema, *status asthmaticus, anaphylaxis, anaphylactoid reactions.*
Systemic effects from high
blood levels of the drug—
**CNS:** anxiety, nervousness,
*seizures* followed by drowsiness.
**CV:** myocardial depression,
hypotension, *arrhythmias,
cardiac arrest.*
**EENT:** blurred vision, tinnitus.
**GI:** nausea, vomiting.
**Respiratory:** *respiratory
arrest.*

---

**etidocaine hydrochloride**
(Duranest)
Dosages given are for the drug without epinephrine
and for adults.
    Dose limit is 4 mg/kg or 300 mg per injection.
When combined with epinephrine, dose limit is 5.5
mg/kg or 400 mg per injection. May be repeated q 2
to 3 hours.
*Peripheral nerve block—*
1% solution: 5 to 40 ml (50 to 400 mg)

**Skin:** dermatologic reactions.
**Other:** edema, *status asthmaticus, anaphylaxis, anaphylactoid reactions.*
Systemic effects from high
blood levels of the drug—
**CNS:** anxiety, apprehension,
nervousness, *seizures* followed by drowsiness.

---

Reactions may be *common,* uncommon, *life-threatening,* or COMMON AND LIFE-THREATENING.

| INTERACTIONS | NURSING CONSIDERATIONS |
|---|---|

*Beta-adrenergic blockers:* enhanced sympathomimetic effects. Avoid concomitant use.
*Chloroprocaine:* may lessen bupivacaine's action. Don't use together.
*Cyclic antidepressants, MAO inhibitors:* severe, sustained hypertension when used with bupivacaine and epinephrine. Use with extreme caution.
*Enflurane, halothane, isoflurane, related drugs:* arrhythmias when used with bupivacaine and epinephrine. Use with extreme caution.

- Contraindicated in children under 12 years and for spinal or topical anesthesia or paracervical block. Some solutions contain sulfites and should be avoided in patients with sulfite hypersensitivity.
- Should not be used for I.V. regional anesthesia (Bier block, Bier's anesthesia).
- The 0.75% solution should not be used for obstetrical surgery; lower concentrations are effective and less hazardous.
- Use cautiously in debilitated, elderly, or acutely ill patients and in patients with severe hepatic disease or drug allergies.
- Use solutions with epinephrine cautiously in patients with CV disorders and in body areas with limited blood supply (ears, nose, fingers, toes).
- Keep resuscitation equipment and drugs available.
- Don't use solution with preservatives for caudal or epidural block.
- Discard partially used vials without preservatives.
- Check solution for particles.
- Protect solutions containing epinephrine from light.

---

None significant.

- Contraindicated in patients with hypersensitivity to procaine, tetracaine, or other PABA derivatives and for spinal or topical anesthesia. Epidural and caudal blocks are contraindicated in patients with CNS disease.
- Use cautiously in debilitated, elderly, or acutely ill patients; in children; and in patients with drug allergies, paracervical block, or CV disease.
- Keep resuscitation equipment and drugs available.
- Don't use solution with preservatives for caudal or epidural block.
- Don't use discolored solution.
- Check solution for particles.
- Discard partially used vials without preservatives.

---

*Cyclic antidepressants, MAO inhibitors, phenothiazines:* severe, sustained hypertension or hypotension with etidocaine and epinephrine. Use with extreme caution.
*Enflurane, halothane, isoflurane, related drugs:* arrhythmias when used with etidocaine and epinephrine. Use with extreme caution.

- Contraindicated in patients with inflammation or infection in puncture region, septicemia, severe hypertension, spinal deformities, or neurologic disorders; in children under 14 years; and for spinal anesthesia. Some solutions contain sulfites and should be avoided in patients with sulfite hypersensitivity.
- Use cautiously in debilitated, elderly, or acutely ill patients; in patients with severe shock, heart block, general drug allergies, or hepatic and renal disease; and as epidural block in obstetric patients.

---

*Liquid form contains alcohol.   **May contain tartrazine.   †Canada only.   ‡Australia only.   ◊OTC.

## Selected local and topical anesthetics (continued)

| DRUG, INDICATIONS, DOSAGE | ADVERSE REACTIONS |
|---|---|

**Local** (continued)

**etidocaine hydrochloride** (continued)
*Central neural block (lower limbs, cesarean section, lumbar, epidural) —*
1% solution: 10 to 30 ml (100 to 300 mg)
1.5% solution: 10 to 20 ml (150 to 300 mg)
*Transvaginal block —*
1% solution: 5 to 20 ml (50 to 200 mg)
*Caudal block —*
1% solution: 10 to 30 ml (100 to 300 mg)

**CV:** myocardial depression, hypotension, **arrhythmias, cardiac arrest.**
**EENT:** blurred vision, tinnitus.
**GI:** nausea, vomiting.
**Respiratory:** *respiratory arrest.*

---

**lidocaine hydrochloride**
**[lignocaine hydrochloride]**
(Dilocaine, Lidoject-1, Lidoject-2, Xylocaine)
Dosages given are for the drug without epinephrine and for adults. Volume listed below refers to the total volume of anesthetic given, sometimes in incremental doses of 2 to 6 ml.
*For anesthesia other than spinal —*
Maximum single dose is 4.5 mg/kg or 300 mg. With epinephrine, maximum dose is 7 mg/kg or 500 mg.
*Caudal (obstetric) or epidural (thoracic) block —*
1% solution: 20 to 30 ml (200 to 300 mg)
*Epidural (lumbar anesthesia) block —*
1.5% solution: 15 to 20 ml (225 to 300 mg)
2% solution: 10 to 15 ml (200 to 300 mg)
*Spinal surgical anesthesia —*
5% (with 7.5% dextrose): 1.5 to 2 ml (75 to 100 mg)
*Caudal (surgery) block —*
1.5% solution: 15 to 20 ml (225 to 300 mg)

**Skin:** dermatologic reactions.
**Other:** edema, ***status asthmaticus, anaphylaxis, anaphylactoid reactions.***
Systemic effects from high blood levels of the drug —
**CNS:** anxiety, nervousness, *seizures* followed by drowsiness.
**CV:** myocardial depression, hypotension, **arrhythmias, cardiac arrest.**
**EENT:** blurred vision, tinnitus.
**GI:** nausea, vomiting.
**Respiratory:** *respiratory arrest.*

---

**procaine hydrochloride**
(Novocain)
*Spinal anesthesia —*
**Adults:** initial dose should not exceed 1 g.
Before using, dilute 10% solution with 0.9% sodium chloride injection, sterile distilled water, or CSF. For hyperbaric technique, use dextrose solution.
*Perineum:* 0.5 ml 10% solution and 0.5 ml diluent injected at the L4 interspace.
*Perineum and lower extremities:* 1 ml 10% solution and 1 ml diluent injected at the L3 or L4 interspace.
*Up to costal margin:* 2 ml 10% solution and 1 ml diluent injected at the L2, L3, or L4 interspace.
*Epidural block —*
1.5% solution: 25 ml (375 mg)
*Peripheral nerve block —*
1% solution: 50 ml (500 mg)
2% solution: 25 ml (500 mg)
*Infiltration —*
350 to 600 mg in a 0.25% to 0.5% solution. Maximum initial dose is 1 g.

**Skin:** dermatologic reactions.
**Other:** edema, ***status asthmaticus, anaphylaxis, anaphylactoid reactions.***
Systemic effects from high blood levels of the drug —
**CNS:** anxiety, nervousness, *seizures* followed by drowsiness.
**CV:** myocardial depression, hypotension, **arrhythmias, cardiac arrest.**
**EENT:** blurred vision, tinnitus.
**GI:** nausea, vomiting.
**Respiratory:** *respiratory arrest.*

---

Reactions may be *common,* uncommon, ***life-threatening,*** or **COMMON AND LIFE-THREATENING.**

| INTERACTIONS | NURSING CONSIDERATIONS |
|---|---|

• Use solutions with epinephrine cautiously in patients with CV disease and in body areas with limited blood supply (ears, nose, fingers, toes).
• Don't use solution with preservatives for caudal or epidural block.
• Keep resuscitation equipment and drugs available.
• Check solution for particles.

---

*Cyclic antidepressants, MAO inhibitors:* severe, sustained hypertension when used with lidocaine and epinephrine. Use with extreme caution.
*Enflurane, halothane, isoflurane, related drugs:* arrhythmias when used with lidocaine and epinephrine. Use with extreme caution.

• Contraindicated in patients with inflammation or infection in puncture region, septicemia, severe hypertension, spinal deformities, and neurologic disorders.
• Use cautiously in debilitated, elderly, or acutely ill patients; in patients with severe shock, heart block, general drug allergies; in obstetric patients; and for paracervical block.
• Dose and interval are increased with epinephrine.
• Use solutions with epinephrine cautiously in patients with CV disorders and in body areas with limited blood supply (ears, nose, fingers, toes).
• Don't use solution with preservatives for spinal, epidural, or caudal block.
• Keep resuscitation equipment and drugs available.
• Discard partially used vials without preservatives.
• Check solution for particles.

---

*Echothiophate iodide:* reduced hydrolysis of procaine. Use together cautiously.
*Succinylcholine:* prolonged neuromuscular blockade. Use together cautiously.

• Contraindicated in patients with traumatized urethras and in those with hypersensitivity to chloroprocaine, tetracaine, or other PABA derivatives.
• Contraindicated for obstetric use in patients with cephalopelvic disproportion, placenta previa, abruptio placentae, floating fetal head, and intrauterine manipulation.
• Use cautiously in hyperexcitable patients; in those with CNS disease, infection at puncture site, shock, profound anemia, cachexia, sepsis, hypertension, hypotension, GI hemorrhage, bowel perforation or strangulation, peritonitis, cardiac decompensation, massive pleural effusion, or increased intra-abdominal pressure; and in obstetric patients.
• Keep resuscitation equipment and drugs available.
• Use solution without preservatives for epidural block.
• Discard partially used vials without preservatives.
• Check solution for particles.

---

*Liquid form contains alcohol.   **May contain tartrazine.   †Canada only.   ‡Australia only.   ◇OTC.

## Selected local and topical anesthetics (continued)

| DRUG, INDICATIONS, DOSAGE | ADVERSE REACTIONS |
|---|---|

**Local** (continued)

**tetracaine hydrochloride**
(Pontocaine)
Dosage for adults varies according to the extent of
the block as follows.
*Low spinal (saddle) block in vaginal delivery* —
2 to 5 mg as hyperbaric solution (in 10% dextrose).
*Perineum and lower extremities:* 5 to 10 mg.
*Up to costal margin:* 15 to 20 mg.

**Skin:** dermatologic reactions.
**Other:** edema, ***status
asthmaticus, anaphylaxis,
anaphylactoid reactions.***
Systemic effects from high
blood levels of the drug —
**CNS:** anxiety, nervousness,
***seizures*** followed by
drowsiness.
**CV:** myocardial depression,
hypotension, ***arrhythmias,
cardiac arrest.***
**EENT:** blurred vision, tinnitus.
**GI:** nausea, vomiting.
**Respiratory:** ***respiratory
arrest.***

---

## Topical

**proparacaine hydrochloride**
(AK-taine, Alcaine, Ophthaine, Ophthetic)
*Anesthesia for tonometry, gonioscopy; removal of
sutures or foreign bodies from cornea* —
**Adults and children:** 1 to 2 drops of 0.5% solution
instilled in eye just before procedure.
*Anesthesia for cataract extraction, glaucoma
surgery* —
**Adults and children:** 1 drop of 0.5% solution
instilled in eye q 5 to 10 minutes for five to seven
doses.

**EENT:** conjunctival redness,
transient eye pain.
**Other:** hypersensitivity
reactions.

---

**tetracaine**
(Pontocaine Eye Ointment)
**tetracaine hydrochloride**
(Pontocaine)
*Anesthesia for tonometry, gonioscopy; removal of
corneal foreign bodies, suture removal from cornea;
other diagnostic and minor surgical procedures* —
**Adults and children:** 1 to 2 drops of 0.5% solution
or a small strip ½" [1.25 to 2.5 cm] of ointment
in eye just before procedure.

**EENT:** transient stinging in
eye 30 seconds after initial
instillation, epithelial damage
in excessive or long-term use.
**Other:** sensitization with
repeated use (allergic skin
rash, urticaria).

---

Reactions may be *common,* uncommon, ***life-threatening,*** or **COMMON AND LIFE-THREATENING.**

| INTERACTIONS | NURSING CONSIDERATIONS |
| --- | --- |
| None significant. | • Contraindicated in patients with infection at injection site or CNS disease and in those with hypersensitivity to procaine or related agents.<br>• Saddle block is contraindicated in patients with cephalopelvic disproportion, placenta previa, abruptio placentae, intrauterine manipulation, and floating fetal head.<br>• Use cautiously in patients with shock, profound anemia, cachexia, hypertension, hypotension, peritonitis, cardiac decompensation, massive pleural effusion, increased intracranial pressure, and infection.<br>• Keep resuscitation equipment and drugs available.<br>• When CSF is added to powdered drug or drug solution during spinal anesthesia, solution may be cloudy. Don't use discolored or crystallized solutions.<br>• Protect from light; store in refrigerator. |
| None significant. | • Use cautiously in patients with cardiac disease and hyperthyroidism.<br>• Not for long-term use; may delay wound healing.<br>• Warn patients not to rub or touch eye while cornea is anesthetized. This may cause corneal abrasion and greater discomfort when anesthesia wears off.<br>• Warn patients with corneal abrasion that pain is relieved only temporarily.<br>• Don't use discolored solution.<br>• Store in tightly closed container. Refrigerate opened containers. |
| *Cholinesterase inhibitors:* prolonged ocular anesthesia and increased risk of toxicity.<br>*Sulfonamides:* interference with sulfonamide antibacterial activity. Wait ½ hour after anesthesia before instilling sulfonamide. | • Contraindicated in patients with hypersensitivity to the drug.<br>• Avoid long-term use.<br>• Does not dilate the pupil, paralyze accommodation, or increase intraocular pressure.<br>• Don't use discolored solution. Keep container tightly closed.<br>• Warn patient not to touch or rub eye while cornea is anesthetized. This may cause corneal abrasion and greater discomfort when anesthesia wears off. |

# Cancer chemotherapy: Acronyms and protocols

Combination chemotherapy is well established for treatment of cancer. The chart below lists commonly used acronyms and protocols, including standard dosages for specific cancers.

| ACRONYM & INDICATION | DRUG | | DOSAGE |
|---|---|---|---|
| | Generic name | Trade name | |
| **AA** (Leukemia — AML, induction) | cytarabine (ara-C) | Cytosar-U | 100 mg/m² daily by continuous I.V. infusion for 7 to 10 days |
| | doxorubicin | Adriamycin | 30 mg/m² I.V., days 1 to 3 |
| **ABVD** (Hodgkin's lymphoma) | doxorubicin | Adriamycin | 25 mg/m² I.V., days 1 and 15 |
| | bleomycin | Blenoxane | 10 units/m² I.V., days 1 and 15 |
| | vinblastine | Velban | 6 mg/m² I.V., days 1 and 15 |
| | dacarbazine | DTIC-Dome | 375 mg/m² I.V., days 1 and 15 *Repeat cycle q 28 days.* |
| **AC** (Multiple myeloma) | doxorubicin | Adriamycin | 30 mg/m² I.V., day 1 |
| | carmustine | BiCNU | 30 mg/m² I.V., day 1 *Repeat cycle q 21 to 28 days.* |
| **AC** (Bony sarcoma) | doxorubicin | Adriamycin | 75 to 90 mg/m² by 96-hour continuous I.V. infusion |
| | cisplatin | Platinol | 90 to 120 mg/m² I.V., day 6 *Repeat cycle q 28 days.* |
| **AC** (Breast cancer) | doxorubicin | Adriamycin | 45 mg/m² I.V., day 1 |
| | cyclophosphamide | Cytoxan | 500 mg/m² I.V., day 1 *Repeat cycle q 28 days.* |
| **AFM** (Breast cancer) | doxorubicin | Adriamycin | 25 mg/m² by continuous I.V. infusion, days 1 to 3 |
| | fluorouracil (5-FU) | Adrucil | 400 mg/m² I.V., days 1 to 5 |
| | methotrexate | Folex | 250 mg/m² I.V., day 18 |
| | leucovorin calcium | Wellcovorin | 15 mg/m² P.O. q 6 hours, days 19 to 20 *Repeat cycle q 21 days for four cycles.* |
| **AP** (Ovarian cancer, epithelial) | doxorubicin | Adriamycin | 50 to 60 mg/m² I.V., day 1 |
| | cisplatin | Platinol | 50 to 60 mg/m² I.V., day 1 *Repeat cycle q 21 days.* |
| **APE (EAP)** (Gastric cancer) | doxorubicin | Adriamycin | 20 mg/m² I.V. daily, days 1 and 7 |
| | cisplatin | Platinol | 40 mg/m² I.V. daily, days 2 and 8 |
| | etoposide (VP-16) | VePesid | 120 mg/m² I.V. daily, days 4, 5, and 6 *Repeat cycle q 8 weeks.* |

# Cancer chemotherapy: Acronyms and protocols (continued)

| ACRONYM & INDICATION | DRUG | | DOSAGE |
|---|---|---|---|
| | **Generic name** | **Trade name** | |
| **ASHAP** (Malignant lymphoma) | doxorubicin | Adriamycin | 10 mg/m² daily by continuous I.V. infusion, days 1 to 4 |
| | cisplatin | Platinol | 25 mg/m² daily by continuous I.V. infusion days 1 to 4 |
| | cytarabine (ara-C) | Cytosar-U | 1,500 mg/m² I.V. immediately after completion of doxorubicin and cisplatin therapy |
| | methylprednisolone | Solu-Medrol | 500 mg I.V. daily, days 1 to 5 *Repeat cycle q 21 to 25 days.* |
| **BACON** (Non-small-cell lung cancer) | bleomycin | Blenoxane | 30 units I.V. q 6 weeks, day 2 |
| | doxorubicin | Adriamycin | 40 mg/m² I.V. q 4 weeks, day 1 |
| | lomustine (CCNU) | CeeNU | 65 mg/m² P.O. q 8 weeks, day 1 |
| | vincristine | Oncovin | 0.75 to 1 mg/m² I.V. q 6 weeks, day 2 |
| | mechlorethamine (nitrogen mustard) | Mustargen | 8 mg/m² I.V. q 4 weeks, day 1 |
| **BACOP** (Malignant lymphoma) | bleomycin | Blenoxane | 5 units/m² I.V. daily, days 15 and 22 |
| | doxorubicin | Adriamycin | 25 mg/m² I.V., days 1 and 8 |
| | cyclophosphamide | Cytoxan | 650 mg/m² I.V., days 1 and 8 |
| | vincristine | Oncovin | 1.4 mg/m² (2 mg maximum) I.V., days 1 and 8 |
| | prednisone | Deltasone | 60 mg/m² P.O., days 15 to 28 *Repeat cycle q 28 days.* |
| **BCP** (Multiple myeloma) | carmustine | BiCNU | 75 mg/m² I.V., day 1 |
| | cyclophosphamide | Cytoxan | 400 mg/m² I.V., day 1 |
| | prednisone | Deltasone | 75 mg P.O., days 1 to 7 *Repeat cycle q 28 days.* |
| **BEP** (Genitourinary cancer) | bleomycin | Blenoxane | 30 units I.V., days 2, 9, and 16 |
| | etoposide (VP-16) | VePesid | 100 mg/m², days 1 to 5 |
| | cisplatin | Platinol | 20 mg/m² I.V., days 1 to 5 *Repeat cycle q 21 days.* |
| **BHD** (Malignant melanoma) | carmustine | BiCNU | 100 to 150 mg/m² I.V. q 6 weeks |
| | hydroxyurea | Hydrea | 1,480 mg/m² P.O. q 3 weeks, days 1 to 5 |
| | dacarbazine | DTIC-Dome | 100 to 150 mg/m² I.V. q 3 weeks, days 1 to 5 |
| **CA** (Breast cancer) | cyclophosphamide | Cytoxan | 200 mg/m² P.O., days 3 to 6 |
| | doxorubicin | Adriamycin | 40 mg/m² I.V., day 1 *Repeat cycle q 21 to 28 days.* |
| **CAE (ACE)** (Small-cell lung cancer) | cyclophosphamide | Cytoxan | 1 g/m² I.V., day 1 |
| | doxorubicin | Adriamycin | 45 mg/m² I.V., day 1 |
| | etoposide (VP-16) | VePesid | 50 mg/m² I.V., day 1 *Repeat cycle q 21 days.* |

*(continued)*

# Cancer chemotherapy: Acronyms and protocols (continued)

| ACRONYM & INDICATION | DRUG | | DOSAGE |
|---|---|---|---|
| | Generic name | Trade name | |
| **CAF (FAC)** (Breast cancer) | cyclophosphamide | Cytoxan | 100 mg/m² P.O., days 1 to 14 |
| | doxorubicin | Adriamycin | 30 mg/m² I.V., days 1 and 8 |
| | fluorouracil (5-FU) | Adrucil | 400 to 500 mg/m² I.V., days 1 and 8 *Repeat cycle q 28 days.* |
| *or* | cyclophosphamide | Cytoxan | 400 to 600 mg/m² I.V., day 1 |
| | doxorubicin | Adriamycin | 40 to 60 mg/m² I.V., day 1 |
| | fluorouracil (5-FU) | Adrucil | 400 to 600 mg/m² I.V., day 1 *Repeat cycle q 21 days.* |
| **CAMP** (Non-small-cell lung cancer) | cyclophosphamide | Cytoxan | 300 mg/m² I.V., days 1 and 8 |
| | doxorubicin | Adriamycin | 20 mg/m² I.V., days 1 and 8 |
| | methotrexate | Folex | 15 mg/m² I.V., days 1 and 8 |
| | procarbazine | Matulane | 100 mg/m² P.O., days 1 to 10 *Repeat cycle q 28 days.* |
| **CAP** (Genitourinary cancer) | cisplatin | Platinol | 60 mg/m² I.V., day 1 |
| | doxorubicin | Adriamycin | 40 mg/m² I.V., day 1 |
| | cyclophosphamide | Cytoxan | 400 mg/m² I.V., day 1 *Repeat cycle q 21 days.* |
| **CAP** (Non-small-cell lung cancer) | cyclophosphamide | Cytoxan | 400 mg/m² I.V., day 1 |
| | doxorubicin | Adriamycin | 40 mg/m² I.V., day 1 |
| | cisplatin | Platinol | 60 mg/m² I.V., day 1 *Repeat cycle q 28 days.* |
| **CAP (PAC)** (Ovarian cancer, epithelial) | cisplatin | Platinol | 50 mg/m² I.V., day 1 |
| | doxorubicin | Adriamycin | 50 mg/m² I.V., day 1 |
| | cyclophosphamide | Cytoxan | 500 mg/m² I.V., day 1 *Repeat cycle q 21 days for eight cycles.* |
| **CAV** (Small-cell lung cancer) | cyclophosphamide | Cytoxan | 1,000 mg/m² I.V., day 1 |
| | doxorubicin | Adriamycin | 50 mg/m² I.V., day 1 |
| | vincristine | Oncovin | 1.4 mg/m² I.V., day 1 *Repeat cycle q 3 weeks.* |
| **CAVE** (Small-cell lung cancer) | cyclophosphamide | Cytoxan | 750 mg/m² I.V., day 1 |
| | doxorubicin | Adriamycin | 50 mg/m² I.V., day 1 |
| | vincristine | Oncovin | 1.4 mg/m² I.V., day 1 |
| | etoposide (VP-16) | VePesid | 60 to 100 mg/m² I.V., days 1 to 3 *Repeat cycle q 21 days.* |
| **CAVe** (Hodgkin's lymphoma) | lomustine (CCNU) | CeeNU | 100 mg/m² I.V., day 1 |
| | doxorubicin | Adriamycin | 60 mg/m² I.V., day 1 |
| | vinblastine | Velban | 5 mg/m² I.V., day 1 *Repeat cycle q 6 weeks for nine cycles.* |

## Cancer chemotherapy: Acronyms and protocols *(continued)*

| ACRONYM & INDICATION | DRUG | | DOSAGE |
|---|---|---|---|
| | Generic name | Trade name | |
| CC (Ovarian cancer, epithelial) | carboplatin | Paraplatin | 300 mg/m² I.V., day 1 |
| | cyclophosphamide | Cytoxan | 600 mg/m² I.V., day 1<br>*Repeat cycle q 28 days.* |
| CD (DC) (Leukemia – ANLL, consolidation) | cytarabine (ara-C) | Cytosar-U | 3,000 mg/m² I.V. q 12 hours for 6 days |
| | daunorubicin | Cerubidine | 30 mg/m² I.V. daily for 3 days, after cytarabine therapy |
| CDC (Ovarian cancer, epithelial) | carboplatin | Paraplatin | 300 mg/m² I.V., day 1 |
| | doxorubicin | Adriamycin | 40 mg/m² I.V., day 1 |
| | cyclophosphamide | Cytoxan | 500 mg/m² I.V., day 1<br>*Repeat cycle q 28 days.* |
| CF (Head and neck cancer) | cisplatin | Platinol | 100 mg/m² I.V., day 1 |
| | fluorouracil (5-FU) | Adrucil | 1,000 mg/m² daily by continuous I.V. infusion, days 1 to 5<br>*Repeat cycle q 21 to 28 days.* |
| *or* | carboplatin | Paraplatin | 400 mg/m² I.V., day 1 |
| | fluorouracil (5-FU) | Adrucil | 1,000 mg/m² daily by continuous I.V. infusion, days 1 to 5<br>*Repeat cycle q 21 to 28 days.* |
| CFL (Head and neck cancer) | cisplatin | Platinol | 100 mg/m² I.V., day 1 |
| | fluorouracil (5-FU) | Adrucil | 600 to 800 mg/m² daily by continuous I.V. infusion, days 1 to 5 |
| | leucovorin calcium | Wellcovorin | 200 to 300 mg/m² I.V. daily, days 1 to 5<br>*Repeat cycle q 21 days.* |
| CFM (Breast cancer) | cyclophosphamide | Cytoxan | 500 mg/m² I.V., day 1 |
| | fluorouracil (5-FU) | Adrucil | 500 mg/m² I.V., day 1 |
| | mitoxantrone | Novantrone | 10 mg/m² I.V., day 1<br>*Repeat cycle q 21 days.* |
| CFPT (Breast cancer) | cyclophosphamide | Cytoxan | 150 mg/m² I.V., days 1 to 5 |
| | fluorouracil (5-FU) | Adrucil | 300 mg/m² I.V., days 1 to 5 |
| | prednisone | Deltasone | 10 mg P.O. t.i.d. for first 7 days of each course |
| | tamoxifen | Nolvadex | 10 mg P.O. b.i.d. (daily through each course)<br>*Repeat cycle q 6 weeks.* |
| CHAP (Ovarian cancer, epithelial) | cyclophosphamide | Cytoxan | 300 to 500 mg/m² I.V., day 1 |
| | altretamine | Hexalen | 150 mg/m² P.O., days 1 to 7 |
| | doxorubicin | Adriamycin | 30 to 50 mg/m² I.V., day 1 |
| | cisplatin | Platinol | 50 mg/m² I.V., day 1<br>*Repeat cycle q 28 days.* |

*(continued)*

## Cancer chemotherapy: Acronyms and protocols (continued)

| ACRONYM & INDICATION | DRUG | | DOSAGE |
|---|---|---|---|
| | Generic name | Trade name | |
| ChlVPP (Hodgkin's lymphoma) | chlorambucil | Leukeran | 6 mg/m² P.O., days 1 to 14 (10 mg/day maximum) |
| | vinblastine | Velban | 6 mg/m² I.V., days 1 to 8 (10 mg/day maximum) |
| | procarbazine | Matulane | 50 mg P.O., days 1 to 14 (150 mg/day maximum) |
| | prednisone | Deltasone | 40 mg/m² P.O., days 1 to 14 (25 mg/m² for child) |
| CHOP (Malignant lymphoma) | cyclophosphamide | Cytoxan | 750 mg/m² I.V., day 1 |
| | doxorubicin | Adriamycin | 50 mg/m² I.V., day 1 |
| | vincristine | Oncovin | 1.4 mg/m² (2 mg maximum) I.V., day 1 |
| | prednisone | Deltasone | 100 mg/m² P.O., days 1 to 5 *Repeat cycle q 21 days.* |
| CHOP-Bleo (Malignant lymphoma) | cyclophosphamide | Cytoxan | 750 mg/m² I.V., day 1 |
| | doxorubicin | Adriamycin | 50 mg/m² I.V., day 1 |
| | vincristine | Oncovin | 2 mg I.V., days 1 and 5 |
| | prednisone | Deltasone | 100 mg P.O., days 1 to 5 |
| | bleomycin | Blenoxane | 15 units I.V., days 1 and 5 *Repeat cycle q 21 days.* |
| CISCA (Genitourinary cancer) | cyclophosphamide | Cytoxan | 650 mg/m² I.V., day 1 |
| | doxorubicin | Adriamycin | 50 mg/m² I.V., day 1 |
| | cisplatin | Platinol | 70 to 100 mg/m² I.V., day 2 *Repeat cycle q 21 to 28 days.* |
| CMF (Breast cancer) | cyclophosphamide | Cytoxan | 100 mg/m² P.O., days 1 to 14, or 400 to 600 mg/m² I.V., day 1 |
| | methotrexate | Folex | 40 to 60 mg/m² I.V., days 1 and 8 |
| | fluorouracil (5-FU) | Adrucil | 400 to 600 mg/m² I.V., days 1 and 8 *Repeat cycle q 28 days.* |
| CMFP (Breast cancer) | cyclophosphamide | Cytoxan | 100 mg/m² P.O., days 1 to 14 |
| | methotrexate | Folex | 60 mg/m² I.V., days 1 and 8 |
| | fluorouracil (5-FU) | Adrucil | 700 mg/m² I.V., days 1 and 8 |
| | prednisone | Deltasone | 40 mg/m² P.O., days 1 to 14 *Repeat cycle q 28 days.* |
| CMFVP (Cooper's) (Breast cancer) | cyclophosphamide | Cytoxan | 2 mg/kg P.O. daily |
| | methotrexate | Folex | 0.75 mg/kg I.V. weekly |
| | fluorouracil (5-FU) | Adrucil | 12 mg/kg I.V. weekly |
| | vincristine | Oncovin | 0.025 mg/kg (2 mg/week maximum) I.V. weekly |
| | prednisone | Deltasone | 0.75 mg/kg P.O. daily, days 1 to 21, then tapered |

# Cancer chemotherapy: Acronyms and protocols *(continued)*

| ACRONYM & INDICATION | DRUG | | DOSAGE |
|---|---|---|---|
| | Generic name | Trade name | |
| **CMFVP (SWOG)** (Breast cancer) | cyclophosphamide | Cytoxan | 60 mg/m² P.O. daily for 1 year |
| | methotrexate | Folex | 15 mg/m² I.V. weekly for 1 year |
| | fluorouracil (5-FU) | Adrucil | 300 mg/m² I.V. weekly for 1 year |
| | vincristine | Oncovin | 0.625 mg/m² I.V. weekly for 1 year |
| | prednisone | Deltasone | 30 mg/m² P.O., days 1 to 14; 20 mg/m², days 15 to 28; 10 mg/m², days 29 to 42 *Repeat cycle q 42 days.* |
| **CMV** (Genitourinary [bladder] cancer) | vinblastine | Velban | 4 mg/m² I.V., days 1 and 8 |
| | methotrexate | Folex | 30 mg/m² I.V., days 1 and 8 |
| | cisplatin | Platinol | 100 mg/m² I.V., 12 hours after methotrexate *Repeat cycle q 21 days.* |
| **COAP** (Leukemia— AML, induction) | cyclophosphamide | Cytoxan | 100 mg/m² I.V. or P.O., days 1 to 5 |
| | vincristine | Oncovin | 2 mg/m² I.V., day 1 |
| | cytarabine (ara-C) | Cytosar-U | 100 mg/m² I.V., days 1 to 5 |
| | prednisone | Deltasone | 100 mg P.O., days 1 to 5 |
| **COB** (Head and neck cancer) | cisplatin | Platinol | 100 mg/m² I.V., day 1 |
| | vincristine | Oncovin | 1 mg I.V., days 2 and 5 |
| | bleomycin | Blenoxane | 30 units by continuous I.V. infusion, days 2 to 5 *Repeat cycle q 21 days.* |
| **CODE** (Small-cell lung cancer) | cisplatin | Platinol | 25 mg/m² I.V. weekly for 9 weeks |
| | vincristine | Oncovin | 1 mg/m² I.V., weeks 1, 2,4, 6, and 8 |
| | doxorubicin | Adriamycin | 25 mg/m² I.V, weeks 1, 3, 5, 7, and 9 |
| | etoposide (VP-16) | VePesid | 80 mg/m² I.V., weeks 1, 3, 5, 7, and 9 |
| **COMLA** (Malignant lymphoma) | cyclophosphamide | Cytoxan | 1,500 mg/m² I.V., day 1 |
| | vincristine | Oncovin | 1.4 mg/m² (2.5 mg maximum) I.V., days 1, 8, and 15 |
| | methotrexate | Folex | 120 mg/m² I.V., days 22, 29, 36, 43, 50, 57, 64, and 71 |
| | leucovorin calcium | Wellcovorin | 25 mg/m² P.O. q 6 hours for four doses, beginning 24 hours after each methotrexate dose |
| | cytarabine (ara-C) | Cytosar-U | 300 mg/m² I.V., days 22, 29, 36, 43, 50, 57, 64, and 71 *Repeat cycle q 21 days.* |
| **COP** (Malignant lymphoma) | cyclophosphamide | Cytoxan | 800 to 1,000 mg/m² I.V., day 1 |
| | vincristine | Oncovin | 1.4 mg/m² (2 mg maximum) I.V., day 1 |
| | prednisone | Deltasone | 60 mg/m² P.O., days 1 to 5 *Repeat cycle q 21 days.* |

*(continued)*

# Cancer chemotherapy: Acronyms and protocols (continued)

| ACRONYM & INDICATION | DRUG | | DOSAGE |
| --- | --- | --- | --- |
| | Generic name | Trade name | |
| COP-BLAM (Malignant lymphoma) | cyclophosphamide | Cytoxan | 400 mg/m² I.V., day 1 |
| | vincristine | Oncovin | 1 mg/m² I.V., day 1 |
| | prednisone | Deltasone | 40 mg/m² P.O., days 1 to 10 |
| | bleomycin | Blenoxane | 15 mg I.V., day 14 |
| | doxorubicin | Adriamycin | 40 mg/m², day 1 |
| | procarbazine | Matulane | 100 mg/m², days 1 to 10 |
| COPE (Small-cell lung cancer) | cyclophosphamide | Cytoxan | 750 mg/m² I.V., day 1 |
| | cisplatin | Platinol | 20 mg/m² I.V., days 1 to 3 |
| | etoposide (VP-16) | VePesid | 100 mg/m² I.V., days 1 to 3 |
| | vincristine | Oncovin | 1.4 mg/m² I.V., day 3 Repeat cycle q 21 days. |
| COPP (Malignant lymphoma) | cyclophosphamide | Cytoxan | 400 to 650 mg/m² I.V., days 1 and 8 |
| | vincristine | Oncovin | 1.4 to 1.5 mg/m² (2 mg maximum) I.V., days 1 and 8 |
| | procarbazine | Matulane | 100 mg/m² P.O., days 1 to 10 or 1 to 14 |
| | prednisone | Deltasone | 40 mg/m² P.O., days 1 to 14 Repeat cycle q 28 days. |
| CP (Ovarian cancer, epithelial) | cyclophosphamide | Cytoxan | 1,000 mg/m² I.V., day 1 |
| | cisplatin | Platinol | 75 mg/m² I.V., day 1 Repeat cycle q 21 days. |
| CV (Small-cell lung cancer) | cisplatin | Platinol | 50 mg/m² I.V., day 1 |
| | etoposide (VP-16) | VePesid | 60 mg/m² I.V., days 1 to 5 Repeat cycle q 21 to 28 days. |
| CV (Non-small-cell lung cancer) | cisplatin | Platinol | 60 to 80 mg/m² I.V., day 1 |
| | etoposide (VP-16) | VePesid | 120 mg/m² I.V., days 4, 6, and 8 Repeat cycle q 21 to 28 days. |
| CVEB (Genitourinary cancer) | cisplatin | Platinol | 40 mg/m² I.V., days 1 to 5 |
| | vinblastine | Velban | 7.5 mg/m² I.V., day 1 |
| | etoposide (VP-16) | VePesid | 100 mg/m² I.V., days 1 to 5 |
| | bleomycin | Blenoxane | 30 units I.V. weekly Repeat cycle q 21 days. |
| CVI (VIC) (Non-small-cell lung cancer) | carboplatin | Paraplatin | 300 mg/m² I.V., day 1 |
| | etoposide (VP-16) | VePesid | 60 to 100 mg/m² I.V., day 1 |
| | ifosfamide | Ifex | 1.5 g/m² I.V., days 1, 3, and 5 |
| | mesna | Mesnex | Dosage is 20% of ifosfamide dose, given immediately before and at 4 and 8 hours after ifosfamide infusion Repeat cycle q 28 days. |

## Cancer chemotherapy: Acronyms and protocols (continued)

| ACRONYM & INDICATION | DRUG | | DOSAGE |
|---|---|---|---|
| | Generic name | Trade name | |
| **CVP** (Leukemia – CLL, blast crisis) | cyclophosphamide | Cytoxan | 300 mg/m² P.O., days 1 to 5 |
| | vincristine | Oncovin | 1.4 mg/m² (2 mg maximum) I.V., day 1 |
| | prednisone | Deltasone | 100 mg/m² P.O., days 1 to 5 *Repeat cycle q 21 days.* |
| **CVP** (Malignant lymphoma) | cyclophosphamide | Cytoxan | 400 mg/m² P.O., days 1 to 5 |
| | vincristine | Oncovin | 1.4 mg/m² (2 mg maximum) I.V., day 1 |
| | prednisone | Deltasone | 100 mg/m² P.O., days 1 to 5 *Repeat cycle q 21 days.* |
| **CVPP** (Hodgkin's lymphoma) | lomustine (CCNU) | CeeNU | 75 mg/m² P.O., day 1 |
| | vinblastine | Velban | 4 mg/m² I.V., days 1 and 8 |
| | procarbazine | Matulane | 100 mg/m² P.O., days 1 to 14 |
| | prednisone | Deltasone | 30 mg/m² P.O., days 1 to 14 (cycles 1 and 4 only) *Repeat cycle q 28 days.* |
| **CYADIC** (Soft-tissue sarcoma) | cyclophosphamide | Cytoxan | 600 mg/m² I.V., day 1 |
| | doxorubicin | Adriamycin | 15 mg/m² by continuous I.V. infusion, days 1 to 4 |
| | dacarbazine | DTIC-Dome | 250 mg/m² by continuous I.V. infusion, days 1 to 4 *Repeat cycle q 21 to 28 days.* |
| **CYVADIC** (Bony sarcoma) | cyclophosphamide | Cytoxan | 600 mg/m² I.V., day 1 |
| | vincristine | Oncovin | 1.4 mg/m² (2 mg maximum) I.V., days 1 and 5 |
| | doxorubicin | Adriamycin | 50 mg/m² I.V., day 1 |
| | dacarbazine | DTIC-Dome | 250 mg/m² I.V., days 1 to 5 *Repeat cycle q 21 days.* |
| **CYVADIC** (Soft-tissue sarcoma) | cyclophosphamide | Cytoxan | 500 mg/m² I.V., day 1 |
| | vincristine | Oncovin | 1.4 mg/m² (2 mg maximum) I.V., days 1 and 5 |
| | doxorubicin | Adriamycin | 50 mg/m² I.V., day 1 |
| | dacarbazine | DTIC-Dome | 250 mg/m² I.V., days 1 to 5 *Repeat cycle q 21 days.* |
| **DC** (Leukemia – pediatric AML, induction) | daunorubicin | Cerubidine | 45 to 60 mg/m² I.V., days 1 to 3 |
| | cytarabine (ara-C) | Cytosar-U | 100 mg/m² I.V. or S.C. q 12 hours for 5 to 7 days |
| **DCPM** (Leukemia – pediatric AML, induction) | daunorubicin | Cerubidine | 25 mg/m² I.V., day 1 |
| | cytarabine (ara-C) | Cytosar-U | 80 mg/m² I.V., days 1 to 3 |
| | prednisone | Deltasone | 40 mg/m² P.O. daily |
| | mercaptopurine (6-MP) | Purinethol | 100 mg/m² P.O. daily |

*(continued)*

# Cancer chemotherapy: Acronyms and protocols (continued)

| ACRONYM & INDICATION | DRUG | | DOSAGE |
|---|---|---|---|
| | Generic name | Trade name | |
| DCT (Leukemia – ANLL, induction) | daunorubicin | Cerubidine | 60 mg/m² I.V., days 1 to 3 |
| | cytarabine (ara-C) | Cytosar-U | 200 mg/m² daily by continuous I.V. days 1 to 5 |
| | thioguanine (6-TG) | | 100 mg/m² P.O. q 12 hours, days 1 to 5 |
| DHAP (Hodgkin's lymphoma) | dexamethasone | Decadron | 40 mg P.O. or I.V., days 1 to 4 |
| | cisplatin | Platinol | 100 mg/m² by continuous I.V. infusion, day 1 |
| | cytarabine (ara-C) | Cytosar-U | 2 g/m² q 12 hours for two doses, day 2 *Repeat cycle q 3 to 4 weeks.* |
| DTIC-ACTD (Malignant melanoma) | dacarbazine | DTIC-Dome | 750 mg/m² I.V., day 1 |
| | dactinomycin (actinomycin D) | Cosmegen | 1 mg/m² I.V., day 1 *Repeat cycle q 28 days.* |
| DVP (Leukemia – ALL, induction) | daunorubicin | Cerubidine | 45 mg/m² I.V., days 1 to 3 and 14 |
| | vincristine | Oncovin | 2 mg/m² (2 mg max.) I.V. weekly for 4 weeks |
| | prednisone | Deltasone | 45 mg/m² P.O., for 28 to 35 days |
| EAP (Gastric cancer) | doxorubicin | Adriamycin | 20 mg/m² I.V., days 1 and 7 |
| | cisplatin | Platinol | 40 mg/m² I.V., days 2 and 8 |
| | etoposide (VP-16) | VePesid | 120 mg/m² I.V., days 4, 5, and 6 *Repeat cycle q 21 days.* |
| EC (Small-cell lung cancer) | etoposide (VP-16) | VePesid | 60 to 100 mg/m² I.V., days 1 to 3 |
| | carboplatin | Paraplatin | 400 mg/m² I.V., day 1 *Repeat cycle q 28 days.* |
| EDAP (Multiple myeloma) | etoposide (VP-16) | VePesid | 100 to 200 mg/m² by continuous I.V. infusion, days 1 to 4 |
| | dexamethasone | Decadron | 40 mg/m² I.V. or P.O., days 1 to 5 |
| | cytarabine (ara-C) | Cytosar-U | 1,000 mg/m² I.V., day 5 |
| | cisplatin | Platinol | 20 mg by continuous I.V. infusion, days 1 to 4 |
| ELF (Gastric cancer) | etoposide (VP-16) | VePesid | 120 mg/m² I.V., days 1 to 3 |
| | fluorouracil (5-FU) | Adrucil | 500 mg/m² I.V., days 1 to 3 |
| | leucovorin calcium | Wellcovorin | 300 mg/m² I.V., days 1 to 3 *Repeat cycle q 21 to 28 days.* |
| EP (Small-cell or non-small-cell lung cancer) | cisplatin | Platinol | 75 to 100 mg/m² I.V., day 1 |
| | etoposide (VP-16) | VePesid | 75 to 100 mg/m² I.V., days 1 to 3 *Repeat cycle q 21 to 28 days.* |
| ESHAP (Malignant lymphoma) | etoposide (VP-16) | VePesid | 60 mg/m² I.V. over 30 to 60 minutes, days 1 to 4 |
| | cisplatin | Platinol | 25 mg/m² daily by continuous I.V., days 1 to 4 |
| | cytarabine (ara-C) | Cytosar-U | 2 g/m² I.V. immediately after completion of etoposide and cisplatin therapy |
| | methylprednisolone | Solu-Medrol | 500 mg I.V. daily, days 1 to 4 *Repeat cycle q 21 to 28 days.* |

## Cancer chemotherapy: Acronyms and protocols *(continued)*

| ACRONYM & INDICATION | DRUG | | DOSAGE |
|---|---|---|---|
| | Generic name | Trade name | |
| **EVA** (Hodgkin's lymphoma) | etoposide (VP-16) | VePesid | 100 mg/m² I.V., days 1 to 3 |
| | vinblastine | Velban | 6 mg/m² I.V., day 1 |
| | doxorubicin | Adriamycin | 50 mg/m² I.V., day 1 *Repeat cycle q 28 days.* |
| **FAC (CAF)** (Breast cancer) | fluorouracil (5-FU) | Adrucil | 500 mg/m² I.V., days 1 and 8 |
| | doxorubicin | Adriamycin | 50 mg/m² I.V., day 1 |
| | cyclophosphamide | Cytoxan | 500 mg/m² I.V., day 1 *Repeat cycle q 21 days.* |
| **FAM** (Colon cancer; gastric cancer) | fluorouracil (5-FU) | Adrucil | 600 mg/m² I.V., days 1, 8, 29, and 36 |
| | doxorubicin | Adriamycin | 30 mg/m² I.V., days 1 and 29 |
| | mitomycin | Mutamycin | 10 mg/m² I.V., day 1 *Repeat cycle q 8 weeks.* |
| **FAM** (Non-small-cell lung cancer) | fluorouracil (5-FU) | Adrucil | 600 mg/m² I.V., days 1, 8, 28, and 36 |
| | doxorubicin | Adriamycin | 30 mg/m² I.V., days 1 and 28 |
| | mitomycin | Mutamycin | 10 mg/m² I.V., day 1 *Repeat cycle q 8 weeks.* |
| **FAM** (Pancreatic cancer) | fluorouracil (5-FU) | Adrucil | 600 mg/m² I.V., days 1, 8, 29, 36, and 57 |
| | doxorubicin | Adriamycin | 30 mg/m² I.V., days 1, 29, and 57 |
| | mitomycin | Mutamycin | 10 mg/m² I.V., days 1 and 57 |
| **FAME** (Gastric cancer) | fluorouracil (5-FU) | Adrucil | 350 mg/m² I.V., days 1 to 5 and 36 to 40 |
| | doxorubicin | Adriamycin | 40 mg/m² I.V., days 1 and 36 |
| | semustine (methyl CCNU) | | 150 mg/m² P.O., day 1 *Repeat cycle q 10 weeks.* |
| **FAMTX** (Gastric cancer) | fluorouracil (5-FU) | Adrucil | 1,500 mg/m² I.V., day 1 |
| | methotrexate | Folex | 1,500 mg/m² I.V., day 1 |
| | doxorubicin | Adriamycin | 30 mg/m² I.V., day 15 |
| | leucovorin calcium | Wellcovorin | 20 to 25 mg P.O. q 6 hours for 8 doses, beginning 24 hours after each methotrexate dose |
| **FCE** (Gastric cancer) | fluorouracil (5-FU) | Adrucil | 900 mg/m² by continuous I.V. infusion, days 1 to 5 |
| | cisplatin | Platinol | 20 mg/m² I.V., days 1 to 5 |
| | etoposide (VP-16) | VePesid | 90 mg/m² I.V., days 1, 3, and 5 *Repeat cycle q 21 days.* |
| **F-CL** (Breast cancer) | fluorouracil (5-FU) | Adrucil | 500 mg/m² I.V. weekly, 1 hour after initiating leucovorin calcium infusion, for 6 weeks |
| | leucovorin calcium | Wellcovorin | 500 mg/m² I.V., over 2 hours, weekly for 6 weeks *Two-week pause, then cycle repeated.* |

*(continued)*

# Cancer chemotherapy: Acronyms and protocols *(continued)*

| ACRONYM & INDICATION | DRUG | | DOSAGE |
|---|---|---|---|
| | Generic name | Trade name | |
| **F-CL** (Colon cancer) | fluorouracil (5-FU) | Adrucil | 370 mg/m² I.V., days 1 to 5 |
| | leucovorin calcium | Wellcovorin | 200 mg/m² daily I.V., days 1 to 5, begun 15 minutes before fluorouracil infusion *Repeat cycle q 28 days.* |
| **5 + 2** (Leukemia—ANLL, consolidation) | cytarabine (ara-C) | Cytosar-U | 100 to 200 mg/m² by continuous I.V. infusion, days 1 to 5 |
| | daunorubicin | Cerubidine | 45 mg/m² I.V., days 1 and 2 |
| **FL** (Genitourinary cancer) *or* | flutamide | Eulexin | 250 mg P.O. t.i.d. |
| | leuprolide acetate | Lupron | 1 mg S.C. daily |
| | flutamide | Eulexin | 250 mg P.O. t.i.d. |
| | leuprolide acetate | Lupron Depot | 7.5 mg I.M. q 28 days |
| **FLe** (Colon cancer) | levamisole | Ergamisol | 50 mg P.O. t.i.d. for 3 days, repeated q 2 weeks for 1 year |
| | fluorouracil (5-FU) | Adrucil | 450 mg/m² I.V. for 5 days, then, after a pause of 4 weeks, 450 mg/m² I.V. weekly for 48 weeks |
| **FMS** (Pancreatic cancer) | fluorouracil (5-FU) | Adrucil | 600 mg/m² I.V., days 1, 8, 29, and 36 |
| | mitomycin | Mutamycin | 10 mg/m² I.V., day 1 |
| | streptozocin | Zanosar | 1 g/m² I.V., days 1, 8, 29, and 36 *Repeat cycle q 8 weeks.* |
| **FMV** (Colon cancer) | fluorouracil (5-FU) | Adrucil | 10 mg/kg I.V., days 1 to 5 |
| | semustine (methyl CCNU) | | 175 mg/m² P.O., day 1 |
| | vincristine | Oncovin | 1 mg/m² (2 mg maximum) I.V., day 1 *Repeat cycle q 35 days.* |
| **FZ** (Genitourinary cancer) | flutamide | Eulexin | 250 P.O. t.i.d. |
| | goserelin acetate | Zoladex | 3.6 mg implant S.C. q 28 days |
| **HDMTX** (high-dose methotrexate) (Bony sarcoma) | methotrexate sodium | Folex | 12 g/m² I.V. (20 g maximum) |
| | leucovorin calcium | Wellcovorin | 15 mg I.V. or P.O. q 6 hours for 10 doses, beginning 24 hours after methotrexate dose (serum methotrexate levels must be monitored) *Repeat cycle q 4 to 16 weeks.* |
| **Hexa-CAF** (Ovarian cancer, epithelial) | altretamine | Hexalen | 150 mg/m² P.O., days 1 to 14 |
| | cyclophosphamide | Cytoxan | 150 mg/m² P.O., days 1 to 14 |
| | methotrexate sodium | Folex | 40 mg/m², days 1 and 8 |
| | fluorouracil (5-FU) | Adrucil | 600 mg/m² I.V., days 1 and 8 *Repeat cycle q 28 days.* |

## Cancer chemotherapy: Acronyms and protocols *(continued)*

| ACRONYM & INDICATION | DRUG | | DOSAGE |
|---|---|---|---|
| | Generic name | Trade name | |
| **HiDAC** (Leukemia – ANLL, consolidation) | cytarabine (ara-C) | Cytosar-U | 3,000 mg/m² I.V. q 12 hours, days 1 to 6 or days 1, 3, and 5 |
| **IMF** (Breast cancer) | ifosfamide | Ifex | 1.5 g/m² I.V., days 1 and 8 |
| | mesna | Mesnex | Dosage is 20% of ifosfamide dose, given immediately before and at 4 and 8 hours after ifosfamide infusion |
| | methotrexate | Folex | 40 mg/m² I.V., days 1 and 8 |
| | fluorouracil (5-FU) | Adrucil | 600 mg/m² I.V., days 1 and 8 *Repeat cycle q 28 days.* |
| **L-VAM** (Genitourinary cancer) | leuprolide acetate | Lupron | 1 mg S.C. daily |
| | vinblastine | Velban | 1.5 mg/m² by continuous I.V. infusion, days 2 to 7 |
| | doxorubicin | Adriamycin | 50 mg/m² by 24-hour continuous I.V. infusion, day 1 |
| | mitomycin | Mutamycin | 10 mg/m² I.V., day 2 *Repeat VAM cycle q 28 days.* |
| **MACC** (Non-small-cell lung cancer) | methotrexate | Folex | 40 mg/m² I.V., day 1 |
| | doxorubicin | Adriamycin | 40 mg/m² I.V., day 1 |
| | cyclophosphamide | Cytoxan | 400 mg/m² I.V., day 1 |
| | lomustine (CCNU) | CeeNU | 30 mg/m² P.O., day 1 *Repeat cycle q 21 days.* |
| **MACOP-B** (Malignant lymphoma) | methotrexate sodium | Folex | 100 mg/m² I.V., weeks 2, 6, and 10; then 300 mg/m² I.V. for 4 hours, weeks 2, 6, and 10 |
| | leucovorin calcium | Wellcovorin | 15 mg P.O.q 6 hours for 6 doses, beginning 24 hours after methotrexate |
| | doxorubicin | Adriamycin | 50 mg/m² I.V., weeks 1, 3, 5, 7, 9, and 11 |
| | cyclophosphamide | Cytoxan | 350 mg/m² I.V., weeks 1, 3, 5, 7, 9, and 11 |
| | vincristine | Oncovin | 1.4 mg/m² I.V. (2 mg maximum), weeks 2, 4, 8, 10, and 12 |
| | bleomycin | Blenoxane | 10 mg/m² I.V., weeks 4, 8, and 12 |
| | prednisone | Deltasone | 75 mg P.O. daily |
| **MAID** (Bony sarcoma) | mesna | Mesnex | Uroprotection 1.5 to 2.5 g/m² by continuous I.V. infusion, days 1 to 4 |
| | doxorubicin | Adriamycin | 15 mg/m² by continuous I.V. infusion, days 1 to 3 |
| | ifosfamide | Ifex | 1.5 to 2.5 g/m² by continuous I.V. infusion, days 1 to 3 |
| | dacarbazine | DTIC-Dome | 250 mg/m² by continuous I.V. infusion, days 1 to 3 *Repeat cycle q 21 to 28 days.* |

*(continued)*

## Cancer chemotherapy: Acronyms and protocols (continued)

| ACRONYM & INDICATION | DRUG | | DOSAGE |
|---|---|---|---|
| | Generic name | Trade name | |
| **MAID** (Soft-tissue sarcoma) | mesna | Mesnex | 1.5 to 2.5 g/m² by continuous I.V. infusion, days 1 to 4 |
| | doxorubicin | Adriamycin | 15 mg/m² by continuous I.V. infusion, days 1 to 3 |
| | ifosfamide | Ifex | 1.5 to 2.5 g/m² by continuous I.V. infusion, days 1 to 3 |
| | dacarbazine | DTIC-Dome | 250 mg/m² by continuous I.V. infusion, days 1 to 3 *Repeat cycle q 21 to 28 days.* |
| **MAP** (Head and neck cancer) | mitomycin | Mutamycin | 8 mg/m² I.V., day 1 |
| | doxorubicin | Adriamycin | 40 mg/m² I.V., day 1 |
| | cisplatin | Platinol | 60 mg/m² I.V., day 1 *Repeat cycle q 28 days.* |
| **m-BACOD** (Malignant lymphoma) | bleomycin | Blenoxane | 4 units/m² I.V., day 1 |
| | doxorubicin | Adriamycin | 45 mg/m² I.V., day 1 |
| | cyclophosphamide | Cytoxan | 600 mg/m² I.V., day 1 |
| | vincristine | Oncovin | 1 mg/m² I.V., day 1 |
| | dexamethasone | Decadron | 6 mg/m² I.V., days 1 to 5 |
| | methotrexate | Folex | 200 mg/m² I.V., days 8 and 15 |
| | leucovorin calcium | Wellcovorin | 10 mg/m² P.O. q 6 hours for 8 doses, beginning 24 hours after each methotrexate dose *Repeat cycle q 21 days.* |
| **m-BACOS** (Malignant lymphoma) | doxorubicin | Adriamycin | 50 mg/m² by 24-hour continuous I.V. infusion, day 1 |
| | vincristine | Oncovin | 1.4 mg/m² (2 mg maximum) I.V., day 1 |
| | bleomycin | Blenoxane | 10 units/m² I.V., day 1 |
| | cyclophosphamide | Cytoxan | 750 mg/m² I.V., day 1 |
| | methotrexate | Folex | 1 g/m² I.V., day 2 |
| | leucovorin calcium | Wellcovorin | 15 mg P.O. q 6 hours for 8 doses starting 24 hours after methotrexate dose |
| | methylprednisolone | Solu-Medrol | 500 mg I.V., days 1 to 3 *Repeat cycle q 21 to 25 days.* |
| **MBC** (Head and neck cancer) | methotrexate | Folex | 40 mg/m² I.M. or I.V., days 1 and 15 |
| | bleomycin | Blenoxane | 10 units I.M. or I.V. weekly |
| | cisplatin | Platinol | 50 mg/m² I.V., day 1 *Repeat cycle q 21 days.* |
| **MC** (Leukemia—ANLL, consolidation) | mitoxantrone | Novantrone | 12 mg/m² I.V. daily, days 1 and 2 |
| | cytarabine (ara-C) | Cytosar-U | 100 mg/m² daily by continuous I.V. infusion, days 1 to 5 *Repeat cycle q 28 days.* |

## Cancer chemotherapy: Acronyms and protocols *(continued)*

| ACRONYM & INDICATION | DRUG | | DOSAGE |
|---|---|---|---|
| | Generic name | Trade name | |
| **MC** (Leukemia – ANLL, induction) | mitoxantrone | Novantrone | 12 mg/m² I.V., days 1 to 3 and 17 to 18 |
| | cytarabine (ara-C) | Cytosar-U | 100 mg/m² daily by continuous I.V. infusion, days 1 to 7 and 17 to 21 |
| **MF** (Head and neck cancer) | methotrexate | Folex | 125 to 250 mg/m² I.V., day 1 |
| | fluorouracil (5-FU) | Adrucil | 600 mg/m² I.V., beginning 1 hour after methotrexate dose |
| | leucovorin calcium | Wellcovorin | 10 mg/m² I.V. or P.O. q 8 hours for 8 doses, beginning 24 hours after methotrexate dose *Repeat cycle weekly.* |
| **MICE (ICE)** (Small-cell and non-small-cell lung cancer) | mesna | Mesnex | Dosage is 20% of ifosfamide dose given I.V. immediately before and at 4 and 8 hours after ifosfamide infusion |
| | ifosfamide | Ifex | 2,000 mg/m² I.V., days 1 to 3 |
| | carboplatin | Paraplatin | 300 to 350 mg/m² I.V., day 1 |
| | etoposide (VP-16) | VePesid | 60 to 100 mg/m² I.V., days 1 to 3 |
| **MINE** (Malignant lymphoma) | mesna | Mesnex | 1.3 to 1.5 g/m² I.V., days 1 to 3 |
| | ifosfamide | Ifex | 1.3 to 1.5 g/m² I.V., days 1 to 3 |
| | mitoxantrone | Novantrone | 8 to 10 mg/m² I.V., day 1 |
| | etoposide (VP-16) | VePesid | 65 to 80 mg/m² I.V., days 1 to 3 |
| **MM** (Leukemia – ALL, maintenance) | mercaptopurine (6-MP) | Purinethol | 50 mg/m² P.O. daily |
| | methotrexate sodium | Folex | 20 mg/m² P.O. or I.V. weekly |
| **MOF** (Colon cancer) | fluorouracil (5-FU) | Adrucil | 10 mg/kg/day I.V., days 1 to 5 |
| | semustine (methyl CCNU) | | 175 mg/m² P.O., day 1 |
| | vincristine | Oncovin | 1 mg/m² (2 mg maximum) I.V., day 1 *Repeat cycle q 35 days.* |
| **MOP** (Pediatric brain tumors) | mechlorethamine (nitrogen mustard) | Mustargen | 6 mg/m² I.V., days 1 and 8 |
| | vincristine | Oncovin | 1.4 mg/m² (2 mg maximum) I.V., days 1 and 8 |
| | procarbazine | Matulane | 100 mg/m² P.O., days 1 to 14 *Repeat cycle q 28 days.* |
| **MOPP** (Hodgkin's lymphoma) | mechlorethamine | Mustargen | 6 mg/m² I.V., days 1 and 8 |
| | vincristine | Oncovin | 1.4 mg/m² (2 mg maximum) I.V., days 1 and 8 |
| | procarbazine | Matulane | 100 mg/m² P.O., days 1 to 14 |
| | prednisone | Deltasone | 40 mg/m² P.O., days 1 to 14 *Repeat cycle q 28 days.* |

*(continued)*

## Cancer chemotherapy: Acronyms and protocols *(continued)*

| ACRONYM & INDICATION | DRUG | | DOSAGE |
|---|---|---|---|
| | Generic name | Trade name | |
| **MP** (Multiple myeloma) | melphalan (L-phenylalanine mustard) | Alkeran | 8 mg/m² P.O., days 1 to 4 |
| | prednisone | Deltasone | 40 mg/m² P.O., days 1 to 7 *Repeat cycle q 28 days.* |
| **m-PFL** (Genitourinary cancer) | methotrexate sodium | Folex | 60 mg/m², day 1 |
| | cisplatin | Platinol | 25 mg/m² by continuous I.V. infusion, days 2 to 6 |
| | fluorouracil (5-FU) | Adrucil | 800 mg/m² by continuous I.V. infusion, days 2 to 6 |
| | leucovorin calcium | Wellcovorin | 500 mg/m² by continuous I.V. infusion, days 2 to 6 *Repeat cycle q 28 days for four cycles.* |
| **M-2** (Multiple myeloma) | vincristine | Oncovin | 0.03 mg/kg (2 mg maximum) I.V., day 1 |
| | carmustine | BiCNU | 0.5 mg/kg I.V., day 1 |
| | cyclophosphamide | Cytoxan | 10 mg/kg I.V, day 1 |
| | melphalan (L-phenylalanine mustard) | Alkeran | 0.25 mg/kg P.O., days 1 to 4 |
| | prednisone | Deltasone | 1 mg/kg, days 1 to 7, then tapered over next 14 days *Repeat cycle q 35 days.* |
| **MV** (Leukemia— AML, induction) | mitoxantrone | Novantrone | 10 mg/m² I.V., days 1 to 5 |
| | etoposide (VP-16) | VePesid | 100 mg/m² I.V., days 1 to 5 |
| **MVAC** (Genitourinary cancer) | methotrexate | Folex | 30 mg/m² I.V., days 1, 15, and 22 |
| | vinblastine | Velban | 3 mg/m² I.V., days 2, 15, and 22 |
| | doxorubicin | Adriamycin | 30 mg/m² I.V., day 2 |
| | cisplatin | Platinol | 70 mg/m² I.V., day 2 *Repeat cycle q 28 days.* |
| **MVP** (Non-small-cell lung cancer) | mitomycin | Mutamycin | 8 mg/m² I.V., days 1, 29, and 71 |
| | vinblastine | Velban | 4.5 mg/m² I.V., days 15, 22, and 29, then q 2 weeks |
| | cisplatin | Platinol | 120 mg/m² I.V., days 1 and 29, then q 6 weeks |
| **MVPP** (Hodgkin's lymphoma) | mechlorethamine (nitrogen mustard) | Mustargen | 6 mg/m² I.V., days 1 and 8 |
| | vinblastine | Velban | 6 mg/m² I.V., days 1 and 8 |
| | procarbazine | Matulane | 100 mg/m² P.O., days 1 to 14 |
| | prednisone | Deltasone | 40 mg/m² P.O., days 1 to 14 *Repeat cycle q 42 days for six cycles.* |

*(continued)*

## Cancer chemotherapy: Acronyms and protocols (continued)

| ACRONYM & INDICATION | DRUG | | DOSAGE |
|---|---|---|---|
| | Generic name | Trade name | |
| **NFL** (Breast cancer) | mitoxantrone | Novantrone | 12 mg/m² I.V., day 1 |
| | leucovorin calcium | Wellcovorin | 300 mg I.V., days 1 to 3 |
| | fluorouracil (5-FU) | Adrucil | 350 mg/m² I.V. given after leucovorin calcium, days 1 to 3 |
| *or* | mitoxantrone | Novantrone | 10 mg/m² I.V., day 1 |
| | leucovorin calcium | Wellcovorin | 100 mg/m² I.V., days 1 to 3 |
| | fluorouracil (5-FU) | Adrucil | 1,000 mg/m² by continuous I.V infusion given after leucovorin calcium, days 1 to 3 *Repeat cycle q 21 days.* |
| **NOVP** (Hodgkin's lymphoma) | mitoxantrone | Novantrone | 10 mg/m² I.V., day 1 |
| | vincristine | Oncovin | 2 mg/m² I.V., day 8 |
| | vinblastine | Velban | 6 mg/m² I.V., day 1 |
| | prednisone | Deltasone | 100 mg P.O., days 1 to 5 *Repeat cycle q 21 days.* |
| **OPEN** (Malignant lymphoma) | vincristine | Oncovin | 2 mg I.V., day 1 |
| | prednisone | Deltasone | 100 mg P.O. daily for 5 days |
| | etoposide (VP-16) | VePesid | 100 mg/m² I.V. daily for 3 days |
| | mitoxantrone | Novantrone | 10 mg/m² I.V., day 1 |
| **PCV** (Pediatric brain tumors) | procarbazine | Matulane | 60 mg/m² P.O., days 18 to 21 |
| | lomustine (CCNU) | CeeNU | 110 mg/m² P.O., day 1 |
| | vincristine | Oncovin | 1.4 mg/m² (2 mg maximum), days 8 and 29 *Repeat cycle q 6 to 8 weeks.* |
| **PFL** (Head and neck cancer; gastric cancer) | cisplatin | Platinol | 25 mg/m² by continuous I.V. infusion, days 1 to 5 |
| | fluorouracil (5-FU) | Adrucil | 800 mg/m² by continuous I.V. infusion, days 2 to 5 |
| | leucovorin calcium | Wellcovorin | 500 mg/m² by continuous I.V. infusion, days 1 to 5 *Repeat cycle q 28 days.* |
| **PFL** (Non-small-cell lung cancer) | cisplatin | Platinol | 25 mg/m² I.V., days 1 and 15 |
| | fluorouracil (5-FU) | Adrucil | 800 mg/m² by continuous I.V. infusion, days 1 to 5 |
| | leucovorin calcium | Wellcovorin | 500 mg/m² by continuous I.V. infusion, days 1 to 5 *Repeat cycle q 28 days.* |
| **PFL + IFN** (Head and neck cancer) | cisplatin | Platinol | 100 mg/m² I.V., day 1 |
| | fluorouracil (5-FU) | Adrucil | 640 mg/m² by continuous I.V. infusion, days 1 to 5 |
| | leucovorin calcium | Wellcovorin | 100 mg P.O. q 4 hours, days 1 to 5 |
| | interferon alfa-2b | Intron A | 2 × 10⁶ units/m² S.C., days 1 to 6 |

*(continued)*

## Cancer chemotherapy: Acronyms and protocols *(continued)*

| ACRONYM & INDICATION | DRUG | | DOSAGE |
|---|---|---|---|
| | Generic name | Trade name | |
| **ProMACE/ MOPP** (Malignant lymphoma) | prednisone | Deltasone | 60 mg/m² P.O., days 1 to 14 |
| | methotrexate | Folex | 1.5 g/m² I.V., day 14 |
| | leucovorin calcium | Wellcovorin | 50 mg/m² I.V. q 6 hours for 5 doses, beginning 24 hours after methotrexate dose |
| | doxorubicin | Adriamycin | 25 mg/m² I.V., days 1 and 8 |
| | cyclophosphamide | Cytoxan | 650 mg/m² I.V., days 1 and 8 |
| | etoposide (VP-16) | VePesid | 120 mg/m² I.V., days 1 and 8 *Repeat cycle q 28 days; MOPP therapy to begin after the required number of ProMACE cycles are completed.* |
| **ProMACE/ cytaBOM** (Malignant lymphoma) | cyclophosphamide | Cytoxan | 650 mg/m² I.V., day 1 |
| | doxorubicin | Adriamycin | 25 mg/m² I.V., day 1 |
| | etoposide (VP-16) | VePesid | 120 mg/m² I.V., day 1 |
| | cytarabine (ara-C) | Cytosar-U | 300 mg/m² I.V., day 8 |
| | bleomycin | Blenoxane | 5 mg/m² I.V., day 8 |
| | vincristine | Oncovin | 1.4 mg/m² I.V., day 8 |
| | methotrexate | Folex | 120 mg/m² I.V., day 8 |
| | leucovorin calcium | Wellcovorin | 25 mg/m² P.O. q 6 hours for 4 doses *Repeat cycle q 28 days.* |
| **(pulse) VAC** (Soft-tissue sarcoma) | vincristine | Oncovin | 1.5 g/m² (2 mg maximum) I.V., day 1 or weekly, starting on day 1 |
| | dactinomycin (actinomycin D) | Cosmegen | 0.4 mg/m² I.V., day 1 |
| | cyclophosphamide | Cytoxan | 1,000 mg/m² I.V., day 1 *Repeat cycle q 3 to 4 weeks.* |
| **PVB** (Testicular cancer) | vinblastine | Velban | 6 mg/m² I.V., days 1 and 2 |
| | bleomycin | Blenoxane | 30 units I.V. weekly |
| | cisplatin | Platinol | 20 mg/m² I.V., days 1 to 5 *Repeat cycle q 21 to 28 days.* |
| **7 + 3 (A + D)** (Leukemia— AML, induction) | cytarabine (ara-C) | Cytosar-U | 100 or 200 mg/m² by continuous I.V. infusion, days 1 to 7 |
| | daunorubicin | Cerubidine | 45 mg/m² I.V., days 1 to 3 |
| **TC** (Leukemia— ANLL, maintenance) | thioguanine (6-TG) | | 40 mg/m² P.O. q 12 hours for 8 doses, days 1 to 4 |
| | cytarabine (ara-C) | Cytosar-U | 60 mg/m² S.C., day 5 *Repeat cycle weekly.* |

## Cancer chemotherapy: Acronyms and protocols *(continued)*

| ACRONYM & INDICATION | DRUG | | DOSAGE |
|---|---|---|---|
| | Generic name | Trade name | |
| **T-10** (Pediatric bony sarcoma) | methotrexate | Folex | 12 g/m² I.V. for 12 or 16 doses |
| | leucovorin calcium | Wellcovorin | 15 mg I.V. or P.O. q 6 hours for 10 doses, each starting 20 hours after methotrexate dose |
| | doxorubicin | Adriamycin | 30 mg/m² I.V. for 2 to 3 days |
| | cisplatin | Platinol | 120 mg/m² I.V. for 1 day |
| | bleomycin | Blenoxane | 15 units/m² I.V. for 2 days |
| | cyclophosphamide | Cytoxan | 600 mg/m² I.V. for 2 days |
| | dactinomycin (actinomycin D) | Cosmegen | 0.6 mg/m² I.V. for 2 days |
| **VA** (Wilms' tumor) | vincristine | Oncovin | 1.5 mg/m² (2 mg maximum) weekly |
| | dactinomycin (actinomycin D) | Cosmegen | 0.4 mg/m² q 2 weeks |
| **VAB** (Genitourinary cancer) | vinblastine | Velban | 4 mg/m² I.V., day 1 |
| | dactinomycin (actinomycin D) | Cosmegen | 1 mg/m² I.V., day 1 |
| | bleomycin | Blenoxane | 30 units I.V. push, then 20 units/m² by continuous I.V. infusion, days 1 to 3 |
| | cisplatin | Platinol | 120 mg/m² I.V., day 4 |
| | cyclophosphamide | Cytoxan | 600 mg/m² I.V., day 1 *Repeat cycle q 21 days.* |
| **VAC** (Small-cell lung cancer) | vincristine | Oncovin | 2 mg I.V., day 1 |
| | doxorubicin | Adriamycin | 50 mg/m² I.V., day 1 |
| | cyclophosphamide | Cytoxan | 750 mg/m² I.V., day 1 *Repeat cycle q 21 days for four cycles.* |
| **VAC** (Ovarian cancer, germ-cell) | vincristine | Oncovin | 1.2 to 1.5 mg/m² (2 mg maximum) I.V. weekly for 10 to 12 weeks, or q 2 weeks for 12 doses |
| | dactinomycin (actinomycin D) | Cosmegen | 0.3 to 0.4 mg/m² I.V., days 1 to 5 |
| | cyclophosphamide | Cytoxan | 150 mg/m² I.V., days 1 to 5 *Repeat cycle q 28 days.* |
| **VAC** (Wilms' tumor) | vincristine | Oncovin | 1.5 mg/m² (2 mg maximum) weekly |
| | dactinomycin (actinomycin D) | Cosmegen | 1.25 g/m² q 3 weeks |
| | cyclophosphamide | Cytoxan | 1,000 mg/m² q 3 weeks |
| **VAD** (Multiple myeloma) | vincristine | Oncovin | 0.4 mg by continuous I.V. infusion, days 1 to 4 |
| | doxorubicin | Adriamycin | 12 mg/m² by continuous I.V. infusion, days 1 to 4 |
| | dexamethasone | Decadron | 40 mg P.O. on days 1 to 4, 9 to 12, and 17 to 20 *Repeat cycle q 25 to 35 days.* |

*(continued)*

# Cancer chemotherapy: Acronyms and protocols (continued)

| ACRONYM & INDICATION | DRUG | | DOSAGE |
|---|---|---|---|
| | Generic name | Trade name | |
| **VAP (VP + A)** (Leukemia – pediatric ALL, induction) | vincristine | Oncovin | 1.5 to 2 mg/m² (2 mg maximum) I.V. weekly for 4 weeks |
| | asparaginase | Elspar | 10,000 units I.M., days 1 and 8 (other doses include 6,000 units/m² I.M. for 3 days/week or 25,000 units/m²) |
| | prednisone | Deltasone | 40 mg/m² P.O., days 1 to 28, then tapered over 7 days |
| **VATH** (Breast cancer) | vinblastine | Velban | 4.5 mg/m² I.V., day 1 |
| | doxorubicin | Adriamycin | 45 mg/m² I.V., day 1 |
| | thiotepa | Thiotepa | 12 mg/m² I.V., day 1 |
| | fluoxymesterone | Halotestin | 30 mg P.O. daily (through each course) *Repeat cycle q 21 days.* |
| **VB** (Genitourinary cancer) | vinblastine | Velban | 3 to 4 mg/m² I.V., day 1 |
| | methotrexate | Folex | 30 to 40 mg/m² I.V., day 1 *Repeat cycle weekly.* |
| **VBAP** (Multiple myeloma) | vincristine | Oncovin | 1 mg I.V., day 1 |
| | carmustine | BiCNU | 30 mg/m² I.V., day 1 |
| | doxorubicin | Adriamycin | 30 mg/m² I.V., day 1 |
| | prednisone | Deltasone | 100 mg P.O., days 1 to 4 *Repeat cycle q 21 days.* |
| **VBC** (Malignant melanoma) | vinblastine | Velban | 6 mg/m² I.V., days 1 and 2 |
| | bleomycin | Blenoxane | 15 units/m² by continuous I.V. infusion, days 1 to 5 |
| | cisplatin | Platinol | 50 mg/m² I.V., day 5 *Repeat cycle q 28 days.* |
| **VBP** (Genitourinary cancer) | vinblastine | Velban | 6 mg/m² I.V., days 1 and 2 |
| | bleomycin | Blenoxane | 30 units I.V. weekly |
| | cisplatin | Platinol | 20 mg/m² I.V., days 1 to 5 *Repeat cycle q 21 to 28 days.* |
| **VC** (Small-cell lung cancer) | etoposide (VP-16) | VePesid | 100 to 200 mg/m² I.V., days 1 to 3 |
| | carboplatin | Paraplatin | 50 to 125 mg/m² I.V., days 1 to 3 *Repeat cycle q 28 days.* |

*(continued)*

## Cancer chemotherapy: Acronyms and protocols *(continued)*

| ACRONYM & INDICATION | DRUG | | DOSAGE |
|---|---|---|---|
| | Generic name | Trade name | |
| **VCAP** (Multiple myeloma) | vincristine | Oncovin | 1 mg I.V., day 1 |
| | cyclophosphamide | Cytoxan | 100 mg/m² P.O., days 1 to 4 |
| | doxorubicin | Adriamycin | 25 mg/m² I.V., day 2 |
| | prednisone | Deltasone | 60 mg/m² P.O., days 1 to 4 *Repeat cycle q 28 days.* |
| **VDP** (Malignant melanoma) | vinblastine | Velban | 5 mg/m² I.V., days 1 and 2 |
| | dacarbazine | DTIC-Dome | 150 mg/m² I.V., days 1 to 5 |
| | cisplatin | Platinol | 75 mg/m² I.V., day 5 *Repeat cycle q 21 to 28 days.* |
| **VIP** (Genitourinary cancer) | vinblastine | Velban | 0.11 mg/kg I.V., days 1 and 2 |
| | ifosfamide | Ifex | 1.2 g/m² I.V., days 1 to 5 |
| | cisplatin | Platinol | 20 mg/m²I.V., days 1 to 5 |
| | mesna | Mesnex | 400 mg I.V. 15 minutes before ifosfamide, then 1.2 g by continuous I.V. infusion, days 1 to 5 *Repeat cycle q 3 weeks for four cycles.* |
| *or* | etoposide (VP-16) | VePesid | 75 mg/m² I.V., days 1 to 5 |
| | ifosfamide | Ifex | 1.2 g/m² I.V., days 1 to 5 |
| | cisplatin | Platinol | 20 mg/m², days 1 to 5 |
| | mesna | Mesnex | 400 mg I.V. 15 minutes before ifosfamide, then 1.2 g by continuous I.V. infusion, days 1 to 5 *Repeat cycle q 3 weeks for four cycles.* |
| **Wayne State** (Head and neck cancer) | cisplatin | Platinol | 100 mg/m² I.V. over 30 minutes, day 1 |
| | fluorouracil (5-FU) | Adrucil | 1,000 mg/m² by continuous I.V. infusion, days 1 to 4 or days 1 to 5 *Repeat cycle q 21 days.* |

# Diagnostic skin tests

## DRUG, INDICATIONS, DOSAGE

### coccidioidin
Spherulin

*Suspected coccidioidomycosis —*
**Adults and children:** 0.1 ml of 1:100 dilution intradermally into flexor surface of forearm. In persons nonreactive to this form, test is repeated using 1:10 dilution.

### histoplasmin
Histolyn-CYL, Histoplasmin Diluted

*To differentiate histoplasmosis from coccidioidomycosis, tuberculosis, sarcoidosis, and other mycotic or bacterial infections —*
**Adults and children:** 0.1 ml intradermally into flexor surface of forearm.

### mumps skin test antigen
MSTA

*To assess T-cell-mediated immunity —*
**Adults and children:** 0.1 ml intradermally into flexor surface of forearm.

### tuberculin purified protein derivative (PPD)
Aplisol, PPD-stabilized Solution (Mantoux test), Tubersol

*Diagnosis of tuberculosis —*
**Adults and children:** initially, 1 TU (for patients suspected of being highly sensitized) or 5 TU (for patients not expected to be highly sensitized) intradermally into flexor surface of forearm. If negative, patient is retested with 250 TU.

### tuberculosis multiple-puncture tests
Aplitest (dried purified protein derivative [PPD]), Mono-Vacc Test (liquid Old Tuberculin [OT]), Sclavo Test (dried PPD), Tine Test (dried OT, dried PPD)

*Screening for tuberculosis —*
**Adults and children:** clean skin thoroughly with alcohol; make skin taut on flexor surface of forearm and press points firmly into selected site. Hold device at injection site for about 3 seconds to ensure depositing of dried tuberculin B in tissue lymph.

---

Reactions may be *common,* uncommon, *life-threatening,* or COMMON AND LIFE-THREATENING.

| ADVERSE REACTIONS | SPECIAL CONSIDERATIONS |
|---|---|
| **Systemic:** hypersensitivity reactions (vesiculation, ulceration, necrosis), *anaphylaxis,* Arthus reaction. | • Pregnancy risk category: NR.<br>• Contraindicated in patients with hypersensitivity to thimerosal or erythema nodosum.<br>• Read test at 24 and 48 hours. |
| **Skin:** urticaria, ulceration, or necrosis in highy sensitive patients.<br>**Systemic:** *anaphylaxis.* | • Pregnancy risk category: NR.<br>• Contraindicated in patients known to be positive reactors.<br>• Read test within 24 to 48 hours. |
| **Systemic:** hypersensitivity reactions (vesiculation, ulceration), *anaphylaxis,* Arthus reaction. | • Pregnancy risk category: NR.<br>• Contraindicated in patients with hypersensitivity to eggs, egg products, or thimerosal.<br>• Read test at 48 and 72 hours. |
| **Skin:** pruritus, vesiculation.<br>**Systemic:** hypersensitivity reactions, *anaphylaxis,* Arthus reaction.<br>**Other:** pain, ulceration, necrosis. | • Pregnancy risk category: C.<br>• Contraindicated in known tuberculin-positive reactors; severe reactions may occur.<br>• Read test within 48 to 72 hours. If repeat test using 250 TU shows no response, patient is nonreactive. |
| **Systemic:** hypersensitivity reactions (vesiculation, ulceration, necrosis), *anaphylaxis.* | • Pregnancy risk category: C.<br>• Contraindicated in known tuberculin-positive reactors.<br>• Read test within 48 to 72 hours. Verify questionable or positive reactions with the Mantoux test. |

# Table of equivalents

## Metric system equivalents

### Metric weight

| | |
|---|---|
| 1 kilogram | = 1,000 grams (g or gm) |
| 1 gram | = 1,000 milligrams (mg) |
| 1 milligram | = 1,000 micrograms ($\mu$g or mcg) |
| 0.6 g | = 600 mg |
| 0.3 g | = 300 mg |
| 0.1 g | = 100 mg |
| 0.06 g | = 60 mg |
| 0.03 g | = 30 mg |
| 0.015 g | = 15 mg |
| .001 g | = 1 mg |

### Metric volume

| | |
|---|---|
| 1 liter (l or L) | = 1,000 milliliters (ml)* |
| 1 milliliter | = 1,000 microliters ($\mu$l) |

### Household | Metric

| | | |
|---|---|---|
| 1 teaspoon (tsp) | = | 5 ml |
| 1 tablespoon (T or tbs) | = | 15 ml |
| 2 tablespoons | = | 30 ml |
| 1 measuring cupful | = | 240 ml |
| 1 pint (pt) | = | 473 ml |
| 1 quart (qt) | = | 946 ml |
| 1 gallon (gal) | = | 3,785 ml |

## Temperature conversions

| FAHRENHEIT DEGREES | CENTIGRADE DEGREES | FAHRENHEIT DEGREES | CENTIGRADE DEGREES | FAHRENHEIT DEGREES | CENTIGRADE DEGREES |
|---|---|---|---|---|---|
| 106.0 | 41.1 | 100.6 | 38.1 | 95.2 | 35.1 |
| 105.8 | 41.0 | 100.4 | 38.0 | 95.0 | 35.0 |
| 105.6 | 40.9 | 100.2 | 37.9 | 94.8 | 34.9 |
| 105.4 | 40.8 | 100.0 | 37.8 | 94.6 | 34.8 |
| 105.2 | 40.7 | 99.8 | 37.7 | 94.4 | 34.7 |
| 105.0 | 40.6 | 99.6 | 37.6 | 94.2 | 34.6 |
| 104.8 | 40.4 | 99.4 | 37.4 | 94.0 | 34.4 |
| 104.6 | 40.3 | 99.2 | 37.3 | 93.8 | 34.3 |
| 104.4 | 40.2 | 99.0 | 37.2 | 93.6 | 34.2 |
| 104.2 | 40.1 | 98.8 | 37.1 | 93.4 | 34.1 |
| 104.0 | 40.0 | 98.6 | 37.0 | 93.2 | 34.0 |
| 103.8 | 39.9 | 98.4 | 36.9 | 93.0 | 33.9 |
| 103.6 | 39.8 | 98.2 | 36.8 | 92.8 | 33.8 |
| 103.4 | 39.7 | 98.0 | 36.7 | 92.6 | 33.7 |
| 103.2 | 39.6 | 97.8 | 36.5 | 92.4 | 33.6 |
| 103.0 | 39.4 | 97.6 | 36.4 | 92.2 | 33.4 |
| 102.8 | 39.3 | 97.4 | 36.3 | 92.0 | 33.3 |
| 102.6 | 39.2 | 97.2 | 36.2 | 91.8 | 33.2 |
| 102.4 | 39.1 | 97.0 | 36.1 | 91.6 | 33.1 |
| 102.2 | 39.0 | 96.8 | 36.0 | 91.4 | 33.0 |
| 102.0 | 38.9 | 96.6 | 35.9 | 91.2 | 32.9 |
| 101.8 | 38.8 | 96.4 | 35.8 | 91.0 | 32.8 |
| 101.6 | 38.7 | 96.2 | 35.7 | 90.8 | 32.7 |
| 101.4 | 38.6 | 96.0 | 35.6 | 90.6 | 32.6 |
| 101.2 | 38.4 | 95.8 | 35.4 | 90.4 | 32.4 |
| 101.0 | 38.3 | 95.6 | 35.3 | 90.2 | 32.3 |
| 100.8 | 38.2 | 95.4 | 35.2 | 90.0 | 32.2 |

## Weight conversions

| | | |
|---|---|---|
| 1 oz = 30 g | 1 lb = 453.6 g | 2.2 lb = 1 kg |

*1 ml = 1 cubic centimeter (cc); however, ml is the preferred measurement term today.

# Nomogram for estimating surface area in children

The surface area (S.A.) is indicated below where the S.A. column intersects the straight line that connects height and weight; or for a child of average size, opposite the child's weight.

**NOMOGRAM**

| For Children of Normal Height and Weight | HEIGHT cm | in | S.A. m² | WEIGHT lb | kg |
|---|---|---|---|---|---|

Behrman, R.E., ed., *Nelson Textbook of Pediatrics*, 15th ed, Philadelphia; W.B. Saunders Co., 1996.

# Index

t refers to a table; **boldface** refers to full-color photoguide

---

t refers to a table; **boldface** refers to full-color photoguide

t refers to a table; **boldface** refers to full-color photoguide

t refers to a table; **boldface** refers to full-color photoguide

t refers to a table; **boldface** refers to full-color photoguide

# About *Nursing97 DrugDisk*

*Nursing97 DrugDisk* lets you:

- take 2 continuing education tests (and earn 9.5 contact hours)
- learn and perform dosage calculations
- print out concise instructions for your patients on more than 700 commonly prescribed drugs.

---

### Minimum system requirements
- IBM-compatible personal computer
- DOS 3.1 or greater
- High-density 3½″ floppy drive
- 640K RAM
- EGA monitor
- 2 MB of available space on hard drive

### Installing and running the program
- Turn on your computer, and insert diskette into drive A (or B). *Note:* This is a DOS program. If you're using Windows, exit Windows to the C:\ > prompt before proceeding.
- At the C:\ > prompt, type *A:\ INSTALL* (or *B:\ INSTALL*), and press Enter. Follow the directions on your monitor to complete installation.
- To run from the C:\ > prompt, type *CD\ SHDRUG*, and press Enter. Then type *start*, and press Enter.
- For technical support, call 1-614-594-5403 Monday through Friday, 9 a.m. to 5 p.m. Eastern Standard Time.

---

The clinical information and tools in *Nursing97 DrugDisk* are based on research and consultation with nursing, medical, and legal authorities. To the best of our knowledge, this program reflects currently accepted practice; nevertheless, it can't be considered absolute and universal. For individual application, all recommendations must be considered in light of the patient's clinical condition and, before administration of new or infrequently used drugs, in light of the latest package-insert information. The authors and publisher disclaim responsibility for any adverse effects resulting directly or indirectly from the suggested procedures, from any undetected errors, or from the reader's misunderstanding of the program.